NATIONAL KIDNEY FOUNDATION'S PRIMER ON KIDNEY DISEASES

Sixth Edition

Scott J. Gilbert, MD

Associate Professor of Medicine, Tufts University School of Medicine
Division of Nephrology, Tufts Medical Center
Boston, Massachusetts

Daniel E. Weiner, MD, MS

Assistant Professor of Medicine, Tufts University School of Medicine
Division of Nephrology, Tufts Medical Center
Boston, Massachusetts

ASSOCIATE EDITORS
Debbie S. Gipson, MD, MS

Associate Professor of Pediatrics,
University of Michigan School of Medicine
Ann Arbor, Michigan

Mark A. Perazella, MD, MS

Professor of Medicine, Yale University School of Medicine
Section of Nephrology, Yale-New Haven Hospital
New Haven, Connecticut

Marcello Tonelli, MD, SM

Professor of Medicine, University of Alberta
Alberta Kidney Disease Network
Edmonton, Alberta, Canada

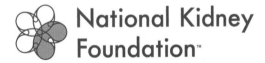

National Kidney
Foundation™

ELSEVIER
SAUNDERS

ELSEVIER
SAUNDERS

1600 John F. Kennedy Blvd.
Ste 1800
Philadelphia, PA 19103-2899

Notices

Knowledge and best practice in this field are constantly changing. As new research and experience broaden our understanding, changes in research methods, professional practices, or medical treatment may become necessary.

Practitioners and researchers must always rely on their own experience and knowledge in evaluating and using any information, methods, compounds, or experiments described herein. In using such information or methods they should be mindful of their own safety and the safety of others, including parties for whom they have a professional responsibility.

With respect to any drug or pharmaceutical products identified, readers are advised to check the most current information provided (i) on procedures featured or (ii) by the manufacturer of each product to be administered, to verify the recommended dose or formula, the method and duration of administration, and contraindications. It is the responsibility of practitioners, relying on their own experience and knowledge of their patients, to make diagnoses, to determine dosages and the best treatment for each individual patient, and to take all appropriate safety precautions.

To the fullest extent of the law, neither the Publisher nor the authors, contributors, or editors assume any liability for any injury and/or damage to persons or property as a matter of products liability, negligence or otherwise, or from any use or operation of any methods, products, instructions, or ideas contained in the material herein.

Library of Congress Cataloging-in-Publication Data

National Kidney Foundation's primer on kidney diseases/[edited by] Scott J. Gilbert, Daniel E. Weiner; associate editors, Debbie S. Gipson, Mark A. Perazella, Marcello Tonelli. – Sixth edition.
    p. ; cm.
  Primer on kidney diseases
  Preceded by (work): Primer on kidney diseases. 5th ed. c2009.
  Includes bibliographical references and index.
  ISBN 978-1-4557-4617-0 (pbk. : alk. paper)
  I. Gilbert, Scott J., editor of compilation. II. Weiner, Daniel E., editor of compilation. III. Gipson, Debbie S., editor. IV. Perazella, Mark A., editor. V. Tonelli, Marcello, editor. VI. National Kidney Foundation. VII. Primer on kidney diseases. Preceded by (work): VIII. Title: Primer on kidney diseases.
  [DNLM: 1. Kidney Diseases. 2. Kidney–pathology. WJ 300]
  RC902
  616.6'1–dc23   2013012338

Senior Content Strategist: Kate Dimock
Senior Content Development Specialist: Janice Gaillard
Publishing Services Manager: Anne Altepeter
Project Managers: Louise King/Jessica Becher
Design Direction: Steve Stave

Printed in China.

Last digit is the print number: 9 8 7 6 5 4 3 2 1

Working together to grow libraries in developing countries

www.elsevier.com • www.bookaid.org

Contributors

Sharon Adler, MD
Professor of Medicine, David Geffen School of Medicine at University of California Los Angeles, Los Angeles, California; Chief, Division of Nephrology and Hypertension, Harbor-University of California Los Angeles Medical Center, Torrance, California
Thrombotic Microangiopathies

Horacio J. Adrogué, MD
Professor of Medicine, Division of Nephrology, Baylor College of Medicine; The Methodist Hospital, Michael E. DeBakey Veterans Affairs Medical Center, Houston, Texas
Respiratory Acidosis and Alkalosis

Michael Allon, MD
Professor of Medicine, Division of Nephrology, University of Alabama at Birmingham, Birmingham, Alabama
Disorders of Potassium Metabolism

Hina Arif-Tiwari, MD
Assistant Professor, Body Section, Department of Medical Imaging, Director, Clinical Ultrasound, University of Arizona College of Medicine, Tucson, Arizona
Kidney Imaging

Vincente Arroyo, MD
Professor of Medicine, Liver Unit, Institute of Digestive and Metabolic Diseases, Hospital Clinic, University of Barcelona, Barcelona, Spain
Hepatorenal Syndrome and Other Liver-Related Kidney Diseases

Robin K. Avery, MD
Professor-at-Rank, Division of Infectious Disease, Johns Hopkins Medicine, Baltimore, Maryland
Infectious Complications of Kidney Transplantation

Carmen Avila-Casado, MD, PhD
Professor of Pathology, Laboratory Medicine Program, University of Toronto; Medical Director, Emergency Medicine Lab, Renal Pathologist and Renal Pathology Consultant, Department of Pathology, Toronto General Hospital, University Health Network, Toronto, Ontario, Canada
Focal Segmental Glomerulosclerosis

Jonathan Barratt, MB ChB (Hons), PhD
Senior Lecturer, Department of Infection, Immunity, and Inflammation, University of Leicester; Honorary Consultant Nephrologist, John Walls Renal Unit, University Hospitals of Leicester, Leicester, United Kingdom
Immunoglobulin A Nephropathy and Related Disorders

Jeffrey S. Berns, MD
Professor of Medicine and Pediatrics, Renal, Electrolyte and Hypertension Division, Perelman School of Medicine at the University of Pennsylvania, Philadelphia, Pennsylvania
Viral Nephropathies: Human Immunodeficiency Virus, Hepatitis C Virus, and Hepatitis B Virus

Andrew S. Bomback, MD, MPH
Assistant Professor of Clinical Medicine, Department of Medicine, Division of Nephrology, Columbia University College of Physicians and Surgeons, New York, New York
Kidney Manifestations of Systemic Lupus Erythematosus

Joseph V. Bonventre, MD, PhD
Samuel A. Levine Professor of Medicine, Renal Division, Brigham and Women's Hospital; Department of Medicine, Harvard Medical School, Boston, Massachusetts
Pathophysiology of Acute Kidney Injury

C. Barrett Bowling, MD
Assistant Professor of Gerontology, Geriatrics, and Palliative Care, University of Alabama at Birmingham; Investigator, Birmingham Veterans Affairs Medical Center, Birmingham/Atlanta Geriatric Research, Education, Clinical Center, Birmingham, Alabama
Kidney Disease in the Elderly

Ursula C. Brewster, MD
Associate Professor of Medicine, Department of Internal Medicine, Section of Nephrology, Yale University School of Medicine, New Haven, Connecticut
Acute Interstitial Nephritis

Josephine P. Briggs, MD
Director, National Center for Complementary and Alternative Medicine, National Institutes of Health, Bethesda, Maryland
Overview of Kidney Function and Structure

Daniel C. Cattran, MD
Professor of Medicine, Division of Nephrology, University of Toronto; Senior Scientist, Toronto General Research Institute, Toronto, Ontario, Canada
Membranous Nephropathy

Sindhu Chandran, MBBS
Clinical Assistant Professor of Medicine, Division of Nephrology, Kidney Transplant Service, University of California San Francisco, San Francisco, California
Immunosuppression in Transplantation

Arlene B. Chapman, MD
Professor of Medicine, Division of Renal Diseases and
  Hypertension, Emory University, Atlanta, Georgia
  Polycystic and Other Cystic Kidney Diseases

Steven G. Coca, DO, MS
Assistant Professor of Medicine, Section of Nephrology, Yale
  University School of Medicine, New Haven, Connecticut
  Acute Tubular Injury and Acute Tubular Necrosis

Peter J. Conlon, MB, MHS
Consultant Nephrologist and Renal Transplant Physician,
  Beaumont Hospital, Royal College of Surgeons in
  Ireland, Dublin, Ireland
  Secondary Hypertension

Lawrence A. Copelovitch, MD
Assistant Professor of Pediatrics, Division of Nephrology,
  The Children's Hospital of Philadelphia, Philadelphia,
  Pennsylvania
  The Kidney in Infants and Children

Gary Curhan, MD, ScD
Professor of Medicine, Harvard Medical School; Professor
  of Epidemiology, Harvard School of Public Health;
  Physician, Medicine, Renal Division and Channing
  Laboratory, Brigham and Women's Hospital, Boston,
  Massachusetts
  Nephrolithiasis

Vivette D. D'Agati, MD
Professor of Pathology, Columbia University College of
  Physicians and Surgeons; Director, Renal Pathology
  Laboratory, Department of Pathology, Columbia
  University Medical Center, New York, New York
  Kidney Manifestations of Systemic Lupus Erythematosus

Jacques R. Daoud, MD, MS
Nephrologist, Department of Medicine, Division of
  Nephrology, Indiana University School of Medicine,
  Indianapolis, Indiana
  *Disorders of Mineral Metabolism: Calcium, Phosphorus,
  and Magnesium)*

Dick de Zeeuw, MD, PhD
Chair and Professor of Clinical Pharmacology, University
  Medical Center Groningen, University of Groningen,
  Groningen, the Netherlands
  *Pathogenesis, Pathophysiology, and Treatment of Diabetic
  Nephropathy*

Paula Dennen, MD
Assistant Professor of Medicine, Divisions of Nephrology
  and Critical Care Medicine, Denver Health, University of
  Colorado, Denver, Colorado
  Hypernatremia

Vimal K. Derebail, MD, MPH
Assistant Professor of Medicine, University of North
  Carolina Kidney Center, Division of Nephrology and
  Hypertension, University of North Carolina at Chapel
  Hill, Chapel Hill, North Carolina
  Sickle Cell Nephropathy

Thomas D. DuBose, Jr., MD
Tinsley R. Harrison Professor and Chair, Department of
  Internal Medicine, Wake Forest School of Medicine,
  Winston-Salem, North Carolina
  Metabolic Alkalosis

Michael Emmett, MD
Professor of Internal Medicine, Texas A&M Health Science
  Center, College of Medicine; Clinical Professor of
  Internal Medicine, University of Texas Southwestern
  School of Medicine; Chief of Internal Medicine, Baylor
  University Medical Center, Dallas, Texas
  Approach to Acid-Base Disorders

Todd Fairhead, MD, MSc
Assistant Professor, Department of Medicine, University of
  Ottawa; Division of Nephrology, The Ottawa Hospital,
  Ottawa, Ontario, Canada
  *Selection of Prospective Kidney Transplant Recipients and
  Donors*

Ronald J. Falk, MD
Professor of Medicine, University of North Carolina Kidney
  Center, Division of Nephrology and Hypertension,
  University of North Carolina at Chapel Hill, Chapel Hill,
  North Carolina
  Glomerular Clinicopathologic Syndromes
  Kidney Involvement in Systemic Vasculitis

John Feehally, DM
Professor of Renal Medicine, Department of Infection,
  Immunity, and Inflammation, University of Leicester;
  Consultant Nephrologist, John Walls Renal Unit,
  University Hospitals of Leicester, Leicester, United
  Kingdom
  Immunoglobulin A Nephropathy and Related Disorders

Javier Fernández, MD, PhD
Staff Physician, Liver Unit, Hospital Clinic, University of
  Barcelona, Barcelona, Spain
  Hepatorenal Syndrome and Other Liver-Related Kidney Diseases

Fernando C. Fervenza, MD, PhD
Professor of Medicine, Division of Nephrology and
  Hypertension, Mayo Clinic, Rochester, Minnesota
  Membranous Nephropathy

Paola Fioretto, MD, PhD
Associate Professor of Medicine, University of Padua,
  Padua, Italy
  *Pathogenesis, Pathophysiology, and Treatment of Diabetic
  Nephropathy*

Manuela Födinger, MD
Associate Professor of Laboratory Medicine, Clinical
  Institute of Laboratory Diagnostics, Sociomedical
  Center South, Kaiser-Franz Josef Spital mit Gottfried von
  Preyer'schem Children's Hospital, Vienna, Austria
  Fabry Disease

Susan L. Furth, MD, PhD
Professor of Pediatrics and Epidemiology, University of
    Pennsylvania School of Medicine; Laffey-Connelly Chair
    in Pediatric Nephrology, Chief, Division of Nephrology,
    The Children's Hospital of Philadelphia, Philadelphia,
    Pennsylvania
The Kidney in Infants and Children

Todd W.B. Gehr, MD
Professor of Medicine, Chairman, Division of Nephrology,
    Virginia Commonwealth University Health System,
    Richmond Virginia
Edema and the Clinical Use of Diuretics

Scott J. Gilbert, MD
Associate Professor of Medicine, Tufts University School of
    Medicine; Division of Nephrology, Tufts Medical Center,
    Boston, Massachusetts

Jagbir S. Gill, MD, MPH
Assistant Professor of Medicine, University of British
    Columbia; Division of Nephrology, St. Paul's Hospital,
    Vancouver; Division of Nephrology, Tufts Medical
    Center, British Columbia, Canada
Posttransplantation Monitoring and Outcomes

Debbie S. Gipson, MD, MS
Associate Professor of Pediatrics, University of Michigan
    School of Medicine, Ann Arbor, Michigan
Focal Segmental Glomerulosclerosis

D. Jordi Goldstein-Fuchs, DSc, APN, RD
Clinical Assistant Professor, Department of Internal
    Medicine, University of Nevada, Reno; Clinical and
    Research Nephrology, Sierra Nevada Nephrology, Reno,
    Nevada
Nutrition and Kidney Disease

Arthur Greenberg, MD
Professor of Medicine, Division of Nephrology, Duke
    University Medical Center, Durham, North Carolina
Urinalysis and Urine Microscopy

Martin C. Gregory, BM, BCh, DPhil
Professor of Medicine, Division of Nephrology, University
    of Utah Health Sciences Center, Salt Lake City, Utah
Alport Syndrome and Related Disorders

Lakshman Gunaratnam, MD, MSc
Assistant Professor of Medicine, Schulich School of
    Medicine and Dentistry, University of Western Ontario;
    Transplant Nephrologist, London Health Sciences
    Center, University Hospital, London, Ontario, Canada
Pathophysiology of Acute Kidney Injury

Raymond M. Hakim, MD, PhD
Clinical Professor of Medicine, Division of Nephrology,
    Vanderbilt University Medical Center, Nashville,
    Tennessee
Hemodialysis

Friedhelm Hildebrandt, MD
Professor of Pediatrics, Harvard Medical School;
    Investigator, Howard Hughes Medical Institute; Director,
    Pediatric Nephrology, Boston Children's Hospital,
    Boston, Massachusetts
Nephronophthisis and Medullary Cystic Kidney Disease

Michelle A. Hladunewich, MD, MSc
Assistant Professor of Medicine, University of Toronto;
    Head, Divisions of Nephrology and Obstetric Medicine,
    Department of Medicine, Sunnybrook Health
    Sciences Centre; Clinical Research Director, Toronto
    Glomerulonephritis Registry, University Health Network,
    Toronto, Ontario, Canada
Focal Segmental Glomerulosclerosis

Jonathan Hogan, MD
Instructor of Clinical Medicine, Department of Medicine,
    Division of Nephrology, Columbia University Medical
    Center; Assistant Director of Nephrology Fellowship,
    New York Presbyterian Hospital, New York, New York
Minimal Change Disease

Susan Hou, MD
Professor of Medicine, Division of Nephrology and
    Hypertension, Loyola University Medical Center,
    Maywood, Illinois
The Kidney in Pregnancy

Andrew A. House, MD, MSc
Professor of Medicine, Schulich School of Medicine and
    Dentistry, University of Western Ontario; Site Chief of
    Nephrology, London Health Sciences Center, University
    Hospital, London, Ontario, Canada
Acute Cardiorenal Syndrome

Yonghong Huan, MD
Renal Hypertension and Electrolyte Division, Perelman
    School of Medicine at the University of Pennsylvania,
    Philadelphia, Pennsylvania
Evaluation and Management of Hypertension

Alastair J. Hutchison, MB ChB, MD
Head, Division of Specialist Medicine, Consultant in
    Renal Medicine, Manchester Institute of Nephrology
    and Transplantation, The Royal Infirmary, Manchester,
    United Kingdom
Peritoneal Dialysis

Lesley A. Inker, MD, MS
Associate Professor of Medicine, Tufts University School of
    Medicine; Division of Nephrology, Tufts Medical Center,
    Boston, Massachusetts
*Assessment of Glomerular Filtration Rate in Acute and Chronic
    Settings*
Staging and Management of Chronic Kidney Disease

Matthew T. James, MD, PhD
Assistant Professor of Medicine, Division of Nephrology,
    Department of Community Health Sciences, University
    of Calgary, Calgary, Alberta, Canada
Management of Acute Kidney Injury

David Jayne, MD
Department of Medicine, University of Cambridge, Cambridge, United Kingdom
Hematuria and Proteinuria

J. Charles Jennette, MD
Brinkhous Distinguished Professor and Chair, Department of Pathology and Laboratory Medicine, University of North Carolina at Chapel Hill, Chapel Hill, North Carolina
Glomerular Clinicopathologic Syndromes
Kidney Involvement in Systemic Vasculitis

Wladimiro Jiménez, PhD
Hormonal Laboratory, Hospital Clinic, University of Barcelona, Barcelona, Spain
Hepatorenal Syndrome and Other Liver-Related Kidney Diseases

Renate Kain, MD, PhD
Associate Professor, Clinical Department of Pathology, Medical University Vienna, Vienna, Austria
Fabry Disease

Kamyar Kalantar-Zadeh, MD, MPH, PhD
Professor and Chief, Division of Nephrology and Hypertension, University of California Irvine, School of Medicine, Orange, California
Outcomes of Kidney Replacement Therapies

Bobby Kalb, MD
Associate Professor of Medical Imaging, Vice Chair, Quality and Safety, Director of Magnetic Resonance Imaging, Chief, Body Section, University of Arizona College of Medicine, Tucson, Arizona
Kidney Imaging

Greg Knoll, MD, MSc
Professor of Medicine, University of Ottawa; Medical Director, Kidney Transplantation, Division of Nephrology, The Ottawa Hospital, Ottawa, Ontario, Canada
Selection of Prospective Kidney Transplant Recipients and Donors

Wilhelm Kriz, MD
Anatomy and Developmental Biology, Medical Faculty Mannheim, University Heidelberg, Mannheim, Germany
Overview of Kidney Function and Structure

Manjula Kurella Tamura, MD, MPH
Associate Professor of Medicine, Veterans Affairs Palo Alto Health Care System, Stanford University School of Medicine, Palo Alto, California
Kidney Disease in the Elderly

Amy Frances LaPierre, RD
Nephrology Dietitian, Liberty South Dialysis, Reno, Nevada
Nutrition and Kidney Disease

Hiddo J. Lambers Heerspink, PhD
Assistant Professor of Clinical Pharmacology, University Medical Center Groningen, University of Groningen, Groningen, the Netherlands
Pathogenesis, Pathophysiology, and Treatment of Diabetic Nephropathy

Andrew S. Levey, MD
Dr. Gerald J. and Dorothy R. Friedman Professor of Medicine, Tufts University School of Medicine; Chief, William B. Schwartz Division of Nephrology, Tufts Medical Center, Boston, Massachusetts
Assessment of Glomerular Filtration Rate in Acute and Chronic Settings
Staging and Management of Chronic Kidney Disease

Edmund J. Lewis, MD
Muehrcke Family Professor of Nephrology, Director, Section of Nephrology, Department of Medicine, Rush University Medical Center, Chicago, Illinois
Pathophysiology of Chronic Kidney Disease

Stuart L. Linas, MD
Professor and Program Director, Nephrology Fellowship Program, Division of Renal Disease and Hypertension, University of Colorado School of Medicine; Chief of Nephrology, Department of Medicine, Denver Health and Hospital Authority, Denver, Colorado
Hypernatremia

Etienne Macedo, MD, PhD
Staff Physician, Division of Nephrology, University of Sao Paulo, Sao Paulo, Brazil
Clinical Approach to the Diagnosis of Acute Kidney Injury

Nicolaos E. Madias, MD
Maurice S. Segal, MD Professor of Medicine, Tufts University School of Medicine; Chairman, Department of Medicine, St. Elizabeth's Medical Center, Boston, Massachusetts
Respiratory Acidosis and Alkalosis

Colm Magee, MD, MPH
Consultant Nephrologist, Beaumont Hospital; Lecturer in Medicine, Royal College of Surgeons in Ireland, Dublin, Ireland
The Kidney in Cancers

Laura H. Mariani, MD
Clinical Lecturer, Nephrology Division, University of Michigan Medical School, Ann Arbor, Michigan
Viral Nephropathies: Human Immunodeficiency Virus, Hepatitis C Virus, and Hepatitis B Virus

Diego R. Martin, MD, PhD
Cosden Professor and Chair, Department of Medical Imaging, University of Arizona College of Medicine, Tucson, Arizona
Kidney Imaging

Gary R. Matzke, PharmD
Professor and Director, Pharmacy Transformation
    Initiatives, Department of Pharmacotherapy and
    Outcomes Science, School of Pharmacy, Virginia
    Commonwealth University, Richmond, Virginia
*Principles of Drug Therapy in Patients with Reduced Kidney
Function*

Rory F. McQuillan, MB, BCh, BAO, MRCPI
Nephrologist, University Health Network, Toronto,
    Ontario, Canada
Secondary Hypertension

Rajnish Mehrotra, MD
Professor of Medicine, Section Head, Nephrology,
    Harborview Medical Center, University of Washington,
    Seattle, Washington
Outcomes of Kidney Replacement Therapies

Ankit N. Mehta, MD
Active Faculty, Internal Medicine and Nephrology, Baylor
    University Medical Center; Assistant Professor of Internal
    Medicine, Texas A&M Health Science Center, College of
    Medicine; Dallas Nephrology Associates, Dallas, Texas
Approach to Acid-Base Disorders

Ravindra L. Mehta, MBBS, MD, DM
Professor of Clinical Medicine, University of California San
    Diego, San Diego, California
Clinical Approach to the Diagnosis of Acute Kidney Injury

Catherine M. Meyers, MD
Director, Office of Clinical and Regulatory Affairs, National
    Center for Complementary and Alternative Medicine,
    National Institutes of Health, Bethesda, Maryland
Chronic Tubulointerstitial Disease

Alain Meyrier, MD, PhD
Professor of Medicine, University of Paris-Descartes; Senior
    Consultant Nephrologist, Department of Nephrology,
    Georges Pompidou Hospital, Public Assistance-Hospitals
    Paris, Paris, France
Postinfectious Glomerulonephritis

Sharon M. Moe, MD
Stuart A. Kleit Professor of Medicine and Director,
    Division of Nephrology, Department of Medicine,
    Indiana University School of Medicine; Chief of
    Nephrology, Roudebush Veterans Administration
    Medical Center, Indianapolis, Indiana
*Disorders of Mineral Metabolism: Calcium, Phosphorus,
and Magnesium*

Cynthia C. Nast, MD
Professor of Pathology, Cedars-Sinai Medical Center, David
    Geffen School of Medicine at University of California
    Los Angeles, Los Angeles, California
Thrombotic Microangiopathies

Lindsay E. Nicolle, MD
Professor of Internal Medicine and Medical Microbiology,
    University of Manitoba, Winnipeg, Manitoba, Canada
Urinary Tract Infection and Pyelonephritis

Thomas D. Nolin, PharmD, PhD
Assistant Professor of Pharmacy and Therapeutics,
    University of Pittsburgh School of Pharmacy; Assistant
    Professor of Medicine, Renal-Electrolyte Division,
    University of Pittsburgh School of Medicine, Pittsburgh,
    Pennsylvania
*Principles of Drug Therapy in Patients with Reduced Kidney
Function*

Ann M. O'Hare, MD, MA
Associate Professor of Medicine, University of Washington;
    Staff Physician, Department of Medicine, Veterans
    Affairs Puget Sound Healthcare System, Seattle,
    Washington
Kidney Disease in the Elderly

John F. O'Toole, MD
Assistant Professor of Nephrology, MetroHealth Medical
    Center, Case Western Reserve University, Cleveland,
    Ohio
Nephronophthisis and Medullary Cystic Kidney Disease

Neesh Pannu, MD, SM
Associate Professor of Medicine, Divisions of Nephrology
    and Critical Care, University of Alberta, Edmonton,
    Alberta, Canada
Management of Acute Kidney Injury

Mark A. Perazella, MD, MS
Professor of Medicine, Yale University School of Medicine;
    Section of Nephrology, Yale-New Haven Hospital,
    New Haven, Connecticut
Kidney Disease Caused by Therapeutic Agents

Charles D. Pusey, DSc
Professor of Medicine, Imperial College London;
    Honorary Consultant Physician, West London Renal
    and Transplant Centre, Imperial College Healthcare
    National Health Service Trust, London, United Kingdom
*Goodpasture Syndrome and Other Antiglomerular Basement
Membrane Diseases*

L. Darryl Quarles, MD
Professor of Medicine, University of Tennessee Health
    Science Center, Memphis, Tennessee
Bone Disorders in Chronic Kidney Disease

Jai Radhakrishnan, MD, MS
Professor of Clinical Medicine, Department of Medicine,
    Division of Nephrology, Columbia University Medical
    Center; Director, Nephrology Fellowship, New York
    Presbyterian Hospital, New York, New York
Minimal Change Disease

Asghar Rastegar, MD
Professor of Medicine, Section of Nephrology, Yale
    University School of Medicine, New Haven, Connecticut
Acute Interstitial Nephritis

Lynn Redahan, MB, BCh, BAO, MRCPI
Nephrology Fellow, Beaumont Hospital, Dublin, Ireland
The Kidney in Cancers

Dana V. Rizk, MD
Associate Professor of Internal Medicine, Division of
    Nephrology, University of Alabama at Birmingham,
    Birmingham, Alabama
Polycystic and Other Cystic Kidney Diseases

Claudio Ronco, MD
Director, Department of Nephrology, San Bortolo Hospital;
    Director, International Renal Research Institute, San
    Bortolo Hospital, Vicenza, Italy
Acute Cardiorenal Syndrome

Norman D. Rosenblum, MD
Professor of Pediatrics, University of Toronto; Pediatric
    Nephrologist, Department of Pediatrics, Senior Scientist,
    Program in Developmental and Stem Cell Biology, The
    Hospital for Sick Children, Toronto, Ontario, Canada
Kidney Development

Alan D. Salama, MBBS, PhD
Reader and Consultant in Nephrology, University College
    London Center for Nephrology, Royal Free Hospital,
    London, United Kingdom
*Goodpasture Syndrome and Other Antiglomerular Basement
    Membrane Diseases*

Paul W. Sanders, MD
Thomas E. Andreoli Professor in Nephrology, Department
    of Medicine, University of Alabama at Birmingham,
    Birmingham, Alabama
Dysproteinemias and Amyloidosis

Mark J. Sarnak, MD, MS
Professor of Medicine, Tufts University School of Medicine;
    Director of Research, Division of Nephrology, Tufts
    Medical Center, Boston, Massachusetts
*Cardiac Function and Cardiovascular Disease in Chronic
    Kidney Disease*

Steven J. Scheinman, MD
President and Dean, The Commonwealth Medical College,
    Scranton, Pennsylvania
Genetically Based Renal Transport Disorders

Jurgen B. Schnermann, MD
Senior Investigator, Branch Chief, Kidney Disease Branch,
    National Institute of Diabetes, Digestive, and Kidney
    Diseases, National Institutes of Health, Bethesda,
    Maryland
Overview of Kidney Function and Structure

Richard C. Semelka, MD
Professor and Vice Chair Quality and Safety, Department of
    Radiology, University of North Carolina at Chapel Hill,
    Chapel Hill, North Carolina
Kidney Imaging

Anushree Shirali, MD
Assistant Professor of Medicine, Department of Internal
    Medicine, Section of Nephrology, Yale University School
    of Medicine, New Haven, Connecticut
Kidney Disease Caused by Therapeutic Agents

Domenic A. Sica, MD
Professor of Medicine and Pharmacology, Chairman,
    Clinical Pharmacology and Hypertension, Division
    of Nephrology, Virginia Commonwealth University,
    Richmond, Virginia
Edema and the Clinical Use of Diuretics

Gere Sunder-Plassmann, MD
Associate Professor of Medicine, Division of Nephrology
    and Dialysis, Department of Medicine III, Medical
    University Vienna, Vienna, Austria
Fabry Disease

Richard W. Sutherland, MD
Associate Professor of Surgery, Division of Urology,
    University of North Carolina School of Medicine,
    Chapel Hill, North Carolina
Obstructive Uropathy

Harold M. Szerlip, MD
Professor and Vice-Chairman, Department of Medicine,
    University of Arizona College of Medicine, Tucson, Arizona
Metabolic Acidosis

Marcello Tonelli, MD, SM
Professor of Medicine, University of Alberta, Alberta
    Kidney Disease Network, Edmonton, Alberta, Canada

Raymond R. Townsend, MD
Professor of Medicine, Perelman School of Medicine at the
    University of Pennsylvania, Philadelphia, Pennsylvania
Evaluation and Management of Hypertension

Howard Trachtman, MD
Professor of Clinical Pediatrics, Department of Pediatrics,
    Director, Division of Nephrology, New York University
    Langone Medical Center, New York, New York
Minimal Change Disease

Jeffrey M. Turner, MD
Assistant Professor of Medicine, Department of Internal
    Medicine, Section of Nephrology, Yale University School
    of Medicine, New Haven, Connecticut
Acute Tubular Injury and Acute Tubular Necrosis

Anand Vardhan, MD
Consultant Nephrologist, Manchester Institute of
    Nephrology and Transplantation, Central Manchester
    University Hospitals, Manchester, United Kingdom
Peritoneal Dialysis

Kavitha Vellanki, MD
Assistant Professor of Medicine, Division of Nephrology
    and Hypertension, Loyola University Medical Center,
    Maywood, Illinois
The Kidney in Pregnancy

Joseph G. Verbalis, MD
Professor of Medicine, Georgetown University;
  Chief, Division of Endocrinology and Metabolism,
  Georgetown University Hospital, Washington, DC
Hyponatremia and Hypoosmolar Disorders

Flavio G. Vincenti, MD
Professor of Clinical Medicine, Kidney Transplant Service,
  University of California San Francisco, San Francisco,
  California
Immunosuppression in Transplantation

Sushrut S. Waikar, MD, MPH
Assistant Professor of Medicine, Harvard Medical School;
  Director, Renal Ambulatory Services, Brigham and
  Women's Hospital, Boston, Massachusetts
Pathophysiology of Acute Kidney Injury

Daniel E. Weiner, MD, MS
Assistant Professor of Medicine, Tufts University School
  of Medicine; Division of Nephrology, Tufts Medical
  Center, Boston, Massachusetts
*Cardiac Function and Cardiovascular Disease in Chronic
Kidney Disease*

Colin T. White, MD
Clinical Associate Professor, Department of Pediatrics,
  University of British Columbia; Pediatric Nephrologist
  and Director of Dialysis, British Columbia's Children's
  Hospital, Vancouver, British Columbia, Canada
The Kidney in Infants and Children

William L. Whittier, MD
Associate Professor of Medicine, Department of Internal
  Medicine, Division of Nephrology, Rush University
  Medical Center, Chicago, Illinois
Pathophysiology of Chronic Kidney Disease

Christopher S. Wilcox, MD, PhD
Chief, Division of Nephrology and Hypertension, Director,
  Center for Hypertension, Kidney and Vascular Health,
  Georgetown University, Washington, DC
Pathogenesis of Hypertension

Jay B. Wish, MD
Professor of Medicine, Case Western Reserve University;
  Medical Director, Dialysis Program, University Hospitals
  Case Medical Center, Cleveland, Ohio
*Anemia and Other Hematologic Complications of Chronic
Kidney Disease*

Vivian Yiu, MB BChir, MRCP
Specialist Registrar, Department of Nephrology, Cambridge
  University Hospitals National Health Service Foundation
  Trust, Cambridge, United Kingdom
Hematuria and Proteinuria

Preface

We are pleased to present the sixth edition of the *Primer on Kidney Diseases*. The *Primer* strives to remain a key resource for students, residents, fellows, and practitioners as they approach clinical challenges in nephrology, electrolyte and acid-base disorders, and hypertensive conditions. Although the text has been completely revised and updated to cover the quickly changing landscape of clinical nephrology, the accessibility and utility that define the *Primer* have been carefully preserved.

This edition brings changes to the *Primer*. The *Primer* was first introduced in 1993, and developed through five editions by Arthur Greenberg and his editorial team of Alfred Cheung, Tom Coffman, Ron Falk, and Charles Jennette. With the sixth edition, the reins have been turned over to a new group, with Debbie Gipson, Mark Perazella, and Marcello Tonelli joining us in this exciting opportunity. Our new team brings a fresh perspective and a wealth of clinical experience to this effort. However, we continue the commitment of our predecessors to the careful selection of content and a diligent editorial process, stressing usability and clinical applicability.

To maintain the *Primer* as a current review of clinical nephrology, we have included new sections that highlight recent advances in nephrology. Chapters on kidney development, assessment of kidney function, onconephrology, and transplant infectious disease have been added, and content on acute kidney injury, transplant medicine, and the kidney in the elderly has been expanded. Specific details on glomerular filtration rate estimation, biomarkers in kidney disease, and recently described pathologic targets in membranous nephropathy, minimal change disease, and viral nephropathies ensure that the *Primer* remains current, accurate, and practical. Suggested readings have been updated to direct readers to additional material.

We are also pleased to offer enhanced online features with this edition of the *Primer*. Access to Expert Consult is available with the activation code provided on the inside front cover. By visiting www.expertconsult.com, readers are able to access the entire *Primer* electronically in a searchable format, download figures and images, and enjoy additional content. The *Primer* will now fit into your pocket on a smartphone or tablet, delivering the information that you seek when you need it.

We are grateful to the authors and editors who diligently compiled a wealth of information into thorough yet concise reviews, ensuring that the *Primer* maintains its clarity and brevity. We are also grateful to the publisher, designers, and copy editors who strove to create an appealing and highly accessible text with illustrative tables and figures to reinforce key messages.

We hope you find the *Primer* to be the same go-to resource clinicians have relied on for the past 20 years.

Scott J. Gilbert, MD
Daniel E. Weiner, MD, MS

Contents

STRUCTURE AND FUNCTION OF THE KIDNEYS AND THEIR CLINICAL ASSESSMENT

1

Overview of Kidney Function and Structure

Josephine P. Briggs | Wilhelm Kriz | Jurgen B. Schnermann

BASIC CONCEPTS

FUNCTIONS OF THE KIDNEY

The main functions of the kidneys can be categorized as follows:

1. *Maintenance of body composition:* The kidney regulates the volume of fluid in the body; its osmolarity, electrolyte content, and concentration; and its acidity. It achieves this regulation by varying the amounts of water and ions excreted in the urine. Electrolytes regulated by changes in urinary excretion include sodium, potassium, chloride, calcium, magnesium, and phosphate.
2. *Excretion of metabolic end products and foreign substances:* The kidney excretes a number of products of metabolism, most notably urea, and a number of toxins and drugs.
3. *Production and secretion of enzymes and hormones:*
    a. Renin is an enzyme produced by the granular cells of the juxtaglomerular apparatus that catalyzes the formation of angiotensin from a plasma globulin, angiotensinogen. Angiotensin is a potent vasoconstrictor peptide that significantly contributes to salt balance and blood-pressure regulation.
    b. Erythropoietin, a glycosylated protein comprising 165 amino acids that is produced by renal cortical interstitial cells, stimulates the maturation of erythrocytes in the bone marrow.
    c. 1,25-Dihydroxyvitamin D_3, the most active form of vitamin D_3, is formed by proximal tubule cells. This steroid hormone plays an important role in the regulation of body calcium and phosphate balance.

In later chapters of this *Primer,* the pathophysiologic mechanisms and consequences of derangements in kidney function are discussed in detail. This chapter reviews the basic anatomy of the kidney, the normal mechanisms for urine formation, and the physiology of sodium, potassium, water, and acid-base balance.

THE KIDNEY AND HOMEOSTASIS

Numerous functions of the body proceed optimally only when body-fluid composition and volume are maintained within an appropriate range. For example,

- Cardiac output and blood pressure are dependent on optimal plasma volume.
- Most enzymes function best over rather narrow ranges of pH and ionic concentrations.

- Cell membrane potential depends on the potassium ion (K^+) concentration.
- Membrane excitability depends on the calcium ion (Ca^{2+}) concentration.

The principal job of the kidneys is the correction of perturbations in the composition and volume of body fluids that occur as a consequence of food in take, metabolism, environmental factors, and exercise. In healthy people, such perturbations are typically corrected within a matter of hours so that, in the long term, body-fluid volume and the concentrations of most ions do not deviate much from normal set points. In many disease states, however, these regulatory processes are disturbed, resulting in persistent deviations in body-fluid volume or ionic concentrations. Understanding these disorders requires an understanding of the normal regulatory processes.

THE BALANCE CONCEPT

A central theme of the physiology of the kidneys is understanding the mechanisms by which urine composition is altered to maintain the body in balance. The maintenance of stable body-fluid composition requires that appearance and disappearance rates of any substance in the body balance each other. Balance is achieved when

$$\text{Ingested amount} + \text{Produced amount} = \\ \text{Excreted amount} + \text{Consumed amount}$$

For a large number of organic compounds, balance is the result of metabolic production and consumption. However, electrolytes are not produced or consumed by the body, so balance can only be achieved by adjusting excretion to match intake. Hence, when a person is in balance for sodium, potassium, and other ions, the amount excreted must equal the amount ingested. Because the kidneys are the principal organs where regulated excretion takes place, urinary excretion of such solutes closely follows the dietary intake.

BODY-FLUID COMPOSITION

To a large extent, humans are composed of water. Adipose tissue is low in water content; therefore, in obese people, the fraction of body weight that is water is lower than in lean individuals. As a consequence of their slightly greater fat content, women contain a lower percentage of water on average than men—about 55% instead of 60%. Useful round numbers to remember for bedside estimates of body-fluid volumes are provided in Table 1.1. Typical values for

Table 1.1 Bedside Estimates of Body-Fluid Compartment Volumes

Remember	Example for 60-kg Patient
TBW = 60% × body weight	60% × 60 kg = 36 L
Intracellular water = ⅔ of TBW	⅔ × 36 L = 24 L
Extracellular water = ⅓ of TBW	⅓ × 36 L = 12 L
Plasma water = ¼ of extracellular water	¼ × 12 L = 3 L
Blood volume = plasma water ÷ (1 – Hct)	3 L ÷ (1 – 0.40) = 5 L

Hct, Hematocrit; *TBW*, total body water.

Table 1.2 Typical Ionic Composition of Plasma and Intracellular Fluid

Constituent	Plasma (mEq/L)	Intracellular Fluid (mEq/L)
Cations		
K^+	4	150
Na^+	143	12
Ca^{2+} (ionized)	2	0.001
Mg^{2+}	1	28
Total cations	150 mEq/L	190 mEq/L
Anions		
Cl^-	104	4
HCO_3^-	24	10
Phosphates	2	40
Protein	14	50
Other	6	86
Total anions	150 mEq/L	190 mEq/L

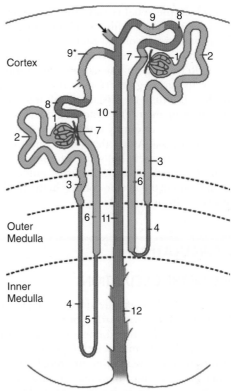

Figure 1.1 Organization of the nephron. The human kidney is made up of approximately one million nephrons, two of which are shown schematically here. Each nephron consists of the following parts: glomerulus (1), proximal convoluted tubule (2), proximal straight tubule (3), thin descending limb of the loop of Henle (4), thin ascending limb (5), thick ascending limb (6), macula densa (7), distal convoluted tubule (8), and connecting tubule (9). Several nephrons coalesce to empty into a collecting duct, which has three distinct regions: the cortical collecting duct (10), the outer medullary collecting duct (11), and the inner medullary collecting duct (12). As shown, the deeper glomeruli give rise to nephrons with loops of Henle that descend all the way to the papillary tips, whereas the more superficial glomeruli have loops of Henle that bend at the junction between the inner and outer medulla.

the ionic composition of the intracellular and extracellular fluid compartments are presented in Table 1.2.

KIDNEY STRUCTURE

The kidneys are two bean-shaped organs that lie in the retroperitoneal space, each weighing about 150 g. The kidney is an anatomically complex organ consisting of many different types of highly specialized cells, which are arranged in a highly organized, three-dimensional pattern. The functional unit of the kidney is the *nephron;* each nephron consists of a glomerulus and a long tubule, which is composed of a single layer of epithelial cells. There are approximately one million nephrons in one human kidney (Fig. 1.1). The nephron is segmented into distinct parts—proximal tubule, loop of Henle, distal tubule, and collecting duct—each with a typical cellular appearance and special functional characteristics.

The nephrons are packed together tightly to make up the kidney parenchyma, which can be divided into regions. The outer layer of the kidney is called the *cortex;* it comprises all of the glomeruli, much of the proximal tubules, and some of the more distal portions as well. The inner section, called the *medulla,* consists largely of the parallel arrays of the loops of Henle and the collecting ducts. The medulla is formed into seven to nine cone-shaped regions, called *pyramids,* that extend into the renal pelvis. The tips of the medullary pyramids are called *papillae.* The medulla is important for concentration of the urine; the extracellular fluid in this region of the kidney has a much higher concentration of solutes than the plasma, with the highest solute concentrations at the papillary tips. The osmolality in the medulla is as much as four times that of the plasma.

The process of urine formation begins in the glomerular capillary tuft, where an ultrafiltrate of plasma is formed. The filtered fluid is collected in Bowman capsule and enters the renal tubule to be carried over a circuitous course, successively modified by exposure to the sequence of specialized tubular epithelial segments with different transport functions. The proximal convoluted tubule, which is located entirely in the renal cortex, absorbs approximately two thirds of the glomerular filtrate. Fluid remaining at the end of the proximal convoluted tubule enters the loop of Henle, which dips down in a hairpin configuration into the medulla. Returning to the cortex, the tubular fluid passes close by its parent glomerulus at the juxtaglomerular apparatus, then it enters the distal convoluted tubule and, finally, the collecting duct. The collecting duct courses back through the medulla, to empty into the renal pelvis at the tip of the renal papilla. Along the tubule, most of the glomerular filtrate is absorbed, but some additional substances are secreted. The final product, the *urine,* enters the renal pelvis and then enters the ureter, collects in the bladder, and is finally excreted from the body.

RENAL CIRCULATION

ANATOMY OF THE CIRCULATION

The renal artery, which enters the kidney at the renal hilum, carries about one fifth of the cardiac output; this represents the highest tissue-specific blood flow of all larger organs in the body (about 350 mL/min per 100 g tissue). As a consequence of this generous perfusion, the renal arteriovenous O_2 difference is much lower than that of most other tissues (and blood in the renal vein is noticeably redder than the blood in other veins). The renal artery bifurcates several times after it enters the kidney and then breaks into the arcuate arteries, which run in an archlike fashion along the border between the cortex and the outer medulla. As shown in Figure 1.2, the arcuate vessels give rise, typically at right angles, to interlobular arteries, which run to the surface of the kidney. The afferent arterioles supplying the glomeruli come off the interlobular vessels.

TWO CAPILLARY BEDS IN SERIES

The renal circulation is unusual in that it breaks into two separate capillary beds: the glomerular bed and the peritubular bed. These two capillary networks are arranged in series, so that all of the renal blood flow passes through both. As blood leaves the glomerulus, the capillaries coalesce into the efferent arteriole, but almost immediately the vessels bifurcate again to form the peritubular capillary network. This second network of capillaries is the site where the fluid reabsorbed by the tubules is returned to the circulation. Pressure in the first capillary bed, that of the glomerulus, is rather high (40 to 50 mm Hg), whereas pressure in the peritubular capillaries is similar to that in capillary beds elsewhere in the body (5 to 10 mm Hg).

About one fourth of the plasma that enters the glomerulus passes through the filtration barrier to become the glomerular filtrate. Blood cells, most of the proteins, and about 75% of the fluid and small solutes stay in the capillary and leave the glomerulus via the efferent arteriole. This postglomerular blood, which has a relatively high concentration of protein and red cells, enters the peritubular capillaries where the high oncotic pressure resulting from the high protein concentration facilitates the reabsorption of fluid. The peritubular capillaries coalesce to form venules and, eventually, the renal vein.

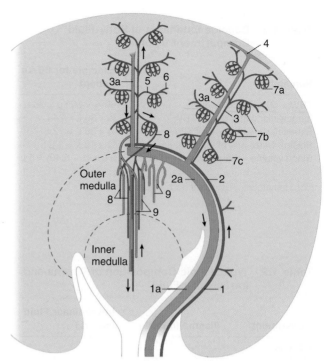

Figure 1.2 Organization of the renal vascular system. The renal artery bifurcates soon after entering the kidney parenchyma and gives rise to a system of arching vessels that run along the border between the cortex and the medulla. In this diagram, the vascular elements surrounding a single renal pyramid are shown. The human kidney typically has seven to nine renal pyramids. Here the arterial supply and glomeruli are shown in red, and the venous system is shown in blue. The peritubular capillary network that arises from the efferent arterioles is omitted for the sake of simplicity. The vascular elements are named as follows: interlobar artery and vein (1 and 1a); arcuate artery and vein (2 and 2a); interlobular artery and vein (3 and 3a); stellate vein (4); afferent arteriole (5); efferent arteriole (6); glomerular capillaries from superficial (7a), midcortex (7b), and juxtamedullary (7c) regions; and juxtamedullary efferent arterioles supplying descending vasa recti (8) and ascending vasa recti (9).

MEDULLARY BLOOD SUPPLY

The blood supplying the medulla is also postglomerular. Specialized peritubular vessels, called vasa recta, arise from the efferent arterioles of the glomeruli nearest the medulla (the juxtamedullary glomeruli). Like medullary renal tubules, these vasa recta form hairpin loops that dip into the medulla.

GLOMERULUS

STRUCTURE

The structure of the glomerulus is shown schematically in Figure 1.3 and in a photomicrograph in Figure 1.4. The glomerulus is a ball consisting of capillaries lined by endothelial cells. The capillaries are held together by a stalk of cells called the *mesangium,* and the outer surface of the capillaries is covered with specialized epithelial cells called *podocytes.* Podocytes are large, highly differentiated cells that form an array of lacelike foot processes over the outer layer of the glomerular capillaries. The foot processes of adjacent podocytes interdigitate, and a thin, membranous structure called the

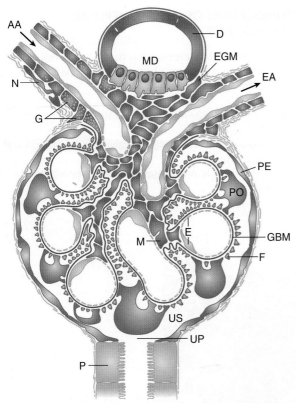

Figure 1.3 Schematic diagram of a section of a glomerulus and its juxtaglomerular apparatus. *AA,* Afferent arteriole; *D,* distal tubule; *E,* endothelial cell; *EA,* efferent arteriole; *EGM,* extraglomerular mesangial cell; *F,* podocyte foot process; *G,* juxtaglomerular granular cell; *GBM,* glomerular basement membrane; *M,* mesangial cell; *MD,* macula densa; *N,* sympathetic nerve endings; *P,* proximal tubule; *PE,* parietal epithelial cell; *PO,* epithelial podocyte; *UP,* urinary pole; *US,* urinary space.

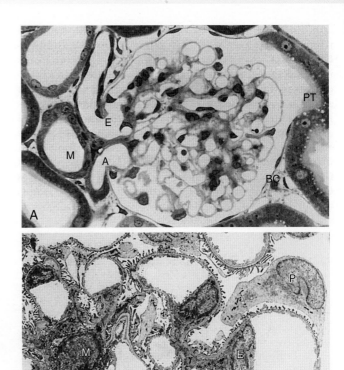

Figure 1.4 Structure of the glomerulus. A, Light micrograph of a glomerulus, showing the afferent arteriole *(A),* efferent arteriole *(E),* macula densa *(M),* Bowman capsule *(BC),* and beginning of the proximal tubule *(PT).* The typical diameter of a glomerulus is approximately 100 to 150 μm, which is just visible to the naked eye (×400). **B,** Higher-power view of glomerular capillary loops, showing the epithelial podocyte *(P),* endothelial cells *(E),* and mesangial cells *(M)* (×4000).

slit diaphragm connects adjacent podocyte foot processes. A structure called *Bowman capsule* acts as a pouch to capture the filtrate and direct it into the beginning of the proximal tubule.

GLOMERULAR FILTRATION BARRIER

Urine formation begins at the glomerular filtration barrier. The glomerular filter through which the ultrafiltrate has to pass consists of three layers: the fenestrated endothelium, the intervening glomerular basement membrane, and the podocyte slit diaphragm (Fig. 1.5). This complex "membrane" is freely permeable to water and small dissolved solutes, but retains most of the proteins and other larger molecules, as well as all blood particles. The main determinant of passage through the glomerular filter is molecular size. A molecule such as inulin (5 kDa) passes freely through the filter. Even a small protein such as myoglobin (16.9 kDa) filters through to a large extent. Substances of increasing size are retained with increasing efficiency until, at a size of approximately 60 to 70 kDa, the amount passing through the filter becomes very small. Some albumin escapes through the glomerular filtration barrier, but it is normally reabsorbed in the proximal tubule.

Proper functioning of the podocyte is critical for maintaining the integrity and selectivity of the glomerular filtration barrier. Podocyte dysfunction causes increased protein excretion in the urine and a condition called *nephrotic syndrome,* which is introduced in Chapter 16. Genetic studies in patients with proteinuria have established the identity of a number of the proteins critical for normal function of the podocyte. The podocyte is a terminally differentiated cell, with little capacity for division or cell repair. Injury to the podocyte is increasingly recognized as a key mechanism in many chronic kidney diseases.

FILTRATION BY THE GLOMERULUS

Filtrate formation in the glomerulus is governed by Starling forces, which are the same forces that determine fluid transport across other blood capillaries. The glomerular filtration rate (GFR) is equal to the product of the net ultrafiltration pressure (P_{net}), the hydraulic permeability (L_p), and the filtration area:

$$GFR = L_p \times Area \times P_{net}$$

The effective filtration pressure (P_{net}) is the difference between the hydrostatic pressure difference and the osmotic pressure difference across the capillary wall:

$$P_{net} = \Delta P - \Delta \Pi = (P_{GC} - P_B) - (\Pi_{GC} - \Pi_B)$$

where P is hydrostatic pressure, Π is osmotic pressure, and the subscripts GC and B refer to the glomerular capillaries and Bowman space, respectively. Changes in GFR can result from changes in product of the permeability and surface area ($L_p \times$ Area) or from changes in P_{net}. One factor influencing P_{net} is the resistance in the afferent and efferent arterioles. An increase in resistance in the afferent arteriole (before blood gets to the glomerulus) decreases P_{GC} and GFR, whereas an increase in resistance as blood exits through the efferent arteriole tends to increase P_{GC} and GFR. Changes in P_{net} can also occur as a result of an increase in renal arterial pressure, which increase P_{GC} and GFR. Obstruction of the tubule increases P_B and decreases GFR, and a decrease in plasma protein concentration tends to increase GFR.

DETERMINATION OF THE GLOMERULAR FILTRATION RATE

GFR is measured by determining the plasma concentration and excretion of a marker substance that meets the following requirements:

1. The substance should be freely filterable across the glomerular membranes.
2. The substance must be neither absorbed nor secreted by the renal tubules.
3. The substance is not metabolized nor produced by the kidneys.

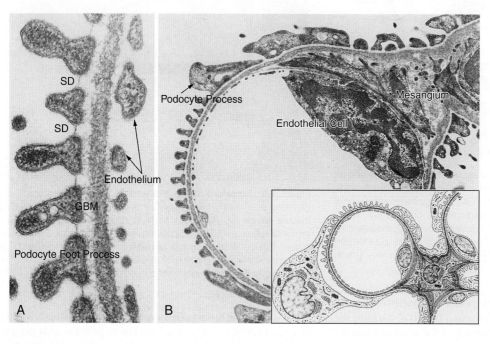

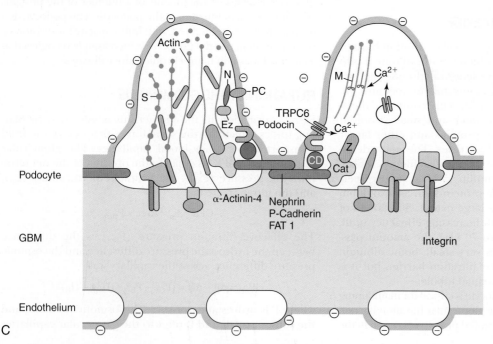

Figure 1.5 Structure of the glomerular capillary loop and the filtration barrier. A, The glomerular filtration barrier consisting of endothelial cells, glomerular basement membrane *(GBM)*, and the slit diaphragms *(SD)* between podocyte foot processes (×34,000). B, A single capillary loop showing the endothelial and foot process layers and the attachments of the basement membrane to the mesangium. Pressure in the glomerular capillary bed is substantially higher than in other capillaries. As shown in the diagrammatic insert, the mesangium provides the structural supports that permit the cells to withstand these high pressures (×13,000). C, Schematic diagram of the filtration barrier. The porous endothelium and the glomerular basement membrane (GBM composed of collagen IV and laminin 521 among others) and the slit diaphragm between two podocyte foot processes are shown. *Cat,* Catenin; *CD,* CD2 associated protein; *Ez,* ezrin; *FAT1,* FAT tumor suppressor homolog 1; *M,* myosin; *N,* NERF2; *PC,* podocalyxin; *S,* synaptopodin; *TRPC 6,* transient receptor potential-channel 6; *Z,* ZO1.

Inulin, a large sugar molecule with a molecular weight of about 5000 Da, meets these requirements and is the classic marker substance infused to measure GFR. It follows from the requirements listed that, if P_{in} is the plasma concentration of inulin, U_{in} is the urinary concentration of inulin, and V is the urine flow rate,

$$\text{Filtered amount of inulin} = GFR \times P_{in}$$
$$\text{Excreted amount of inulin} = U_{in} \times V$$

Because the filtered amount of inulin is equal to the excreted amount of inulin,

$$GFR \times P_{in} = U_{in} \times V$$

Therefore,

$$GFR = \frac{U_{in} \times V}{P_{in}}$$

Other molecules with similar properties have been developed, including iothalamate and iohexol, and these compounds can be administered to patients to measure GFR. Creatinine is an endogenous substance that, although not a perfect GFR marker, is handled by the kidney in a similar way so that its plasma concentration can be used to estimate GFR. The clearance of creatinine is slightly greater than GFR (15% to 20%) because some creatinine is secreted; therefore, the excreted amount exceeds the amount filtered. Cystatin is another endogenous substance that is cleared by the kidney roughly in proportion to the level of GFR; plasma levels of cystatin have also been used to estimate GFR. The estimation of GFR is discussed in more detail in Chapter 3.

GFR is dependent on body size, age, and physiologic state. Typical normal values for GFR in adults are 100 mL/min for women and 120 mL/min for men. Values in children increase with growth and depend on age. A high-protein diet and high salt intake increase GFR, and GFR increases markedly with pregnancy (see Chapter 51). GFR decreases with a low-protein diet and declines steadily with age (see Chapter 52).

JUXTAGLOMERULAR APPARATUS

Tightly adherent to every glomerulus, in between the entry and the exit of the arterioles, is a plaque of distal tubular cells called the *macula densa*. Part of the juxtaglomerular apparatus, this cell plaque is at the very terminal end of the thick ascending limb of the loop of Henle just before its transition to the distal convoluted tubule. This is a special position along the nephron, because at this site the salt concentration is quite variable. Low tubular flow rates result in a very low concentration of NaCl at this site, 15 mEq/L or less, whereas at higher flow rates the salt concentration increases to 40 to 60 mEq/L. The NaCl concentration at this site regulates glomerular function through a mechanism called *tubuloglomerular feedback:* changes in luminal salt concentration produced by changes in loop of Henle flow rate regulate afferent arteriolar resistance in a way that causes inverse changes in glomerular blood flow and filtration rate.

The other unique cells that make up the juxtaglomerular apparatus are the renin-containing juxtaglomerular granular cells. Renin secretion is also regulated locally by salt concentration in the tubule at the macula densa. In addition, the granular cells have extensive sympathetic innervation, and renin secretion is further controlled by the sympathetic nervous system.

TUBULAR FUNCTION: BASIC PRINCIPLES

EPITHELIAL TRANSPORT ALONG THE RENAL TUBULE

The glomerular filtrate undergoes a series of modifications before becoming urine. These changes consist of removal (reabsorption) and addition (secretion) of solutes and fluid (Fig. 1.6).

1. *Reabsorption,* the movement of solute or water from tubular lumen to blood, is the predominant process in the renal handling of Na^+, Cl^-, H_2O, bicarbonate (HCO_3^-), glucose, amino acids, protein, phosphates, Ca^{2+}, Mg^{2+}, urea, uric acid, and other molecules. Reabsorption can occur both across the cell membranes (transcellular pathway) or between cells (paracellular pathway). Transcellular transport depends on the presence of specific transport proteins in the membrane, whereas paracellular transport across the tight junctions depends on the characteristics of a family of tight junction proteins called claudins.

2. *Secretion,* the movement of solute from blood or cell interior to tubular lumen, is important in the renal handling of H^+, K^+, ammonium ion (NH_4^+), and a number of organic acids and bases.

Many specialized membrane proteins participate in the movement of substances across cell membranes along the renal tubule. Some of the important membrane transport mechanisms, together with examples of substances that use these mechanisms and proteins involved, are listed in

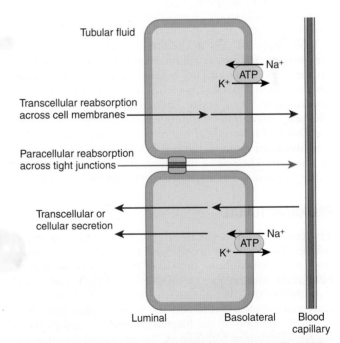

Figure 1.6 General scheme for epithelial transport. The driving force for solute movement is primarily generated by the action of sodium-potassium adenosine triphosphatase (Na^+,K^+-ATPase) in the basolateral membrane. Solutes and water can move either through a paracellular pathway between cells *(red arrows)* or through a transcellular transport pathway *(blue arrows)*, which requires movement across both luminal and basolateral membranes. *ATP,* Adenosine triphosphate.

Table 1.3   Types of Membrane Transport Mechanisms Used in the Kidney

Mechanism	Examples of Substances	Examples of Transport Protein
Facilitated or carrier-mediated	Glucose, urea	GLUT1 carrier, urea carrier
Active transport (pumps)	Na^+, K^+, H^+, Ca^{2+}	Na^+ K^+-ATPase, H^+-ATPase, Ca^{2+}-ATPase
Coupled transport		
Cotransport	Cl^-, glucose, amino acids, formate, phosphates	NKCC2, SGLT, NaPi II
Countertransport	Bicarbonate, H^+	Cl^-/HCO_3^- exchanger (AE1), Na^+/H^+ anti-porter (NHE3)
Osmosis	H_2O	Water channels (aquaporins)

ATPase, Adenosine triphosphatase; *GLUT1,* glucose transporter 1; *NaPi II,* sodium phosphate cotransporter type II; *NKCC2,* Na^+-K^+-$2Cl^-$ cotransporter; *SGLT,* sodium-linked glucose transporter.

Table 1.3. A variety of mechanisms exist to regulate the activity of membrane proteins. Transport proteins may undergo alterations in physical confirmation, triggered for example by phosphorylation or dephosphorylation, resulting in changed channel activity or transport affinity. A consequence of these changes may be insertion or removal of the transport protein from the membrane, which are processes known, respectively, as endocytosis and exocytosis. As shown in Figures 1.7 through 1.10, one of the more striking characteristics of the renal tubule is its dramatic cellular heterogeneity. Early renal anatomists recognized that there are marked differences in the appearance of the cells of the proximal tubule, loop of Henle, and distal tubule. We now know that these nephron segments also differ markedly in function, distribution of important transport proteins, and responsiveness to drugs such as diuretics.

Most epithelial cells in the kidney and in other organs possess a single primary cilium. New attention has focused on the importance of cilia because of the discovery that genetic defects in cilial proteins are associated with the development of renal cysts. There is growing evidence that cilia play a role in determining epithelial shape and in the regulation of intracellular cell calcium by shear stress. Cilia may also participate in the regulation of tubular function by flow rate. The role of the cilium in cystic diseases of the kidney is discussed in more detail in Chapters 42 and 43.

PROXIMAL TUBULE

The proximal tubules reabsorb the bulk of filtered small solutes. These solutes are present at the same concentration in proximal tubular fluid as in plasma. Approximately 60% of the filtered Na^+, Cl^-, K^+, Ca^{2+}, and H_2O, and more than 90% of the filtered HCO_3^-, are reabsorbed along the proximal tubule. This is also the segment that normally reabsorbs virtually all the filtered glucose and amino acids via Na^+-dependent cotransport. An additional function of the proximal tubule is phosphate transport, which is regulated by parathyroid hormone. The proximal tubule is an example of an epithelium with low transepithelial resistance ("leaky" epithelium). Leakiness is the result of a tight junction protein (claudin-2) that is permeable to cations and water. In addition to these reabsorption functions,

secretion of solutes also occurs along the proximal tubule. The terminal portion of the proximal tubule, the S3 segment or pars recta, is the site of secretion of numerous organic anions and cations, a mechanism used by the body for elimination of many drugs and toxins.

The proximal tubule (Fig. 1.7) has a prominent brush border, extensive interdigitated basolateral infoldings, and large prominent mitochondria, which supply the energy for sodium-potassium adenosine triphosphatase (Na^+,K^+-ATPase).

LOOP OF HENLE

The loop of Henle consists of the terminal or straight portion of the proximal tubule, thin descending and ascending limbs, and a thick ascending limb. It is important for generation of a concentrated medulla and for dilution of the urine. The thick ascending limb is often called the diluting segment, because transport along this water-impermeable segment results in the development of a dilute tubular fluid. The thick ascending limb is also the site of paracellular reabsorption of divalent cations such as Ca^{++} and Mg^{++}. The principal luminal transporter expressed in this segment is the Na^+-K^+-$2Cl^-$ cotransporter (NKCC2), which is the target of loop diuretics such as furosemide. The morphology of the loop of Henle epithelia is illustrated in Figure 1.8.

DISTAL NEPHRON

The distal nephron, which includes the distal convoluted tubule, the connecting tubule, and the cortical and medullary collecting duct, is the portion of the nephron where final adjustments in urine composition, tonicity, and volume are made. Distal segments are the sites where critical regulatory hormones such as aldosterone and vasopressin regulate acid and potassium excretion and also determine final urinary concentrations of K^+, Na^+, and Cl^-. Both the distal convoluted tubule and the connecting tubule have well-developed basolateral infoldings with abundant mitochondria, like the proximal tubule. They are easily distinguished from the latter by the lack of brush border (Fig. 1.9). The distal convoluted tubule is the principal site of action of thiazide diuretics.

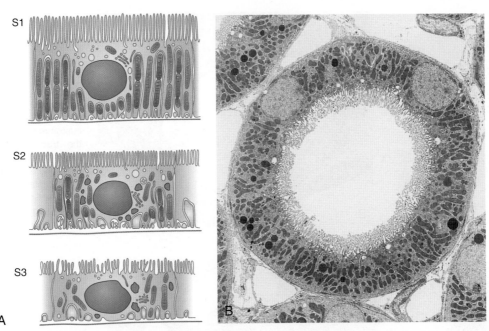

Figure 1.7   Proximal tubule. The proximal tubule consists of three segments: S1, S2, and S3. **A,** Schematic diagrams of the typical cells from these three segments. **B,** A cross-section of the S1 segment. The S1 begins at the glomerulus and extends for several millimeters before the transition to the S2 segment. The S3 segment, which is also called the proximal straight tubule, descends into the inner medulla. The proximal tubule is characterized by a prominent brush border, which increases the membrane surface area about fortyfold. The basolateral infoldings, which are lined with mitochondria, are interdigitated with the basolateral infoldings of adjacent cells (in the diagrams, processes that come from adjacent cells are shaded). These adaptations are most prominent in the first parts of the proximal tubule and are less developed further along the proximal tubule (×2300).

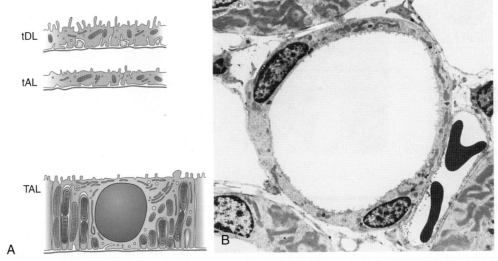

Figure 1.8   Loop of Henle. The loop of Henle makes a hairpin loop within the medulla. Segments included in the loop are the terminal portion of the proximal tubule, the thin descending (tDL) and thin ascending (tAL) limbs, and the thick ascending limb (TAL). **A,** Schematic drawings of cell morphology. **B,** A cross-section through the tDL in the outer medulla. The thin limbs, as their names suggest, are shallow epithelia without the prominent mitochondria of more proximal segments. The thick limb, in contrast, is a taller epithelium with basolateral infoldings and well-developed mitochondria. This segment is water impermeable; transport along this segment is important for generation of interstitial solute gradients (×3000).

The collecting duct cells are cuboidal, and their basolateral folds do not interdigitate extensively. When there is a sizable osmotic gradient and water moves across this epithelium, the spaces between cells widen. The collecting duct changes its appearance as it travels from the cortex to the papillary tip (Fig. 1.10). In the cortex, there are two different cell types in the collecting duct: principal cells and intercalated cells. Principal cells are the main site of salt and water transport, and intercalated cells are the key site for acid-base regulation. The medullary collecting duct, in its most terminal portions, comes increasingly to resemble the tall cells typical of the transitional epithelium that lines the bladder.

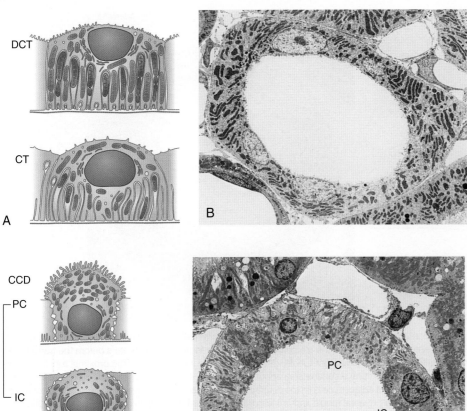

Figure 1.9 Distal convoluted tubule. The distal convoluted tubule is customarily divided into two parts: the true distal convoluted tubule (DCT) and the connecting tubule (CT), where cell morphology is somewhat similar to that of the collecting duct. **A,** Schematic diagrams of cell morphology. **B,** Cross-section of DCT (×3000).

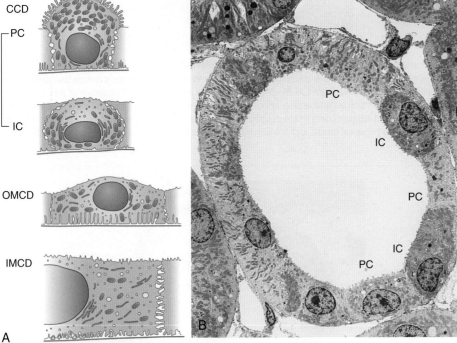

Figure 1.10 Collecting duct. A, Schematic appearance of cell morphology. **B,** Cross-section. The collecting duct changes its morphology as it travels from cortex to the medulla. In the cortex there are two cell types: principal cells (PC) and intercalated cells (IC). *CCD,* Cortical collecting duct; *IMCD,* inner medullary collecting duct; *OMCD,* outer medullary collecting duct (×3000).

SALT AND VOLUME REGULATION

ABSORPTION OF SODIUM

Because of its high extracellular concentration, large amounts of Na^+ and its accompanying anions are present in the glomerular filtrate, and the absorption of this filtered Na^+ is, in a quantitative sense, the dominant work performed by the renal tubules. The amount of Na^+ absorbed by the tubules is the difference between the amount of Na^+ filtered and the amount excreted:

$$Na^+\ absorption = Filtered\ Na^+ - Excreted\ Na^+$$

or

$$Na^+\ absorption = (GFR \times P_{Na}) - (V \times U_{Na})$$

where U_{Na} is the urinary Na^+ concentration and P_{Na} is the plasma Na^+ concentration. With a GFR of 120 mL/min and a plasma Na^+ concentration of 145 mEq/L, 17.4 mEq of Na^+ is filtered every minute, or about 25,000 mEq (575 g) of Na^+ per day. Because only about 100 to 250 mEq of Na^+ is excreted per day (this reflects the average intake provided by a typical Western diet), one can estimate that the tubule reabsorbs somewhat more than 99% of the filtered Na^+. The fractional excretion of Na^+ (FE_{Na}) is defined as the fraction of filtered Na^+ excreted in the urine. Using creatinine as a GFR estimate, FE_{Na} is calculated as follows:

$$FE_{Na} = \frac{Excreted\ Na^+}{Filtered\ Na^+} = \frac{U_{Na} \times V}{P_{Na} \times GFR}$$
$$= \frac{U_{Na} \times V}{P_{Na} \times (U_{Cr}/P_{Cr} \times V)} = \frac{U_{Na}/P_{Na}}{U_{Cr}/P_{Cr}}$$

where U_{Cr} and P_{Cr} are the urinary and plasma concentrations of creatinine, respectively.

FE_{Na} is usually less than 1%. However, this value depends on Na^+ intake and can vary physiologically from almost 0% at extremely low intakes to about 2% at extremely high intakes. FE_{Na} can also exceed 1% in disease states in which the tubular transport of Na^+ is impaired (e.g., in most cases of acute kidney injury).

MECHANISMS OF SODIUM ION ABSORPTION

Tubular Na^+ absorption is a primary active transport process driven by the enzyme Na^+,K^+-ATPase. In renal epithelial cells, as in most cells of the body, this pump translocates Na^+ out of cells (and K^+ into cells), thereby lowering intracellular Na^+ concentration (and elevating intracellular K^+ concentration). A key for the generation of net Na^+ movement from the tubular lumen to the blood is the asymmetrical distribution of this enzyme; it is present exclusively in the basolateral membrane (the blood side) of all nephron segments. Delivery of Na^+ to the pump sites is maintained by Na^+ entry across the luminal side of the cells along a favorable electrochemical gradient. Because Na^+ permeability of the luminal membrane is much higher than that of the basolateral membrane, Na^+ entry is fed from the luminal Na^+ pool. The asymmetrical permeability results from the presence of a variety of transport proteins and channels located exclusively in the luminal membrane.

A number of these luminal transporters are the target molecules for diuretic action. Principal entry mechanisms for Na^+ and Cl^- in the various nephron segments are as follows:

1. *Early proximal tubule:* Na^+-dependent cotransporter, Na^+/H^+ exchanger (NHE3)
2. *Late proximal tubule:* Na^+/H^+ exchanger, Cl^--anion exchanger
3. *Thick ascending limb:* NKCC2 cotransporter (furosemide-sensitive carrier)
4. *Distal convoluted tubule:* Na^+/Cl^- cotransporter (NCCT) (thiazide-sensitive carrier)
5. *Collecting duct:* epithelial Na^+ channel (ENaC) (amiloride-sensitive channel)

REGULATION OF SALT EXCRETION

Because Na^+ salts are the most abundant extracellular solutes, the amount of sodium in the body (the total body sodium) determines the extracellular fluid volume. Therefore, excretion or retention of Na^+ salts by the kidneys is critical for the regulation of extracellular fluid volume. Disturbance in volume regulation, particularly enhanced salt retention, is common in disease states. The sympathetic nervous system, the renin-angiotensin-aldosterone system, atrial natriuretic peptide, and vasopressin represent the four main regulatory systems that change their activity in response to changes in body-fluid volume. These changes in activity mediate the effects of body-fluid volume on urinary Na^+ excretion.

SYMPATHETIC NERVOUS SYSTEM

A change in extracellular fluid volume is sensed by stretch receptors on blood vessels, principally those located on the low-pressure side of the circulation in the thorax (e.g., vena cava, cardiac atria, pulmonary vessels). A decreased firing rate in the afferent nerves from these volume receptors enhances sympathetic outflow from cardiovascular medullary centers. Increased renal sympathetic tone enhances renal salt reabsorption and can decrease renal blood flow at higher frequencies. In addition to its direct effects on kidney function, increased sympathetic outflow promotes the activation of another salt-retaining system, the renin-angiotensin system.

RENIN-ANGIOTENSIN SYSTEM

Renin is an enzyme that is formed by and released from granular cells in the wall of renal afferent arterioles near the entrance to the glomerulus. These granular cells are part of the juxtaglomerular apparatus (see Fig. 1.3). Renin cleaves angiotensin I from angiotensinogen, a large circulating protein made principally in the liver. Angiotensin I, a decapeptide, is converted by angiotensin-converting enzyme to the biologically active angiotensin II. Renin catalyzes the rate-limiting step in the production of angiotensin II, and therefore it is the plasma level of renin that determines the concentration of angiotensin II in plasma. There are three principal mechanisms that control renin release:

1. *Macula densa mechanism:* The term "macula densa" refers to a group of distinct epithelial cells located in the wall of the thick ascending limb of the loop of Henle where it makes contact with its own glomerulus. At this location, the NaCl concentration is between 30 and 40 mEq/L and varies as a direct function of tubular fluid flow rate (i.e., it increases when the flow rate is high and decreases when it is low). A decrease in NaCl concentration at the macula densa strongly stimulates renin secretion, and an increase inhibits it. The connection to the regulation of body-fluid volume results from the dependence of the flow rate past the macula densa cells on the body sodium content. The flow rate is high in states of sodium excess and low in sodium depletion.
2. *Baroreceptor mechanism:* Renin secretion is stimulated by a decrease in arterial pressure, an effect believed to be mediated by a "baroreceptor" in the wall of the afferent arteriole that responds to pressure, stretch, or shear stress.
3. *β-Adrenergic stimulation:* An increase in renal sympathetic activity or in circulating catecholamines stimulates renin release through β-adrenergic receptors on the juxtaglomerular granular cells.

Angiotensin II has direct and indirect effects that promote salt retention. It enhances Na^+ reabsorption in the proximal tubule (through stimulation of Na^+/H^+ exchange). Angiotensin II affects salt balance indirectly by stimulating the production and release of the steroid hormone aldosterone from the zona glomerulosa of the adrenal gland.

ALDOSTERONE

Aldosterone acts on the collecting duct to augment salt reabsorption, largely by increasing the activity of the sodium channel, ENaC, and thereby increasing salt absorption. A second important action of aldosterone in the kidney is the stimulation of K^+ secretion. This effect is not dependent on angiotensin; rather, high K^+ stimulates the secretion of aldosterone directly. In the distal nephron, these two effects of aldosterone are not always coupled, and recent evidence suggests that a family of kinases, called WNK kinases, may participate in switching the distal nephron response to allow either maximal NaCl reabsorption (in hypovolemia) or maximal K^+ secretion (in hyperkalemia). The first evidence that these kinases are important functional molecular switches came from genetic studies in patients with a Mendelian form of hypertension accompanied by hyperkalemia called pseudohypoaldosteronism type II.

ATRIAL NATRIURETIC PEPTIDE

Atrial natriuretic peptide (ANP) is a hormone that is synthesized by atrial myocytes and is released in response to increased atrial distention. As a result, ANP secretion is increased in volume expansion and is inhibited in volume depletion. ANP produces an increase in salt excretion primarily by inhibiting Na^+ reabsorption along the collecting duct.

VASOPRESSIN OR ANTIDIURETIC HORMONE

Vasopressin, or antidiuretic hormone (ADH), is regulated primarily by body-fluid osmolarity. However, in states of intravascular volume depletion, the set point for vasopressin release is shifted so that for any given plasma osmolarity, vasopressin levels are higher than they would be normally. This shift promotes water retention to aid in restoration of body-fluid volumes.

WATER AND OSMOREGULATION

REGULATION OF BODY-FLUID OSMOLARITY

When water intake is low or water is lost from the body (e.g., in hypotonic fluids such as sweat), the kidneys conserve water by producing a small volume of concentrated urine. In dehydration, urine production is less than 1 L/day (<0.5 mL/min) and the osmotic concentration of the urine (U_{osm}) may reach 1200 mOsm/kg H_2O. When water intake is high, urine flow may increase to as much as 14 L/day (10 mL/min), with an osmolality substantially lower than that of plasma (75 to 100 mOsm/kg). These wide variations in urine volume and osmotic concentration do not obligatorily affect the excretion of the daily solute load. For example, the daily solute excess of about 1200 mOsm may be excreted in 12 L of urine (U_{osm} = 100 mOsm/L) or in 1 L (U_{osm} = 1200 mOsm/L). The hormone responsible for the regulatory changes in urine volume and tonicity is ADH (vasopressin).

ROLE OF ANTIDIURETIC HORMONE IN OSMOLARITY REGULATION

ADH is a nonapeptide produced by neurons located in the supraoptic and paraventricular nuclei of the hypothalamus. It is stored in and released from granules in nerve terminals

that are located in the posterior pituitary (neurohypophysis). The release of ADH is exquisitely sensitive to changes in plasma osmolality (P_{osm}), with increases in P_{osm} above a threshold of about 285 mOsm/kg leading to increases in ADH secretion and plasma ADH concentration. As has been pointed out, the actual set point for release depends on body-fluid volume as well.

The most important function of ADH is the regulation of the water permeability of the distal portions of the nephron, particularly the collecting duct. As shown schematically in Figure 1.11, ADH binds to specific receptors (V2 receptors) in the basolateral membrane of collecting duct cells activating adenylate cyclase to form cyclic adenosine monophosphate (cAMP). Activation of cAMP-dependent protein kinase triggers fusion of membrane vesicles that contain aquaporin-2 water channels. The result is a rapid increase in water permeability of the luminal membrane of collecting duct cells. When ADH levels fall, water channels are quickly removed from the luminal membrane by endocytosis.

TUBULAR WATER ABSORPTION

At each point along the nephron, the osmotic pressure of the tubular fluid is lower than that in the interstitial space. This transtubular osmotic pressure difference provides the driving force for tubular water reabsorption. The rate of fluid absorption in a given nephron segment is determined by the magnitude of this gradient and the water permeability of the segment. Even though the osmotic pressure difference across the proximal tubule epithelium is small (3 to 4 mOsm/L), the rate of fluid absorption is high, because this segment has very high water permeability. In contrast, osmotic gradients across the thick ascending limb may be as high as 250 mOsm/L, and yet virtually no water flows across this segment, because it is highly water

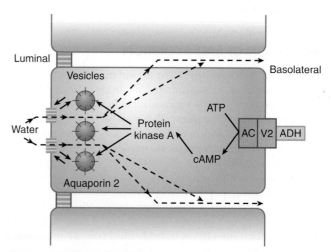

Figure 1.11   Mechanism of action of antidiuretic hormone (ADH) on the collecting duct. ADH combines with a basolateral receptor (V2), which is coupled with adenylate cyclase (AC). Generation of cyclic adenosine monophosphate (cAMP) leads to activation of protein kinase A, which in turn phosphorylates the water channel, aquaporin 2. The vesicles containing aquaporin are then inserted into the luminal membrane, increasing water permeability. *ATP,* Adenosine triphosphate.

impermeable. This segment dilutes the urine as it absorbs Na^+ and Cl^- without water.

In contrast to the constancy of water conductivity in the proximal tubule and the thick ascending limb, water permeability in the collecting duct is highly variable and controlled by ADH. When ADH is absent, water permeability and water absorption are low, and the hypotonicity generated in the thick ascending limb persists along the collecting duct. As a consequence, a dilute urine is excreted. When ADH is present, the collecting duct becomes quite water permeable, and water is reabsorbed until the tubular fluid in the collecting duct equilibrates with the hypertonic interstitium. In this situation, the final urine is osmotically concentrated and has a low volume.

MEDULLARY HYPERTONICITY

To allow osmotically driven water absorption, the osmotic concentration in the medullary interstitium must be slightly higher than that in the collecting duct lumen. For example, when a final urine with an osmolality of 1200 mOsm/kg is excreted, the medullary interstitium at the tips of the papillae must be a little higher than 1200 mOsm/kg. The generation of such a unique extracellular environment is achieved by the countercurrent multiplication system of the renal medulla, which consists of the countercurrent arrangement of descending and ascending limbs of the loops of Henle.

COUNTERCURRENT MULTIPLICATION

By passing through two adjacent tubes with flow in opposite directions, the tubular fluid can attain an osmotic concentration difference in the longitudinal axis of the system that

by far exceeds that seen at each level along it. This principle of countercurrent multiplication requires energy expenditure and the presence of unique differences in membrane characteristics between the two limbs of the system.

The countercurrent multiplier represented by the loops of Henle is believed to generate an osmotic gradient for the following reasons:

1. Active NaCl transport across the ascending limb (the so-called single effect of the countercurrent system) generates an osmotic difference between the tubular fluid and the surrounding local interstitium.
2. Low water permeability in the ascending limb prevents dissipation of this gradient.
3. High water permeability in the descending limb permits equilibration of descending limb contents with the surrounding local interstitium.

The mechanism by which such a system can result in progressive increases in osmotic concentration along the corticopapillary axis is shown in Figure 1.12. In step 1 (time zero), the fluid in the descending and ascending limbs and in the interstitium is isoosmotic to plasma. In step 2, NaCl is absorbed from the ascending limb into the interstitium until a gradient of 200 mOsm/kg is reached. In step 3, the fluid in the descending limb equilibrates osmotically with the interstitium by water movement out of the tubule. In step 4, the hypertonic fluid is presented to the thick ascending limb with an increased solute concentration in the region near the tip of the system. Active NaCl transport along the ascending limb again establishes a 200 mOsm/kg gradient (step 5), thereby increasing the interstitial concentration and (by water abstraction) the descending limb concentration (step 6). Note that concentrations near the tip are now higher than those near the base. Continued operation of such

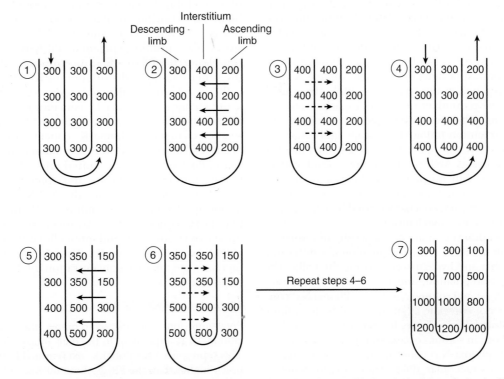

Figure 1.12   The process of countercurrent multiplication. (From Koeppen BM, Stanton BA: *Renal physiology.* St. Louis, CV Mosby, 1992.)

a mechanism gradually results in the generation of a gradient of hypertonicity, with the highest osmolarities at the papillary tip (step 7). The tubular fluid leaving the ascending limb of the loop of Henle countercurrent multiplier is hypotonic, but the medullary interstitium has been osmotically "charged."

Because the collecting ducts on their way to the papillary tip return through the hypertonic medullary environment, their content can be concentrated by water flow along an osmotic gradient.

ROLE OF UREA IN THE COUNTERCURRENT MECHANISM

In addition to Na^+ and Cl^-, urea is the other major solute concentrated in the renal medulla. Urea enters the medulla by reabsorption across the collecting duct. Marked differences in permeability to urea allow reabsorption to proceed only across the terminal portions of the medullary collecting duct. In the early portions of the collecting duct, urea permeability is low, and reabsorption of urea cannot occur. Because water leaves the tubule under the influence of ADH, the urea staying behind is progressively concentrated. As a consequence, a substantial urea gradient develops, providing the driving force for urea reabsorption when the permeability to urea permits it. The contribution of urea accumulation to osmotic water absorption along the inner medullary collecting duct must be sizable, because urea accounts for about half of inner medullary tonicity. Therefore, a reduction in urea synthesis due to reduced protein intake markedly impairs the concentrating ability of the kidneys.

COMPARISON BETWEEN VOLUME REGULATION AND OSMOREGULATION

Osmoregulation is under the control of a single hormonal system, ADH, whereas volume regulation is under the control of a set of redundant and overlapping control mechanisms. Lack or excess of ADH results in defined and rather dramatic clinical syndromes of excess water loss or water retention. In contrast, a defect in a single volume regulatory mechanism generally results in more subtle abnormalities because of the redundant regulatory capacity from the other mechanisms. Therefore, excess aldosterone results in a mild volume retention followed by escape and return to normal Na^+ excretion, due to the action of the other mechanisms. Similarly, excess ANP produces only a modest decrement in volume, with no persistent abnormality in Na^+ excretion. Severe salt-retaining states, such as liver cirrhosis or congestive heart failure, are characterized by activation of all the volume regulatory mechanisms.

Finally, the symptoms that are characteristic of disorders of osmoregulation and of volume regulation are different, with hyponatremia and hypernatremia being the hallmarks of deranged osmoregulation, and edema or hypovolemia resulting from deranged volume regulation. Plasma Na^+ concentration does not correlate at all with total body sodium or the extracellular fluid volume. In fact, a low serum Na^+ may be found both in sodium excess and sodium deficiency states. However, plasma Na^+ concentration is the principal determinant of extracellular fluid osmolarity. In general, abnormalities in Na^+ concentration arise from defects in osmoregulation, not volume regulation.

REGULATION OF BODY-FLUID POTASSIUM AND ACIDITY

Both potassium and hydrogen ions are present in body fluids at low concentrations, about 4 to 5 mEq/L for K^+ and about 40 nEq/L for H^+. Both ions show a number of features:

1. Relatively small deviations in either the K^+ or the H^+ concentration can be life-threatening, and therefore the regulation of K^+ and H^+ requires control systems with high sensitivity and precision.
2. Constancy of both the K^+ and the H^+ concentration over the long term is achieved by regulated excretion of these ions in the urine. However, in both cases, other mechanisms exist that provide immediate protection against excessive deviations of plasma concentrations from normal.
3. Regulation in the renal excretion of both K^+ and H^+ is caused to a large extent by variation in the secretion of these ions by collecting ducts. The principal cell of the collecting duct is responsible for regulated K^+ secretion; the intercalated cell is responsible for H^+ secretion (see Fig. 1.10).
4. The rate of both K^+ secretion and H^+ secretion is increased by aldosterone.
5. A primary derangement of K^+ balance can cause an acidity disturbance, and a primary acidity disturbance can derange K^+ homeostasis.

REGULATION OF BODY-FLUID POTASSIUM

DISTRIBUTION OF POTASSIUM ION IN THE BODY

K^+ is primarily an intracellular ion owing to the presence of Na^+,K^+-ATPase in virtually all cell membranes. Of the 3500 mEq of body potassium, only about 1% to 2% is present in the extracellular space, where it has a concentration of 4 to 5 mEq/L. The remainder (about 98%) is intracellular. This distribution poses a potential risk in that the release of even a small amount of K^+ from intracellular stores (e.g., insulin deficiency, cell lysis, severe exercise) can elevate the plasma K^+ concentration substantially. On the other hand, the distribution of K^+ between the extracellular and intracellular spaces serves as a means to buffer acute changes in plasma K^+ concentration. For example, the administration of an acute oral K^+ load induces much smaller changes in plasma K^+ concentration than would occur if all absorbed K^+ were to remain in the extracellular space. Potassium ions are shifted into cells under the stimulatory influence of insulin and epinephrine. The effect of either hormone activates the Na^+,K^+-ATPase. Another important factor in determining K^+ distribution is the plasma H^+ concentration. An increase in H^+ ions causes uptake of H^+ into cells and intracellular buffering, to some extent, in exchange for K^+. Therefore, acidosis tends to increase the plasma concentration of K^+, and alkalosis tends to decrease it.

RENAL HANDLING OF POTASSIUM

Potassium ion homeostasis requires the excretion of an amount of K^+ equivalent to the daily intake (50 to 150 mEq). This represents a fractional K^+ excretion (FE_K) of about 10%, much higher than the FE_{Na}. About 60% to 70% of filtered K^+ is absorbed along the proximal tubule, and further reabsorption of K^+ takes place in the thick ascending limb of the loop of

Henle; only about 10% of filtered K$^+$ enters the distal tubule. Along the collecting duct, K$^+$ is both secreted and absorbed. Collecting duct K$^+$ secretion increases when dietary K$^+$ intake is elevated. When dietary intake is low, collecting duct K$^+$ secretion virtually ceases, and absorption is dominant. Therefore, although K$^+$ absorption along the proximal tubule and the loop of Henle does not change very much depending on intake, collecting duct K$^+$ secretion is variable. This variability accounts almost completely for the variation in urinary K$^+$ excretion.

MECHANISMS OF POTASSIUM ION SECRETION

K$^+$ secretion across the collecting duct epithelium uses the transcellular route. K$^+$ uptake across the basolateral membrane is driven by Na$^+$,K$^+$-ATPase, which elevates the intracellular K$^+$ concentration to a level above electrochemical equilibrium. K$^+$ can then move along a favorable gradient from cell interior to tubule lumen using potassium channels in the luminal membrane.

Three major variables determine the rate at which K$^+$ is secreted by collecting duct cells:

1. Changes in the activity of Na$^+$,K$^+$-ATPase affect K$^+$ uptake across the basolateral membrane and thereby intracellular K$^+$ concentration. An increase in pump activity increases intracellular K$^+$ levels and tends to stimulate K$^+$ secretion.
2. Changes in the electrochemical gradient affect the driving force for K$^+$ movement across the luminal membrane. Either an increase in intracellular K$^+$ concentration or in the transepithelial potential difference (lumen-negative) will increase the driving force for K$^+$ secretion.
3. Changes in the permeability of the luminal membrane determine the amount of K$^+$ that can be secreted for a given driving force. An increase in luminal K$^+$ conductance increases K$^+$ secretion.

REGULATION OF POTASSIUM ION EXCRETION

Plasma K$^+$ Concentration

One important determinant of K$^+$ excretion is the plasma K$^+$ concentration. For example, the change in K$^+$ excretion that occurs after an increase in dietary K$^+$ intake is mediated by an increase in plasma K$^+$. The effect of plasma K$^+$ on secretion is induced in part by a direct effect on the intracellular K$^+$ concentration.

Aldosterone

At any level of plasma K$^+$, the secretion of K$^+$ also depends on the plasma aldosterone level. Aldosterone enhances K$^+$ secretion by activation of Na$^+$,K$^+$-ATPase and by an increase in permeability of the luminal membrane to K$^+$. Aldosterone is partly responsible for the diet-induced increase in K$^+$ excretion, because its production and secretion are directly stimulated by the plasma K$^+$ concentration. This effect is independent of angiotensin.

Tubular Flow Rate

An increase in tubular flow rate past the principal cells stimulates K$^+$ secretion, and a decrease reduces K$^+$ secretion. The K$^+$ concentration gradient across the luminal membrane increases when delivery of fluid increases. In addition, increased flow has been found to increase K$^+$ permeability, perhaps mediated by changes in the deflection of the cilia on tubular cells.

Distal Sodium Delivery

When more Na$^+$ is delivered to the distal nephron and reabsorption increases, the net electrical charge in the lumen becomes more negative. This favorable electrochemical gradient tends to increase urinary K$^+$ secretion.

Hydrogen Ions

A decrease in H$^+$ concentration in alkalemic states stimulates K$^+$ secretion. This effect is mediated by the increase in intracellular K$^+$ concentration that occurs in alkalemia.

DIURETICS AND POTASSIUM ION EXCRETION

Diuretics increase the tubular flow rate. Agents such as loop diuretics and thiazides that inhibit absorption of NaCl and water in segments that precede the collecting duct (NaCl in the loop of Henle and water in the distal tubule) increase the flow of fluid past the collecting duct cells, which causes increased K$^+$ secretion. In addition, diuretics cause volume depletion, which stimulates aldosterone secretion.

REGULATION OF BODY-FLUID ACIDITY

BASIC CONSIDERATIONS

Maintenance of the extracellular pH at approximately 7.4 depends on the operation of buffer systems that accept protons (H$^+$) when they are produced and liberate protons when they are consumed. The state of the demand on total body buffering can be determined by assessing the behavior of the HCO$_3^-$/CO$_2$ system, which is the major extracellular buffer. The law of mass action for this buffer system states the following:

$$pH = 6.1 + \log\frac{[HCO_3^-]}{[CO_2]}$$

where brackets indicate the concentration of a substance, HCO$_3^-$ in mEq/L and CO$_2$ in mmHg. Because the [CO$_2$] equals the solubility coefficient multiplied by the partial pressure of carbon dioxide (PCO$_2$), the equation can be rewritten as:

$$pH = 6.1 + \log\frac{[HCO_3^-]}{0.03 \times PCO_2}$$

This, the familiar Henderson-Hasselbalch equation, tells us that pH constancy depends on a constant ratio between the concentrations of the two buffer components. If this ratio increases, because either HCO$_3^-$ increases or CO$_2$ decreases, the pH will increase (alkalosis). If the ratio decreases, because either HCO$_3^-$ decreases or CO$_2$ increases, the pH will decrease (acidosis). Regulation of HCO$_3^-$ is mainly a function of the kidneys, and regulation of CO$_2$ is a respiratory function.

The regulation of HCO$_3^-$ concentration by the kidneys consists of two main components:

1. *Absorption of HCO$_3^-$:* Because of the high GFR and plasma HCO$_3^-$ concentrations (24 mEq/L), large amounts of HCO$_3^-$ are filtered. Retrieval of this filtered HCO$_3^-$ is essential for acid-base balance. This process of renal HCO$_3^-$ absorption does not add new HCO$_3^-$ to the blood but merely prevents a loss of filtered HCO$_3^-$ into the urine. Therefore, renal HCO$_3^-$ absorption cannot correct an existing metabolic acidosis.

2. *Excretion of H⁺:* Under normal dietary conditions, approximately 40 to 80 mmol of H^+ is generated daily (mostly sulfuric acid from the metabolism of sulfur-containing amino acids). This H^+ is buffered and therefore consumes HCO_3^-. The kidneys must excrete this H^+ to regenerate the HCO_3^- pool; this second task can therefore be viewed as generation of "new" HCO_3^-.

MECHANISMS OF BICARBONATE ABSORPTION

Filtered HCO_3^- (about 4300 mEq/day) is efficiently absorbed by the renal tubules, predominantly the proximal tubules, and under normal acid-base conditions very little HCO_3^- is found in the urine. As a rule, all tubular HCO_3^- absorption is the consequence of H^+ secretion and not of direct absorption of HCO_3^- ions. H^+ is continuously generated inside cells from the dissociation of H_2O (or from the reaction of CO_2 with H_2O) and transported into the lumen. In the lumen, secreted H^+ combines with filtered HCO_3^- to form carbonic acid, which is broken down to CO_2 and H_2O in a reaction that is catalyzed by a carbonic anhydrase located in the luminal brush border membrane. CO_2 and H_2O are then absorbed passively. The OH^- generated in the cell during this process combines with CO_2 to form HCO_3^-, a reaction catalyzed by a cytosolic carbonic anhydrase. HCO_3^- exits across the basolateral side of the cell and returns to the blood in association with Na^+. The net balance of this process can be expressed as follows:

Cl^-/HCO_3^- exchanger (equivalent to the band 3 protein of red cells, AE1).

BICARBONATE SECRETION

Although net HCO_3^- transport for the whole kidney is always in the reabsorptive direction, certain intercalated cells in the cortical portion of the collecting duct can actually secrete HCO_3^-. These bicarbonate-secreting cells have a polarity that is the reverse of the proton-secreting cells; that is, they possess a basolateral H^+-ATPase and probably a luminal Cl^-/HCO_3^- exchanger. HCO_3^- secretion may be important during consumption of a diet providing base equivalents and for the correction of metabolic alkalosis.

EXCRETION OF PROTONS (FORMATION OF NEW BICARBONATE IONS)

Urinary acid excretion cannot, to any significant extent, occur as free H^+. The minimum urinary pH in humans is about 4.5, corresponding to an H^+ concentration of only 0.03 mEq/L. Because some 40 to 80 mEq of H^+ must be excreted each day, it is clear that most H^+ ions must be excreted in a bound or buffered form. Excretion of bound H^+ is achieved in two ways: by the titration of luminal nonbicarbonate buffers and by the renal synthesis and excretion of ammonium ions.

Titratable Acidity

Binding of secreted H^+ to filtered nonbicarbonate buffer anions leads to the formation and excretion of urinary titrat-

$$H_2O + CO_2 \leftarrow H_2CO_3 \leftarrow HCO_3^- + H^+ \leftarrow H_2O \rightarrow OH^- + CO_2 \rightarrow HCO_3^- + Na^+$$

| tubular lumen | cell interior | blood |

Specific transport proteins in renal epithelial cells cause the H^+ and HCO_3^- to move in the right directions. Two different mechanisms, both located in the luminal membrane, are responsible for the movement of protons into the tubular fluid.

1. The first mechanism is a Na^+/H^+ exchanger (NHE3) driven by the Na^+ gradient and found in the proximal tubule. In terms of milliequivalents transported, it contributes the most to HCO_3^- absorption.
2. The second mechanism is primary active transport of H^+. An H^+-ATPase has been found in the luminal membrane of one class of intercalated collecting duct cells. There is also some evidence for the presence of a similar H^+,K^+-ATPase in parietal cells of the gastric mucosa. Active H^+ transport is responsible for the secretion of smaller amounts of H^+ than Na^+/H^+ exchange, but it can proceed against a steeper gradient.

There are also at least two mechanisms for the transport of HCO_3^- across the basolateral membrane. The major exit mechanism in the proximal tubule is the coupling of the movement of HCO_3^- and Na^+. In the collecting duct, HCO_3^- exit occurs predominantly through a basolateral

able acidity. (Titratable acidity is defined as the number of moles of NaOH that must be added to bring the urine pH back to 7.4.) The ability to buffer H^+ depends on the dissociation constant (pK) and the quantity of a buffer. Under normal conditions, only the $HPO_4^{2-}/H_2PO_4^-$ buffer is present in amounts sufficient to act as an intratubular H^+ acceptor. This buffer pair has a pH of 6.8, and it is excreted at a daily rate of about 50 mmol. Applying the Henderson-Hasselbalch equation for the phosphate buffer (pH = 6.8 + log $[HPO_4^{2-}]/[H_2PO_4^-]$), and considering only that fraction of total phosphate that is actually excreted (about 25% to 30% of the filtered phosphate load), the relationships shown in Table 1.4 can be calculated.

This tabulation shows that the buffer capacity of HPO_4^{2-} can be fully utilized if the intratubular pH is lowered sufficiently. In some situations, other urinary buffers become important. In diabetic ketoacidosis, large amounts of β-hydroxybutyrate are excreted (e.g., 300 mmol/L). Even though this buffer component has a pK of 4.8, it carries up to 150 mmol H^+ per liter.

Ammonium Excretion

The second form of bound H^+ in the urine is ammonium. The excretion of NH_4^+ is equivalent to generation

Table 1.4 Effect of Tubular Acidification on Buffering Capacity

Location	pH	HPO_4^{2-} (mmol/day)	$H_2PO_4^-$ (mmol/day)	H^+ Buffered (mmol/day)
Filtrate	7.4	40	10	0
End of proximal tubule	6.8	25	25	15
Urine	4.8	0.5	49.5	39.5

of HCO_3^- or excretion of H^+. The major source of urinary ammonium is glutamine, which is synthesized in the liver from glutamate and extracted from the blood by uptake mechanisms in the luminal and basolateral membranes of renal proximal tubule cells. Ammonium is generated in the proximal tubule by a metabolic pathway that degrades glutamine to glutamate, and further to α-ketoglutarate; this yields $2NH_4^+$ and $2HCO_3^-$ (rather than NH_3, CO_2, and H_2O). Whereas the NH_4^+ ions are secreted through distinct transport pathways into the lumen of the proximal tubule, the new HCO_3^- ions are added to the blood HCO_3^- pool.

It is essential for the NH_4^+ formed by renal proximal tubules to be preferentially secreted into the tubular lumen and then to be excreted in the urine. If the generated NH_4^+ is reabsorbed by the renal tubular epithelium (or secreted preferentially into the blood), it would then form urea (H_2NCONH_2). Ureagenesis forms protons that consume the produced bicarbonate and thereby negates the net base production. This is shown in the following reactions:

$$2NH_4^+ + CO_2 \rightarrow urea + H_2O + 2H^+$$

or

$$2NH_4^+ + 2HCO_3^- \rightarrow urea + CO_2 + 3H_2O$$

Urinary H^+ excretion in the form of NH_4^+ is on the order of 40 to 50 mmol/day, and is greatly enhanced in metabolic acidosis. Failure of the proximal tubules to generate adequate NH_4^+ is the main reason that metabolic acidosis occurs in chronic kidney disease.

REGULATION OF PROTON SECRETION

Intracellular pH

Systemic pH changes, whether caused by changes in plasma HCO_3^- (metabolic) or by changes in P_{CO2} (respiratory), alter H^+ secretion (and therefore HCO_3^- absorption). Intracellular acidification (e.g., in acidosis) stimulates H^+ secretion, and intracellular alkalinization (alkalosis) inhibits it.

Aldosterone

In addition to affecting Na^+ absorption and K^+ secretion, aldosterone stimulates H^+ secretion by the collecting ducts.

Potassium

Changes in plasma K^+ concentration can affect H^+ secretion, in part by changing the intracellular pH. For example, hypokalemia increases intracellular acidity and stimulates H^+ ion secretion. Although the effect of hypokalemia alone is relatively small, a marked stimulation of H^+ secretion results when hypokalemia occurs with high plasma aldosterone levels. In this situation, which occurs in primary hyperaldosteronism or after administration of diuretics, metabolic alkalosis may be generated by the kidneys.

RENAL HANDLING OF GLUCOSE AND AMINO ACIDS

An important function of the renal tubule is retrieval of the glucose and amino acids that are present in glomerular filtrate and would be lost to the body if they were not reabsorbed. To a large extent, this is a function of the proximal tubule, and disordered glucose and amino acid transport is characteristic of diseases that disturb proximal tubular function.

Glucose transport by the proximal tubule occurs via a transport protein present in the luminal membrane that carries a glucose molecule together with a sodium ion, the glucose-sodium cotransporter. This transporter uses the sodium concentration gradient (the concentration of Na^+ is higher outside the cell) to drive the movement of glucose across the luminal membrane into the cell. Glucose then diffuses out of the cell across the basolateral membrane, a process facilitated by a second carrier protein. The resulting reabsorption process is highly efficient. In normal circumstances, almost all of the filtered glucose is removed from the proximal tubule fluid, and, as a result, glucose is virtually absent from urine.

When the plasma glucose concentration rises, increasing amounts of glucose are filtered. At a certain point, the filtered load of glucose exceeds the capacity of the proximal transport mechanisms. This maximum reabsorption rate is called the *tubular transport maximum for glucose* (T_{mG}). When glucose delivery exceeds the T_{mG}, the excess glucose is excreted in the urine (Fig. 1.13).

Many of the same principles apply to the reabsorption of amino acids. Amino acid absorption is also highly effective with less than 1% of most filtered amino acids escaping into the urine. A number of different luminal and basolateral transport proteins are needed to remove the amino acids from the glomerular filtrate. A specific transporter carries the dibasic amino acids, L-arginine and L-lysine, and another carrier is responsible for removal of the acidic amino acids from the tubular fluid. There also are luminal transporters that, like the sodium-glucose cotransporter, exploit the sodium concentration gradient for cotransport. Other carrier molecules in the basolateral membrane facilitate the exit of amino acids from the cell.

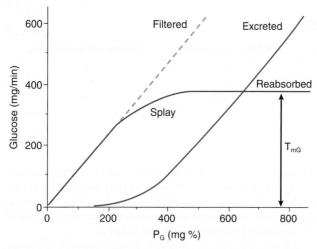

Figure 1.13   A typical filtration curve for renal glucose reabsorption. At plasma glucose concentrations less than approximately 200 mg/dl, the filtered glucose is completely reabsorbed, and no glucose is excreted in the urine. When the plasma glucose concentration exceeds this level, the filtered load of glucose exceeds the transport capacity of the tubule, and glucose appears in the urine. P_G, Plasma glucose; T_{mG}, tubular transport maximum for glucose.

BIBLIOGRAPHY

Aronson PS, Giebisch G: Effects of pH on potassium: new explanations for old observations, *J Am Soc Nephrol* 22:1981-1989, 2011.

Bindels RJ: Minerals in motion: from new ion transporters to new concepts, *J Am Soc Nephrol* 21:1263-1269, 2009.

Brater DC: Diuretic therapy, *N Engl J Med* 339:387-395, 1998.

Castrop H, Hocherl K, Kurtz A, et al: Physiology of kidney renin, *Physiol Rev* 90:607-673, 2010.

D'Agati VD, Kaskel FJ, Falk RJ: Focal segmental glomerulosclerosis, *N Engl J Med* 365:2398-2411, 2011.

Fenton RA, Knepper MA: Mouse models and the urinary concentrating mechanism in the new millennium, *Physiol Rev* 87:1083-1112, 2007.

Giebisch G, Windhager E: The urinary system. In Boron WF, Emile L, Boulpaep EL, editors: *Medical physiology: a cellular and molecular approach. section VI*, Philadelphia, 2003, WB Saunders, pp 735-875.

Greka A, Mundel P: Cell biology and pathology of podocytes, *Annu Rev Physiol* 74:299-323, 2012.

Guyton AC, Hall JE: Unit V: the body fluids and kidney. In Guyton AC, Hall JE, editors: *Textbook of medical physiology*, ed 11, Philadelphia, 2006, Elsevier.

Jefferson JA, Shankland SJ: The molecular mechanisms of proteinuria. In Mount DB, Pollak MR, editors: *Molecular and genetic basis of renal disease*, Philadelphia, PA, 2007, Saunders Elsevier.

Lifton RP: Genetic dissection of human blood pressure variation: common pathways from rare phenotypes, *Harvey Lect* 100:71-101, 2004.

Schrier RW: The sea within us: disorders of body water homeostasis, *Curr Opin Investig Drugs* 8:304-311, 2007.

Stevens LA, Coresh J, Greene T, et al: Assessing kidney function: measured and estimated glomerular filtration rate, *N Engl J Med* 354:2473-2483, 2006.

Zhou J: Polycystins and primary cilia: primers for cell cycle progression, *Annu Rev Physiol* 71:83-113, 2009.

Kidney Development

Norman D. Rosenblum

DEVELOPMENT OF THE MAMMALIAN KIDNEY

OVERVIEW OF KIDNEY DEVELOPMENT

The metanephros constitutes the permanent mammalian kidney. Establishment of the metanephric kidney is preceded by formation of two other mesenchyme-derived kidney-like structures—the pronephros and the mesonephros. Both are transient kidney-like paired structures that do not contribute to the permanent kidney. The pronephros is the more anterior of these structures and degenerates in mammals. The more posterior structure, the mesonephros, gives rise to male reproductive organs including the rete testis, efferent ducts, epididymis, vas deferens, seminal vesicle, and prostate. In females, the mesonephric portion of the Wolffian duct degenerates.

The metanephric kidney is composed of the metanephric mesenchyme and the ureteric bud, both of which are derived from the intermediate mesoderm (Fig. 2.1). Metanephric mesenchyme is the tissue source of all epithelial cell types comprising the mature nephron. The ureteric bud originates as an epithelial outgrowth of the caudal portion of the Wolffian duct (also termed the mesonephric or nephric duct) (see Fig. 2.1A). Reciprocal inductive interactions between the metanephric mesenchyme and the ureteric bud result in: (1) nephrogenesis, defined as formation of the glomerulus and all tubules proximal to the collecting ducts, and (2) branching morphogenesis, defined as growth and branching of the ureteric bud and subsequent formation of the renal collecting system, which is constituted by the cortical and medullary collecting ducts, the renal calyces, and the renal pelvis.

DEVELOPMENT OF THE RENAL COLLECTING SYSTEM

The ureteric bud arises from the Wolffian duct in response to signals elaborated by the adjacent metanephric mesenchyme at week 5 of human fetal gestation. Failure to induce ureteric bud outgrowth results in renal agenesis, whereas outgrowth of more than one ureteric bud can result in renal malformations including a double collecting system and duplication of the ureter. The position at which the ureteric bud arises from the Wolffian duct relative to the metanephric mesenchyme is critical to the nature of the interactions between the ureteric bud and the metanephric mesenchyme and is controlled by a regulatory gene network. Ectopic positioning of the ureteric bud is associated with renal tissue malformation

(dysplasia), which may result from abnormal ureteric bud-metanephric mesenchyme interactions. Ectopic positioning of the ureteric bud is also thought to contribute to the integrity of the ureterovesical junction. Consistent with this hypothesis, mutations in *BMP4*, which controls ureteric bud outgrowth, are associated with vesicoureteral reflux in humans (Table 2.1).

Branching of the ureteric bud occurs immediately following invasion of the metanephric mesenchyme by the ureteric bud. The number of ureteric bud branches is a major determinant of final nephron number, because ureteric bud branch tips induce discrete subsets of metanephric mesenchyme cells to undergo nephrogenesis. Repetitive branching events (see Fig. 2.1C) result in the formation of approximately 15 branch generations, and, in humans, the first 9 branch generations are formed by approximately the fifteenth week of gestation. Concomitant with formation of these branches, new nephrons are induced by reciprocal inductive interactions between newly formed ureteric branch tips and surrounding metanephric mesenchyme. By the twentieth to twenty-second week of gestation, ureteric branching is completed. Thereafter, collecting duct development occurs by extension of peripheral branch segments, and new nephrons predominantly form around the tips of terminal collecting duct branches. Ureteric branching is positively regulated by genetic factors. For example, humans with inactivating mutations in *PAX2*, a positive regulator of ureteric branching, exhibit renal-coloboma syndrome and renal hypoplasia (see Table 2.1).

Between the twenty-second and thirty-fourth weeks of gestation, the peripheral (cortical) and central (medullary) domains of the developing kidney are established. The renal cortex, which represents 70% of total kidney volume at birth, becomes organized as a relatively compact, circumferential rim of tissue surrounding the periphery of the kidney. The renal medulla, which represents 30% of total kidney volume at birth, has a modified cone shape with a broad base contiguous with cortical tissue. The apex of the cone is formed by convergence of collecting ducts in the inner medulla and is termed the *papilla*. Distinct morphologic differences emerge between collecting ducts located in the medulla compared to those located in the renal cortex. Medullary collecting ducts are organized into elongated, relatively unbranched linear arrays, which converge centrally in a region devoid of glomeruli. In contrast, collecting ducts located in the renal cortex continue to induce metanephric mesenchyme. The most central segments of the collecting duct system, formed from the first five generations of ureteric bud branching, undergo remodeling by increased growth and dilatation of these tubules to form

19

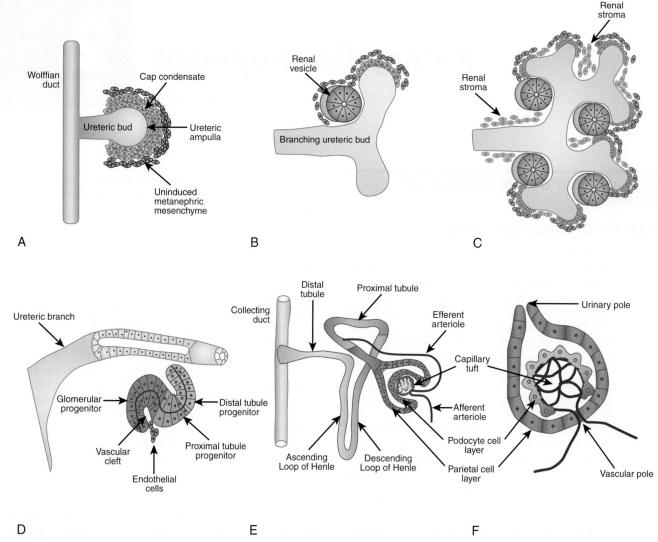

Figure 2.1   Stages of kidney formation. A, Induction of the metanephric mesenchyme by the ureteric bud promotes aggregation of mesenchyme cells around the tip of the ureteric bud. **B,** Mesenchyme-epithelial transformation. Polarized renal vesicles are formed. **C,** Branching morphogenesis. Stromal cells secrete factors that influence nephrogenesis and branching morphogenesis. **D,** S-shaped body. Formation of the S-shaped body involves the formation of a proximal cleft that is invaded by angioblasts. **E,** The complete nephron is joined to the collecting duct. **F,** Glomerulus demonstrating organization of the capillary tuft, podocytes, and parietal epithelial cells.

the pelvis and calyces. The integrity of medullary collecting ducts is dependent on control of cell proliferation. In Simpson-Golabi-Behmel syndrome, mutations in Glypican-3 *(GPC3)* result in cystic formation within medullary collecting ducts. Medullary dysplasia also occurs in humans with mutations in p57$^{\text{KIP2}}$, an inhibitor of cell proliferation, and in Beckwith-Wiedemann syndrome.

FORMATION OF THE NEPHRON

Nephrons arise from metanephric mesenchyme cells via a process termed *nephrogenesis.* Cells adjacent to the invading ureteric bud are induced to undergo a mesenchymal-to-epithelial transformation. Initially, mesenchyme cells aggregate to form a layer that is four to five cells thick, termed a *cap condensate,* around the ampulla of the advancing ureteric bud (see Fig. 2.1A). Near the interface of the ampulla and its adjacent ureteric branch, a cluster of cells separates

from the cap condensate and forms an oval mass called a *pretubular aggregate* (see Fig. 2.1B). An internal cavity forms within the pretubular aggregate, at which point the structure is called a *renal vesicle.* Multipotential precursors residing in renal vesicles give rise to all the epithelial cell types of the nephron. Nephron segmentation into glomerular and tubular domains is initiated by the sequential formation of two clefts in the renal vesicle. Creation of a lower cleft, termed the *vascular cleft,* precedes formation of the comma-shaped body. Generation of an upper cleft in the comma-shaped body precedes formation of an S-shaped body, which is characterized by three segments or limbs (see Fig. 2.1D). The middle limb gives rise to the proximal convoluted tubule and the upper limb to the descending and ascending limbs of the loops of Henle and the distal convoluted tubule.

Formation of the glomerulus begins as the vascular cleft broadens and deepens and as the lower limb of the S-shaped

Table 2.1   Human Gene Mutations Exhibiting Defects in Renal Morphogenesis

Primary Disease	Gene	Kidney Phenotype
Alagille syndrome	*JAGGED1*	Cystic dysplasia
Apert syndrome	*FGFR2*	Hydronephrosis
Bardet-Biedl syndrome	*BBS1*	Cystic dysplasia
Beckwith-Wiedemann syndrome	*p57^KIP2*	Medullary dysplasia
BOR syndrome	*EYA1, SIX1*	Unilateral or bilateral agenesis/dysplasia, hypoplasia, collecting system anomalies
Campomelic dysplasia	*SOX9*	Dysplasia, hydronephrosis
Duane radial ray (Okihiro) syndrome	*SALL4*	UNL agenesis, VUR, malrotation, crossfused ectopia, pelviectasis
Fraser syndrome	*FRAS1*	Agenesis, dysplasia
HDR syndrome	*GATA3*	Dysplasia
Kallmann syndrome	*KAL1, FGFR1, PROK2, PROK2R*	Agenesis
Mammary-ulnar syndrome	*TBX3*	Dysplasia
Meckel-Gruber syndrome	*MKS1, MKS3, NPHP6, NPHP8*	Cystic dysplasia
Nephronophthisis	*CEP290, GLIS2, RPGRIP1L, NEK8, SDCCAG8, TMEM67, TTC21B*	Cystic dysplasia
Pallister-Hall syndrome	*GLI3*	Dysplasia
Renal-coloboma syndrome	*PAX2*	Hypoplasia, vesicoureteral reflux
Renal hypoplasia, isolated	*BMP4, RET*	Hypoplasia
RTD	*RAS* components	Tubular dysplasia
Renal cysts and diabetes syndrome	*HNF1b*	Dysplasia, hypoplasia
Rubinstein-Taby syndrome	*CREBBP*	Agenesis, hypoplasia
Simpson-Golabi-Behmel syndrome	*GPC3*	Medullary dysplasia
Smith-Lemli-Opitz syndrome	7-hydroxy-cholesterol reductase	Agenesis, dysplasia
Townes-Brocks syndrome	*SALL1*	Hypoplasia, dysplasia, VUR
Zellweger syndrome	*PEX1*	VUR, cystic dysplasia

BOR, Branchio-oto-renal; *HDR,* hypoparathyroidism, sensorineural deafness, and renal anomalies; *RTD,* renal tubular dysgenesis; *UNL,* unilateral; *VUR,* vesicoureteral reflux.

body forms a cup-shaped unit (see Fig. 2.1D and F). Epithelial cells lining the inner wall of this cup will comprise the visceral glomerular epithelium, or podocyte layer. Cells lining the outer wall of the cup will form parietal glomerular epithelium, which lines Bowman capsule (see Fig. 2.1F). The glomerular capillary tuft is formed via recruitment and proliferation of endothelial and mesangial cell precursors. Recruitment of angioblasts and mesangial precursors into the vascular cleft results in deformation of the lower S-shaped body limb into a cuplike structure (see Fig. 2.1E). A primitive vascular plexus forms at this capillary loop stage. Podocytes of capillary loop stage glomeruli lose mitotic capacity and begin to form actin-based cytoplasmic extensions, or foot processes, and specialized intercellular junctions, termed *slit diaphragms.* Subsequent development of the glomerular capillary tuft involves extensive branching of capillaries and formation of endothelial fenestrae. Mesangial cells, in turn, populate the core of the tuft and provide structural support to capillary loops through the deposition of extracellular matrix. The full complement of glomeruli in the fetal human kidney is attained between 32 and 34 weeks, when nephrogenesis ceases. At birth, superficial glomeruli, the last glomeruli that are formed, are significantly smaller than juxtamedullary glomeruli, which are the earliest formed glomeruli. Subsequent glomerular development involves hypertrophy, and glomeruli reach adult size by 3½ years of age.

RENAL MALFORMATION

DEFINITION AND OVERVIEW

Kidney and lower urinary tract malformations are the most frequently detected abnormalities during intrauterine life (0.1 to 0.7 pregnancies) and are the major cause of childhood kidney failure. Because formation of the kidney and lower urinary tract begins and ends during intrauterine life, these malformations are, by definition, congenital. Renal-urinary tract malformations occur in combination with nonrenal malformations as part of a genetic syndrome in 30% of affected patients. At least 70 distinct syndromes feature some type of kidney and urinary tract malformation (Box 2.1).

A classification of kidney and urinary tract malformations follows:

- Aplasia (agenesis): congenital absence of kidney tissue.
- Simple hypoplasia: kidney length more than two standard deviations below the mean for age, with a reduced nephron number but normal kidney architecture.
- Dysplasia ± cysts: malformation of tissue elements.
- Isolated dilatation of the renal pelvis ± ureters (collecting system).
- Anomalies of position including the ectopic and fused (horseshoe) kidney.

Box 2.1   Syndromes, Chromosomal Abnormalities, and Metabolic Disorders With Renal or Urinary Tract Malformation

Syndromes

Beckwith-Wiedemann
Cerebro-oculo-renal
CHARGE
DiGeorge
Ectrodactyly, ectodermal dysplasia and cleft lip/palate
Ehlers Danlos
Fanconi pancytopenia
Fraser
Fryns
Meckel
Marfan
MURCS Association
Oculo-auriculo-vertebral (Goldenhar)
OFD
Pallister-Hall
Renal cyst and diabetes
SGBS
Tuberous sclerosis
Townes-Brocks

VATER
WAGR
Williams Beuren
Zellweger (cerebrohepatorenal)

Chromosomal Abnormalities

Trisomy 21
Klinefelter
DiGeorge, 22q11
45, X0 (Turner)
(XXY) Klinefelter
Tri 9 mosaic, Tri 13, Tri 18, del 4q, del 18q, dup3q, dup 10q
Triploidy

Metabolic Disorders

Peroxysomal
Glycosylation defect
Mitochondriopathy
Glutaric aciduria type II
Carnitine palmitoyl transferase II deficiency

CHARGE, Coloboma, heart defect, atresia choanae, retarded growth and development, genital hypoplasia, ear anomalies/deafness; *MURCS,* Mullerian hypoplasia/aplasia, renal agenesis and cervicothoracic somite dysplasia; *OFD,* oculo-facial-digital; *SGBS,* Simpson-Golabi-Behmel; *VATER,* vertebrae, anus, trachea, esophagus, and renal; *WAGR,* Wilms tumor, aniridia, genitourinary anomalies, and mental retardation.

Kidney and urinary tract malformations may be unilateral or bilateral. Anomalies of the kidney are associated with structural abnormalities of the lower urinary tract in 50% of affected patients. These structural abnormalities include vesicoureteral reflux (25% of cases), ureteropelvic junction obstruction (11% of cases), and ureterovesical junction obstruction (11% of cases). Renal dysplasia is a polymorphic disorder characterized at the microscopic level by abnormal differentiation of mesenchymal and epithelial elements, decreased nephron number, loss of the demarcating zone between the cortex and the medulla, and metaplastic transformation of mesenchyme to cartilage and bone. Dysplastic kidneys range in size from large distended kidneys with multiple large cysts to small kidneys with or without cysts. A small dysplastic kidney without macroscopic cysts, imaged by ultrasonography, is classified as hypoplastic/dysplastic in the absence of a pathologic examination, which distinguishes between simple hypoplasia and dysplasia. The multicystic dysplastic kidney (MCDK) is an extreme form of renal dysplasia.

As a group, renal-urinary tract malformations are classified under the overall term *congenital anomalies of the kidney and urinary tract* (CAKUT). Use of this clinical classification is supported by the observation that multiple structures within the kidney and urinary tract may be malformed within any given affected individual (e.g., the kidney and vesicoureteric junction), mutation in a particular gene is associated with different urinary tract anomalies in different affected individuals (e.g., renal-coloboma syndrome is characterized by a spectrum of kidney anomalies in association with vesicoureteral reflux), and mutations in different genes give rise to similar renal and lower urinary tract phenotypes

(e.g., renal hypoplasia is associated with mutations in EYA1 in Townes-Brocks syndrome and with mutations in PAX2 in renal-coloboma syndrome).

ETIOLOGY OF HUMAN RENAL-URINARY TRACT MALFORMATION

Congenital anomalies of the kidney and urinary tract (CAKUT) most often occur in a sporadic manner. In the majority of affected children, neither a syndrome nor a Mendelian pattern of inheritance is obvious. In probands with bilateral renal agenesis or bilateral renal dysgenesis and without evidence of a genetic syndrome or a family history, 9% of first-degree relatives show some type of malformation in the kidney and/or lower urinary tract apparent on ultrasonography. In approximately 30% of CAKUT, renal and/or urinary tract malformation occurs as part of a genetic syndrome, a chromosomal disorder, or an inborn error of metabolism (see Box 2.1). More than 30 genes have been identified as mutant in multiorgan syndromes with CAKUT (see Table 2.1).

CAKUT is caused by prenatal exposure to a variety of prescription and nonprescription drugs (Box 2.2). Angiotensin converting enzyme inhibitors and angiotensin II receptor blockers cause a particular form of CAKUT termed *renal tubular dysgenesis* (RTD), which is a severe perinatal disorder characterized by absence or paucity of differentiated proximal tubules, early severe oligohydramnios, and perinatal death. Kidney appearance on the antenatal renal ultrasound in RTD is characteristically normal. RTD may also be caused by mutations in the genes that encode renin, angiotensinogen, angiotensin converting enzyme, and angiotensin II receptor type 1.

CLINICAL MANAGEMENT OF CONGENITAL ANOMALIES OF THE KIDNEY AND URINARY TRACT

MAJOR CONSIDERATIONS DURING THE ANTENATAL PERIOD

The sensitivity of prenatal ultrasonography screening for CAKUT at week 23 of gestation is approximately 80%. Assessment of amniotic fluid volume is a key element of the antenatal evaluation. Fetal urine production begins at 9 weeks of gestation and makes a significant contribution to amniotic fluid volume by the onset of the second trimester. By 20 weeks of gestation, 90% of the amniotic fluid volume is determined by fetal urine production. Thus, a decrease in amniotic fluid volume, termed *oligohydramnios*, at or beyond the twentieth week of gestation is a surrogate marker of fetal kidney dysfunction. When two kidneys exist, oligohydramnios is observed in bilateral renal agenesis or severe dysgenesis, bilateral ureteric obstruction, or obstruction of the bladder outlet or urethra. When a solitary kidney exists, oligohydramnios is caused by renal dysgenesis or obstruction of urinary outflow. Poor postnatal outcome is suggested by the presence of severe oligohydramnios and small and hyperechogenic kidneys.

MANAGEMENT AFTER BIRTH

The clinical presentation of renal malformation in the postnatal period is dependent on the amount of functioning renal mass, the presence of bilateral urinary tract obstruction, and the occurrence of urinary tract infection. Bilateral renal agenesis or severe dysplasia is likely to present soon after birth due to decreased kidney function that may be accompanied by oliguria or polyuria. Alternatively, patients may present with a flank mass or an asymptomatic abnormality detected by kidney imaging.

A detailed history and careful physical examination should be performed on all infants with antenatally detected CAKUT (see Box 2.2), specifically evaluating teratogen exposure. Physical examination focuses on the pulmonary system with careful attention to possible pneumothorax associated with pulmonary hypoplasia. Examination of the abdomen may show a mass, which represents a MCDK, an obstructed kidney, or an obstructed bladder as in posterior urethral valves. A single umbilical artery is associated with CAKUT, particularly vesicoureteral reflux. A male infant with prune belly syndrome will have deficient abdominal wall musculature and undescended testes. Physical examination may also show abnormalities that occur in multiorgan syndromes characterized by CAKUT. Some of the more frequently observed abnormalities include abnormal positioning of the anal orfice, abnormal external genitalia, periauricular pits, and coloboma.

Urine output should be carefully documented. Ultrasonography of the upper and lower urinary tract should be performed within the first 24 hours of life in newborns with a history of oligohydramnios, progressive antenatal hydronephrosis, a distended bladder on antenatal sonograms, or bilateral severe hydroureteronephrosis. In male infants, a distended bladder and bilateral hydroureteronephrosis may be secondary to posterior urethral valves, a condition that requires immediate renal imaging and clinical intervention. In general, unilateral anomalies do not require urgent investigation after birth. Renal ultrasonography for unilateral hydronephrosis is not recommended within the first 72 hours of life, because urine output gradually increases during the first 24 to 48 hours of life as renal plasma flow and glomerular filtration rate increase. Thus, the degree of urinary tract dilatation can be underestimated during this period of transition.

Measurement of serum creatinine should be considered in the postnatal period when there is bilateral renal disease or an affected solitary kidney. However, measurement should be delayed until after the first 24 hours of life, because levels in the first 24 hours are reflective of maternal serum creatinine (usually ≤1.0 mg/dl [88 µmol/L]). Newborn serum creatinine declines to 0.3 to 0.5 mg/dl [27 to 44 µmol/L] within approximately 1 week in term infants and 2 to 3 weeks in preterm infants.

CLINICAL APPROACH TO SPECIFIC MALFORMATIONS

FETAL ECHOGENIC KIDNEY

Increased echogenicity of one or both kidneys is a frequent presentation of kidney disease in the fetus. Deletions in *TCF2* are the most frequent mutations identified in the fetal echogenic kidney. Other genetic causes include autosomal dominant and autosomal recessive forms of polycystic kidney disease. Mutations in *TCF2* are also associated with other renal malformations such as renal hypoplasia and dysplasia, MCDK, renal agenesis, horseshoe kidney, and pelviureteric junction obstruction. Newborns with an antenatal history of hyperechoic kidneys should be studied with renal ultrasonography to define the phenotype further. At this point, polycystic kidney disease may be obvious. A genetic metabolic disorder may be indicated by nonrenal findings. In the absence of such findings, a careful physical examination and pelvic ultrasonography should be performed to rule out genital abnormalities.

UNILATERAL RENAL AGENESIS

A diagnosis of unilateral renal agenesis requires verification that a second kidney does not exist. Such a "second" kidney may reside in the pelvis or some other ectopic location. A diagnosis of unilateral renal agenesis is supported by compensatory hypertrophy in the normally positioned kidney. Unilateral agenesis is associated with contralateral urinary tract abnormalities including ureteropelvic junction obstruction and vesicoureteral reflux in 20% to 40% of cases. Thus, imaging of the existing kidney and lower urinary tract is important and should consist of ultrasonography and a voiding cystourethrogram (VCUG). Management of affected patients involves determining the functional status of the existing kidney; if serum creatinine is normal, the long-term prognosis is excellent. However, some studies have shown that a substantial proportion of patients ultimately will develop proteinuria and hypertension; accordingly, it is reasonable to propose that individuals with a single functioning kidney should have their blood pressure measured and their urine tested for protein periodically.

RENAL DYSPLASIA

The dysplastic kidney is most commonly small for the age because of decreased nephrogenesis, and it may be termed a *hypodysplastic kidney*. However, a large dysplastic kidney may exist in at least two clinical circumstances. First, cystic elements can generate a large kidney, the most extreme example being the MCDK. Second, larger dysplastic kidneys are a feature of somatic overgrowth syndromes including Beckwith-Wiedemann syndrome and Simpson-Golabi-Behmel syndrome. During the antenatal period, a unilateral dysplastic kidney is likely to be discovered as an incidental finding. This may also be the case for bilateral renal dysplasia unless it is associated with oligohydramnios. After birth, bilateral renal dysplasia is associated with a variable degree of decreased kidney function proportional to the severity of the dysplasia. Postnatal ultrasonography of the dysplastic kidney shows increased echogenicity, loss of corticomedullary differentiation, and cortical cysts. Clinical follow-up involves serial measurement of kidney function. Because renal dysplasia is associated with lower urinary tract abnormalities including vesicoureteric reflux, imaging of the lower urinary tract should be performed via a VCUG.

MULTICYSTIC DYSPLASTIC KIDNEY

Multicystic dysplastic kidney is a severe form of renal dysplasia that may present as a flank mass. Renal ultrasonography demonstrates a large cystic mass in the renal fossa with a paucity of intervening solid tissue; this appearance is commonly described as a "cluster of grapes." The MCDK is nonfunctional and usually unilateral. If bilateral, it gives rise to Potter syndrome. Complications of MCDK include hypertension and urinary tract infection, but these are rare. Wilms tumor and renal cell carcinoma have also been described in MCDK, but the incidence of malignant complications is not

significantly different from the general population. Contralateral urinary tract abnormalities are detected in approximately 25% of cases and include rotational or positional anomalies, renal hypoplasia, vesicoureteric reflux, and ureteropelvic junction obstruction.

The natural history of MCDK is gradual reduction in kidney size. By 2 years of life, 60% of kidneys will decrease in size and 20% to 25% will not be detectable by ultrasonography. Increase in the size of the MCDK, an unusual event, should prompt consideration of removal to rule out malignant transformation. Ultrasonography shows compensatory hypertrophy in the contralateral kidney. Because of the risk of associated anomalies in the contralateral kidney, the possibility of vesicoureteroreflux should be evaluated, and blood pressure should be measured. Renal ultrasonography is generally recommended at an interval of 3 months for the first year of life and then every 6 months up to involution of the mass, or at least up to 5 years. Nephrectomy should be considered when a MCDK is increasing in size and when hypertension occurs during infancy or early childhood.

RENAL ECTOPIA

Renal ectopy is defined as an abnormally located kidney. Normally, the kidneys lie in the retroperitoneal fossa on either side of the spine in the lumbar region. Rapid caudal growth during embryogenesis results in migration of the developing kidney from the pelvis to the retroperitoneal renal fossa. As the kidney ascends, it rotates 90 degrees such that the renal hilum is directed medially after ascent is complete. Migration and rotation are complete by 8 weeks of gestation.

The most common presentation of renal ectopy is a pelvic kidney. Less commonly, the kidney may lie on the contralateral side of the body, a state that is termed *crossed ectopy*. Clinical presentation can be asymptomatic or symptomatic. Diagnosis of the ectopic kidney may occur during a routine antenatal ultrasonography. Alternatively, a pelvic mass may be palpated on physical examination. Renal ectopia is commonly associated with lower urinary tract anomalies, and vesicoureteral reflux is most common, occurring in 20% of crossed renal ectopia, 30% of simple renal ectopia, and 70% of bilateral simple renal ectopia. Other associated urologic abnormalities include contralateral renal dysplasia (4%), cryptorchidism (5%), and hypospadias (5%). Female genital anomalies such as agenesis of the uterus and vagina or unicornuate uterus have also been associated with ectopic kidneys. Other described anomalies include adrenal, cardiac, and skeletal anomalies.

Identification of an ectopic kidney should prompt a careful physical examination for other anomalies. A serum creatinine should be obtained to track kidney function. A VCUG should be performed to rule out vesicoureteral reflux, which occurs with a greater incidence in affected patients and which may be associated with urinary tract infection, and a 99mTc–dimercaptosuccinic acid scan is also recommended to assess for differential renal functions. A normal appearing contralateral kidney and no evidence of hydronephrosis in the ectopic kidney suggests that no further evaluation is required, whereas elevated serum creatinine or abnormal appearing contralateral kidney indicates a need for continued follow-up. If the ectopic kidney is severely hydronephrotic, and the VCUG examination is normal, then a diuretic renogram with a mercaptoacetyltri-glycine or diethylenetriaminepentaacetic acid scan should be performed to further assess the degree of obstruction; in mild or moderate hydronephrosis, serial ultrasonography is suggested.

RENAL FUSION

Renal fusion is defined as the fusion of two kidneys. The most common fusion anomaly is the horseshoe kidney, in which fusion occurs at one pole of each kidney, usually the lower pole. The fused kidney may lie in the midline (symmetric horseshoe kidney), or the fused part may lie lateral to the midline (asymmetric horseshoe kidney). In a crossed fused ectopic kidney, the kidney from one side has crossed the midline to fuse with the kidney on the other side. Fusion is thought to occur before the kidneys ascend from the pelvis to their normal dorsolumbar position. As a result, fusion anomalies seldom assume the normal ana-tomic position. Because of the failure of ascent, the renal blood supply may be derived from vessels such as the iliac arteries.

Other associated urologic anomalies include ureteral duplication, ectopic ureter, and retrocaval ureter. Genital anomalies such as bicornuate and/or septate uterus, hypo-spadias, and undescended testis have also been described. Associated nonrenal anomalies involve the gastrointestinal tract (anorectal malformations such as imperforate anus, malrotation, and Meckel diverticulum), the central nervous system (neural tube defects), and the skeleton (rib defects, clubfoot, or congenital hip dislocation).

Most patients with a horseshoe kidney are asymptomatic and are diagnosed incidentally; however, some patients present with pain and/or hematuria from hydronephrosis with or without obstruction or infection. Causes of hydro-nephrosis include vesicoureteral reflux or obstruction of the collecting system due to renal calculi, ureteropelvic junction obstruction, or external ureteric compression by an aberrant vessel. Infection and calculi likely are caused by increased urinary stasis.

Antenatal detection of a horseshoe kidney requires that postnatal ultrasonography be performed to confirm the diagnosis and to identify any associated urogenital abnor-malities. A VCUG is indicated to rule out vesicoureteral reflux, and, if obstruction is observed, serum creatinine should be measured.

ACKNOWLEDGMENTS

This work was supported by research operating grants from the Canadian Institute of Health Research and the Kidney Foundation of Canada and a Canada Research Chair in Developmental Nephrology (to N.D.R.).

BIBLIOGRAPHY

Abdelhak S, Kalatzis V, Heilig R, et al: A human homologue of the *Drosophila eyes absent* gene underlies Branchio-Oto-Renal (BOR) syn-drome and identifies a novel gene family, *Nat Genet* 15:157-164, 1997.

Barbaux S, Niaudet P, Gubler M-C, et al: Donor splice-site mutations in WT1 are responsible for Frasier syndrome, *Nat Genet* 17:467-470, 1997.

Bamshad M, Lin RC, Law DJ, et al: Mutations in human TBX3 alter limb, apocrine and genital development in ulnar-mammary syn-drome, *Nat Genet* 16:311-315, 1997.

Cain JE, Di Giovanni V, Smeeton J, et al: Genetics of renal hypoplasia: insights into mechanisms controlling nephron endowment, *Pediatr Res* 68:91-98, 2010.

Cano-Gauci DF, Song HH, Yang H, et al: Glypican-3-deficient mice exhibit the overgrowth and renal abnormalities typical of the Simpson-Golabi-Behmel syndrome, *J Cell Biol* 146:255-264, 1999.

Cheng HT, Kim M, Valerius MT, et al: Notch2, but not Notch1, is required for proximal fate acquisition in the mammalian nephron, *Development* 134:801-811, 2007.

Cullen-McEwen LA, Caruana G, Bertram JF: The where, what and why of the developing renal stroma, *Nephron Exp Nephrol* 99:e1-e8, 2005.

Franco B, Guioli S, Pragliola A, et al: A gene deleted in Kallmann's syndrome shares homology with neural cell adhesion and axonal path-finding molecules, *Nature* 353:529-536, 1991.

Hatada I, Ohashi H, Fukushima Y, et al: An imprinted gene p57KIP2 is mutated in Beckwith Wiedemann syndrome, *Nat Genet* 14:171-173, 1996.

Kang S, Graham JM Jr, Olney AH, et al: GLI3 frameshift mutations cause autosomal dominant Pallister-Hall syndrome, *Nat Genet* 15:266-268, 1997.

Kohlhase J, Wischermann A, Reichenbach H, et al: Mutations in the SALL1 putative transcription factor gene cause Townes-Brocks syn-drome, *Nat Genet* 18:81-83, 1998.

Kreidberg JA: Podocyte differentiation and glomerulogenesis, *J Am Soc Nephrol* 14:806-814, 2003.

Mackie GG, Stephens FD: Duplex kidneys: a correlation of renal dys-plasia with position of the ureteral orifice, *J Urol* 114:274-280, 1975.

McGregor L, Makela V, Darling SM, et al: Fraser syndrome and mouse blebbed phenotype caused by mutations in FRAS1/Fras1 encoding a putative extracellular matrix protein, *Nat Genet* 34:203-208, 2003.

Oda T, Elkahloun AG, Pike BL, et al: Mutations in the human Jagged1 gene are responsible for Alagille syndrome, *Nat Genet* 16:235-242, 1997.

Piscione TD, Rosenblum ND: The molecular control of renal branch-ing morphogenesis: current knowledge and emerging insights, *Differentiation* 70:227-246, 2002.

Porteous S, Torban E, Cho N-P, et al: Primary renal hypoplasia in humans and mice with PAX2 mutations: evidence of increased apop-tosis in fetal kidneys of Pax2[1Neu] +/- mutant mice, *Hum Mol Genet* 9:1-11, 2000.

Sakaki-Yumoto M, Kobayashi C, Sato A, et al: The murine homolog of SALL4, a causative gene in Okihiro syndrome, is essential for embry-onic stem cell proliferation, and cooperates with Sall1 in anorectal, heart, brain and kidney development, *Development* 133:3005-3013, 2006.

Weber S, Moriniere V, Knuppel T, et al: Prevalence of mutations in renal and developmental genes in children with renal hypodysplasia: results of the ESCAPE study, *J Am Soc Nephrol* 17:2864-2870, 2006.

Weber S, Taylor JC, Winyard P, et al: SIX2 and BMP4 mutations associ-ate with anomalous kidney development, *J Am Soc Nephrol* 19:891-903, 2008.

3 Assessment of Glomerular Filtration Rate in Acute and Chronic Settings

Lesley A. Inker | Andrew S. Levey

Excretory function of the kidney is performed by glomerular filtration of plasma volume and then by selective tubular reabsorption or secretion of water and solutes to maintain homeostasis. As glomerular filtration rate (GFR) is generally considered the best overall assessment of kidney function, this chapter will focus on GFR and its assessment, with other functions of the kidney reviewed elsewhere in the *Primer*.

GLOMERULAR FILTRATION RATE

Glomerular filtration rate is the product of the average filtration rate of each single nephron (the filtering unit of the kidneys) multiplied by the number of nephrons in both kidneys. The normal level for GFR varies considerably according to age, sex, body size, physical activity, diet, pharmacologic therapy, and physiologic states such as pregnancy. To standardize the function of the kidney for differences in kidney size (kidney size is proportional to body size), GFR is adjusted for body surface area, which is computed from height and weight, and GFR is then expressed per 1.73 m² surface area, which is the mean body surface area of young men and women. Normal average GFR values are approximately 130 and 120 mL/min/1.73 m² for young men and women, respectively.

Reductions in GFR can be due either to a decline in the nephron number or a decline in the single nephron GFR (SNGFR) resulting from either physiologic or hemodynamic alterations. However, an increase in SNGFR due to increased filtration pressure (for example, increased glomerular capillary pressure) or surface area (for example, glomerular hypertrophy) can compensate for decreases in nephron number; therefore, the level of GFR may not reflect the loss of nephrons. As a result, there may be substantial kidney damage before GFR decreases.

MEASUREMENT OF THE GLOMERULAR FILTRATION RATE

Glomerular filtration rate cannot be measured directly. Instead, "measured" GFR is determined from the urinary clearance of an ideal filtration marker. This clearance is calculated as the product of the urinary flow rate (V) and the urinary concentration (U_x) divided by the plasma concentration (P_x). Urinary excretion of a substance depends on filtration, tubular secretion, and tubular reabsorption. Substances that are filtered but neither secreted nor reabsorbed

by the tubules are ideal filtration markers, because their urinary clearance can be used as a measure of GFR. The ideal filtration marker for GFR measurement is inulin. Alternative exogenous substances include iothalamate, iohexol, ethylenediamine tetraacetic acid, and diethylenetriamine pentaacetic acid, which often are chelated to radioisotopes for ease of detection. Urinary clearance requires a timed urine collection for measurement of urine volume, and special care must be taken to avoid incomplete urine collections, which will limit the accuracy of the clearance calculation. Plasma clearance is an alternative method to measure GFR and has the advantage of avoiding the need for a timed urine collection but is also affected by extrarenal elimination. All of these considerations mean that measured GFR differs from the physiologic property, which we will refer to as "true" GFR. Understanding the strengths and limitations of each alternative marker and each clearance method facilitates interpretation of measured GFR.

ESTIMATION OF THE GLOMERULAR FILTRATION RATE

ENDOGENOUS FILTRATION MARKERS

Because of the difficulties in measuring GFR, GFR is often estimated from the serum concentration of endogenous filtration markers. Creatinine is the most commonly used endogenous filtration marker in clinical practice. In the past, urea was widely used, and cystatin C currently shows great promise. For all of these markers, the plasma level of the marker is related to the reciprocal of the level of GFR, but the plasma level is also influenced by generation, tubular secretion and reabsorption, and extrarenal elimination; these are collectively termed "non-GFR determinants" of the plasma concentration (Fig. 3.1). In the steady state, a constant plasma level is maintained, because generation is equal to urinary excretion and extrarenal elimination. Estimating equations incorporate demographic and clinical variables as surrogates for the non-GFR determinants and provide a more accurate estimate of GFR than the reciprocal of the plasma concentration alone. Estimated GFR may differ from measured GFR in the nonsteady state or if there is a discrepancy between the true and average value for the relationship of the surrogate to the non-GFR determinants of the filtration marker. Other sources of errors include measurement error in the filtration marker (including failure to calibrate the assay for the filtration marker to the

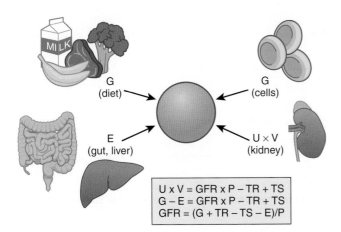

$$U \times V = GFR \times P - TR + TS$$
$$G - E = GFR \times P - TR + TS$$
$$GFR = (G + TR - TS - E)/P$$

Figure 3.1   Determinants of the serum level of endogenous filtration markers. The serum level (P) of an endogenous filtration marker is determined by its generation (G) from cells and diet, extrarenal elimination (E) by gut and liver, and urinary excretion (U × V) by the kidney. Urinary excretion is the sum of filtered load (GFR × P), tubular secretion (TS), and reabsorption (TR). In the steady state, urinary excretion equals generation and extrarenal elimination. By substitution and rearrangement, GFR can be expressed as the ratio of the non-GFR determinants (G, TS, TR, and E) to the serum level. (Adapted from Stevens LA, Levey AS: Use of measured GFR as a confirmatory test, *J Am Soc Nephrol* 20:2305-2313, 2009.)

assay used in the development of the equation) or measurement error in GFR in developing the equation. In principle, the magnitude of all these errors likely is greater at higher measured GFR, although such errors may be more clinically significant at lower measured GFR. The concepts discussed later are relevant for children as well as for adults; however, the specifics of the following discussion focus on estimating GFR in adults. Table 3.1 includes the two most commonly used GFR estimating equations for children.

CREATININE

Metabolism and Excretion

Creatinine is an end product of muscle catabolism, with a molecular mass of 113 Da. It is derived by the metabolism of phosphocreatine in muscle, and generation can be increased by creatine intake in meat or dietary supplements. Advantages of creatinine are that it is freely filtered and is easily measured at low cost. The main disadvantage is the large number of non-GFR determinants (see Fig. 3.1), leading to a wide range of GFR for a given serum creatinine level (Table 3.2). The effect of tubular secretion and extrarenal elimination on the serum level of creatinine is greater in patients with reduced GFR. Clinically, it can be difficult to distinguish a rise in serum creatinine due to inhibition of creatinine secretion or extrarenal elimination from a decline in GFR, but these causes should be suspected if the serum urea nitrogen remains unchanged. Another limitation is the variation in creatinine assay methods across laboratories, especially at low serum concentrations. This latter problem has been improved in recent years by the development of an international standard.

Creatinine Clearance

Creatinine clearance is usually computed from the creatinine excretion in a 24-hour urine collection and a single measurement of serum creatinine in the steady state. In a complete collection, creatinine excretion should be approximately 20 to 25 and 15 to 20 mg/kg/day in healthy young men and women, respectively, and deviations from these expected values can provide some indication of errors in timing or completeness of urine collection. Creatinine clearance systematically overestimates GFR because of tubular creatinine secretion. In the past, the amount of creatinine excreted due to tubular secretion at normal levels of GFR was thought to be relatively small (10% to 15%), but newer, more accurate assays suggest that this difference may be greater than previously suspected. In the nonsteady state (for example, in acute kidney disease or between dialysis treatments), it is necessary to obtain additional blood samples during the urine collection for more accurate estimation of the average serum concentration.

Equations for Estimating the Glomerular Filtration Rate from Serum Creatinine

Glomerular filtration rate can be estimated from serum creatinine by the use of equations that consider age, sex, race, and body size as surrogates for creatinine generation (see Table 3.1). Despite substantial advances in the accuracy of estimating equations based on creatinine during the past several years, all equations are limited by variation in non-GFR determinants of serum creatinine (see Fig. 3.1). In particular, none of these equations is expected to perform well in patients with extreme levels for creatinine generation, such as amputees, large or small individuals, patients with muscle-wasting conditions, or people with high or low levels of dietary meat intake (see Table 3.2). Because of differences of body compositions, it is unlikely that equations developed in one racial or ethnic group will be accurate in multiethnic populations. Later, we describe the three most commonly used equations in adults.

Cockcroft-Gault Formula. The Cockcroft-Gault formula (see Table 3.1) estimates creatinine clearance from age, sex, and body weight in addition to serum creatinine. There is an adjustment factor for women based on a theoretical assumption of 15% lower creatinine generation because of lower muscle mass. Comparison to normative values for creatinine clearance requires computation of body surface area and adjustment to 1.73 m². Because of the inclusion of a term for weight in the numerator, this formula systematically overestimates creatinine clearance in patients who are edematous or obese, and, because of the function of age, the estimated values sharply decline with age. The formula systematically overestimates GFR because of creatinine secretion, but more important, because it was derived using older assay methods for serum creatinine, it also systematically overestimates creatinine clearance. For all these reasons, the Cockcroft-Gault formula is less accurate than newer formulas described later.

Modification of Diet in Renal Disease Study Equation. The Modification of Diet in Renal Disease (MDRD) Study equation was originally expressed as a six-variable equation using serum creatinine, urea, and albumin concentrations in addition to age, sex, and race (black vs. white or other) to estimate GFR as measured by urinary clearance of ^{125}I-iothalamate. The revised four-variable equation has

Table 3.1   Equations for Estimating Glomerular Filtration Rate

Creatinine-Based Equations

Cockcroft-Gault Formula

C_{cr} (mL/min) = (140-age) × weight/72 × Scr × 0.85 [if female]

MDRD Study Equation for Use with Standardized Serum Creatinine (Four-Variable Equation)

GFR (mL/min/1.73 m^2) = 175 × $S_{Cr}^{-1.154}$ × age$^{-0.203}$ × 0.742 [if female] × 1.210 [if black]

CKD-EPI Equation for Use with Standardized Serum Creatinine

GFR (mL/min/1.73 m^2) = 141 × min(Scr/κ, 1)^α × max(Scr/κ, 1)$^{1.209}$ × 0.993^{Age} × 1.018 [if female] × 1.157 [if black]
where κ is 0.7 for females and 0.9 for males, α is –0.329 for females and –0.411 for males, min indicates the minimum of Scr/κ or 1, and max indicates the maximum of Scr/κ or 1.

Female	≤0.7 →	GFR = 144 × (Scr/0.7)$^{-0.329}$		
	>0.7 →	GFR = 144 × (Scr/0.7)$^{-1.209}$	× (0.993)^{Age}	× 1.157 [if black]
Male	≤0.9 →	GFR = 141 × (Scr/0.9)$^{-0.411}$		
	>0.9 →	GFR = 141 × (Scr/0.9)$^{-1.209}$		

Schwartz Formula (Younger than 18 Years of Age)

GFR = 0.413 × ht/Scr
eGFR = 40.7 × [HT/Scr]$^{0.640}$ × [30/BUN]$^{0.202}$

Cystatin C-Based Equations

CKD-EPI Cystatin C equation 2012

133 × min(Scys/0.8, 1)$^{-0.499}$ × max(Scys/0.8, 1)$^{-1.328}$ × 0.996^{Age} × 0.932 [if female]
where Scys is serum cystatin C, min indicates the minimum of Scr/κ or 1, and max indicates the maximum of Scr/κ or 1.

Female	≤0.8	GFR = 133 × (Scys/0.8)$^{-0.499}$ × 0.996^{Age} × 0.932
	>0.8	GFR = 133 × (Scys/0.8)$^{-1.328}$ × 0.996^{Age} × 0.932
Male	≤0.8	GFR = 133 × (Scys/0.8)$^{-0.499}$ × 0.996^{Age}
	>0.8	GFR = 133 × (Scys/0.8)$^{-1.328}$ × 0.996^{Age}

Creatinine-Cystatin C-Based Equations

CKD-EPI Creatinine-Cystatin C equation 2012

135 × min(Scr/κ, 1)^α × max(Scr/κ, 1)$^{-0.601}$ × min(Scys/0.8, 1)$^{-0.375}$ × max(Scys/0.8, 1)$^{-0.711}$ × 0.995^{Age} × 0.969 [if female] × 1.08 [if black]
where Scr is serum creatinine, Scys is serum cystatin C, κ is 0.7 for females and 0.9 for males, α is –0.248 for females and –0.207 for males, min indicates the minimum of Scr/κ or 1, and max indicates the maximum of Scr/κ or 1.

Female	≤0.7	≤0.8	GFR = 130 × (Scr/0.7)$^{-0.248}$ × (Scys/0.8)$^{-0.375}$ × 0.995^{Age} × 1.08 [if black]
		>0.8	GFR = 130 × (Scr/0.7)$^{-0.248}$ × (Scys/0.8)$^{-0.711}$ × 0.995^{Age} × 1.08 [if black]
	>0.7	≤0.8	GFR = 130 × (Scr/0.7)$^{-0.601}$ × (Scys/0.8)$^{-0.375}$ × 0.995^{Age} × 1.08 [if black]
		>0.8	GFR = 130 × (Scr/0.7)$^{-0.601}$ × (Scys/0.8)$^{-0.711}$ × 0.995^{Age} × 1.08 [if black]
Male	≤ 0.9	≤0.8	GFR = 135 × (Scr/0.9)$^{-0.207}$ × (Scys/0.8)$^{-0.375}$ × 0.995^{Age} × 1.08 [if black]
		>0.8	GFR = 135 × (Scr/0.9)$^{-0.207}$ × (Scys/0.8)$^{-0.711}$ × 0.995^{Age} × 1.08 [if black]
	>0.9	≤0.8	GFR = 135 × (Scr/0.9)$^{-0.601}$ × (Scys/0.8)$^{-0.375}$ × 0.995^{Age} × 1.08 [if black]
		>0.8	GFR = 135 × (Scr/0.9)$^{-0.601}$ × (Scys/0.8)$^{-0.711}$ × 0.995^{Age} × 1.08 [if black]

Schwartz Formula (Less than 18 Years of Age)

39.1 × (HT/Scr)$^{0.516}$ × (1.8/cysC)$^{0.294}$ × (30/BUN)$^{0.169}$ × (HT/1.4)$^{0.188}$ × 1.099 [if male]

Age in years; weight in kg. *ht,* Height in cm; *HT,* height in m; *Scr,* serum creatinine in mg/dl. SCr refers to standardized creatinine for all equations except the Cockcroft-Gault formula. For use of the MDRD Study equation without standardized creatinine, use 186 as the intercept.

now been reexpressed for use with standardized serum creatinine (see Table 3.1). This equation has been validated in African Americans, people with diabetic kidney disease, and kidney transplant recipients. The MDRD Study equation is more accurate than the Cockcroft-Gault formula, but it underestimates GFR in populations with higher levels of GFR. The MDRD Study equation is widely reported, but because of limitations in accuracy at higher levels, it has been recommended to report GFR estimates as a numeric value only if the GFR estimate is less than 60 mL/min/1.73 m^2 and as "greater than 60 mL/min/1.73 m^2" for higher values.

Table 3.2   Factors Affecting Serum Creatinine Concentration

Factor	Effect on Serum Creatinine	Mechanism/Comment
Age		
	Decrease	Reduced creatinine generation due to age-related decline in muscle mass
Female Sex		
	Decrease	Reduced creatinine generation due to reduced muscle mass
Race		
African American	Increase	Higher creatinine generation rate due to higher average muscle mass in African Americans; not known how muscle mass in other races compared to that of African Americans or Caucasians
Diet		
Vegetarian diet	Decrease	Decrease in creatinine generation
Ingestion of cooked meats and creatine supplements	Increase	Transient increase in creatinine generation; however, this may be blunted by transient increase in GFR
Body Habitus		
Muscular	Increase	Increased muscle generation due to increased muscle mass ± increased protein intake
Malnutrition/muscle wasting/amputation	Decrease	Reduced creatinine generation due to reduced muscle mass ± reduced protein intake
Obesity	No change	Excess mass is fat, not muscle mass, and does not contribute to increased creatinine generation
Medications		
Trimethoprim, cimetidine, fibric acid derivatives other than gemfibrozil	Increase	Reduced tubular secretion of creatinine
Ketoacids, some cephalosporins	Increase	Interference with alkaline picrate assay for creatinine
Antibiotics	Increase	Destroying intestinal flora, thereby interfering with extrarenal elimination

From Stevens LA, Levey AS: Measurement of kidney function, Med Clin North Am *89:457-473, 2005.*

Modifications of the MDRD Study equation have now been reported in racial and ethnic populations other than black and white. In general, these modifications improve the accuracy of the MDRD Study equation in the study population, but there is some uncertainty because of inconsistencies among studies.

Chronic Kidney Disease Epidemiology Equation. The chronic kidney disease epidemiology (CKD-EPI) equation (see Table 3.1) was recently developed using a large database of subjects from research studies and patients from clinical populations with diverse characteristics, including people with and without kidney disease, diabetes, and a history of organ transplantation. The equation is based on the same four variables as the MDRD Study equation, but uses a two-slope "spline" to model the relationship between GFR and serum creatinine; this partially corrects the underestimation of GFR at higher levels seen with the MDRD Study equation. As a result, the CKD-EPI equation is more accurate than the MDRD Study equation at eGFR >60 mL/min/1.73 m² and only slightly less accurate at lower levels (Fig. 3.2). The

CKD-EPI equation is more accurate than the MDRD Study across a wide range of characteristics, including age, sex, race, body mass index, and presence or absence of diabetes or history of organ transplantation. With the CKD-EPI equation, it is now reasonable to report eGFR across the entire range of values without substantial bias, and some clinical laboratories have begun to do so.

UREA

The serum urea concentration (expressed as urea nitrogen concentration in the United States) has limited value as an index of GFR because of widely variable non-GFR determinants, primarily urea generation and tubular reabsorption. Urea is an end product of protein catabolism by the liver with a molecular mass of 60 Da. Urea is freely filtered by the glomerulus and then passively reabsorbed in both the proximal and distal nephrons. Owing to tubular reabsorption, urinary clearance of urea underestimates GFR. Reduced kidney perfusion and states of antidiuresis (such as volume depletion or heart failure) are associated with increased urea reabsorption. This leads to a greater decrease in urea clearance than

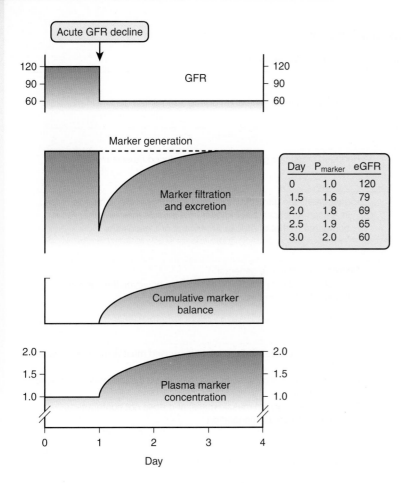

Day	P_{marker}	eGFR
0	1.0	120
1.5	1.6	79
2.0	1.8	69
2.5	1.9	65
3.0	2.0	60

Figure 3.2   Effect of an acute GFR decline on generation, filtration, excretion, balance, and serum level of endogenous filtration markers. After an acute GFR decline, generation of the marker is unchanged, but filtration and excretion are reduced, resulting in retention of the marker (a rising positive balance) and a rising plasma level (nonsteady state). During this time, estimated GFR (eGFR) is lower than measured GFR (mGFR). Although GFR remains reduced, the rise in plasma level leads to an increase in filtered load (the product of GFR times the plasma level) until filtration equals generation. At that time, cumulative balance and the plasma level plateau at a new steady state. In the new steady state, eGFR approximates mGFR. GFR is expressed in units of mL/min/1.73 m². Tubular secretion and reabsorption and extrarenal elimination are assumed to be zero. (Adapted from Stevens LA, Levey AS: Use of measured GFR as a confirmatory test, *J Am Soc Nephrol* 20:2305-2313, 2009. Original permission from Kassirer JP: Clinical evaluation of kidney function—glomerular function, *N Engl J Med* 285:385-389, 1971.)

the concomitant decrease in GFR. When measured GFR is less than approximately 20 mL/min/1.73 m², the overestimation of GFR by creatinine clearance due to creatinine secretion is approximately equal to the underestimation of GFR by urea clearance due to urea reabsorption; accordingly, the average of the urea clearance and the creatinine clearance provides a reasonable approximation of the measured GFR. Factors associated with the increased generation of urea include protein loading from hyperalimentation or absorption of blood after gastrointestinal hemorrhage. Catabolic states due to infection, corticosteroid administration, or chemotherapy also increase urea generation. Decreased urea generation is seen in severe malnutrition and liver disease.

CYSTATIN C

Metabolism and Excretion

Cystatin C is a 122 amino acid protein with a molecular mass of 13 kDa. Cystatin C has been thought of as produced at a constant rate by a "housekeeping" gene expressed in all nucleated cells. Cystatin C is freely filtered at the glomerulus because of its small size and basic pH. After filtration, approximately 99% of the filtered cystatin C is reabsorbed and catabolized by the proximal tubular cells. There is some evidence for the existence of tubular secretion as well as extrarenal elimination, which has been estimated at 15% to 21% of renal clearance.

Because cystatin C is not excreted in the urine, it is difficult to study its generation and renal handling. Thus,

understanding determinants of cystatin C other than GFR relies on epidemiological associations. In two studies, key factors that led to higher levels of cystatin C after adjusting for creatinine clearance or measured GFR were older age, male gender, fat mass, white race, diabetes, higher C-reactive protein and white blood cell count, and lower serum albumin. Other studies have suggested that inflammation, adiposity, thyroid diseases, certain malignancies, smoking, and use of glucocorticoids may increase cystatin C levels. Altogether, these studies suggest that factors other than GFR must be considered when interpreting cystatin C levels.

Equations for Estimating the Glomerular Filtration Rate from Serum Cystatin C

Some studies show that higher levels of cystatin C are a better predictor of the risk of cardiovascular disease and total mortality than an estimated GFR based on serum creatinine. Whether this is due to its superiority as a filtration marker or due to confounding by non-GFR determinants of both cystatin C and creatinine remains to be determined.

Several studies have compared accuracy of serum cystatin C and creatinine in relation to measured GFR, with the majority finding that serum cystatin C levels are a better estimate of GFR. However, cystatin C itself or equations based on cystatin C alone are not more accurate than creatinine-based estimating equations (see Table 3.1); rather, it is the combination of the two markers that results in the most accurate estimate in populations with and without CKD.

As with creatinine, variations in the assay used to measure cystatin C can lead to differences in estimated GFR. The CKD-EPI has recently published equations developed with or reexpressed for assays that are standardized to higher order reference materials. Most recently, the CKD-EPI creatinine-cystatin and CKD-EPI cystatin C equations (see Table 3.1) were developed from a large database of subjects with diverse characteristics, including people with and without CKD and diabetes. The CKD-EPI creatinine-cystatin C equation performed better than equations with either marker alone (Fig. 3.3). As standardized cystatin C becomes available for clinical use, the new CKD-EPI creatinine-cystatin C equation could be used as a confirmatory test for low estimated GFR from creatinine.

In certain populations, such as in children, the elderly, transplant recipients, and patients with neuromuscular diseases or liver disease, cystatin C has been hypothesized to be a more accurate estimate, but this hypothesis has not been rigorously evaluated. In patients with acute kidney injury (AKI), serum cystatin C increases more rapidly than serum creatinine. More data are required to establish whether cystatin C is a more sensitive indicator of a rapid GFR than creatinine.

CLINICAL APPLICATION OF ESTIMATED GLOMERULAR FILTRATION RATE

CHRONIC KIDNEY DISEASE

The level of GFR is used to define and stage chronic kidney disease (CKD). Therefore, estimation of GFR is necessary for the detection, evaluation, and management of CKD. Current guidelines recommend testing patients at increased risk of CKD by the use of albuminuria as a marker of kidney damage and serum creatinine to estimate GFR. Using serum creatinine alone can lead to misclassification of CKD and delays in detection. Use of estimating equations allows for reporting of GFR estimates by clinical laboratories whenever the marker is measured, facilitating interpretation of the result.

ACUTE KIDNEY DISEASE

Acute kidney injury is defined and staged according to the rate of rise in serum creatinine rather than the level of GFR. AKI is one of a number of acute kidney diseases in which GFR may be changing and serum creatinine concentrations are not in the steady state. In the nonsteady state, there is a lag before the rise in serum level because of the time required for retention of an endogenous filtration marker (Fig. 3.4). Conversely, following recovery of GFR, there is a lag before the excretion of the retained marker. During this time, neither the serum level of the marker (nor the corresponding estimate of GFR) accurately reflect the measured GFR. Nonetheless, a change in the estimated GFR in the nonsteady state can be a useful indication of the magnitude and direction of the change in measured GFR. If the estimated GFR is falling, the decline in estimated GFR is less than the decline in measured GFR. Conversely, if the estimated GFR is rising, the rise in estimated GFR is greater than the rise in measured GFR. The more rapid the change in estimated GFR, the larger the change in measured GFR.

DRUG DOSAGE ADJUSTMENT

The Cockcroft-Gault formula has been widely used to assess pharmacokinetic properties of drugs in people with impaired kidney function, and it remains the most commonly used method for drug dosage adjustment in this setting. There is current interest in using GFR estimates from the MDRD Study or CKD-EPI equations for drug dosing, because these estimates and equations are reported in clinical laboratories. Regardless of which equation is used, the variation in creatinine assays in past pharmacokinetic studies is likely to lead to unpredictable variations in dosage adjustment when applied in current clinical settings, As such, the continued use of the Cockcroft-Gault equation is not likely to lead to better drug dosage assignments than newer, more accurate equations. In fact, one recent study suggests that drug dosage adjustment, guided by the Cockcroft-Gault formula, is slightly less accurate than adjustments based on the MDRD Study equation. Accordingly, a recent Kidney Disease Improving Global Outcomes (KDIGO) controversies conference on drug dosing in patients with CKD recommends using the most accurate assessment of kidney function when assigning a drug dose.

NEED FOR CONFIRMATORY TEST

All creatinine-based estimating equations will be less accurate in people with factors affecting serum creatinine other than GFR (see Fig. 3.1). In these situations, a more accurate GFR estimate would require a clearance measurement, using either an exogenous filtration marker or a timed urine collection for creatinine clearance. In the future, improved estimating equations using the combination of creatinine and cystatin C, and potentially other novel endogenous markers, will allow more accurate GFR estimates that are less dependent on non-GFR determinants of any one marker. Ideally, it would be possible to estimate the GFR from a combination of endogenous markers that is as accurate as measured GFR.

KEY BIBLIOGRAPHY

Earley A, Miskulin D, Lamb EJ, et al: Estimating equations for glomerular filtration rate in the era of creatinine standardization: a systematic review, *Ann Intern Med* 156:785-795, 2012.

Inker LA, Eckfeldt J, Levey AS, et al: Expressing the CKD-EPI (Chronic Kidney Disease Epidemiology Collaboration) cystatin C equations for estimating GFR with standardized serum cystatin C values, *Am J Kidney Dis* 58:682-684, 2011.

Inker LA, Lafayette R, Upadhyay A, et al. In: Schrier RW, editor: *Diseases of the kidney & urinary tract*, ed 9, New York, 2012, Lippincott Williams & Wilkins.

Inker LA, Schmid CH, Tighiouart H, et al: Estimating glomerular filtration rate from creatinine and cystatin C, *N Engl J Med* 367:20-29, 2012.

Ix JH, Wassel CL, Stevens LA, et al: Equations to estimate creatinine excretion rate: the CKD epidemiology collaboration, *Clin J Am Soc Nephrol* 6:184-191, 2011. Epub 2010.

Knight EL, Verhave JC, Spiegelman D, et al: Factors influencing serum cystatin C levels other than renal function and the impact on renal function measurement, *Kidney Int* 65:1416-1421, 2004.

Kottgen A, Selvin E, Stevens LA, et al: Serum cystatin C in the United States: the Third National Health and Nutrition Examination Survey (NHANES III), *Am J Kidney Dis* 51:385-394, 2008.

Levey AS, Deo A, Jaber BL: Filtration markers in acute kidney injury, *Am J Kidney Dis* 56:619-622, 2010.

Levey AS, Stevens LA, Schmid CH, et al: A new equation to estimate glomerular filtration rate, *Ann Intern Med* 150:604-612, 2009.

Peralta CA, Shlipak MG, Judd S, et al: Detection of chronic kidney disease with creatinine, cystatin C, and urine albumin-to-creatinine ratio and association with progression to end-stage renal disease and mortality, *JAMA* 305:1545-1552, 2011.

Rule AD, Teo BW: GFR estimation in Japan and China: what accounts for the difference? *Am J Kidney Dis* 53:932-935, 2009.

Schwartz GJ, Munoz A, Schneider MF, et al: New equations to estimate GFR in children with CKD, *J Am Soc Nephrol* 20:629-637, 2009.

Schwartz GJ, Work DF: Measurement and estimation of GFR in children and adolescents, *Clin J Am Soc Nephrol* 4:1832-1843, 2009.

Stevens LA, Coresh J, Greene T, et al: Assessing kidney function—measured and estimated glomerular filtration rate, *N Engl J Med* 354:2473-2483, 2006.

Stevens LA, Coresh J, Schmid CH, et al: Estimating GFR using serum cystatin C alone and in combination with serum creatinine: a pooled analysis of 3,418 individuals with CKD, *Am J Kidney Dis* 51:395-406, 2008.

Stevens LA, Levey AS: Measured GFR as a confirmatory test for estimated GFR, *J Am Soc Nephrol* 20:2305-2313, 2009.

Stevens LA, Levey AS: Use of the MDRD study equation to estimate kidney function for drug dosing, *Clin Pharmacol Ther* 86:465-467, 2009.

Stevens LA, Nolin TD, Richardson MM, et al: Comparison of drug dosing recommendations based on measured GFR and kidney function estimating equations, *Am J Kidney Dis* 54:33-42, 2009.

Stevens LA, Padala S, Levey AS: Advances in glomerular filtration rate-estimating equations, *Curr Opin Nephrol Hypertens* 19:298-307, 2010.

Stevens LA, Schmid CH, Greene T, et al: Factors other than glomerular filtration rate affect serum cystatin C levels, *Kidney Int* 75:652-660, 2009.

Full bibliography can be found on www.expertconsult.com.

Urinalysis and Urine Microscopy

Arthur Greenberg

The relatively simple chemical tests performed during routine urinalysis rapidly provide important information about a number of primary kidney and systemic disorders. The microscopic examination of the urine sediment is an indispensable part of the evaluation of patients with impaired kidney function, proteinuria, hematuria, urinary tract infection, or nephrolithiasis. The urine sediment provides valuable clues about the renal parenchyma. Dipstick tests can be automated, and flow cytometry can be used to identify some cells in the urine. Because mechanized tests cannot detect unusual cells or distinguish among casts, there is still no substitute for careful examination of the urine under the microscope. This task must not be delegated; it should be performed personally as experience in examining the urine is essential. Studies show both that a urinalysis performed by a nephrologist is more likely to aid in reaching a correct diagnosis than a urinalysis reported by a clinical chemistry laboratory and that urinalysis performed by physicians without special training is inaccurate. The features of a complete urinalysis are listed in Box 4.1.

SPECIMEN COLLECTION AND HANDLING

Urine should be collected with a minimum of contamination. A clean-catch midstream sample is preferred. If this is not feasible, bladder catheterization is appropriate in adults; the risk of contracting a urinary tract infection after a single catheterization is negligible. Suprapubic aspiration is used in infants. In the uncooperative male patient, a clean, freshly applied condom catheter and urinary collection bag may be used. Urine in the collection bag of a patient with an indwelling bladder catheter is subject to stasis, but a sample suitable for examination may be collected by withdrawing urine from above a clamp placed on the tube that connects the catheter to the drainage bag.

The chemical composition of the urine changes with standing, and the formed elements degenerate over time. The urine is best examined when fresh, but a brief period of refrigeration is acceptable. Because bacteria multiply at room temperature, bacterial counts from unrefrigerated urine are unreliable. High urine osmolality and low pH favor cellular preservation. These two characteristics of the first-voided morning urine give it particular value in cases of suspected glomerulonephritis.

PHYSICAL AND CHEMICAL PROPERTIES OF THE URINE

APPEARANCE

Normal urine is clear with a faint yellow tinge because of the presence of urochromes. As the urine becomes more concentrated, its color deepens. Bilirubin, other pathologic metabolites, and a variety of drugs may discolor the urine or change its smell. Suspended erythrocytes, leukocytes, or crystals may render the urine turbid. Conditions associated with a change in the appearance or odor of the urine are listed in Table 4.1.

SPECIFIC GRAVITY

The specific gravity of a fluid is the ratio of its weight to the weight of an equal volume of distilled water. The urine specific gravity is a conveniently determined but inaccurate surrogate for osmolality. Specific gravities of 1.001 to 1.035 correspond to an osmolality range of 50 to 1000 mOsm/kg. A specific gravity near 1.010 connotes isosthenuria, with a urine osmolality matching that of plasma. Relative to osmolality, the specific gravity is elevated when dense solutes such as protein, glucose, or radiographic contrast agents are present.

Three methods are available for specific gravity measurement. The hydrometer is the reference standard, but it requires a sufficient volume of urine to float the hydrometer and equilibration of the specimen to the hydrometer-calibrated temperature. The second method is based on the well-characterized relationship between urine specific gravity and refractive index. Refractometers calibrated in specific gravity units are commercially available and require only a drop of urine. Finally, the specific gravity may also be estimated by dipstick.

The specific gravity is used to determine whether the urine is or can be concentrated. During a solute diuresis accompanying hyperglycemia, diuretic therapy, or relief of obstruction, the urine is isosthenuric. In contrast, with a water diuresis caused by overhydration or diabetes insipidus, the specific gravity is typically 1.004 or lower. In the absence of proteinuria, glycosuria, or iodinated contrast administration, a specific gravity of more than 1.018 implies preserved concentrating ability. Measurement of specific gravity is useful in differentiating between prerenal azotemia and acute tubular necrosis (ATN), and in assessing the significance of proteinuria observed in a random voided urine sample. Because the protein indicator strip responds to the concentration of protein, the significance of a borderline reading depends on the overall urine concentration.

ROUTINE DIPSTICK METHODOLOGY

The urine dipstick is a plastic strip to which paper tabs impregnated with chemical reagents have been affixed. The reagents in each tab are chromogenic. After timed development, the color on the paper segment is compared with a chart. Some reactions are highly specific. Others are affected by the presence of interfering substances or extremes of pH. Discoloration of the urine with bilirubin or blood may obscure the color changes.

pH

Test pads for pH tests use indicator dyes that change color with pH. The physiologic urine pH ranges from 4.5 to 8. The determination is most accurate if performed promptly, because growth of urea-splitting bacteria and loss of carbon dioxide raise the pH. In addition, bacterial metabolism of glucose may produce organic acids that lower pH. These strips are not sufficiently accurate to be used for the diagnosis of renal tubular acidosis.

PROTEIN

Protein measurement uses the protein-error-of-indicators principle. The pH at which some indicators change color varies with the protein concentration of the bathing solution. Protein indicator strips are buffered at an acid pH near their color change point. Wetting them with a protein-containing specimen induces a color change. The protein reaction may be scored from trace to 4+, or by concentration. Their equivalence is as follows: trace, 5 to 20 mg/dl; 1+, 30 mg/dl; 2+, 100 mg/dl; 3+, 300 mg/dl; 4+, greater than 2000 mg/dl. Highly alkaline urine, especially after contamination with quaternary ammonium skin cleansers, may produce false-positive reactions.

Protein strips are highly sensitive to albumin but less so to globulins, hemoglobin, or light chains. If light-chain proteinuria is suspected, more sensitive assays should be used. With acid precipitation tests, an acid that denatures protein is added to the urine specimen, and the density of the precipitate is related to the protein concentration. Urine that is negative by dipstick but positive by sulfosalicylic acid precipitation is highly suspicious for light chains. Tolbutamide, high-dose penicillin, sulfonamides, and radiographic

---

Box 4.1   Routine Urinalysis

Appearance

Specific Gravity

Chemical Tests (Dipstick)

pH
Protein
Glucose
Ketones
Blood
Urobilinogen
Bilirubin
Nitrites
Leukocyte esterase

Microscopic examination (formed elements)

Crystals: urate; calcium phosphate, oxalate, or carbonate; triple phosphate; cystine; drugs
Cells: leukocytes, erythrocytes, renal tubular cells, oval fat bodies, transitional epithelium, squamous cells
Casts: hyaline, granular, red blood cell, white blood cell, tubular cell, degenerating cellular, broad, waxy, lipid-laden
Infecting organisms: bacteria, yeast, *Trichomonas*, nematodes
Miscellaneous: spermatozoa, mucous threads, fibers, starch, hair, and other contaminants

---

Table 4.1   Selected Substances That May Alter the Physical Appearance or Odor of the Urine

Color Change	Substances
White	Chyle, pus, calcium phosphate crystals
Pink/red/brown	Erythrocytes, hemoglobin, myoglobin, porphyrins, beets, senna, cascara, levodopa, methyldopa, deferoxamine, phenolphthalein and congeners, food colorings, metronidazole, phenacetin, anthraquinones, doxorubicin, phenothiazines
Yellow/orange/brown	Bilirubin, urobilin, phenazopyridine urinary analgesics, senna, cascara, mepacrine, iron compounds, nitrofurantoin, riboflavin, rhubarb, sulfasalazine, rifampin, fluorescein, phenytoin, metronidazole
Brown/black	Methemoglobin, homogentisic acid (alcaptonuria), melanin (melanoma), levodopa, methyldopa
Blue or green, green/brown	Biliverdin, *Pseudomonas* infection, dyes (methylene blue and indigo carmine), triamterene, vitamin B complex, methocarbamol, indican, phenol, chlorophyll, propofol, amitriptyline, triamterene
Purple	Infection with *Escherichia coli*, *Pseudomonas*, *Enterococcus*, others
Odor	**Substance or Condition**
Sweet or fruity	Ketones
Ammoniac	Urea-splitting bacterial infection
Maple syrup	Maple syrup urine disease
Musty or mousy	Phenylketonuria
"Sweaty feet"	Isovaleric or glutaric acidemia, or excess butyric or hexanoic acid
Rancid	Hypermethioninemia, tyrosinemia

contrast agents may yield false-positive turbidimetric reactions. More sensitive and specific tests for light chains, such as immunoelectrophoresis or immunoprecipitation, are preferred.

If the urine is very concentrated, the presence of a modest protein reaction is less likely to correspond to significant proteinuria in a 24-hour collection or when assessed by spot urine protein:creatinine ratio. Even so, it is unlikely that a 3+ or 4+ reaction would be seen solely because of a high urine concentration or, conversely, that the urine would be dilute enough to yield a negative reaction despite significant proteinuria. The protein indicator used for routine dipstick analysis is not sensitive enough to detect microalbuminuria.

BLOOD

Reagent strips for blood rely on the peroxidase activity of hemoglobin to catalyze an organic peroxide with subsequent oxidation of an indicator dye. Free hemoglobin produces a homogeneous color. Intact red cells cause punctate staining. False-positive reactions occur if the urine is contaminated with other oxidants such as povidone-iodine, hypochlorite, or bacterial peroxidase. Ascorbate yields false-negative results. Myoglobin is also detected, because it has intrinsic peroxidase activity. A urine sample that is positive for blood by dipstick analysis, but shows no red cells on microscopic examination, is suspect for myoglobinuria or hemoglobinuria. Pink discoloration of serum may occur with hemolysis, but free myoglobin is seldom present in a concentration sufficient to change the color of plasma. A specific assay for urine myoglobin confirms the diagnosis.

SPECIFIC GRAVITY

Specific gravity reagent strips actually measure ionic strength using indicator dyes with ionic strength-dependent dissociation constants (pKa). They do not detect glucose or nonionic radiographic contrast agents.

GLUCOSE

Dipstick reagent strips are specific for glucose, relying on glucose oxidase to catalyze the formation of hydrogen peroxide, which then reacts with peroxidase and a chromogen to produce a color change. High concentrations of ascorbate or ketoacids reduce test sensitivity. However, the degree of glycosuria occurring in diabetic ketoacidosis is sufficient to prevent false-negative results despite ketonuria.

KETONES

Ketone reagent strips depend on the development of a purple color after acetoacetate reacts with nitroprusside. Some strips can also detect acetone, but none react with β-hydroxybutyrate. False-positive results may occur in patients who are taking levodopa or drugs such as captopril or mesna that contain free sulfhydryl groups.

UROBILINOGEN

Urobilinogen is a colorless pigment that is produced in the gut from the metabolism of bilirubin. Some is excreted in feces, and the rest is reabsorbed and excreted in the urine. In obstructive jaundice, bilirubin does not reach the bowel,

and urinary excretion of urobilinogen is diminished. In other forms of jaundice, urobilinogen is increased. The urobilinogen test is based on the Ehrlich reaction in which diethylaminobenzaldehyde reacts with urobilinogen in acid medium to produce a pink color. Sulfonamides may produce false-positive results, and degradation of urobilinogen to urobilin may yield false-negative results. Better tests are available to diagnose obstructive jaundice.

BILIRUBIN

Bilirubin reagent strips rely on the chromogenic reaction of bilirubin with diazonium salts. Conjugated bilirubin is not normally present in the urine. False-positive results may be observed in patients receiving chlorpromazine or phenazopyridine. False-negative results occur in the presence of ascorbate.

NITRITE

The nitrite screening test for bacteriuria relies on the ability of gram-negative bacteria to convert urinary nitrate to nitrite, which activates a chromogen. False-negative results occur with infection with enterococcus or other organisms that do not produce nitrite, when ascorbate is present, or when urine has not been retained in the bladder long enough (approximately 4 hours) to permit sufficient production of nitrite from nitrate.

LEUKOCYTES

Granulocyte esterases can cleave pyrrole amino acid esters, producing free pyrrole that subsequently reacts with a chromogen. The test threshold is 5 to 15 white blood cells per high-power field (WBCs/HPF). False-negative results occur with glycosuria, high specific gravity, cephalexin or tetracycline therapy, or excessive oxalate excretion. Contamination with vaginal material may yield a positive test result without true urinary tract infection.

MICROALBUMIN DIPSTICKS

Albumin-selective dipsticks are available for screening microalbuminuria in patients with incipient diabetic nephropathy. The most accurate screening occurs when first morning specimens are examined, because exercise can increase albumin excretion. One type of dipstick uses colorimetric detection of albumin bound to gold-conjugated antibody. Normally, the urine albumin concentration is less than the 20 mcg/L detection threshold for these strips. Unless the urine is very dilute, a patient with no detectable albumin by this method is unlikely to have microalbuminuria. Because urine concentration varies widely, however, this assay has the same limitations as any test that only measures concentration. This strip is useful only as a screening test, and more formal testing is required if albuminuria is found.

A second type of dipstick has tabs for measurement of both albumin and creatinine concentration that permits calculation of the albumin-to-creatinine ratio. In contrast to the other dipstick tests described in this chapter, these strips cannot be read by simple visual comparison with a color chart. An instrument is required, but this system is suitable for point-of-care testing. When present on more than one determination, an albumin-to-creatinine ratio of 30 to 300 mcg/mg signifies microalbuminuria. Details on the interpretation of microalbuminuria are provided in Chapters 5 and 25.

MICROSCOPIC EXAMINATION OF THE SPUN URINARY SEDIMENT

SPECIMEN PREPARATION AND VIEWING

The contents of the urine are reported as the number of cells or casts per HPF (×400) after resuspension of the centrifuged pellet in a small volume of urine. The accuracy and reproducibility of this semiquantitative method depends on using the correct volume of urine. Twelve milliliters of urine should be spun in a conical centrifuge tube for 5 minutes at 1500 to 2000 rpm (450 g). After centrifugation, the tube is inverted and drained. The pellet is resuspended in the few drops of urine that remain in the tube after inversion by flicking the base of the tube gently with a finger or with the use of a pipette. Care should be taken to suspend the pellet fully without excessive agitation.

A drop of urine is poured or transferred by pipette onto a microscope slide. The drop should be of sufficient size so that a standard 22 × 22 mm coverslip just floats on the urine with a thin rim of urine at the edges. If too little is used, the specimen rapidly dries. If an excess of urine is applied, it will spill onto the microscope objective or stream distractingly under the coverslip. Rapid commercial urine stains, or the Papanicolaou stain, may be used to enhance detail. Most nephrologists prefer the convenience of viewing unstained urine. Subdued light is necessary. The condenser and diaphragm are adjusted to maximize contrast and definition. When the urine is dilute and few formed elements are present, detection of motion of objects suspended in the urine ensures that the focal plane is correct. One should scan the urine at low power (×100) to obtain a general impression of its contents before moving to high power (×400) to look at individual fields. It is useful to scan large areas at low power and then move to high power when a structure of interest is located. Cellular elements should be quantitated by counting or estimating the number in at least 10 representative HPFs. Casts may be quantitated by counting the number per low-power field, although most observers use less specific terms, such as rare, occasional, few, frequent, and numerous.

CELLULAR ELEMENTS

The principal formed elements of the urine are listed (see Box 4.1). The figures in this chapter constitute an atlas of selected formed elements.

ERYTHROCYTES

Red blood cells (RBCs) (Fig. 4.1A and B) may find their way into the urine from any source between the glomerulus and the urethral meatus. The presence of more than two to three erythrocytes per HPF is considered pathologic. Erythrocytes are biconcave disks 7 μm in diameter. They become crenated in hypertonic urine. In hypotonic urine, they swell or burst, leaving ghosts. Erythrocytes originating in the renal parenchyma are dysmorphic, with spicules, blebs, submembrane cytoplasmic precipitation, membrane folding, and

vesicles. Those originating in the collecting system retain their uniform shape. Experienced observers report success differentiating renal parenchymal from collecting system bleeding by systematic examination of erythrocytes using phase contrast microscopy. Use of conventional microscopy to make this differentiation is unreliable.

LEUKOCYTES

Polymorphonuclear leukocytes (PMNs) (Fig. 4.1C) are approximately 12 μm in diameter and are most readily recognized in a fresh urine sample before their multilobed nuclei or granules have degenerated. Swollen PMNs with prominent granules displaying Brownian motion are termed "glitter" cells. PMNs may indicate urinary tract inflammation, intraparenchymal diseases such as glomerulonephritis or interstitial nephritis, or upper or lower urinary tract infection. Periureteral inflammation, as in regional ileitis or acute appendicitis, may also cause pyuria.

RENAL TUBULAR EPITHELIAL CELLS

Tubular cells (Fig. 4.1D) are larger than PMNs, ranging from 12 to 20 μm in diameter. Proximal tubular cells are oval- or egg-shaped and tend to be larger than the cuboidal distal tubular cells. However, because size varies with urine osmolality, these cells cannot be reliably differentiated. In hypotonic urine, it may be difficult to distinguish tubular cells from swollen PMNs. A few tubular cells may be seen in a normal urine sample. More commonly, these cells indicate tubular damage or inflammation from ATN or interstitial nephritis.

OTHER CELLS

Squamous cells (Fig. 4.1E) of urethral, vaginal, or cutaneous origin are large, flat cells with small nuclei. Transitional epithelial cells (Fig. 4.1F) line the renal pelvis, ureter, bladder, and proximal urethra. They are rounded cells several times the size of leukocytes and often occur in clumps. In hypotonic urine, they may be confused with swollen tubular epithelial cells.

CASTS AND OTHER FORMED ELEMENTS

Based on their shape and origin, casts are appropriately named. Immunofluorescence studies demonstrate that they consist of a matrix of Tamm-Horsfall urinary glycoprotein (uromodulin) in the shape of the distal tubular or collecting duct segment from where they were formed. The matrix has a straight margin that is helpful in differentiating casts from clumps of cells or debris.

HYALINE CASTS

Hyaline casts (Fig. 4.2A) consist of protein alone. Because their refractive index is close to that of urine, they may be difficult to see, requiring subdued light and careful manipulation of the iris diaphragm to increase diffraction and visual contrast. Hyaline casts are nonspecific. They occur in concentrated urine from healthy individuals as well as in numerous pathologic conditions.

GRANULAR CASTS

Granular casts (Fig. 4.2B) consist of finely or coarsely granular material. Immunofluorescence studies show that the fine granules are derived from altered serum proteins. Coarse granules may result from degeneration of embedded cells.

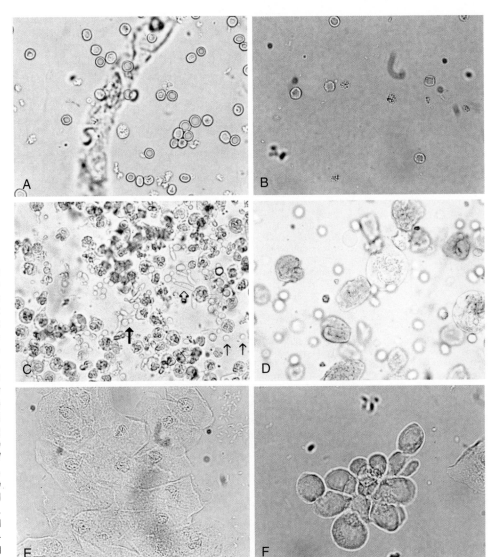

Figure 4.1 Cellular elements in the urine. In this and subsequent figures, all photographs were made from unstained sediments and, except as specified, were photographed at ×400 original magnification. **A,** Non-dysmorphic red blood cells. They appear as uniform, biconcave disks. **B,** Dysmorphic red blood cells from a patient with IgA nephropathy. Their shape is irregular, with membrane blebs and spicules. **C,** Urine obtained from a patient with an indwelling bladder catheter. Innumerable white blood cells as well as individual *(small arrows)*, budding *(single thick arrow)*, and hyphal *(open arrow)* forms are present. **D,** Renal tubular epithelial cells. Note the variability of shape. The erythrocytes in the background are much smaller. **E,** Squamous epithelial cells. **F,** Transitional epithelial cells in a characteristic clump.

Granular casts are nonspecific but usually pathologic. They may be seen after exercise or with simple volume depletion, and as a finding in ATN, glomerulonephritis, or tubulointerstitial disease.

WAXY CASTS

Waxy casts or broad casts (Fig. 4.2C) are made of hyaline material with a much greater refractive index than hyaline casts—hence, their waxy appearance. They behave as though they are more brittle than hyaline casts, and they frequently have fissures along their edges. Broad casts form in tubules that have become dilated and atrophic, and from their presence one can infer that the patient has chronic parenchymal disease.

RED BLOOD CELL CASTS

Red blood cell casts indicate intraparenchymal bleeding. The hallmark of glomerulonephritis, they are seen less frequently with tubulointerstitial disease. RBC casts have been described along with hematuria in healthy individuals after exercise. Fresh RBC casts (Fig. 4.2D) retain their brown pigment and consist of readily discernible erythrocytes in a tubular cast matrix. Over time, the heme color is lost,

along with the distinct cellular outline. With further degeneration, RBC casts are difficult to distinguish from coarsely granular casts. RBC casts may be diagnosed by the company they keep; they appear in a background of hematuria with dysmorphic red cells, granular casts, and proteinuria. Occasionally, the evidence for intraparenchymal bleeding is a hyaline cast with embedded red cells. These have the same pathophysiologic implication as RBC casts.

WHITE BLOOD CELL CASTS

White blood cell casts consist of WBCs in a protein matrix. They are characteristic of pyelonephritis, and they are useful in distinguishing that disorder from lower urinary tract infection. They may also be seen with interstitial nephritis and other tubulointerstitial disorders.

TUBULAR CELL CASTS

Tubular cell casts (Fig. 4.2E) can consist either of a few tubular cells in a hyaline matrix or a dense agglomeration of sloughed tubular cells. They occur in concentrated urine, but are more characteristically seen with the sloughing of tubular cells that occurs with ATN.

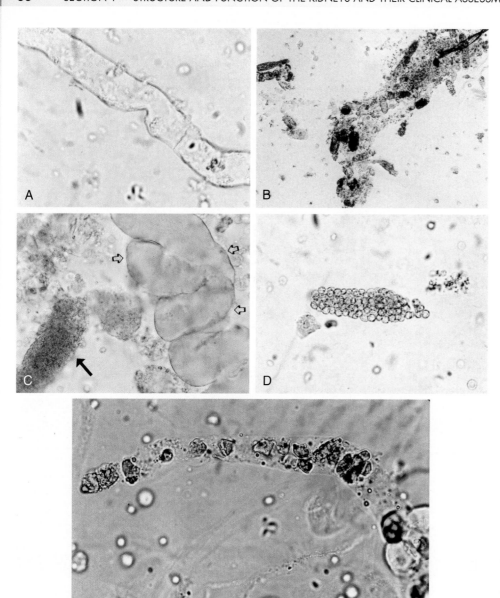

Figure 4.2   Casts. A, Hyaline cast. **B,** Muddy brown granular casts and amorphous debris from a patient with acute tubular necrosis (original magnification ×100). **C,** Waxy cast *(open arrows)* and granular cast *(solid arrow)* from a patient with lupus nephritis and a telescoped sediment. Note background hematuria. **D,** Red blood cell cast. Background hematuria is also present. **E,** Tubular cell cast. Note the hyaline cast matrix.

BACTERIA, YEAST, AND OTHER INFECTIOUS AGENTS

Bacillary or coccal forms of bacteria may be discerned even on an unstained urine sample. Examination of a Gram stain preparation of unspun urine allows estimation of the bacterial count. One organism per HPF of unspun urine corresponds to 20,000 organisms per cubic millimeter. Individual and budding yeasts and hyphal forms occur with Candida infection or colonization. Candida organisms are similar in size to erythrocytes, but are greenish spheres, not biconcave disks. When budding forms or hyphae are present, yeast cells are obvious (see Fig. 4.1C). Trichomonas organisms are identified by their teardrop shape and motile flagellum.

LIPIDURIA

In the nephrotic syndrome with lipiduria, tubular cells reabsorb luminal fat. Sloughed tubular cells containing fat droplets are called oval fat bodies. Fatty casts contain lipid-laden tubular cells or free lipid droplets. By light microscopy, lipid droplets appear round and clear with a green tinge. Cholesterol esters are anisotropic, cholesterol-containing droplets that rotate polarized light to produce a "Maltese cross" appearance. Triglycerides appear similar by light microscopy, but they are isotropic. Crystals, starch granules, mineral oil, and other urinary contaminants are also anisotropic. Before concluding that anisotropic structures are lipid, the observer must compare polarized and bright-field views of the same object (Fig. 4.3).

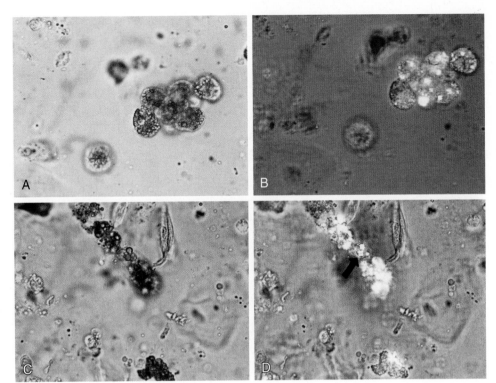

Figure 4.3   Lipid. A, Oval fat bodies, as seen by bright-field illumination. **B,** Same field as in **A,** viewed under polarized light. **C,** Lipid-laden cast, bright-field illumination. **D,** Same field as in **C,** viewed under polarized light. *Arrow* points to characteristic Maltese cross.

TABLE 4.2	Common Urinary Crystals	
DESCRIPTION	**COMPOSITION**	**COMMENT**
Crystals Found in Acid Urine		
Amorphous	Uric acid	Cannot be distinguished from amorphous phosphates except by urine pH; may be orange tinted by urochromes.
	Sodium urate	
Rhomboid prisms	Uric acid	
Rosettes	Uric acid	
Bipyramidal	Calcium oxalate	Also termed "envelope-shaped."
Dumbbell-shaped	Calcium oxalate	
Needles	Uric acid	Clinical history provides useful confirmation
	Sulfa drugs	Sulfa may resemble sheaves of wheat; urate and contrast crystals
	Radiographic contrast material	are thicker.
Hexagonal plates	Cystine	Presence may be confirmed with nitroprusside test.
Crystals Found in Alkaline Urine		
Amorphous	Phosphates	Indistinguishable from urates except by pH.
"Coffin lid" (beveled rectangular prisms)	Triple (magnesium ammonium) phosphate	Seen with urea-splitting infection and bacteriuria.
Granular masses or dumbbells	Calcium carbonate	Larger than amorphous phosphates.
Yellow-brown masses with or without spicules	Ammonium biurate	
Platelike rectangles, fan-shaped, starburst	Indinavir	Causes nephrolithiasis or renal colic. In vitro solubility increased at very low pH. The lowest urine pH achievable in vivo may not actually be acid enough to lessen crystalluria.

CRYSTALS

Crystals may be present spontaneously, or may precipitate with refrigeration of a specimen. They can be difficult to identify, because they have similar shapes; the common urinary crystals are described in Table 4.2. The pH is an important clue to identity, because the solubility of many urinary constituents is pH dependent. The three most distinctive crystal forms are cystine, calcium oxalate, and magnesium ammonium (triple) phosphate. Cystine crystals (Fig. 4.4A) are hexagonal plates that resemble benzene rings. Calcium oxalate crystals (see Fig. 4.4A) are classically

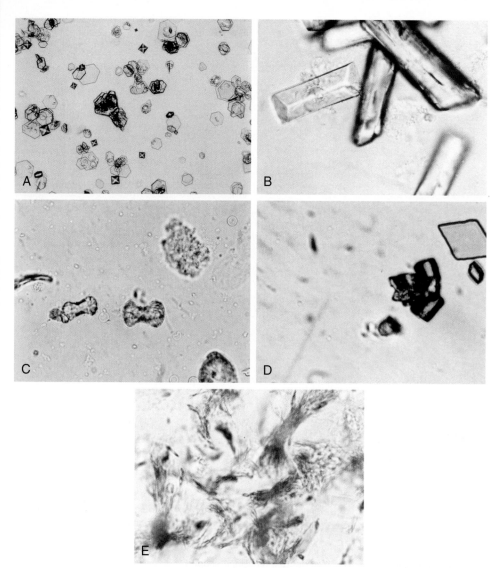

Figure 4.4   Crystals. A, Hexagonal cystine and bipyramidal or envelope-shaped oxalate. **B,** Coffin-lid–shaped triple phosphate. **C,** Dumbbell-shaped oxalate. **D,** Rhomboid urate. **E,** Needle-shaped urate. (**A,** Courtesy Dr. Thomas O. Pitts.)

described as "envelope shaped," but when viewed as they rotate in the urine under the microscope appear bipyramidal. Coffin-lid–shaped triple phosphates (Fig. 4.4B) are rectangular with beveled ends. Oxalate (Fig. 4.4C) may also occur in dumbbell-shaped crystals. Urate may have several forms, including rhomboids (Fig. 4.4D) or needles (Fig. 4.4E).

CHARACTERISTIC URINE SEDIMENTS

The urine sediment is a rich source of diagnostic information. Occasionally, a single finding (for example, cystine crystals) is pathognomonic. More often, the sediment must be considered as a whole and interpreted in conjunction with clinical and other laboratory findings. Several patterns bear emphasis.

In the acute nephritic syndrome, the urine may be pink or pale brown and turbid. Blood and moderate proteinuria are detected by dipstick analysis. The microscopic examination shows dysmorphic RBCs and RBC casts as well as granular and hyaline casts; WBC casts are rare. In the nephrotic syndrome, the urine is clear or yellow.

Foaminess may be noted because of the elevated protein content altering the urine surface tension. In comparison with the sediment of nephritic patients, the nephrotic sediment is bland. Hyaline casts and lipiduria with oval fat bodies or lipid-laden casts predominate. Granular casts and a few tubular cells may also be present, along with a few RBCs. With some forms of chronic glomerulonephritis, a "telescoped" sediment is observed (see Fig. 4.2C). This term refers to the presence of the elements of a nephritic sediment together with broad or waxy casts, the latter indicative of tubular atrophy. Dipstick findings of heavy proteinuria may be present. In pyelonephritis, WBC casts and innumerable WBCs are present, along with bacteria. In lower tract infections, WBC casts are absent. The sediment in ATN (see Fig. 4.2B) shows tubular cells, tubular cell casts, and muddy brown granular casts. Recently, a urine sediment score, derived by totaling points given for the number of renal tubular epithelial cells observed per HPF and the number of granular casts observed per low-power field, has been found in a single-center study to be useful in differentiating ATN from other etiologies of AKI. At least one other similar index has been proposed.

This quantitative approach shows promise, but no scoring system has yet been widely validated or has yet gained general acceptance. The typical urinary findings in individual kidney disorders are discussed in their respective chapters.

BIBLIOGRAPHY

Birch DF, Fairley KF, Becker GJ, et al: *A color atlas of urine microscopy*, New York, 1994, Chapman & Hall.

Canaris CJ, Flach SD, Tape TG, et al: Can internal medicine residents master microscopic urinalysis? Results of an evaluation and teaching intervention, *Acad Med* 78:525-529, 2003.

Claure-Del Granado R, Macedo E, Mehta RL: Urine microscopy in acute kidney injury: time for a change, *Am J Kidney Dis* 57:657-660, 2011.

Fairley KF, Birch DF: Hematuria: simple method for identifying glomerular bleeding, *Kidney Int* 21:105-108, 1982.

Fassett RG, Owen JE, Fairley J, et al: Urinary red-cell morphology during exercise, *Br Med J* 285:1455-1457, 1982.

Fogazzi GB, Cameron JS: Urinary microscopy from the seventeenth century to the present day, *Kidney Int* 50:1058-1068, 1996.

Fogazzi GB, Ponticelli C, Ritz E: *The urinary sediment: an integrated view*, ed 2, Oxford, 1999, Oxford University Press.

Fogazzi GB, Verdesca S, Carigali G: Urinalysis: core curriculum 2008, *Am J Kidney Dis* 51:1052-1067, 2008.

Foot CL, Fraser JF: Uroscopic rainbow: modern matula medicine, *Postgrad Med* 82:126-129, 2006.

Graff L: *A handbook of routine urinalysis*, Philadelphia, 1983, JB Lippincott.

Kincaid-Smith P: Haematuria and exercise-related haematuria, *Br Med J* 285:1595-1597, 1982.

Kopp JB, Miller KD, Mican JM, et al: Crystalluria and urinary tract abnormalities associated with indinavir, *Ann Intern Med* 127:119-125, 1997.

Perazella MA, Coca SG: Traditional urinary biomarkers in the assessment of hospital-acquired AKI, *Clin J Am Soc Nephrol* 7:167-174, 2012.

Raymond JR, Yarger WE: Abnormal urine color: differential diagnosis, *South Med J* 81:837-841, 1988.

Rutecki GJ, Goldsmith C, Schreiner GE: Characterization of proteins in urinary casts: fluorescent-antibody identification of Tamm-Horsfall mucoprotein in matrix and serum proteins in granules, *N Engl J Med* 284:1049-1052, 1971.

Schumann GB, Harris S, Henry JB: An improved technic for examining urinary casts and a review of their significance, *Am J Clin Pathol* 69:18-23, 1978.

Stamey TA, Kindrachuk RW: *Urinary sediment and urinalysis: a practical guide for the health professional*, Philadelphia, 1985, WB Saunders.

Tsai JJ, Yeun JY, Kumar VA, et al: Comparison and interpretation of urinalysis performed by a nephrologist versus a hospital-based clinical laboratory, *Am J Kidney Dis* 46:820-829, 2005.

Voswinckel P: A marvel of colors and ingredients: the story of urine test strips, *Kidney Int* 46(Suppl):3-7, 1994.

5 Hematuria and Proteinuria

David Jayne | Vivian Yiu

Hematuria and proteinuria are signs of disease in the kidney or urinary tract. Their presence is often asymptomatic, so serendipitous testing of urine with dipsticks can be an important first clue indicating underlying disease. Certain populations at higher risk for kidney disease, such as patients with diabetes mellitus, undergo regular urine testing, because early detection of kidney disease is vital to prevent progression to end-stage renal disease (ESRD).

Detection of hematuria and/or proteinuria should trigger further investigation and referral to the appropriate specialist (nephrologist or urologist). An understanding of the techniques of urine testing and the pathophysiology of hematuria and proteinuria, coupled with a systematic approach to the patient, are required to achieve a definitive diagnosis.

HEMATURIA

DEFINITION

Hematuria is the presence of erythrocytes in the urine. It can be grossly visible (macroscopic hematuria/visible hematuria) or only detectable on urine dipstick testing (microscopic hematuria/nonvisible hematuria). The degree of color change does not necessarily reflect the amount of blood in the urine, because as little as 1 mL of blood/L of urine can induce a color change. Centrifugation is the first step in analyzing red-brown urine, as hematuria is present only in the sediment. If the supernatant is red-brown, the presence of hemoglobin or myoglobin in the urine should be tested with dipsticks. Hemoglobin and myoglobin can be more accurately assessed by urinary electrophoresis. If testing is negative for heme, rare causes of urine discoloration, including porphyria, beetroot ingestion, or the use of drugs such as rifampicin, should be considered.

Erythrocytes appear in low numbers in healthy individuals, but it is prudent to avoid urine testing for a few days after strenuous exertion ("jogger's nephritis") or menstruation. Urethral catheterization and bladder trauma can also increase the number of erythrocytes in the urine. Microscopic hematuria is defined as the presence of two or more erythrocytes per high-powered (400x) field on light microscopy in the centrifuged sediment, or less than 13,000/mL of uncentrifuged urine. Hematuria is present in up to 3% to 6% of healthy individuals, but interestingly it is present in 5% to 10% of relatives of patients with chronic kidney disease.

ETIOLOGY

Macroscopic hematuria, especially if brisk and associated with clots, is most commonly associated with extraglomerular processes that vary with age. The most common causes include infection or inflammation of the prostate and bladder, or kidney stones. In patients over the age of 40, malignancy should be evaluated and excluded (Fig. 5.1).

The American Urological Association best practice policy listed several risk factors for urologic malignancy:

1. Age greater than 40 years.
2. Smoking history (higher risk with increased exposure).
3. Occupational exposure to benzene or amine dyes (printers, painters).
4. History of gross hematuria.
5. History of chronic cystitis.
6. History of pelvic irradiation.
7. Previous cyclophosphamide use.
8. History of analgesic abuse.

Damage or injury to the glomerular basement membrane (GBM) can allow the passage of red blood cells (RBCs) from the glomerular capillaries into Bowman capsule. This is often due to inflammatory conditions (glomerulonephritis—particularly IgA nephropathy and crescentic glomerulonephritis), when infiltrating leukocytes, immune complexes, or activated glomerular cells alter or rupture the GBM. It can also be a result of noninflammatory causes such as Alport syndrome, thin basement membrane disease, or diabetic nephropathy. Plasma proteins that are normally retained by the GBM often also appear in the urine, leading to associated proteinuria. Inflammation of the tubules can result in the transit of RBCs from peritubular capillaries into the tubular lumen (often accompanied by modest amounts of proteinuria) in tubulointerstitial nephritis or acute tubular necrosis, for example.

Macroscopic hematuria of glomerular origin occurs in IgA nephropathy, renal vasculitis, and as a complication of anticoagulation. It can also result from secondary renal tubular damage and acute kidney injury (AKI).

Persistent, isolated hematuria of glomerular origin is of prognostic significance in epidemiologic studies and confers an increased risk of ESRD. This is likely a result of four main causes:

1. IgA nephropathy, which can be associated with macroscopic hematuria and a positive family history.
2. Alport syndrome, often associated with deafness, corneal disorders, and a positive family history.
3. Mesangioproliferative glomerulonephritis without IgA deposits.
4. Thin basement membrane disease, with a positive family history and autosomal dominant pattern of inheritance.

Rare causes of hematuria include hereditary hemorrhagic telangiectasia, schistosomiasis (most notably in endemic

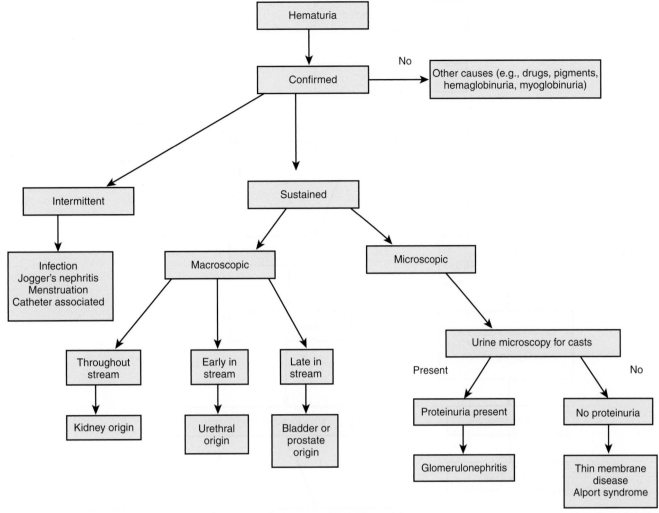

Figure 5.1   Causes of hematuria.

areas), and radiation cystitis. Arteriovenous malformations (AVMs) can be congenital or acquired and can cause macroscopic hematuria. They are often demonstrable on computed tomography (CT) scanning or angiography, where a therapeutic embolization procedure can be performed. Nutcracker syndrome, where the left renal vein is compressed between the aorta and the proximal superior mesenteric artery, can cause left flank pain, orthostatic proteinuria, and hematuria. Treatment can involve stenting of the left renal artery, or transposition of the artery. Loin pain hematuria syndrome is associated with dysmorphic RBCs and loin pain (which can be severe), but usually normal kidney function.

DETECTION

A variety of findings on urinalysis favor a diagnosis of glomerular bleeding: red blood cell (RBC) casts, proteinuria exceeding 500 mg/day, and dysmorphic RBCs. These are assessed by microscopy, which can also detect other abnormalities including leukocyturia and microorganisms. A fresh urine sample should always be used, because storage can lead to erythrocyte damage. Phase-contrast microscopy or supravital staining with Eosin-Y or the Steinheimer-Malbin

stain can improve the quality of the assessment. If these techniques are unavailable, RBC morphology is best assessed using reduced illumination and adjustment of the microscope condenser to increase diffraction. Prolonged centrifugation tends to disrupt the casts, reducing the likelihood of their positive identification (Fig. 5.2).

RBCs tend to be uniform and round in extrarenal sources of bleeding (normomorphic), but appear dysmorphic after traveling through the tubule in glomerular or tubular sources. In severe glomerular bleeding (i.e., IgA nephropathy or crescentic glomerulonephritis), there may be a mixture of dysmorphic and normomorphic RBCs. Very dilute urine causes osmotic lysis of RBCs forming "ghost cells." Acanthyocytes are dysmorphic RBCs with multiple spine or bubblelike projections, typically of glomerular origin. Laboratory analysis of RBCs can quantify results (in RBCs/mL) and assess mean corpuscular volume (less than 70 fl is typical of dysmorphic hematuria). The presence of granular casts, oval fat bodies, and waxy casts together with RBC casts imply an underlying kidney lesion.

Urine dipsticks impregnated with orthotolidine are very sensitive to low levels of RBCs in the urine (2 cells per high-powered field) so a positive result should be confirmed by microscopy. False positives can occur with the presence of

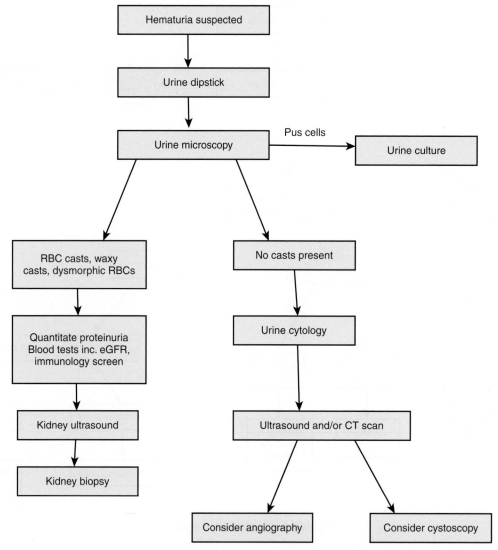

Figure 5.2 Investigation of hematuria.

hemoglobin or myoglobin. False negatives can occur if the dipsticks have been incorrectly stored or are expired, as well as in patients who consume large quantities of vitamin C.

Hematuria is quantified by the number of RBCs in a spun urine sediment (RBC/high-powered field) or by counting RBCs in a hemocytometer chamber (RBCs/mL), such as the Fychs-Rosenthal chamber. The chamber avoids the loss of RBCs that may stick to the tube during centrifugation or may be discarded in the supernatant. However, there are no simple techniques to control for urine concentration.

ASSESSMENT OF THE PATIENT WITH HEMATURIA

HISTORY

Certain points in the patient's history may be helpful in indicating the source of the hematuria (Table 5.1). The timing of macroscopic hematuria may provide information. Bladder lesions (e.g., schistosomiasis) tend to cause terminal hematuria, whereas urethral bleeding causes hematuria at the start of micturition. Blood from a kidney source tends to persist throughout the urinary stream. Glomerular bleeding often results in a smoky brown appearance of the urine

("Coca-Cola urine"), whereas bladder or prostate bleeding typically results in bright red blood.

The duration of hematuria, either transient or persistent, also provides important clues to etiology. Associated dysuria and frequency may suggest infection but can also be associated with acute hemorrhagic cystitis or bladder malignancy. Unilateral flank pain may indicate obstruction, either by calculus or clot (especially if the pain radiates to the groin), but can also be a sign of malignancy. Rarely it can be caused by loin pain hematuria syndrome. Hesitancy, terminal dribbling, or poor stream is indicative of prostatic obstruction in older male patients, as the new vessels formed in benign prostatic hypertrophy are fragile.

A recent upper respiratory tract infection and macroscopic hematuria raise the possibility of IgA nephropathy or postinfectious glomerulonephritis. A travel history should be taken, especially to areas endemic for schistosomiasis or tuberculosis. Recent trauma, strenuous exercise, and menstruation should be excluded as causes of hematuria. Associated symptoms of edema, proteinuria ("frothy urine"), hypertension, and reduced glomerular filtration rate (GFR) suggest a glomerular cause. Previous or current symptoms

Table 5.1   Causes of Hematuria

Glomerular Hematuria

Primary glomerulonephritis	Membranoproliferative glomerulonephritis
	Mesangioproliferative glomerulonephritis
	Crescentic glomerulonephritis
	Anti-GBM disease
	Focal segmental glomerulosclerosis
	Membranous glomerulopathy (less than 30%)
	Minimal change disease (less than 20%)
	Fibrillary glomerulopathy
			Infection
			  Pyelonephritis
			  Tuberculosis
			  BK nephropathy
			Hereditary
			  Polycystic kidney disease
			  Medullary sponge kidney
			Trauma
			Idiopathic hematuria

Multisystem or autoimmune disorder	SLE
	Vasculitis
	Scleroderma glomerulopathy
	Thrombotic microangiopathy
		Urinary tract origin	Malignancy
			  Transitional cell carcinoma
			  Carcinoma of the bladder/prostate
			Vascular
			  Malformations/nevi
			Infection
			  Cystitis
			  Prostatitis
			  Tuberculosis
			  Schistosomiasis

Other	Hereditary (Alport syndrome, Fabry disease, thin basement membrane disease)
	Infection associated glomerulonephritis
			Calculi
			Inflammatory
			  Retroperitoneal fibrosis/aortitis
			  Endometriosis
			  Diverticulitis/Crohn's disease
			  Hypersensitivity cystitis

Nonglomerular Hematuria

Kidney origin	Tubulointerstitial nephritis
	Hypersensitivity tubulointerstitial nephritis
	TINU
	Sjögren syndrome
	Vascular disorder
	  Malignant hypertension
	  Renal artery or vein thrombosis
	  AVM
	  Scleroderma renal crisis
	  Polyarteritis nodosa
	Papillary necrosis
	Malignancy
	  Renal cell carcinoma
	  Wilms tumor
	  Lymphoma/leukemia
	  Metastatic disease
		Other	Vasculitis
			  Churg-Strauss angiitis
			  Polyarteritis nodosa
			Drugs
			  Cyclophosphamide
			Trauma/foreign body
			Loin pain hematuria syndrome
			Acquired cystic disease of kidney failure
			Coagulation disorder
			Factitious

Anti-GBM, Antiglomerular basement membrane; *AVM,* arteriovenous malformation; *SLE,* systemic lupus erythematosus; *TINU,* tubulointerstitial nephritis with uveitis.

suggestive of vasculitis, diabetes mellitus, or malignancy are also useful indicators of cause.

A thorough medication history to look for potential causes of nephritis, anticoagulation, or risk factors for malignancy (such as cyclophosphamide) should be obtained. A family history is important in the diagnosis of polycystic kidney disease, sickle cell anemia, and thin basement membrane disease.

INVESTIGATION OF NONGLOMERULAR HEMATURIA

Urine microscopy and culture enable diagnosis of most bacterial (and parasitic) infections, although sterile pyuria can occur with renal tuberculosis. If this is suspected, multiple early morning urine specimens are required for culture, as well as serum T-spot or QuantiFERON testing. Renal calculi are visible on plain radiography or noncontrast CT scanning. If stones are found, the patient requires further metabolic screening with 24-hour urine collections to identify hypercalciuria, hyperuricosuria, or hyperoxaluria. In older men, prostate-specific antigen tests and

urine cytology will help identify a malignant cause, but cystoscopy should be performed, especially if the patient is passing blood clots.

The preferred imaging strategy for patients with unexplained nonglomerular hematuria is CT scanning—ideally combining conventional scanning CT with CT urography. Images of the kidney and urinary tract taken precontrast, in the renal parenchymal phase, and in the excretory phase provide a global view to look for kidney masses and transitional cell carcinomas. Ultrasonography is useful in characterizing smaller renal tumors, and angiography can be used in cases of suspected AVMs.

If no cause is found, rarer diagnoses such as factitious macroscopic hematuria (which can be excluded by testing a sample voided under direct observation) or loin-pain-hematuria syndrome should be considered. Unexplained persistent hematuria requires ongoing follow-up in case serious underlying pathology emerges. Patients who have had a urothelial tumor should have screening for additional lesions in the rest of the urothelial tract.

Table 5.2   Laboratory Investigation of Glomerular Hematuria

Diagnosis	Relevant Abnormal Investigations
MPGN	C3/4, C3 nephritic factor, cryoglobulins, hepatitis B/C
Anti-GBM disease	Anti-GBM antibodies, chest radiography
Fibrillary and immunotactoid glomerulopathy	Serum and urine electrophoresis, C3/C4, calcium, bone marrow biopsy, skeletal survey
SLE	ANA, anti-dsDNA, ENAs, C3/4, anticardiolipin antibody
Vasculitis (granulomatosis with polyangitis [Wegener], microscopic polyangiitis, Churg-Strauss angiitis)	ANCA: c-ANCA/PR3-ANCA or p-ANCA/MPO-ANCA
Thrombotic microangiopathy	Anticardiolipin antibody, lupus anticoagulant
Hereditary	
Alport disease	Audiometry
Fabry disease	Plasma α-galactosidase A activity
Infection Associated Glomerulonephritis	
HIV nephropathy	HIV
Poststreptococcal glomerulonephritis	ASO, anti-DNAase, C3/4, rheumatoid factor
Infective endocarditis	Echocardiography, C3/4, rheumatoid factor

Anti-GBM, Antiglomerular basement membrane; *ANA,* antinuclear antibody; *ANCA,* antineutrophil cytoplasmic antibody; *ASO,* antistreptolysin O *ENAs,* extractable nuclear antigens; *HIV,* human immunodeficiency virus; *MPGN,* membranoproliferative glomerulonephritis; *SLE,* systemic lupus erythematosus.

INVESTIGATION OF GLOMERULAR HEMATURIA

Glomerular hematuria can be caused by primary glomerulonephritis or multisystem autoimmune disorders, such as systemic lupus erythematosus (SLE), vasculitis, scleroderma, and thrombotic microangiopathies. Other causes include inherited disorders (Alport syndrome, Fabry disease, thin basement membrane disease) or infection (human immunodeficiency virus [HIV]-associated nephropathy, infective endocarditis). Investigation is aimed at eliciting the severity of kidney disease, looking for extrarenal manifestations of inflammatory disease, and identifying the underlying cause (Table 5.2).

Proteinuria should be quantified and urine microscopy performed to identify RBC casts. Blood tests should include a C-reactive protein (CRP), which is elevated in acute glomerulonephritis and infections. An infection screen looking for the presence of HIV and hepatitis B and C should be included if risk factors are present. In children with suspected poststreptococcal glomerulonephritis, a raised antistreptolysin O (ASO) titer and elevated anti-DNAase antibodies are usually found. A transesophageal echocardiogram to look for endocarditis and a CT scan to look for occult abscesses should also be considered if the infective source is unclear. Genetic screening is available in the case of Alport syndrome, and measurement of plasma α-galactosidase will confirm a diagnosis of Fabry disease.

Immunologic investigations for patients with glomerular hematuria of unknown cause should include antinuclear antibodies (ANAs), antineutrophil cytoplasmic antibodies (ANCAs), complement levels, protein electrophoresis, and antiglomerular basement membrane (anti-GBM) antibodies if there is associated pulmonary hemorrhage, RBC casts, or deteriorating kidney function. If ANA testing is positive, a further screen to look for related autoantibodies should be performed (see Table 5.2). Crescentic glomerulonephritis typically presents with microscopic hematuria, proteinuria greater than 100 mg/dl (2+) on urine dipstick testing, and deteriorating kidney function (Fig. 5.3).

Ultrasonography is the first imaging modality used to define kidney anatomy (often as a prelude to kidney biopsy), exclude mass lesions, and demonstrate corticomedullary differentiation in acute inflammatory conditions. Doppler examination should be performed to exclude renal vein thrombosis (a cause of nonglomerular hematuria).

A definitive diagnosis often requires a kidney biopsy, with samples being processed for light microscopy, immunofluorescence, and electron microscopy. The risks of the procedure need to be weighed against the benefits of a histologic diagnosis. For patients with isolated glomerular hematuria (in the absence of proteinuria or elevated serum creatinine), biopsy is usually not indicated, because the management of patients is rarely influenced by the result. The most likely diagnoses in such scenarios are IgA nephropathy or thin basement membrane disease, and specific therapy is often not warranted in the absence of adverse features.

PROTEINURIA

The prevalence of proteinuria in the general population is approximately 2%, and it is higher in older individuals and those with comorbidities. Proteinuria is a marker of kidney disease, and it plays a role in screening, diagnosis, and monitoring. Large epidemiologic studies have shown that proteinuria is an independent risk factor for cardiovascular events and progressive kidney disease.

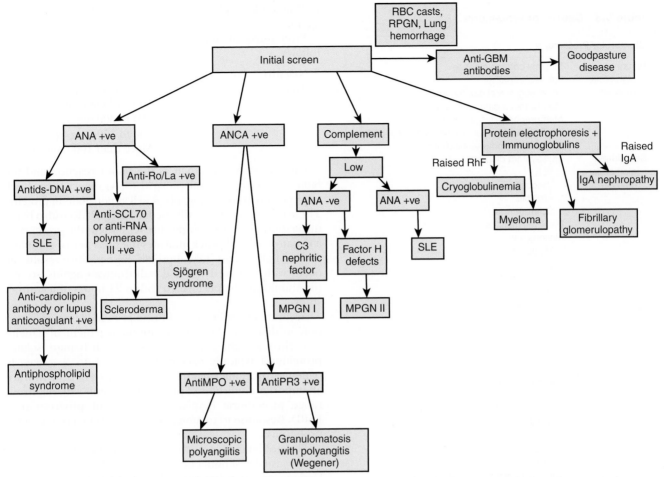

Figure 5.3   Immunologic tests. *ANA,* Antinuclear antibody; *ANCA,* antineutrophil cytoplasm antibody; *anti-GBM,* anti-glomerular basement membrane; *MPGN,* membranoproliferative glomerulonephritis; *RPGN,* rapidly progressive glomerulonephritis; *SLE,* systemic lupus erythematosus.

DEFINITION

Normal urinary protein excretion in an adult is less than 100 mg/24 h. Higher levels of excretion (more than 200 mg/24 h) suggest that glomerular pathology allows the passage of macromolecules such as albumin, which are not normally filtered. Excretion rates tend to increase on standing, during exertion, or with fever. Pressor agents such as angiotensin and norepinephrine tend to increase proteinuria (Table 5.3).

Proteinuria is usually asymptomatic and detected by dipstick testing during routine medical examinations (e.g., with participation in high-school athletics, on entry to armed forces, or at antenatal visits). Patients often report "frothy urine" if excretion rates are high, and this is associated with hypoalbuminemia and edema as part of the nephrotic syndrome. Other causes of frothy urine include bilirubinuria, retrograde ejaculation, and pneumaturia. Protein excretion rates greater than 3000 mg/24 h are termed *nephrotic range proteinuria* (Fig. 5.4).

In health, proteinuria results from tubular protein excretion, particularly Tamm-Horsfall protein. Albumin is the predominant protein filtered by the glomerulus, and therefore it is the most consistent marker of glomerular pathology. In health, albumin contributes little to urinary proteinuria (around 12 mg/24 h), as proteins crossing the GBM are mainly reabsorbed and degraded via receptor-mediated endocytosis. This process shows a preference for cationic proteins and only a limited capacity for albumin, resulting in even minor glomerular abnormalities raising albuminuria. Microalbuminuria refers to albumin excretion in the range of 30 to 300 mg/24 h (20 to 200 µg/min). This equates to a urinary albumin-creatinine ratio (ACR) of 17 to 250 mg/g for men and 25 to 355 mg/g for women. Albumin and its ligands, megalin and cubulin, induce inflammatory and fibrogenic mediators, such as TGFβ, that cause tubular injury.

DETECTION AND QUANTIFICATION

Urine testing using a standard dipstick relies on a colorimetric reaction between albumin and an indicator dye (such as tetrabromophenol blue or bromocrescol green) to produce a semiquantitative grading of the degree of proteinuria. As nonalbumin proteins, such as immunoglobulin light chains, are not detected, dipsticks will underestimate urine proteinuria in their presence, and dilute urine (specific gravity less than 1.005) will yield falsely low results. False positive results also occur if the urine is strongly alkaline, with pH greater than 8, thereby overwhelming the buffer on the dipstick. Inaccuracies are also seen in the presence of certain drugs

Table 5.3   Causes of Proteinuria

Glomerular Proteinuria

Primary glomerular disease	Minimal change disease
	IgA nephropathy
	Focal segmental glomerulosclerosis
	Membranous glomerulonephritis
	Membranoproliferative glomerulopathy
	Fibrillary and immunotactoid glomerulopathy
	Crescentic glomerulonephritis
Secondary glomerular disease	Multisystem disease
	SLE
	Vasculitis
	Amyloid
	Scleroderma
	Diabetes mellitus
	Malignancy
	Myeloma
	Leukemia
	Solid tumors
	Infection
	Bacterial
	Viral
	Fungal
	Parasitic
	Drugs
	Gold
	Penicillamine
	Lithium
	Nonsteroidals
	Familial
	Alport syndrome
	Nephronopthisis
	Fabry disease
	Congenital nephrotic syndrome
	Other
	Preeclampsia
	Transplant glomerulopathy
	Reflux nephropathy
Other	Febrile proteinuria
	Exercise-induced proteinuria (rare beyond 30 years of age)
	Orthostatic proteinuria

Tubular Proteinuria

Drugs and toxins	Luminal injury
	Light chain nephropathy
	Lysozyme (myelogenous leukemia)
	Exogenous
	Heavy metals (lead, cadmium)
	Aristolochic acid (Balkan nephropathy)
	Tetracycline
Tubulointerstitial nephritis	Hypersensitivity (drugs, toxin)
	Systemic disease
	SLE
	Sjögren syndrome
	Tubulointerstitial nephritis with uveitis
Other	Fanconi syndrome

Overflow Proteinuria

Monoclonal gammopathies	Myeloma
	Light chain disease
Amyloidosis	
Hemoglobinuria	
Myoglobinuria	

SLE, Systemic lupus erythematosus.

(tolbutamide, cephalosporins) and iodinated radiocontrast agents.

Proteinuria on dipstick is graded from trace to 4+ as follows:

Negative	
Trace	15 to 30 mg/dl
1+	30 to 100 mg/dl
2+	100 to 300 mg/dl
3+	300 to 1000 mg/dl
4+	More than 1000 mg/dl

Laboratory testings such as the biuret reaction and turbidimetry using sulfosalicylic acid (SSA) detect lower levels of proteinuria (up to 5 mg/dl) as well as nonalbumin proteins. These testings are primarily used in cases of AKI with a bland urine dipstick. A strongly positive SSA test in the presence of a negative urine dipstick indicates the presence of globulins, such as light chains. Like dipsticks, false positive results can occur with certain drugs and radiocontrast agents, so testing should not be performed within 24 hours of a contrast study.

Accurate quantification of urine protein is important not only in diagnosis, but also in the management of patients with chronic kidney disease. Patients with benign isolated proteinuria typically excrete less than 1 to 2 g/day. In patients with glomerular disease, the degree of proteinuria is an important indicator of prognosis; patients with nephrotic range proteinuria have a higher risk of progression to ESRD. Response to treatment often results in a reduction in proteinuria.

The gold-standard method of quantification has been a timed (usually 24 hour) urine collection. However, these collections are often fraught with inaccuracies, and it is cumbersome to transport large volumes of urine, particularly for patients with persistent proteinuria who need regular monitoring. An alternative is the use of a smaller urine volume adjusted for urinary concentration by calculating the spot protein-creatinine ratio (PCR, mg/mg or g/g). This ratio correlates with daily protein excretion expressed as $g/1.73 \, m^2$ of body surface area. The most consistent results are obtained from a midstream urine specimen collected during the first urine void in the morning, but the ratio can also be applied to a random clinic sample. ACR has greater sensitivity for low-level proteinuria; however, both PCR and ACR have correlated well with 24-hour measurements in clinical trials. The normal ranges for PCR and ACR are less than 300 mg/g and less than 30 mg/g, respectively.

As mentioned earlier, standard dipstick testing for protein is highly specific but not very sensitive, and it is therefore unable to detect microalbuminuria. There are specifically designed test strips for this purpose, and these should be used in screening diabetic patients as well as those with hypertension and systemic diseases such as SLE. The presence of proteinuria is an independent risk factor for the development of ESRD in patients with cardiovascular disease or a reduced GFR. However, there is currently no evidence for routine population screening, although this is performed in some countries.

ETIOLOGY

Two thirds of urinary protein is filtered (glomerular proteinuria), and the remaining third is secreted (tubular

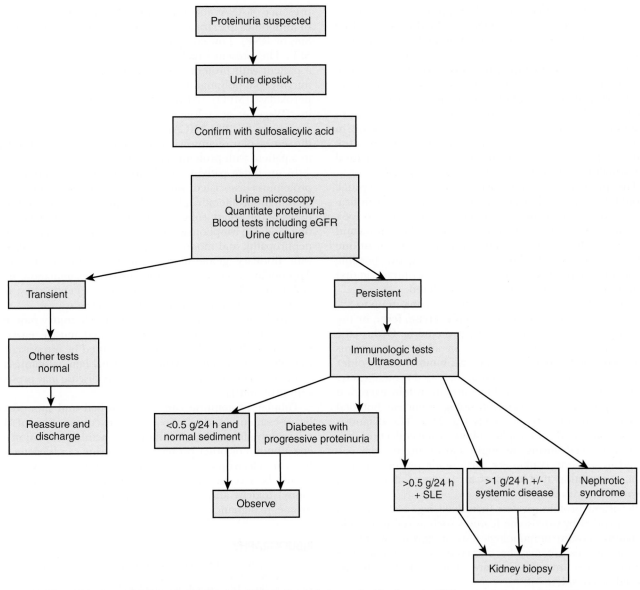

Figure 5.4   Investigation of proteinuria. *eGFR,* Estimated glomerular filtration rate; *SLE,* systemic lupus erythematosus.

proteinuria). Glomerular proteinuria is the only type detected on urine dipsticks and is responsible for most cases of persistent proteinuria. It occurs when excess protein crosses the GBM and overwhelms the tubular reabsorption capacity. The GBM is a high-capacity ultrafiltration membrane with proteins passing across by convection or by diffusion down a concentration gradient. Mutations of podocyte cell surface proteins (such as nephrin or podocin) or of podocyte intracellular proteins that contribute to the integrity of the membrane result in proteinuria. The membrane is negatively charged because of heparin sulfates in the glomerular endothelial wall that prevent similarly charged proteins (such as albumin) from passing across. Any glomerular pathology that impairs the ability of the GBM to maintain its charge results in proteinuria. Selective proteinuria occurs when there is minimal glomerular injury (such as minimal change nephropathy), but as more damage to the GBM occurs, larger molecules contribute to proteinuria.

Tubular pathology such as Dent disease, Lowe syndrome, tubulointerstitial nephritis, and heavy-metal poisoning leads to a failure to reabsorb smaller proteins normally filtered or secreted by the renal tubules. These include α-globulins and β-globulins, (e.g., α-microglobulin and β2-microglobulin) which are detectable by urine protein electrophoresis. Proteinuria in the range of 200 to 2000 mg/24 h is seen, although mixed glomerular and tubular pathologies can coexist.

Overflow proteinuria occurs when there is increased production of low molecular weight proteins that exceeds the reabsorptive capacity of the proximal tubule. The quantity of the excreted protein reflects the severity of the underlying pathology. In cases of hemolytic anemia, free hemoglobin not bound to haptoglobin appears in the urine. In rhabdomyolysis, greatly increased levels of myoglobin result in myoglobinuria.

ASSESSMENT OF THE PATIENT WITH PROTEINURIA

A careful history may suggest underlying systemic or kidney disease, such as diabetes mellitus, heart failure, or previous glomerular injury that can result in proteinuria. Examination should include measurement of blood pressure, fluid balance, and cardiac status, and an evaluation for signs of vasculitis or other systemic disease. A complete set of laboratory blood tests, including blood counts (with white cell differential) and biochemical studies for kidney function, electrolytes, albumin, globulins, cholesterol, calcium, phosphate, liver function tests, and uric acid should be sent. In addition, an immunology screen and virology testing in those patients deemed at risk is indicated. A kidney ultrasound is necessary to evaluate kidney sizes and structural abnormalities before a kidney biopsy is performed.

The presence of proteinuria on a screening dipstick should be confirmed by laboratory analysis and quantification. Urine microscopy should also be performed to look for other signs of glomerular disease such as hematuria and RBC casts. The dipstick should be repeated on at least one other occasion, and if subsequent tests are negative, possible causes of false-positive results (such as radiocontrast agents) or transient proteinuria should be considered.

Transient proteinuria is common, occurring in up to 4% of men and 7% of women. Vigorous exercise, fever, or the use of pressor agents can increase proteinuria. Orthostatic proteinuria should be considered in adolescent patients (frequency of 2% to 5%), but it is uncommon in those older than 30 years. It is characterized by increased protein excretion in an upright position but normal protein excretion when supine. The exact pathophysiology is unclear, but total protein excretion rarely exceeds 1 g/24 h. The diagnosis can be confirmed with a split 24-hour urine collection with urine produced during the night and during the day collected in separate containers. Orthostatic proteinuria is a benign condition that requires no further follow-up and often abates with time.

Persistent proteinuria less than 2000 mg/24 h and not accompanied by worrisome features such as reduced GFR, hematuria, positive immunologic tests, or signs and symptoms of systemic disease may be observed for several months before further investigations are planned. Kidney biopsy should be considered if:

- Proteinuria is of glomerular or tubular origin without a clear cause.
- Progressive proteinuria is accompanied by rise in plasma creatinine.
- Nephrotic range proteinuria exists.
- Persistent proteinuria exists greater than 500 mg/24 h in patients with a history of SLE.
- There is suspicion of vasculitis.

In patients with longstanding diabetes and progressive microalbuminuria, a kidney biopsy is not justified. However, it is more difficult to evaluate a diabetic patient who suddenly develops nephrotic range proteinuria, because a minority will have other glomerular pathologies. Similarly, hypertensive patients often have low-level proteinuria, but sudden onset nephrotic syndrome often has another cause.

Immunologic testing identifies circulating autoantibodies, abnormal complement levels, and pathologic immunoglobulins or immune complexes. SLE is suggested by the presence of ANAs and antidouble stranded DNA antibodies or antibodies to extractable nuclear antigens (especially Ro, Sm, or RNP). Low complement levels typically accompany SLE. The presence of hematuria and a positive ANCA in a patient with proteinuria strongly suggests a diagnosis of microscopic polyangiitis (confirmed with a positive myeloperoxidase [MPO]-ANCA) or granulomatosis with polyangiitis (Wegener granulomatosis) (confirmed with a positive proteinase 3 [PR3]-ANCA). A positive rheumatoid factor in the setting of proteinuria is associated with cryoglobulinemia in a patient with proteinuria (see Fig. 5.3).

In an older patient, occult malignancy may present as proteinuria associated with membranous nephropathy or membranoproliferative glomerulonephritis (commonly carcinoma of the breast, colon, stomach, and lung). Hodgkin and non-Hodgkin lymphomas are associated with minimal change nephropathy, and monoclonal gammopathies are associated with fibrillary glomerulopathy and overflow proteinuria. Appropriate screening with bone marrow examination, skeletal survey, CT scanning, gastrointestinal tract endoscopy, and mammography should be instigated as necessary.

Myoglobinuria in the absence of muscle injury requires evaluation for drug toxicity or inherited muscle enzyme deficiency. Hemoglobinuria can be caused by intravascular hemolysis (such as paroxysmal nocturnal hemoglobinuria). Other inherited disorders such as Fabry disease may present with proteinuria.

Tubular proteinuria can be quantified and monitored by assessment of the ratio of the excretion rate of β2-microglobulin to that of albumin. Factitious addition of egg albumin or other proteins to the urine can be detected by urine electrophoresis. Patients with tubular proteinuria should be screened for heavy metal (cadmium, lead, antimony) toxicity and also for systemic disease (Sjögren syndrome, malignancy).

BIBLIOGRAPHY

Cohen RA, Brown RS: Microscopic hematuria, *N Engl J Med* 348:2330-2338, 2003.

Fairley K, Birch DF: A simple method for identifying glomerular bleeding, *Kidney Int* 21:105-108, 1982.

Fogazi GB, Ponticelli C, Ritz E: *The urinary sediment: an integrated view*, ed 2, Oxford, 1999, Oxford University Press.

Gaspari F, Perico N, Remuzzi G: Timed urine collections are not needed to measure urine protein excretion in clinical practice, *Am J Kidney Dis* 47:8-14, 2006.

Grossfeld GD, Litwin MS, Wolf JS, et al: Evaluation of asymptomatic microscopic haematuria in adults: The American Urological Association best practice policy. Part 1: Definition, detection, prevalence and etiology, *Urology* 57:599-603, 2001.

Grossfeld GD, Litwin MS, Wolf JS, et al: Evaluation of asymptomatic microscopic haematuria in adults: The American Urological Association best practice policy. Part 2: Patient evaluation, cytology, voided markers, imaging, cystoscopy, nephrology evaluation and follow-up, *Urology* 57:604-610, 2001.

Hogg RJ, Furth S, Lemley KV: National Kidney Foundation's Kidney Disease Outcomes Quality Initiative Clinical Practice Guidelines for Chronic Kidney Disease in children and adolescents: evaluation, classification and stratification, *Pediatrics* 111:1416-1421, 2003.

National Kidney Foundation: Clinical Practice Guidelines for Chronic Kidney Disease: Evaluation Classification and Stratification. Part 4: Definition and classification of stages of chronic kidney disease, *Am J Kidney Dis* 39(Suppl 1):46-75, 2002.

Kidney Imaging 6

Hina Arif-Tiwari | Bobby Kalb | Richard C. Semelka | Diego R. Martin

There has been an impressive evolution and development of diagnostic imaging methods in recent years, expanding the array of techniques that can be used to understand and diagnose kidney disease. Imaging modalities range from conventional fluoroscopic studies to nuclear medicine techniques to cross-sectional methods based on ultrasound, computed tomography (CT), or magnetic resonance imaging (MRI). Optimal patient care depends on an understanding of potential imaging applications and the benefits and risks related to these diagnostic imaging techniques. This is a task made more challenging because of continuing and rapid changes in the technology.

IMAGING MODALITIES

ABDOMINAL RADIOGRAPHY AND INTRAVENOUS UROGRAPHY

Plain radiography and intravenous urography (IVP) had been the preliminary tools for evaluation of kidney disease; however, these conventional methods provide limited sensitivity and specificity for most important urological pathologies. Cross-sectional techniques have now superseded plain radiography and IVP to diagnose focal or diffuse renal parenchymal pathologies and nephrolithiasis.

ULTRASONOGRAPHY

Ultrasonography (US) is a nonionizing technique that produces images in real time. It is a powerful initial kidney imaging modality that is safe, noninvasive, portable, and widely available with a lower initial test cost compared to CT or MRI. Additionally, US can be performed in patients with kidney failure as iodinated contrast is not required, and it can readily differentiate between obstructive (surgical) and nonobstructive (medical) causes of kidney failure. However, image quality and detail are limited by a patient's body habitus and the operator's skills.

US is valuable in kidney imaging as it can provide information about kidney size, cortical thickness, and echogenicity (Fig. 6.1). It can easily distinguish between solid and cystic renal masses; however, characterization and differentiation between complex renal cysts and cystic renal tumors is limited by its soft-tissue resolution. Generally, focal lesions identified on US require further imaging evaluation with CT or MRI. US is useful in detecting the presence or absence of hydronephrosis. Sensitivity for renal calculi is generally restricted to calculi greater than 3 to 5 mm located within the renal pelvis, with relative insensitivity to ureteric calculi. Gray scale ultrasound can be combined with color Doppler duplex imaging to assess patency and flow in renal vasculature, particularly in the transplant kidney.

COMPUTED TOMOGRAPHY

In the United States, CT is commonly used for imaging the kidneys. CT provides good spatial resolution, with detailed anatomy of the renal parenchyma, vasculature, and the excretory system. In contrast to the other imaging techniques, CT provides the highest sensitivity for detecting fine calcifications within the kidney parenchyma and throughout the collecting system, making unenhanced CT the optimal test for detecting stone disease.

Contrast-enhanced multiphase CT has been used to evaluate kidney masses. Although CT provides high spatial resolution, a relative limitation is soft-tissue contrast. This necessitates more complex diagnostic algorithms for assessing complex cystic kidney lesions that entail measurement of density units before and after contrast administration. Multiphase CT increases the radiation dose to the patient proportionate to the number of phases used. CT for urologic indications represents the source of greatest diagnostic radiation exposures in our population; three to four CT exams, or phases within one exam, will approximate the radiation exposure determined to cause increased cancer risk in atomic bomb survivors. Contrast allergies are relatively common, and contrast-induced nephropathy (CIN) is a well characterized risk of iodinated CT contrast. Patients with even moderately impaired kidney function are at risk for CIN, with other risk factors including advanced age, diabetes, hypertension, heart failure, and volume depletion.

Dual-energy computed tomography (DECT) is a recent advancement in CT hardware that provides information about how substances behave at different energies. The ability to generate virtual unenhanced datasets and improved detection of iodine-containing substances on low-energy images are promising grounds for continued research and development in DECT, targeting the achievement of radiation dose reductions. Potential applications of DECT include distinguishing hyperdense kidney cysts from renal cell carcinoma, identifying renal calculi within contrast-filled renal collecting systems, and characterizing the composition of renal calculi, including the differentiation of uric acid stones from nonuric acid stones. Iterative reconstruction image postprocessing is another recent application in CT that may also lead to significant radiation dose reduction.

RENAL SCINTIGRAPHY

Radionuclide studies of the kidney have been used to provide imaging-based qualitative assessment of kidney function. However, these techniques suffer from low spatial

51

resolution and do not provide detailed analysis of both structure and function. The test is based on time resolved imaging of the kidney after intravenous administration of a radiopharmaceutical that is either filtered (Technetium-diethylene triamine pentacetic acid, Tc-DTPA) or secreted by the tubule (Technetium-mercapto acetyl triglycine, Tc-MAG3). The use of radioactive tracers, particularly in monitoring applications where the study will be repeated, raises the concern of radiation risk, which is increased in younger patients.

MAGNETIC RESONANCE IMAGING

MRI is evolving as a robust imaging technique for comprehensive evaluation of the kidneys and the collecting system (Fig. 6.2). Excellent intrinsic tissue contrast and high spatial resolution of MRI results in more sensitive detection and specific characterization of focal and diffuse kidney pathologies, including complex cystic lesions considered problematic on CT or US. Because there is no ionizing radiation, MRI is an ideal imaging technique for assessment of kidney masses, particularly in younger

patients or in patients requiring serial studies. In patients with impaired kidney function, gadolinium-chelate–based contrast agents (GBCA) have been associated with nephrogenic systemic fibrosis (NSF), which will be discussed separately.

Advantages of MRI include multiplanar imaging, multiphase contrast-enhanced imaging, and acquisition of multiple types of soft-tissue contrast using an array of sequences. This ensures optimal soft-tissue contrast for detection and characterization of disease. This array of image contrast may be obtained using the most up-to-date, fast imaging techniques that allow for a total scan time of less than 20 minutes, yet without any concern for radiation dose accumulation as with CT.

Multiple sequences that yield specific tissue information can be used. Fluid-sensitive T2W images (half-Fourier acquisition single-shot echo train, HASTE) and T2-like sequences (true free induction with steady-state free precision, TFISP) are helpful in evaluating the collecting system by virtue of the intrinsic high-signal intensity of urine. Precontrast and dynamic postcontrast T1W three-dimensional (3D) gradient echo fat suppressed images in arterial, capillary, venous,

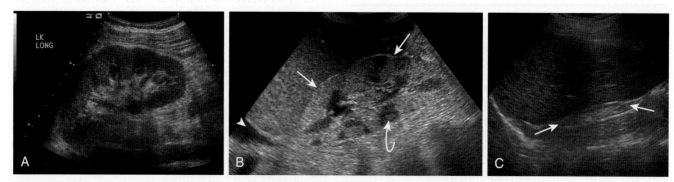

Figure 6.1   Sonographic imaging of normal and abnormal kidneys. Longitudinal axis sonographic images in: **A,** Normal patient: right kidney demonstrates normal corticomedullary differentiation (CMD). **B,** Acute renal parenchymal disease: increased renal cortical echogenicity resulting in accentuated CMD *(arrows)* in a patient with pyelonephritis. Note additional focal regions of decreased cortical echogenicity that likely represent small, evolving abscesses *(curved arrow).* Also note the small right pleural effusion *(arrowhead).* **C,** Chronic kidney disease: marked parenchymal atrophy and scarring with loss of normal CMD *(arrows).*

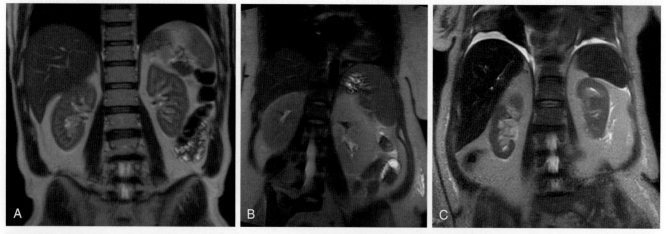

Figure 6.2   Magnetic resonance imaging of normal and abnormal kidneys. Coronal T2-weighted MRI in: **A,** Normal patient: corticomedullary differentiation on T2W imaging; the renal medulla, by virtue of increased water content, appears brighter than the renal cortex. **B,** Acute renal parenchymal disease: enlarged kidneys with diffuse parenchymal edema demonstrating abnormal elevated T2 signal and resultant loss of CMD in a patient with acute kidney injury. **C,** Chronic kidney disease: diffuse parenchymal atrophy and loss of normal CMD.

and delayed phases demonstrate improved spatial resolution vital for resolving masses and vascular anatomy. Arterial phase can also be optimized for evaluation of renal artery anatomy.

Functional data analysis with magnetic resonance nephrourography (MRNU) allows for evaluation of renal physiology in a manner that was not previously possible. Both structural and functional data can be extracted in a single examination, with measurements of renal blood flow (RBF) and glomerular filtration rate (GFR).

STRUCTURAL IMAGING

T2W and steady-state magnetization (TFISP) imaging offer excellent structural evaluation of the kidneys and can display collecting system morphology, even in a nondistended system, by virtue of the bright signal of native urine. Focal lesions, filling defects, and obstructive causes of urinary tract dilation can be identified even in the absence of contrast excretion.

FUNCTIONAL IMAGING

Like inulin, gadolinium chelates are freely filtered at the glomerulus and are neither secreted nor absorbed by the renal tubules. Therefore, the rate of gadolinium uptake in the kidney is related to the renal blood flow. Accelerated 3D volumetric T1W gradient echo sequence facilitates imaging of the gadolinium contrast as it arrives through the feeding renal artery and perfuses the renal parenchyma. Rapid increase in concentration of gadolinium is seen as it enters the renal parenchyma equivalent to the blood perfusion through the kidney. Although a portion of the perfused contrast leaves the kidney through the renal vein, another portion remains in the kidney as a result of glomerular filtration. Assessments of renal parenchymal volume, and calculations of renal perfusion in terms of RBF and GFR, are made by semiautomated methods based on mathematical modeling.

MRNU can identify the cause of obstruction in the renal collecting system, including congenital anomalies such as ureteropelvic junction obstruction (Fig. 6.3), and acquired conditions such as stone disease, transitional cell carcinoma of the upper and lower tract, and extrinsic compression from retroperitoneal fibrosis, to name a few. Preoperative assessment of kidney function using MRNU in cases of renal cell carcinoma may direct surgical planning toward a potential nephron-sparing procedure. Comprehensive imaging can be obtained for kidney transplant donor and recipient evaluation, discussed later in this chapter.

RISKS AND BENEFITS OF IMAGING CONTRAST IN KIDNEY DISEASE

In patients with reduced kidney function, including those on dialysis, the choice of contrast-enhanced CT or MR should be based on the expected diagnostic benefits.

NSF is a systemic fibrotic disorder that occurs in patients with advanced CKD or severe acute kidney injury who were exposed to one or more doses of certain GBCAs. Delayed excretion and prolonged tissue exposure to circulating free GBCA is likely a key factor in the relationship between reduced GFR and NSF. The largest subset of cases has occurred in dialysis-dependent patients (on either hemo dialysis or peritoneal dialysis) who had a delay between contrast exposure and dialysis. On average, the affected NSF patients have been exposed to multiple GBCA doses or a large single dose, and the majority of documented cases have been associated with gadobenate dimeglumine (Gadodiamide). Available data from both clinical reports and animal studies support the conclusion that different GBCA formulations have different relative risks of NSF, with the risk associated with the relative agent chemical stability. Recommended guidelines to minimize the risk of NSF include use of macrocyclic GBCAs, because of their relatively stable structure, or stable linear GBCAs with higher relaxivity. Relaxivity is a measure of signal generated by the GBCA, with the higher relaxivity of an agent resulting in a lower required dose. Regardless of the GBCA used, the objective is to administer the minimum dose necessary to achieve a diagnostic MRI. Hemodialysis is effective at lowering the serum concentrations of GBCAs, and hemodialysis should be performed within 24 hours after GBCA administration. Dialysis is advocated only in patients who are on dialysis before the MRI as the mortality and morbidity risk of hemodialysis is much greater than the risk of developing NSF following the exposure to stable GBCAs. Precautions to reduce NSF risk include selection of more stable GBCA, use of lowest possible dose, and postprocedure dialysis for patients who are dialysis-dependent. Following the institution of these precautions and more judicious use of GBCA in patients with kidney disease, no new cases of NSF have been described in the United States since 2010, and the risk of NSF with more stable GBCAs appears low. Centers have more recently reported that NSF incidence has diminished after observing these precautions, while continuing to employ MRI with selected GBCA enhancement even in patients who are on dialysis when warranted.

Contrast-induced nephropathy (CIN) is defined as an acute decrease in kidney function after exposure to iodinated contrast agents (ICAs) in the absence of another explanation. This is the third most common cause of hospital-acquired acute kidney injury. Multiple risk factors are associated with CIN, including reduced GFR, volume depletion, diabetes, congestive cardiac failure, advanced age, and type and dose of ICA. Evidence suggests that ICA osmolarity and viscosity may relate to CIN risk. For patients on dialysis, preservation of residual kidney function is associated with improved outcomes, and ICAs may jeopardize residual kidney function in these patients.

The selection of contrast, specifically GBCAs versus ICAs versus no contrast, should be individualized based on a careful risk–benefit assessment. Consideration of alternative studies, including nonenhanced exam protocols, should always be assessed. Generally, there are more unenhanced options available for the evaluation of soft tissues and blood vessels using MRI than CT. If a contrast-enhanced CT or MRI is warranted, the most diagnostic test with impact on management should represent a predominant factor to minimize the risk of delayed or missed diagnosis, or the need for study repetition.

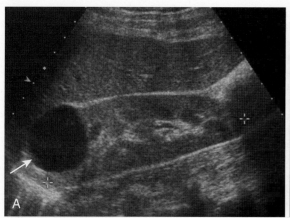
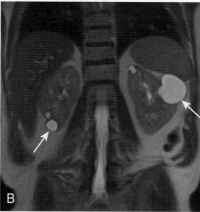

Figure 6.4   **Simple renal cortical cysts.** Longitudinal US **(A)** shows a simple, uncomplicated, exophytic cyst arising from the superior pole, consistent with Bosniak Category I cyst *(arrow)*. Coronal ssT2W image **(B)** in another patient depicting multiple simple cortical renal cysts, showing simple internal fluid, no septations, and a thin wall *(arrows)*.

CYSTIC RENAL LESIONS

RENAL CYSTS

Renal cysts represent the most common focal kidney lesion in adults. Cysts in the kidney have been classified and characterized by Bosniak into four categories: *Category I:* Simple benign cysts with negligible likelihood of malignancy; *Category II:* Benign cystic lesions that are minimally complicated; *Category IIF* (*F* for follow-up): Cysts less complex than category III and likely to be benign, which given their complexity require follow-up studies to prove their nature; *Category III:* More complicated cystic lesions that require follow-up imaging and/or surgical excision; *Category IV:* Masses that are clearly malignant cystic carcinomas.

IMAGING FEATURES

Ultrasonography is the preferred method to differentiate cystic from solid lesions because of its ease of performance and lower cost. It is also accurate in differentiating simple renal cysts (Fig. 6.4) from complex cystic renal masses. Although CT is widely used for characterization of cystic renal masses, it should be noted that kidney lesions are best evaluated with triple-phase multidetector row CT (that is, unenhanced, arterial phase, and nephrographic phase) with increasing radiation risk. Enhancing thick septations, solid components, or change in attenuation between 10 and 15 Hounsfield units (HU) after intravenous administration of contrast material are considered suspicious. Cystic angiomyolipomas, oncocytomas, and infections may also show enhancement, whereas hypovascular papillary cancers may demonstrate less enhancement. MR imaging with better soft-tissue contrast resolution is 100% sensitive and 95% specific for distinguishing benign and malignant renal cysts. Precontrast T1W images can easily identify intracyst hemorrhage in Bosniak Category IIF, which is challenging on CT. Signal intensity changes in dynamic postcontrast 3D T1-weighted gradient echo sequences (GRE) can delineate septae, solid elements, and nodules within a fluid-filled cyst or its wall. T2-weighted sequences also complement the 3D T1W GRE sequences for accurate characterization of renal cysts (see Fig. 6.4).

AUTOSOMAL DOMINANT POLYCYSTIC KIDNEY DISEASE

Autosomal dominant polycystic kidney disease (ADPKD) is the most common hereditary renal cystic disease, and the third most common cause of end-stage renal disease. Imaging features of ADPKD may differ according to the severity of the disease. An inverse linear correlation exists between kidney volume and GFR.

IMAGING FEATURES

As ADPKD progresses, both kidneys enlarge massively with architectural distortion and display numerous cysts of varying sizes (Fig. 6.5). Cysts can be seen on US, although because of the large size of the kidneys, the utility of US is severely limited in reproducibility in follow-up examinations. Unenhanced CT can evaluate cyst hemorrhage and calcifications. Extrarenal cysts in the liver and pancreas can be identified by either CT or MRI. The Consortium for Radiologic Imaging Studies of Polycystic Kidney Disease (CRISP) favors MRI-based correlation of kidney and cyst volume measurements that can be used as indicators of disease progression or treatment response. Accurate RBF estimations can be obtained on MR imaging when disease progression parallels the increase in kidney volume and declining GFR. Although there is no increased risk of renal cell carcinoma (RCC) in ADPKD, MRI remains the preferred method of assessing a solid mass amid multiple cysts.

ACQUIRED CYSTIC DISEASE OF DIALYSIS

Acquired cystic disease of dialysis occurs in maintenance dialysis patients. Over time, the atrophic kidneys develop multiple small cortical, typically exophytic, cysts. These cysts are at increased risk of hemorrhage and development of RCC.

IMAGING FEATURES

The kidneys appear small and echogenic on US and may demonstrate multiple cysts. US may also be used to screen for potential complications of intracyst hemorrhage and evolution of RCC in asymptomatic patients. Unenhanced CT can detect cyst hemorrhage and renal or ureteric stones. Multiphase pre- and postcontrast-enhanced CT is required for comprehensive evaluation of cystic kidneys and for the evaluation of possible RCC. MR is well suited for evaluating cystic disease of dialysis (Fig. 6.6). Differentiation between nonenhancing hemorrhagic cysts (bright on precontrast T1W images) and vascularized renal cell cancer can safely and easily be achieved after administration of a stable and/or high-relaxivity GBCA.

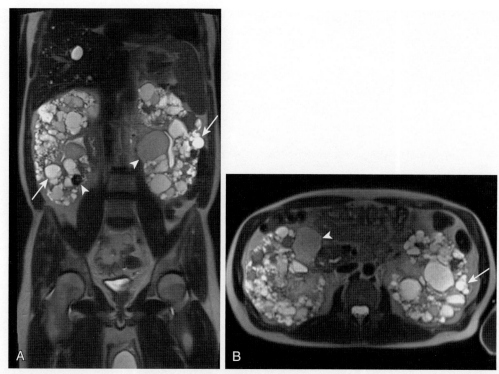

Figure 6.5 Autosomal dominant polycystic kidney disease (ADPKD). Coronal **(A)** and axial **(B)** ssT2W images. The kidneys are markedly enlarged with numerous cysts. The majority of cysts demonstrate increased T2 signal consistent with simple internal fluid *(arrows)*, but a sizable fraction have varying signal suggestive of blood products of differing age *(arrowheads)*. Note the presence of cystic disease in the liver **(A)**, although to a lesser extent.

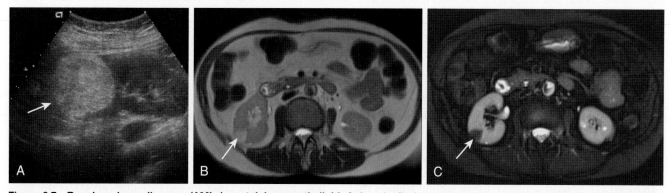

Figure 6.7 Renal angiomyolipomas (AMLs) containing mostly lipid. A, Longitudinal sonogram shows a well marginated, echogenic renal mass *(arrow)*; fatty tissue demonstrates increased echogenicity with sonographic imaging. **B,** Axial ssT2W image without fat suppression in a different patient shows a small subcapsular lesion in the right kidney *(arrow)*. This lesion loses signal on **C,** which shows the axial, fat suppressed ssT2W image *(arrow)*, in keeping with another lipid containing AML.

SOLID KIDNEY MASSES

ANGIOMYOLIPOMA

Angiomyolipoma (AML) is a benign renal tumor composed of variable amounts of smooth muscle, blood vessels, and mature adipocytes. Diagnosis is usually based on detection of fat. Eighty percent of angiomyolipomas are isolated and sporadic, whereas 20% occur in patients with tuberous sclerosis and are often bilateral and multiple. Larger AMLs present the risk of hemorrhage.

IMAGING FEATURES

On US, AML appears as solid echogenic mass with echogenicity comparable to the renal sinuses. CT can identify AML based on an attenuation value of −10 or less, predicting the presence of fat. Being vascular lesions, AML may enhance and must be differentiated from RCC by the presence and distribution of fat. This can be depicted on ssT2W sequences and pre- and postcontrast fat-saturated T1W GRE MR images, where areas of signal drop-out represent focal macroscopic fat in the lesion confirming the diagnosis of AML (Fig. 6.7).

RENAL CELL CARCINOMA

Improved imaging of kidney masses by US, CT, and MRI has led to smaller average size of neoplasm at time of initial detection. Currently, approximately 30% of all RCCs are incidentally identified on imaging studies performed for other reasons.

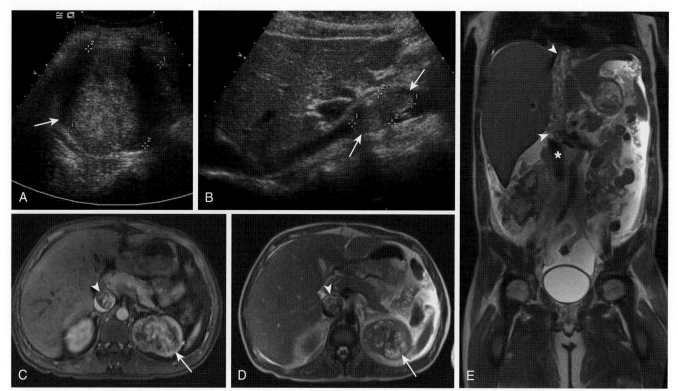

Figure 6.8   Renal cell carcinoma with inferior vena cava (IVC) invasion. Longitudinal sonogram of left kidney **(A)** shows an exophytic, heterogeneous solid renal mass *(arrow)*. Sagittal US image **(B)** demonstrates tumor thrombus in the IVC *(arrows)*. Early phase T1W fat suppressed gadolinium-enhanced GRE image **(C)** in a different patient shows a heterogeneously enhancing left renal cell cancer *(arrow)*. Enhancing tumor thrombus is also seen in the IVC *(arrowhead)*. The left renal tumor and IVC thrombus are also demonstrated on axial **(D)** and coronal **(E)** ssT2W images, a noncontrast and motion-insensitive technique. High-signal tumor thrombus is seen extending into the IVC to the level of the diaphragm, with loss of the dark flow void *(asterisk)* that is normally seen in patent vessels on single-shot MR images.

IMAGING FEATURES

US can delineate kidney masses larger than 25 mm. Sensitivity of US decreases to about 25% for smaller lesions. US is limited in differentiating between benign and malignant solid kidney masses. Extension into the renal vein and inferior vena cava can be evaluated on duplex Doppler (Fig. 6.8). CT can characterize kidney masses larger than 10 mm, and the nephrographic phase of dynamic contrast-enhanced CT is most sensitive for detecting tumors that appear as heterogeneous enhancing solid mass with or without cystic/necrotic changes. Vascular extension and potential metastases can be assessed for treatment planning. The superior soft-tissue detail and multiphase and multiplanar capabilities of MRI aid in sensitive detection and staging of RCC (see Fig. 6.8), although multiphase CT exposes patients to higher radiation risk. Pre- and post-contrast T1W 3D-GRE images can distinguish cystic and hypovascular RCC from other benign kidney lesions, even when less than 2 cm. Subtraction imaging may further increase sensitivity in hemorrhagic or proteinaceous cystic masses.

NEPHROLITHIASIS AND OBSTRUCTIVE UROPATHY

Acute flank pain is a frequent clinical presentation in the emergency department (ED). Nearly 22% of all CT examinations performed for the evaluation of acute abdominal pain in the ED are for clinical suspicion of urolithiasis.

IMAGING FEATURES

Plain radiograph KUB (kidney, ureter, and bladder) and IVP are no longer the preferred method of diagnosis of kidney stone disease. US is a rapid, safe, and readily available tool for evaluation of renal colic. Although US has limited sensitivity for small kidney stones and ureteric stones, obstructive hydronephrosis can easily be detected (Fig. 6.9). US is useful in young patients, pregnant women, and those requiring multiple follow-up examinations. Unenhanced CT is the most sensitive (95% to 98%) and specific (96% to 98%) test for urolithiasis (see Fig. 6.9). Identification of the number, size, and location of calculi, and the presence of hydronephrosis, can be routinely made. The role of MRI is still evolving in the evaluation of acute abdominal pain in the emergency setting. Calcium fails to generate MR signal thereby limiting the sensitivity of MRI to detect kidney stones; however, MRI can detect perirenal fluid as an indicator of acute renal obstruction, as well as other abdominal pathologies.

KIDNEY INFECTION

Pyelonephritis and kidney abscess usually result from an ascending infection in the urinary tract. In uncomplicated cases, routine radiologic imaging is not usually required for diagnosis or treatment.

IMAGING FEATURES FOR ACUTE PYELONEPHRITIS

US is not sensitive for diagnosis of acute pyelonephritis, although changes in echogenicity due to edema (hypoechoic),

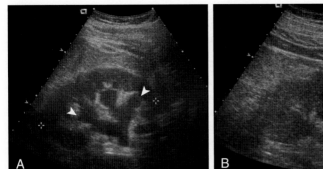
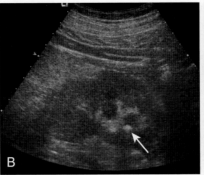
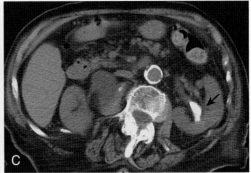

Figure 6.9 Nephrolithiasis and hydronephrosis. Longitudinal US image **(A)** shows moderate distension of the renal collecting system, representing hydronephrosis *(arrowheads)*. A nonobstructing hyperechoic stone is present in a lower pole calyx **(B,** *arrow)*. Unenhanced axial CT in a different patient demonstrates a hyperdense calculus **(C,** *black arrow)* in the left kidney.

hemorrhage (hyperechoic), and hypoperfusion (visible with duplex Doppler) can sometimes be seen in the renal parenchyma with associated hydronephrosis (Fig. 6.10). Renal scintigraphy using radiolabeled white blood cells or gallium can be used to locate renal infection, because photopenic areas of focal or global reduced uptake are seen with tubular radiotracer agent (Tc DMSA). Infected kidneys show alternating bands of enhancement (striated nephrogram) and perinephric inflammatory changes in Gerota's fascia on contrast-enhanced CT or MRI (see Fig. 6.10).

IMAGING FEATURES FOR RENAL ABSCESS

Renal abscess on US appears as a hypoechoic mass with through transmission that lacks internal flow on duplex Doppler images, differentiating it from solid masses. A hypoattenuating area with peripheral enhancement is seen on contrast-enhanced CT. Extraparenchymal collections can be identified on either CT or MRI. Mixed signal on T1 and T2W MR images is seen with increased peripheral inflammatory edema. Postgadolinium T1W images show nonenhancing central core with marked perinephric enhancement (Fig. 6.11).

RENAL ARTERY STENOSIS

Renovascular hypertension (RVH) is a leading cause of potentially correctable secondary hypertension, and early diagnosis of renal artery stenosis (RAS) may alleviate the hypertension and arrest the loss of kidney function. Overall, renal vascular disease is responsible for 1% to 5% of cases of hypertension. At least two thirds of these cases are caused by atherosclerosis, whereas fibromuscular dysplasia accounts for most of the remaining cases. Although catheter angiography is the reference standard test for RAS, CT and MR angiography are noninvasive alternative tools that have comparable diagnostic performance using the latest generation technologies.

IMAGING FEATURES

Duplex Doppler is a moderately accurate, cost-effective, operator-dependent technique for initial evaluation of RAS. Peak systolic velocity greater than 100 to 200 cm/sec is considered indicative of RAS. ACE inhibitor scintigraphy may be used to demonstrate impaired kidney function in

patients with RVH; important information about kidney size, perfusion, and excretory capacity can be obtained from scintigraphic images and computer-generated time-activity curves. Two major agents have been employed: Technetium-DTPA, a filtered agent; or MAG-3, a tubular excreted agent. Using these techniques, renal artery stenosis can be diagnosed based on two criteria: (1) asymmetry of kidney size and function, and (2) specific captopril-induced changes in the renogram. However, overall sensitivity and specificity of scintigraphy for RAS-induced RVH has been questioned.

CT angiography (CTA) is an excellent examination for obtaining information about the arterial anatomy and for evaluation of stenosis. High spatial resolution CTA is now routinely combined with sophisticated image postprocessing software that can produce 3D volume renderings to provide images that are interpreted more easily. Advancement in MR technology now offers detailed evaluation of vascular anatomy. Additionally, MRI techniques have been developed to provide kidney functional assessment including measures of perfused renal parenchymal volume, blood flow, and GFR. Renal artery imaging has been routinely obtained using GBCA enhanced MR angiography. Newer methods using flow-sensitive balanced fast-field echo technique are providing alternatives to GBCA. For detection of greater than 50% narrowing of the renal artery, most studies have shown excellent correlation between conventional angiography and MR angiography (sensitivity >95% and specificity >90%). Earlier reports have indicated that limitations of MR angiography include overestimation of moderate stenosis, but the latest generation MR technologies are significantly improving the capacity to generate higher quality images reliably. Catheter angiography remains the reference standard, but this is an invasive test that requires direct administration of concentrated iodinated contrast into the kidneys, which has been associated with significant acute and long-term kidney dysfunction in at-risk patients.

INTERVENTION

Therapeutic procedures are fundamentally based on techniques including balloon angioplasty and stent placement. Unfortunately both short-term and long-term results have not been found to correlate with the degree of stenosis, whether unilateral or bilateral. The ability to predict good long-term response to renal angioplasty and stenting remains an active area of investigation.

RENAL PARENCHYMAL DISEASE AND KIDNEY TRANSPLANTATION

DIFFUSE RENAL PARENCHYMAL DISEASE

Diffuse renal parenchymal diseases are common medical conditions. A variety of disease processes may involve the parenchyma and be classified into the following broad categories: glomerular disease, acute and chronic tubulointerstitial disease, diabetic nephropathy and nephrosclerosis, other forms of microvascular disease, ischemic nephropathy caused by disease of the main renal arteries, obstructive nephropathy, and infectious kidney disease. Radiologic techniques have limited specificity in the diagnosis of various types of diffuse renal parenchymal disease, because imaging features are overlapping in these pathologies. Nevertheless, there remains a growing clinical need for accurate, reproducible, and noninvasive measures of kidney function.

IMAGING FEATURES

Obstructive and nonobstructive causes of kidney failure may be differentiated using US as the initial imaging test. Kidney size and parenchymal thickness are useful parameters to assess chronicity. Enlarged kidneys usually indicate an acute parenchymal process, but they can be seen with chronic infiltrative kidney disease, diabetic nephropathy, and HIV-associated nephropathy. Contracted, small kidneys suggest a chronic disease (see Figs. 6.1 and 6.2). Increased renal cortical echogenicity may be useful in suggesting the presence of renal parenchymal disease. Kidney failure poses restriction to the use of nephrotoxic iodinated contrast, and noncontrast CT fails to provide additional diagnostic information. Scintigraphic techniques have been the mainstay of kidney function measurements for assessment of GFR. These methods require timed blood sampling and have been shown to have decreased precision with diminished GFR, especially when lower than 30 mL/min. MRI with MRNU can confirm the findings of US in cases of diminished corticomedullary differentiation and can offer detailed anatomic information about the renal parenchymal and collecting system. It also provides quantitative measures of kidney function that may be applied to each kidney.

KIDNEY TRANSPLANTATION

Kidney transplantation has emerged as the treatment of choice for end-stage renal disease (ESRD) patients, on average providing improved quality of life and lower healthcare costs compared with dialysis. Given the importance of kidney transplantation and the limitation of available donor kidneys, detailed analysis of factors that affect transplant survival is critical (Fig. 6.12).

IMAGING FEATURES

Ultrasonography is the principal imaging test that can be used in the bedside examination of perioperative patients for assessment of complications including perinephric fluid collections, hematomas, and urinoma. In addition,

Doppler duplex US is used to evaluate renal vein thrombosis and to measure the renal artery resistive index (RI). An elevated RI (>0.80) in the main renal artery and its branches has been considered predictive of transplant failure. Ultrasound lacks ionizing radiation and may be used safely for follow-up longitudinal studies. US is also frequently used for image-guided biopsy of the transplant kidney.

Preoperative CT angiography of potential donors can depict variant arterial and venous anatomy, vascular disorders, and other unexpected abnormalities. Ionizing radiation remains a limitation in both the donor and recipient, and the added risk of CIN may preclude the use of iodinated contrast in CT imaging in some kidney transplant recipients. Noncontrast CT imaging is limited in its ability to evaluate pelvic soft tissues, the transplanted kidney and collecting system, and the renal vasculature.

Impaired transplant function on radionucleotide study is attributed to either obstruction of urine outflow or to other causes. No additional information can be obtained on nuclear medicine exams to delineate between the causes of kidney failure.

MAGNETIC RESONANCE NEPHROUROGRAPHY

Magnetic resonance imaging benefits from excellent soft-tissue details even in absence of gadolinium, and avoids radiation. It may be used for preoperative imaging evaluation for both potential kidney donors and recipients. Comprehensive pretransplant evaluation of the kidney donor can be performed, with assessment of renal parenchymal, arterial, venous, and ureteric anatomy, as well as measurement of differential kidney function.

In posttransplant recipient evaluation, comprehensive structural and functional analysis can be performed.

- *Anatomic imaging:* T2W HASTE sequences and T2W-like TFISP images offer morphologic details of the collecting system based on the bright signal of urine, allowing identification of causes of obstruction such as stenosis, extrinsic compression, or anastomotic fibrosis of transplant ureter.
- *Functional imaging:* Postoperative hematomas and proteinaceous debris or hemorrhage in the collecting system can be identified as high signal on precontrast T1W images. Gadolinium perfusion technique can be used to extract renal functional volume, RBF, and GFR. Dynamic postcontrast 3D GRE T1W images can assist in accurately delineating postoperative complications and causes of transplant failure.

This modality can be useful in the evaluation of a number of posttransplant conditions, including:

1. *Vascular disorders:*
   a. Renal artery thrombosis or stenosis: Narrowing or abrupt cut-off in the main renal artery or its branch is seen in the angiographic phase. Segmental lack of perfusion in renal artery territory can be depicted by functional imaging.
   b. Renal vein thrombosis: T2W images demonstrate thrombus as loss of patent dark vascular lumen.

2. *Intrinsic kidney disorders:*
   a. Acute tubular necrosis (ATN): Normal cortical enhancement with markedly delayed medullary perfusion and excretion is shown, similar to the scintigraphic appearance of ATN.

b. Hyperacute and accelerated acute rejection: Intrinsic graft dysfunction with ischemic microvascular injury manifests as striated nephrogram.

c. Acute rejection: Blood oxygen level dependent (BOLD) MRI can detect changes in hemoglobin oxygenation, and thus assesses kidney tissue oxygenation. It can help differentiate ATN from acute rejection.

d. Chronic rejection: Loss of renal corticomedullary differentiation on T2 and T1W images is seen. This is a nonspecific finding that depicts impaired kidney function.

SUMMARY

Medical imaging plays a critical role in the diagnosis and management of kidney disease, and this role is continuing to evolve with new advances in diagnostic techniques. US provides a valuable first-line tool for the evaluation of most localized renal pathologies, including the detection of solid masses, characterization of cystic masses, detection of hydronephrosis, and diagnosis of renal calculi. CT provides the greatest sensitivity for calcifications within the kidney or urinary tract, including renal calculi. CT has been used to detect and characterize kidney masses, but cystic lesions require more challenging multiphase contrast-enhanced methodology combined with quantitative density measurements. MRI has developed technically, and currently provides an alternative to ultrasound and CT for better detection and characterization of solid and cystic masses. In addition, MRI techniques are developing to provide qualitative and quantitative assessment of diffuse parenchymal disease and measures of kidney function, including RBF, parenchymal perfusion, and glomerular filtration. Both CT and MRI use contrast agents with potential toxic effects in the setting of impaired kidney function, although these risks can be managed. An understanding of iodinated and gadolinium-chelate–based contrast agents is imperative. Overall, excessive use of CT is increasingly raised as a safety concern because of radiation exposure risks. US and MRI provide alternatives with high levels of safety.

KEY BIBLIOGRAPHY

Craig W, Wagner B, Travis M: Pyelonephritis: Radiologic-Pathologic Review, *RadioGraphics* 28:255-276, 2008.

Escobar GA, Campbell DN: Randomized trials in angioplasty and stenting of the renal artery: tabular review of the literature and critical analysis of their results, *Ann Vasc Surg* 26(3):434-442, 2012.

Hartman D, Choyke P, Hartman M: A practical approach to the cystic renal mass, *RadioGraphics* 24:S101-S115, 2004.

Heinz-Peer G, Schoder M, Rand T, et al: Prevalence of acquired cystic kidney disease and tumors in native kidneys of renal transplant recipients: a prospective us study, *Radiology* 195:667-671, 1995.

Kalb B, Sharma P, Salman K: Acute abdominal Pain – Is there a potential role for MRI in the setting of the Emergency Department in a patient with renal calculi? *J Magn Reson Imaging* 32(5):1012-1023, 2010.

Kalb B, Vatow J, Salman K, et al: Magnetic resonance nephrourography: current and developing techniques, *Radiol Clin North Am* 46:11-24, 2008.

Martin DR: Nephrogenic system fibrosis: A radiologist's practical perspective, *Eur J Radiol* 66:220-224, 2008.

Martin DR, Brown M, Semelka R: *Primer on MR imaging of the abdomen and pelvis*, ed 1, 2005, New York, John Wiley & Sons, pp 153-222.

Martin DR, Kalb B, Salman K, et al: Kidney transplantation: structural and functional evaluation using mr nephro-urography, *J Magn Reson Imaging* 28:805-822, 2008.

Martin DR, Krishnamoorthy S, Kalb B, et al: Decreased incidence of nsf in patients on dialysis after changing gadolinium contrast-enhanced mri protocols, *J Magn Reson Imaging* 31:440-446, 2010.

Martin DR, Semelka R, Chapman A, et al: Nephrogenic systemic fibrosis versus contrast-induced nephropathy: risks and benefits of contrast-enhanced mr and ct in renally impaired patients, *J Magn Reson Imaging* 30:1350-1356, 2009.

Martin DR, Sharma P, Salman K, et al: Individual kidney blood flow measured by contrast enhanced magnetic resonance first-pass perfusion imaging, *Radiology* 246:241-248, 2008.

Michaely H, Schoenberg S, Oesingmann N: Renal artery stenosis—functional assessment with dynamic mr perfusion measurements—feasibilty study, *Radiology* 238:586-596, 2006.

Mousa AY, Campbell JE, Stone PA, et al: Short- and long-term outcomes of percutaneous transluminal angioplasty/stenting of renal fibromuscular dysplasia over a ten-year period, *J Vasc Surg* 55:421-427, 2012.

Prando A, Prando D, Prando P: Renal Cell Carcinoma: Unusual Imaging Manifestations, *RadioGraphics* 26:233-244, 2006.

Radermacher J, Mengel M, Ellis S, et al: The renal arterial resistance index and renal allograft survival, *N Engl J Med* 349:115-124, 2003.

Semelka RC, Shoenut JP, Magro CM, et al: Renal cancer staging: comparison of contrast-enhanced ct and gadolinium-enhanced fat-suppressed spin-echo and gradient-echo mr imaging, *J Magn Reson Imaging* 3:597-602, 1993.

Silva A, Morse B, Hara Robert B, et al: Dual-energy (spectral) ct: applications in abdominal imaging, *RadioGraphics* 31:1031-1046, 2011.

Soulez G, Pasowicz M, Benea G, et al: Renal artery stenosis evaluation: diagnostic performance of gadobenate dimeglumine–enhanced mr angiography—comparison with DSA, *Radiology* 273-285, 2008.

Williams G, Macaskill P, Chan SF, et al: Comparative accuracy of renal duplex sonographic parameters in the diagnosis of renal artery stenosis: paired and unpaired analysis, *AJR* 188:798-811, 2007.

Full bibliography can be found on www.expertconsult.com.

ACID-BASE, FLUID, AND ELECTROLYTE DISORDERS

7 Hyponatremia and Hypoosmolar Disorders

Joseph G. Verbalis

The incidence of hyponatremia depends on the patient population screened and the criteria used to define the disorder. Hospital incidences of 15% to 22% are common if hyponatremia is defined as any serum sodium concentration ($[Na^+]$) of less than 135 mEq/L, but in most studies only 1% to 4% of patients have a serum $[Na^+]$ lower than 130 mEq/L, and fewer than 1% have a value lower than 120 mEq/L. Recent studies have confirmed prevalences from 7% in ambulatory populations up to 38% in acutely hospitalized patients. The elderly are particularly susceptible to hyponatremia, with reported incidences as high as 53% among institutionalized geriatric patients. Although most cases are mild, hyponatremia is important clinically because (1) acute severe hyponatremia can cause substantial morbidity and mortality; (2) mild hyponatremia can progress to more dangerous levels during management of other disorders; (3) general mortality is higher in hyponatremic patients across a wide range of underlying diseases; and (4) overly rapid correction of chronic hyponatremia can produce severe neurologic complications and death.

DEFINITIONS

Hyponatremia is of clinical significance only when it reflects corresponding plasma hypoosmolality. Plasma osmolality (P_{osm}) can be measured directly by osmometry, and is expressed as milliosmoles per kilogram of water (mOsm/kg H_2O). P_{osm} can also be calculated from the serum $[Na^+]$, measured in milliequivalents per liter (mEq/L), and the glucose and blood urea nitrogen (BUN) levels, both expressed as milligrams per deciliter (mg/dl) as follows:

$$P_{osm} = (2 \times \text{Serum } [Na^+]) + \text{Glucose}/18 + \text{BUN}/2.8$$

Because the glucose term and the BUN terms are normally dwarfed by the sodium term, osmolality can be estimated simply by doubling the serum $[Na^+]$. All three methods produce comparable results under most conditions. However, total osmolality is not always equivalent to *effective osmolality*, which is sometimes referred to as the *tonicity* of the plasma. Solutes that are predominantly compartmentalized in the extracellular fluid (ECF) are effective solutes because they create osmotic gradients across cell membranes and lead to osmotic movement of water from the intracellular fluid (ICF) to ECF compartments. In contrast, solutes that freely permeate cell membranes (e.g., urea, ethanol, methanol) are not effective solutes, because they do not create osmotic gradients across cell membranes, and therefore they are not associated with secondary water shifts. Only the concentration of effective solutes in plasma should be used to determine whether clinically significant hypoosmolality is present. In most cases, these effective solutes include sodium, its associated anions, and glucose (but only in the presence of insulin deficiency, which allows the development of an ECF/ICF glucose gradient); importantly, they do not include urea, a solute that freely penetrates cells.

Hyponatremia and hypoosmolality are usually synonymous, but with two important exceptions. First, *pseudohyponatremia* can be produced by marked elevation of serum lipids or proteins. In such cases, the concentration of Na^+ per liter of serum water is unchanged, but the concentration of Na^+ per liter of serum is artifactually decreased because of the increased relative proportion occupied by lipid or protein. Although measurement of serum or plasma $[Na^+]$ by ion-specific electrodes, currently used by most clinical laboratories, is less influenced by high concentrations of lipids or proteins than is measurement of serum $[Na^+]$ by flame photometry, such errors nonetheless still occur. However, because direct measurement of P_{osm} is based on the colligative properties of only the solute particles in solution, increased lipids or proteins will not affect the measured P_{osm}. Second, high concentrations of effective solutes other than Na^+ can cause relative decreases in serum $[Na^+]$ despite an unchanged P_{osm}; this commonly occurs with hyperglycemia. Misdiagnosis can be avoided again by direct measurement of P_{osm} or by correcting the serum $[Na^+]$ by 1.6 mEq/L for each 100 mg/dl increase in blood glucose concentration greater than 100 mg/dl (although recent studies have suggested that 2.4 mEq/L may be a more accurate correction factor, especially when the glucose is very high).

PATHOGENESIS

The presence of significant hypoosmolality indicates excess water relative to solute in the ECF. Because water moves freely between the ICF and ECF, this also indicates an excess of total body water relative to total body solute. Imbalances between water and solute can be generated initially either by *depletion* of body solute more than body water or by *dilution* of body solute because of increases in body water more than body solute (Box 7.1). However, this distinction represents an oversimplification, as most hypoosmolar states include variable contributions of both solute depletion and water retention. For example, isotonic solute losses occurring during an acute hemorrhage do not produce hypoosmolality until the subsequent retention of water from ingested or infused hypotonic fluids causes a secondary dilution of the remaining ECF solute. Nonetheless, this concept has proved useful because it provides a framework for understanding the diagnosis and treatment of hypoosmolar disorders.

Box 7.1 Pathogenesis of Hypoosmolar Disorders

Depletion (Primary Decreases in Total Body Solute + Secondary Water Retention)[*]

Renal Solute Loss

Diuretic use
Solute diuresis (glucose, mannitol)
Salt-wasting nephropathy
Mineralocorticoid deficiency

Nonrenal Solute Loss

Gastrointestinal (diarrhea, vomiting, pancreatitis, bowel obstruction)
Cutaneous (sweating, burns)
Blood loss

Dilution (Primary Increases in Total Body Water ± Secondary Solute Depletion)[†]

Impaired Renal Free Water Excretion

Increased proximal reabsorption
    Hypothyroidism
Impaired distal dilution
    SIADH
    Glucocorticoid deficiency
Combined increased proximal reabsorption and impaired distal dilution
    Congestive heart failure
    Cirrhosis
    Nephrotic syndrome
Decreased urinary solute excretion
    Beer potomania

Excess Water Intake

Primary polydipsia
Dilute infant formula

Modified from Verbalis JG: The syndrome of inappropriate antidiuretic hormone secretion and other hypoosmolar disorders. In Schrier RW, editor: Diseases of the kidney, Philadelphia, 2007, Lippincott Williams & Wilkins, pp 2214-2248.

SIADH, Syndrome of inappropriate antidiuretic hormone secretion.

[*]Virtually all disorders of solute depletion are accompanied by some degree of secondary retention of water by the kidneys in response to the resulting intravascular hypovolemia; this mechanism can lead to hypoosmolality even when the solute depletion occurs via hypotonic or isotonic body fluid losses.

[†]Disorders of water retention primarily cause hypoosmolality in the absence of any solute losses, but in some cases of SIADH, secondary solute losses occur in response to the resulting intravascular hypervolemia and can further aggravate the hypoosmolality. (However, this pathophysiology probably does not contribute to the hyponatremia of edema-forming states such as congestive heart failure and cirrhosis, because in these cases, multiple factors favoring sodium retention result in an increased total body sodium load.)

DIFFERENTIAL DIAGNOSIS

The diagnostic approach to hypoosmolar disorders should include a careful history (especially concerning medications and diet); physical examination with emphasis on clinical assessment of ECF volume status and a thorough neurologic evaluation; measurement of serum or plasma electrolytes, glucose, BUN, creatinine, and uric acid; calculated and/or directly measured P_{osm}; and determination of simultaneous urine sodium and osmolality. Although prevalences vary according to the population being studied, a sequential analysis of hyponatremic patients who were admitted to a large university teaching hospital showed that approximately 20% were hypovolemic, 20% had edema-forming states, 33% were euvolemic, 15% had hyperglycemia-induced hyponatremia, and 10% had kidney failure. Consequently, euvolemic hyponatremia generally constitutes the largest single group of hyponatremic patients found in this setting. A definitive diagnosis is not always possible at the time of presentation, but an initial categorization based on the patient's clinical ECF volume status allows selection of an appropriate initial therapy in most cases (Fig. 7.1).

DECREASED EXTRACELLULAR FLUID VOLUME (HYPOVOLEMIA)

Clinically detectable hypovolemia, determined most sensitively by careful measurement of orthostatic changes in blood pressure and pulse rate, usually indicates some degree of solute depletion. Elevations of the BUN and uric acid concentrations are useful laboratory correlates of decreased ECF volume. Even isotonic or hypotonic volume losses can lead to hypoosmolality if water or hypotonic fluids are ingested or infused as replacement. A low urine sodium concentration (U_{Na}) in such cases suggests a nonrenal cause of solute depletion, whereas a high U_{Na} suggests renal causes of solute depletion (see Box 7.1). Diuretic use is the most common cause of hypovolemic hypoosmolality, and thiazides are more commonly associated with severe hyponatremia than are loop diuretics such as furosemide.

Although diuretics represent a prime example of solute depletion, the pathophysiologic mechanisms underlying diuretic-associated hypoosmolality are complex and have multiple components, including free water retention. Many patients do not manifest clinical evidence of marked hypovolemia, in part because ingested water has been retained in response to nonosmotically stimulated secretion of arginine vasopressin (AVP), as is generally true for all disorders of solute depletion. To complicate diagnosis further, the U_{Na} may be high or low depending on when the last diuretic dose was taken. Consequently, any suspicion of diuretic use mandates careful consideration of this diagnosis. A low serum $[K^+]$ is an important clue to diuretic use, as few other disorders that cause hyponatremia and hypoosmolality also produce appreciable hypokalemia. Whenever the possibility of diuretic use is suspected in the absence of a positive history, a urine screen for diuretics should be performed.

Most other causes of renal or nonrenal solute losses resulting in hypovolemic hypoosmolality will be clinically apparent, although some cases of salt-wasting nephropathies (e.g., chronic interstitial nephropathy, polycystic kidney disease, obstructive uropathy, Bartter syndrome) or mineralocorticoid deficiency (e.g., Addison's disease) can be challenging to diagnose during the early phases of the disease.

NORMAL EXTRACELLULAR FLUID VOLUME (EUVOLEMIA)

Virtually any disorder associated with hypoosmolality can manifest with an ECF volume status that appears normal

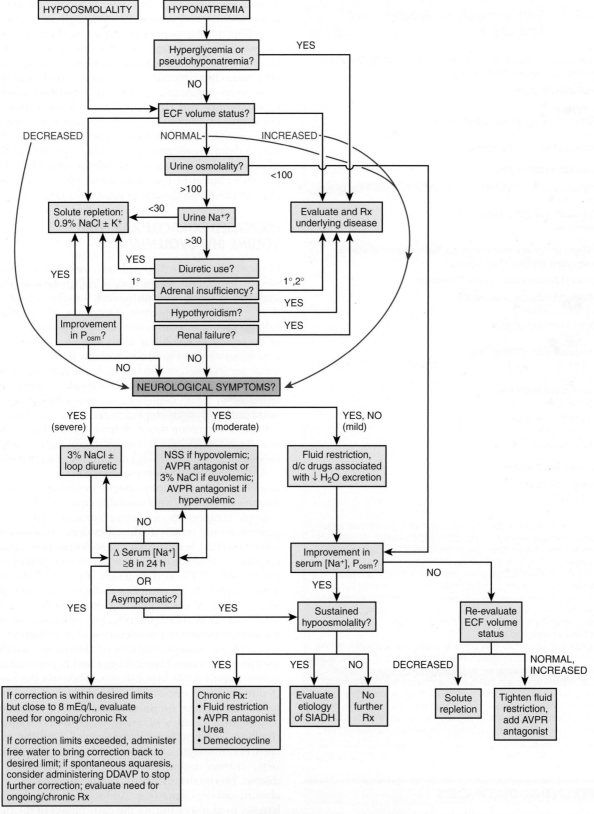

Figure 7.1   Algorithm for evaluation and treatment of hypoosmolar patients. The *red arrow* in the center emphasizes that the presence of central nervous system dysfunction resulting from hyponatremia should always be assessed immediately, so that appropriate therapy can be started as soon as possible in significantly symptomatic patients, even while the outlined diagnostic evaluation is proceeding. Values for osmolality are in mOsm/kg H_2O, and those referring to serum Na^+ concentration are in mEq/L. Δ, Change (in concentration); *1°*, Primary; *2°*, secondary; *AVPR*, arginine vasopressin receptor; *d/c*, discontinue; *DDAVP*, desmopressin; *ECF*, extracellular fluid volume; P_{osm}, plasma osmolality; *Rx*, treatment; *SIADH*, syndrome of inappropriate antidiuretic hormone secretion. (Modified from Verbalis JG: The syndrome of inappropriate antidiuretic hormone secretion and other hypoosmolar disorders. In Schrier RW, editor: *Diseases of the kidney,* Philadelphia, 2007, Lippincott Williams & Wilkins, pp 2214-2248.)

by standard methods of clinical evaluation. Because clinical assessment of ECF volume status is not very sensitive, normal or low levels of serum BUN and uric acid are helpful laboratory correlates of relatively normal ECF volume.

Conversely, a low U_{Na} suggests a depletional hypoosmolality secondary to ECF losses with subsequent volume replacement by water or other hypotonic fluids; as discussed earlier, such patients may appear euvolemic by all the usual clinical parameters used to assess ECF volume status. Primary dilutional disorders are less likely in the presence of a low U_{Na} (less than 30 mEq/L), although this pattern can occur in hypothyroidism as well.

A high U_{Na} ($\geq$30 mEq/L) generally indicates a dilutional hypoosmolality such as the *syndrome of inappropriate antidiuretic hormone secretion* (SIADH) (see Box 7.1). SIADH is the most common cause of euvolemic hypoosmolality in clinical medicine. The criteria necessary for a diagnosis of SIADH remain essentially unchanged since defined by Bartter and Schwartz in 1967 (Box 7.2), but several points deserve emphasis. First, true hypoosmolality must be present, and hyponatremia secondary to pseudohyponatremia or hyperglycemia must be excluded. Second, the urinary osmolality (U_{osm}) must be inappropriate for the low P_{osm}. This does not require that the U_{osm} be greater than P_{osm}, but merely that the urine not be maximally dilute (i.e., U_{osm} greater than 100 mOsm/kg H_2O in adults). U_{osm} need not be inappropriately elevated at all levels of P_{osm}, but simply at some level of P_{osm} less than 275 mOsm/kg H_2O. This is evident in patients with a reset osmostat who suppress AVP secretion at some level of P_{osm}, resulting in maximal urinary dilution and free water excretion at plasma osmolalities falling below this level. Although some consider a reset osmostat to be a separate disorder rather than a variant of SIADH, such cases nonetheless illustrate that some hypoosmolar patients can exhibit an appropriately dilute urine at some, although not all, plasma osmolalities. Third, clinical euvolemia must be present to diagnose SIADH, and this diagnosis cannot be made in a hypovolemic or significantly edematous patient. Importantly, this does not mean that patients with SIADH cannot become hypovolemic for other reasons, but in such cases it is impossible to diagnose the underlying SIADH until the patient is rendered euvolemic. The fourth criterion, renal salt wasting, has probably caused the most confusion regarding SIADH. The importance of this criterion lies in its usefulness in differentiating hypoosmolality caused by a decreased effective intravascular volume (in which case renal Na^+ conservation occurs) from dilutional disorders in which urinary Na^+ excretion is normal or increased because of ECF volume expansion. However, U_{Na} can also be high in renal causes of solute depletion, such as diuretic use or Addison's disease, and, conversely, patients with SIADH can have a low urinary Na^+ excretion if they subsequently become hypovolemic or solute depleted, conditions sometimes produced by imposed salt and water restriction. Consequently, although high urinary Na^+ excretion is generally the rule in patients with SIADH, its presence does not necessarily confirm this diagnosis, nor does its absence exclude it. The final criterion emphasizes that SIADH remains a diagnosis of exclusion, and the absence of other potential causes of hypoosmolality must always be verified. Glucocorticoid deficiency and SIADH can be especially difficult to distinguish, because either primary or secondary hypocortisolism can cause elevated plasma AVP levels and, in addition, can have direct renal effects to prevent maximal urinary dilution. Therefore, no patient with chronic hyponatremia should be diagnosed as having SIADH without a thorough evaluation of adrenal function, preferably via a rapid adrenocorticotropin (ACTH) stimulation test (acute hyponatremia of obvious origin, such as postoperative or in association with pneumonitis, may be treated without adrenal testing as long as there are no other clinical signs or symptoms suggestive of adrenal dysfunction). Many different disorders have been associated with SIADH, and these can be divided into several major etiologic groups (Box 7.3).

Some cases of euvolemic hyponatremia do not fit particularly well into either a dilutional or a depletional category. Chief among these is the hyponatremia that occurs in patients who ingest large volumes of beer with little food intake for prolonged periods, called *beer potomania*. Even though the volume of fluid ingested may not seem sufficiently excessive to overwhelm renal diluting mechanisms, in these cases free water excretion is limited by very low urinary solute excretion, resulting in water retention and dilutional hyponatremia. However, because such patients have very low sodium intakes as well, it is likely that relative depletion of body Na^+ stores also contributes to the hypoosmolality in some cases.

Box 7.2 Criteria for the Diagnosis of Syndrome of Inappropriate Antidiuretic Hormone Secretion

Essential Criteria

1. Decreased effective osmolality of the ECF (P_{osm} less than 275 mOsm/kg H_2O)
2. Inappropriate urinary concentration (U_{osm} greater than 100 mOsm/kg H_2O with normal kidney function) at some level of plasma hypoosmolality
3. Clinical euvolemia, as defined by the absence of signs of hypovolemia (orthostasis, tachycardia, decreased skin turgor, dry mucous membranes) or hypervolemia (subcutaneous edema, ascites)
4. Elevated urinary sodium excretion despite a normal salt and water intake
5. Normal thyroid, adrenal, and kidney function

Supplemental Criteria

6. Abnormal water load test (inability to excrete at least 80% of a 20 mL/kg water load in 4 h and/or failure to dilute U_{osm} to less than 100 mOsm/kg H_2O)
7. Plasma vasopressin (AVP) level inappropriately elevated relative to plasma osmolality
8. No significant correction of serum sodium concentration ([Na^+]) with volume expansion but improvement after fluid restriction

---

Modified from Verbalis JG: The syndrome of inappropriate antidiuretic hormone secretion and other hypoosmolar disorders. In Schrier RW, editor: Diseases of the kidney, Philadelphia, 2007, Lippincott Williams & Wilkins, pp 2214-2248.
AVP, Arginine vasopressin; ECF, extracellular fluid; P_{osm}, plasma osmolality; U_{osm}, urinary osmolality.

INCREASED EXTRACELLULAR FLUID VOLUME (HYPERVOLEMIA)

The presence of hypervolemia, as detected clinically by the presence of significant edema and/or ascites, indicates whole-body sodium excess, and hypoosmolality in these patients suggests a relatively decreased effective intravascular volume or pressure leading to water retention as a result of both elevated plasma AVP levels and decreased distal delivery of glomerular filtrate. Such patients usually have a low U_{Na} because of secondary hyperaldosteronism, but under certain conditions the U_{Na} may be elevated (e.g., glucosuria in diabetics, diuretic therapy). Hyponatremia generally does not occur until fairly advanced stages of diseases such as congestive heart failure, cirrhosis, and nephrotic

---

Box 7.3   Common Causes of Syndrome of Inappropriate Antidiuretic Hormone Secretion

Tumors

Pulmonary/mediastinal (bronchogenic carcinoma, mesothelioma, thymoma)
Nonchest (duodenal carcinoma, pancreatic carcinoma, ureteral/prostate carcinoma, uterine carcinoma, nasopharyngeal carcinoma, leukemia)

Central Nervous System Disorders

Mass lesions (tumors, brain abscesses, subdural hematoma)
Inflammatory diseases (encephalitis, meningitis, systemic lupus, acute intermittent porphyria, multiple sclerosis)
Degenerative/demyelinative diseases (Guillain-Barré, spinal cord lesions)
Miscellaneous (subarachnoid hemorrhage, head trauma, acute psychosis, delirium tremens, pituitary stalk section, transphenoidal adenomectomy, hydrocephalus)

Drugs

Stimulated AVP release (nicotine, phenothiazines, tricyclic antidepressants)
Direct renal effects and/or potentiation of AVP antidiuretic effects (desmopressin, oxytocin, prostaglandin synthesis inhibitors)
Mixed or uncertain actions (ACE inhibitors, carbamazepine and oxcarbazepine, chlorpropamide, clofibrate, clozapine, cyclophosphamide, 3,4-methylenedioxymethamphetamine ["Ecstasy"], omeprazole, serotonin reuptake inhibitors, vincristine)

Pulmonary Diseases

Infections (tuberculosis, acute bacterial or viral pneumonia, aspergillosis, empyema)
Mechanical/ventilatory (acute respiratory failure, COPD, positive-pressure ventilation)

Other

AIDS and AIDS-related complex
Prolonged strenuous exercise (marathon, triathlon, ultra-marathon, hot-weather hiking)
Postoperative state
Senile atrophy
Idiopathic

Modified from Verbalis JG: The syndrome of inappropriate antidiuretic hormone secretion and other hypoosmolar disorders. In Schrier RW, editor: Diseases of the kidney, Philadelphia, 2007, Lippincott Williams & Wilkins, pp 2214-2248.
ACE, Angiotensin-converting enzyme; *AIDS,* acquired immunodeficiency syndrome; *AVP,* arginine vasopressin; *COPD,* chronic obstructive pulmonary disease.

---

syndrome, so the diagnosis is usually not difficult. Kidney failure can also cause retention of both sodium and water, but in this case, the factor limiting excretion of excess body fluid is not decreased effective circulating volume but rather decreased glomerular filtration.

It should be remembered that even though many edema-forming states have secondary increases in plasma AVP levels as a result of decreased effective arterial blood volume, they are nonetheless not classified as SIADH because they fail to meet the criterion of clinical euvolemia (see Box 7.2). Although it can be argued that this distinction is semantic, this criterion remains important because it allows segregation of identifiable etiologies of hyponatremia that are associated with different methods of evaluation and therapy.

Several situations can cause hyponatremia because of acute water loading in excess of renal excretory capacity. Primary polydipsia can cause hypoosmolality in a small subset of patients with some degree of underlying SIADH, particularly psychiatric patients with longstanding schizophrenia who are taking neuroleptic drugs or, rarely, patients with normal kidney function in whom the volumes ingested exceed the maximum renal free water excretory rate of approximately 500 to 1000 mL/h.

Endurance exercising, such as marathon or ultramarathon racing, has been associated with sometimes fatal hyponatremia, primarily as a result of ingestion of excessive amounts of hypotonic fluids during the exercise that exceed the water excretory capacity of the kidney. This has been called *exercise-associated hyponatremia* (EAH). Many athletes with EAH have met diagnostic criteria for SIADH immediately following prolonged exercise, which serves to decrease further their free water excretory capacity both during and following exercise. Although the stimuli for AVP secretion during endurance excise have not been fully elucidated, potential candidates include baroreceptor activation, nausea, cytokine release from muscle rhabdomyolysis, and exercise itself. Most cases of EAH are associated with weight gain reflecting the excess water retention, but patients are usually classified as clinically euvolemic, because water retention alone without sodium excess, as observed in these patients, does not generally produce clinical manifestations of hypervolemia such as edema or ascites.

CLINICAL MANIFESTATIONS OF HYPONATREMIA

Hypoosmolality is associated with a broad spectrum of neurologic manifestations, ranging from mild, nonspecific symptoms (e.g., headache, nausea) to more significant deficits (e.g., disorientation, confusion, obtundation, focal neurologic deficits, seizures). In the most severe cases, death can result from respiratory arrest after tentorial herniation with subsequent brainstem compression. This neurologic symptom complex, termed *hyponatremic encephalopathy*, primarily reflects brain edema resulting from osmotic water shifts into the brain caused by the decreased effective P_{osm}. Significant symptoms generally do not occur until the serum [Na^+] falls to less than 125 mEq/L, and the severity of symptoms can be roughly correlated with the degree of hypoosmolality. However, individual variability is marked, and the level of serum [Na^+] at which symptoms will appear cannot be accurately predicted for any individual patient.

Furthermore, several factors other than the severity of the hypoosmolality also affect the degree of neurologic dysfunction. Most important is the acuity over which hypoosmolality develops. Rapid development of severe hypoosmolality is frequently associated with marked neurologic symptoms, whereas gradual development during several days or weeks is often associated with relatively mild symptomatology despite achievement of an equivalent degree of hypoosmolality. This occurs because the brain can counteract osmotic swelling by secreting intracellular solutes, both electrolytes and organic osmolytes, via a process called *brain volume regulation*. Because this is a time-dependent process, rapid development of hypoosmolality can result in brain edema before adaptation can occur; with slower development of hypoosmolality, brain cells can deplete solute sufficiently to prevent the development of brain edema and subsequent neurologic dysfunction.

Underlying neurologic disease also can significantly affect the level of hypoosmolality at which central nervous system symptoms appear. For example, moderate hypoosmolality is usually not of major concern in an otherwise healthy patient, but it can precipitate seizure activity in a patient with underlying epilepsy. Nonneurologic metabolic disorders (e.g., hypoxia, hypercapnia, acidosis, hypercalcemia) similarly can also affect the level of P_{osm} at which central nervous system symptoms occur. Recent studies have indicated that some patients may be susceptible to a vicious cycle in which hypoosmolality-induced brain edema causes noncardiogenic pulmonary edema, and the resulting hypoxia and hypercapnia then further impair the ability of the brain to volume-regulate, leading to more brain edema, neurologic deterioration, and death in some cases. Other clinical studies have suggested that menstruating women and young children may be particularly susceptible to the development of neurologic morbidity and mortality during hyponatremia, especially in the acute postoperative setting. The true clinical incidence and underlying pathophysiologic mechanisms responsible for these sometimes catastrophic outcomes remain to be determined.

Finally, the issue of whether mild-to-moderate hyponatremia is truly "asymptomatic" has been challenged by studies showing subtle defects in cognition and gait stability in hyponatremic patients that appear to be reversed by correction of the disorder. The functional significance of the gait instability was illustrated in a study of Belgian patients with a variety of levels of hyponatremia, all judged to be "asymptomatic" at the time of presentation to an emergency department (ED). These patients demonstrated a markedly increased incidence of falls, despite being apparently "asymptomatic." The clinical significance of the gait instability and fall data has been further evaluated by multiple independent studies that have shown increased bone fractures in hyponatremic subjects. More recently published studies have shown that hyponatremia is associated with increased bone loss in experimental animals, and a significant increase in odds ratio for osteoporosis of the femur in humans older than 50 years in the NHANES III database. Thus, the major clinical significance of chronic hyponatremia may lie in the increased morbidity and mortality associated with falls and fractures in the elderly population. Confirmation of these findings in larger numbers of subjects would have significant import for the management of chronic hyponatremia.

TREATMENT

Despite continuing controversy about the optimal speed of correction of osmolality in hyponatremic patients, there is now a relatively uniform consensus about appropriate therapy in most cases (see Fig. 7.1). If any degree of clinical hypovolemia is present, the patient should be considered to have a solute depletion–induced hypoosmolality and should be treated with isotonic (0.9%) NaCl at a rate appropriate for the estimated volume depletion. If diuretic use is known or suspected, fluid therapy should be supplemented with potassium (30 to 40 mEq/L) even if the serum [K$^+$] is not low because of the propensity of such patients to have total body potassium depletion. Patients with diuretic-induced hyponatremia usually respond well to isotonic NaCl and do not require 3% NaCl unless they exhibit severe symptoms. However, such patients often have an electrolyte-free water diuresis after their ECF volume deficit has been corrected, as correction of the ECF volume removes the hypovolemic stimulus to AVP secretion, resulting in a more rapid correction of the serum [Na$^+$] than that predicted from the rate of saline infusion.

Most often, the hypoosmolar patient is clinically euvolemic, but several situations dictate a reconsideration of potential solute depletion even in the patient without clinically apparent hypovolemia. These include a decreased U_{Na} (less than 30 mEq/L), any history of recent diuretic use, and any suggestion of primary adrenal insufficiency. Whenever a reasonable likelihood of depletion, rather than dilution, hypoosmolality exists, it is appropriate to treat initially with isotonic NaCl. If the patient has SIADH, no significant harm will have been done with a limited (1 to 2 L) saline infusion, because such patients will excrete excess NaCl without markedly changing their P_{osm}. However, this therapy should be abandoned if the serum [Na$^+$] does not improve, because longer periods of continued isotonic NaCl infusion can worsen the hyponatremia by virtue of cumulative water retention.

Treatment of euvolemic hypoosmolality varies depending on the presentation. If all criteria for SIADH are met except that the U_{osm} is low, the patient should simply be observed, because this presentation may represent spontaneous reversal of a transient form of SIADH. If there is any suspicion of either primary or secondary adrenal insufficiency, glucocorticoid replacement should be started immediately after completion of a rapid ACTH stimulation test. Prompt water diuresis after initiation of glucocorticoid treatment strongly supports glucocorticoid deficiency, but the absence of a quick response does not exclude this diagnosis, because several days of glucocorticoid therapy may be necessary for normalization of P_{osm}.

Hypervolemic hypoosmolality is usually treated initially with diuresis and other measures directed at the underlying disorder. Such patients rarely require any therapy to increase P_{osm} acutely, but often benefit from varying degrees of sodium and water restriction to reduce body fluid retention. However, worsened hyponatremia as a result of aggressive loop diuretic therapy in combination with continued or increased fluid intake and/or ineffectiveness of fluid restriction sometimes necessitates additional treatment of the hyponatremia, particularly using vasopressin receptor antagonists (vaptans) as saline administration will worsen the fluid retention.

In any case of significant hyponatremia, one is faced with the question of how quickly the P_{osm} should be corrected. Although hyponatremia is associated with a broad spectrum of neurologic symptoms, sometimes leading to death in severe cases, too rapid correction of severe hyponatremia can produce the osmotic demyelination syndrome, a brain demyelinating disease that also can cause substantial neurologic morbidity and mortality. Clinical and experimental results suggest that optimal treatment of hyponatremia must entail balancing the risks of hyponatremia against the risks of correction for each patient. Several factors should be considered: the severity of the hyponatremia, the duration of the hyponatremia, and the patient's symptom burden. Neither sequelae from hyponatremia itself nor myelinolysis after therapy is very likely in a patient whose serum $[Na^+]$ is greater than 125 mEq/L, although in some cases significant symptoms can develop even with serum $[Na^+]$ greater than 125 mEq/L if the rate of fall of serum $[Na^+]$ has been rapid. The importance of the duration and symptom burden of hyponatremia relate to how well the brain has volume regulated in response to the hyponatremia, and, consequently, relate to the degree of risk for demyelination with rapid correction. Cases of acute hyponatremia (arbitrarily defined as hyponatremia of 48 hours' duration or less) are usually symptomatic if the hyponatremia is severe (i.e., less than 125 mEq/L). These patients are at greatest risk from neurologic complications caused by the hyponatremia itself, and the serum $[Na^+]$ should be corrected to higher levels promptly, most often with the use of 3% NaCl unless the patient is undergoing a spontaneous aquaresis, in which case the correction will occur without intervention. Conversely, patients with more chronic hyponatremia (greater than 48 hours in duration) who have mild-to-moderate neurologic symptoms are at little risk from complications of hyponatremia itself, but can develop demyelination after overly rapid correction. There is no indication to correct the serum $[Na^+]$ in these patients rapidly, and slower-acting therapies, such as fluid restriction or vaptans, which correct serum $[Na^+]$ over 24 to 48 hours, should be used rather than 3% NaCl.

Although these extreme situations have clear treatment indications, most patients have hyponatremia of indeterminate duration and varying degrees of neurologic impairment. This group presents the most challenging treatment decision, because the hyponatremia has been present sufficiently long to allow some degree of brain volume regulation but not long enough to prevent an element of brain edema and neurologic symptoms. Most authors recommend prompt treatment for such patients because of their symptoms, but with methods that allow a controlled and limited correction of their hyponatremia. Reasonable correction parameters consist of a rate of correction of serum $[Na^+]$ in the range of 0.5 to 2 mEq/L/h, as long as the total magnitude of correction does not exceed 12 mEq/L during the first 24 hours and 18 mEq/L throughout the first 48 hours of correction. However, maximum correction rates should be even lower (no more than 8 mEq/L in 24 hours) if certain

risk factors for the development of osmotic demyelination are present, including alcoholism, liver disease, malnutrition, hypokalemia, and a very low serum $[Na^+]$ ($\leq$105 mEq/L). Treatments for individual patients should be chosen within these limits, depending on their symptoms. For patients who are only moderately symptomatic, one should proceed at the lower recommended limit of 0.5 mEq/L/h; in those who manifest more severe neurologic symptoms, initial correction at a rate of 1 to 2 mEq/L/h is appropriate.

Controlled corrections of hyponatremia can be accomplished with hypertonic (3%) NaCl solution administered via continuous infusion, because patients with euvolemic hypoosmolality (e.g., SIADH) usually will not respond to isotonic NaCl. An initial infusion rate can be estimated by multiplying the patient's body weight (in kilograms) by the desired rate of increase in serum $[Na^+]$ in milliequivalents per liter per hour. For example, in a 70-kg patient, an infusion of 3% NaCl at 70 mL/h will increase serum $[Na^+]$ by approximately 1 mEq/L/h, whereas infusing 35 mL/h will increase serum $[Na^+]$ by approximately 0.5 mEq/L/h.

Furosemide (20 to 40 mg IV) can be used to treat volume overload occurring as a result of 3% NaCl, in some cases anticipatorily, in patients at risk of volume overload as a result of sodium administration. Alternatively, vaptans can be used to increase the serum $[Na^+]$ by stimulating renal free water excretion, or *aquaresis*, thereby leading to increased serum $[Na^+]$ in the majority of patients with hyponatremia resulting from SIADH, congestive heart failure, or cirrhosis. Although the optimal use of AVP receptor antagonists in any setting has not yet been fully determined, the U.S. Food and Drug Administration (FDA) has now approved two vaptans for the treatment of euvolemic and hypervolemic hyponatremia.

Conivaptan is FDA-approved for euvolemic and hypervolemic hyponatremia in hospitalized patients. It is available only as an intravenous preparation, and is administered as a 20-mg loading dose over 30 minutes, followed by a continuous infusion of 20 or 40 mg/day. Generally, the 20-mg continuous infusion is used for the first 24 hours to gauge the initial response. If the correction of serum $[Na^+]$ is felt to be inadequate (e.g., less than 5 mEq/L), then the infusion rate can be increased to 40 mg/day. Therapy is limited to a maximum duration of 4 days because of drug interactions with other agents metabolized by the CYP3A4 hepatic isoenzyme. Importantly, for conivaptan and all other vaptans, it is critical that the serum $[Na^+]$ concentration is measured frequently during the active phase of correction of the hyponatremia (a minimum of every 6 to 8 hours, but more frequently in patients with risk factors for development of osmotic demyelination syndrome). If the correction approaches 12 mEq/L in the first 24 hours, the infusion should be stopped and the patient monitored on a fluid restriction. If the correction exceeds 12 mEq/L, consideration should be given to administering sufficient water, either orally or as intravenous D_5W, to bring the overall correction below 12 mEq/L. The maximum correction limit should be reduced to 8 mEq/L during the first 24 hours in patients with risk factors for development of osmotic demyelination as described previously. The most common adverse effects include injection-site reactions, which are generally mild and usually do not lead to treatment discontinuation, headache, thirst, and hypokalemia.

Tolvaptan, an oral AVP receptor antagonist, is FDA-approved for treatment of dilutional hyponatremias. In contrast to conivaptan, oral administration allows it to be used for both short- and long-term treatment of hyponatremia. Similar to conivaptan, tolvaptan treatment must be initiated in the hospital so that the rate of correction can be monitored carefully. Patients with a serum [Na$^+$] less than 125 mEq/L are eligible for therapy with tolvaptan as primary therapy; if the serum [Na$^+$] is ≥125 mEq/L, tolvaptan therapy is only indicated if the patient has symptoms that could be attributable to the hyponatremia and the patient is resistant to attempts at fluid restriction. The starting dose of tolvaptan is 15 mg on the first day, and the dose can be titrated to 30 mg and 60 mg at 24-hour intervals if the serum [Na$^+$] remains less than 135 mEq/L or the increase in serum [Na$^+$] has been ≤5 mEq/L in the previous 24 hours. As with conivaptan, it is essential that the serum [Na$^+$] concentration be measured frequently during the active phase of correction of the hyponatremia (a minimum of every 6 to 8 hours, but more frequently in patients with risk factors for development of osmotic demyelination). Limits for safe correction of hyponatremia and methods to compensate for overly rapid corrections are the same as described previously for conivaptan. One additional factor that helps to avoid overly rapid correction with tolvaptan is the recommendation that fluid restriction not be used during the active phase of correction, thereby allowing the patient's thirst to compensate for an overly vigorous aquaresis. Side effects include dry mouth, thirst, increased urinary frequency, dizziness, and nausea.

Because inducing increased renal fluid excretion via either a diuresis or an aquaresis can cause or worsen hypotension in patients with hypovolemic hyponatremia, vaptans are contraindicated in this patient population. Clinically significant hypotension was not observed in either the conivaptan or tolvaptan clinical trials in euvolemic and hypervolemic hyponatremic patients, although orthostatic hypotension as a result of the aquaresis has been reported. Although vaptans are not contraindicated with decreased kidney function, these agents generally will not be effective if the serum creatinine is greater than 2.5 mg/dl.

Regardless of the method or initial rate of correction chosen, acute treatment should be interrupted after any of three endpoints is reached: (1) the patient's symptoms are abolished, (2) a safe serum [Na$^+$] (typically, 125 mEq/L) has been reached, or (3) a total magnitude of correction of 16 to 18 mEq/L has been achieved. It follows from these recommendations that serum [Na$^+$] levels must be carefully monitored at frequent intervals during the active phases of treatment (every 2 to 4 hours for 3% NaCl administration; every 6 to 8 hours for vaptan administration) to adjust therapy so that the correction stays within accepted guidelines. It cannot be emphasized too strongly that it is necessary to correct the P$_{osm}$ acutely only to a safe range, rather than to normal levels. As a practical point, after an acute correction has reached 8 mEq, the need for continued acute therapy should be carefully assessed, because ongoing correction may result in an overcorrection by the time the next serum [Na$^+$] is available (see Fig. 7.1). In some situations, patients may spontaneously correct their hyponatremia via a water diuresis. If the hyponatremia is acute (e.g., psychogenic polydipsia with water intoxication), such patients do not appear at risk for demyelination. However, if the hyponatremia has been chronic (e.g., hypocortisolism, diuretic therapy), intervention should be considered to limit the rate and magnitude of correction of serum [Na$^+$], such as administration of desmopressin 1 to 2 μg IV or infusion of hypotonic fluids to match urine output, using the same therapeutic endpoints as for active corrections.

Some patients will benefit from continued treatment of hyponatremia following discharge from the hospital. One important exception is those patients with the reset osmostat syndrome; because the hyponatremia of such patients is not progressive but rather fluctuates around their reset level of serum [Na$^+$], no therapy is generally required. For most other cases of mild-to-moderate SIADH, fluid restriction represents the least toxic therapy and is the treatment of choice. It should usually be tried as the initial therapy, with pharmacologic intervention reserved for refractory cases in which the degree of fluid restriction required to avoid hypoosmolality is so severe that the patient is unable, or unwilling, to maintain it. In general, the higher the urine solute concentration, as reflected by either U$_{osm}$ or the sum of urine Na$^+$ and K$^+$, the less likely it is that fluid restriction will be successful because of lower renal electrolyte free water excretion.

If pharmacologic treatment is necessary, the choices include urea, furosemide in combination with NaCl tablets, demeclocycline, and the vasopressin receptor antagonists. Although each of these treatments can be effective in individual circumstances, the only drugs currently approved by the FDA for treatment of hyponatremia are the vasopressin receptor antagonists. For patients who have responded to either conivaptan or tolvaptan in the hospital, consideration should be given to continuing tolvaptan as an outpatient after discharge. In patients with established chronic hyponatremia, tolvaptan has been shown to be effective at maintaining a normal [Na$^+$] for as long as 4 years on continued daily therapy. However, many patients with hospitalized hyponatremia have a transient form of SIADH without the need for long-term therapy. In the conivaptan open-label study, approximately 70% of patients treated as an inpatient for 4 days had normal serum [Na$^+$] concentrations 7 and 30 days after cessation of the vaptan therapy in the absence of chronic therapy for hyponatremia. Deciding which patients with hospitalized hyponatremia are selected as candidates for long-term therapy should be based on the etiology of the SIADH, because patients with some causes of SIADH are more likely to experience persistent hyponatremia that may benefit from long-term treatment with tolvaptan following discharge. Nonetheless, for any individual patient this simply represents an estimate of the likelihood of requiring long-term therapy. In all cases, consideration should be given to a trial of stopping the drug at 2 to 4 weeks following discharge to see if hyponatremia recurs. Seven days is a reasonable period of tolvaptan cessation to evaluate the presence of continued SIADH, because this period was sufficient to demonstrate recurrence of hyponatremia in the tolvaptan SALT clinical trials. Serum [Na$^+$] should be monitored every 2 to 3 days following cessation of tolvaptan so that the drug can be resumed as quickly as possible in those patients with recurrent hyponatremia, since the longer the patient is hyponatremic the greater the risk of subsequent osmotic demyelination with overly rapid correction of the low serum [Na$^+$].

Guidelines for the appropriate treatment of hyponatremia, and particularly the role of vaptans, are still evolving and will likely change substantially during the next several years. Of special interest will be studies to assess whether more effective treatment of hyponatremia can reduce the incidence of falls and fractures in elderly patients, the use of healthcare resources for both inpatients and outpatients with hyponatremia, and the markedly increased morbidity and mortality of patients with hyponatremia across multiple disease states. A potential role for vaptans in the treatment of heart failure has already been studied; a large trial (EVEREST) demonstrated short-term improvement in dyspnea, but no long-term survival benefit. However, this trial was not powered to evaluate the outcomes of hyponatremic patients with heart failure. Consequently, the potential therapeutic role of vaptans in the treatment of water-retaining disorders must await further studies specifically designed to assess the outcomes of hyponatremic patients, as well as clinical experience that better delineates efficacies as well as potential toxicities of all treatments for hyponatremia. Nonetheless, it is abundantly clear that the vaptans have ushered in a new era in the management of hyponatremic disorders.

BIBLIOGRAPHY

Berl T, Quittnat-Pelletier F, Verbalis JG, et al: Oral tolvaptan is safe and effective in chronic hyponatremia, *J Am Soc Nephrol* 21:705-712, 2010.

Fenske W, Stork S, Koschker AC, et al: Value of fractional uric acid excretion in differential diagnosis of hyponatremic patients on diuretics, *J Clin Endocrinol Metab* 93:2991-2997, 2008.

Greenberg A, Verbalis JG: Vasopressin receptor antagonists, *Kidney Int* 69:2124-2130, 2006.

Hawkins RC: Age and gender as risk factors for hyponatremia and hypernatremia, *Clin Chim Acta* 337:169-172, 2003.

Hoorn EJ, Rivadeneira F, van Meurs JB, et al: Mild hyponatremia as a risk factor for fractures: the Rotterdam Study, *J Bone Miner Res* 26:1822-1828, 2011.

Kovesdy CP, Lott EH, Lu JL, et al: Hyponatremia, hypernatremia, and mortality in patients with chronic kidney disease with and without congestive heart failure, *Circulation* 125:677-684, 2012.

Renneboog B, Musch W, Vandemergel X, et al: Mild chronic hyponatremia is associated with falls, unsteadiness, and attention deficits, *Am J Med* 119:71-78, 2006.

Rosner MH, Kirven J: Exercise-associated hyponatremia, *Clin J Am Soc Nephrol* 2:151-161, 2007.

Schrier RW, Gross P, Gheorghiade M, et al: Tolvaptan, a selective oral vasopressin V2-receptor antagonist, for hyponatremia, *N Engl J Med* 355:2099-2112, 2006.

Sterns RH, Nigwekar SU, Hix JK: The treatment of hyponatremia, *Semin Nephrol* 29:282-299, 2009.

Verbalis JG: The syndrome of inappropriate antidiuretic hormone secretion and other hypoosmolar disorders. In Schrier RW, editor: *Diseases of the kidney*, Philadelphia, 2007, Lippincott Williams & Wilkins, pp 2214-2248.

Verbalis JG, Barsony J, Sugimura Y, et al: Hyponatremia-induced osteoporosis, *J Bone Miner Res* 25:554-563, 2010.

Verbalis JG, Goldsmith SR, Greenberg A, et al: Hyponatremia treatment guidelines 2007: expert panel recommendations, *Am J Med* 120:S1-S21, 2007.

Wald R, Jaber BL, Price LL, et al: Impact of hospital-associated hyponatremia on selected outcomes, *Arch Intern Med* 170:294-302, 2010.

Hypernatremia

8

Paula Dennen | Stuart L. Linas

Dysnatremias, or abnormalities of serum sodium concentration, include both hyponatremia and hypernatremia. These electrolyte abnormalities occur in a wide spectrum of patient populations, ranging from infants to the elderly and from outpatients to the critically ill. Their occurrence is common, and prompt diagnosis and appropriate management of these disorders can decrease the associated morbidity and mortality. This chapter focuses on hypernatremia.

It is important to recognize that a patient's fluid and electrolyte balance is dynamic, and therefore management must include frequent assessment of the individual's response to therapy. Close monitoring can facilitate early recognition of unanticipated clinical changes and can avoid potential complications of treatment.

DEFINITIONS

Normal serum sodium concentration ([Na$^+$]) is 135 to 145 mEq/L. This range is generally maintained despite large individual variations in salt and water intake. Hypernatremia is defined as a [Na$^+$] greater than 145 mEq/L and reflects cellular dehydration. It is *always* a water problem and sometimes a salt problem as well. There is no predictable relationship between serum [Na$^+$] (a measure of osmolality and tonicity) and total body salt or volume status. To be more specific, whereas hypernatremia confirms the presence of a relative water deficit, the isolated laboratory finding of a serum [Na$^+$] greater than 145 mEq/L does not reveal anything about a person's volume status. Hypernatremia can occur in the context of hypovolemia, euvolemia, or hypervolemia.

DEHYDRATION AND VOLUME DEPLETION

Although the term "dehydration" is commonly used to describe a person's volume status, this use is incorrect. Dehydration does not equal volume depletion. In fact, *dehydration* is a description of water balance, whereas *volume depletion* refers to a person's sodium balance. Although these two clinical scenarios may coexist, they should not be confused, and it is important that the two terms are not used interchangeably. In hypernatremia, cells become dehydrated and shrink because of water movement from the intracellular to the extracellular space.

HYPEROSMOLALITY AND HYPERTONICITY

Hypernatremia always reflects a hyperosmolar state, whereas the reverse is not always true. For example, hyperosmolality may also be a consequence of severe hyperglycemia or elevated blood urea nitrogen (BUN), as is seen in acute or chronic kidney failure. Furthermore, hyperosmolality does not necessarily mean hypertonicity. For example, uremia is a hyperosmolar but not a hypertonic state. Urea can freely cross cell membranes, unlike sodium, and therefore contributes to osmolality but not to tonicity. In contrast to urea, sodium, which is unable to cross cell membranes freely, is an effective osmole and is the primary electrolyte that affects plasma osmolality (P$_{osm}$). In hypernatremia, which is a hypertonic state, sodium is an effective osmole causing water to flow from the intracellular to the extracellular space.

BACKGROUND

Hypernatremia is all about water. A more accurate term for hypernatremia might be "hypoaquaremia," because it literally means a state in which there is too little water in the intravascular space and, as a consequence, in the intracellular space. To begin any discussion of hypernatremia (or hyponatremia), it is important to understand that dysnatremias are actually disorders of water homeostasis.

Water distributes throughout all body compartments, two thirds in the intracellular and one third in the extracellular compartment. Three quarters of the water in the extracellular compartment is located in the interstitial space, and one quarter is in the intravascular space. Water is lost (or gained) in the same proportions as it is distributed throughout all body compartments. Pure water loss does not affect plasma volume status or hemodynamics significantly until very late because of the normal distribution of water throughout all body compartments. For example, for every 1 L of water deficit, only approximately 80 mL is lost from the intravascular (plasma) compartment.

EPIDEMIOLOGY

The incidence of hypernatremia in all hospitalized patients ranges from less than 1% to approximately 3%. However, in critically ill patients the overall prevalence of hypernatremia ranges between 9% and 26% and is hospital acquired in ≤80% of cases. Hypernatremia in adults that is present at the time of hospital admission is primarily a disease of the elderly and of those with mental illness or impaired sensorium. Most patients with hypernatremia on admission to the hospital have concomitant infections. Hypernatremia that is present on hospital admission is generally treated earlier than hypernatremia that develops during the hospital course, most likely because of increased attention paid to individual laboratory values and volume status on hospital admission.

71

In contrast, hospital-acquired hypernatremia is typically seen in patients who are younger than those with hypernatremia on admission, with an age distribution similar to that of the general hospitalized population. Hospital-acquired hypernatremia is largely iatrogenic from inadequate and/or inappropriate fluid prescription, and therefore is largely preventable. It results from a combination of decreased access to water and disease processes that may increase insensible losses or interfere with the thirst mechanism. About half of patients with hospital-acquired hypernatremia are intubated and therefore have no free access to water. Of the remaining 50%, most have altered mental status.

Patients at highest risk for hospital-acquired hypernatremia are those at the extremes of age (infants and the elderly), those with altered mental status, and those without access to water (i.e., intubated or debilitated patients). Furthermore, in addition to the impaired thirst and decreased urinary concentrating ability that accompany advanced age, elderly patients have a lower baseline total body water content, making smaller changes more clinically relevant.

CLINICAL MANIFESTATIONS

SIGNS

Signs of hypernatremia depend, in part, on its cause and severity. Abnormal subclavicular and forearm skin turgor and altered sensorium are commonly found in patients with hypovolemic or euvolemic hypernatremia, whereas patients with hypervolemic hypernatremia typically have classic signs of volume overload, such as elevated neck veins and edema.

SYMPTOMS

Clinical symptoms related to hypernatremia can be attributed to cellular dehydration (cell shrinkage) due to the loss of intracellular water. Loss of intracellular water occurs throughout the body, but the primary symptoms are neurologic. The severity of neurologic symptoms is more dependent on the rate of rise in serum [Na+] than on the absolute value. Polyuria and polydipsia are frequently the presenting symptoms of diabetes insipidus (DI), with or without the presence of hypernatremia.

Neurologic symptoms comprise a continuum that begins with fatigue, lethargy, irritability, and confusion, and progresses to seizures and coma. Additional symptoms of hypernatremia include anorexia, nausea, vomiting, and generalized muscle weakness. Altered mental status can be both a cause and an effect of hypernatremia, and consequently can be difficult to distinguish clinically. Additionally, cellular dehydration (cell shrinkage) can lead to rupture of cerebral veins because of traction, which results in focal intracerebral and subarachnoid hemorrhages; this occurs more often in infants than in adults.

PATHOPHYSIOLOGY

A sound understanding of the normal physiology of water and salt balance is integral to the understanding and management of dysnatremias. The intracellular and extracellular body compartments exist in osmotic equilibrium. The development of hypernatremia is most commonly the result of increased water losses in the setting of inadequate intake, but it may also occur as a consequence of excessive sodium intake.

Regulation of plasma [Na+] is dependent on changes in water balance. Sodium is the primary determinant of P_{osm}. Normal P_{osm} is between 285 and 295 mOsm/kg. If the P_{osm} varies by 1% to 2% in either direction, normal physiologic mechanisms are in place to return the P_{osm} to normal. In the case of hypernatremia or hyperosmolality, receptor cells in the hypothalamus detect increases in P_{osm}; in response, they stimulate thirst to increase water intake and simultaneously stimulate antidiuretic hormone (ADH) release to limit renal water losses (by increasing water reabsorption in the collecting duct). Under normal conditions, the body is able to maintain the serum osmolality under tight control. The goal of "normonatremia" is to avoid changes in cellular volume and thereby prevent potential disruptions in cellular structure and function. The body's normal physiologic defense against hypernatremia is twofold: renal conservation of water and an endogenous thirst stimulus.

As with other electrolyte disturbances, the pathophysiology of hypernatremia can be easily categorized into two phases, an initiation phase and a maintenance phase. Simply stated, the initiation, or generation, phase must be caused by a net water loss or, less commonly, a net sodium gain. For hypernatremia to exist as anything more than a transient state, there must be a maintenance phase, defined necessarily by inadequate water intake.

Water metabolism is controlled primarily by arginine vasopressin (AVP) or ADH, as it is commonly termed. ADH is produced in the hypothalamus (supraoptic and paraventricular nuclei) and is stored in and secreted by the posterior pituitary. ADH release can be stimulated by either increases in P_{osm} or decreases in mean arterial pressure or blood volume. In the setting of hypernatremia, the primary stimulus for the release of ADH comes from osmoreceptors located in the hypothalamus. ADH acts on the vasopressin type-2 (V_2) receptors in the collecting duct to cause increased water reabsorption from the tubular lumen via insertion of aquaporin-2 channels.

The kidney's primary role in hypernatremia is to concentrate the urine maximally, preventing further loss of electrolyte-free fluid. For the kidney to do so, the following must occur: (1) development of a concentrated medullary interstitium, (2) presence of ADH to insert aquaporin-2 channels into the apical membranes of the collecting duct, and (3) ability of the collecting duct cells to respond to ADH.

In a steady state, water intake must equal water output. Obligatory renal water loss is directly dependent on solute excretion and urinary concentrating ability. If a person has to excrete, for example, 700 mOsm of solute per day (primarily Na+, K+, and urea), and the maximum urinary osmolality (U_{osm}) is 100 mOsm/kg, then the minimum urine output requirement will be 7 L. However, if the kidney is able to concentrate the urine to a U_{osm} of 700 mOsm/kg, urine output would need to be only 1 L.

Thirst, on the other hand, is an ADH-independent mechanism of defense against hypertonicity. Like ADH release, thirst is triggered by osmoreceptors located in the hypothalamus. The intense thirst stimulated by hypernatremia may

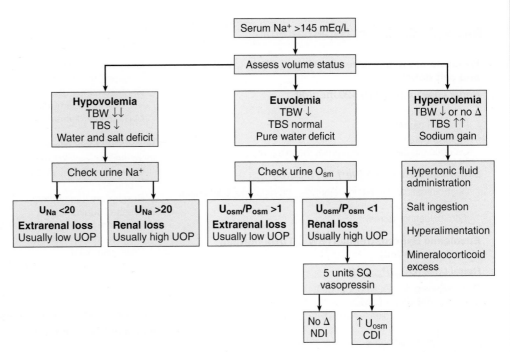

Figure 8.1 Diagnostic approach to hypernatremia. Refer to Box 8.1 for further details on the specific causes of hypernatremia in each category. *Δ,* Change; *CDI,* central diabetes insipidus; *NDI,* nephrogenic diabetes insipidus; P_{osm}, plasma osmolality; *SQ,* subcutaneous; *TBS,* total body salt; *TBW,* total body water; U_{Na}, random urine sodium concentration; *UOP,* urine output; U_{osm}, urine osmolality.

be impaired or absent in patients with altered mental status or hypothalamic lesions, and in the elderly. It is important to note that patients with moderate to severe increases in electrolyte-free water losses may maintain eunatremia because of the powerful thirst mechanism. For example, a patient with partial nephrogenic DI due to a history of lithium use will have a normal serum [Na$^+$] if given free access to water, but may become quite symptomatic (with marked hypernatremia) if circumstances prevent this free access (e.g., acute hospitalization for altered mental status or mechanical ventilation).

Although ADH activity is a pivotal physiologic defense against hyperosmolality, only an increase in water intake can replace a water deficit. An increase in ADH activity in collecting tubules can only help to decrease ongoing water losses but cannot replace water that has already been lost. Therefore, it is the combination of both ADH-dependent and ADH-independent mechanisms that is integral to the body's efforts to protect against hypernatremia or hyperosmolality.

The brain has multiple defense mechanisms designed to protect it from the adverse effects of cellular dehydration. As the serum [Na$^+$] rises, water moves from the intracellular to the extracellular space to return the serum osmolality to the normal range. Almost immediately, there is an increase in the net leak of serum electrolytes (primarily Na$^+$ and K$^+$) into the intracellular space, which increases intracellular osmolality. Additionally, there is an increased production of cerebrospinal fluid, with movement into the interstitial areas of the brain. Within the subsequent approximately 24 hours, the brain cells produce organic solutes (e.g., amino acids, trimethylamines, myoinositol), referred to as *osmolytes* or *idiogenic osmoles,* in an effort to draw water back into the cells. The increase in intracellular osmolality restores intracellular volume, thereby decreasing the adverse clinical impact of hypernatremia (i.e., cellular dehydration). The increase in transcellular transport of electrolytes is somewhat transient, because over time, it interferes with

normal cellular function. Cellular adaptation by the production of idiogenic osmoles requires days to reach full effect. Idiogenic osmoles clearly serve a protective role, but their removal is also slow (days) when isotonicity has been reestablished. The clinical implication of the slow removal of these idiogenic osmoles is that correction of hypernatremia (hypertonicity) must be gradual to avoid cellular swelling or cerebral edema.

DIAGNOSTIC APPROACH AND PATHOGENESIS

Hypernatremia most commonly results from the combination of increased water loss and decreased water intake. Any clinical condition associated with increased water loss or decreased water intake predisposes to hypernatremia. Generally speaking, for hypernatremia to occur, the rate of water excretion must exceed that of water intake. An exception to this basic principle, occurring less commonly, is hypernatremia secondary to sodium loading. Insensible losses include any water loss from the skin or respiratory tract. Examples of conditions that lead to increases in insensible losses include fever, burns, open wounds, and hyperventilation.

Although hypernatremia is due to an imbalance of water homeostasis, there may also be a concomitant salt disturbance. After taking a thorough clinical history and doing a complete physical examination, the first decision point in the evaluation of any patient with hypernatremia is to determine the patient's volume status (Fig. 8.1). Hypernatremia can be seen in patients who are hypovolemic, euvolemic, or hypervolemic.

HYPOVOLEMIC HYPERNATREMIA

Hypovolemic hypernatremia describes the individual who is both salt and water depleted because of the loss of hypotonic

Box 8.1   Causes of Hypernatremia

Hypovolemic Hypernatremia (TBW ⇊, TBNa ↓, water and salt deficit)

Renal Loss (urine [Na⁺] >20 mEq/dl)

Loop diuretics
Post-AKI diuresis
Postobstructive diuresis
Osmotic diuresis (hyperglycemia, mannitol, urea)

Extrarenal Loss (urine [Na⁺] <20 mEq/dl)

Gastrointestinal (vomiting, diarrhea, nasogastric suctioning, enterocutaneous fistula)
Skin (sweating, burns)

Euvolemic Hypernatremia (TBW ↓, TBNa normal, pure water deficit)

Renal Loss (U_{osm}/P_{osm} <1)

Diabetes Insipidus (ADH-dependent mechanism)
Central diabetes insipidus
    Lack of ADH release, complete or partial (see Box 8.2 for causes)
Nephrogenic diabetes insipidus (hereditary)
    X-linked recessive (defect in vasopressin V2 receptor or aquaporin channel)
    Unresponsive to ADH, complete or partial
Gestational diabetes insipidus
    Peripheral degradation of ADH
    Vasopressinase-mediated
Acquired Nephrogenic Diabetes Insipidus (urinary concentrating defect, ADH-independent)
Electrolyte disturbances (hypercalcemia, hypokalemia)

Drug-induced (lithium, demeclocycline, amphotericin B, foscarnet, methoxyflurane, V2 receptor antagonists)
Chronic kidney disease (e.g., medullary cystic disease, sickle cell disease, amyloidosis, Sjögren syndrome)
Malnutrition (decreased medullary gradient)

Extrarenal Loss (U_{osm}/P_{osm} >1)

Increased Insensible Loss
    Cutaneous (fever, sweating, increased ambient temperature, burns)
    Respiratory (tachypnea)
Decreased Intake
    Primary hypodipsia (hypothalamic or osmoreceptor dysfunction, advanced age)
Reset osmostat
Decreased access to water (altered mental status, iatrogenic)
Shift
    Water Loss into Cells (seizures, severe exercise)

Hypervolemic Hypernatremia TBW ↓ or no Δ, TBNa ⇈

Increased Sodium Intake

Excessive Na⁺ administration (saline or bicarbonate)
Hyperalimentation (total parenteral nutrition)
Salt ingestion
Inadvertent substitution of salt for sugar in infant formula
Mineralocorticoid excess
Hypertonic dialysis

ADH, Antidiuretic hormone; *AKI,* acute kidney injury; *P_{osm},* plasma osmolality; *TBNa,* total body sodium; *TBW,* total body water; *U_{osm},* urine osmolality.

---

fluids (Box 8.1). These individuals have sustained losses of both sodium and water but with a relatively greater loss of water. They usually manifest typical signs of volume depletion, such as tachycardia and orthostatic hypotension. Determination of the urine sodium concentration (U_{Na}) can help distinguish between renal losses, such as from diuretics or osmotic diuresis (U_{Na} >20 mEq/dl), and extrarenal losses, such as from diarrhea or vomiting (U_{Na} <20 mEq/dl).

EUVOLEMIC HYPERNATREMIA

Euvolemic hypernatremia refers to those conditions associated with a loss of electrolyte-free fluid, or pure water (see Box 8.1). These patients have a normal total body sodium (and are therefore euvolemic), but they are depleted in total body water. As in the evaluation of hypovolemic hypernatremia, euvolemic hypernatremia can be further categorized into renal and extrarenal causes. In this case, urine osmolality (U_{osm}) is often more helpful than U_{Na}. U_{osm} reflects ADH levels and function. A low U_{osm} is consistent with renal losses and therefore with low ADH levels or function (DI), whereas a high U_{osm} suggests extrarenal losses of free water and intact secretion of and response to ADH.

Etiologies of DI may be central (Box 8.2), nephrogenic, or gestational. The key diagnostic step in determining a central versus a nephrogenic cause is based on the response

Box 8.2   Central Diabetes Insipidus

Congenital (autosomal dominant or recessive)
Trauma
Neurosurgery
Primary or secondary CNS tumors
Infiltrative disorders (e.g., sarcoidosis, tuberculosis)
Hypoxic encephalopathy (postcardiac arrest, Sheehan's syndrome)
Bleeding
Infection (meningitis, encephalitis)
Aneurysm
Idiopathic

CNS, Central nervous system.

to exogenous hormone replacement (i.e., vasopressin). A finding of no change in U_{osm} after administration of exogenous vasopressin is diagnostic of nephrogenic DI. However, it is important to remember that central or nephrogenic DI may be partial: either ADH is present but in insufficient quantity (partial central DI) or there is an incomplete response to ADH in the collecting duct (partial nephrogenic DI).

One rare form of DI is gestational, or pregnancy-related, DI, which is caused by production of placental vasopressinase. Gestational DI should be evident from the clinical history. The manifestations are similar to those of nephrogenic DI in that there is no change in U_{osm} with exogenous vasopressin; however gestational DI responds to desmopressin acetate (dDAVP), a synthetic analogue of ADH which is unaffected by vasopressinase.

Nephrogenic DI can be either hereditary (genetic defect of the V_2 receptor gene or aquaporin water channel) or acquired. Acquired nephrogenic DI may be reversible and includes any clinical condition in which the kidney is unable to maximally concentrate the urine. The most common cause of acquired nephrogenic DI is chronic lithium use. The mechanism of lithium-induced nephrogenic DI includes both a decrease in density of V_2 receptors and decreased expression of aquaporin-2 channels. Hypercalcemia, hypokalemia, and severe malnutrition are other common examples of reversible nephrogenic DI. Hypercalcemia can induce a reversible nephrogenic DI through inhibition of sodium reabsorption in the loop of Henle, which impairs the generation of an adequate medullary gradient and reduces concentrating ability. Additionally, dysregulation of the aquaporin-2 channel can be seen with hypercalcemia. Hypokalemia causes nephrogenic DI by decreasing collecting tubule responsiveness to ADH. Decreased protein intake leads to decreased urea production and, therefore, a decreased medullary gradient with inability to maximally concentrate the urine.

A high U_{osm} suggests extrarenal losses as the cause of euvolemic hypernatremia. To generate a high U_{osm}, the kidney must be able to concentrate the urine, an ability that requires intact ADH-dependent mechanisms. Insensible losses are the primary source of electrolyte-free water loss in this subgroup of patients. Increased insensible losses occur via the skin (burns, sweat), respiratory tract (tachypnea), or both.

Finally, patients with hypodipsia or adipsia may develop euvolemic hyponatremia. Most often, they have normally functioning kidneys but lack adequate water intake. These patients typically have a high U_{osm} and low urine output. Idiopathic hypodipsia occurs, but identification of an impaired thirst mechanism as the primary disorder causing hypernatremia should lead to a more thorough neurologic investigation to rule out the presence of hypothalamic tumors or disorders. An impaired thirst mechanism or limited access to water in the setting of DI can result in severe hypernatremia and can be life threatening.

HYPERVOLEMIC HYPERNATREMIA

Hypervolemic hypernatremia is caused by sodium gain, and it is the least common type of hypernatremia (see Box 8.1). Total body sodium is uniformly increased, but total body water may be increased or unchanged, depending on the cause. An increase in extracellular volume should be readily identifiable on clinical examination. This clinical presentation is usually iatrogenic, resulting from hypertonic fluid administration (saline or bicarbonate), and it reflects a gain of sodium without an appropriate gain of water. Excess mineralocorticoid activity can also cause hypervolemic hypernatremia and, in the absence of typical iatrogenic risk factors, should alert the clinician to evaluate for potential causes of mineralocorticoid excess.

Box 8.3 Approach to the Treatment of Hypernatremia

Step 1. Determine volume status.
Step 2. Calculate free water deficit.
Step 3. Choose a replacement fluid.
Step 4. Determine rate of repletion.
Step 5. Estimate ongoing "sensible" losses.
Step 6. Estimate ongoing "insensible" losses.
Step 7. Determine underlying cause, if possible.

An example of *relative* hypervolemic hypernatremia is the hemodynamically stable hypernatremic patient with acute respiratory distress syndrome (ARDS) and an elevated central venous pressure. This *relative* hypervolemic hypernatremic state reflects an imbalance of both water and salt. Commonly, the physician might be concerned that administration of the free water necessary to correct the serum [Na+] (e.g., 3 L) would cause the patient to become fluid overloaded. This would be in direct contrast to the goal of a net negative fluid balance for optimal management of ARDS. However, because of the normal distribution of water, <10% of the administered water, either intravenously or enterally (i.e., <300 mL for administration of 3 L), would remain in the vascular space; therefore, the fluid administration would not materially impact the patient's volume status. Additionally, it is imperative to understand that further diuresis to obtain a net negative sodium balance will exacerbate the hypernatremia by increasing free water urinary losses, and therefore it must be considered in calculating the free water deficit.

TREATMENT

Treatment goals of hypernatremia include both replacement of the free water deficit and prevention or reduction of ongoing water loss. The amount, route, and rate of replacement depend on the severity of symptoms, rate of onset, concurrent clinical conditions, and volume status. Volume resuscitation is always a priority, no matter how severe the hypernatremia. Depletion of extracellular fluid in the setting of hemodynamic instability should always be corrected with normal saline before the water deficit is addressed. Once hemodynamically stable, it is important to focus on the treatment of hypernatremia, because the complications of hypernatremia frequently result not from the electrolyte disturbance itself but from its inappropriate correction or treatment. Management of hypernatremia should include identification of the underlying cause in addition to correction of the hypertonic state. Treatment of hypernatremia can, most often, be broken down into the following seven steps (Box 8.3).

Step 1. Determine Volume Status. Evaluation of the patient's volume status is a critical first step for both appropriate diagnosis and treatment of hypernatremia. This information should be obtained through a thorough history and physical examination.

Box 8.4

Formula 1   Water deficit $= TBW \times ($plasma $[Na^+]/140 - 1)$
$= (0.5$ or $0.4) \times$ lean body weight
$\times ($Plasma $[Na^+]/140 - 1$

Formula 2 $\Delta [Na^+]_s = \dfrac{[Na^+]_{inf} - [Na^+]_s}{TBW + 1}$

Formula 3   Urine output $= C_{electrolytes} + C_{electrolyte\text{-}free}$
or
$C_{electrolyte\text{-}free} = V \times \left[1 - \dfrac{U_{Na} + U_K}{P_{Na}} \right]$

Step 2. Calculate Free Water Deficit (Box 8.4). Before initiating therapy, it is both prudent and appropriate to quantify the deficit and develop a treatment plan for the individual patient. Calculation of the water deficit represents only a snapshot in time. If it were possible to prevent any further water losses, insensible or otherwise, the calculated water deficit would be the amount that must be administered to normalize the serum $[Na^+]$, as shown in Box 8.4, Formula 1:

$$Water\ deficit = TBW \times (plasma[Na^+]/140 - 1)$$
$$= (0.5\ or\ 0.4) \times lean\ body\ weight \times (Plasma\ [Na^+]/140 - 1)$$

where the lean body weight is expressed in kilograms. Total body water (TBW) is generally considered to be 60% of lean body weight in men and 50% in women. The final term in the equation, (Plasma $[Na^+]/140 - 1$), may be replaced by the target serum $[Na^+]$. For example, if the current $[Na^+]$ is 160 mEq/L and the goal is to reduce this concentration by 10 mEq/L in 24 hours, then 150 mEq/L may be substituted. This method may be used to calculate the water deficit for any target serum $[Na^+]$.

Step 3. Choose a Replacement Fluid. The choice of fluid for repletion of a free water deficit depends on the clinical assessment of volume status. Specifically, a key determination is whether the deficit is the result of a pure water loss, requiring only water repletion, or a hypotonic fluid loss, which requires both water and salt repletion. Generally, patients with a pure water loss should be repleted with the use of enteral free water (oral or nasogastric tube) or by intravenous administration of D_5W. Hypovolemic hypernatremic patients should be repleted with a combination of salt and water. This correction may be accomplished by the administration of 0.2% or 0.45% saline or with the use of separate intravenous solutions, one for water repletion and one for correction of the salt deficit. The potential advantage of using two separate infusions is the avoidance of continued salt repletion after the volume deficit has been corrected.

The route of repletion must also be determined. As with nutritional repletion, the enteral route for repletion of free water is preferable; however, it is not always an option, because patients commonly have altered mental status. Water can be repleted through a nasogastric tube if gut function is not compromised. One reason that the enteral route is preferable for repletion of free water is to avoid administration of the dextrose that is required to provide water through the intravenous route. Dextrose has the potential to increase serum osmolality via hyperglycemia, and this can contribute to additional unwanted renal clearance of electrolyte-free water because of an osmotic diuresis. Most commonly, correction of the free water deficit will be done, at least initially, via the intravenous route.

Step 4. Determine Rate of Repletion. The rate of correction of serum $[Na^+]$ is recommended to be approximately 0.5 mEq/L/h, or a decrease of 10 to 12 mEq/L in a 24-hour period. No human studies have been performed to substantiate the appropriateness of this rate. However, based on animal studies, this reflects the observed rate of cerebral de-adaptation, or the rate at which the brain is able to shed electrolytes and idiogenic osmoles acquired in the adaptive response to cellular dehydration. An important exception to this recommended rate of correction occurs in acutely symptomatic patients who have seizures or acute obtundation, potentially requiring intubation for airway protection. In these circumstances, the rate of correction can be 1 to 2 mEq/L/h initially, with the overall rate still not to exceed the recommended 10 to 12 mEq/L in 24 hours. Furthermore, acute symptoms suggest that the hypernatremia developed rapidly and, consequently, the brain has not had time to adapt. If adaption to hypernatremia has not yet occurred, the risk that cerebral edema will complicate rapid correction is minimal. If the duration of hypernatremia is unknown, the clinician should err on the side of caution and avoid rapid correction. However, if the onset is known to be acute (i.e., developing within the last 12 hours), the serum $[Na^+]$ can be corrected more quickly, because brain adaptation does not occur this rapidly.

The calculation of water deficit shown in Step 2 (see Formula 1) is particularly useful for hypernatremia caused by pure water losses. However, in multiple observational studies hypovolemia is present in more than 50% of cases of hypernatremia. For this reason, it is frequently necessary to replace both water and sodium deficits, and the use of 0.2% or 0.45% saline may be appropriate. (Table 8.1 lists the sodium concentrations of commonly used intravenous fluids.) Formula 2 can be clinically useful for predicting the change in serum $[Na^+]$ that will occur with infusion of 1 L of a particular fluid, and, accordingly, choosing an appropriate rate of infusion.

$$\Delta [Na^+]_s = \frac{[Na^+]_{inf} - [Na^+]_s}{TBW + 1}$$

where TBW is the ideal body weight times 60% (for men) or 50% (for women), expressed in liters (L) (see note in Step 2 for explanation), $\Delta[Na^+]_s$ is the change in serum $[Na^+]$ per L of fluid infused, $[Na^+]_{inf}$ is the concentration of sodium in the infusate, and $[Na^+]_s$ is the patient's current concentration of sodium.

Step 5. Estimate Ongoing "Sensible" Losses. The formulas presented for calculation of the water deficit (see Step 2) and estimation of the impact of a particular infusate on serum $[Na^+]$ (see Step 4) both assume a closed system. They do not account for any ongoing renal or extrarenal losses. In patients with DI or an osmotic diuresis due to hyperglycemia or administration of mannitol, ongoing urinary water losses can be significant. Formula 3 is clinically useful in

Table 8.1 Distribution of Commonly Used Fluids*

Fluid	Infusate [Na⁺] (mEq/L)	% ECF Distribution*	% Intravascular Distribution*
D_5W	0	33 (⅓)	8 (¼ × ⅓)
0.225% NaCl in D_5W	38.5	50	12.5
0.45% NaCl	77	62.5	15.5
Ringer's lactate	130	100	25
0.9% NaCl in water	154	100	25

D_5W, 5% Dextrose in water; *ECF*, extracellular fluid; *[Na⁺]*, sodium ion concentration, *NaCl*, sodium chloride.
*The distribution of water is assumed to be ⅔ intracellular and ⅓ extracellular, with the extracellular distribution being ¼ intravascular and ¾ interstitial.

estimating the amount of ongoing renal water losses, based on clearance (C) of the electrolyte and electrolyte-free components of the urinary fluid:

$$\text{Urine output} = C_{electrolytes} + C_{electrolyte\text{-}free}$$

or

$$C_{electrolyte\text{-}free} = V \times \left[1 - \frac{(U_{Na} + U_K)}{P_{Na}}\right]$$

where U_{Na} is the urine sodium concentration, U_K is the urine potassium concentration, and P_{Na} is the plasma sodium concentration, all expressed in milliequivalents per liter (mEq/L). Volume (V) may be expressed in any increment of time, with subsequent extrapolation to a 24-hour period.

The following example illustrates the utility of this free water clearance formula. If the random U_{Na} = 25 mEq/L, U_K = 15 mEq/L, and P_{Na} = 160 mEq/L, then 25% of the urine output can be attributed to the clearance of electrolytes, and 75% is electrolyte-free water. In the setting of a serum [Na⁺] of 160 mEq/L, urine with 75% electrolyte-free water clearance is inappropriate. The urine osmolality can help distinguish whether the high free water clearance represents an osmotic diuresis or DI. A high urine osmolality would be consistent with an osmotic diuresis (from glucose, urea, or mannitol), whereas a low urine osmolality would be consistent with DI.

Step 6. Estimate Ongoing "Insensible" Losses. Ongoing losses include urine and stool output as well as insensible losses from the skin and respiratory tracts. It is usually reasonable to assume that insensible losses are 10 to 15 mL/kg/day for women and 15 to 20 mL/kg/day for men, with factors such as fever, ambient temperature, infection, burns, open wounds, and tachypnea causing an increase in insensible losses.

Step 7. Determine Underlying Cause, if Possible. Although the mainstay of treatment of hypernatremia is repletion of the water deficit, attempts to prevent additional losses should be undertaken. In central DI, for example, treatment with a V_2 antagonist (i.e., desmopressin) is critical. Nephrogenic DI is considerably more difficult to treat, but treatment can include administration of a thiazide diuretic to create a mildly volume-depleted state and, consequently, decreased water delivery to the collecting ducts. Low-protein and low-sodium diets can also help to decrease the

Box 8.5 Special Considerations for Treatment of Hypernatremia

Hypovolemic Hypernatremia

Correct water and salt deficit
Treat underlying condition (e.g., hyperglycemia, urinary obstruction)

Euvolemic Hypernatremia

Correct water deficit
CDI: dDAVP, correct underlying disorder
GDI: dDAVP, vasopressinase does not cleave dDAVP
NDI (reversible): remove offending medication, correct electrolyte abnormality
NDI (irreversible): thiazide diuretic, NSAIDs, decrease salt intake
NDI (lithium-related): amiloride

Hypervolemic Hypernatremia

Correct water deficit and volume (salt) overload
Diuretics
Dialysis if concurrent kidney failure is present

CDI, Central diabetes insipidus; *dDAVP*, desmopressin; *GDI*, gestational diabetes insipidus; *NDI*, nephrogenic diabetes insipidus; *NSAIDs*, nonsteroidal antiinflammatory drugs.

amount of obligatory solute clearance and thereby decrease the urine output. See Box 8.5 for further condition-specific treatment recommendations.

The treatment approach described earlier applies primarily to hypovolemic and euvolemic hypernatremia. Treatment of hypervolemic hypernatremia is quite different and relies primarily on correction of the hypervolemic state with diuretics. An important consideration in this clinical scenario is that, although gain of sodium is the primary disturbance, there is still a relative lack of water. Diuresis in the absence of water repletion will exacerbate the hypernatremia. Loop diuretics interfere with the concentrating mechanism of the kidneys and therefore cause an inappropriate loss of electrolyte-free water in addition to the desired natriuresis. For this reason, it is imperative to replete the free water deficit in these patients and to calculate their ongoing losses using Formula 3 (see Step 5) to achieve adequate repletion. This is of particular concern in those patients who are without free access to water, such as intubated patients.

Common mistakes encountered in the treatment of hypernatremia include both undercorrection and overcorrection. Undercorrection is most commonly caused by underestimation of ongoing sensible and insensible losses. Formula 3 allows the clinician to obtain a more accurate reflection of ongoing renal electrolyte-free water loss. Additionally, it is important to identify and account for insensible losses applicable to the individual patient. Overcorrection, or overly rapid correction, poses the greater danger. Because the formulas described here are only a guide and lack precision for individual patients, it is critical that serum chemistry values be checked frequently to ensure that the expected and actual rates of correction are similar. The clinician can then adjust the treatment decisions as needed and avoid the potentially devastating neurologic complications of overcorrection.

All formulas used to facilitate treatment of hypernatremia have limitations. As mentioned earlier, they do not factor in ongoing sensible or insensible losses. Furthermore, a key component of both Formula 1 and Formula 2 is TBW, which itself is an imprecise term providing only rough estimates of the impact of age and gender. These formulas should be considered as adjunctive tools, but should in no way replace sound clinical judgment. The isolated use of these formulas to guide therapy could prove deleterious to the patient if used in lieu of appropriate clinical assessment. For these reasons, it is critical that serum [Na$^+$] be measured frequently (typically, every 2 hours initially) to assess whether the patient is responding as predicted. This is particularly important for patients with significant unmeasurable losses (e.g., diarrhea, burns) and for those patients with particularly high ongoing water losses (as frequently occurs with central DI).

A patient's volume status must be determined at the bedside, and it plays a critical role in both diagnosis and the appropriate selection of fluids. Additionally, determination of the rate of correction is dependent, in part, on the clinical symptoms. For example, seizures or severely altered mental status should alert the clinician to the need to correct the serum [Na$^+$] more rapidly. In contrast, if the patient is relatively asymptomatic despite a serum [Na$^+$] greater than 170 mEq/L, rapid correction can significantly increase the complication rate, and, therefore, careful attention must be paid to slow correction.

COMPLICATIONS OF HYPERNATREMIA

In several large observational studies, hypernatremia is independently associated with both an increased length of stay and an increased mortality. These observational studies have confirmed mortality rates ranging from 40% to greater than 60%, but it remains unclear whether hypernatremia is simply a marker of illness severity or whether it itself truly contributes to an increase in mortality. Acute (≤24 hours) hypernatremia with serum [Na$^+$] levels greater than 160 mEq/L is associated with a 75% mortality rate in adults, whereas chronic hypernatremia is associated with a much lower rate of approximately 10%. Even modest hospital-acquired hypernatremia has been associated with increased mortality in patients with serum [Na$^+$] greater than 150 mEq/L, demonstrating a severity of illness-adjusted relative

---

Box 8.6 Hypernatremia Key Points

- Hypernatremia always reflects a hyperosmolar state.
- Hypernatremia is always a water problem and sometimes a salt problem.
- Patients must have a defect in their thirst mechanism or limited access to free water for hypernatremia to persist.
- The sodium concentration itself does not provide any information about total body salt or volume status.
- A calculation of the water deficit represents only a snapshot in time.
- Failure to consider ongoing sensible and insensible losses is the most common cause of undercorrection.

---

risk of 2.6 for death. The increased mortality and increased length of stay seen in patients with hypernatremia have been demonstrated across a broad spectrum of patient populations, including postcardiac surgery and medical and general surgical ICU patients. A decreased level of consciousness occurring as a complication of hypernatremia is an important prognostic indicator associated with mortality. Even though the mechanism of the high mortality is not known, it is clear that a judicious approach to diagnosis and treatment of hypernatremia is imperative (Box 8.6). Detailed clinical examples showing the step-by-step approach to hypernatremia are shown in Cases 8.1 to 8.3.

As discussed earlier, neurologic sequelae can occur both with hypernatremia and with its correction. Decreased cell volume impairs tissue function, and overly rapid correction can cause cerebral edema if adaptation has occurred. In addition to the adverse central nervous system effects, hypernatremia also inhibits insulin release and increases insulin resistance, thereby predisposing patients to hyperglycemia. Hypernatremia also decreases hepatic gluconeogenesis, lactate clearance, and cardiac function. A patient's level of consciousness, rather than the absolute serum [Na$^+$], is the one prognostic indicator of mortality.

Adverse sequelae associated with hypernatremia are often underappreciated and frequently lead to a delay in treatment. Studies have shown that fewer than 50% of patients with hospital-acquired hypernatremia receive free water replacement within 24 hours of the first identified elevated serum [Na$^+$], and the majority take longer than 72 hours to treat. Furthermore, patients whose hypernatremia is corrected within 72 hours had a lower mortality than those whose hypernatremia was not corrected within 72 hours. In light of the significant associations with adverse physiologic sequelae, increased length of stay, and increased mortality seen with hospital-acquired hypernatremia, hypernatremia should not be viewed as an incidental or negligible electrolyte abnormality in the ICU patient.

BIBLIOGRAPHY

Adler SM, Verbalis JG: Disorders of body water homeostasis in critical illness, *Endocrinol Metab Clin North Am* 35:873-894, 2006.

Adrogue HA, Madias NE: Aiding fluid prescription for the dysnatremias, *Intensive Care Med* 23:309-316, 1997.

Adrogue HJ, Madias NE: Hypernatremia. *N Engl J Med* 342:1493-1499, 2000.

Alshayeb HM, Showkat A, Babar F, et al: Severe hypernatremia correction rate and mortality in hospitalized patients, *Am J Med Sci* 341: 356-360, 2011.

Berl T, Robertson G: Pathophysiology of water metabolism. In Brenner BM, editor: *The Kidney*, ed 6, Philadelphia, 2000, WB Saunders, pp 866-893.

Chassagne P, Druesne L, Capet C, et al: Clinical presentation of hypernatremia in elderly patients: a case control study, *J Am Geriatr Soc* 54:1225-1230, 2006.

Darmon M, Timsit J, Francais A, et al: Association between hypernatraemia acquired in the ICU and mortality: a cohort study, *Nephrol Dial Transplant* 25:2502-2510, 2010.

Funk G, Lindner G, Druml W, et al: Incidence and prognosis of dysnatremias present on ICU admission, *Intensive Care Med* 36:304-311, 2010.

Hall JB, Schmidt GA, Wood LDH: Electrolyte disorders in critical care. In Hall JB, Schmidt GA, Wood LDH, editors: *Principles of Critical Care*, ed 3, New York, 2005, McGraw-Hill, pp 1161-1166.

Hoorn EJ, Betjes M, Weigel J, et al: Hypernatraemia in critically ill patients: too little water and too much salt, *Nephrol Dial Transplant* 23:1562-1568, 2008.

Liamis G, Kalogirou M, Saugos V, et al: Therapeutic approach in patients with dysnatraemias, *Nephrol Dial Transplant* 21:1564-1569, 2006.

Lien YH, Shapiro JI, Chan L: Effect of hypernatremia on organic brain osmoles, *J Clin Invest* 85:1427-1435, 1990.

Lindner G, Funk G, Lassnigg A, et al: Intensive care-acquired hypernatremia after major cardiothoracic surgery is associated with increased mortality, *Intensive Care Med* 36:1718-1723, 2010.

Lindner G, Funk G, Schwarz C, et al: Hypernatremia in the critically ill is an independent risk factor for mortality, *Am J Kidney Dis* 50:952-957, 2007.

Nguyen MK, Kurtz I: Analysis of current formulas used for treatment of the dysnatremias, *Clin Exp Nephrol* 8:12-16, 2004.

Palevsky PM: Hypernatremia. *Semin Nephrol* 18:20-30, 1998.

Palevsky PM, Bhagrath R, Greenberg A: Hypernatremia in hospitalized patients, *Ann Intern Med* 124:197-203, 1996.

Polderman K, Schreuder W, van Schijndel R, et al: Hypernatremia in the intensive care unit: an indicator of quality of care? *Crit Care Med* 27:1105-1108, 1999.

Rose BD, Post TW: *Clinical Physiology of Acid-Base and Electrolyte Disorders*, ed 3, New York, 2001, McGraw-Hill, pp 775-784.

Shoker AS: Application of the clearance concept to hyponatremic and hypernatremic disorders: a phenomenological analysis, *Clin Chem* 40:1220-1227, 1994.

Stelfox HT, Ahmed SB, Khandwala F, et al: The epidemiology of intensive care unit-acquired hyponatraemia and hypernatraemia in medical-surgical intensive care units, *Crit Care* 12:1-9, 2008.

9 Edema and the Clinical Use of Diuretics

Domenic A. Sica | Todd W.B. Gehr

Chlorothiazide, which became available in 1958, ushered in the modern era of diuretic therapy, initially for the treatment of edematous states and shortly thereafter for the treatment of hypertension. As such, diuretics remain important therapeutic tools. First, they are capable of reducing blood pressure (BP) while simultaneously decreasing the morbidity and mortality that attends the inadequately treated hypertensive state. Diuretics are currently recommended as a first-line therapy for the treatment of hypertension by the Joint National Commission on Detection, Evaluation, and Treatment of Hypertension of the National High Blood Pressure Education Program. In addition, they remain an important element of the treatment regimen for volume overload states, such as nephrotic syndrome, cirrhosis, and heart failure, because they improve the congestive symptomatology that typifies these disease states. This chapter reviews the various diuretic classes and the physiologic adaptations that accompany their use, and establishes the basis for their use in the treatment of volume overload and hypertension.

INDIVIDUAL CLASSES OF DIURETICS

The predominant nephron sites of action of the various diuretic classes are depicted in Figure 9.1. Inter- and intraclass differences exist for all diuretic classes. Diuretic classes of note include proximal tubular, distal tubular, and loop diuretics, potassium (K^+)–sparing agents, and osmotic diuretics.

PROXIMAL TUBULAR DIURETICS

The administration of a carbonic anhydrase (CA) inhibitor ordinarily results in a brisk alkaline diuresis. By inhibiting CA, these compounds decrease the generation of intracellular H^+, which is a prerequisite for the absorption of sodium (Na^+) (see Fig. 9.1). Although CA inhibitors work at the proximal tubule level where the bulk of Na^+ reabsorption occurs, their final diuretic effect is typically muted by reabsorption in more distal nephron segments. Acetazolamide is currently the only CA inhibitor employed primarily for its diuretic properties; others are used topically for treatment of glaucoma. Acetazolamide is readily absorbed and is eliminated by tubular secretion ($\approx 50\%$). Its use is constrained by its transient action and because prolonged use results in a metabolic acidosis. Notably, acetazolamide at doses of 250 to 500 mg daily can correct the metabolic alkalosis that sometimes occurs with thiazide or loop diuretic therapy. Acetazolamide should be used cautiously in patients with advanced kidney failure since it accumulates systemically with repeat

dosing and may have neurologic side effects. In addition, intravenous acetazolamide may reduce the glomerular filtration rate (GFR); however, the dose-dependency of this effect is poorly worked out. The anticonvulsant topiramate also inhibits carbonic anhydrase and therein can cause metabolic acidosis. Unless other treatment options do not exist, patients with a history of renal calculi or known renal tubular acidosis should not receive topiramate except with caution.

DISTAL CONVOLUTED TUBULE DIURETICS

The major site of action of the thiazide diuretics is the early distal convoluted tubule (DCT), where they inhibit the coupled reabsorption of Na^+ and chloride (Cl^-). The water-soluble thiazides such as hydrochlorothiazide (HCTZ) also inhibit CA and, at high doses, further increase Na^+ excretion by this mechanism. Thiazides also inhibit NaCl and fluid reabsorption in the medullary-collecting duct. In addition to these varied effects on Na^+ excretion, thiazide diuretics impair urinary diluting capacity without affecting urinary concentrating mechanisms, reduce calcium (Ca^{++}) and urate excretion, and increase magnesium (Mg^{++}) excretion. The most widely prescribed drug in this class is HCTZ, although chlorthalidone is also commonly used. The onset of diuresis with HCTZ occurs within 2 hours, peaks between 3 and 6 hours, and dose-dependently continues for as long as 12 hours. The half-life (T1/2) of HCTZ is prolonged in patients with decompensated heart failure and/or kidney failure. Doses of thiazide diuretics in the HCTZ equivalent range of 100 to 200 mg/day will initiate a diuresis in patients with chronic kidney disease (CKD), although the natriuretic response is a function of the GFR and filtered Na^+ load.

The concept of "class effect" is debated relative to the actions of DCT diuretics, applied both to BP reduction and cardiovascular (CVR) outcomes. Much of the recent debate on diuretic class effect has centered on the differences between chlorthalidone and HCTZ. Although chlorthalidone and HCTZ are structurally similar, they are quite different pharmacokinetically: chlorthalidone has a lengthier T1/2 (40 to 60 hr) compared with HCTZ (3.2 to 13.1 hr) as well as a larger volume of distribution by virtue of its extensive partitioning into red blood cells. This latter feature creates a depot for chlorthalidone streaming (red cell → plasma → tubular secretion). This plasma half-life difference correlates with a more extended effect of chlorthalidone on diuresis and BP reduction and is a probable explanation for the series of studies now showing chlorthalidone to be a better mg-for-mg antihypertensive than HCTZ.

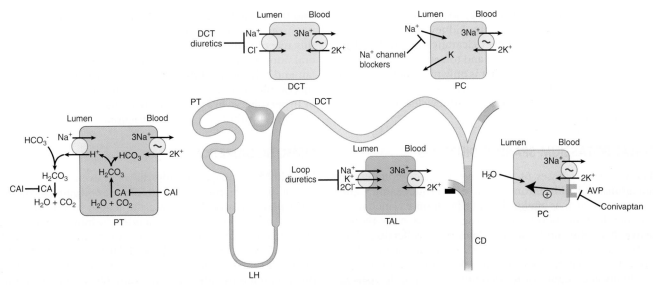

Figure 9.1 **Predominant sites and mechanisms of action of clinically important diuretic drugs.** Color patterns identify sites of action along the nephron and corresponding cell types affected. The proximal tubule (PT, *purple segment*) is represented by a typical PT cell, shown in purple. The loop of Henle (LH) includes a thick ascending limb (TAL, *green segment*) and a typical TAL cell shown in green. The distal convoluted tubule (DCT, *blue segment*) is represented by a typical DCT cell in blue. The collecting duct (CD, *yellow and orange segments*) includes principal cells (PC), both shown in yellow. Note that, for clarity, two principal cells are shown. Both water and salt pathways exist in the same cells. Both intracellular and luminal actions of carbonic anhydrase (CA) inhibitors in suppressing CA are important in their ability to reduce sodium (Na^+) reabsorption by the renal proximal tubule. Note that Na^+ channel blockers probably act along the last half of the DCT and in the connecting tubule as well as in the CD. Spironolactone and eplerenone (not shown) are competitive mineralocorticoid receptor antagonists and act primarily in the cortical collecting tubule. Aquaretics, such as conivaptan, inhibit water reabsorption by PC by blocking the action of arginine vasopressin on V_2 receptors. V_2 receptors facilitate insertion of aquaporin-2 water channels in the apical membrane.

LOOP DIURETICS

Loop diuretics act predominantly at the apical membrane in the thick ascending limb (TAL) of the loop of Henle, where they compete with Cl^- for binding to the $Na^+/K^+/2Cl^-$ cotransporter, thereby inhibiting Na^+ and Cl^- reabsorption. Loop diuretics also have qualitatively minor effects on Na^+ reabsorption within other nephron segments. Other clinically relevant effects of loop diuretics include a decrease in both free water (H_2O) excretion and absorption during H_2O loading and dehydration, respectively; a 30% increase in fractional Ca^{2+} excretion; a significant increase in Mg^{2+} excretion; and a brief increase followed by a more prolonged decrease in uric acid excretion. Loop diuretics also stimulate renal prostaglandin synthesis, particularly that of the vasodilatory prostaglandin E_2 (PGE_2). Angiotensin-II generated following the administration of intravenous loop diuretics and increased synthesis of PGE_2 are the likely reasons for the shift in renal blood flow (RBF) from the inner to the outer cortex of the kidney with these drugs; however, both total RBF and GFR are maintained when loop diuretics are given to normal subjects.

Available loop diuretics include bumetanide, ethacrynic acid, furosemide, and torsemide. These agents are highly bound to albumin; therefore, to gain access to their site of action in the tubular lumen, they must undergo secretion (the same applies to thiazide-type diuretics), which occurs via probenecid-sensitive organic anion transporters localized to the proximal tubule (PT). Tubular secretion of loop diuretics may be impeded by elevated levels of endogenous organic acids, as occur in CKD, and by drugs that share the same transporter, such as salicylates and nonsteroidal

antiinflammatory drugs (NSAIDs). Uremic toxins and fatty acids decrease loop diuretic protein binding and therein alter diuretic pharmacokinetics.

Diuretic excretion rates approximate drug delivery to the medullary TAL and correspond to the observed natriuretic response. The relationship between the urinary loop diuretic excretion rate and natriuresis is that of an S-shaped sigmoidal curve. A normal dose-response relationship, as is typically seen in the untreated patient with hypertension, can be skewed (downward and rightward shifted) by a variety of clinical conditions, ranging from volume depletion to disease-state alterations (heart failure or nephrotic syndrome). As an example of the latter, NSAIDs modify this dose-response relationship by inhibiting prostaglandin synthesis, blunting the expected diuretic effect. Finally, the binding of loop diuretics to urinary protein seems not to be the basis for the blunted diuretic effect in the setting of nephrotic syndrome.

Furosemide is the most widely used loop diuretic. The coefficient of variation for absorption ranges from 25% to 43% for different oral furosemide products, and the bioavailability is equally broad, ranging from 10% to 100%; thus exchanging one oral furosemide formulation for another will not standardize patient response. Notably, both bumetanide and torsemide are better absorbed than is furosemide. The consistency of torsemide's absorption and its longer duration of action are features to consider when loop diuretic therapy is needed in patients with chronic heart failure. Loop diuretics are commonly used in patients with CKD, although kidney clearance of these drugs is reduced in parallel with the level of reduction in the GFR. In general, furosemide's pharmacokinetic profile is more significantly affected in CKD than that of other loop diuretics because furosemide is metabolized by the kidney. Therefore both its renal metabolism and intact clearance are reduced in CKD. Alternatively, bumetanide and torsemide undergo significant hepatic metabolism that is only marginally affected by CKD; thus in CKD their pharmacokinetic profiles only change as the result of decreased kidney clearance of the intact molecules.

DISTAL POTASSIUM-SPARING DIURETICS

There are two classes of K+-sparing diuretics: competitive antagonists of aldosterone, such as spironolactone, and compounds such as amiloride and triamterene, which work independent of aldosterone. Drugs in this class reduce active Na+ absorption in the late DCT/collecting duct (CD). In so doing, basolateral Na+, K+-ATPase activity falls off, intracellular K+ concentration decreases, and the electrochemical gradient for K+ secretion is lowered. K+-sparing diuretics also reduce Ca2+ and Mg2+ excretion, which is a useful feature in heart failure patients. Since K+-sparing diuretics are only modestly natriuretic, their clinical utility resides more in their K+-sparing capacity, particularly when more proximally acting diuretics increase distal Na+ delivery, or in the instance of either primary or secondary hyperaldosteronism.

Spironolactone is a highly protein-bound and well-absorbed, lipid-soluble K+-sparing diuretic with a 20-hour half-life. The onset of action for spironolactone is characteristically slow, with peak response 48 hours or more after the initial dose. 7α-thiomethylspirolactone and canrenone are the two main metabolites of spironolactone, and they account for a substantial portion of its mineralocorticoid receptor blocking activity. Spironolactone, unlike amiloride and triamterene, remains active as a diuretic and antihypertensive agent in advanced kidney failure because its site of action is basolateral; thus it does not require glomerular filtration to gain access to its site of action. Eplerenone is a mineralocorticoid receptor antagonist that is highly selective for the aldosterone receptor. Because of a much lower affinity for androgen and progesterone receptors, its use is associated with considerably less gynecomastia than spironolactone. Eplerenone is at best a very mild diuretic, and its antihypertensive effects originate from nondiuretic aspects of its action.

Amiloride and triamterene are K+-sparing diuretics that block epithelial Na+ channels (ENaC) in the luminal membrane of the CD. Both drugs are actively secreted by cationic transporters that reside in the proximal tubule, and each has only a modest natriuretic effect. They are seldom used in heart failure other than for their K+ and Mg2+-sparing properties. Amiloride and triamterene are both extensively cleared by the kidney and will accumulate with repetitive dosing (unlike spironolactone) in the setting of a reduced GFR.

Arginine vasopressin (AVP), also called antidiuretic hormone (ADH), regulates H$_2$O excretion in a manner largely independent of NaCl handling. The molecular target for ADH is the vasopressin 2 (V$_2$) receptor, located on the basolateral membrane of principal cells of the connecting tubule and the cortical and medullary CD. When ADH binds to V$_2$ receptors, aquaporin 2 channels are subsequently inserted into the apical membrane of epithelial cells along the distal nephron, resulting in increased water absorption. Blocking this receptor therefore increases free water clearance. Several vasopressin antagonists are available, including conivaptan and tolvaptan. These compounds have each been used successfully to increase serum Na+ values in either euvolemic or hypervolemic hyponatremic patients. As such, they are an effective substitute for water restriction.

OSMOTIC DIURETICS

Mannitol is a polysaccharide diuretic given intravenously that is freely eliminated by glomerular filtration. Mannitol is poorly reabsorbed along the length of the nephron and thereby exerts a dose-dependent osmotic effect. This osmotic effect traps water and solutes in the tubular fluid, thus increasing Na+, K+, Cl−, and HCO$_3$− excretion. The plasma T1/2 of mannitol depends on the level of kidney function but is usually between 30 and 60 minutes, resulting in a transient diuresis. Although mannitol historically has been used to reduce the incidence of acute kidney injury (AKI) in patients undergoing cardiopulmonary bypass, experiencing rhabdomyolysis, or following exposure to contrast media, findings from clinical trials in these settings do not support its use. Because mannitol also expands extracellular fluid (ECF) volume and can precipitate pulmonary edema in patients with heart failure, it should be used cautiously in these patients. Moreover, excessive mannitol administration, particularly in the setting of a reduced GFR, can cause dilutional hyponatremia, hyperkalemia, and/or kidney failure. The latter is dose-dependent, relates to afferent arteriolar vasoconstriction, and commonly corrects with the elimination of excess mannitol, as may be achieved with hemodialysis.

ADAPTATION TO DIURETIC THERAPY

Diuretic-induced inhibition of Na+ reabsorption in one nephron segment elicits important adaptations in other segments, which not only limit their antihypertensive and fluid-depleting action but also contribute to the development of side effects. Although a portion of this diuretic resistance is a normal consequence of diuretic use, disease-state related diuretic resistance is often encountered in patients with clinical disorders such as heart failure, cirrhosis, and kidney failure.

The initial dose of a diuretic normally produces a brisk diuresis, which is quickly followed by a new equilibrium state in which daily fluid and electrolyte excretion either matches or is less than intake with body weight stabilization. In nonedematous patients given either a thiazide or a loop diuretic, this adaptation, called braking phenomenon, occurs within 1 to 2 days and limits net weight loss to 1 to 2 kg. This braking phenomenon is most evident in normal subjects given a loop diuretic. For example, furosemide administered orally to subjects ingesting a high-Na+ diet (270 mmol/24 hr) produces an initial brisk natriuresis, which results in a negative Na+ balance over the ensuing 6 hours. This is followed by an 18-hour period when Na+ excretion is reduced to levels well below the prescribed Na+ intake, resulting in a positive Na+ balance. This postdiuresis Na+ retention

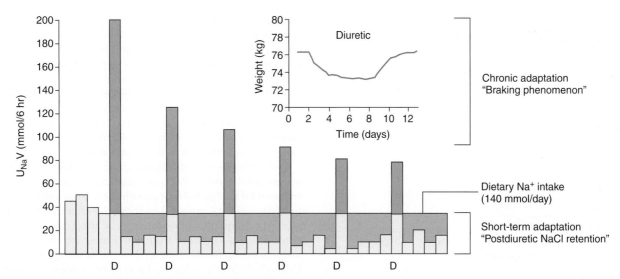

Figure 9.2   Effects of a loop diuretic on urinary sodium (Na⁺) excretion. Each bar represents a 6-hour time interval. Purple bars indicate periods during which urinary Na⁺ excretion ($U_{Na}V$) exceeds dietary intake. *D* indicates administration of a loop diuretic. Blue areas indicate periods of postdiuretic NaCl retention, during which dietary Na⁺ intake exceeds urinary Na⁺ excretion. The horizontal black line indicates dietary Na⁺ intake per 24-hour period. Changes in the magnitude of the natriuretic response over several days are reflective of the braking phenomenon. Inset shows the effect of diuretics on weight (and extracellular fluid volume) during several days of diuretic administration. (Data redrawn from Wilcox CS, Mitch WE, Kelly RA et al: Response of the kidney to furosemide: I. Effects of salt intake and renal compensation, *J Lab Clin Med* 102:450-458, 1983.)

matches the initial natriuresis, with the result being a neutral Na⁺ balance state and no weight loss. After 3 successive days of furosemide administration, a similar pattern of Na⁺ loss and retention is demonstrated each day (Fig. 9.2). This phenomenon is quite reproducible, being evident after even a month of furosemide administration. However, if Na⁺ intake is kept very low, balance can remain negative after a single dose of furosemide, even though there is some blunting of the initial natriuretic response.

The mechanism for the braking phenomenon is complex. The relationship between natriuresis and the rate of furosemide excretion is shifted to the right in subjects receiving a low-salt diet, which denotes a blunting of the tubular response. The importance of ECF volume depletion in postdiuretic Na⁺ retention has been clearly shown, although there is an ECF volume-independent component to this process. The latter appears to be unrelated to aldosterone, because spironolactone therapy has little effect on the Na⁺ retention. Structural hypertrophy in the distal nephron occurs in rats receiving prolonged infusions of loop diuretics. These structural changes are marked by increased distal nephron Na⁺ and Cl⁻ absorption and K⁺ secretion, phenomena which are aldosterone independent. These structural adaptations may contribute to postdiuretic Na⁺ retention and to diuretic tolerance in humans, potentially explaining the Na⁺ retention that persists for up to 2 weeks after loop diuretic therapy is stopped.

NEUROHUMORAL RESPONSE TO DIURETICS

Plasma renin activity (PRA) and plasma aldosterone concentrations rise within minutes of receiving an intravenous diuretic, a process that is independent of volume loss and/or sympathetic nervous system (SNS) activation. This rise in PRA is caused by inhibition of NaCl reabsorption at the macula densa in conjunction with loop-diuretic stimulation of renal prostaglandin release. This first wave of neurohumoral effects,

although transient, recognizably increases afterload and for a short period of time may lessen the efficacy of a loop diuretic. Shortly after this initial rise in PRA, diuretics cause a more sustained increase in PRA and aldosterone arising from an increase in SNS activity (β-agonism) and a fall in ECF volume. The increased renal prostaglandin production is the likely explanation for the preload reduction and decrease in ventricular filling pressures that occur within 15 minutes of loop diuretic administration.

DIURETIC TREATMENT OF EDEMA

The pathophysiology of Na⁺ and H₂O retention in patients with edema is characterized by a complex interchange of hemodynamic and neurohumoral factors. For example, systemically perceived arterial underfilling sets into motion related Na⁺ and H₂O retention in patients with heart failure. The level of neurohormonal activation, the magnitude of renal vasoconstriction, and the extent to which kidney perfusion is reduced moderates this process. In other instances, such as in patients with reduced GFR and/or nephrotic syndrome, Na⁺ and H₂O retention is derived from a more primary set of kidney processes. In each instance, however, efforts should be directed toward correcting the underlying disease state even as diuretic use is being contemplated.

Two important factors should be considered before and/or concurrent with initiation of diuretic therapy: restriction of dietary Na⁺ intake (to 2-4 g per day) and dose minimization or elimination of drugs that foster Na⁺ retention such as NSAIDs, nonspecific vasodilators such as hydralazine and minoxidil, and thiazolidinediones used in the treatment of diabetes. The initial choice of drug and dosage is often a rather arbitrary process, centering on the etiology and severity of the edema. A hierarchy exists among the thiazide diuretics, with longer-acting compounds, such as chlorthalidone, favored in edematous patients. Chlorthalidone can be quite effective at doses of 25 to 50 mg/day in mild to moderate

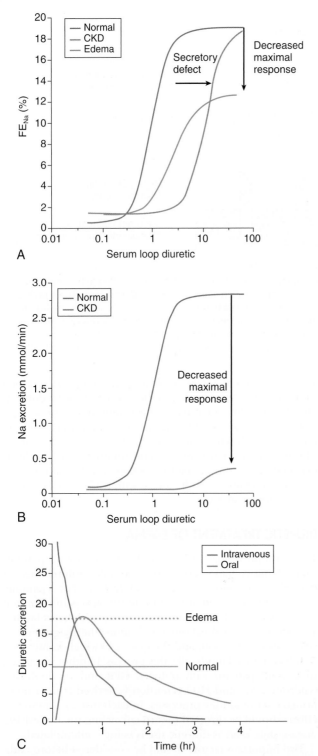

edematous states. When edema becomes more severe, usually when the underlying disease state has worsened and/or dietary Na⁺ restriction cannot be satisfactorily maintained, conversion to a loop diuretic-based regimen is prudent. Combination diuretic therapy can be considered when the severity of the edema requires the "sequential nephron blockade" that marks multidiuretic therapy and/or the underlying disease state is particularly sensitive to non-loop diuretic medications, as is the case for spironolactone (50 to 400-mg/day range) in patients with cirrhosis and ascites.

Determining the threshold dose for diuretic effect is an essential clinical exercise, particularly in patients with reduced GFR (Fig. 9.3). Gradually increasing a diuretic dose until a response is seen will establish the effective dose; thereafter, the frequency of dosing can be determined based on clinical need. The dose from which dose escalation starts is influenced by the GFR as well as the severity of edema. If kidney function is reduced, the dose-response curve shifts to the right, and the maximal effectiveness, based on absolute Na⁺ excretion, can be significantly reduced, making dietary Na⁺ restriction of the utmost importance. In a significantly edematous patient with CKD, furosemide 40 mg, torsemide 10 mg, or bumetanide 1-2 mg given twice daily could be considered an initial doses that is gradually increased until the desired effect is achieved. Often, the dose that elicits an increase in urine output can be continued indefinitely, unless the underlying disease state worsens and/or dietary Na⁺ intake becomes excessive. Of note, once euvolemia is reached, diuretic dose can occasionally be reduced if an Na⁺-restricted diet can be followed.

DIURETIC RESISTANCE: CAUSES AND TREATMENT

Control of ECF volume expansion in most edematous patients is an attainable goal, albeit one that requires systematic application of the principles of diuretic therapy. Diuretic-resistant patients are common in both outpatient and hospital settings. In the latter, diuretic resistance is linked to the complexity of the volume-retaining state, with multiple organ systems often implicated and the acuity of illness being a major driver. In outpatients, dietary Na⁺ indiscretion is a key factor that often is overlooked. What constitutes a "dry" or "target" weight in the edematous patient frequently is defined by symptom relief, patient preference, level of comorbid illness, and the determination of realistic goals with available therapies. An organized and systematic approach to diuretic therapy can usually result in a safe and effective regimen (Fig. 9.4).

As discussed, poorly regulated Na⁺ intake can limit the net negative Na⁺ balance that might otherwise occur with an appropriate diuretic regimen. A 24-hour urine Na⁺ excretion higher than 100 mmol/day is a reasonable marker of adequate diuretic action; however, obtaining a complete 24-hour urine collection can prove cumbersome. An alternative approach to assessing the adequacy of diuretic action is to obtain an FE_{Na} 1 to 2 hours after oral ingestion of a well-absorbed loop diuretic, such as torsemide, and, if this value is above 2%, "true" diuretic resistance is unlikely. The slow rate and variable extent of diuretic absorption, as is the case with furosemide, can create the impression that diuretic resistance is present when the "resistance" is more a reflection of altered pharmacokinetics. This is a less common issue at higher furosemide doses (>80-120 mg/day).

Figure 9.3 A, Comparison of effects of chronic kidney disease (CKD) and edematous conditions (edema) on the loop diuretic dose response, expressed as the fractional Na⁺ excretion (FE_{Na}). Diuretic delivery via secretion into the lumen is impaired in CKD (pharmacokinetic abnormality), whereas the response to delivered drug is diminished with edema (pharmacodynamic defect). **B,** Effect of CKD on the absolute response to a loop diuretic (compare with panel **A**). **C,** Pharmacokinetics of intravenous and oral loop diuretics. The diuretic thresholds for normal and edematous individuals are shown as horizontal lines. Whereas a normal individual responds appropriately to either an intravenous or oral diuretic, some edematous individuals achieve threshold levels only with intravenous diuretic administration.

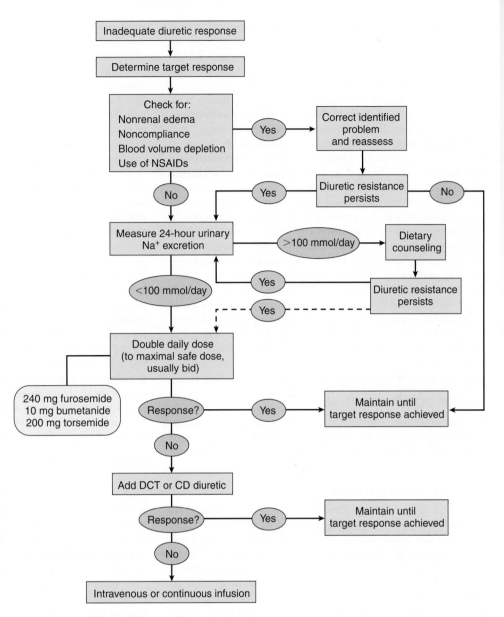

Figure 9.4 Sample algorithm for the approach to treatment of a diuretic-resistant patient. Combination diuretic regimens are addressed in the text. Maximal recommended loop diuretic doses given as monotherapy are provided in the yellow box. Note that higher doses are recommended for patients with acute kidney injury. Larger doses may improve the natriuretic response because of a lengthier duration of action; however, this can occur at the cost of increased side effects. *CD,* Collecting duct; *DCT,* distal convoluted tubule; *NSAIDs,* nonsteroidal antiinflammatory drugs. (Modified with permission from Wilcox CS: Diuretics. In Brenner B, editor: *Brenner and Rector's the kidney,* ed 5, Philadelphia, WB Saunders, 1996.)

Impaired renal clearance of a diuretic may be a factor in attenuating diuretic response. In CKD, the tubular secretion of loop diuretics is slowed, requiring higher doses to achieve sufficient serum levels to overcome the pathologic impediment to luminal drug delivery. Conversion from an intravenous loop diuretic to an orally administered one is an unpredictable process. In the instance of furosemide, approximately twice as much diuretic must be given orally to match what might have been given intravenously. However, when the diuretic is orally administered, the uncertain process of absorption may lend itself to the notion that the patient is diuretic resistant when in reality the oral dose was too low or administration was too infrequent.

Nephrotic syndrome often presents as a diuretic-resistant state. Alterations in both the pharmacokinetics and pharmacodynamics of loop diuretics account for their blunted effect. Loop diuretic delivery is impaired in hypoalbuminemic individuals because the renal secretion of diuretics is strongly dependent on the plasma albumin concentration. In patients with nephrotic syndrome, the dose-response relationship for diuretic effect is shifted to the right (higher threshold for effect) and downwards (reduction in maximal response or decreased sensitivity). Diuretics can bind to albumin in the tubular fluid, decreasing the amount of unbound, active drug available for interaction with its tubular receptor. When urinary albumin concentrations are greater than 4 g/L, as much as 65% of the diuretic reaching the tubular fluid is bound to albumin. Consequently, starting doses of two to three times higher than the normal dose are recommended to ensure delivery of adequate amounts of free drug to the site of action. Accordingly, strategies to reduce proteinuria may aid diuresis in nephrotic individuals. The cornerstone of therapy for nephrotic syndrome–related edema is restricting Na^+ intake, an approach that usually needs to be supported by diuretic therapy. However, the "reduced" response often requires more frequent dosing of a loop diuretic. Other therapies include concurrent administration of loop diuretics and albumin. Hemodynamic factors may also impact diuretic resistance, particularly in systolic heart failure. In this setting, positive inotropes, such as dobutamine, can improve renal blood flow and, therefore, diuretic action. Allowing BP to drift up by limiting inhibition of renin-angiotensin-aldosterone system (RAAS) can also help restore diuretic action by potentially reducing systemic hypotension and renal hypoperfusion.

Other approaches to diuretic therapy in patients with diuretic resistance include high-dose oral loop diuretic therapy, diuretic rotation, combination diuretic therapy, continuous infusions, admixed albumin/furosemide, admixed high-dose loop diuretic/hypertonic saline, admixed nesiritide/loop diuretic therapy, and vasopressin receptor antagonists. These approaches are not mutually exclusive and, for the most part, are employed with limited supporting scientific data. When the previously mentioned principles of therapy are applied, most diuretic-resistant patients respond to therapy, albeit in a variable fashion; however, a major limiting factor in "diuresing" volume-overloaded patients is the ensuing reduction in GFR. Accordingly, obtaining effective control of ECF volume excess requires a certain artfulness, with careful timing of the ongoing diuresis to avoid subsequent response-limiting reductions in GFR and often preventable electrolyte complications. As such, when the principles of diuretic therapy are carefully applied to the management of the volume-overloaded patient, more times than not a patient can be safely and effectively diuresed.

DIURETIC DOSING STRATEGIES

Not uncommonly, simple approaches to diuretic resistance may fail (see Fig 9.4). Several strategies can be used to control edema in such patients, including the very simple maneuver of increasing the frequency of diuretic administration.

High-Dose Oral Loop Diuretics

Very high doses of loop diuretics have been suggested as an alternative for the management of diuretic resistance, although this approach has been employed with some hesitancy, presumably because of concern for toxicity. Nevertheless, in one outpatient advanced heart failure cohort, oral administration of furosemide (dosage range 700 to 1000 mg/day) was both safe and effective. With regard to toxicity, furosemide absorption is typically both delayed and incomplete, in part relating to gut wall edema, which lowers the peak systemic concentrations that can be reached with such a therapeutic approach.

Diuretic Rotation

Rotation from one diuretic class to another and, occasionally, rotation within a class may induce diuresis in a patient previously unresponsive to the diuretic effects of a different compound. This practice has not been critically examined and, at best, remains hearsay. If response varies among orally administered diuretics within the same class, it likely reflects differences in the rate of drug absorption and the positive effect garnered from a more efficient time course for urinary drug delivery. Also, better hemodynamics may exist when a diuretic is "switched" that may prove the basis for a "recovered" response.

Combination Diuretic Therapy

The use of diuretic combinations in diuretic resistant states such as nephrotic syndrome or heart failure is predicated on the ability of diuretics of different classes to effect sequential nephron blockade, thereby generating an additive response. Another consideration relates to the ability of thiazide diuretic to negate the effect of distal tubular cell hypertrophy that is induced by loop diuretic therapy to increase Na^+ absorption. Although all permutations of diuretic combination have been tried, the use of a thiazide and a loop diuretic with or without a potassium-sparing diuretic is most common in clinical practice. Although a loop diuretic and metolazone are commonly used, the diuretic response to these drugs may be unpredictable owing to the erratic pattern of absorption for metolazone. Achieving adequate systemic concentrations of metolazone to effect synergy with a loop diuretic may require multiple doses and thus several hours to days of dosing. If an intravenous DCT diuretic is required, chlorothiazide (500-1000 mg) may be used with a loop diuretic. In the outpatient setting, when circumstances are typically less pressing, a starting dose of 2.5 to 5 mg of metolazone daily or every other day can be given with a loop diuretic. With the initiation of combination therapy, the dosage of loop diuretic is generally kept constant until a response is evident. Once a diuretic response occurs, the frequency of administration of metolazone can be decreased; often, the loop diuretic dose can also be lowered. In all instances, careful monitoring of the achieved diuretic response is warranted in order to avoid overdiuresis and significant electrolyte depletion. If either occurs, both drugs should be discontinued and therapeutic measures instituted in anticipation of continuing diuresis, because the plasma half-life of metolazone is prolonged, particularly in the setting of reduced GFR.

Diuretic Infusions

Pharmacokinetic and pharmacodynamic studies suggest potential advantages to continuous infusion of loop diuretics in diuretic-resistant patients. However, in a recently published study in acute decompensated heart failure comparing bolus with intravenous furosemide, those receiving a continuous infusion of furosemide fared no better in terms of global symptom assessment or change in serum creatinine than those who received furosemide by bolus. Accordingly, the use of loop diuretic infusions becomes a matter of personal preference.

Admixed Albumin and Furosemide

In patients with edema and hypoalbuminemia, options include administering albumin and furosemide as separate infusions or premixed in a syringe. Whether these approaches reproducibly generate a meaningful diuretic response is untested. If separate albumin infusions and intravenous furosemide are contemplated, this should probably be limited to severely hypoalbuminemic patients in whom aggressively applied traditional approaches have failed to elicit an adequate diuresis. A premixed infusion of loop diuretic and albumin was studied in cirrhotic patients with ascites (40 mg of furosemide and 25 g of albumin premixed ex vivo versus 40 mg of furosemide alone); it failed to improve the natriuretic response, rendering this a less advisable approach.

Hypertonic Saline and Loop Diuretic Therapy

This combination may seem counterintuitive based on the presence of an already volume-expanded state. However, the hypertonic saline appears to temporarily compensate for the "underfilling" related to the disease state, improving systemic and renal hemodynamics and therefore the likelihood of response to an administered diuretic. One such regimen used furosemide (250-1000 mg twice daily IV) plus hypertonic saline (150 mL H_2O with NaCl 1.4-4.6%) and was shown to be a safe and effective alternative to repeated paracentesis when treating hospitalized patients with cirrhosis and refractory ascites.

Nesiritide and Loop Diuretic Therapy

Although nesiritide may enhance the effect of loop diuretic therapy, relating to its generally favorable effect on cardiac hemodynamics as well as its positive effects on the neurohormonal profile characteristic of heart failure, recent studies in stable heart failure patients showed that nesiritide and furosemide used together afford no incremental benefit for Na^+ excretion compared with furosemide alone. This may be related to BP reductions and accompanying decreased tubular delivery of furosemide. Nesiritide should be reserved as a last step to potentially enhance diuretic action in the patient who has CKD and a high enough BP that any ensuing reduction is not effect limiting.

Vasopressin Receptor Antagonists

These aquaretic agents have been added to loop diuretic regimens to augment diuretic effect. In that regard, without adversely affecting hemodynamic variables, neurohormones, renal blood flow, or GFR, conivaptan increased both the diuretic and natriuretic response to furosemide in patients with chronic heart failure; however, the combination of a vasopressin receptor antagonist and a loop diuretic is at an early stage of maturation in its clinical use and should not be viewed as a routine clinical option in the patient with diuretic resistance.

SPECIAL CONSIDERATIONS IN EDEMA MANAGEMENT

ISOLATED ULTRAFILTRATION

In some patients with ECF volume expansion and resistant edema, isolated peripheral venovenous ultrafiltration (UF) may be of some use, particularly in the patient with volume overload and acute decompensated heart failure. This approach can now occur at the bedside with simplified technology and not overly complicated staff training. Small studies suggest that UF may allow for more effective fluid removal compared with diuretic therapy, resulting in improved quality of life, more rapid symptomatic improvement, and reduced rehospitalization rates in acute decompensated heart failure. Questions with this approach include whether the beneficial effects, such as the improvement in volume status and the observed decrease in neurohormonal activation, are sustainable following UF therapy and whether diuretic responsiveness is restored in patients whose basis for UF therapy was extreme diuretic resistance. Further investigation is needed to define the role of UF in decompensated heart failure.

DIALYSIS

In dialysis patients, interdialytic weight gain may be substantial. If sufficient residual GFR exists to permit a meaningful diuretic response, loop diuretic therapy can be considered. Patients with residual kidney function (urine output of ≥200 mL/24 hr) on diuretic therapy have been shown to be almost twice as likely to retain urine output after 1 year as were patients not receiving diuretics. Because of the high plasma protein binding common to all loop diuretics, less than 10% of the total body stores of any loop diuretic are eliminated during a routine hemodialysis session; accordingly, diuretic dosing can occur without any impact from the dialysis process.

DIURETIC-RELATED ADVERSE EFFECTS

Diuretic-related side effects can be divided into those with recognizable mechanisms, such as electrolyte and metabolic abnormalities, and those that are more obscure mechanistically, such as impotence and idiosyncratic drug reactions. Electrolyte changes are the most common side effects of diuretics and ostensibly most noticeable with the more potent loop diuretics. However, the strength of a diuretic is likely not as critical as is its duration of action. For example, long-acting thiazide-type diuretics, such as chlorthalidone and metolazone, although considerably less potent than a loop diuretic, can still cause significant hypokalemia and hypomagnesemia.

HYPONATREMIA

Hyponatremia is a potentially serious complication of diuretic therapy. Thiazide diuretics are more apt to cause hyponatremia than are loop diuretics because they increase Na^+ excretion and preclude maximal urine dilution while preserving the kidney's inherent concentrating ability. Older adult women treated with thiazide diuretics are most frequently affected, and the onset of hyponatremia is usually within the first few weeks of therapy. Treatment for mild, asymptomatic hyponatremia can include withholding diuretics, restricting free H_2O intake, and normalizing serum K^+ values if hypokalemia exists. Severe, symptomatic hyponatremia, complicated by seizures, requires emergent correction (see Chapter 7).

HYPOKALEMIA AND HYPERKALEMIA

Hypokalemia is a common finding in patients treated with loop and/or thiazide diuretics. Mechanisms that contribute to hypokalemia with diuretic use include augmented flow-dependent K^+ secretion in the distal nephron, a fall in luminal Cl^- concentration in the distal tubule, metabolic alkalosis, and stimulation of aldosterone and/or vasopressin release, both of which promote distal K^+ secretion. It is unusual for serum K^+ values to drop below 3.0 mmol/L in diuretic-treated outpatients, apart from a high dietary Na^+ intake and/or when a long-acting diuretic is being given (as is the case with chlorthalidone). Although mild degrees of diuretic-induced hypokalemia can be associated with increased ventricular ectopy and altered glucose homeostasis, the clinical significance of diuretic-induced hypokalemia is still argued. Profound degrees of hypokalemia with serum K^+ concentrations less than 2.5 mmol/L, however, can lead to generalized muscle weakness and, at the extremes, rhabdomyolysis and AKI.

Potassium-sparing diuretics (such as triamterene and amiloride) and mineralocorticoid-receptor antagonists (such as spironolactone and eplerenone) are used for their ability to conserve K^+ when it might otherwise be lost with thiazide and loop diuretic therapy. In certain instances, K^+ retention occurs such that hyperkalemia develops with these compounds. Hyperkalemia with K^+-sparing diuretics is usually encountered in patients with an existing reduction in their GFR, those who develop acute-on-chronic kidney failure, persons treated with an angiotensin converting enzyme (ACE) inhibitor/angiotensin receptor blocker and/or an NSAID, or with other situations that predispose to hyperkalemia, such as metabolic acidosis, hyporeninemic hypoaldosteronism, and administration of trimethoprim-sulfamethoxazole or heparin therapy (including subcutaneous heparin regimens).

ACID-BASE CHANGES

Mild metabolic alkalosis is a common feature of thiazide diuretic therapy, particularly at higher doses, whereas severe metabolic alkalosis may be seen with loop diuretic use. The generation of a metabolic alkalosis with diuretic therapy is mainly due to contraction of the ECF space caused by urinary losses of a relatively HCO_3^--free fluid. Diuretic-induced metabolic alkalosis is corrected with K^+ and/or Na^+ chloride, although the latter may be unworkable in volume-expanded patients (such as those with heart failure). In this setting, a K^+-sparing diuretic or a CA inhibitor, such as acetazolamide, may be considered. Metabolic alkalosis also impairs the natriuretic response to loop diuretics, a factor that may be relevant in diuretic resistance. All K^+-sparing diuretics can cause metabolic acidosis, an occurrence of some significance to older adults and patients with CKD.

HYPOMAGNESEMIA

Loop diuretics inhibit Mg^{2+} reabsorption in the loop of Henle, the site where approximately 30% of the filtered load of Mg^{2+} is reabsorbed. All K^+-sparing diuretics diminish the magnesuria that derives from thiazide or loop diuretic use. Cellular Mg^{2+} depletion occurs in 20% to 50% of patients during thiazide therapy and can be present even in the setting of a normal serum Mg^{2+} concentration. Hypomagnesemia-related symptoms include depression, muscle weakness, refractory hypokalemia, hypocalcemia, and atrial/ventricular arrhythmias. Many of these abnormalities, particularly refractory hypokalemia and hypocalcemia, correct promptly with even modest amounts of Mg^{2+}.

HYPERURICEMIA

Thiazide diuretic therapy dose-dependently increases serum urate concentrations by as much as 35%, an effect related to decreased renal clearance of urate and one that is most prominent in those with the highest pretherapy urate clearance values. Decreased urate clearance may be linked to increased urate reabsorption secondary to diuretic-related ECF volume depletion and competition for its tubular secretion, because both diuretics and urate undergo tubular secretion by the same organic anion transporter pathway.

Hyperuricemia itself has been linked to new-onset hypertension, cardiovascular events, and perhaps the development and progression of CKD. It is unclear what relationship these items have to hyperuricemia stemming from diuretic therapy.

HYPERGLYCEMIA

Prolonged thiazide diuretic therapy impairs glucose tolerance and occasionally precipitates diabetes mellitus. Hyperglycemia has been linked to diuretic-induced hypokalemia, which inhibits insulin secretion by β cells. Diuretic-associated glucose intolerance appears to be dose-related, less common with loop diuretics, and, in many instances, reversible on withdrawal of the agent (although the data on reversibility in HCTZ-treated patients appear conflicting). In sum, long-term thiazide therapy can be expected to cause only small changes, if any, in fasting serum glucose concentration, an effect that might be reversed with the simultaneous use of a K^+-sparing diuretic.

HYPERLIPIDEMIA

Short-term thiazide diuretic therapy can dose-dependently elevate serum total cholesterol levels, modestly increase low-density lipoprotein cholesterol levels, and raise triglyceride levels, while minimally changing high-density lipoprotein cholesterol concentrations. All diuretics, including loop diuretics, cause these lipid changes, with the possible exception of indapamide. The mechanism of diuretic-induced dyslipidemia remains uncertain, but has been attributed to insulin resistance and/or reflex activation of the RAAS and SNS in response to volume depletion.

OTOTOXICITY

Loop diuretics are well established as ototoxic agents. Loop diuretics are direct inhibitors of the $Na^+/K^+/2Cl^-$ cotransport system, which also exists in the marginal and dark cells of the stria vascularis to secrete endolymph. Thus the ototoxicity of these agents may be indirect, as a result changes in ionic composition and fluid volume within the endolymph. Loop diuretic–induced ototoxicity usually occurs within 20 minutes of infusion and is typically reversible, although permanent deafness has been reported, particularly with ethacrynic acid. Ototoxicity is related both to the rate of infusion and to peak serum concentrations of a diuretic, and its risk appears to be higher with furosemide than bumetanide. In general, the rate of furosemide infusion should not exceed 4 mg/minute and serum concentrations should be maintained below 40 mcg/mL Patients with kidney failure and those receiving concomitant aminoglycoside therapy are at greatest risk for developing ototoxicity.

DRUG ALLERGY

Photosensitivity dermatitis occurs rarely during thiazide or furosemide therapy. Hydrochlorothiazide more commonly causes photosensitivity than do the other thiazides. Acute allergic interstitial nephritis with fever, rash, and eosinophilia, although an uncommon complication of diuretics, can cause permanent kidney failure if the drug exposure is protracted.

It may occur abruptly or months after therapy is begun with a thiazide diuretic or, less commonly, with furosemide. The chemical structure of ethacrynic acid differs from that of the other loop diuretics, making it a safe replacement in patients having experienced diuretic-related allergic complications.

ADVERSE DRUG–DRUG INTERACTIONS

Loop diuretics can potentiate aminoglycoside nephrotoxicity. By causing hypokalemia, diuretics increase digitalis toxicity. Plasma lithium (Li$^+$) concentrations can increase with diuretic therapy if significant volume contraction occurs. Lithium levels should be closely monitored in all patients being administered Li$^+$ in conjunction with diuretics. NSAIDs can both antagonize the effects of diuretics and predispose diuretic-treated patients to a reversible form of AKI. The combination of indomethacin and triamterene may be particularly hazardous in that prolonged AKI can occur. Triamterene can also crystallize, forming kidney stones, a phenomenon unique to triamterene. A reversible reduction in GFR may also develop when excessive diuresis occurs in patients treated with RAAS inhibitors.

BIBLIOGRAPHY

Brater DC: Diuretic therapy, *N Engl J Med* 339:387-395, 1998.

Chalasani N, Gorski JC, Horlander JC, et al: Effects of albumin/furosemide mixtures on responses to furosemide in hypoalbuminemic patients, *J Am Soc Nephrol* 12:1010-1016, 2001.

Costanzo MR, Ronco C: Isolated ultrafiltration in heart failure patients, *Curr Cardiol Rep* 14:254-264, 2012.

Felker GM, Lee KL, Bull DA, et al: NHLBI Heart Failure Clinical Research Network: Diuretic strategies in patients with acute decompensated heart failure, *N Engl J Med* 364:797-805, 2011.

Fliser D, Schröter M, Neubeck M, et al: Co-administration of thiazides increases the efficacy of loop diuretics even in patients with advanced renal failure, *Kidney Int* 46:482-488, 1994.

Freda BJ, Slawsky M, Mallidi J, et al: Decongestive treatment of acute decompensated heart failure: cardiorenal implications of ultrafiltration and diuretics, *Am J Kidney Dis* 58:1005-1017, 2011.

Goldsmith SR, Gilbertson DT, Mackedanz SA, et al: Renal effects of conivaptan, furosemide, and the combination in patients with chronic heart failure, *J Card Fail* 17:982-989, 2011.

Hari P, Bagga A: Co-administration of albumin and furosemide in patients with the nephrotic syndrome, *Saudi J Kidney Dis Transpl* 23:371-372, 2012.

Hix JK, Silver S, Sterns RH: Diuretic-associated hyponatremia. *Semin Nephrol* 31:553-566, 2011.

Karadsheh F, Weir MR: Thiazide and thiazide-like diuretics: an opportunity to reduce blood pressure in patients with advanced kidney disease, *Curr Hypertens Rep* 14, 2012. 416–320.

Rosner MH, Gupta R, Ellison D, et al: Management of cirrhotic ascites: physiological basis of diuretic action, *Eur J Intern Med* 17:8-19, 2006.

Shankar SS, Brater DC: Loop diuretics: from the Na-K-2Cl transporter to clinical use, *Am J Physiol Renal Physiol* 284:F11-F21, 2003.

Sica DA, Gehr TW: Diuretic combinations in refractory oedema states: pharmacokinetic-pharmacodynamic relationships, *Clin Pharmacokinet* 30:229-249, 1996.

Sica DA, Gehr TW: Diuretic use in stage five chronic kidney disease and end-stage renal disease, *Curr Opinion Nephrol Hypertens* 12:483-490, 2003.

Sica DA: Diuretic use in chronic kidney disease, *Nat Rev Nephrol* 8:100-109, 2011.

Tuttolomondo A, Pinto A, Parrinello G, et al: Intravenous high-dose furosemide and hypertonic saline solutions for refractory heart failure and ascites, *Semin Nephrol* 31:513-522, 2011.

Wilcox CS: New insights into diuretic use in the patient with chronic renal disease, *J Am Soc Nephrol* 13:798-805, 2002.

Zillich AJ, Garg J, Basu S, et al: Thiazide diuretics, potassium, and the development of diabetes: a quantitative review, *Hypertension* 48:219-224, 2006.

10 Disorders of Potassium Metabolism

Michael Allon

MECHANISMS OF POTASSIUM HOMEOSTASIS

Total body potassium is about 3500 mmol. Approximately 98% of the total is intracellular, primarily in skeletal muscle, and to a lesser extent in liver. The remaining 2% (about 70 mmol) is in the extracellular fluid. Two homeostatic systems help to maintain potassium homeostasis. The first system regulates potassium excretion (kidney and intestine). The second regulates potassium shifts between the extracellular and intracellular fluid compartments.

EXTERNAL POTASSIUM BALANCE

The average American diet contains about 100 mmol of potassium per day. Dietary potassium intake may vary widely from day to day. To stay in potassium balance, it is necessary to increase potassium excretion when dietary potassium increases and to decrease potassium excretion when dietary potassium decreases. Normally, the kidneys excrete 90% to 95% of dietary potassium, with the remaining 5% to 10% excreted by the gut. Potassium excretion by the kidney is a relatively slow process, taking 6 to 12 hours to excrete an acute potassium load.

RENAL HANDLING OF POTASSIUM

To understand the physiologic factors that determine renal excretion of potassium, it is critical to review the main features of tubular potassium handling. Plasma potassium is freely filtered across the glomerular capillary into the proximal tubule. It is subsequently completely reabsorbed by the proximal tubule and loop of Henle. In the distal tubule and the collecting duct, potassium is secreted into the tubular lumen. For practical purposes, urinary excretion of potassium reflects potassium secretion into the lumen of the distal tubule and collecting duct. Thus, any factor that stimulates potassium secretion increases urinary potassium excretion; conversely, any factor that inhibits potassium secretion decreases urinary potassium excretion.

PHYSIOLOGIC REGULATION OF RENAL POTASSIUM EXCRETION

Five major physiologic factors stimulate distal potassium secretion and increase excretion: aldosterone; high distal sodium delivery; high urine flow rate; high [K+] in tubular cell; and metabolic alkalosis. Aldosterone directly increases the activity of the Na,K-ATPase in the collecting duct cells, increasing intracellular potassium content and facilitating secretion of potassium into the tubular lumen. Medical

conditions that impair aldosterone production or secretion (e.g., diabetic nephropathy, chronic interstitial nephritis) or drugs that inhibit aldosterone production or action (e.g., nonsteroidal antiinflammatory drugs [NSAIDs], angiotensin converting enzyme [ACE] inhibitors, angiotensin receptor blockers [ARBs], heparin, spironolactone) decrease potassium secretion by the kidney. Conversely, medical conditions associated with increased aldosterone levels (primary aldosteronism, secondary aldosteronism caused by diuretics or vomiting) increase potassium excretion by the kidney. Although there is profound secondary hyperaldosteronism in congestive heart failure and cirrhosis, each of these conditions may be associated with hyperkalemia because of decreased delivery of sodium to the distal nephron. Many diuretics increase urinary potassium excretion by a number of mechanisms, including high distal sodium delivery, high urine flow rate, metabolic alkalosis, and hyperaldosteronism from volume depletion. Poorly controlled diabetes commonly increases urinary potassium excretion because of osmotic diuresis with high urinary flow rate and high distal delivery of sodium.

Reabsorption of sodium in the collecting duct occurs through selective sodium channels. This creates an electronegative charge within the tubular lumen relative to the tubular epithelial cell, which in turn promotes secretion of cations (K+ and H+) into the lumen. Therefore, drugs that block the sodium channel in the collecting duct decrease potassium secretion. Conversely, in Liddle syndrome, a rare genetic disorder, this sodium channel is constitutively open, resulting in avid sodium reabsorption and excessive potassium secretion.

ADAPTATION IN CHRONIC KIDNEY DISEASE

In patients with chronic kidney disease (CKD), the kidney compensates by increasing the efficiency of potassium excretion. Clearly, there is a limit to renal compensation, and a significant loss of kidney function impairs the ability to excrete potassium, thereby predisposing to a positive potassium balance and a tendency to hyperkalemia. In most patients with CKD overt hyperkalemia does not occur until the creatinine clearance falls below 10 mL/min. Serum aldosterone levels are elevated in many patients with CKD. Aldosterone stimulates the activity of both Na,K-ATPase and H,K-ATPase, thereby promoting secretion of potassium in the collecting duct and defending against hyperkalemia. These adaptive mechanisms are less effective in patients with acute kidney injury (AKI) as compared to those with CKD. Moreover, patients with AKI are often hypotensive, resulting in tissue hypoperfusion and release of potassium from ischemic limbs. For these reasons, severe hyperkalemia occurs more frequently in patients with AKI than it does in those with CKD.

A subset of patient with CKD develops hyperkalemia at moderately reduced GFRs (< 50 ml/min). This results from a failure to appreciably increase aldosterone levels, typically in association with hyperchloremic, normal anion gap metabolic acidosis (Type IV renal tubular acidosis). This condition is most commonly associated with diabetic nephropathy and chronic interstitial nephritis. Moreover, administration of drugs that inhibit aldosterone production or secretion (e.g., ACE inhibitors, ARBs, NSAIDs, heparin) may provoke hyperkalemia in patients with mild to moderate CKD.

INTESTINAL POTASSIUM EXCRETION

Similar to the renal collecting duct, the small intestine and colon secrete potassium in response to aldosterone. In normal individuals, intestinal potassium excretion plays a minor role in potassium homeostasis. However, in patients with advanced CKD, intestinal potassium secretion is increased three- to fourfold, thereby contributing significantly to potassium homeostasis. This adaptation is limited and is inadequate to compensate for the loss of excretory function in patients with kidney failure.

INTERNAL POTASSIUM BALANCE

OVERVIEW

Extracellular fluid [K] is ~4 mEq/L, whereas the intracellular [K] is ~150 mEq/L. Because of the uneven distribution of potassium between the fluid compartments, a relatively small net shift of potassium from the intracellular to the extracellular fluid compartment produces marked increases in plasma potassium. Conversely, a relatively small net shift from the extracellular to the intracellular fluid compartment produces a marked decrease in plasma potassium. Whereas renal excretion of potassium requires several hours, potassium shift between the extracellular and intracellular fluid compartment (also referred to as extrarenal potassium disposal) is extremely rapid, occurring within minutes.

Clearly, in patients with advanced CKD whose capacity to excrete potassium is marginal, extrarenal potassium disposal plays a critical role in the prevention of life-threatening hyperkalemia following potassium-rich meals. The following example will illustrate this important principle. Suppose that a 70-kg dialysis patient with serum potassium of 4.5 mmol/L eats one cup of pinto beans (~35 mmol potassium). Initially, the dietary potassium is absorbed into the extracellular fluid compartment ($0.2 \times 70 = 14$ L). This amount of dietary potassium will increase the serum potassium by 2.5 mmol/L (35 mmol/14 L). In the absence of extrarenal potassium disposal, the patient's serum potassium would rise acutely to 7.0 mmol/L, a level frequently associated with serious ventricular arrhythmias. In practice, the increase in serum potassium is much smaller as a result of efficient physiologic mechanisms that rapidly promote potassium shifts into the intracellular fluid compartment.

EFFECTS OF INSULIN AND CATECHOLAMINES ON EXTRARENAL POTASSIUM DISPOSAL

The two major physiologic factors that stimulate transfer of potassium from the extracellular to the intracellular fluid compartments are insulin and epinephrine. The stimulation of extrarenal potassium disposal by insulin and β2-adrenergic agonists are both mediated by the Na,K-ATPase activity, primarily in skeletal muscle cells. Interference with these two physiologic mechanisms (insulin deficiency or β2-adrenergic blockade, respectively) predisposes to hyperkalemia. On the other hand, excessive insulin or epinephrine levels predispose to hypokalemia.

The potassium-lowering effect of insulin is dose-related within the physiologic range of plasma insulin and is independent of its effect on plasma glucose. Even the low physiologic levels of insulin present during fasting promote extrarenal potassium disposal. In nondiabetic individuals, hyperglycemia stimulates endogenous insulin secretion, thereby decreasing the serum potassium. In insulin-dependent diabetics, endogenous insulin production is limited, and significant hyperglycemia may occur. Hyperglycemia results in plasma hypertonicity, which promotes potassium shifts out of the cells and produces paradoxic hyperkalemia.

The potassium-lowering action of epinephrine is mediated by β2-adrenergic stimulation, and it is blocked by nonselective β-blockers, but not by selective β1-adrenergic blockers. Alpha-adrenergic stimulation promotes shifts of potassium out of cells into the extracellular fluid compartment, tending to increase serum potassium. Epinephrine is a mixed alpha- and β-adrenergic agonist, such that its net effect on serum potassium reflects the balance between its β-adrenergic (potassium-lowering) and alpha-adrenergic (potassium-raising) effects. In normal individuals the β-adrenergic effect of epinephrine predominates over the alpha-adrenergic effect, and the result is a fall in the serum potassium. In contrast, the alpha-adrenergic effect of epinephrine on potassium shifts is more prominent in patients with kidney failure; as a result, dialysis patients are refractory to the potassium-lowering effect of epinephrine.

EFFECT OF ACID-BASE DISORDERS ON EXTRARENAL POTASSIUM DISPOSAL

Acid-base disorders produce internal potassium shifts in a less predictable manner. As a general rule, metabolic alkalosis shifts potassium into the cells, whereas metabolic acidosis shifts potassium out of the cells. However, the nature of the metabolic acidosis determines its effect on serum potassium. Cells are relatively impermeable to chloride. With inorganic acidosis, entry of protons (but not chloride) into the cell results in a reciprocal extrusion of potassium out of the cell to maintain electric neutrality. In contrast, cells are highly permeable to organic anions. The addition of an organic acid to the extracellular fluid results in parallel shifts of protons and organic anions into the cells with no net change in the electric balance; as a result, potassium is not extruded from the cells. Thus, mineral acidosis (i.e., hyperchloremic, normal anion gap metabolic acidosis) typically results in hyperkalemia, whereas organic metabolic acidosis (e.g., lactic acidosis) does not affect the serum potassium concentration. Bicarbonate administration to individuals with normal kidney function decreases serum potassium, but this effect is largely due to enhanced urinary excretion of potassium. In contrast, bicarbonate administration to dialysis patients (in whom the capacity for urinary potassium excretion is negligible) does not lower plasma potassium acutely. Moreover, bicarbonate administration does not potentiate the potassium-lowering effects of insulin or albuterol in dialysis patients.

LABORATORY TESTS TO EVALUATE POTASSIUM DISORDERS

DIFFERENTIAL DIAGNOSIS OF HYPOKALEMIA AND HYPERKALEMIA

The clinical history, review of medications, family history, and physical examination are sufficient to develop a rapid differential diagnosis of the etiology of most potassium disorders. In selected patients, the etiology of hypokalemia or hyperkalemia is not apparent, and additional specialized laboratory tests may be needed. Measurements of the fractional excretion of potassium (FE_K) and transtubular potassium gradient (TTKG) are useful in distinguishing between renal and nonrenal etiologies of hyperkalemia and hypokalemia. The general principle underlying these tests is that the kidney compensates for hyperkalemia by increasing potassium excretion, and it compensates for hypokalemia by decreasing potassium excretion. In contrast, when potassium excretion is inappropriate for the serum potassium, this suggests a renal etiology. The optimal use of FE_K or TTKG in the differential diagnosis requires that these values be obtained before the potassium abnormality (hyperkalemia or hypokalemia) is corrected.

FRACTIONAL EXCRETION OF POTASSIUM

FE_K is the percent of potassium filtered into the proximal tubule that appears in the urine. It represents potassium clearance corrected for GFR, or Cl_K/Cl_{Cr}:

$$FE_K = Cl_K/Cl_{Cr}$$

Because the clearance of any substance can be calculated from UV/P, the ratio Cl_K/Cl_{Cr} can be algebraically transformed to:

$$FE_K = \frac{(V \times U_K/S_K)}{(V \times U_{Cr}/S_{Cr})} \times 100\%$$

The V in the numerator and denominator cancel out, yielding the simplified formula:

$$FE_K = \frac{U_K/S_K}{U_{Cr}/S_{Cr}} \times 100\%$$

where U_K and U_{Cr} are the concentrations of potassium and creatinine in the urine, and S_K and S_{Cr} are the corresponding serum concentrations. For an individual with normal kidney function with average dietary potassium intake, the FE_K is approximately 10%. When hypokalemia is a result of extrarenal causes (low potassium diet, GI losses, potassium shifts into cells), the kidney conserves potassium and the FE_K is low. In contrast, hypokalemia due to renal potassium losses is associated with an increased FE_K. Similarly, in the setting of hyperkalemia, a high FE_K suggests an extrarenal etiology, whereas a low FE_K is consistent with a renal etiology. If a urine creatinine measurement is not available, one can often use U_K alone to differentiate between renal and extrarenal causes of hyperkalemia. Specifically, in a hypokalemic patient, $U_K > 20$ mEq/L suggests a renal etiology, whereas $U_K < 20$ mEq/L suggests an extrarenal etiology.

TRANSTUBULAR POTASSIUM GRADIENT

The TTKG is a formula that estimates the potassium gradient between the urine and the blood in the distal nephron. It is calculated from:

$$TTKG = \left[U_K \div (U_{osm}/P_{osm}) \right] \div P_K$$

where U_{osm} and P_{osm} are the urine and plasma osmolalities. The U_{osm}/P_{osm} term is included to correct for the rise in U_K that is due purely to water abstraction and concentration of urine. TTKG values have been derived from empiric measurements in normal individuals under a variety of physiologic conditions. In a normal individual under normal circumstances, the TTKG is about 6 to 8. Hypokalemia with a high TTKG suggests excessive renal potassium losses, whereas hypokalemia with a low TTKG suggests an extrarenal etiology. Similarly, hyperkalemia with a low TTKG suggests a renal etiology, whereas hyperkalemia with a high TTKG is consistent with an extrarenal etiology.

Several factors limit the utility of the FE_K and TTKG in the differential diagnosis of potassium disorders. The FE_K and TTKG are increased when dietary potassium is increased, and they are decreased when dietary potassium is decreased. Furthermore, in patients with CKD, there is an adaptive increase in potassium excretion per functioning nephron such that FE_K and TTKG increase. This means that the "normal" value for a given individual can vary substantially, making it difficult to determine the significance of a high or low FE_K or TTKG.

HYPOKALEMIA

HYPOKALEMIA VERSUS POTASSIUM DEFICIENCY

It is important to distinguish between potassium deficiency and hypokalemia. Potassium deficiency is the state resulting from a persistent negative potassium balance, that is, potassium excretion exceeding potassium intake. Hypokalemia refers to a low plasma potassium concentration. Hypokalemia can be due either to potassium deficiency (inadequate potassium intake or excessive potassium losses) or to net potassium shifts from the extracellular to the intracellular fluid compartment. A patient may have severe potassium deficiency without manifesting hypokalemia. An important example is a patient presenting with diabetic ketoacidosis. Such patients typically have severe hyperglycemia with osmotic diuresis for several days, leading to high levels of renal potassium excretion and potassium deficiency. However, as a result of insulin deficiency and hyperosmolality, there is a concomitant shift of potassium out of the cells into the extracellular fluid compartment. At presentation to the hospital, such patients are frequently normokalemic or even hyperkalemic. After they are treated with exogenous insulin, there is a rapid shift of potassium back into the cells, and within a few hours the patients develop significant hypokalemia. Conversely, patients hospitalized with an acute myocardial infarction commonly have hypokalemia as a result of stress-induced catecholamine release and enhanced extrarenal potassium disposal, even though they have a normal external potassium balance.

CLINICAL DISORDERS ASSOCIATED WITH HYPOKALEMIA

Box 10.1 provides a list of the most common causes of hypokalemia. The kidney can avidly conserve potassium, such

---

Box 10.1   Causes of Hypokalemia

Inadequate Potassium Intake (Severe Malnutrition)

Extrarenal Potassium Losses
Vomiting
Diarrhea

Hypokalemia Due to Urinary Potassium Losses
Diuretics (loop diuretics, thiazides, acetazolamide)
Osmotic diuresis (e.g., hyperglycemia)

Hypokalemia with Hypertension
   Primary aldosteronism
   Glucocorticoid remediable hypertension
   Malignant hypertension
   Renovascular hypertension
   Renin-secreting tumor
   Essential hypertension with excessive diuretics
   Liddle syndrome
   11β-Hydroxysteroid dehydrogenase deficiency
      Genetic
      Drug induced (chewing tobacco, licorice, some French wines)
      Congenital adrenal hyperplasia

Hypokalemia with a Normal Blood Pressure
   Distal renal tubular acidosis (type I)
   Proximal renal tubular acidosis (type II)
   Bartter syndrome
   Gitelman syndrome
   Hypomagnesemia (cis-platinum, alcoholism, diuretics)

Hypokalemia Due to Potassium Shifts
Insulin administration
Catecholamine excess (acute stress)
Familial periodic hypokalemic paralysis
Thyrotoxic hypokalemic paralysis

---

that hypokalemia caused by inadequate potassium intake is a rare event requiring prolonged starvation ("tea and toast diet"). Therefore, hypokalemia is usually caused by excessive potassium losses from the gut or the kidney, or by potassium shifts from the extracellular to the intracellular fluid compartments. Prolonged vomiting causes potassium losses, in part due to potassium present in gastric secretions (~10 mEq/L), but primarily due to renal losses because of secondary aldosteronism from volume depletion. Severe diarrhea, either due to disease or laxative abuse, results in significant potassium excretion in the stool.

Excessive renal potassium loss is the cause of hypokalemia in a number of clinical syndromes. Conceptually, it is useful to classify hypokalemia as associated with elevated or normal blood pressure (Fig. 10.1). When hypokalemia is associated with hypertension, measurements of plasma renin and aldosterone may be helpful in the differential diagnosis. Several physiologic observations are relevant in this regard: (1) Aldosterone, a mineralocorticoid, stimulates sodium reabsorption and potassium secretion in the collecting duct. (2) The physiologic stimulus for aldosterone secretion is activation of the renin-angiotensin axis. Moreover, aldosterone-induced sodium retention suppresses the renin-angiotensin axis by negative feedback. (3) Glucocorticoids at high concentrations bind to mineralocorticoid receptors and mimic their physiologic actions. (4) Glucocorticoids are stimulated by adrenocorticotropic hormone (ACTH), and glucocorticoids suppress ACTH production by negative feedback.

Primary aldosteronism is caused by autonomous (non–renin-mediated) secretion of aldosterone by the adrenal cortex. This results in avid sodium retention and potassium secretion by the distal nephron. Patients with this condition present with volume-dependent hypertension, hypokalemia, and metabolic alkalosis. Biochemical evaluation shows a high serum aldosterone level and suppressed plasma renin activity. Abdominal CT scan shows either a unilateral adrenal adenoma or a bilateral adrenal hyperplasia. The former is treated surgically and the latter with spironolactone.

Glucocorticoid-remediable aldosteronism (GRA) is a rare, autosomal dominant condition in which there is fusion of the 11β-hydroxylase and aldosterone synthase genes. As a result, ACTH stimulates aldosterone secretion. Abnormally high levels of aldosterone result from stimulation by ACTH, but can be suppressed by dexamethasone. Patients with GRA have a similar clinical presentation to those with primary aldosteronism (volume-dependent hypertension,

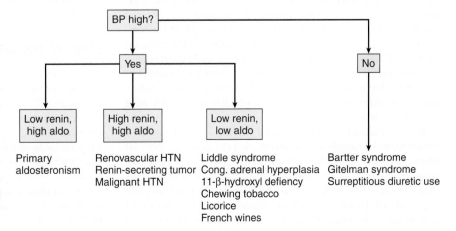

Figure 10.1   Differential diagnosis of hypokalemia according to blood pressure, renin activity, and aldosterone levels. *Aldo,* Aldosterone; *BP,* blood pressure; *HTN,* hypertension.

hypokalemia, high serum aldosterone, and low plasma renin activity), except that they are younger and have a family history of hypertension.

Patients with renovascular hypertension, renin-secreting tumors, and severe malignant hypertension may also present with severe hypertension and hypokalemia. In contrast to patients with primary aldosteronism, these patients have secondary aldosteronism, with high plasma renin activity and aldosterone levels. Of course, patients with essential hypertension may also have hypokalemia and high plasma renin and aldosterone levels if they are treated with loop or thiazide diuretics.

Patients with *11β-hydroxysteroid dehydrogenase deficiency*, a rare genetic disorder, have a defect in the conversion of cortisol to cortisone in the peripheral tissues. This results in high tissue cortisol levels that activate the mineralocorticoid receptors, producing hypokalemia and hypertension. Such patients have low plasma renin activity and aldosterone levels. Chewing tobacco, certain brands of licorice, and some French red wines contain glycyrrhizic acid, which inhibits 11β-hydroxysteroid dehydrogenase. Ingestion of these substances may produce hypokalemia, volume-dependent hypertension, and low plasma renin activity and aldosterone levels similar to the clinical presentation of congenital 11β-hydroxysteroid dehydrogenase deficiency.

Patients with *congenital adrenal hyperplasia* have a deficiency of 11β-hydroxylase, an enzyme required in the common synthetic pathways for mineralocorticoids and glucocorticoids. These patients have low plasma renin activity and aldosterone levels, high levels of desoxycorticosterone acetate (DOCA, a mineralocorticoid), and high levels of androgen. Males have early puberty, and females exhibit virilization with hirsutism and clitoromegaly. This condition improves with ACTH suppression by exogenous corticosteroids.

Liddle syndrome is a rare autosomal dominant disorder caused by a defect of the sodium channel of the distal nephron, such that there is increased sodium absorption and potassium secretion. Patients present with hypokalemia, hypertension, and volume overload. Their biochemical profile reveals a low plasma renin activity and aldosterone level. The patients' blood pressure and serum potassium improve dramatically with inhibitors of the sodium channel, such as amiloride.

Hypokalemia due to excessive renal potassium excretion is also seen in a number of clinical conditions in which hypertension is infrequent. Both distal (Type I) and proximal (Type II) renal tubular acidosis (RTA) are associated with kaliuresis and hypokalemia, in addition to normal anion gap metabolic acidosis. *Distal RTA* is frequently associated with hypercalciuria and calcium oxalate kidney stones. *Proximal RTA* is rare in adults, and is often associated with a generalized defect in proximal tubular function, manifesting with glycosuria (with a normal serum glucose), hypophosphatemia with phosphaturia, and a low serum uric acid with uricosuria.

Bartter syndrome is a rare familial disease characterized by hypokalemia, metabolic alkalosis, hypercalciuria, normal blood pressure, and high plasma renin activity and aldosterone levels. It has been associated with a number of mutations that inhibit active sodium reabsorption in the thick ascending limb of Henle, including mutations in the Na-K-2Cl transporter, ClC-Kb, and outer medullary potassium channel

(ROMK) (see Chapter 40). These patients act as if they are chronically ingesting loop diuretics, and for this reason they are difficult to distinguish clinically from patients with surreptitious diuretic ingestion. Patients with *Gitelman syndrome* differ in that they have hypocalciuria and hypomagnesemia. Gitelman syndrome has been linked to a mutation in the renal thiazide-sensitive Na-Cl transporter. These patients act as if they are chronically ingesting thiazide diuretics.

Familial hypokalemic periodic paralysis is a rare, autosomal dominant disorder in which affected individuals develop periodic episodes of severe muscle weakness in association with profound hypokalemia. This is due to rapid shifts of potassium from the extracellular to the intracellular fluid compartment. Interestingly, even when the patient has complete paralysis, the diaphragm and bulbar muscles are spared, allowing the patient to breathe, swallow, talk, and blink. The paralysis resolves within hours of potassium ingestion. The patients are asymptomatic with a normal serum potassium level between acute episodes. *Thyrotoxic hypokalemic paralysis* is an unusual manifestation of hyperthyroidism that is seen primarily in Asian patients. The clinical presentation is similar to that of hypokalemic periodic paralysis, except that the paralytic episodes cease when the hyperthyroidism is corrected.

DRUG-INDUCED HYPOKALEMIA

A number of drugs have the potential to cause hypokalemia, either by stimulating renal potassium excretion or by blocking extrarenal disposal. Exogenous mineralocorticoids mimic the effects of aldosterone, thereby stimulating distal potassium secretion. High doses of glucocorticoids possess some mineralocorticoid activity and have a similar effect. Most diuretics, including loop diuretics, thiazide diuretics, and acetazolamide, increase renal potassium excretion. Other drugs, including alcohol, diuretics, and cis-platinum, cause renal magnesium wasting and hypomagnesemia. For reasons that are not well understood, hypomagnesemia impairs renal potassium conservation. These patients may thus experience associated hypokalemia that is refractory to potassium supplementation until the magnesium deficit is corrected.

Drugs that promote extrarenal potassium disposal may also result in hypokalemia. This phenomenon can be seen after the administration of an acute dose of insulin. Similarly, β2-agonists (either intravenous or nebulized), including albuterol and terbutaline, frequently result in acute hypokalemia.

CLINICAL MANIFESTATIONS OF HYPOKALEMIA

Hypokalemia may produce electrocardiographic abnormalities, including a flattened T wave and a U wave (Fig. 10.2). Hypokalemia also appears to increases the risk of ventricular arrhythmias in patients with ischemic heart disease or patients taking digoxin. Severe hypokalemia is associated with variable degrees of skeletal muscle weakness, even to the point of paralysis. On rare occasions, diaphragmatic paralysis from hypokalemia can lead to respiratory arrest. Ileus or urinary retention can result from decreased motility of smooth muscle. Rarely, severe hypokalemia may cause rhabdomyolysis.

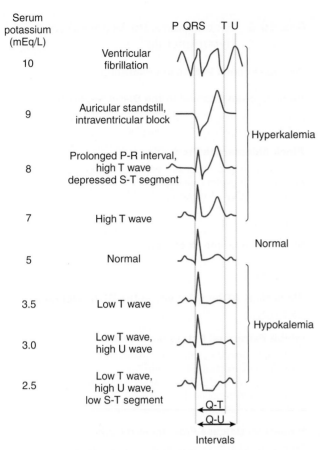

Figure 10.2 Typical electrocardiographic changes associated with hypokalemia and hyperkalemia. (With permission from Seldin DW, Giebisch G, editors: *The regulation of potassium balance*, New York, 1989, Raven.)

Severe hypokalemia also interferes with the urinary concentrating mechanism in the distal nephron, resulting in nephrogenic diabetes insipidus. Such patients have a low urine osmolality in the face of high serum osmolality, and are refractory to vasopressin.

TREATMENT OF HYPOKALEMIA

The acute treatment of hypokalemia requires potassium supplementation. This can be administered either intravenously or orally. The correlation between serum potassium and total potassium deficit in hypokalemic patients is poor. A particular patient's serum potassium is a reflection of both external potassium balance and transcellular potassium shifts. The percentage of administered exogenous potassium that remains in the extracellular fluid compartment is variable. It is thus difficult to predict how much potassium replacement will be required for a particular patient. If the patient is hypokalemic in the setting of potassium deficiency, a large amount of potassium replacement is needed. In contrast, hypokalemia that is primarily due to transcellular potassium shifts requires relatively little potassium repletion. Without adequate monitoring, it is possible to administer too much potassium, which can result in hyperkalemia. Therefore, one should give multiple small doses of potassium with frequent checks of serum potassium values.

Oral potassium administration is safer than the intravenous route, and it is less likely to produce an overshoot in the serum potassium. Each oral dose should not exceed 20 to 40 mEq of potassium. Intravenous KCl should be reserved for severe, symptomatic hypokalemia (<3.0 mEq/L) or for patients who cannot ingest oral potassium. Intravenous KCl should not be administered more quickly than 10 mmol/h in the absence of continuous ECG monitoring. The serum potassium should be rechecked every 2 to 3 hours to confirm a clinical response and to avoid an overshoot.

Treatment of the underlying medical condition may prevent recurrence of hypokalemia after its correction. If the patient has a chronic condition associated with persistent urinary potassium losses, such that hypokalemia is likely to recur, the patient should be encouraged to increase the intake of foods high in potassium (especially fresh fruits, nuts, and legumes). In some patients, chronic oral potassium supplementation may be necessary.

HYPERKALEMIA

Pseudohyperkalemia is a factitious elevation of the serum potassium due to in vitro release of potassium from blood cells. It may be seen with in vitro hemolysis, thrombocytosis, or severe leukocytosis. Pseudohyperkalemia due to hemolysis is readily apparent because the serum is pink. Pseudohyperkalemia due to severe thrombocytosis or leukocytosis can be confirmed by drawing simultaneous blood samples in tubes with and without anticoagulant; if potassium in the latter (serum) is higher than in the former (plasma), the diagnosis is confirmed.

True hyperkalemia is caused by positive potassium balance (increased potassium intake or decreased potassium excretion) or an increase in net potassium shift from the intracellular to the extracellular fluid compartment. Box 10.2 provides a list of the most common causes of hyperkalemia. In practice, most patients who develop severe hyperkalemia have multiple contributory factors. For example, a patient with moderate CKD due to diabetic nephropathy medicated with an ACE inhibitor may have mild hyperkalemia. However, when he is started on indomethacin for acute gouty arthritis, the patient rapidly develops severe hyperkalemia.

DRUG-INDUCED HYPERKALEMIA

A large number of drugs have the potential to cause hyperkalemia, either by inhibiting renal potassium excretion or by blocking extrarenal disposal (Box 10.3). Most individuals taking these drugs will not develop hyperkalemia. Patients with advanced CKD are at the highest risk, especially if they have a high dietary potassium intake or are taking additional medication that predispose to hyperkalemia. Most diuretics (loop diuretics, thiazide diuretics, acetazolamide) increase urinary potassium excretion and tend to cause hypokalemia. However, potassium-sparing diuretics inhibit urinary potassium excretion and predispose to hyperkalemia by one of two mechanisms. *Spironolactone* and *eplerenone* are competitive inhibitors of aldosterone that bind to the aldosterone receptors in the collecting duct, inhibiting Na,K-ATPase activity and indirectly limiting potassium

---

Box 10.2   Causes of Hyperkalemia

Pseudohyperkalemia

Hemolysis
Thrombocytosis
Severe leukocytosis
Fist clenching

Decreased Renal Excretion

Acute or chronic kidney disease
Aldosterone deficiency (e.g., type IV renal tubular acidosis) that
    is frequently associated with diabetic nephropathy, chronic
    interstitial nephritis, or obstructive nephropathy
Adrenal insufficiency (Addison disease)
Drugs that inhibit potassium excretion (see Box 10.3)
Kidney diseases that impair distal tubule function
    Sickle cell anemia
    Systemic lupus erythematosis

Abnormal Potassium Distribution

Insulin deficiency
β-blockers
Metabolic or respiratory acidosis
Familial hyperkalemic periodic paralysis

Abnormal Potassium Release From Cells

Rhabdomyolysis
Tumor lysis syndrome

Box 10.3   Mechanisms for Drug-Induced Hyperkalemia

Decrease Renal Potassium Excretion

Block Sodium Channel in the Distal Nephron

Potassium-sparing diuretics: amiloride, triamterene
Antibiotics: trimethoprim, pentamidine

Block Aldosterone Production

ACE inhibitors (e.g., captopril, enalapril, lisinopril, benazepril)
Angiotensin receptor blockers
NSAIDs and COX-2 inhibitors
Heparin
Tacrolimus

Block Aldosterone Receptors

Spironolactone
Eplerenone

Block Na,K-ATPase Activity in the Distal Nephron

Cyclosporine

Inhibit Extrarenal Potassium Disposal

Block β2-adrenergic mediated extrarenal potassium dis-
    posal: nonselective β-blockers
Block Na,K-ATPase activity in skeletal muscles: digoxin over-
    dose (not therapeutic doses)
Inhibit insulin release (e.g., somatostatin)

Potassium Release From Injured Cells

Drug-induced rhabdomyolysis (e.g., lovastatin, cocaine)
Drug-induced tumor lysis syndrome (chemotherapy agents in
    acute leukemias, high-grade lymphomas)
Depolarizing paralytic agents (e.g., succinylcholine)

Drug-Induced Acute Kidney Injury

ACE, Angiotensin converting enzyme; *NSAIDs,* nonsteroidal antiin-
    flammatory drugs.

---

secretion. Interestingly, the immunosuppressant drug *cyclosporine* also blocks Na,K-ATPase activity in the distal nephron. Two other potassium-sparing diuretics, *amiloride* and *triamterene*, bind to the sodium channel in the collecting duct. This inhibits sodium reabsorption in the distal nephron and limits the electrochemical gradient required for potassium secretion. Two antibiotics, *trimethoprim* (one of the components of Bactrim) and *pentamidine*, have also been shown to block the sodium channel in the collecting duct, predisposing patients to hyperkalemia. In addition, trimethoprim has been shown to inhibit H,K-ATPase in the collecting tubule.

Because aldosterone plays an important role in enhancing renal potassium excretion in patients with kidney failure, drugs that inhibit aldosterone production (either directly or indirectly) predispose such patients to hyperkalemia. Angiotensin II is a potent stimulator of aldosterone production in the adrenal cortex. ACE inhibitors inhibit the production of angiotensin II, thereby decreasing aldosterone levels. Similarly, angiotensin II receptor blockers also inhibit aldosterone production. Prostaglandins directly stimulate renin production, and prostaglandin inhibitors (nonsteroidal antiinflammatory drugs) inhibit the production of renin, thereby indirectly decreasing aldosterone production. This effect is seen even with "renal-sparing NSAIDs," such as sulindac (a nonselective COX-1 and COX-2 inhibitor). Hyperkalemia may also be caused by selective COX-2 inhibitors. Heparin has been shown to inhibit directly the production of aldosterone in the renal cortex, primarily by decreasing the number and affinity of angiotensin II receptors in the zona glomerulosa. This effect occurs even with the low doses of subcutaneous

heparin used for prophylaxis of venous thrombosis in hospitalized patients (e.g., 5000 units every 12 hours). *Tacrolimus,* an immunosuppressant drug, causes hyperkalemia by inhibiting aldosterone synthesis. Oral contraceptives containing drospirenone (a progestin) inhibit renal potassium excretion and may provoke hyperkalemia in women with CKD.

Given the stimulation of extrarenal potassium disposal by β-adrenergic agonists, it is not surprising that β2-antagonists can predispose to hyperkalemia. This effect is seen primarily with nonselective β-blockers (e.g., propranolol and nadolol), rather than β-selective blockers (e.g., atenolol, metoprolol). There is significant systemic absorption of topical β-blockers, and severe hyperkalemia may rarely be provoked by timolol eye drops. Drugs inhibiting endogenous insulin release, such as somatostatin, have been implicated rarely as a cause of hyperkalemia in patients with renal failure. Presumably, long-acting somatostatin analogs, such as octreotide, would have a similar effect on serum potassium. Digoxin overdose causes inhibition of Na,K-ATPase activity in skeletal muscle cells, and may manifest as hyperkalemia. This effect is rarely seen at therapeutic doses of the drug. Depolarizing paralytic agents used for general anesthesia, such as succinylcholine, can occasionally produce hyperkalemia by causing potassium to leak out of the cells.

Finally, drugs can also induce hyperkalemia indirectly by causing the release of intracellular potassium from injured cells (e.g., rhabdomyolysis with statins and cocaine, or tumor lysis syndrome when chemotherapy is administered in patients with acute leukemia or high-grade lymphoma). Moreover, drug-induced AKI may be associated with secondary hyperkalemia.

A common clinical dilemma occurs when patients with CKD develop hyperkalemia after starting an ACE inhibitor or ARB. One would like to continue this drug because of its renoprotective benefit. Therapeutic options for this scenario include reducing the dose of ACE inhibitor or ARB, starting or increasing the dose of a loop or thiazide diuretic, discontinuing other medications that promote hyperkalemia, and reinforcing a dietary potassium restriction. Fludrocortisone (0.1 to 0.2 mg daily) can be tried in refractory cases, although it may promote sodium retention resulting in peripheral edema and hypertension. Finally, the patient should be questioned about constipation, as the addition of laxatives may promote fecal potassium excretion.

FASTING HYPERKALEMIA IN DIALYSIS PATIENTS

Prolonged fasting decreases plasma insulin concentrations, thereby promoting potassium shifts from the intracellular to the extracellular fluid compartments. In normal individuals, the excess potassium is excreted in the urine to maintain constant plasma potassium levels. In dialysis patients, the potassium entering the extracellular fluid compartment during fasting cannot be excreted, resulting in progressive hyperkalemia. The phenomenon of fasting hyperkalemia may be clinically significant in dialysis patients who fast longer than 8 to 12 hours before a surgical or radiologic procedure. Occasionally, such patients develop life-threatening hyperkalemia in these instances. The hyperkalemia can be prevented by the administration of intravenous dextrose (to stimulated endogenous insulin secretion) for the duration of the fast. If the patient is diabetic, insulin must be added to the dextrose infusion to prevent paradoxic hyperkalemia.

CLINICAL MANIFESTATIONS OF HYPERKALEMIA

Hyperkalemia may produce progressive electrocardiographic abnormalities, including peaked T waves, flattening or absence of P waves, widened QRS complexes, and sine waves (see Fig. 10.2). The major risk of severe hyperkalemia is the development of life-threatening ventricular arrhythmias.

Severe hyperkalemia, like severe hypokalemia, can cause skeletal muscle weakness, even to the point of paralysis and respiratory failure. Hyperkalemia impairs urinary acidification by decreasing collecting tubule apical H,K-ATPase, which may result in a renal tubular acidosis (Type IV RTA). Hyperkalemia stimulates endogenous aldosterone secretion, but not insulin secretion.

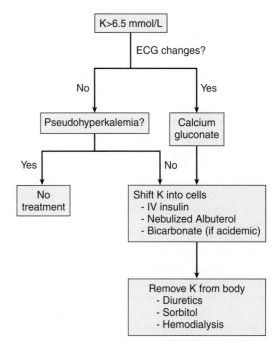

Figure 10.3   Approach to treatment of hyperkalemia. (Reproduced from Shingarev R, Allon M: A physiologic approach to the treatment of acute hyperkalemia. *Am J Kidney Dis* 56:578-584, 2010.)

TREATMENT OF HYPERKALEMIA

Severe hyperkalemia associated with electrocardiographic changes is a life-threatening state requiring emergent intervention (Fig. 10.3). If the patient's ECG is suspicious for hyperkalemia, one should initiate therapy without waiting for laboratory confirmation. If the patient has kidney failure, urgent dialysis is required for removal of potassium from the body. Because of the inevitable delay in initiating dialysis, the following temporizing measures must be initiated promptly:

1. *Stabilize the myocardium.* Acute administration of intravenous calcium gluconate does not change plasma potassium, but does transiently improve the ECG. The effect is almost immediate after administering 10 mL of 10% calcium gluconate over 1 minute. If there is no improvement in the ECG appearance within 3 to 5 minutes, the dose should be repeated.

2. *Shift potassium* from the extracellular to the intracellular fluid, rapidly decreasing the serum potassium. This involves administration of insulin and a β2-agonist.

   a. *Intravenous insulin* is the fastest way to lower the serum potassium. The plasma potassium starts to decrease within 15 minutes. Intravenous glucose is administered concurrently to prevent hypoglycemia. One should give 10 units of regular insulin and 50 mL of 50% dextrose (one ampule of D_{50}) as a bolus, followed by a continuous infusion of 5% dextrose at 100 mL/h to prevent late hypoglycemia. In diabetic patients, the serum glucose should be measured with a glucometer; if it is >300 mg/dl, one can administer the intravenous insulin alone (without concomitant 50% dextrose). One should never administer dextrose without insulin for the acute treatment of hyperkalemia; in patients with inadequate endogenous insulin production, the resulting hyperglycemia and hyperosmolality can produce a paradoxical increase in serum potassium.

b. *β-agonists.* One should administer 20 mg of albuterol (a β2-agonist) by inhalation over 10 minutes, with an onset of action within 30 minutes. The concentrated form of albuterol (5 mg/mL) should be used to minimize the inhalation volume. The dose required to lower plasma potassium is considerably higher than that used to treat asthma, because only a small fraction of nebulized albuterol is absorbed systemically. Thus, 0.5 mg of intravenous albuterol (not available in the USA) produces a comparable change in plasma potassium to that seen after 20 mg of nebulized albuterol. The potassium-lowering effect of albuterol is additive to that of insulin.

c. *Sodium bicarbonate.* In patients with CKD who are not yet on dialysis, bicarbonate administration can lower serum potassium by enhancing renal potassium excretion. However, bicarbonate administration is of dubious value for treatment of hyperkalemia in patients without residual kidney function. It takes at least 3 to 4 hours for the serum potassium to start to decrease after bicarbonate administration to dialysis patients, so this modality is not useful for the acute management of hyperkalemia. Moreover, bicarbonate administration does not enhance the potassium-lowering effects of insulin or albuterol. Bicarbonate administration is still indicated in cases of severe metabolic acidosis (serum bicarbonate <10 mmol/L).

3. After the previous temporizing measures have been performed, further interventions are necessary for removing potassium from the body.

a. *Diuretics.* These only work if the patient has adequate kidney function.

b. *Kayexalate.* This resin-exchanger removes potassium from the blood and moves it into the gut, in exchange for an equal amount of sodium. It is relatively slow acting, requiring 1 to 2 hours before plasma potassium decreases. Each gram of Kayexalate removes 0.5 to 1.0 mmol of potassium. Kayexalate should be administered as 50 g in 30 mL sorbitol by mouth, or 50 g in a retention enema. The rectal route is faster and more reliable. A recent study suggested that a single standard oral dose of Kayexalate may not decrease the serum potassium within 4 hours in normokalemic hemodialysis patients despite a documented increase in potassium excretion by the gut. Whether this treatment is effective in hyperkalemic dialysis patients, or when administered in multiple doses, remains to be determined. However, given this uncertainty, frequent monitoring of plasma potassium in patients treated with Kayexalate is warranted. The use of Kayexalate has been associated with colonic necrosis in rare cases.

c. *Hemodialysis.* This is the definitive treatment for patients with advanced kidney failure and severe hyperkalemia.

For patients with moderate hyperkalemia not associated with electrocardiographic changes, it is frequently sufficient to discontinue the drugs predisposing to hyperkalemia.

Table 10.1 Potassium Content of Selected Foods

Food	Potassium (mg)	Potassium (mEq)
Pinto beans (1 cup)	1370	35
Raisins (1 cup)	1106	28
Honeydew (1/2 melon)	939	24
Nuts (1 cup)	688	18
Black-eyed peas (1 cup)	625	16
Collard greens (1 cup)	498	13
Banana (1 medium)	440	11
Tomato (1 medium)	366	9
Orange (1 large)	333	9
Milk (1 cup)	351	9
Potato chips (10)	226	6

To prevent a recurrence of hyperkalemia after the acute treatment has been provided, the following measures are useful:

1. Counsel the patient on dietary potassium restriction, 40 to 60 mEq per day (Table 10.1).
2. Avoid medications that interfere with renal excretion of potassium (see Box 10.3). ACE inhibitors and ARBs play a major role in slowing the progression of CKD. For this reason, when patients on these medications develop hyperkalemia, one should first attempt to decrease dietary potassium intake, treat constipation if present to maximize gastrointestinal excretion of potassium, stop other drugs contributing to hyperkalemia, add a diuretic, or reduce the dose of ACE inhibitor or ARB. Only if all other measures fail to control the hyperkalemia should the ACE inhibitor or ARB be discontinued.
3. Avoid drugs that interfere with potassium shifts from the extracellular to the extracellular compartments, (e.g., nonselective β-blockers).
4. When hemodialysis patients are fasted in preparation for surgery or a radiologic procedure, administer intravenous 10% dextrose at 50 mL/h to prevent hyperkalemia. If the patient is diabetic, add 10 units of regular insulin to each liter of 10% dextrose.
5. In selected patients, chronic medication with loop diuretics can be used to stimulate urinary potassium excretion.
6. Specific therapy may be indicated for the underlying etiology, when available. For example, patients with adrenal insufficiency require replacement with exogenous glucocorticoids and mineralocorticoids. In patients with hyperkalemic periodic paralysis (a rare, autosomal dominant disorder in which affected individuals develop periodic episodes of severe muscle weakness in association with profound hyperkalemia), prophylactic aerosolized albuterol can prevent both exercise-induced hyperkalemia and muscle weakness.

BIBLIOGRAPHY

Allon M: Hyperkalemia in end-stage renal disease: mechanisms and management, *J Am Soc Nephrol* 6:1134-1142, 1995.

Allon M: Treatment and prevention of hyperkalemia in end-stage renal disease, *Kidney Int* 43:1197-1209, 1993.

Allon M, Takeshian A, Shanklin N: Effect of insulin-plus-glucose infusion with or without epinephrine on fasting hyperkalemia, *Kidney Int* 43:212-217, 1993.

DuBose TD: Hyperkalemic hyperchloremic metabolic acidosis: pathophysiologic insights, *Kidney Int* 51:591-602, 1997.

Ethier JH, Kamel KS, Magner PO, et al: The transtubular potassium concentration in patients with hyperkalemia and hypokalemia, *Am J Kidney Dis* 15:309-315, 1990.

Farese RV, Biglieri EG, Shackleton CHL, et al: Licorice-induced hypermineralocorticoidism, *N Engl J Med* 325:1223-1227, 1991.

Gruy-Kapral C, Emmett M, Santa Ana CA, et al: Effect of single dose resin-cathartic therapy on serum potassium concentration in patients with end-stage renal disease, *J Am Soc Nephrol* 9:1924-1930, 1998.

Kamel KS, Halperin ML, Faber MD, et al: Disorders of potassium balance. In Brenner BM, editor: *The Kidney*, 1996, WB Saunders Co, pp 999-1037.

Kamel KS, Wei C: Controversial issues in the treatment of hyperkalemia, *Nephrol Dial Transplant* 18:2215-2218, 2003.

Krishna GG, Steigerwalt SP, Pikus R, et al: Hypokalemic states. In Narins RG, editor: *Clinical disorders of fluid and electrolyte metabolism*, 1994, McGraw-Hill, pp 659-696.

Kurtz I: Molecular pathogenesis of Bartter's and Gitelman's syndromes, *Kidney Int* 54:1396-1410, 1998.

Lifton RP, Dluhy RG, Powers M, et al: A chimaeric 11 beta-hydroxylase/aldosterone synthase gene causes glucocorticoid-remediable aldosteronism and human hypertension, *Nature* 355:262-265, 1992.

Putcha N, Allon M: Management of hyperkalemia in dialysis patients, *Semin Dial* 20:431-439, 2007.

Salem MM, Rosa RM, Batlle DC: Extrarenal potassium tolerance in chronic renal failure: implications for the treatment of acute hyperkalemia, *Am J Kidney Dis* 18:421-440, 1991.

Shimkets RA, Warnock DG, Bositis CM, et al: Liddle's syndrome: heritable human hypertension caused by mutations in the beta subunit of the epithelial sodium channel, *Cell* 79:407-414, 1994.

11

Disorders of Mineral Metabolism: Calcium, Phosphorus, and Magnesium

Sharon M. Moe | Jacques R. Daoud

Disorders of mineral metabolism, specifically calcium, phosphorus, and magnesium homeostasis, are common in patients with chronic kidney disease (CKD). The homeostatic regulation of calcium, phosphorus, and magnesium maintains normal serum levels, normal intracellular levels, and optimal mineral content in bone. This regulation occurs in three major target organs (intestine, kidney, and bone) via the complex integration of three hormones (parathyroid hormone [PTH], vitamin D and its derivatives, and fibroblast growth factor 23 [FGF23]). An understanding of normal physiology is necessary to accurately diagnose and treat disorders of calcium, phosphorus, and magnesium.

NORMAL PHYSIOLOGY

PARATHYROID HORMONE

Parathyroid hormone is released in response to hypocalcemia (Fig. 11.1) and maintains calcium homeostasis by three mechanisms: (1) increasing bone mineral dissolution, thus releasing calcium and phosphorus; (2) increasing renal reabsorption of calcium and excretion of phosphorus; and (3) enhancing the gastrointestinal absorption of both calcium and phosphorus indirectly through its effects on the synthesis of $1,25(OH)_2D_3$. In healthy individuals, the increase in serum PTH level in response to hypocalcemia effectively restores serum calcium levels while maintaining normal serum phosphorus levels.

Parathyroid hormone enhances the conversion of 25(OH)-vitamin D [calcidiol] to $1,25(OH)_2$-vitamin D [calcitriol], which in turn decreases PTH secretion at the level of the parathyroid glands, completing a typical endocrine feedback loop. In primary hyperparathyroidism, PTH is secreted autonomously from adenomatous glands without regard to physiologic stimuli. In contrast, in secondary hyperparathyroidism, the glands initially respond appropriately; however, after a prolonged period of CKD and secondary hyperparathyroidism, the hyperplastic glands become adenomatous and therefore unresponsive to stimuli that would normally suppress PTH secretion. After entering the circulation, PTH binds to PTH receptors that are located throughout the body. Therefore, disorders of PTH excess or insufficiency not only affect serum levels of calcium and phosphorus, but also lead to bone, cardiac, skin, neurologic, and other manifestations.

Parathyroid hormone is cleaved from a precursor preprohormone to an 84-amino-acid protein in the parathyroid gland, where it is stored with other PTH-protein fragments in secretory granules for release. After release, the circulating 1-84 amino-acid protein has a half-life of 2 to 4 minutes. It is then further cleaved into N-terminal, C-terminal, and midregion fragments of PTH, which are finally metabolized in the liver and kidneys. PTH secretion can be triggered by hypocalcemia, hyperphosphatemia, or calcitriol deficiency, whereas profound hypomagnesemia can reduce PTH release. The extracellular concentration of ionized calcium is the most important determinant of minute-to-minute PTH levels. Active secretion of PTH from stored granules in response to hypocalcemia is controlled by the calcium-sensing receptor (CaSR), and mutations of the CaSR gene can lead to syndromes of hypercalcemia or hypocalcemia through dysregulated PTH release. The CaSR is expressed in thyroid C-cells and in the kidney, where it controls renal excretion of calcium in the thick ascending limb of the loop of Henle in response to changes in serum calcium concentration.

Through the years, a succession of increasingly sensitive assays has been developed to measure PTH. A major difficulty in measuring PTH accurately is cross-reactivity with inactive, circulating PTH-protein fragments that may accumulate in CKD. Early assays targeted the C-terminus, but were inaccurate in patients with kidney disease because of accumulation of these fragments. Subsequent N-terminus assays resulted in similar problems. Accuracy was improved by the development of a two-site antibody test (commonly called "INTACT" assay) to detect full-length (1-84, or active) PTH molecules. In this assay, a capture antibody binds to the N-terminus and a second antibody binds to the C-terminus. However, because the N-terminal antibody is at amino acid 7 instead of amino acid 1, this intact assay still detects some retained C-terminal fragments (although less than the older assays). These fragments accumulate in CKD, leading to falsely elevated values in assays of intact PTH such that values above the normal range are associated with complications of hypoparathyroidism at the level of bone. In addition, there are normal minute-to-minute oscillations in PTH secretion that account for some of the variability in measurements in patients. Despite these limitations, the intact PTH assay is currently the most widely used assay in clinical care.

VITAMIN D

Vitamin D is called a "vitamin," because it is an essential nutrient that must come from an exogenous source if it

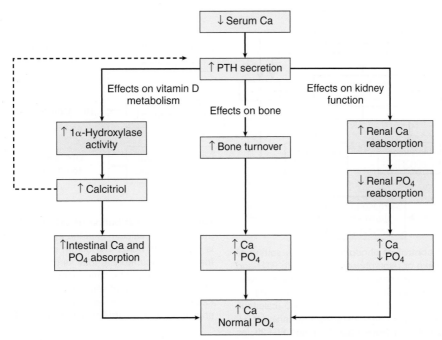

Figure 11.1   Normal homeostatic response to hypocalcemia. In the presence of hypocalcemia, secretion of parathyroid hormone (PTH) is increased. PTH acts on three target organs. PTH works at the intestine indirectly by first increasing the 1α-hydroxylase activity in the kidney; this enzyme converts calcidiol to calcitriol, which increases intestinal absorption of both calcium and phosphorus. Calcitriol then negatively feeds back on the parathyroid glands to suppress PTH release *(dotted line)*. In bone, PTH increases bone turnover, resulting in a release of calcium and phosphorus. Last, PTH works directly on the kidney to increase renal calcium reabsorption and to decrease renal phosphorus reabsorption. The net effect is a rise in serum calcium but no net change in serum phosphorus. The blue boxes indicate homeostatic steps in the kidney that are abnormal in people with chronic kidney disease. Because of diminished kidney mass, conversion of calcidiol to calcitriol and phosphorus excretion are impaired.

cannot be manufactured in humans in sufficient quantity; however, this is a misnomer, because vitamin D can be synthesized in the skin, and in actuality is a hormone. Vitamin D_2 (ergocalciferol) from plants and vitamin D_3 (cholecalciferol) primarily from oily fish are the main exogenous sources in a Western diet outside of supplementation in food products. In the skin, 7-dehydrocholesterol is converted to vitamin D_3 in response to sunlight, a process that is inhibited by sunscreen of skin protection factor (SPF) 8 or greater. After entering the blood, vitamins D_2 and D_3 from diet or skin bind to vitamin D–binding protein and are carried to the liver, where they are hydroxylated to yield 25(OH)D, often called calcidiol; accordingly, blood calcidiol levels are a direct assessment of the nutritional (dietary) intake and skin conversion of vitamin D. Some clinical assays measure hydroxylated forms of both D_2 and D_3, whereas others measure the total level of 25(OH)D (D_2 + D_3). 25(OH)D (calcidiol) is then converted in the kidney to $1,25(OH)_2D$ (calcitriol) by the action of 1α-hydroxylase (the CYP27B1 isoenzyme of the cytochrome P-450 system). In the kidney, CYP27B1 activity is affected by almost every hormone involved in calcium homeostasis. Its activity is stimulated by PTH, estrogen, calcitonin, prolactin, growth hormone, low serum calcium, and low serum phosphorus, and inhibited by calcitriol and fibroblast growth factor 23 (FGF23).

Calcitriol circulates in the bloodstream bound to vitamin D–binding protein. The free form of $1,25(OH)_2D$ enters the target cell, where it interacts with its nuclear vitamin D receptor (VDR). This complex then combines with the retinoic acid X receptor to form a heterodimer, which in turn interacts with the vitamin D response element (VDRE) on the target gene. The major functions of $1,25(OH)_2D$ are carried out in three target organs: (1) the small intestine, where it regulates the intestinal absorption of calcium and, to a lesser degree, phosphorus and possibly magnesium; (2) the parathyroid gland, where it inhibits PTH synthesis at the level of messenger RNA transcription; and (3) the osteoblast/osteocytes in bone, where it directly stimulates the secretion of FGF23. Importantly, the kidney CYP27B1 is essential for the feedback loops between calcitriol and both PTH and FGF23.

In addition to the role of vitamin D in mineral metabolism, the VDR is expressed in multiple organs, and 1α-hydroxylase activity can be detected in extrarenal tissues including immune cells, muscle cells, and myocardiocytes. Both 25(OH)D and $1,25(OH)_2D$ can be taken up by extrarenal cells, with the former then converted intracellularly to $1,25(OH)_2D$. These features may mediate autocrine or paracrine effects of vitamin D outside its classic target tissues, especially effects on cell differentiation and proliferation and immune function. Recent studies in both normal and CKD patients have demonstrated widespread vitamin D insufficiency and deficiency. Low levels of this precursor to calcitriol are associated with hyperparathyroidism, falls, fractures, cardiovascular disease, mortality, and cancers in the general population.

FGF23

Fibroblast growth factor 23 is a phosphatonin, which is a group of proteins that were identified from the study of

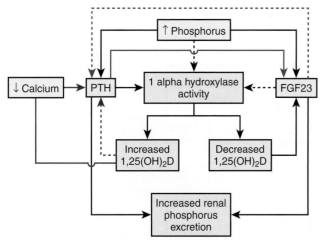

Figure 11.2 Hormonal control of phosphorus. In the setting of increased phosphorus intake or hyperphosphatemia, both PTH and FGF23 are stimulated and induce renal phosphorus excretion. However, these hormones have opposing effects on the CYP27B1 (1-alpha hydroxylase) to increase and decrease 1,25(OH)$_2$D (calcitriol) production. The increased calcitriol then feeds back to inhibit PTH, and the decreased calcitriol then feeds back to inhibit FGF23 (as calcitriol normally stimulates FGF23). The *solid lines* represent an increase in levels, the *dotted lines* represent a decrease or inhibition of levels. (Adapted from Moe SM, Sprague SM. Chronic kidney disease–mineral bone disorder. In Taal MW, Chertow GM, Marsden PA, Skorecki K, Yu ASL, Brenner BM, editors: *Brenner and Rector's The Kidney,* ed 9, Philadelphia, 2012, Elsevier Saunders, p. 2023.)

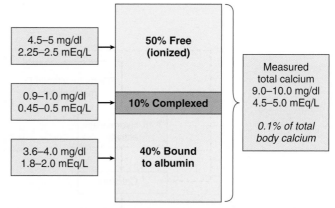

Figure 11.3 Distribution of extracellular calcium. Only 0.1% of the total body calcium is in the extracellular space; the other 99.9% is localized in bone. The serum calcium concentration reported by the clinical laboratory is total serum calcium. However, only 50% of this total calcium is the physiologically active ionized component. The 50% bound fraction of serum calcium comprises the 10% of the total calcium that is complexed to anions such as bicarbonate, phosphate, and citrate and the 40% that is bound to albumin.

genetic disorders characterized by hypophosphatemia due to urinary phosphate wasting, and from cases of tumor-induced osteomalacia associated with urinary phosphate wasting. FGF23 is made by osteocytes, a subgroup of osteoblasts that are interconnected through a series of cannuliculi within cancellous (trabecular) bone. FGF23 directly inhibits the conversion of 25(OH)D to 1,25(OH)$_2$D through downregulation of the CP27B1 in the kidney. FGF23 also inhibits PTH, while 1,25(OH)D and PTH stimulate FGF23, completing a feedback loop (Fig. 11.2). Thus, FGF23 provides the key PTH-bone link and kidney-bone link. Levels of FGF23 are elevated in patients with CKD, presumably because of net phosphate retention or a deficiency in 1,25(OH)$_2$D, and higher FGF23 levels in CKD patients are associated with left ventricular hypertrophy and increased mortality. In the kidney, FGF23 acts through the FGF receptor and its coreceptor klotho; however, in cardiomyocytes, FGF23 acts independently of klotho. In addition to FGF23, there are other phosphatonins, such as matrix extracellular phosphoglycoprotein (MEPE), that may provide an intestine-kidney link.

CALCIUM

Serum calcium levels are tightly controlled within a narrow range, usually 8.5 to 10.5 mg/dl (2.1 to 2.6 mmol/L). However, the serum calcium level is a poor reflection of overall total body calcium, because the intravascular space contains only 0.1% to 0.2% of extracellular calcium, which in turn represents only 1% of total body calcium, with nearly all total body calcium stored in bone. Only ionized calcium, approximately 50% of total serum calcium, is physiologically active, with the remaining 50% of total serum calcium

bound to albumin or anions such as citrate, bicarbonate, and phosphorus (Fig. 11.3).

Reduced serum levels of ionized calcium stimulate PTH secretion, an effect that helps restore normal levels of ionized calcium (see Fig. 11.1). PTH increases bone resorption, renal calcium reabsorption, and the conversion of 25(OH)D$_3$ to 1,25(OH)$_2$D$_3$ in the kidney, thereby stimulating gastrointestinal calcium absorption. In individuals with intact kidneys, net calcium balance varies with age. Children and young adults are usually in a slightly positive net calcium balance, because bone accrual accompanies skeletal growth; after age 25 to 35 years, when bones stop growing, the calcium balance tends to be neutral. Normal individuals are protected against calcium overload by hormonal controls, which increase urinary calcium excretion and decrease intestinal calcium absorption.

Calcium absorption across the intestinal epithelium occurs via both a vitamin D–dependent mechanism and a passive, concentration-dependent pathway that is independent of calcitriol. The duodenum is the major site of calcium absorption, although the other segments of the small intestine and the colon also contribute to net calcium absorption. In addition, there is an obligatory secretion of calcium into the gut. Individuals on a calcium-free diet will have a net loss of calcium from the body in stool resulting in a negative calcium balance. In the kidney, the majority (60% to 70%) of calcium is reabsorbed passively in the proximal tubule, driven by a gradient that is generated by reabsorption of sodium and water. In the thick ascending limb, another 20% to 30% of calcium is reabsorbed via paracellular transport driven by the lumen positive net charge. The remaining 10% of calcium reabsorption occurs in the distal convoluted tubule, the connecting tubule, and the initial portion of the cortical collecting duct. The final regulation of urinary calcium excretion is carried out in these distal segments.

Calcium enters epithelial cells in the intestine and kidney through specialized channels called transient receptor potential (TRP) cation channels TRPV5 and TRPV6; it is then transported through the cell by a protein called calbindin and ultimately extruded through the basolateral side by the Na^+/Ca^{2+} exchanger (NCX1) or the calcium–adenosine triphosphatase (Ca^{2+}-ATPase) pump (PMCA1b). Genetic defects in these various transporters lead to a variety of rare disorders of calcium homeostasis. Calcitriol actively regulates all of these channels and transporters, and vitamin D deficiency leads to impaired intestinal calcium absorption. At the level of the kidney, vitamin D and PTH work together to control calcium excretion.

PHOSPHORUS

Inorganic phosphorus is critical for numerous normal physiologic functions, including skeletal development, cell membrane phospholipid content and function, cell signaling, platelet aggregation, and energy transfer through mitochondrial metabolism. Normal homeostasis maintains serum concentrations between 2.5 and 4.5 mg/dl (0.81 to 1.45 mmol/L). The terms *phosphorus* and *phosphate* are often used interchangeably, but, strictly speaking, "phosphate" refers to the inorganic form that is in equilibrium (pK = 6.8) between HPO_4^{2-} and $H_2PO_4^-$ at physiologic pH in a ratio of about 4:1. For that reason, phosphorus is usually expressed in millimoles (mmol) rather than milliequivalents (mEq) per liter (L); however, as most laboratories report this inorganic component as "phosphorus," we will use this term in the remainder of this chapter. Levels are highest in infants and decrease throughout growth, reaching adult levels in the late teenage years.

Total adult body stores of phosphorus are approximately 700 g, of which 85% is contained in bone. Of the remainder, 14% is intracellular, and only 1% is extracellular. Of this extracellular phosphorus, 70% is organic and contained within phospholipids, and 30% is inorganic. Of the latter, 15% is protein-bound, and the remaining 85% is either complexed with sodium, magnesium, or calcium, or is circulating as the free monohydrogen or dihydrogen forms. Accordingly, only 0.15% of total body phosphorus (15% of extracellular phosphorus) is freely circulating, and this is the portion that is measured. Therefore, as with calcium, serum measurements reflect only a small fraction of total body phosphorus and do not accurately indicate total body stores in the setting of abnormal homeostasis (e.g., CKD).

The average American diet contains approximately 1000 to 1400 mg of phosphorus per day, and the recommended daily allowance (RDA) is 800 mg/day. Approximately two thirds of the ingested phosphorus is excreted in the urine and the remaining third in stool. In general, high-protein foods and dairy products contain the most phosphorus, whereas fruits and vegetables contain the least. In addition, grain-based (e.g., soy) protein contains phosphorus bound with phytate, making it less bioavailable. Many prepackaged and fast foods contain extra phosphorus as a preservative, which may not be identified on food labels. Therefore, it is difficult to predict accurately the dietary intake based on food type alone. Between 60% and 70% of dietary phosphorus is absorbed by the gut, in all intestinal segments. Medications that bind dietary phosphorus can decrease the net amount of phosphorus absorbed by decreasing the amount of free phosphorus available for absorption. In patients with CKD, these agents are used to compensate for the loss of renal excretion.

Passive enteric absorption (which is dependent on the luminal phosphorus concentration) occurs via the epithelial brush border sodium-phosphate cotransporter (NPT2b), driven by the sodium gradient created by the energy-using basolateral sodium-potassium ATPase transporter. The NPT2b sits in the terminal web, just below the brush border in "ready-to-use" vesicles that traffic to the brush border in response to acute and chronic changes in phosphorus concentration. Calcitriol can upregulate the NPT2b and thereby actively increase phosphorus absorption.

Most inorganic phosphorus is freely filtered by the glomerulus. Approximately 70% to 80% of the filtered load is reabsorbed in the proximal tubule, the primary site of regulated phosphorus reabsorption in the kidney, with the remaining 20% to 30% reabsorbed in the distal tubule. Hypophosphatemia stimulates CYP27B1, thereby increasing conversion of calcidiol to calcitriol, which in turn increases intestinal phosphorus absorption. Calcitriol also stimulates renal tubular phosphorus reabsorption, leading to a reduction in urinary phosphorus excretion. In the presence of hyperphosphatemia, there is a rapid increase in urinary excretion of phosphorus, mediated by the serum phosphorus level, PTH, and FGF23. Although the effects are more minor, renal phosphorus excretion is also increased by volume expansion, metabolic acidosis, glucocorticoids, and calcitonin, and is decreased by growth hormone and thyroid hormone. Because of the capacity of the kidney to increase urinary phosphorus excretion, sustained hyperphosphatemia is not seen clinically without impairment of kidney function.

MAGNESIUM

Magnesium plays an important role in neuromuscular function, control of cardiac excitability and vasomotor tone, mitochondrial function and energy metabolism, and DNA and protein synthesis. Magnesium is also a cofactor for many transporters involved in the regulation of sodium, potassium, and calcium. Normal magnesium levels are 0.7 to 1.1 mmol/L (1.4 to 2.2 mEq/L). Similar to calcium and phosphorus, a minority (1%) of total body magnesium is located in the extracellular space, whereas the majority of magnesium (approximately 60%) is in bone. Magnesium is the second most abundant cation in the intracellular fluid after potassium, with 20% of total body stores located in the intracellular compartments of muscle and 20% in other soft tissues. As a consequence (and similar to calcium and phosphorus), the serum magnesium level is a poor indicator of the total body stores.

There are no known hormones that specifically regulate magnesium homeostasis or balance. Magnesium transport is linked to carbohydrate-dependent active transport. Insulin, vitamin B_6, and 1,25 OH vitamin D favor magnesium entry into cells. Approximately 30% of the dietary magnesium is absorbed, mostly in the small intestine with a smaller contribution in the colon. Absorption is controlled by the transient receptor membrane potential 6 channel (TRMP6), which is downregulated by increased intracellular magnesium. High dietary phosphate inhibits magnesium intestinal absorption, whereas vitamins D and B_6 may enhance it. Magnesium enters cells through specific channels, TRMP6 and TRPM7. TRMP7 is ubiquitous, controlling magnesium balance in individual cells affecting their growth, whereas TRMP6 is localized to the distal convoluted tubule of the nephron and the gastrointestinal tract.

About 10% to 20% of filtered magnesium is reabsorbed in the proximal convoluted tubule, and reabsorption decreases with extracellular volume expansion in parallel with that of sodium and calcium. Unlike other divalent ions, the majority (75%) of magnesium is reabsorbed passively in the thick ascending limb of the loop of Henle, driven by a lumen-positive voltage in a specific cation-permeable channel formed by the tight junction proteins Claudin-16 (formerly called paracellin) and Claudin-19. Mutations of the latter proteins have a role in the development of familial hypomagnesemia with hypercalciuria and nephrocalcinosis. About 5% to 10% of magnesium is reabsorbed in the distal convoluted tubule, driven primarily by the luminal membrane potential established by the voltage-gated potassium channel and facilitated by TRMP6, which is located at the luminal membrane of the distal convoluted tubule.

BONE

The majority of the total body stores of calcium and phosphorus are located in bone in the form of hydroxyapatite $[Ca_{10}(PO_4)_6(OH)_2]$. Trabecular (cancellous) bone is 15% to 20% calcified. Trabecular bone is located predominately in the epiphyses of the long bones and serves a metabolic function. There is a relatively rapid exchange of calcium between trabecular bone and plasma (days to weeks), as evidenced by a short turnover rate of the radioisotope[45] calcium. In contrast, cortical (compact) bone is located in the shafts of long bones and is 80% to 90% calcified. This bone serves primarily a protective and mechanical function, and it has a calcium turnover rate of months. The nonmineral component of bone consists principally (90%) of highly organized cross-linked fibers of type I collagen; the remainder consists of proteoglycans and "noncollagen" proteins such as osteopontin, osteocalcin, osteonectin, and alkaline phosphatase. The predominant cell types involved in bone turnover are osteoclasts, the bone-resorbing cells derived from circulating hematopoietic cells, and osteoblasts, the bone-forming cells derived from the marrow. These cells are important in bone remodeling, which occurs in response to hormones, cytokines, and changes in mechanical forces, and can in turn affect calcium and phosphorus homeostasis.

DISORDERS OF MINERAL METABOLISM

HYPERCALCEMIA

Ionized calcium represents the biologically active fraction of total serum calcium. In the presence of hypoalbuminemia, there is a proportionate increase in ionized calcium relative to total calcium, so that measurements of total serum calcium in patients with hypoalbuminemia may underestimate the amount of physiologically active (ionized) calcium. A commonly used formula to estimate ionized calcium from total serum calcium is to add 0.8 mg/dl to the total calcium value for every 1 mg/dl decrease in serum albumin below 4 mg/dl. In certain circumstances, such as the presence of

increased concentrations of proteins capable of binding calcium (e.g., phosphate and citrate), paraproteinemias, or abnormally high or low blood pH, direct measurement of serum ionized calcium is essential, especially if intravenous calcium infusion is contemplated.

CLINICAL MANIFESTATIONS OF HYPERCALCEMIA

The severity of symptoms caused by hypercalcemia depends on the degree and rate of rise in serum calcium. Gastrointestinal symptoms such as nausea, vomiting, constipation, abdominal pain, and, rarely, peptic ulcer disease may occur. Neuromuscular involvement includes altered mentation, impaired concentration, fatigue, lethargy, and muscle weakness. Hypercalcemia can impair renal water handling by inducing nephrogenic diabetes insipidus and sodium wasting. The resulting diuresis worsens the hypercalcemia, because volume depletion limits the protective hypercalciuria and exacerbates the volume dependent proximal tubule reabsorption of calcium. In addition, volume depletion may lead to acute kidney injury, which further limits calcium excretion and favors an additional increase in serum calcium. The hypercalciuria associated with prolonged hypercalcemia can rarely lead to nephrolithiasis and nephrocalcinosis. Cardiovascular effects include hypertension and shortening of the QT interval on the electrocardiogram. Although cardiac arrhythmias are uncommon, hypercalcemia can trigger digitalis toxicity.

DIFFERENTIAL DIAGNOSIS OF HYPERCALCEMIA

The most common causes of hypercalcemia are malignancy and hyperparathyroidism; in most series, these two diagnoses account for more than 80% of cases. The remaining causes are listed in Box 11.1, with key causes discussed in more detail in the following paragraphs.

Box 11.1 Causes of Hypercalcemia

Malignancy
  Local osteolytic hypercalcemia
  Humoral hypercalcemia of malignancy (PTHrp)
  Hematologic malignancies such as lymphoma where there is ectopic calcitriol synthesis
Hyperparathyroidism
Thyrotoxicosis
Granulomatous diseases (sarcoidosis, histoplasmosis, tuberculosis)
Drug-induced
  Vitamin D
  Thiazide diuretics
  Estrogens and antiestrogens
  Androgens (breast cancer therapy)
  Vitamin A
  Lithium
Immobilization
Total parenteral nutrition
Impaired kidney function (AKI or CKD), usually from medications such as calcium-containing phosphate binders or calcitriol or its analogues

AKI, Acute kidney injury; *CKD,* chronic kidney disease; *PTHrp,* parathyroid hormone–related peptide.

Malignancy

Malignancy is the most common cause of hypercalcemia, and the presence of hypercalcemia in cancer patients confers a poor prognosis. Hypercalcemia can result from direct invasion of bone by metastatic disease (local osteolytic hypercalcemia [LOH]). In LOH, tumor cells within the bone marrow space produce a variety of inflammatory cytokines, collectively termed osteoclast-activating factors, which lead to net bone resorption and hypercalcemia. PTH levels are suppressed in response to the hypercalcemia. This mechanism is common with hypercalcemia resulting from breast cancer or multiple myeloma. Hypercalcemia can also result from the production of circulating factors that stimulate osteoclastic resorption of bone. Humoral hypercalcemia of malignancy is caused by secretion of parathyroid hormone–related peptide (PTHrp) by tumor cells. PTHrp bears similarity to PTH only in the initial 8-amino-acid sequence, but this homology permits binding to the PTH receptor, leading to increased bone turnover and hypercalcemia. Specific assays are available to distinguish circulating PTHrp from PTH. Finally, hypercalcemia in malignancy can result from increased production of calcitriol, which stimulates gastrointestinal absorption of calcium. Various lymphoid tumors, most notably Hodgkin's lymphoma, have been shown to synthesize large quantities of calcitriol.

Hyperparathyroidism

The incidence of *primary hyperparathyroidism* has declined during the last 30 years, but it is still the second most common cause of hypercalcemia. In most cases, primary hyperparathyroidism is caused by a benign adenoma of a single parathyroid gland that autonomously secretes PTH. The disorder may be sporadic, familial, or inherited as a component of the constellation of multiple endocrine neoplasia (MEN). The elevation in PTH results in increased intestinal absorption of calcium through stimulation of calcitriol production, increased osteoclastic bone resorption, and increased renal tubular reabsorption of calcium. However, because of the elevation in serum calcium, the filtered load of calcium exceeds the ability of the kidney to reabsorb calcium, leading to hypercalciuria and potentially to nephrolithiasis. *Secondary hyperparathyroidism* is caused by diffuse hyperplasia of all four glands in response to ongoing stimuli such as hypocalcemia or hyperphosphatemia. Iatrogenic hypercalcemia may occur in patients with secondary hyperparathyroidism treated with calcium-based phosphate binders or calcitriol and its derivatives. Secondary hyperparathyroidism can also cause hypercalcemia via increased bone resorption when the glands become adenomatous and no longer respond to the change in calcium—a stage often called *tertiary hyperparathyroidism.*

Lithium may interfere with the CaSR, leading to a "resetting" of the parathyroid gland sensitivity such that higher levels of calcium are needed to decrease PTH. Clinically, these patients may appear to have hyperparathyroidism, but hypercalcemia resolves when lithium is stopped.

Vitamin D Excess

Hypercalcemia from excessive exogenous intake of native vitamin D supplements (ergocalciferol and cholecalciferol) is rare, because 1α-hydroxylase (CHYP27B1) activity is tightly regulated by calcium levels. In contrast, the excessive administration of calcitriol or of other active vitamin D analogues, such as paricalcitol or doxercalciferol, which bypass this regulatory step at the level of the kidney, can lead to hypercalcemia. These drugs are commonly used in the treatment of secondary hyperparathyroidism in CKD. An endogenous source of excess calcitriol is production by nonkidney tissue. Lymphomas and granulomatous diseases such as sarcoidosis, tuberculosis, and leprosy likely cause hypercalcemia via increased production of calcitriol by monocytes and macrophages that possess 1α-hydroxylase activity.

Familial Hypocalciuric Hypercalcemia

Inactivating mutations of the CaSR cause familial hypocalciuric hypercalcemia (FHH), a rare hereditary disease with autosomal dominant transmission. Calcium is unable to activate the mutant receptor, leading to increased renal reabsorption of calcium into the blood from the tubular fluid and hypocalciuria, usually with urine calcium excretion <100 mg/day. Because this mutation may also affect the receptor at the level of the parathyroid gland, PTH may be slightly elevated out of proportion to the degree of hypercalcemia. Other clues pointing to this diagnosis include a family history of asymptomatic hypercalcemia. Probands are often discovered after parathyroidectomy fails to correct hypercalcemia.

APPROACH TO THE PATIENT WITH HYPERCALCEMIA

Clinicians may approach patients with hypercalcemia by reviewing the list in Box 11.1. An alternative approach is to formulate a differential diagnosis based on the physiology of calcium homeostasis (Fig. 11.4), tailoring diagnostic studies to the suspected pathophysiology.

Parathyroid Glands

The normal response to hypercalcemia is suppression of PTH secretion. Interpretation of a PTH level (normal: 10 to 65 pg/mL) must always be performed in conjunction with a simultaneously measured calcium level. For example, if the serum calcium level is 11.5 mg/dl and the PTH is 50 pg/mL, the circulating level of PTH is inappropriately high, suggesting hyperparathyroidism. Conversely, if the calcium is 8.5 mg/dl and the PTH is 70 pg/mL, then the elevated PTH is appropriate. Because PTH increases urinary phosphorus excretion, a normal or high-normal PTH level with hypercalcemia and a low or low-normal phosphorus level is essentially diagnostic of primary hyperparathyroidism. Radionuclide sestamibi imaging may be helpful in localizing an adenomatous gland; however, there is a high risk of false-negative scans, and an experienced parathyroid surgeon can usually locate the enlarged gland. Rarely, glands are found in the mediastinum. Parathyroid cancers secrete excess PTH, leading to severe hyperparathyroidism, and marked hypercalcemia may be present.

Bone

Hypercalcemia of bony origin occurs either because of enhanced bone turnover (osteoclast activity greater than osteoblast activity, or net bone resorption greater than bone formation) caused by local tumor invasion or as a result of increased secretion of hormonal factors by tumor cells (PTHrp, calcitriol, and PTH). Alternatively, immobilization may lead to the release of calcium from the bone, especially in the setting

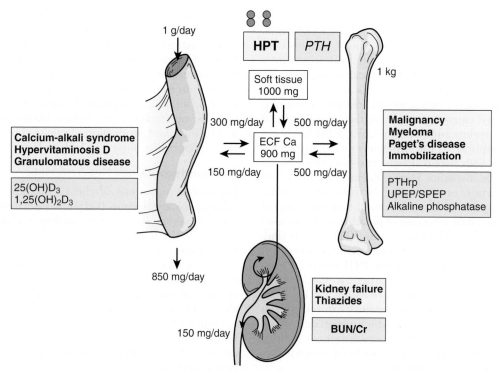

Figure 11.4   Approach to a patient with hypercalcemia. The normal daily calcium balance is shown, demonstrating the fluxes between the serum compartment and intestine and bone as well as the excretion of calcium. The patient with hypercalcemia must have an abnormality at the parathyroid glands *(top)*, intestine *(left)*, bone *(right)*, or kidney *(bottom)*. The *yellow boxes* represent causes of hypercalcemia that are associated with abnormalities at each of these target organs. The *blue boxes* indicate diagnostic tests that may be abnormal in these disorders. *BUN,* Blood urea nitrogen; *Cr,* creatinine; *ECF,* extracellular fluid; *HPT,* hyperparathyroidism; *PTH,* parathyroid hormone; *PTHrp,* parathyroid hormone–related peptide; *SPEP,* serum protein electrophoresis; *UPEP,* urine protein electrophoresis.

of excess turnover. Diagnostic studies for bone-induced hypercalcemia include PTH, PTHrp, urine and serum protein electrophoresis and immunofixation (to diagnose myeloma), and alkaline phosphatase. The latter is markedly elevated in Paget's disease and other high bone turnover states.

Intestine

Enhanced intestinal absorption of calcium can occur in conditions that result in elevated circulating levels of calcidiol or calcitriol. This can occur as a result of vitamin D toxicity with very high calcidiol levels, calcitriol therapy in patients with secondary hyperparathyroidism, calcitriol-producing granulomatous diseases and lymphomas, and hyperparathyroidism, which in turn increases calcitriol synthesis. In addition, excess calcium ingestion, especially with alkali, can lead to hypercalcemia. This is referred to as *calcium-alkali syndrome,* but in the past this was called *milk-alkali syndrome,* named for the combination of therapies used to treat peptic ulcer disease before the advent of proton pump blockers. To detect vitamin D toxicity, levels of both 25(OH)vitD (calcidiol) and 1,25(OH)$_2$vitD (calcitriol) should be measured. In the setting of exogenous vitamin D intake, calcidiol levels will be high and calcitriol levels normal to high. In the setting of granulomatous production of calcitriol, calcitriol levels will be high; calcidiol levels are nondiagnostic but will usually be low-normal.

Kidneys

With volume depletion, serum calcium levels rise and mild hypercalcemia can result. Thiazide diuretics, by blocking

distal tubular sodium reabsorption, enhance the sodium-calcium exchanger. This results in a reduction in urinary calcium excretion and hypercalcemia. These effects are used to advantage in the treatment of hypercalciuria in patients with nephrolithiasis. In most cases, the rise in serum calcium in response to thiazide diuretics does not result in clinical hypercalcemia. When thiazides induce hypercalcemia, there may be underlying hyperparathyroidism. PTH acts at the kidney to increase tubular reabsorption of calcium. Even so, patients with hypercalcemia from hyperparathyroidism tend to have an elevated urine calcium excretion, because the filtered load of calcium is so high. In primary hyperparathyroidism, the urinary calcium/creatinine ratio is usually greater than 0.2 (mg/mg), whereas, in patients with FHH, the urinary calcium/creatinine ratio is less than 0.01 mg/mg. Ideally, a 24-hour urine collection should be measured, but a spot collection may differentiate primary hyperparathyroidism from FHH.

TREATMENT OF HYPERCALCEMIA

The ultimate goal of therapy is to remedy the underlying cause of hypercalcemia; however, patients who present with acute symptoms of hypercalcemia require immediate treatment to reduce the serum levels. The safest and most effective treatment in patients with normal cardiac and kidney function is intravenous volume expansion with normal saline, which reduces proximal tubular reabsorption of sodium, water, and calcium. Most patients with symptomatic hypercalcemia are volume depleted at presentation because of the polyuria and natriuresis induced by hypercalcemia.

Table 11.1   Treatments for Hypercalcemia

Agent	Mode of Action	Dose
IV hydration with saline	Increases tubular flow and excretion of calcium	Hydration based on patient's cardiovascular status and level of kidney function; 200-500 mL/h
IV furosemide or loop diuretics	Block NKCC2 channel in loop of Henle, thus reducing positive electrochemical gradient for passive calcium reabsorption	20-40 mg intravenously after rehydration; dose may need to be adjusted based on level of kidney function
IV bisphosphonates	Inhibit osteoclastic activity	Pamidronate, 60-90 mg over 4 h Zoledronate, 4-8 mg over 15 min
Calcitonin	Inhibits bone resorption and enhances calcium excretion	4-12 IU/kg IM/SQ every 12 h
Glucocorticoids	Inhibit conversion of 25(OH)D to 1,25(OH)$_2$D	Hydrocortisone, 200 mg/day IV for 3 days Prednisone, 60 mg/day PO for 10 days
Cinacalcet	Allosteric activator of CaSR, mimicking increased calcium to reduce PTH	30 mg daily to twice daily, to a maximum dose of 90 mg twice daily; give with food to reduce nausea

CaSR, Calcium-sensing receptor; *IV*, intravenous; *NKCC2*, Na^{2+}/K$^+$/2Cl^{2-} cotransporter; *PTH*, parathyroid hormone.

In severe cases, very aggressive volume resuscitation may be required, with close attention to the patient's cardiopulmonary status to avoid volume overload. After volume expansion is achieved, calcium reabsorption can be further reduced with intravenous loop diuretics, such as furosemide, that block the Na$^+$-K$^+$-2Cl$^-$ cotransporter in the thick ascending limb, thereby disrupting the favorable electrochemical gradient for passive (paracellular) calcium reabsorption. As patients must be adequately hydrated before the diuretic is administered to avoid worsening hypovolemia and hypercalcemia, accurate assessment of intake and output is critical to optimize this treatment approach.

If these conservative treatments fail to restore normocalcemia, other pharmacologic options should be used (Table 11.1). Because the response to these agents is not immediate, their use in patients with severe symptoms of hypercalcemia may be appropriate early in the course of management. In the United States, the bisphosphonates pamidronate and zoledronic acid are approved for the treatment of malignancy-associated hypercalcemia. These agents block osteoclast-mediated bone resorption by inducing osteoclast apoptosis. Typically, a clinical response is seen within 2 to 4 days, with a nadir in serum calcium within 4 to 7 days. Caution is required, because acute kidney injury has been reported with rapid administration of bisphosphonates or in settings of volume depletion. Calcitonin has the advantage of rapid reduction of serum calcium, but its use is limited by a short duration of action and tachyphylaxis. Glucocorticoids are effective first-line agents, along with saline diuresis, when the hypercalcemia is mediated by elevated circulating levels of calcitriol due to granulomatous disorders or lymphoma. Mild hypercalcemia is usually not symptomatic and may not require aggressive therapy.

The approach to patients with hyperparathyroidism is more controversial. In primary hyperparathyroidism, intervention may be indicated only if symptoms (nephrolithiasis, lethargy, fatigue) are present. A National Institutes of Health consensus conference recommended that patients undergo surgical removal of the enlarged parathyroid gland if any of the following conditions are satisfied: (1) serum calcium 1.0 mg/dl greater than the laboratory upper limit of normal; (2) urine calcium excretion greater than 400 mg/day;

(3) creatinine clearance reduced by ≥30%; (4) dual-energy X-ray absorptiometry (DEXA) T-score of −2.5 present at any major site; and (5) age <50 years. An alternative to surgical parathyroidectomy is the use of cinacalcet, a calcimimetic. This agent is an allosteric activator of the CaSR that "mimics" higher levels of calcium, thereby decreasing PTH secretion and serum calcium. For primary hyperparathyroidism, the dose is usually 30 mg twice daily, titrating up to 90 mg twice daily.

HYPOCALCEMIA

With true hypocalcemia, the ionized calcium concentration is low; however, in patients with hypoalbuminemia, there is a decrease in total calcium but not necessarily a decrease in ionized calcium. In patients with excess citrate (from blood transfusions) or acute administration of bicarbonate, the percentage of calcium that is bound to these negatively charged ions increases; this reduces the free ionized calcium, usually with only a minimal change in total calcium. Acute respiratory alkalosis also lowers the ionized calcium. A decrease in the hydrogen ion concentration leads to protons dissociating from binding sites on other proteins. This increases protein binding of ionized calcium, thereby decreasing ionized calcium. Because the actual magnitude of any change in these circumstances may be hard to predict, the ionized calcium concentration is best measured directly.

CLINICAL MANIFESTATIONS OF HYPOCALCEMIA

Symptoms only occur with changes in the free ionized calcium, and most patients with mild hypocalcemia exhibit very few symptoms. Large or abrupt changes in ionized calcium may lead to symptoms including perioral numbness and spasms of the hands and feet. In some patients, progression to tetany or seizures occurs. This increased neuromuscular reactivity can be demonstrated by eliciting Chvostek sign or Trousseau sign. Chvostek sign is tested by tapping on the facial nerve near the temporal mandibular joint and watching for grimacing caused by spasm of the facial muscles. Trousseau sign is tested by inflating a blood pressure cuff to a pressure greater than the systolic blood pressure for

3 minutes and watching for spasm of the outstretched hand. Of these two signs, Trousseau is more specific. If these clinical signs are positive, hypocalcemia should be confirmed by measurement of ionized calcium.

DIFFERENTIAL DIAGNOSIS OF HYPOCALCEMIA

The causes of hypocalcemia are best organized mechanistically.

Vitamin D Deficiency

Vitamin D, once activated to calcitriol, is the primary determinant of intestinal calcium absorption. Individuals may be deficient in vitamin D because of poor absorption from dietary sources (e.g., malabsorption, short bowel, poor nutrition); lack of sun exposure; abnormal conversion of calcidiol to calcitriol in the liver (cirrhosis, some drugs); or decreased renal conversion of calcidiol to calcitriol (CKD). These patients have low levels of vitamin D and an increase in PTH.

Hypoparathyroidism

Deficiency or inactivity of PTH results in hypocalcemia. This may be caused by inadvertent removal of the parathyroid glands during thyroid surgery or by radiation therapy, congenital defects, or autoimmune disease. These patients have an inappropriately low PTH for their low calcium levels. In the absence of PTH, the only mechanism to increase serum calcium is via intestinal absorption stimulated by the administration of vitamin D (usually in the active form, calcitriol) and oral calcium. Hypomagnesemia may also cause resistance to PTH as well as suppression of PTH release.

Pseudohypoparathyroidism

The term *pseudohypoparathyroidism* describes a group of disorders that are characterized by hypocalcemia and hypophosphatemia, elevated PTH levels, and lack of tissue responsiveness to PTH. The magnesium and calcidiol levels are normal. A PTH infusion test can confirm the tissue resistance. Intravenous administration of PTH normally results in increased urinary cyclic adenosine monophosphate (cAMP) and phosphorus excretion, but patients with pseudohypoparathyroidism lack this response. The most common form of pseudohypoparathyroidism is type Ia, Albright's hereditary osteodystrophy, which is also associated with short stature, round facies, obesity, brachydactyly, and other defects.

Tissue Consumption of Calcium

Hypocalcemia may result from the precipitation of calcium into extraskeletal tissue, such as occurs in pancreatitis. In addition, excess bone formation in some malignancies with blastic bone metastases may cause the bone to take up excess calcium acutely. After parathyroidectomy, there is an acute drop in serum calcium and phosphorus because of the "hungry bone syndrome," wherein calcium and phosphorus are rapidly taken up because of the sudden reduction in PTH. This phenomenon is more severe and more protracted in patients with kidney failure who are undergoing parathyroidectomy as a treatment for severe secondary hyperparathyroidism. In acute hyperphosphatemia caused by rhabdomyolysis or tumor lysis syndrome, phosphorus binds to calcium leading to a fall in ionized calcium.

Similarly, the infusion of citrate, a preservative in blood and plasma transfusions, can reduce ionized calcium as discussed earlier. Last, sepsis is also associated with hypocalcemia, although the mechanism is not clear.

TREATMENT OF HYPOCALCEMIA

Intravenous calcium infusions are indicated only in the setting of symptomatic hypocalcemia, and they should not be administered to patients with severe hyperphosphatemia because of the risk of ectopic precipitation of calcium phosphate. Intravenous calcium comes in two forms: calcium gluconate (10 mL vial = 94 mg elemental calcium) and calcium chloride (10 mL vial = 273 mg elemental calcium). Calcium chloride is typically used only during cardiopulmonary resuscitation because its infusion is painful and can cause vein sclerosis. Importantly, patients who are not symptomatic should be repleted with oral, not intravenous, calcium. The most common oral supplement is calcium carbonate, starting with 1 to 2 g of elemental calcium three times daily (1250 mg calcium carbonate = 500 mg elemental calcium), given apart from meals. The amount of calcium absorbed will be increased if calcitriol (0.25 µg twice daily to start) is administered with the calcium. Any hypomagnesemia should be treated concomitantly, and, if appropriate, patients may be changed from loop to thiazide diuretics to decrease urinary calcium excretion.

HYPERPHOSPHATEMIA

Hyperphosphatemia can result from increased intestinal absorption, from cellular release or rapid shifts of phosphorus from the intracellular to the extracellular compartment, or from decreased renal excretion. Persistent hyperphosphatemia (>12 hours) occurs almost exclusively in the setting of impaired kidney function. Increased intestinal absorption is usually caused either by the use of phosphate-containing oral purgatives or enemas, or by vitamin D overdoses. Increased tissue release of phosphorus is commonly seen in acute tumor lysis syndrome, rhabdomyolysis, hemolysis, hyperthermia, profound catabolic stress, or acute leukemia. These disorders can also lead to acute kidney injury, limiting renal phosphate excretion and further exacerbating the hyperphosphatemia. Rarely, thyrotoxicosis or acromegaly leads to hyperphosphatemia. Acute hyperphosphatemia usually does not cause symptoms unless there is a significant reciprocal reduction of serum calcium. The treatment of acute hyperphosphatemia includes volume expansion, dialysis, and administration of phosphate binders. In the setting of normal kidney function, or even mild to moderate kidney disease, hyperphosphatemia is usually self limited because of the capacity of the kidney to excrete a phosphorus load. Sequelae and treatment of hyperphosphatemia related to CKD, including bone disease and cardiovascular disease, is discussed in detail in Chapter 56.

HYPOPHOSPHATEMIA

Hypophosphatemia can occur with decreased phosphorus intake (decreased intestinal absorption or increased gastrointestinal losses) or with excess renal wasting because of renal tubular defects or hyperparathyroidism. In addition, low serum phosphorus levels may also occur in the setting

---

Box 11.2   Causes of Hypophosphatemia

Decreased Intestinal Absorption

Antacid abuse or excessive calcium supplement use
Malabsorption and chronic diarrhea
Vitamin D deficiency
Starvation or anorexia
Alcoholism

Increased Urinary Losses

Primary hyperparathyroidism
Following kidney transplantation
Extracellular volume expansion
Glucosuria (after treatment of DKA)
Postobstructive or resolving ATN diuresis
Acetazolamide
Fanconi syndrome
X-linked and vitamin D–dependent rickets
Oncogenic osteomalacia

Redistribution

Respiratory alkalosis
Alcohol withdrawal
Severe burns
Postfeeding syndrome
Leukemic blast crisis
Treatment of hyperglycemia

ATN, Acute tubular necrosis; *DKA,* diabetic ketoacidosis.

---

of extracellular-to-intracellular shifts. In the case of cellular shifts, total body phosphorus may not be depleted. By convention, hypophosphatemia is often graded as mild (<3.5 mg/dl), moderate (<2.5 mg/dl), or severe (<1.0 mg/dl). Moderate and severe hypophosphatemia usually occur only if there are multiple causes (Box 11.2).

CLINICAL MANIFESTATIONS OF HYPOPHOSPHATEMIA

Hypophosphatemia is fairly common, observed in approximately 3% of all hospitalized patients, 10% of hospitalized alcoholic patients, and 70% of mechanically ventilated patients. Symptoms, including muscle weakness (and difficulty weaning from the ventilator), hemolysis, impaired platelet and white blood cell function, rhabdomyolysis, and, in moderate-to-severe cases, neurologic disorders. Hypophosphatemia is probably overtreated in the intensive care unit, where the "difficult to wean" patient may be given phosphorus when the low phosphorus levels are actually caused by cellular shifts due to respiratory alkalosis. A careful review of the trend in serum phosphorus with arterial blood pH can help discern which patients need to be treated.

DIFFERENTIAL DIAGNOSIS OF HYPOPHOSPHATEMIA

The differential diagnosis and treatment approach are based on the cause and site of phosphate loss. The cause is usually clinically apparent, but if it is not, the simplest test is measurement of the 24-hour urine phosphorus excretion. The expected renal response to hypophosphatemia is avid reabsorption. If the urinary excretion is less than 100 mg/24 h, then the kidney is responding appropriately to hypophosphatemia, and the cause must be impaired

intake, gastrointestinal losses, or extracellular-to-intracellular shifts.

Decreased Oral Intake

The average American diet contains excessive amounts of phosphorus. All proteins and dairy products contain phosphorus, and phosphorus is used as a preservative in most processed foods. Decreased intake of phosphorus is usually seen only with generalized poor oral intake, gastrointestinal losses from diarrhea and malabsorption, or alcoholism. Occasionally, patients abuse antacids or take excessive calcium supplements, both of which bind phosphorus.

Redistribution

Approximately 15% of the extraskeletal phosphorus is intracellular, and hypophosphatemia may result from a shift to intracellular stores. In most situations, this shift is not clinically detectable; however, if there is underlying phosphate depletion, more profound hypophosphatemia may be observed. The most common clinical cause of this form of hypophosphatemia is hyperglycemia with or without ketoacidosis. The glucose-induced osmotic diuresis results in a net deficit of phosphorus, whereas cellular glucose uptake stimulated by insulin during treatment further causes a shift of the extracellular phosphorus into cells as glycogen stores are repleted. In this setting, hypophosphatemia is usually transient and, in general, should not be treated. In patients who are malnourished, sudden "refeeding" may shift phosphorus into cells. Respiratory, but not metabolic, alkalosis also increases the intracellular flux of phosphorus. Even in normal subjects, severe hyperventilation (to a carbon dioxide tension [PCO_2] of <20 mm Hg) may lower serum phosphorus concentrations to <1.0 mg/dl. Therefore, in ventilated patients, arterial blood gases may be helpful in differentiating shifts resulting from true phosphorus depletion. Last, in hungry bone syndrome after parathyroidectomy (described earlier), there is increased bone uptake of phosphorus and resultant hypophosphatemia.

Increased Urinary Losses

Phosphorus clearance by the kidney is primarily determined by the phosphorus concentration, urinary flow, PTH, and FGF23 and other phosphatonins. Patients who are overly volume expanded exhibit less proximal tubular reabsorption of phosphorus in parallel with reduced proximal sodium and water reabsorption. Similarly, patients with glucosuria and postobstructive diuresis experience increased urinary flow and phosphorus losses. In primary hyperparathyroidism, there is increased urinary phosphorus excretion caused by elevated PTH levels. Both congenital and acquired Fanconi syndrome are characterized by increased urinary phosphorus excretion because of defects in proximal tubule reabsorption, together with renal glucosuria, hypouricemia, aminoaciduria, and, potentially, proximal renal tubular acidosis (Type 2). Acquired forms of Fanconi syndrome may be seen in multiple myeloma and after administration of some chemotherapy drugs (cisplatin, ifosfamide, and 6-mercaptopurine), outdated tetracycline, or the antiretroviral agent tenofovir.

Rickets and Osteomalacia

Hypophosphatemia can lead to impaired bone mineralization. Several genetic disorders are associated with hypophosphatemia and rickets in children, including autosomal dominant hypophosphatemic rickets (ADHR) and X-linked hypophosphatemic rickets (XLH). These patients present with phosphaturia, hypophosphatemia, inappropriately low calcitriol levels, normal to slightly elevated PTH, and normocalcemia. The defective gene in XLH is an endopeptidase called PHEX. In XLH, it has been postulated that PHEX abnormalities may lead to altered FGF23 metabolism, but this remains speculative. In ADHR, FGF23 is mutated, resulting in abnormal clearance of the protein and prolonged and inappropriate hypophosphaturia (see also Chapter 40). In tumor-induced osteomalacia, tumors of mesenchymal origin secrete phosphatonins such as FGF23, matrix extracellular phosphoglycoprotein (MEPE), or FRP4, which upregulate the renal sodium phosphate cotransporter with resultant renal phosphate wasting.

TREATMENT OF HYPOPHOSPHATEMIA

Treatment is usually necessary for patients with moderate to severe hypophosphatemia. Increasing oral phosphorus intake is the preferred treatment, because intravenous administration of phosphate complexes with calcium and can lead to extraskeletal calcifications. Oral supplementation can be given with skim milk (1000 mg/quart), whole milk (850 mg/quart), Neutra-Phos K capsules (250 mg/capsule; maximum dose, 3 tabs every 6 hours), or Neutra-Phos solution (128 mg/mL). Oral phosphorus may induce or exacerbate diarrhea. Milk is much better tolerated, is a source of nutrition, and is cheaper! The concomitant administration of vitamin D will enhance its absorption. If necessary, phosphorus may be replaced intravenously as potassium phosphate (3 mmol/mL of phosphorus, 4.4 mEq/mL of potassium) or sodium phosphate (3 mmol/mL of phosphorus, 4.0 mEq/mL of sodium) in a single administration, usually mixed in 50 mL of normal saline.

HYPERMAGNESEMIA

Hypermagnesemia is present when the serum level is >2.9 mg/dl, although clinical manifestations typically do not occur until serum levels are >4 mg/dl. Signs and symptoms include hyporeflexia (usually the first sign) and weakness that may progress to paralysis and can involve the diaphragm. Cardiac findings are bradycardia, hypotension, and cardiac arrest. ECG findings include prolonged PR, QRS, and QT intervals, and complete heart block may occur when the levels are as high as 15 mEq/L. Of note, moderate hypermagnesemia can inhibit the secretion of PTH, which may lead to hypocalcemia and subsequent prolonged QT interval.

DIFFERENTIAL DIAGNOSIS OF HYPERMAGNESEMIA

Because hypermagnesemia appears to stimulate renal excretion, it is "self regulating," and prolonged hypermagnesemia generally occurs only when there is reduced kidney function. Hypermagnesemia is usually iatrogenic from laxatives, antacids, or intravenous magnesium. Levels will be purposefully elevated in the treatment of ecclampsia, but they resolve quickly with cessation of therapy due to renal excretion. Other causes of a mild elevation of magnesium include theophylline intoxication, tumor lysis syndrome, acromegaly, familial hypocalciuric hypercalcemia, and adrenal insufficiency.

TREATMENT OF HYPERMAGNESEMIA

Treatment begins with avoiding magnesium-containing medications, including some laxatives and antacids in patients with reduced kidney function. In the presence of normal kidney function, asymptomatic hypermagnesemia will resolve, and no treatment is indicated. If hypermagnesemia is symptomatic, administration of calcium gluconate (~90 to 180 mg of elemental calcium) over 10 to 20 minutes will help antagonize the effect of the excessive magnesium. Supportive therapy may include mechanical ventilation and the placement of a temporary pacemaker. With adequate kidney function, volume expansion with intravenous saline facilitates renal excretion of magnesium. In the case of kidney failure, dialysis is required.

HYPOMAGNESEMIA

Serum magnesium <0.65 mmol/L (1.3 mEq/L) defines hypomagnesemia. Similar to calcium and phosphorus, a minority of magnesium is in the extracellular space; however, unlike calcium there is no "ionized" magnesium measurement available. Therefore, when blood magnesium levels are normal, this does not exclude magnesium deficiency. On the other hand, when there is severe magnesium deficiency, there is almost always hypomagnesemia. In patients with normal magnesium levels but clinical suspicion of hypomagnesemia, urine magnesium should be checked. If low, this confirms magnesium depletion.

Renal wasting of magnesium can be diagnosed in the presence of hypomagnesemia if there is more than 2 mEq (or >24 mg) of magnesium in the 24-hour urine collection, or if the fractional excretion of magnesium is >2%. The fractional excretion of magnesium is calculated as follows:

$$FE_{Mg} = \frac{U_{Mg}/(0.7 \times P_{Mg})}{U_{Cr}/P_{Cr}} \times 100$$

where U and P are urinary and plasma concentrations of magnesium (Mg) and creatinine (Cr).

CLINICAL MANIFESTATIONS OF HYPOMAGNESEMIA

Hypomagnesemia is seen in 10% of hospitalized patients and 20% of patients in the ICU. Forty percent of patients with hypomagnesemia will have hypokalemia, and 20% will have hypocalcemia, hypophosphatemia, or hyponatremia. Notably, hypokalemia may appear refractory to potassium replacement until the magnesium is repleted, suggesting that magnesium levels should be evaluated in hypokalemia. Patients with severe hypomagnesemia may have clinical neurologic or cardiovascular abnormalities. Symptoms include muscle cramps, generalized fatigue, and ileus. With more severe depletion, confusion, ataxia, nystagmus, tremor, hyperreflexia, fasciculations, tetany, and seizures may occur. Cardiac arrhythmia may occur, particularly with patients on digoxin, with ECG changes including prolonged PR and QT intervals with a widened QRS complex. Torsades de pointes is the other classic finding.

DIFFERENTIAL DIAGNOSIS OF HYPOMAGNESEMIA

Hypomagnesemia may be caused by: (1) decreased intake, as in chronic alcoholism and malabsorption syndromes; (2) increased gastrointestinal losses; (3) increased renal

Box 11.3   Causes of Hypomagnesemia

Decreased Intake

Prolonged fasting
Chronic alcoholism
Protein-calorie malnutrition
Inadequate parenteral nutrition

Gastrointestinal Losses

Chronic diarrhea
Laxative abuse
Malabsorption syndromes
Massive resection of the small intestine
Neonatal hypomagnesemia

Renal Losses

Drugs
    Diuretics
    Amphotericin B
    Aminoglycosides
    Cisplatin
    Pentamidine
    Proton pump inhibitors
    Cyclosporine
    Tacrolimus
    Foscarnet
    Cetuximab
High Urinary Output States
    Postobstructive diuresis
    Diuretic phase of acute tubular necrosis
    Posttransplantation polyuria
Inherited Hypomagnesemia
    Gitelman syndrome
    Bartter syndrome
    Other genetic transient receptor potential abnormalities
Primary hyper aldosteronism
Hypercalcemic states
Phosphate depletion
Chronic metabolic acidosis
Idiopathic renal wasting

Miscellaneous

Acute pancreatitis
Hungry bone syndrome
Diabetic ketoacidosis
Acute intermittent porphyria

Table 11.2   Examples of Magnesium Supplementation

Source	Mass of Elemental Magnesium*
Mag-Ox 400 PO (mg oxide)	240 mg per tablet = 20 mEq per tablet
Uro-Mag 140 PO (mg oxide)	85 mg = 7 mEq
Magnesium Gluconate 500 (tablet or liquid)	27 mg = 2.3 mEq
Slow-Mag PO (mg chloride)	64 mg = 5.3 mEq
MagTab SR (84 mg elemental mg per tab)	84 mg tablet = 7 mEq
Magnesium Sulfate 1 g IV	96 mg = 8 mEq

IV, Intravenous.
*mg of magnesium per tablet = mEq magnesium per tablet.

intracellular space can occur, particularly with treatment of diabetic ketoacidosis and alcohol withdrawal. In contrast to the rapid shifts of calcium and phosphorus from bone to maintain serum levels, this potential compensatory mechanism for magnesium may take weeks, and thus is not a factor in acute homeostasis of blood levels.

TREATMENT OF HYPOMAGNESEMIA

Magnesium should be administered cautiously in the presence of kidney dysfunction. In asymptomatic hypomagnesemia, up to 720 mg of oral elemental magnesium can be given per day, although oral magnesium salts are associated with gastrointestinal symptoms including diarrhea. In some cases, amiloride may be effective in reducing renal wasting. In severe symptomatic hypomagnesemia, 1 to 2 g of intravenous magnesium sulfate may be administered over 15 to 30 minutes, followed by an infusion of 5 to 6 g over 24 hours, with levels checked daily to avoid overrepletion. As only a portion of intravenously administered magnesium is retained, repeat magnesium levels several days later are needed to determine the efficacy of repletion. Dosing for intravenous and oral administration of magnesium is presented in Table 11.2.

BIBLIOGRAPHY

Aloia JF: Clinical review: the 2011 report on dietary reference intake for vitamin D: where do we go from here? *J Clin Endocrinol Metab* 96(10):2987-2996, 2011 Oct.

Atsmon J, Dolev E: Drug-induced hypomagnesaemia: scope and management, *Drug Saf* 28:763-788, 2008.

Glaudemans B, Knoers NB, Hoenderop JG, et al: New molecular players facilitation Mg(2+) reabsorption in the distal convoluted tubule, *Kidney Int* 77:17-22, 2010.

Herroeder S, Schonherr ME, De Hert SG, et al: Magnesium—essentials for anesthesiologists, *Anesthesiology* 114:971-993, 2011.

Hoenderop JG, Bindels RJ: Calciotropic and magnesiotropic TRP channels, *Physiology* 23:32-40, 2008.

Huang CL, Kuo E: Mechanism of hypokalemia in magnesium deficiency, *J Am Soc Nephrol* 18:2649-2652, 2007.

Juppner H: Phosphate and FGF-23, *Kidney Int* 79(Suppl 121):524-527, 2011.

Kuro OM: Phosphate and klotho, *Kidney Int Suppl* S20-S23, 2011.

Makariou S, Liberopoulos EN, Elisaf M, et al: Novel roles of vitamin D in disease: what is new in 2011? *Eur J Intern Med* 22(4):355-362, 2011 Aug.

losses; or (4) intravascular chelation and extravascular deposition, as seen with hypocalcemia (Box 11.3). The latter can occur when substances that complex with magnesium become available, such as fatty acids released in acute pancreatitis and citrate. It also occurs in the hungry bone syndrome following parathyroidectomy. Renal losses occur in the presence of hypercalcemia (where calcium competes with magnesium to be reabsorbed in the thick ascending limb), osmotic diuresis, volume expansion (because of the decreased magnesium reabsorption associated with the increased tubular flow), and genetic disorders or drugs that that lead to defects in tubular magnesium transport. Culprit drugs include diuretics, aminoglycosides, amphotericin B, cisplatin, and cyclosporine, making it important to monitor magnesium blood levels when these drugs are used. Similar to calcium and phosphorus, shifts from the extracellular to

Marcocci C, Cetani F: Primary hyperparathyroidism, *N Engl J Med* 365:2389-2397, 2011.

Renkema KY, Alexander RT, Bindels RJ, et al: Calcium and phosphate homeostasis: concerted interplay of new regulators, *Ann Med* 40: 82-91, 2008.

Romani AM: Cellular magnesium homeostasis, *Arch Biochem Biophys* 512:1-23, 2011.

Santarpia L, Koch CA, Sarlis NJ: Hypercalcemia in cancer patients: pathobiology and management, *Horm Metab Res* 42(3):153-164 Mar.

Vucinic V, Skodric-Trifunovic V, Ignajatovic S: How to diagnose and manage difficult problems of calcium metabolism in sarcoidosis: an evidence-based review, *Curr Opin Pulm Med* 17:297-302, 2011.

Ward DT, Riccardi D: New concepts in calcium-sensing receptor pharmacology and signaling, *Br J Pharmacol* 165:35-48, 2011.

Approach to Acid-Base Disorders

12

Ankit N. Mehta | Michael Emmett

Acid-base disorders can have major clinical and diagnostic implications. If they generate extreme acidemia or alkalemia, then the abnormal pH itself may result in pathophysiologic consequences. For example, the tertiary structure of proteins is altered by extreme pH conditions, potentially affecting the activity of enzymes and ion transport systems. Consequently, every metabolic pathway may be impacted by acidemia or alkalemia. In addition, extreme acidemia can depress cardiac function, impair the vascular response to catecholamines, and cause arteriolar vasodilation and venoconstriction, with resultant systemic hypotension and pulmonary edema. Insulin resistance; reduced hepatic lactate uptake, and accelerated protein catabolism are other effects of acidemia. Alkalemia can generate cardiac arrhythmias, produce neuromuscular irritability, and contribute to tissue hypoxemia. In alkalemic patients, cerebral and myocardial blood flow falls, and respiratory depression occurs. Potassium disorders, a common accompaniment of acid-base perturbations, also contribute to the morbidity.

Although mild and moderate acid-base disorders may not directly affect physiologic function, the identification of such disorders may be an important diagnostic clue to the existence of serious medical conditions. Whenever an acid-base disorder is identified, the underlying cause should be sought. This diagnostic imperative often overrides the importance of any therapeutic intervention directed at the pH itself. The situation is analogous to the discovery of fever or hypothermia. Although very high or very low temperatures can themselves be dangerous and require aggressive therapy directed at restoration of a more normal temperature, often more important is the effort to identify and treat the underlying cause of the abnormal temperature. Similarly, the recognition of an acid-base disorder must generate a search for its clinical cause or causes, and recognition of a mixed acid-base disorder should trigger an investigation to determine the etiology of each component.

The acid-base status of the extracellular fluid (ECF) is carefully regulated to maintain the arterial pH in a narrow range between 7.36 and 7.44 (hydrogen ion concentration [H^+] 44 to 36 nEq/L). The pH is stabilized by multiple buffer systems in the ECF, cells, and bone. The CO_2 tension (pCO_2), primarily under neurorespiratory control, and the serum bicarbonate concentration ($[HCO_3^-]$), primarily under renal/metabolic regulation, are the most important variables in this complex system of buffers.

Currently three different methodologic approaches are widely used to describe normal acid-base status and simple and mixed acid-base disorders.

1. The physiologic or "Boston" method uses measurements of arterial pH, pCO_2, and $[HCO_3^-]$ together with an analysis of the anion gap (AG) and a set of compensation rules.
2. The Base Excess (BE) or "Copenhagen" method uses measurements of arterial pH and pCO_2, and calculation of the BE and the AG.
3. The physicochemical or "Stewart" method uses measurements of arterial pH and pCO_2 together with the calculated apparent (SIDa) and effective (SIDe) "Strong Ion Difference," the "Strong Ion Gap" (SIG = SIDa-SIDe), and the total concentration of plasma weak acids (Atot).

Each of these approaches can be effectively used to characterize acid-base disorders, each has its vocal proponents and detractors, and each has certain unique characteristics that may be particularly helpful under certain conditions. We believe the physiologic, or "Boston," approach is the most straightforward and the easiest model to understand and use. It is generally acceptable in most clinical circumstances, and will be the method we use in this chapter.

The physiologic approach to the elucidation of acid-base disorders uses the following information:

1. Recognition of diagnostic clues provided by the patient's history and physical examination.
2. Analysis of the serum $[HCO_3^-]$, arterial pH, and pCO_2 (although a blood gas analysis is not always necessary to make a diagnosis, it is generally required for complicated cases).
3. Knowledge of the predicted compensatory response to simple acid-base disorders.
4. Calculation of the AG, with consideration of the expected "baseline" AG for each patient.
5. Analysis of the degree of change (Δ) in AG and the degree of Δ in $[HCO_3^-]$ to see if the magnitude of these respective changes is reciprocal. This has been dubbed the Delta/Delta or $\Delta[AG]/\Delta[HCO_3^-]$.

ACIDEMIA, ALKALEMIA, ACIDOSIS, AND ALKALOSIS

The normal arterial blood pH range is between 7.36 and 7.44 ($[H^+]$ between 44 and 36 nEq/L). Acidemia is defined as an arterial pH <7.36 ($[H^+]$ >44 nEq/L) and may result from a primary elevation in pCO_2, a fall in $[HCO_3^-]$, or both. Alkalemia is defined as an arterial pH >7.44 ($[H^+]$ <36 nEq/L). Alkalemia may result from a primary increase in $[HCO_3^-]$, a fall in pCO_2, or both.

The relationship between pH, pCO_2, and HCO_3^- concentrations is described by the familiar Henderson-Hasselbalch equation*:

$$pH = 6.1 + \log\left(\frac{[HCO_3^-]}{0.03 \times P_{CO_2}}\right)$$

Acidosis and alkalosis are pathophysiologic processes that, if unopposed by therapy or complicating disorders, would cause acidemia or alkalemia, respectively.

SIMPLE (SINGLE) ACID-BASE DISTURBANCES AND COMPENSATION

The simple acid-base disorders are divided into primary metabolic and primary respiratory disturbances. Each of these simple, or single, acid-base disorders generates a compensatory response that acts to return the blood pH back toward the normal range. By convention, the physiologic approach to acid-base analysis considers the compensatory response to a simple acid-base disorder to be an integral component of that disorder. Hence there are four primary simple acid-base disturbances (six if each respiratory disorder is divided into an acute and chronic phase):

- *Metabolic acidosis:* The underlying pathophysiology tends to reduce the serum bicarbonate concentration [HCO_3^-].* Causes include excess generation of metabolic acids, excessive exogenous acid intake, reduced kidney excretion of acid, or excessive exogenous loss of HCO_3^- (usually in stool or urine). Metabolic acidosis reduces the arterial plasma pH and generates a hyperventilatory compensatory response, which reduces the arterial pCO_2 and blunts the degree of acidemia.
- *Metabolic alkalosis:* The underlying pathophysiology tends to increase the [HCO_3^-]. Causes include exogenous intake of HCO_3^- salts (or salts that can be converted to HCO_3^-) and/or endogenous generation of HCO_3^-. Regardless of the origin of the HCO_3^-, the pathology must also include reduced or impaired renal HCO_3^- excretion. Metabolic alkalosis increases the arterial plasma pH and generates a hypoventilatory compensatory response, which increases the arterial pCO_2 and blunts the degree of alkalemia.
- *Respiratory acidosis:* The underlying pathophysiology tends to increase the arterial pCO_2. The compensatory response is an increase of the plasma [HCO_3^-] due to rapid generation from buffers and, over a period of days, renal HCO_3^- generation and retention.
- *Respiratory alkalosis:* The underlying pathophysiology tends to decrease the arterial pCO_2. The compensatory response reduces the plasma [HCO_3^-]. This occurs acutely as H^+ is released from buffers and chronically, over a period of days, as the kidneys excrete HCO_3^- and/or retain acid.

The magnitude of each compensatory response is proportional to the severity of the primary disturbance. Generally, respiratory responses to primary metabolic acid-base disorders occur rapidly (within an hour) and are fully developed within 12 to 36 hours. In contrast, the compensatory metabolic alterations triggered by the primary respiratory disorders are divided into two phases. A chemical buffering response occurs within minutes (acute), whereas the quantitatively more significant kidney response takes several days (chronic) to develop fully. Hence, each primary respiratory disorder is subdivided into an acute and a chronic disorder to differentiate the expected compensatory response.

The expected degree of compensation for each simple disorder has been determined by studying patients with isolated simple disorders and normal subjects with experimentally induced acid-base disorders. These data have been used to create various graphic acid-base nomograms, simple mathematical relationships, and a number of mnemonic methods for predicting expected compensation ranges. Figure 12.1 and Table 12.1 provide some of these "compensation rules." Appropriate compensation should generally be present in all patients with an acid-base disorder, and when it is not identified, a complex, or mixed, acid-base disorder must be considered.

In general, with one exception, compensatory responses return the pH toward the normal range but do not completely normalize the pH. The exception is chronic respiratory alkalosis, wherein compensation results in a pH that is normal. With all other disorders, some degree of acidemia or alkalemia remains, even after full compensation. Compensatory responses result in the pCO_2 moving in the same direction as the primary [HCO_3^-] change in case of metabolic acid-base disorder, and the [HCO_3^-] moving in the same direction as the primary pCO_2 change in case of respiratory acid-base disorder (see Table 12.1). If the pCO_2 and [HCO_3^-] are deranged in opposite directions (i.e., the pCO_2 or [HCO_3^-] is increased and the other variable is decreased), then a mixed disturbance must exist.

ANION GAP

The ion profile of normal serum is depicted in Figure 12.2A. In any solution, the total cation charge concentration must be equal to the total anion charge concentration (all measured in units of electrical charge concentration, i.e., mEq/L). Now consider only the three serum electrolytes that are at the highest concentration, namely Na^+, Cl^-, and HCO_3^-. The cation charge concentration [Na^+] normally exceeds the sum of the anion charge concentrations [Cl^-] and [HCO_3^-]. If the sum of the two anions is subtracted from [Na], an "anion gap" (AG) is noted (see Fig. 12.2B).

$$AG = [Na^+] - ([Cl^-] + [HCO_3^-])$$

This AG is of course a function of the decision to consider only the three "major" serum electrolytes and not other ions that normally exist in serum. Nevertheless, the AG, defined in this fashion, is a very useful diagnostic tool.

The normal value of the AG varies among laboratories as a result of the wide variety of analyte measurement technologies and unique normal ranges for each instrument.

---

*Although we refer to serum bicarbonate here, it is often directly measured as total CO_2, which includes bicarbonate (HCO_3^-), carbonic acid (H_2CO_3), and dissolved CO_2. The latter two components account for a very small fraction of the total (roughly 1.2 mEq/L at normal pCO_2). Therefore, for clinical purposes total CO_2 is equated to the serum bicarbonate (HCO_3^-).

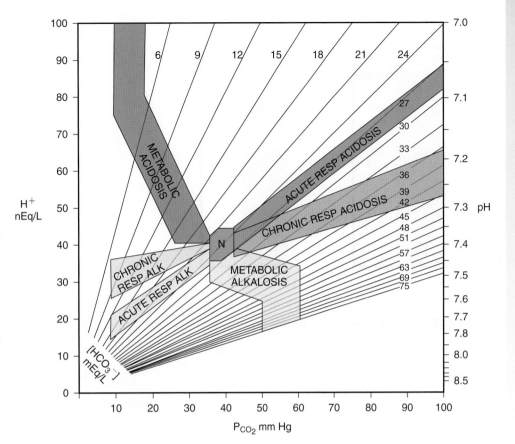

Figure 12.1   The acid-base map. Shaded areas represent the 95% confidence limits for zones of compensation for the simple acid-base disorders. Numbered diagonal lines represent isopleths of plasma bicarbonate concentration ($[HCO_3^-]$). Laboratory values that fall within a colored zone are consistent with the simple acid-base disorder as shown. If the values fall outside a colored zone, a mixed acid-base disorder is likely. *ALK,* Alkalosis; *N,* normal range; *RESP,* respiratory. (Modified and updated from Goldberg M, Green SB, Moss ML, Marhacli MS, Garfinkel D: Computer-based instruction and diagnosis of acid-base disorders. *JAMA* 223:269-275, 1973.)

Table 12.1   "Acid-Base Rules": Changes in pH, Pco_2, and $[HCO_3^-]$ and Expected Compensatory Responses in Simple Disturbances

Primary Disorder	pH	Initial Chemical Change	Compensatory Response	Expected Compensation
Metabolic acidosis	Low	↓ $[HCO_3^-]$	↓ Pco_2	$Pco_2 = (1.5 \times [HCO_3^-]) + 8 \pm 2$
				$Pco_2 = [HCO_3^-] + 15$
				$Pco_2 = $ decimal digits of pH
Metabolic alkalosis*	High	↑ $[HCO_3^-]$	↑ Pco_2	Pco_2 variably increased
				$Pco_2 = (0.9 \times [HCO_3^-]) + 9$
Respiratory acidosis				$Pco_2 = (0.7 \times [HCO_3^-]) + 20$
Acute	Low	↑ Pco_2	↑ $[HCO_3^-]$	$[HCO_3^-]$ increases 1 mEq/L for every 10 mm Hg increase in Pco_2
Chronic	Low	↑ Pco_2	further ↑ $[HCO_3^-]$	$[HCO_3^-]$ increases 3-4 mEq/L for every 10 mm Hg increase in Pco_2
Respiratory alkalosis				
Acute	High	↓ Pco_2	↓ $[HCO_3^-]$	$[HCO_3^-]$ decreases 2 mEq/L for every 10 mm Hg decrease in Pco_2
Chronic	High	↓ Pco_2	further ↓ $[HCO_3^-]$	$[HCO_3^-]$ decreases 5 mEq/L for every 10 mm Hg decrease in Pco_2

$[HCO_3^-]$, Serum bicarbonate concentration; *Pco_2,* arterial partial pressure of carbon dioxide.
*Compensation formulas for metabolic alkalosis have wide confidence limits because the Pco_2 of individuals with this disorder vary greatly at any given $[HCO_3^-]$.

Typically, the normal AG range is considered to be 8 to 12 mEq/L. The normal AG is primarily comprised of anionic albumin, and to a lesser degree, other proteins, sulfate, phosphate, urate, and various organic acid anions such as lactate. In general, if the concentration of these "unmeasured" anions increases, the AG increases. Conversely, the AG falls when the concentration of unmeasured anions is reduced. For example, hypoalbuminemia is a common cause of a reduced AG, with the AG falling about 2.5 mEq/L for each 1 g/dl reduction of albumin below the normal range.

The disorders that produce metabolic acidosis can be subdivided on the basis of an increased or normal AG. An examination of the AG equation reveals that the only way the $[HCO_3^-]$ can fall while the AG remains normal is for the $[Cl^-]$ to increase relative to the $[Na^+]$. Consequently, all

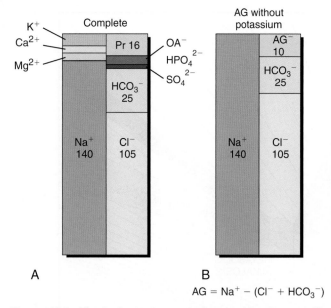

$$AG = Na^+ - (Cl^- + HCO_3^-)$$

Figure 12.2 The ionic anatomy of plasma. All units are milli-equivalents per liter (mEq/L). **A,** Ion profile of normal serum. **B,** Calculation of the anion gap (AG) using the concentrations of sodium, chloride, and bicarbonate concentrations only. *OA,* Organic acid; *Pr,* Protein.

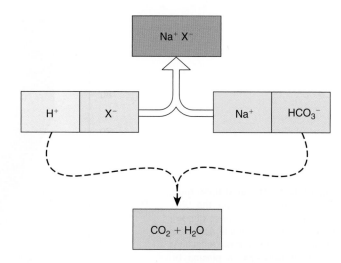

		METABOLIC ACIDOSIS	
	NORMAL	HYPERCHLOREMIC	HIGH AG
Na$^+$	140	140	140
Cl$^-$	105	115	105
HCO$_3^-$	25	15	15
AG	10	10	20
ΔHCO$_3^-$	0	−10	−10
ΔAG	0	0	+10
Lactate	1	1	11

Figure 12.3 Pathogenesis of a metabolic acidosis. If any relatively strong acid, HX (where X$^-$ is an anion), is added to a solution containing NaHCO$_3$, there is decomposition of some HCO$_3^-$ and an equivalent increase of the X$^-$ concentration. If HX is HCl, then a hyperchloremic, or normal anion-gap, acidosis develops. If HX is any acid other than HCl, such as lactic acid or a keto acid, then a high anion-gap acidosis develops.

"non-AG" metabolic acidoses must be hyperchloremic metabolic acidoses. This is shown graphically in Figure 12.3.

Most often, an elevated AG indicates the presence of a metabolic acidosis. However, exceptions include:

- Dehydration, with loss of water in excess of salts, increases the concentration of all electrolytes, including albumin and other unmeasured ions, thereby increasing the AG.
- Rapid infusion, and short-lived accumulation, of metabolizable sodium salts such as lactate, acetate, citrate, etc. To the extent these salts are metabolized, they generate NaHCO$_3$, and the AG does not increase; if metabolic conversion is delayed, the AG increases.
- Infusion of nonmetabolizable sodium salts, other than sodium chloride or bicarbonate. For example, anionic antibiotics such as carbenicillin and penicillin G may be infused as sodium (or potassium) salts and, to the extent that they accumulate, increase the AG.
- Metabolic alkalosis causes a small increase in AG (usually less than 3 to 4 mEq/L) as a result of (1) increased concentrations of the anions of organic acids (mainly lactate), which accumulate because of metabolic stimulation of production, and (2) increased concentration of albumin, due to extracellular fluid volume contraction.
- Laboratory error, or measurement artifact, of one or more analytes.

MIXED ACID-BASE DISTURBANCES

A mixed acid-base disturbance is the simultaneous occurrence of two or more simple acid-base disturbances. Mixed acid-base disorders may develop concurrently or sequentially.

The disorders may be additive, with each process having a similar directional effect on pH. Alternatively they may oppose each other, having offsetting effects on pH. Sometimes three simultaneous acid-base disorders, or a triple acid-base disturbance, can be identified.

Recognition of mixed acid-base disorders is important for several reasons. First, when these disorders are additive (i.e., concurrent metabolic and respiratory acidosis or concurrent metabolic and respiratory alkalosis), the pH excursions may become severe with toxic consequences. When offsetting disorders coexist, the pH may be normal or near normal. Nonetheless, their identification serves as an important diagnostic clue to the underlying pathophysiology. Mixed disorders often suggest specific clinical derangements. For example, concurrent high AG metabolic acidosis and respiratory alkalosis is typical of salicylate poisoning, whereas patients with diabetic ketoacidosis often vomit and may present with concurrent high AG metabolic acidosis and metabolic alkalosis.

INADEQUATE OR "EXCESSIVE" COMPENSATION

The expected compensatory responses shown in the acid-base nomogram (see Fig. 12.1) and described in Table 12.1 are used to determine whether respiratory compensation for a metabolic disorder, or metabolic compensation for a respiratory disorder, is quantitatively appropriate, inadequate, or excessive. The arterial pH,

pCO_2, and $[HCO_3^-]$ values are required for this determination; therefore, a blood gas analysis is necessary for complete characterization of the acid-base disturbance. If a patient with a metabolic acidosis has a pCO_2 that is lower than the expected compensatory response, a respiratory alkalosis also exists; conversely, a pCO_2 that is too high indicates a complicating respiratory acidosis. Analogously, if a primary respiratory acid-base disorder is identified, then the measured $[HCO_3^-]$ should be in the range predicted by the nomogram or compensation rules (see Fig. 12.1 and Table 12.1). It should be noted that the determination of the appropriate compensation range for any primary respiratory disorder also requires the classification of that disorder as acute (from minutes to 1 to 2 days) or chronic (>2 days), a decision that is usually based on the patient's history and physical exam. If the measured $[HCO_3^-]$ is higher than the compensatory range expected with a respiratory acidosis, then a coexistent metabolic alkalosis should be considered; conversely, if the $[HCO_3^-]$ is too low, a coexistent metabolic acidosis should be considered. Examples of such mixed acid-base disorders are provided in Tables 12.2 through 12.5, and they are discussed later in this Chapter (see Clinical Examples).

THE DELTA/DELTA (ΔAG/ΔHCO$_3^-$)

Another group of mixed acid-base disorders are those caused by coexistent metabolic acidosis and metabolic alkalosis. For example, patients with diabetic ketoacidosis (an AG metabolic acidosis) often develop nausea and vomiting, generating a complicating metabolic alkalosis. The final pH may be acid, alkaline, or normal, depending on the relative severity of each disorder. This mixed metabolic acidosis and alkalosis disorder should be suspected when the magnitude of the increased AG exceeds the decrement in HCO_3^- (or the ΔAG/Δ HCO$_3^-$). This relationship is described later.

Whenever an AG metabolic acidosis exists as a single acid-base disorder, the magnitude of the increase in AG should be quantitatively similar to the magnitude of reduction in $[HCO_3^-]$. If the AG increases by 10 mEq/L as a result of an accumulation of ketoacids that have titrated the serum bicarbonate, then the $[HCO_3^-]$ should also decrease by about 10 mEq/L (see Fig. 12.3). The absolute value of each change should be equivalent, such that $\Delta [AG] = \Delta [HCO_3^-]$.

If the increase in AG above its baseline (the ΔAG) exceeds the fall in $[HCO_3^-]$ from its baseline of 24 mEq/L (the ΔHCO$_3^-$), then the presence of an additional acid-base disorder that has elevated the $[HCO_3^-]$ is suggested. Two situations usually cause this discrepancy. Most often, it is the result of a coexistent metabolic alkalosis (see Table 12-6). Another possibility is a coexistent chronic respiratory acidosis for which compensation has increased the $[HCO_3^-]$ to a value greater than the normal range (Fig. 12.4). The resulting arterial pH and pCO_2 should allow the clinician to readily distinguish between these possibilities.

Conversely, if the increase of the AG is smaller than the fall in $[HCO_3^-]$ from a normal baseline of about 24 mEq/L (i.e., ΔAG < ΔHCO$_3^-$), the $[Cl^-]$ must be increased relative

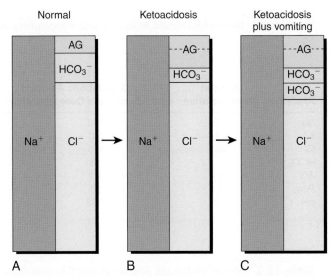

Figure 12.4   The effect of ketoacidosis plus vomiting on the ionic profile of blood. A, The normal electrolyte pattern. **B,** The development of a typical anion gap (AG) metabolic acidosis. **C,** The superimposed effect of vomiting, which causes proton loss without the loss of any organic acid anions. This results in a decrease in the serum chloride concentration and an increase in the bicarbonate concentration. The latter normalizes the $[HCO_3^-]$, but the AG remains large because the keto acid concentration is unchanged by the vomiting.

to $[Na^+]$. The presence of relative hyperchloremia usually indicates the existence of a hyperchloremic metabolic acidosis, or compensation for chronic respiratory alkalosis. Again, the resulting arterial pH and pCO_2 should allow one to readily distinguish between these possibilities.

These ΔAG/ΔHCO$_3^-$ comparisons usually assume that the AG has started in the normal range. If the initial AG is abnormally low to begin (e.g., if the patient has a very low albumin concentration), then the excursion (or Δ) must begin from this lower baseline.

CLINICAL EXAMPLES

CLINICAL EXAMPLE 1

A patient becomes septic and develops lactic acidosis. If that same patient also develops acute respiratory distress syndrome (ARDS), then mild or severe respiratory acidosis may occur as well (Table 12.2).

CLINICAL EXAMPLE 2

A patient with chronic obstructive pulmonary disease (COPD) may show a pattern of chronic respiratory acidosis, as depicted in the first chronic respiratory acidosis column of Table 12.3, whereas a patient receiving loop diuretic therapy may develop metabolic alkalosis as shown in the next column of Table 12.3. If a patient with COPD is treated with a loop diuretic, the pattern in the last column of the table may develop. Note that a chronic pCO_2 of 55 mm Hg should raise the $[HCO_3^-]$ to about 31 mEq/L, so the $[HCO_3^-]$ of 34 mEq/L is too high. Also note that this has resulted in a pH of 7.41, which is too high. Patients with chronic respiratory acidosis should not have a pH in the midnormal range; their pH should remain slightly acidic, even after full compensation.

Table 12.2   Mixed Metabolic Acidosis and Respiratory Acidosis (Clinical Example 1)

| | | | Mixed High AG Metabolic Acidosis and Respiratory Acidosis | |
| | | | Mixed High AG Metabolic Acidosis and Mild Respiratory Acidosis | Mixed High AG Metabolic Acidosis and Severe Respiratory Acidosis |
Analyte	Normal Concentration	High AG Metabolic Acidosis with Appropriate Compensation		
Na+	140	140	140	140
K+	4.0	5.0	5.0	5.0
Cl-	105	105	105	105
HCO3-	25	15	15	15
AG	10	20	20	20
Pco2	40	30	40	50
pH	7.42	7.32	7.20	7.10

Table 12.3   Mixed Metabolic Alkalosis and Chronic Respiratory Acidosis (Clinical Example 2)

Analyte	Normal Concentration	Chronic Respiratory Acidosis with Appropriate Compensation	Metabolic Alkalosis with Appropriate Compensation	Mixed Chronic Respiratory Acidosis and Metabolic Alkalosis
Na+	140	140	140	140
K+	4.0	5.0	3.4	3.5
Cl-	105	98	98	90
HCO3-	25	32	31	37
AG	10	10	12	13
Pco2	40	60	43	60
pH	7.42	7.35	7.47	7.41

Table 12.4   Mixed Metabolic Acidosis and Respiratory Alkalosis (Clinical Example 3)

| | | | Mixed Metabolic Acidosis and Respiratory Alkalosis | |
Analyte	Normal Concentration	High AG Metabolic Acidosis with Appropriate Compensation	Mild Respiratory Alkalosis	Severe Respiratory Alkalosis
Na+	140	140	140	140
K+	4.0	5.0	5.0	5.0
Cl-	105	105	105	105
HCO3-	25	15	15	15
AG	10	20	20	20
Pco2	40	30	25	20
pH	7.42	7.32	7.4	7.5

AG, Anion gap; *Pco2*, arterial carbon dioxide tension.

CLINICAL EXAMPLE 3

Patients with uncomplicated AG metabolic acidosis will have a reduced [HCO3-], an appropriately reduced pCO2, and an acidic pH. Superimposed respiratory alkalosis will further reduce the PCO2 and raise the pH toward normal, or even enough to generate alkalemia (Table 12.4). Patients with aspirin overdose will often present with this mixed acid-base pattern. Inhibition of normal oxidative metabolic reactions causes an accumulation of multiple organic acidosis and, hence, the AG metabolic acidosis. Acetylsalicylic acid itself also contributes to the large AG. Simultaneously, the toxic levels of salicylate stimulate central hyperventilation.

The pattern in the last column of Table 12.4 is typically seen in adults with this disorder. Infants with salicylate poisoning more typically present with less marked respiratory alkalosis, so their arterial pH is generally acidic.

CLINICAL EXAMPLE 4

Metabolic alkalosis raises the [HCO3-], and compensation should increase the pCO2. Respiratory alkalosis decreases the pCO2, and compensation should decrease the [HCO3-]. Hence, in simple alkaloses, both components should deviate in the same direction. If the [HCO3-] is increased and the pCO2 is decreased, then metabolic alkalosis and respiratory

Table 12.5 Simple and Mixed Metabolic and Respiratory Alkalosis (Clinical Example 4)

Analyte	Normal Concentration	Simple Alkalosis		Mixed Metabolic and Chronic Respiratory Alkalosis	
		Metabolic Alkalosis with Appropriate Compensation	Chronic Respiratory Alkalosis with Appropriate Compensation	Mild Metabolic Alkalosis	Severe Metabolic Alkalosis
Na^+	140	140	140	140	140
K^+	4.0	3.2	3.4	3.1	2.9
Cl^-	105	96	108	103	96
HCO_3^-	25	32	19	23*	29
AG	10	12	12	14	15
Pco_2	40	44	30	30	30
pH	7.42	7.48	7.42	7.51	7.61

AG, Anion gap; *Pco₂*, arterial carbon dioxide tension.
*Note that a lack of metabolic compensation—the serum [HCO_3^-] has not decreased—in the presence of chronic respiratory alkalosis is consistent with coexisting metabolic alkalosis. This pattern could also exist in simple *acute* respiratory alkalosis.

Table 12.6 Mixed Metabolic Acidosis and Metabolic Alkalosis (Clinical Example 5)

Analyte	Normal Concentration	High AG Metabolic Acidosis with Appropriate Compensation	Normal AG Metabolic Acidosis with Appropriate Compensation	Mixed Metabolic Alkalosis and Metabolic Acidosis	
				High AG Metabolic Acidosis and Metabolic Alkalosis	Normal AG Metabolic Acidosis and Metabolic Alkalosis
Na^+	140	140	140	140	140
K^+	4.0	5.0	3.8	4.0	4.0
Cl^-	105	105	115	95	105
HCO_3^-	25	15	15	25	25
AG	10	20	10	20	10
Pco_2	40	30	30	40	40
pH	7.42	7.32	7.32	7.42	7.42

AG, Anion gap; *Pco₂*, arterial carbon dioxide tension.

alkalosis coexist (Table 12.5). This mixed acid-base disorder is often seen in patients with severe liver disease. Chronic respiratory alkalosis is extremely common as a result of diaphragmatic elevation, A-V shunting, and a deranged hormonal milieu that stimulates ventilation. Nausea and vomiting occur frequently, and nasogastric suction is often employed. These disorders and treatments generate metabolic alkalosis, which complicates the chronic respiratory alkalosis. Combined, these disorders can generate extreme alkalemia.

CLINICAL EXAMPLE 5

The combination of mixed metabolic acidosis with high AG and metabolic alkalosis can develop in different ways.

1. A large AG metabolic acidosis may develop in a patient with preexisting metabolic alkalosis. In this situation, the [HCO_3^-] falls from a supranormal level as AG develops.
2. Metabolic alkalosis may develop in a patient with a large AG metabolic acidosis. The metabolic alkalosis raises the [HCO_3^-] while AG remains large.
3. AG metabolic acidosis and metabolic alkalosis can develop simultaneously.

In each of these scenarios, the elevated AG remains as a residual marker of the metabolic acidosis. However, the magnitude of increase of the AG is greater than the [HCO_3^-] fall from its baseline. This relationship can be expressed as the Delta/Delta or Δ[AG]/Δ[HCO_3^-], which will be increased above 1 (the Δ[AG] > Δ[HCO_3^-]).

Patients with diabetic ketoacidosis have metabolic acidosis with a large AG. If nausea and vomiting occur, they generate a simultaneous or sequential metabolic alkalosis through loss of acidic gastric fluids. Although the final arterial pH is typically acid, it may sometimes become normal or even alkaline if the alkalosis is more severe than the acidosis. Regardless of the resultant pH and [HCO_3^-], the large AG remains a major chemical clue to the presence of a metabolic acidosis. A similar pattern is seen when uremic patients develop nausea and vomiting.

However, when patients develop mixed hyperchloremic (non-AG) acidosis and metabolic alkalosis, there is no residual AG clue to the presence of this mixed disorder (Table 12.6). This mixed acid-base disorder may be suspected based on the clinical history and physical exam (see next section).

Table 12.7 Metabolic Acidosis, Metabolic Alkalosis, and Respiratory Alkalosis: A Triple Acid-Base Disturbance

Analyte	Normal Concentrations	Case 1: Metabolic Alkalosis with Appropriate Compensation	Case 2: High AG Metabolic Acidosis with Appropriate Compensation	Case 3: Mixed Metabolic Acidosis and Metabolic Alkalosis	Case 4: Mixed Metabolic Acidosis, Metabolic Alkalosis, and Respiratory Alkalosis
Na^+	140	140	140	140	140
K^+	4.0	3.4	4.5	4.5	4.5
Cl^-	105	89	105	92	92
HCO_3^-	25	38	12	25	25
AG	10	13	23	23	23
Pco_2	40	46	26	40	30
pH	7.42	7.54	7.29	7.42	7.54

AG, Anion gap; *Pco₂*, arterial carbon dioxide tension.

OTHER MIXED ACID-BASE DISORDERS

The combination of a hyperchloremic metabolic acidosis and metabolic alkalosis may be more difficult to diagnose. In these patients, there is no residual AG increase to indicate that an underlying metabolic acidosis exists. Instead, the hyperchloremic acidosis reduces the $[HCO_3^-]$ and increases the $[Cl^-]$, whereas the metabolic alkalosis increases the $[HCO_3^-]$ and decreases the $[Cl^-]$. If the two disorders are of similar intensity, the final $[HCO_3^-]$ and $[Cl^-]$ may be restored to their normal ranges with a normal AG. This mixed disorder can be suspected on the basis of the history, clinical setting, and physical exam. For example, a patient with gastroenteritis who has a history of both watery diarrhea and vomiting may have this mixed acid-base disorder despite a normal pH, pCO_2, $[HCO_3^-]$, AG, and $[Cl^-]$. Marked hypokalemia may be present. If the vomiting improves but the diarrhea continues, overt hyperchloremic metabolic acidosis and acidemia may be revealed.

Other forms of mixed acid-base disorders are combinations of different metabolic acidosis disorders or, much less commonly, metabolic alkalosis disorders. For example, it is not uncommon for ketoacidosis to coexist with lactic acidosis; similarly, hyperchloremic acidosis caused by diarrhea or renal tubular acidosis may present in conjunction with lactic acidosis or uremic acidosis. Some patients with nausea and vomiting may medicate themselves with baking soda. The vomiting generates HCO_3^- and the baking soda is a form of exogenous sodium bicarbonate.

Mixed respiratory acid-base disorders can also develop, and they are usually suspected on the basis of the history and clinical setting rather than any specific laboratory results. The patient with chronic obstructive lung disease, who presents with recent pulmonary deterioration caused by a mucus plug or pneumonia, may have chronic respiratory acidosis and a superimposed acute respiratory acidosis. A pregnant woman with underlying hyperventilation who ingests an overdose of sedating drugs and develops respiratory depression will have chronic respiratory alkalosis and a superimposed acute respiratory acidosis.

TRIPLE ACID-BASE DISTURBANCES

A relatively common, and the most readily diagnosed type of triple acid-base disturbance, is that due to the combination of AG metabolic acidosis, metabolic alkalosis, and either respiratory acidosis or respiratory alkalosis. The offsetting effects of the coexistent metabolic acidosis and alkalosis result in a low, normal, or elevated $[HCO_3^-]$. Regardless of the $[HCO_3^-]$, there is a large ΔAG which exceeds the $\Delta[HCO_3^-]$. This is the clue to the double disorder of metabolic acidosis and metabolic alkalosis. The final $[HCO_3^-]$ that results from these two disorders is the parameter that should determine the degree of respiratory compensation and pCO_2. If the pCO_2 is lower than expected, a third disorder, respiratory alkalosis, exists. If the pCO_2 is higher than expected, the third disorder is respiratory acidosis.

A clinical example is shown in Table 12.7. Case 1 is a patient who vomits and develops metabolic alkalosis. The $[HCO_3^-]$ increases to 38 mEq/L, the pCO_2 increases to 46 mm Hg, and the AG increases slightly. Case 2 illustrates the findings expected with high AG metabolic acidosis, such as lactic acidosis. The $[HCO_3^-]$ has fallen by 13 mEq/L and the AG has increased by the same amount. If the patient represented by Case 1 develops severe extracellular fluid volume depletion, then lactic acidosis may ensue (Case 3). Accordingly, the HCO_3^- falls, in this example from 38 to 25 mEq/L (a ΔHCO_3^- of 13 mEq/L), and the AG also increases by a Δ of 23 mEq/L. Evaluating the chemistries shown as Case 3 shows a normal $[HCO_3^-]$ despite an AG of 23 mEq/L. The discrepancy between the normal HCO_3^- and the large AG is the major clue to this mixed acid-base disorder. The normal HCO_3^-, which is the result of equally severe degrees of metabolic acidosis and metabolic alkalosis, should be associated with a normal pCO_2. The last column (Case 4) shows an example of a pCO_2 that is too low, indicating that a third disorder, respiratory alkalosis, is also present. If the pCO_2 had been 50 mm Hg, then respiratory acidosis, metabolic alkalosis, and metabolic acidosis would be the triple disturbance.

The flow charts in Figures 12.5 and 12.6 show one general approach to the diagnostic work-up of a patient with either acidemia or alkalemia.

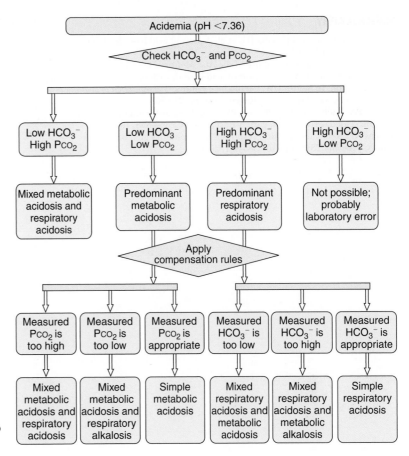

Figure 12.5 A flowchart showing one approach to the diagnostic work-up of a patient with acidemia.

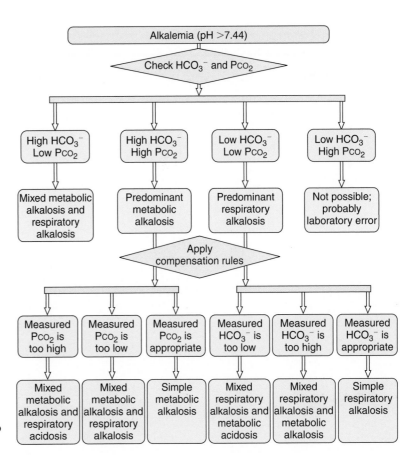

Figure 12.6 A flowchart showing one approach to the diagnostic work-up of a patient with alkalemia.

BIBLIOGRAPHY

Adrogué HJ, Gennari FJ, Galla JH, et al: Assessing acid-base disorders, *Kidney Int* 76:1239-1247, 2009.

Emmett M, Narins R: Clinical use of the AG, *Medicine* 56:38-54, 1977.

Emmett M, Seldin DW: Evaluation of acid-base disorders from plasma composition. In Seldin DW, Giebisch G, editors: *The regulation of acid-base balance*, New York, 1989, Raven Press, pp 213-263.

Gabow PA, Kaehny WD, Fennessey PV, et al: Diagnostic importance of an increased serum anion gap, *N Engl J Med* 303:854-858, 1980.

Madias NE: Renal acidification responses to respiratory acid-base disorders, *J Nephrol* 23(Suppl 16):S85-S91, 2010.

Madias NE, Adrogué HJ: Respiratory alkalosis and acidosis. In Seldin DW, Giebisch G, editors: *The kidney: physiology and pathophysiology*, ed 3, Philadelphia, 2000, Lippincott/Williams & Wilkins, pp 2131-2166.

Narins RG, Emmett M: Simple and mixed acid-base disorders: a practical approach, *Medicine* 59:161-187, 1980.

Palmer BF, Alpern RJ: Metabolic alkalosis, *J Am Soc Nephrol* 8:1462-1469, 1997.

Rastegar A: Use of the Delta AG/DeltaHCO3⁻ ratio in the diagnosis of mixed acid-base disorders, *J Am Soc Nephrol* 18:2429-2431, 2007.

Metabolic Acidosis

13

Harold M. Szerlip

Metabolic acidosis describes a process in which nonvolatile acids accumulate in the body. For practical purposes, this can result from either the addition of protons or the loss of base. The consequence of this process is a decline in the major extracellular buffer, bicarbonate, and, if unopposed, a decrease in extracellular pH. However, depending on the existence and the magnitude of other acid-base disturbances, the extracellular pH may be low, normal, or even high. Normal blood pH is between 7.36 and 7.44, corresponding to a hydrogen ion concentration of 44 to 36 nmol/L.

Because the body tightly defends against changes in pH, decreased pH sensitizes peripheral chemoreceptors, and that triggers an increase in minute ventilation. This compensatory respiratory alkalosis helps offset what would otherwise be a marked fall in pH. Because increased ventilation is a compensatory mechanism stimulated by acidemia, increased ventilation never returns the pH to normal. The expected partial pressure of carbon dioxide (PCO_2) for any given degree of metabolic acidosis can be predicted using Winter's formula:

$$P_{CO_2} = \left(1.5 \times \left[HCO_3^-\right]\right) + 8 \pm 2.$$

OVERVIEW OF ACID-BASE BALANCE

To maintain extracellular pH within the normal range, the entire daily production of acid must be excreted from the body (Fig. 13.1). The vast majority of acid production results from the metabolism of dietary carbohydrates and fats. Complete oxidation of these metabolic substrates produces CO_2 and water. The 15,000 mmol of CO_2 produced daily are efficiently exhaled by the lungs, and are therefore known as volatile acid. As long as ventilatory function remains normal, this volatile acid does not contribute to changes in acid-base balance. Nonvolatile, or fixed, acids are produced by the metabolism of sulfate- and phosphate-containing amino acids. In addition, incomplete oxidation of fats and carbohydrates results in the production of small quantities of lactate and other organic anions, which, when excreted in the urine, represent loss of base. Individuals consuming a typical meat-based diet produce approximately 1 mmol/kg/day of hydrogen ions. Fecal excretion of a small amount of base also contributes to total daily acid production.

The kidney is responsible not only for the excretion of the daily production of fixed acid, but also for the reclamation of the filtered bicarbonate. Bicarbonate reclamation occurs predominantly in the proximal tubule, mainly through the Na^+-H^+ exchanger. Active transporters in the distal tubule secrete hydrogen ion against a concentration gradient. Although urinary pH can be as low as 4.5, if there were no urinary buffers, this would account for very little acid excretion. For example, excretion of 100 mmol of H^+ into unbuffered urine at a minimum urine pH of 4.5 would require a daily urine volume of 5000 L. Fortunately, proton acceptors, including urinary phosphate and creatinine, help buffer these protons, allowing the kidney to excrete approximately 40% to 50% of the daily fixed acid load as titratable acid (TA), so called because these acids are quantitated by titrating the urine pH back to the 7.4 pH of plasma. In addition to TA, renal excretion of acid is supported by ammoniagenesis. NH_3 is generated in the proximal tubule by the deamidation of glutamine to glutamate, which is subsequently deaminated to yield NH_3 and α-ketoglutarate. The enzymes responsible for these reactions are upregulated by acidosis and hypokalemia. Hyperkalemia, on the other hand, reduces ammoniagenesis. NH_3 builds up in the renal interstitium and passively diffuses into the tubule lumen along the length of the collecting duct where it is trapped by H^+.

Under conditions of increased acid production, the normal kidney primarily increases acid excretion by augmenting NH_3 production. Renal acid excretion varies directly with the rate of acid production. Net renal acid excretion (NAE) is equal to the sum of TA and NH_4^+ minus any secreted HCO_3^-

$$\text{Net renal acid excretion} = \left(TA + NH_4^+\right) - HCO_3^-$$

Thus, the etiology of a metabolic acidosis can be divided into four broad categories: (1) overproduction of fixed acids, (2) increased extrarenal loss of base, (3) decrease in the kidney's ability to secrete hydrogen ions, and (4) inability of the kidney to reclaim the filtered bicarbonate (Fig. 13.2).

EVALUATION OF URINARY ACIDIFICATION

The cause of metabolic acidosis is often evident from the clinical situation. However, because the kidney is responsible for both the reclamation of filtered HCO_3^- and the excretion of the daily production of fixed acid, to evaluate a metabolic acidosis it may be necessary to assess whether the kidney is appropriately able to reabsorb HCO_3^-, secrete H^+ against a gradient, and excrete NH_4^+ (Box 13.1). The simplest test is to measure urine pH. Although urine pH can be measured using a dipstick, the lack of precision of this technique prevents it from being useful in clinical decision-making. Ideally the urine should be collected under oil and the pH measured using a pH electrode. Under conditions of acid loading, urine pH should be below 5.5. A pH higher than 5.5 usually reflects impaired distal hydrogen ion secretion. Measuring the pH after challenging the patient with

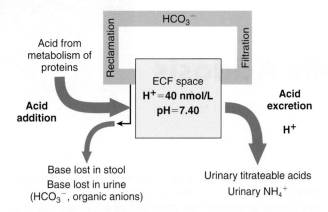

Figure 13.1 **Maintenance of acid-base homeostasis requires that the addition of acid to the body is balanced by excretion of acid.** Production of fixed nonvolatile acid occurs mainly through the metabolism of proteins. A small quantity of base is also lost in the stool and urine. Acid excretion occurs in the kidney through the secretion of H^+ buffered by titratable acids and NH_4^+. Bicarbonate filtration and reclamation by the kidney is normally a neutral process. *ECF,* Extracellular fluid.

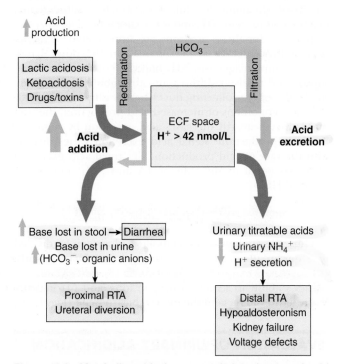

Figure 13.2 **Metabolic acidosis can result from increased acid production, increased loss of base in stool or urine, or decreased H^+ secretion in the distal tubule.** The causes of these processes are shown. *ECF,* Extracellular fluid; *RTA,* renal tubular acidosis.

Box 13.1 Tests of Renal Acid Excretion

Urine pH (Enhanced by Furosemide)
NH_4^+ Excretion
   Urine NH_4^+
   Urine anion gap
   Urine osmol gap
Urine Pco_2 with Bicarbonate Loading
Fractional Excretion of HCO_3^-

---

the loop diuretic, furosemide, will increase the sensitivity of this test by providing Na^+ to the distal tubule for reabsorption. The reabsorption of Na^+ creates a negative electrical potential in the lumen and enhances H^+ secretion. It is important, however, to rule out urinary infections with urea-splitting organisms, which will increase pH. An elevated urine pH may also be misleading in conditions associated with volume depletion and hypokalemia, as can occur in diarrhea. In contradistinction to furosemide, volume depletion with decreased sodium delivery to the distal tubule impairs distal H^+ secretion. Furthermore, hypokalemia, by enhancing ammoniagenesis, raises the urine pH.

Because renal excretion of NH_4^+ accounts for the majority of acid excretion, measurement of urine NH_4^+ provides important information. Urinary NH_4^+ excretion can be decreased by a variety of mechanisms, including a primary decrease in ammoniagenesis by the proximal tubule as seen in chronic kidney disease (CKD), or by decreased trapping in the distal tubule either secondary to decreased H^+ secretion or increased delivery of HCO_3^-, which will preferentially buffer H^+, making it unavailable to form NH_4^+. Although direct measurement of NH_4^+ is becoming more readily available in clinical laboratories and is the true gold standard, many laboratories still do not perform this assay. Fortunately, an estimate of NH_4^+ excretion is easily obtained by calculating the urine anion gap (UAG) or urine osmole gap. If, as is usual, the anion balancing the charge of the NH_4^+ is Cl^-, then

$$UAG = (Na^+ + K^+) - Cl^-$$

should be negative, because the chloride is greater than the sum of Na^+ and K^+ (Fig. 13.3). Although the measurement of the UAG in conditions of acid loading is often reflective of NH_4^+ excretion, the presence of anions other than Cl^- (such as keto anions or hippurate) makes it a less reliable assessment of NH_4^+ than the urine osmole gap. The urine osmole gap, from the measured urine osmolality, is calculated as follows:

$$\text{Urine osmole gap} = U_{osm} - \left[2(Na^+ + K^+) + \text{Urea nitrogen}/2.8 + \text{Glucose}/18 \right] \Big/ 2$$

The osmole gap is composed primarily of NH_4^+ salts. Thus, half of the gap represents NH_4^+. An osmole gap greater than 100 mmol/L signifies normal NH_4^+ excretion.

Another test of distal H^+ ion secretory ability is measurement of urine Pco_2 during bicarbonate loading. Distal delivery of HCO_3^- in the presence of normal H^+ secretory capacity results in elevated Pco_2 in the urine. When there is a secretory defect, urine Pco_2 does not increase. Accurate measurement of urine Pco_2 requires that the urine be collected under oil to prevent the loss of CO_2 into the air.

COMPLICATIONS OF ACIDOSIS

Although most accept that a decrease in extracellular pH has detrimental effects on numerous physiologic parameters and should be aggressively treated, this dogma has been challenged. The proponents of treatment argue that

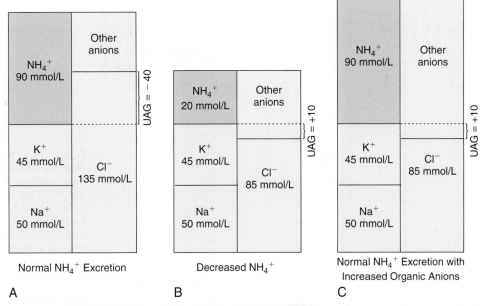

Figure 13.3 In the presence of acidemia, the kidney increases NH$_4^+$ excretion. The urine anion gap (UAG) is an indirect method for estimating urine NH$_4^+$. **A,** Normal NH$_4^+$ excretion. If the accompanying anion is chloride, the UAG (Na$^+$ + K$^+$ − Cl$^-$) will be negative, reflecting the large quantity of NH$_4^+$ in the urine. **B,** Decreased NH$_4^+$ excretion. A decrease in NH$_4^+$ secretion occurs when ammoniagenesis is diminished, H$^+$ secretion is impaired, or HCO$_3^-$ is delivered to the distal tubule. In these cases, the UAG will be inappropriately positive. **C,** Normal NH$_4^+$ excretion with increased organic anions. If anions other than Cl$^-$ are excreted (e.g., ketones, hippurate), the UAG will be positive despite increased NH$_4^+$ excretion, because these anions are not used in calculation of the gap.

acidemia depresses cardiac contractility, blocks activation of adrenergic receptors, and inhibits the action of key enzymes. However, uncontrolled clinical studies are not easy to interpret because of the difficulties in separating the effects of the acidosis from the effects of the underlying illness, and most controlled studies investigating the role of acidosis on cellular processes have been undertaken in isolated cells or organs; therefore, the effects of acidemia on whole-body physiology and their applicability to humans are unclear.

The effect of pH on cardiac function has been strongly debated. Cardiac output is determined by multiple components, and it is the sum of the effects on these individual components that determines the net effect of acidemia on cardiac function. Myocardial contractile strength and changes in vascular tone determine cardiovascular performance, and the relative contributions of each in the context of acidemia remain to be clarified. Because of differing effects of acidemia on contractile force, vascular tone, and sympathetic discharge, it is difficult to predict what happens to cardiac output from studies using isolated myocytes or perfused hearts. In one study, during continuous infusion of lactic acid, cardiac output increased; however, this was not confirmed in other studies. Notably, fractional shortening of the left ventricle as assessed by transthoracic echocardiography appears normal even in cases of severe acidemia, with the pH at which cardiac output and blood pressure fall remaining unclear.

APPROACH TO ACID-BASE DISORDERS

Complete evaluation of acid-base status requires a routine electrolyte panel, measurement of serum albumin, and arterial blood gas analysis (see Chapter 12). The traditional approach to the diagnosis of metabolic acidosis relies on the calculation of the anion gap (AG) and subsequent separation of metabolic acidosis into those with an elevated AG and those where the AG is normal, or so-called hyperchloremic metabolic acidosis (HCMA; Fig. 13.4). The AG is defined as the difference between the concentration of sodium, the major cation, and the sum of the concentrations of chloride and bicarbonate, and the major anions

$$AG = \left[Na^+\right] - \left(\left[Cl^-\right] + \left[HCO_3^-\right]\right)$$

Because the concentration of potassium changes minimally, its contribution is ignored for convenience. Because electrical neutrality must exist, the sum of the anions must equal the sum of the cations. The AG occurs because the unmeasured anions, such as sulfate, phosphate, organic anions, and especially the weak acid proteins, particularly albumin, are greater than the unmeasured cations, such as potassium, calcium, and magnesium. Thus, on examination of the results from a basic chemistry panel, it appears that cations exceed anions, creating an AG. The normal AG is 10 ± 2 mEq/L, and any increase in the AG even in the face of a normal or frankly alkalemic pH represents the accumulation of acids and the presence of an acidosis. In many cases, the anions that make up the gap are not easily identifiable.

One caveat in using the AG is to recognize that the normal gap is predominantly composed of the negative charge on albumin. When hypoalbuminemia is present, the AG must be corrected for the serum albumin. For each 1 g/dl decrease in the serum albumin, the calculated AG should be increased by 2.5 mEq/L. Thus, the corrected AG (AG$_c$) is

$$AG_c = AG + 2.5\left(4 - \text{Serum albumin}\right)$$

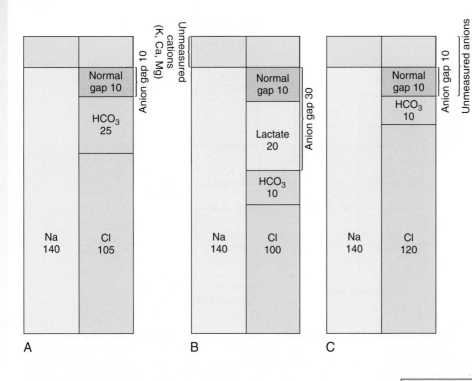

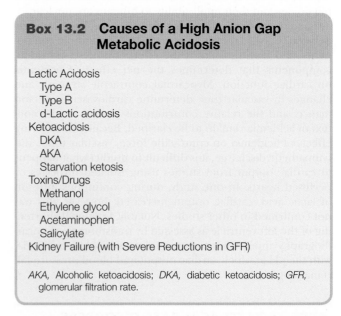

Figure 13.4 Normal anion gap (AG), AG acidosis, and hyperchloremic acidosis. A, In a normal case, the AG is equal to $[Na^+] - ([Cl^-] + [HCO_3^-])$, which is equal to the unmeasured anions minus the unmeasured cations. **B,** In an AG acidosis there is a decrease in $[HCO_3^-]$ and an increase in organic anions (e.g., lactate), which results in an elevated AG. **C,** In a hyperchloremic acidosis, there is a decrease in $[HCO_3^-]$ and an increase in $[Cl^-]$ with no change in the AG.

If the AG is not corrected, the presence of a metabolic acidosis may be masked. This is especially true in critically ill patients who typically have decreased serum albumin.

ANION GAP ACIDOSIS

As previously described, an increased AG represents the accumulation of nonchloride acids. The mnemonic GOLD MARK is a useful tool that helps to identify the causes of an AG acidosis (Fig. 13.5). AG acidosis can be divided into four major categories (Box 13.2): (1) lactic acidosis, (2) ketoacidosis, (3) toxins/drugs, and (4) severe kidney failure. In all but kidney failure, the accumulation of acids is caused by their overproduction. These acids dissociate into protons, which are quickly buffered by HCO_3^- and their respective conjugate bases, the unmeasured anions. As long as these anions are retained in the body and not excreted, they contribute to the elevation in the AG.

LACTIC ACIDOSIS

Lactic acidosis is a common AG acidosis, and it is by far the most serious of all AG acidoses. Anaerobic metabolism of glucose (glycolysis) occurs in the extramitochondrial cytoplasm and produces pyruvate as an intermediary. If this were the end of the glycolytic process, there would be a net production of two protons and a metabolically unsatisfactory reduction of nicotinamide adenine dinucleotide (NAD) to NADH (reduced form). Fortunately, pyruvate rapidly undergoes one of two metabolic fates: (1) under anaerobic conditions, because of the high NADH/NAD ratio, pyruvate is quickly reduced by lactate dehydrogenase to lactate, releasing energy, consuming a proton, and decreasing the NADH/NAD ratio, thus allowing for continued glycolysis; or (2) in the presence of oxygen, pyruvate diffuses into the mitochondria, and, after oxidation by the pyruvate dehydrogenase (PDH) complex, enters the tricarboxylic acid cycle,

- Glycols
- Oxoproline (pyroglutamic acid – acetaminophen)
- L-lactate
- D-lactate

- Methanol
- Aspirin
- Renal failure
- Ketoacidosis

Figure 13.5   GOLD MARK is a useful mnemonic to remember the common causes of an anion gap metabolic acidosis.

Box 13.2   Causes of a High Anion Gap Metabolic Acidosis

Lactic Acidosis
  Type A
  Type B
  d-Lactic acidosis
Ketoacidosis
  DKA
  AKA
  Starvation ketosis
Toxins/Drugs
  Methanol
  Ethylene glycol
  Acetaminophen
  Salicylate
Kidney Failure (with Severe Reductions in GFR)

AKA, Alcoholic ketoacidosis; *DKA*, diabetic ketoacidosis; *GFR*, glomerular filtration rate.

where it is completely oxidized to CO_2 and water. Neither of these pathways results in the production of H^+. During glycolysis, glucose metabolism produces two molecules of lactate and two molecules of adenosine triphosphate (ATP). It is the hydrolysis of ATP (ATP = ADP + H^+ + Pi) that releases protons. Therefore, the acidosis does not occur because of the production of lactate, but rather because, under hypoxic conditions, the hydrolysis of ATP is greater than ATP production. Thus, the buildup of lactate is a surrogate marker for ATP consumption during hypoxic states.

Although lactate production averages about 1300 mmol/day, serum lactate levels are normally less than 1 mmol/L because lactate is either reoxidized to pyruvate and enters the tricarboxylic acid cycle or is used by the liver and kidney via the Cori cycle for gluconeogenesis. An increased concentration of lactate can therefore result from decreased oxidative phosphorylation, increased glycolysis, or decreased gluconeogenesis. Lactate levels between 2 and 3 mmol/L are frequently found in hospitalized patients. Some of these patients will go on to develop frank acidosis, but others will experience no adverse events. Lactic acidosis is defined as the presence of a lactate level greater than 5 mmol/L.

There is a poor correlation among arterial pH, calculated AG, and serum lactate levels, even in those patients with a serum lactic acid level greater than 5 mmol/L. Approximately 25% of patients with serum lactate levels between 5 and 9.9 mmol/L have a pH greater than 7.35, and as many as half have AGs less than 12.

Lactic acidosis has been traditionally divided into types A and B (Box 13.3). Type A, or hypoxic lactic acidosis, results from an imbalance between oxygen supply and oxygen demand. In type B lactic acidosis, oxygen delivery is normal, but oxidative phosphorylation is impaired. This is seen in patients who have inborn errors of metabolism or who have ingested drugs or toxins. It is increasingly clear that lactic acidosis is often caused by the simultaneous existence of both hypoxic and nonhypoxic factors, and, in many cases, it is difficult to separate one from the other. For example, hereditary partial defects in mitochondrial metabolism as well as age-related declines in cytochrome IV complex activity may result in lactic acidosis with a lesser degree of hypoxia than in patients without such defects. Even in cases of shock in which tissue oxygen delivery is obviously inadequate, decreased portal blood flow and reduced hepatic clearance of lactate contribute to the acidosis. Similarly, in sepsis there is a decrease in both tissue perfusion and in the ability to use oxygen. Therefore, this dichotomy into type A and type B, based solely on cause, is largely of historical and conceptual interest.

The presence of lactic acidosis is considered a poor prognostic sign. Studies have shown that, as lactate levels increase above 4 mmol/L, the probability of survival decreases precipitously. However, it remains unclear whether the blood lactate level is an independent contributor to mortality or whether it is a marker of the severity of the patient's illness. Just as important to prognosis is the body's ability to metabolize lactate after restoration of tissue perfusion. Patients able to reduce their lactate by half within 18 hours of resuscitation have a significantly greater chance of survival. In all likelihood, the inability to metabolize lactate is a surrogate marker for organ dysfunction.

TYPE A LACTIC ACIDOSIS

Lactic acidosis is commonly observed in conditions where oxygen delivery is inadequate, such as low cardiac output, hypotension, severe anemia, and carbon monoxide poisoning. States of hypoperfusion are more prone to the accumulation of lactate than hypoxemic states. In the latter state, tissue

---

Box 13.3 Types and Causes of Lactic Acidosis

Type A

Generalized seizure
Extreme exercise
Shock
Cardiac arrest
Low cardiac output
Severe anemia
Severe hypoxemia
Carbon monoxide poisoning

Type B

Sepsis
Thiamine deficiency
Uncontrolled diabetes mellitus
Malignancy
Hypoglycemia
Drugs/toxins
  Ethanol
  Metformin
  Reverse transcriptase inhibitors (e.g., Zidovudine)
  Salicylate
  Linezolid
  Propofol
  Niacin
  Isoniazid
  Nitroprusside
  Cyanide
  Catecholamines
  Cocaine
  Acetaminophen
  Streptozotocin
  Sorbitol/fructose
Pheochromocytoma
Malaria
Inborn errors of metabolism

Other

Hepatic failure
Respiratory or metabolic alkalosis
Propylene glycol
d-Lactic acidosis

---

oxygenation is often preserved because of compensatory mechanisms such as increased cardiac output, augmented red blood cell production, and a reduced affinity of hemoglobin for oxygen. In all cases of type A lactic acidosis, oxygen is unavailable to the mitochondria, and pyruvate, unable to enter the tricarboxylic acid cycle, is reduced to lactate.

TYPE B LACTIC ACIDOSIS

Sepsis

Although sepsis is frequently associated with hypotension and thus with type A lactic acidosis, type B lactic acidosis may also develop during sepsis, even when oxygen delivery and tissue perfusion appear unimpeded. In fact, in the right clinical setting, a lactate level greater than 4 mmol/L has become a surrogate marker for severe sepsis independent of hypotension, so-called compensated shock. It has been postulated that in sepsis there is both an overproduction of pyruvate and an inhibition of PDH activity (the rate-limiting state in oxidative phosphorylation). Because of the increased NADH/NAD ratio, pyruvate is rapidly reduced to lactate. In septic patients with lactic acidosis, dichloroacetate, an activator of the PDH complex, lowers lactate levels significantly, suggesting that tissue oxygenation is adequate to support oxidative phosphorylation and therefore is not the limiting factor.

Drugs

Numerous drugs and toxins can cause lactic acidosis. The *biguanide* derivatives *phenformin* and *metformin* are recognized causes of lactic acidosis. Notably, phenformin was withdrawn from the U.S. market in 1976 because of the high frequency of lactic acidosis associated with its use. Both of these agents bind to complex 1 of the mitochondrial respiratory chain, inhibiting its activity. Metformin, a newer biguanide, has a markedly lower incidence of lactic acidosis, possibly because it is less lipid soluble and thus has limited ability to cross the mitochondrial membrane and bind to the mitochondrial complex. Almost all reported cases of metformin-associated lactic acidosis have occurred in patients with underlying CKD. It has been suggested that the present incidence of lactic acidosis in diabetics is no greater than the incidence of lactic acidosis before the introduction of metformin, and thus the association of metformin with lactic acidosis is more "guilt by association." A causative role, however, is suggested by the observations that, in isolated mitochondria, metformin inhibits the respiratory chain, and that the incidence of lactic acidosis approaches zero when the drug is prescribed according to recommendations.

Lactic acidosis is increasingly recognized in patients with human immunodeficiency virus infection who are taking nucleoside reverse-transcriptase inhibitors. These agents, including *stavudine, zidovudine, didanosine, abacavir,* and *lamivudine,* have been associated with severe lactic acidosis, often with concomitant hepatic steatosis. Nucleoside analogues inhibit mitochondrial DNA polymerase-γ. This causes mitochondrial toxicity and a decrease in oxidative phosphorylation, resulting in both lipid accumulation within the liver and decreased oxidation of pyruvate. Of note, hyperlactatemia without frank lactic acidosis is often present in patients on these medications. What converts these mild elevations in lactate levels into frank lactic acidosis remains unknown.

Salicylate intoxication often produces lactic acidosis. This occurs both because the salicylate-induced respiratory alkalosis stimulates lactate production and because of the inhibitory effects of salicylates on oxidative metabolism. Ethanol ingestion may cause mild elevations in lactate levels secondary to impaired hepatic conversion of lactate to glucose. In addition, the metabolism of ethanol increases the NADH/NAD ratio, favoring the conversion of pyruvate to lactate. Concomitant thiamine deficiency, as is often seen in alcohol abusers, may exacerbate the acidosis. *Linezolid,* an oxazolidinone antibiotic approved for use against methicillin and vancomycin-resistant gram-positive organisms, is reportedly associated with lactic acidosis. The presumed mechanism is mitochondrial toxicity.

Vitamin Deficiency

Deficiency of thiamine, a cofactor for PDH, also can result in lactic acidosis. Patients requiring total parental nutrition may develop thiamine deficiency if not supplemented with this vitamin. During a national shortage of parenteral vitamin preparations, numerous cases of lactic acidosis were reported because of inadequate thiamine supplementation.

Systemic Disease

Diabetes is often associated with lactic acidosis. Even under basal conditions, patients with diabetes experience mildly elevated lactate levels. This is thought to be secondary to decreased PDH activity caused by free fatty acid oxidation by liver and muscle. Lactate levels increase even more during diabetic ketoacidosis (DKA), possibly secondary to decreased hepatic clearance. This accumulation of lactate contributes to the elevated AG present in ketoacidosis.

Malignancy

Lactic acidosis has been detected in patients with acute rapidly progressive hematologic malignancies such as leukemia or lymphoma. Lactate levels usually parallel disease activity. The increased blood viscosity and microvascular aggregates that are frequently found in acute leukemia cause regional hypoperfusion. Overproduction of lactate may also result from a large tumor burden and rapid cell lysis.

Alternate Sugars

The use of intravenous sorbitol or fructose, as irrigants during prostate surgery or in tube feedings, can cause lactic acidosis. The metabolism of these sugars consumes ATP, inhibits gluconeogenesis, and stimulates glycolysis, leading to the accumulation of excess lactate.

Propylene Glycol

Propylene glycol is a common vehicle for many drugs, including topical silver sulfadiazine and intravenous preparations of nitroglycerin, diazepam, lorazepam, phenytoin, etomidate, and trimethoprim-sulfamethoxazole, among others. Although it is considered relatively safe, multiple case reports have verified the association of propylene glycol with lactic acidosis. Approximately 40% to 50% of administered propylene glycol is oxidized by alcohol dehydrogenase to lactic acid. Toxic patients commonly develop an unexplained AG acidosis with increased serum osmolality. Considering that patients who frequently receive many of the medications solubilized with propylene glycol have other possible causes for their acidosis, it is important to be aware of this iatrogenic cause of lactic acidosis. Correction of the metabolic abnormalities quickly occurs quickly following discontinuation of the medication.

d-LACTIC ACIDOSIS

This unusual form of AG acidosis is the result of the accumulation of the d-isomer of lactate. Unlike the lactate produced by glycolysis in animals, which is the l-isomer, colonic bacteria produce both the l- and the d-isomers. Overproduction of d-lactate occurs in patients with short-bowel syndrome and is usually precipitated by high carbohydrate intake, with increased colonic delivery of carbohydrate due to the shortened bowel along with bacterial overgrowth responsible for overproduction of d-lactate. Mammalian clearance of d-lactate is far less efficient than that of l-lactate, and the increased d-lactate produced within the gut accumulates in the blood. Because d-lactate is not detected on routine lactic acid assays, which measure only l-lactate, diagnosis requires a high clinical suspicion. Patients typically present with mental status changes, ataxia, and nystagmus. Treatment consists of an oral fast with intravenous nutrition and restoration of gut flora to normal through the administration of oral antibiotics. In severe cases, hemodialysis can decrease the concentration of d-lactate.

TREATMENT OF LACTIC ACIDOSIS

The treatment of lactic acidosis is fraught with controversy. The most important step is correction of the underlying cause. In sepsis, restoring oxygenation via mechanical ventilation and restoring perfusion via vasopressors or inotropes are of paramount importance, although these interventions do not always improve the lactic acidosis. In some patients with medication-induced lactic acidosis, withdrawal of the offending agent may be sufficient to correct the problem. There are anecdotal case reports of successful use of riboflavin or l-carnitine to treat lactic acidosis associated with nucleoside analogues in patients with acquired immunodeficiency syndrome.

Often these measures fail, and the clinician is faced with the decision of whether or not to give sodium bicarbonate in an effort to increase serum pH. There are several potential problems with this approach. First, as previously discussed, it is not clear to what extent acidosis is deleterious and therefore whether normalizing pH is of any benefit. Also, increasing pH may actually increase lactic acid production. Sodium bicarbonate is often administered as a hypertonic solution, which can lead to hyperosmolality and cellular dehydration. Perhaps most important is the possibility that the administration of HCO_3^- can cause a paradoxical decrease in intracellular pH despite an increase in extracellular pH. Bicarbonate combines with hydrogen to form carbonic acid, which is then converted to CO_2 and water. Thus, PCO_2 increases with the titration of acid by bicarbonate and rapidly diffuses into cells, causing acidification, whereas bicarbonate remains extracellular. Thus, it is difficult to recommend the use of bicarbonate for the treatment of a low-serum pH alone. However, if the serum pH is less than 7.1, many clinicians, despite the lack of supporting data, opt for treatment, because a further small decline in serum bicarbonate can have a profound effect on serum pH.

Other buffers may be better tolerated insofar as they buffer hydrogen ions without increasing CO_2. One such buffer is tris-hydroxymethyl aminomethane (THAM), a biologically inert amino acid that can buffer both CO_2 and protons. It does not lead to production of CO_2 and thus works well in a closed system. The protonated molecule is excreted by the kidney and should be used cautiously in patients with kidney failure. Potential side effects include hyperkalemia, hypoglycemia, ventilatory depression, and hepatic necrosis in neonates. Despite its having been available for many years, there are no studies demonstrating improved outcomes with the use of THAM. The acute dose in milliliters of 0.3 mol/L solution can be derived using the following formula: dose in milliliters = lean body weight (kg) × decrease in HCO_3^- from normal (mmol/L). The first 25% to 50% of the dose is administered over 5 minutes, and the remainder during 1 hour. Alternatively, a steady infusion of no more than 3.5 L/day can be administered for several days.

Dichloroacetate has also been used in the treatment of lactic acidosis. This agent stimulates the activity of PDH, increasing the rate of pyruvate oxidation and thereby decreasing lactate levels. A large multicenter trial in humans showed a reduction in serum lactate, an increase in pH, and an increase in the number of patients able to resolve their hyperlactatemia. Despite these favorable changes, no improvement in hemodynamic parameters or mortality was found.

Various modes of kidney replacement therapy have been used in the treatment of lactic acidosis. Standard bicarbonate hemodialysis treats acidosis primarily by diffusion of bicarbonate from the bath into the blood, and it is thus another form of bicarbonate administration, albeit with several advantages. In contrast to intravenous administration of bicarbonate, hyperosmolality and volume overload are not a concern with hemodialysis. Also, hemodialysis, in addition to adding bicarbonate, removes lactate. Although the removal of lactate does not increase serum pH, there is some evidence that the lactate ion itself is harmful. Unfortunately, there are no randomized, prospective trials demonstrating the benefit of dialysis in lactic acidosis, and its use in the absence of other indications cannot be routinely recommended.

Several studies have shown that high-volume hemofiltration using either lactate or bicarbonate-buffered replacement fluid can rapidly correct metabolic acidosis. These studies have been small, and the degree and type of acidosis have been poorly characterized. In addition, other treatment measures have usually been instituted, making it difficult to draw conclusions about the effectiveness of this treatment. Nevertheless, hemofiltration remains a viable therapeutic option.

Peritoneal dialysis has also been used in the treatment of metabolic acidosis. Although there are case reports of success using this modality, a randomized study comparing lactate-buffered peritoneal dialysis to continuous hemofiltration showed that hemofiltration corrected acidosis more quickly and more effectively than peritoneal dialysis. Whether newer bicarbonate-buffered peritoneal dialysis solution is more efficacious remains to be determined.

KETOACIDOSIS

DIABETIC KETOACIDOSIS

Diabetic ketoacidosis is another common cause of a high AG acidosis. Although DKA may be the initial presentation of diabetes mellitus, patients more commonly have a known diagnosis of diabetes and either were noncompliant with their insulin regimen or have some other precipitating factor such as infection. Patients are generally polyuric and polydipsic, but, if volume depletion becomes severe enough, polyuria may not be seen. Although DKA classically occurs in type 1 diabetes, it can also occur in patients with type 2 diabetes. DKA results from insulin deficiency and concomitant increase in counterregulatory hormones such as glucagon, epinephrine, and cortisol. This hormonal milieu leads to an inability of cells to use glucose, causing them to oxidize fatty acids as fuel, and it results in the production of large amounts of ketoacids. A diagnosis of DKA requires a pH less than 7.35, elevated AG, positive serum ketones of at least 1:2 dilutions, and decreased serum bicarbonate; however, not all patients with DKA meet these criteria. Ketones (anions) are rapidly excreted by the kidney in place of chloride if kidney perfusion and glomerular filtration rate (GFR) are well maintained. With the loss of these anions in the urine, the AG acidosis may be replaced by a mixed AG/hyperchloremic acidosis, or even with a pure hyperchloremic acidosis. Furthermore, an increase in the NADH/NAD ratio, which frequently occurs during DKA, causes ketones to shift from acetoacetate to β-hydroxybutyrate, which is not detected on the standard nitroprusside test used to identify serum and urinary ketones. If this occurs, serum ketones may appear negative or only trace positive. Finally, vomiting may result in a metabolic alkalosis, which would raise the serum bicarbonate toward the normal range. In this case, the serum AG would almost certainly be elevated and the astute clinician would not be fooled.

Treatment

The treatment of DKA consists of three parts: fluid resuscitation, insulin administration, and correction of potassium deficits. Patients with DKA often experience profound deficits of both sodium and free water. Hypovolemia, as demonstrated by hemodynamic compromise, should always be treated first. Patients should rapidly receive 1 to 2 L of 0.9% saline until their blood pressure has stabilized. Thereafter, hypotonic fluids in the form of 0.45% saline should be administered to correct free water deficits while continuing to provide volume. Insulin should be administered only after fluid resuscitation is well under way. If insulin is administered precipitously, the rapid uptake of glucose by the cells will cause water to follow because of the fall in extracellular osmolality, potentially resulting in cardiovascular collapse. A regular insulin bolus of 0.1 unit/kg intravenously is provided, followed by a continuous infusion of 0.1 unit/kg/h. If the glucose does not decline by 50 to 100 mg/dl/h, the infusion should be increased by 50%. As tissue perfusion improves, β-hydroxybutyrate is converted to acetoacetate, and serum ketones paradoxically increase, but then should decrease. Serum glucose usually approaches normal before ketosis is resolved. When glucose is less than 250 mg/dl, intravenous fluids should be changed to 5% dextrose to avoid hypoglycemia while awaiting resolution of ketogenesis. The insulin infusion should be continued until the AG closes, the HCO_3^- rises above 14 mmol/L, and the patient is taking food orally. Although the American Diabetes Association recommends continuing the insulin infusion until the HCO_3^- is greater than 18 mmol/L, regeneration of HCO_3^- may take up to 24 hours after the termination of ketogenesis, and this process is not hastened by insulin. A subcutaneous insulin dose should be given at least 1 hour before stopping the intravenous insulin infusion to avoid rebound ketosis.

Most patients with DKA have total-body potassium depletion. Nevertheless, their serum potassium may be normal or high because of a shift from cell stores caused by the profound insulinopenia. When insulin is restored, extracellular potassium is rapidly taken up by cells, and severe hypokalemia may ensue. Therefore, the addition of potassium to the intravenous fluids is recommended at a concentration of 10 to 20 mEq/L as soon as serum potassium falls below 4.5 mEq/L. Needless to say, this management algorithm requires frequent laboratory tests.

Although bicarbonate therapy has been used in severe DKA, this use is not supported by the literature. In fact,

bicarbonate administration even in patients with pH less than 7.0 has not been shown advantageous. In almost all cases, the acidosis rapidly improves with appropriate management without the use of bicarbonate. Thus, the administration of sodium bicarbonate to patients with DKA cannot be routinely recommended. However, it is important that these patients be closely monitored with frequent analyses of arterial blood gases and electrolytes.

ALCOHOLIC KETOACIDOSIS

Alcoholic ketoacidosis (AKA) usually presents with an AG acidosis and ketonemia, but without significant hyperglycemia. The classic presentation is that of a patient who has been on an alcohol binge, who develops nausea and vomiting, and stops eating. The patient typically presents 24 to 48 hours after the cessation of oral intake and may also complain of abdominal pain and shortness of breath. Alcohol levels are low or even immeasurable by the time AKA develops. AKA is similar to DKA in that it is a state of insulinopenia and increased counterregulatory hormones; in fact, the levels of these hormones are similar in both disorders. In AKA, normo- to hypoglycemia is usually observed despite a hormonal milieu favoring hyperglycemia, because decreased NAD curtails hepatic gluconeogenesis and starvation depletes glycogen stores. However, patients with AKA can occasionally present with hyperglycemia, and in those cases distinguishing it from DKA can be difficult. AKA almost always presents with a high AG, but acidemia is less universal. Patients often have concurrent metabolic alkalosis from vomiting or respiratory alkalosis from liver disease. Thus, patients with AKA may not be acidemic and rarely have a simple metabolic acidosis. Because of the increased NADH/NAD ratio, the primary ketoacid present is β-hydroxybutyrate, and thus serum ketones may be reported as negative. This ratio also favors the formation of lactic acid. Finally, electrolyte disorders, including hypokalemia, hypophosphatemia, and hypomagnesemia, are common.

Treatment

Therapy for AKA is straightforward and consists of volume repletion, provision of glucose (except for those patients with hyperglycemia), and correction of electrolyte abnormalities. Patients are often volume depleted from vomiting combined with poor oral intake. Thiamine must be provided before or concurrently with glucose to avoid precipitating Wernicke encephalopathy. Acidosis resolves as insulin increases and counterregulatory hormones are turned off in response to glucose infusion. The clinician must maintain a high degree of suspicion for this disorder, because the acid-base disturbance may be subtle on routine laboratory analyses, with patients often demonstrating only an elevated AG. Chronic alcoholics often have hypoalbuminemia, which can further obscure the interpretation of the AG. Any patient with nausea and vomiting with a recent history of alcohol abuse should considered for treatment of presumptive AKA until the diagnosis is excluded.

STARVATION KETOSIS

During prolonged fasting, insulin levels are suppressed, whereas glucagon, epinephrine, growth hormone, and cortisol levels are increased. This hormonal milieu results in increased lipolysis with release of free fatty acids into the blood and stimulation of hepatic ketogenesis. The concentrations of both β-hydroxybutyrate and acetoacetate increase during the course of several weeks, resulting in a mild AG metabolic acidosis.

TOXINS AND DRUGS

ETHYLENE GLYCOL

Ingestion of various toxins can cause severe metabolic acidosis with an increased AG and should always be suspected in these cases. Ethylene glycol is a sweet liquid that is found in antifreeze. Ingestion of 100 mL or more can be fatal. Ethylene glycol is metabolized by alcohol dehydrogenase into glycolic acid and subsequently into oxalic acid. This generates NADH, which encourages the formation of lactic acid. The AG acidosis results from the accumulation of the various acid metabolites of ethylene glycol as well as lactic acidosis. Diagnosis can be difficult, because ethylene glycol is not detected on routine toxicology assays. It should be suspected in anyone who presents with intoxication, a low blood alcohol level, and a markedly increased AG metabolic acidosis without ketonemia. The serum osmolar gap may help detect ethylene glycol. The serum osmolar gap is the difference between the calculated serum osmolarity $[([Na^+] * 2) + (glucose/18) + (BUN/2.8)]$ and the actual serum osmolality as measured by the laboratory. A difference greater than about 10 to 15 mOsm/kg suggests the presence of an unmeasured, osmotically active substance, which in the right clinical setting could be a toxin. However, it is important to understand the limitations of this approach. Some laboratories measure serum osmolality using vapor pressure methodology rather than freezing point depression, and volatile substances such as alcohols may not be detected. As the osmotically active alcohol is metabolized into the various acids, the osmolar gap disappears. Thus, early after ingestion, the osmolar gap is elevated without a significant increase in the AG. As the alcohol is metabolized, the osmolar gap decreases while the AG increases. Examination of the urine may show calcium oxalate crystals, a finding that can be considered pathognomonic; however, the absence of these crystals does not rule out the ingestion of ethylene glycol. Precipitation of calcium oxalate may occasionally cause hypocalcemia. Because fluorescein is added as a colorant to antifreeze, the urine of a patient with antifreeze ingestion may fluoresce under a Wood lamp.

METHANOL

Methanol is an alcohol often found in solvents or as an adulterant in alcoholic beverages. Toxicity is usually caused by ingestion of as little as 30 mL, and toxicity has also been reported after inhalation. Methanol is metabolized by alcohol dehydrogenase to formaldehyde and then to formic acid, resulting in an elevated AG acidosis. As with ingestions of other alcohols, NAD depletion favors the production of lactate. Methanol is less intoxicating than either ethanol or ethylene glycol. The most characteristic symptom of methanol toxicity is blurry vision. Blindness may occur because of optic nerve involvement, and pancreatitis may be seen in up to two thirds of patients. As described previously, early after ingestion an osmolar gap may be found. The diagnosis of both ethylene glycol and methanol poisoning can be confirmed by specific toxicologic assays, but treatment should never be delayed while awaiting these results.

Treatment of Toxic Alcohol Ingestions

Treatment of both ethylene glycol and methanol toxicity is based on the fact that it is the metabolites of these alcohols that are actually harmful and that both substances are metabolized by alcohol dehydrogenase; therefore, blocking the activity of this enzyme will prevent the metabolic acidosis and will allow the alcohol to be excreted by the kidneys or to be removed by dialysis. Because alcohol dehydrogenase has a much higher affinity for ethanol than for either ethylene glycol or methanol, the use of ethanol as a competitive inhibitor is the traditional treatment. Ethanol is supplied as a 10% solution in 5% dextrose in water (D5W). A loading dose of 0.8 to 1.0 g/kg body weight followed by an infusion of 100 mg/kg/h should be sufficient to maintain a blood alcohol level of 100 to 150 mg/dl. However, in some patients with marked ethanol tolerance this rate will need to be doubled. Fomepizole (4-methylpyrazole), a competitive inhibitor of alcohol dehydrogenase, has replaced ethanol as the treatment of choice. Fomepizole is a more potent inhibitor of alcohol dehydrogenase than ethanol, and it does not lead to central nervous system (CNS) depression. An initial loading dose of 15 mg/kg body weight is followed 12 hours later by 10 mg/kg every 12 hours for four doses, then 15 mg/kg every 12 hours for four more doses. Although fomepizole, because of its potency, has begun to call into question the need for dialysis, until more studies are available it is recommended that dialysis be instituted in all patients with suspected ingestions of ethylene glycol or methanol who have end-organ damage (kidney failure or visual impairment) and whose pH is less than 7.2. Both compounds can be rapidly removed by hemodialysis. Hemodialysis can also help improve the acidosis by providing a source of bicarbonate. It is important to double the rate of any ethanol infusion or to increase the dose of fomepizole while the patient is receiving hemodialysis. For either ingestion, gastric lavage with charcoal should be performed when ingestion has occurred within the preceding 2 to 3 hours.

SALICYLATE TOXICITY

The ingestion of salicylates is an important cause of mixed acid-base disturbances, producing both a respiratory alkalosis and a metabolic acidosis. Salicylate is a direct respiratory stimulant. Metabolic acidosis results from the accumulation of both lactic and ketoacids, whereas salicylic acid itself accounts for only a small quantity of the acid load. The common presenting sign of salicylate toxicity is tachypnea. The patient may also complain of tinnitus when serum concentrations of salicylic acid reach 20 to 45 mg/dl or higher. Other CNS manifestations are agitation, seizures, and even coma. Both noncardiogenic pulmonary edema and upper gastrointestinal bleeding may occur. Hypoglycemia occurs in children but is rare in adults. Other symptoms include nausea, vomiting, and hyperpyrexia.

In the setting of salicylate overdose, peak serum concentrations are achieved 4 to 6 hours after ingestion. The severity of the ingestion can be predicted by the Done nomogram, which plots the toxic salicylate level at varying points following ingestion. This nomogram cannot be used with chronic ingestions or with the ingestion of enteric-coated aspirin.

The treatment of salicylate toxicity consists of supportive care, removal of unabsorbed compounds using charcoal lavage, administration of bicarbonate, and hemodialysis if necessary. Because the dissociation constant (pK) of salicylic acid is 3.0, alkalinization keeps the drug in its polar dissociated form, preventing diffusion into the CNS. In addition, because tissue salicylic acid is in equilibrium with the nondissociated compound in the plasma, alkalinization also decreases tissue levels. Concurrent alkalinization of the urine traps salicylate in the tubule, promoting its excretion. Hemodialysis is indicated in all patients with altered mental status, kidney failure that decreases renal excretion, volume overload that prevents the administration of bicarbonate, or salicylate levels greater than 100 mg/dl.

PYROGLUTAMIC ACIDOSIS

It is becoming increasingly recognized that glutathione depletion can cause an AG acidosis. This underreported acidosis occurs in patients who usually have underlying infections and are treated with acetaminophen even at therapeutic doses. Glutathione depletion decreases the negative feedback inhibition on γ-glutamylcysteine synthetase, resulting in an increase in pyroglutamic acid (5-oxoproline). Measurement of 5-oxoproline levels in the urine will confirm the diagnosis.

KIDNEY FAILURE

Kidney failure is a well-recognized cause of metabolic acidosis. With the reduction in nephron mass that occurs in CKD, there is decreased ammoniagenesis in the proximal tubule. Many patients with diminished kidney function may also have specific acidification defects in the form of a renal tubular acidosis (RTA). As the GFR declines, the kidney is unable to secrete the daily production of fixed acid. Serum bicarbonate may begin to decline when the GFR falls below 40 mL/min/1.73 m².

The acidosis of kidney failure can be associated with either an elevated AG or a normal AG. With mild-to-moderate reductions in GFR, the anions that comprise the gap are excreted normally, and the acidosis reflects decreased ammoniagenesis and is therefore hyperchloremic. As kidney failure worsens, the kidney loses its ability to filter and excrete various anions, and the accumulation of sulfate, phosphate, and other anions produce an elevated AG. Because of the better control of phosphorus, more intensive

dietary modifications, and earlier initiation of dialysis provided today, even patients who are beginning kidney replacement therapy will often not manifest an increased AG.

Despite daily net positive acid balance, it is unusual for HCO_3^- to fall below 15 mmol/L. Why the acidosis of CKD is rarely severe is unclear. Whether this lack of severity is secondary to buffering of the retained protons in bone, or to retention of organic anions usually lost in the urine that are instead subsequently converted to HCO_3^-, is controversial. The buffering of protons by bone results in the loss of calcium and negative calcium balance. In addition, chronic acidosis causes protein breakdown, muscle wasting, and negative nitrogen balance. Maintaining acid-base balance close to normal can prevent these consequences.

The metabolic acidosis commonly found in patients with CKD can easily be corrected by prescribing oral bicarbonate. Usually two 650-mg (7.8 mEq) tablets three times daily will keep the serum bicarbonate in the normal range. It is rare for maintenance hemodialysis to be initiated solely for the purpose of correcting acidosis.

HYPERCHLOREMIC METABOLIC ACIDOSIS

Acidosis associated with a normal AG, HCMA, has a limited number of causes (Fig. 13.6). HCMA can occur in CKD when reduced ammoniagenesis impairs the kidney's ability to excrete the daily acid load. In individuals with normal or near normal kidney function, it can be divided into cases caused by the kidney's failure to reabsorb HCO_3^- or secrete the daily fixed load of H^+, commonly known as RTAs, and those in which renal acid-base handling is normal. In contrast to AG acidosis, most cases of HCMA are easily treated with a supplemental base.

RENAL CAUSES OF HYPERCHLOREMIC METABOLIC ACIDOSIS

Renal tubular acidoses represent a heterogeneous cause of HCMA in which the kidney is unable to maintain acid-base balance despite preservation of normal or near-normal kidney function (normal GFR). There is often confusion regarding the RTAs, because no standard nomenclature exists, numerous diverse transport defects have been identified, and the literature often presents contradictory information. A grasp of the underlying pathophysiology makes

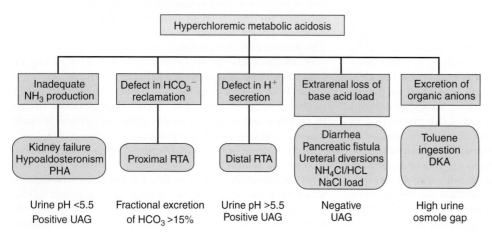

Figure 13.6 The etiology of hyperchloremic metabolic acidosis with useful diagnostic tools. *AG,* Anion gap; *DKA,* diabetic ketoacidosis; *PHA,* pseudohypoaldosteronism; *RTA,* renal tubular acidosis; *UAG,* urine anion gap.

the approach to these disorders more comprehensible. The RTAs can be divided into four major categories: (1) primary defects in ammoniagenesis, (2) hypoaldosteronism, (3) disorders of the proximal tubule, and (4) disorders of the distal tubule. The distal tubule defects can be further divided into those with hypokalemia and those with hyperkalemia (Fig. 13.7).

DEFECTIVE AMMONIAGENESIS

One of the most common causes of an HCMA is the inability of the kidney to generate ammonia because of CKD. By definition, RTA refers to a specific acid excretory defect occurring despite the presence of normal or near-normal kidney function. Thus, it bears emphasis that the HCMA of CKD is not classified as RTA. As the number of nephrons decreases with CKD, there is a proportional decrease in the production of ammonia. As mentioned in the section on AG acidosis, when GFR falls below 40 mL/min/1.73 m², the kidney is unable to excrete the daily acid load, and HCO_3^- begins to decline with a concomitant increase in the serum Cl^-, producing HCMA. Only when the GFR falls below 15 to 20 mL/min/1.73 m² does the kidney lose the ability to secrete anions, thus converting this HCMA into an AG acidosis. It needs to be stressed that the acidosis in kidney failure, whether manifested by hyperchloremia or an AG, is primarily caused by defective ammoniagenesis. As such, the UAG will be positive because of the decrease in ammonia excretion, whereas urine pH will be less than 5.5.

HYPOALDOSTERONISM

Primary or secondary hypoaldosteronism is a common disorder causing hyperkalemia and metabolic acidosis (Box 13.4). Hyporeninemic hypoaldosteronism (type IV RTA) is the most frequently encountered variety of this disorder, which is most common in patients with diabetes and mild CKD. The precise cause of hyporeninemia has not been clearly defined, but the findings that hypertension is frequently present and that the disorder may be partly reversed with chronic furosemide use suggest that renin suppression may be secondary to chronic volume overload. Neither has the cause of the hypoaldosteronism been fully explained. Renin suppression alone should not cause hypoaldosteronism,

because hyperkalemia is a potent stimulus of aldosterone secretion and anephric individuals still secrete aldosterone. The acidosis is primarily caused by decreased ammoniagenesis as a result of the associated hyperkalemia induced by the aldosterone deficiency. Hypoaldosteronism, by diminishing distal sodium reabsorption, also results in a less negative lumen potential, thus decreasing the rate of H^+ secretion but not the electromotive force of the pump. Because the hydrogen pump is not defective, urine pH is usually less than 5.5.

Patients with type IV RTA are usually asymptomatic, with only minor laboratory abnormalities (mild hyperkalemia and decreased HCO_3^-). However, when renal potassium handling is further perturbed by various stressors, marked hyperkalemia ensues with a decline in ammoniagenesis. These stressors include sodium depletion, which decreases delivery of sodium to the distal tubule; high potassium diet; and potassium-sparing diuretics or medications that further decrease renin and aldosterone levels, such as angiotensin-converting enzyme inhibitors, angiotensin receptor blockers, nonsteroidal antiinflammatory drugs, or heparin. Most patients can be treated by removing the insult to potassium homeostasis, restricting potassium intake, and providing supplemental bicarbonate. Proving that type IV RTA is present requires the demonstration of low renin and aldosterone

---

Box 13.4   Causes of Hypoaldosteronism

Primary

Addison disease
Congenital enzyme defects
Drugs
   Heparin
   Angiotensin converting enzyme inhibitors
   Angiotensin receptor blockers

Hyporeninemic Hypoaldosteronism (Type IV RTA)

PHA I (Autosomal Dominant)—Mineralocorticoid Resistance

PHA, Pseudohypoaldosteronism; *RTA*, renal tubular acidosis.

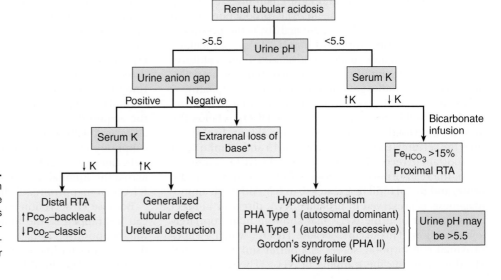

Figure 13.7 Evaluation of RTA. *Extrarenal loss of base is not a form of RTA. Findings shown, because the use of this algorithm may lead to its diagnosis. FE_{HCO_3}, Fractional excretion of bicarbonate; *PHA*, pseudohypoaldosteronism; *RTA*, renal tubular acidosis.

levels after sodium depletion. Because of practical considerations, these tests are rarely ordered, and most patients will be treated empirically.

Autosomal-dominant pseudohypoaldosteronism (PHA) type I is an uncommon disorder caused by a mutation in the renal mineralocorticoid receptor, which results in decreased affinity for aldosterone. This genetic disorder presents in childhood with hyperaldosteronism, hyperkalemia, metabolic acidosis, salt wasting, and hypotension. Autosomal-dominant PHA type I becomes less severe with age. Carbenoxolone and glycyrrhizic acid (found in true licorice) both inhibit 11-β-hydroxysteroid dehydrogenase, the enzyme in the kidney that converts cortisol, which binds the mineralocorticoid receptor, to cortisone, which does not bind to the mineralocorticoid receptor. They can be used to treat this disorder by increasing the intrarenal supply of mineralocorticoid.

PROXIMAL RENAL TUBULAR ACIDOSIS

Proximal RTA, often called type II RTA (because it was the second type described), is a defect in the ability of the proximal tubule to reclaim filtered HCO_3^- (Box 13.5). In type II RTA, the proximal tubule has a diminished threshold (approximately 15 mmol/L instead of the normal 24 mmol/L) for HCO_3^- reabsorption. When plasma HCO_3^- falls below this threshold, complete reabsorption occurs. Proximal RTA can be congenital or acquired, and it may exist as an isolated defect in HCO_3^- reabsorption or as part of a more generalized transport defect known as Fanconi syndrome, in which there is diminished reabsorption of other solutes across the proximal tubule. Patients with proximal RTA from Fanconi syndrome, in addition to the loss of HCO_3^-, inappropriately excrete amino acids, glucose, phosphorus, and uric acid in their urine.

As would be expected, mutations in the Na^+-H^+ exchanger on the luminal membrane, the Na^+-HCO_3^- cotransporter on the basolateral membrane, and cytosolic carbonic anhydrase have all been implicated in the isolated hereditary and sporadic forms of proximal RTA. Several drugs that block carbonic anhydrase, including the diuretic acetazolamide and the anticonvulsant topiramate, also cause isolated HCO_3^- wasting. Proximal RTA with Fanconi syndrome is frequently found in patients with cystinosis, Wilson disease, Lowe syndrome, multiple myeloma, and light chain disease, among other conditions. A decrease in ATP production, which reduces basolateral Na^+-K^+-ATPase activity, is the presumed etiology of this global transport defect. Drugs, particularly the cyclophosphamide analogue ifosfamide, and cidofovir, used in the treatment of cytomegalovirus retinitis, have also been associated with a generalized proximal tubulopathy.

Because distal H^+ excretion is normal, urine pH during steady state will be less than 5.5 when the HCO_3^- is below the lowered threshold and bicarbonaturia is absent. In this setting, the serum HCO_3^- will be between 15 and 18 mEq/L. It is important to recognize that whenever the HCO_3^- increases above the reabsorptive threshold, HCO_3^- will appear in the urine, and the pH will be greater than 6.5. Although ammoniagenesis is preserved in proximal RTA, direct or indirect measurement of urine NH_4^+ may show an inappropriately low excretion. This occurs because HCO_3^-, which escapes proximal reabsorption, serves as a buffer sink for secreted H^+, thus reducing the trapping of NH_4^+. The diagnosis of

---

Box 13.5   Causes of Proximal Renal Tubular Acidosis

Isolated Defects in HCO_3 Reabsorption
  Carbonic anhydrase inhibitors
  Acetazolamide
  Topiramate
  Sulfamylon
  Carbonic anhydrase deficiency
Generalized Defects in Proximal Tubular Transport
  Cystinosis
  Wilson disease
  Lowe syndrome
  Galactosemia
  Multiple myeloma
  Light chain disease
  Amyloidosis
  Vitamin D deficiency
  Ifosfamide
  Cidofovir
  Lead
  Aminoglycosides

---

proximal RTA is established by demonstrating a fractional excretion of HCO_3^- greater than 15% when supplemental bicarbonate is administered in an attempt to increase the serum bicarbonate to normal.

Treatment of proximal RTA is difficult, because administered base is rapidly excreted in the urine. Extremely large amounts of base (10 to 15 mmol/kg/day) are frequently needed, and therefore compliance is limited. The increased delivery of HCO_3^- to the distal nephron induces or exacerbates hypokalemia. It is recommended that frequent doses of a mixture of Na and K salts of bicarbonate and citrate be used.

DISTAL RENAL TUBULAR ACIDOSIS

Classic Distal Renal Tubular Acidosis with Hypokalemia

Distal RTA, also known as type I RTA, represents the inability of the distal tubule to acidify the urine (Box 13.6). As with proximal RTA, the distal variety can be congenital or acquired. Abnormalities have been identified in both the luminal H^+-ATPase and the basolateral Cl^--HCO_3^- exchanger. The acquired form is associated with autoimmune diseases, especially systemic lupus erythematosus and Sjögren syndrome, dysproteinemia, and kidney transplant rejection. Immunocytochemical studies have shown decreased staining of the H^+-ATPase and Cl^--HCO_3^- exchanger in patients with the acquired form of distal RTA. Ifosfamide, which is also associated with a proximal RTA, can cause a distal defect. Amphotericin, which disrupts membrane-forming ion channels, causes a distal RTA by allowing the backleak of protons across the luminal membrane. The classic finding in type I RTA is an inappropriately high urine pH (greater than 5.5).

Because H^+ secretion is defective in distal RTA, less NH_4^+ can be trapped in the lumen of the tubule, and the UAG will be positive, reflecting this decrease in NH_4^+ excretion. Besides having an inappropriately high urine pH and a positive UAG, distal RTA can be further characterized by

---

Box 13.6   Causes of Distal Renal Tubular Acidosis With Hypokalemia

Familial
  Defective HCO_3^--Cl^- exchanger (autosomal dominant)
  Defective H^+-ATPase (autosomal recessive)
Endemic
  Thai endemic distal RTA
Drugs
  Amphotericin
  Toluene
  Lithium
  Ifosfamide
  Foscarnet
  Vanadium
Systemic disorders
  Sjögren syndrome
  Cryoglobulinemia
  Systemic lupus erythematosus
  Kidney transplant rejection

RTA, Renal tubular acidosis.

Box 13.7   Causes of Distal Renal Tubular Acidosis With Hyperkalemia

Lupus Nephritis
Obstructive Nephropathy
Sickle Cell Anemia
Voltage Defects
Familial
  PHA type I (autosomal recessive)
  PHA type II (autosomal recessive)—Gordon syndrome
Drugs
  Amiloride
  Triamterene
  Trimethoprim
  Pentamidine

PHA, Pseudohypoaldosteronism.

---

measuring urine PCO_2 during an HCO_3^- infusion. Distal delivery of HCO_3^- in the presence of a normal H^+ secretory capacity results in elevated pCO_2 in the urine. When there is a H^+ secretory defect, urine pCO_2 will not increase. As would be expected, in amphotericin-induced RTA where H^+ ion secretion is unaffected, urine pCO_2 increases normally. Occasionally it may be difficult to distinguish HCMA induced by diarrhea from a distal RTA. Diarrhea results in HCMA and hypokalemia. Because the hypokalemia increases renal ammoniagenesis, urine pH may be inappropriately elevated. Thus, on the surface, both forms of acidosis appear similar. However, measurement of the UAG will easily distinguish the markedly elevated urine NH_4^+ with its negative AG found in diarrheal illness from the low NH_4^+ excretion and positive AG found with distal RTA. The one caveat is that sodium must be delivered to the distal tubule as indicated by urine Na^+ that is greater than 20 mmol/L.

Classic distal RTA is associated with hypokalemia (due to augmented distal K^+ secretion in lieu of H^+ secretion in exchange for Na^+ reabsorption), hypocitraturia (from enhanced proximal tubule cell reabsorption), hypercalciuria (from the buffering of H^+ in bone and loss of calcium), and nephrocalcinosis. The treatment of distal RTA is simply to supply enough base (2 to 3 mmol/kg/day) to counter the daily fixed production of acid. This can be administered as a mixture of sodium and potassium salts of either bicarbonate or citrate.

Distal Renal Tubular Acidosis with Hyperkalemia

Distal RTA with hyperkalemia can be further divided into two broad general categories: (1) a generalized defect of both distal tubular H^+ and K^+ secretion, or (2) a primary defect in Na^+ transport, often referred to as a "voltage defect" (Box 13.7).

Generalized Distal Tubule Defect

Unlike classic distal RTA, a more generalized defect of the distal tubule can occur in which both H^+ and K^+ secretion is impaired. This has been best characterized in cases of ureteral obstruction and in patients with interstitial kidney disease resulting from sickle cell anemia or systemic lupus erythematosus. In animals with ureteral obstruction, immunocytochemical staining has shown loss of the apical H^+-ATPase. Why hyperkalemia occurs is less clear. Because K^+ excretion cannot be augmented by diuretics, a primary defect in K^+ transport is likely. Similar to classic distal RTA, urine pH is greater than 5.5.

Distal Sodium Transport Defects

Several disorders have been characterized by defective sodium transport in the distal tubule. The reabsorption of Na^+ by the distal tubule generates a lumen-negative potential. This electrical negativity helps promote the secretion of K^+ and H^+. Any drug or disorder that interferes with the creation of this lumen-negative potential will diminish both K^+ and H^+ secretion. These are commonly classified as voltage defects. Autosomal-recessive PHA type I is a syndrome in which there is loss of function of the epithelial sodium channel (ENaC) in the distal tubule. Numerous mutations have been described in various subunits of this channel. This disease manifests in childhood with marked hyperkalemia, metabolic acidosis, hyperaldosteronism, and salt wasting. Because the ENaC also exists in other tissue, including the lung, colon, and sweat glands, patients with this disorder often have defects related to these organs. Treatment consists of providing a high salt intake. Drugs that block ENaC produce a similar metabolic picture. These include the potassium-sparing diuretics amiloride and triamterene, as well as trimethoprim and pentamidine.

Another well-recognized disorder of distal transport is PHA type II, also known as Gordon syndrome (see Chapters 39 and 67). Individuals with this condition have mild volume overload with suppressed renin and aldosterone, hypertension, hyperkalemia, and metabolic acidosis. Mutations in two members of a family of serine-threonine kinases, WNK1 and WNK4, have been shown as the cause of this syndrome. These kinases appear to play an important role in the regulation of Cl^- transport in numerous different tissues. It appears that defects in these kinases result in an increase in the number of neutral NaCl transporters (NCCT) and thus increase NaCl transport across the distal convoluted tubule. Less delivery of sodium to the more distal tubule segments for reabsorption curtails the generation of the lumen-negative potential. This results in decreased H^+ and K^+ secretion. Supporting this hypothesis is the fact that PHA type II can be treated with thiazide-type diuretics, which block the NCCT.

The acidosis in all of these sodium transport disorders is secondary to decreased H^+ secretion caused by an unfavorable electrical gradient in the distal tubule as well as decreased ammoniagenesis caused by the hyperkalemia. Whether the urine pH is less than 5.5 depends on how severely H^+ secretion is affected.

COMBINED PROXIMAL AND DISTAL RENAL TUBULAR ACIDOSIS

Combined proximal and distal renal tubular acidosis is an extremely uncommon disorder, which has been called type 3 RTA. As would be expected, both proximal HCO_3^- reabsorption and distal H^+ secretion are impaired. Mutations in the gene for cytosolic carbonic anhydrase results in such a defect. As already discussed, ifosfamide can also cause a combined defect.

INCOMPLETE DISTAL RENAL TUBULAR ACIDOSIS

Patients with incomplete distal RTA typically come to medical attention because of calcium stone disease and nephrocalcinosis. Serum HCO_3^- is normal, but urine pH never falls below 5.5, even after acid loading with NH_4Cl or $CaCl_2$. This disorder likely represents a milder form of distal RTA. Frank metabolic acidosis may become evident when patients are stressed by diarrhea or other conditions that require compensation by augmented renal proton secretion.

EXTRARENAL CAUSES OF HYPERCHLOREMIC METABOLIC ACIDOSIS

EXTRARENAL BICARBONATE LOSS

Loss of base during episodes of diarrhea or with overzealous use of laxatives is associated with HCMA. Loss of HCO_3^- can also occur with pancreatic fistulae or following pancreas transplantation if drainage of the pancreatic duct occurs into the bladder. Ureteral diversions using an isolated sigmoid loop were frequently associated with bicarbonate loss because of $Cl-HCO_3^-$ exchange in the bowel loop. These ureteral-sigmoidostomies have largely been replaced with ureteral diversions using ileal conduits, which have less surface area and contact time for loss of HCO_3^- to occur; however, if these become obstructed, HCMA can still develop.

ACID LOAD

An obvious cause of an HCMA is ingestion or infusion of a chloride salt of an acid. Both NH_4Cl and $CaCl_2$ can result in a metabolic acidosis and can be used as a provocative test to assess urinary acidification. In addition, total parenteral nutrition using hydrochloric acid salts of various amino acids can produce a metabolic acidosis if an insufficient quantity of base (usually acetate) is added to the infusion mixture. Another form of acid load is saline (NaCl). Volume resuscitation with 0.9% NaCl will often produce an HCMA, referred to as a *dilutional acidosis*. This occurs because of "dilution" of the plasma HCO_3^- by the more acidic saline solution (pH 7.0) and because volume expansion diminishes proximal HCO_3^- reabsorption.

URINARY LOSS OF ANIONS

As previously discussed, if organic anions are excreted in the urine, they represent a source of base lost from the body. Although involving the kidney, this cannot be viewed as being caused by an intrinsic kidney defect. Because of the low renal threshold for the excretion of ketoacids, patients with DKA, if they are able to maintain their intravascular volume or are volume resuscitated, will excrete these anions in place of Cl^-, resulting in HCMA. A similar metabolic disturbance exists after toluene exposure. Toluene is a common solvent found in paint products and glues. Exposure is generally by inhalation, either accidental or intentional. Toluene is rapidly absorbed through the skin and mucous membranes and is metabolized to hippuric acid. Hippurate is quickly excreted by the kidney, leaving behind an HCMA. Although hippurate is not a base, its rapid excretion into the urine conceals the AG origins of this disturbance. Both of these disorders are usually easily discovered after an adequate history has been obtained.

KEY BIBLIOGRAPHY

Adrogue HJ, Madias NE: Management of life-threatening acid-base disorders, *N Engl J Med* 338:26-34, 1998, and 107-111.

Alper SL: Genetic diseases of acid-base transporters, *Annu Rev Physiol* 64:899-923, 2002.

Bonny O, Rossier B: Disturbances of Na/K balance: pseudohypoaldosteronism revisited, *J Am Soc Nephrol* 13:2399-2414, 2002.

Brent J, McMartin K, Phillips S, et al: Fomepizole for the treatment of methanol poisoning, *N Engl J Med* 344:424-429, 2001.

Carlisle EJ, Donnelly SM, Vasuvattakul S, et al: Glue-sniffing and distal renal tubular acidosis: sticking to the facts, *J Am Soc Nephrol* 1:1019-1027, 1991.

Chang CT, Chen YC, Fang JT, et al: Metformin-associated lactic acidosis: case reports and literature review, *J Nephrol* 15; 398-394, 2002.

Claessens YE, Cariou A, Monchi M, et al: Detecting life-threatening lactic acidosis related to nucleoside-analog treatment of human immunodeficiency virus-infected patients, and treatment with l-carnitine, *Crit Care Med* 31:1042-1047, 2003.

Dargan PI, Wallace CI, Jones AL: An evidence based flowchart to guide the management of acute salicylate (aspirin) overdose, *Emerg Med J* 19:206-209, 2002.

DuBose TD Jr, Mcdonald GA: Renal tubular acidosis. In Dubose TD, Hamm LL Jr, editors: *Acid-base and electrolyte disorders: a companion to Brenners and Rector's The Kidney*, Philadelphia, 2002, WB Saunders, pp 189-206.

Figge J, Jabor A, Kazda A: Anion gap and hypoalbuminemia, *Crit Care Med* 26:1807-1810, 1998.

Fraser AD: Clinical toxicologic implications of ethylene glycol and glycolic acid poisoning, *Ther Drug Monit* 24:232-238, 2002.

Han J, Kim G-H, Kim J, et al: Secretory-defect distal renal tubular acidosis is associated with transporter defect in H+-ATPase and anion exchanger-1, *J Am Soc Nephrol* 13:1425-1432, 2002.

Hood VL, Tannen RL: Protection of acid-base balance by pH regulation of acid production, *N Engl J Med* 339:819-826, 1998.

Igarashi T, Sekine T, Inatomi J, et al: Unraveling the molecular pathogenesis of isolated proximal renal tubular acidosis, *J Am Soc Nephrol* 13:2171-2177, 2002.

Ishihara K, Szerlip HM: Anion gap acidosis, *Semin Nephrol* 18:83-89, 1998.

Izzedine H, Launay-Vacher V, Isnard-Bagnis C, et al: Drug-induced Fanconi's syndrome, *Am J Kidney Dis* 41:292-309, 2003.

Karet FE: Inherited distal renal tubular acidosis, *J Am Soc Nephrol* 13:2178-2184, 2002.

Kirschbaum B, Sica D, Anderson F: Urine electrolytes and the urine anion and osmolar gaps, *J Lab Clin Med* 133:597-604, 1999.

Lemann J Jr, Bushinsky DA, Hamm LL: Bone buffering of acid and base in humans, *Am J Physiol Renal Physiol* 285:F811-F832, 2003.

Levraut J, Grimaud D: Treatment of metabolic acidosis, *Curr Opin Crit Care* 9:260-265, 2003.

Full bibliography can be found on www.expertconsult.com.

Metabolic Alkalosis 14

Thomas D. DuBose, Jr.

PATHOGENESIS

The pathogenesis of metabolic alkalosis requires two processes: (1) generation and (2) maintenance. Generation occurs as a result of net gain of bicarbonate ions (HCO_3^-) or net loss of nonvolatile acid (usually HCl by vomiting) from the extracellular fluid. "New" bicarbonate may be generated as a result of both renal and extrarenal disturbances.

The kidneys have an impressive capacity to excrete HCO_3^- under normal circumstances. In the maintenance stage of metabolic alkalosis, however, the kidneys fail to excrete HCO_3^- because of volume contraction, a low glomerular filtration rate (GFR), or depletion of chloride (Cl^-) or potassium (K^+). Maintenance of metabolic alkalosis, therefore, represents a failure of the kidneys to eliminate HCO_3^- in the usual manner. Retention, rather than excretion, of excess alkali by the kidney is promoted when: (1) volume deficiency, Cl^- deficiency, and K^+ deficiency exist in combination with a reduced GFR, or (2) hypokalemia prevails because of autonomous hyperaldosteronism. In the first example, alkalosis is corrected by administration of NaCl and KCl, whereas, in the latter example, it is necessary to repair the alkalosis by pharmacologic or surgical intervention rather than saline administration.

In assessing a patient with metabolic alkalosis, two questions should be considered: (1) What is the source of alkali gain (or acid loss) that generated the alkalosis? and (2) What renal mechanisms are operating to prevent excretion of excess HCO_3^-, thereby maintaining, rather than correcting, the alkalosis?

DIFFERENTIAL DIAGNOSIS

To establish the cause of metabolic alkalosis (Box 14.1), it is necessary to assess the extracellular fluid volume (ECV) status, the recumbent and upright blood pressure, the serum potassium concentration ($[K^+]$), and the renin-angiotensin system. For example, the presence of chronic hypertension and chronic hypokalemia in an alkalotic patient suggests either mineralocorticoid excess or a hypertensive patient receiving diuretics. Low plasma renin activity and urine $[Na^+]$ and $[Cl^-]$ values greater than 20 mEq/L in a patient not taking diuretics are consistent with a primary mineralocorticoid excess syndrome.

The combination of hypokalemia and alkalosis in a normotensive, nonedematous patient can pose a difficult problem. Possible causes include Bartter or Gitelman syndromes, magnesium deficiency, vomiting, exogenous alkali, and diuretic ingestion. Determination of urine electrolytes (especially $[Cl^-]$) and screening of the urine for diuretics may be helpful. When the urine chloride concentration is measured (Table 14.1), it should be considered in context with assessment of the ECV status of the patient. A low urine $[Cl^-]$ (i.e., <10 mEq/L) indicates avid Cl^- retention by the kidney and denotes ECV depletion even if the urine Na^+ is high (i.e., >15 mEq/L), whereas a high urine $[Cl^-]$ in the absence of concurrent diuretic use suggests inappropriate chloruresis resulting from a tubular defect or mineralocorticoid excess. If the urine is alkaline, with an elevated $[Na^+]$ and $[K^+]$ but a urine $[Cl^-]$ lower than 10 mEq/L, the diagnosis is usually either vomiting (overt or surreptitious) or alkali ingestion. If the urine is relatively acid and has low concentrations of Na^+, K^+, and Cl^-, the most likely possibilities are previous vomiting, the posthypercapnic state, or previous diuretic ingestion. If, on the other hand, neither the urine $[Na^+]$, $[K^+]$, nor $[Cl^-]$ is depressed, magnesium deficiency, Bartter or Gitelman syndromes, or active diuretic use should be considered. Gitelman syndrome is distinguished from Bartter syndrome by the presence of hypocalciuria and, on occasion, hypomagnesemia in Gitelman syndrome.

METABOLIC ALKALOSIS DUE TO EXOGENOUS BICARBONATE LOADS

ALKALI ADMINISTRATION

Administration of base to individuals with normal kidney function rarely causes alkalosis, because the kidney has a high capacity for HCO_3^- excretion. Nevertheless, in patients with coexistent hemodynamic disturbances, alkalosis may develop, because either the normal capacity to excrete HCO_3^- has been exceeded, or there is enhanced reabsorption of HCO_3^-. Examples include patients receiving oral or intravenous HCO_3^-, acetate loads (parenteral hyperalimentation solutions), citrate loads (transfusions, continuous renal replacement therapy, or infant formula), or antacids plus cation-exchange resins (aluminum hydroxide and sodium polystyrene sulfonate).

In patients with acute kidney injury or advanced chronic kidney disease, overt alkalosis can develop after alkali administration, because the capacity to excrete HCO_3^- is exceeded or coexistent hemodynamic disturbances have caused enhanced HCO_3^- reabsorption. In this regard, baking soda use should be suspected in CKD patients, especially when baking soda is used as a home remedy for dyspepsia. The use of tube feedings in elderly patients in long-term

Box 14.1   Causes of Metabolic Alkalosis

Exogenous HCO₃⁻ Loads

Acute alkali administration
Milk-alkali syndrome
Use of NaOH in "freebasing" of crack cocaine or street cocaine "cut" with baking soda
Baking soda pica in pregnancy
Bicarbonate precursors (citrate, acetate) in chronic or acute kidney disease
Skilled nursing home patients on nasogastric tube feeding

Effective ECV Contraction, Normotension, K⁺ Deficiency, and Secondary Hyperreninemic Hyperaldosteronism

Gastrointestinal origin

Vomiting
Gastric aspiration
Congenital chloridorrhea
Villous adenoma
Combined administration of sodium polystyrene sulfonate (Kayexalate) and aluminum hydroxide
Cystic fibrosis and volume depletion
Gastrocystoplasty
Chronic laxative abuse
Cl⁻ deficient infant formula

Renal origin

Diuretics (remote use of thiazides and loop diuretics)
Edematous states
Posthypercapnic state
Hypercalcemia–hypoparathyroidism
Recovery from lactic acidosis or ketoacidosis
Nonreabsorbable anions (e.g., penicillin, carbenicillin)
Mg²⁺ deficiency
K⁺ depletion
Bartter syndrome
Gitelman syndrome
Carbohydrate refeeding after starvation
Pendred syndrome (during thiazide diuretic use or intercurrent illness)

ECV Expansion, Hypertension, K⁺ Deficiency, and Hypermineralocorticoidism

Associated with high renin

Renal artery stenosis
Accelerated hypertension
Renin-secreting tumor
Estrogen therapy

Associated with low renin

Primary aldosteronism
  Adenoma
  Hyperplasia
  Carcinoma
  Glucocorticoid suppressible
Adrenal enzymatic defects
  11β-Hydroxylase deficiency
  17α-Hydroxylase deficiency
Cushing syndrome or disease
  Ectopic corticotropin
  Adrenal carcinoma
  Adrenal adenoma
  Primary pituitary

Other

Licorice
Carbenoxolone
Chewing tobacco (containing glycyrrhizinic acid)
Lydia Pinkham tablets

Gain-of-Function Mutation of ENaC with ECV Expansion, Hypertension, K⁺ Deficiency, and Hyporeninemic Hypoaldosteronism

Liddle syndrome

ECV, Extracellular fluid volume; *ENaC*, epithelial sodium channel.

Table 14.1   Diagnosis of Metabolic Alkalosis

Low Urinary [Cl⁻] (<10 mEq/L)	High or Normal Urinary [Cl⁻] (>15-20 mEq/L)
Normotensive	**Hypertensive**
Vomiting, nasogastric	Primary aldosteronism
Aspiration	Cushing syndrome
Diuretics	Renal artery stenosis
Posthypercapnia	Renal failure plus alkali therapy
Bicarbonate treatment of organic acidosis	
K⁺ deficiency	**Normotensive or Hypotensive**
	Mg²⁺ deficiency
Hypertensive	Severe K⁺ deficiency
Liddle syndrome	Bartter syndrome
	Gitelman syndrome
	Diuretics

care facilities has been associated with metabolic alkalosis, because tube feeding preparations in the elderly are a common and underappreciated source of alkali loads. Plasma electrolytes should be monitored more frequently in these patients. Other examples of acute metabolic alkalosis resulting from alkali ingestion include the association of a pica for baking soda in pregnancy. Additionally, the use of crack cocaine has been described as a cause of severe alkalosis in patients undergoing hemodialysis, as "freebasing" involves the addition of alkali (NaOH as drain cleaner) to cocaine hydrochloride.

MILK-ALKALI SYNDROME

A long-standing history of excessive ingestion of milk and antacids, termed milk-alkali syndrome, is an historically important cause of metabolic alkalosis. However, because ingestion of calcium carbonate and vitamin D has become common for the treatment of osteoporosis, there has been a resurgence of milk-alkali syndrome since the 1990s. The majority of patients with this form of milk-alkali syndrome are asymptomatic women with incidental hypercalcemia, previously unappreciated CKD, and hypophosphatemia. Older women on diuretics and ACE inhibitors appear to be at higher risk. Both hypercalcemia and vitamin D excess increase renal HCO_3^- reabsorption. A critical component of this syndrome is reduced GFR. Patients with this disorder are prone to developing nephrocalcinosis, kidney function impairment, and metabolic alkalosis. Discontinuation of alkali ingestion is usually sufficient to correct the alkalosis, but the kidney disease may be irreversible if nephrocalcinosis is advanced.

CITRATE-BASED CONTINUOUS RENAL REPLACEMENT THERAPY

If citrate is used for regional anticoagulation in continuous renal replacement therapy, metabolic alkalosis can be expected. The metabolism of citrate by the liver and skeletal muscle results in a net gain of HCO_3^-. Strategies have been advanced to reduce the complications of regional trisodium citrate anticoagulation (hypocalcemia, metabolic alkalosis, use of 0.1 N HCl, and subsequent hyponatremia) by using anticoagulant citrate dextrose formula A.

METABOLIC ALKALOSIS ASSOCIATED WITH EXTRACELLULAR FLUID VOLUME CONTRACTION, K+ DEPLETION, AND SECONDARY HYPERRENINEMIC HYPERALDOSTERONISM

GASTROINTESTINAL ORIGIN

Gastrointestinal loss of H^+, Cl^-, Na^+, and K^+ from vomitus or gastric aspiration results in retention of HCO_3^-. The loss of fluid and electrolytes results in contraction of the ECV and stimulation of the renin-angiotensin system. Volume contraction causes a reduction in GFR and an enhanced capacity of the renal tubule to reabsorb HCO_3^-. Excess angiotensin II stimulates Na^+/H^+ exchange in the proximal tubule. During active vomiting, there is continued addition of HCO_3^- to plasma in exchange for Cl^-, and the plasma $[HCO_3^-]$ exceeds the reabsorptive capacity of the proximal tubule. Aldosterone and endothelin also stimulate the proton-transporting adenosine triphosphatase (H^+-ATPase) in the distal nephron, resulting in enhanced capacity for distal nephron HCO_3^- absorption and, paradoxically, aciduria. When the excess $NaHCO_3$ reaches the distal tubule, potassium secretion is enhanced by aldosterone and the delivery of the poorly reabsorbed anion, HCO_3^-. Thus the predominant cause of the hypokalemia is renal loss of K^+, and not gastrointestinal potassium wasting.

Hypokalemia has selective effects on renal bicarbonate absorption and ammonium production that are counterproductive to metabolic alkalosis. Hypokalemia dramatically increases the activity of the proton pump (H^+,K^+-ATPase)

in the cortical collecting tubule for reabsorbing K^+, but this occurs at the expense of both enhanced net acid excretion and HCO_3^- absorption. Hypokalemia also increases ammonium production independently of acid-base status, which, in the face of enhanced H^+ secretion, results in increased ammonium production and excretion; this in turn adds new bicarbonate to the systemic circulation (increase in net acid excretion). Therefore, hypokalemia plays an important role in the seemingly maladaptive response of the kidney to maintain the alkalosis. Because of contraction of the ECV and hypochloremia, Cl^- is avidly conserved by the kidney. This can be recognized clinically by a low urinary chloride concentration (see Table 14.1). Correction of the contracted ECV with isotonic NaCl and repletion of the K^+ deficit correct the acid-base disorder.

CONGENITAL CHLORIDORRHEA

Congenital chloridorrhea, a rare autosomal-recessive disorder, causes metabolic alkalosis by an extrarenal mechanism of severe diarrhea, fecal acid loss, and HCO_3^- retention. The disease is the result of mutations in the *SLC26A3* gene that disrupt the ileal and colonic Cl^-/HCO_3^- anion exchange mechanism so that Cl^- cannot be reabsorbed. The parallel Na^+/H^+ ion exchanger remains functional, allowing Na^+ to be reabsorbed and H^+ to be secreted. Therefore, the stool has high concentrations of H^+ and Cl^-, causing Na^+ and HCO_3^- retention in the extracellular fluid. The alkalosis is sustained by concomitant ECV contraction, hyperaldosteronism, and K^+ deficiency. Delivery of Cl^- to the distal nephron is low because of volume contraction. As in cystic fibrosis, this low delivery of HCO_3^- results in impaired HCO_3^- secretion by the β-intercalated cell. Therapy consists of oral supplementation of sodium and potassium chloride. Recently, the use of proton pump inhibitors has been advanced as a means of reducing chloride secretion by the parietal cells and thus reducing the diarrhea. The long-term outcome is good with daily supplementation of NaCl and KCl.

VILLOUS ADENOMA

Metabolic alkalosis has been described in cases of villous adenoma. K^+ depletion probably induces the alkalosis, because colonic secretion is alkaline.

RENAL ORIGIN

The generation of metabolic alkalosis through renal mechanisms involves three processes for increasing distal nephron H^+ secretion and enhancing net acid excretion (ammonium) excretion: (1) high delivery of Na^+ salts to the distal nephron, (2) excessive elaboration of mineralocorticoids, and (3) K^+ deficiency (Fig. 14.1).

DIURETICS

Drugs that induce distal delivery of sodium salts, such as thiazides and loop diuretics (furosemide, bumetanide, torsemide, and ethacrynic acid), diminish ECV without altering total body bicarbonate content. Consequently, the serum $[HCO_3^-]$ increases. The chronic administration of diuretics generates a metabolic alkalosis by increasing distal salt delivery, such that the secretion of K^+ and H^+ by the collecting

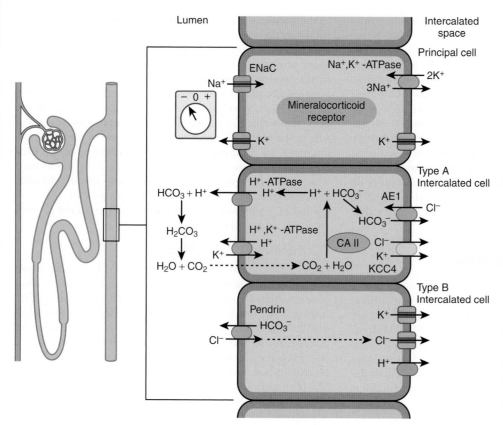

Figure 14.1 Contribution of distal nephron to maintenance of metabolic alkalosis. Extracellular volume depletion maintains metabolic alkalosis by increasing the activity of the epithelial sodium channel in principal cells (*top cell*, labeled ENaC) through enhanced elaboration of mineralocorticoid (secondary hyperaldosteronism); which further aggravates potassium wasting by increasing the negative transepithelial potential. Similarly, secondary hyperaldosteronism enhances H^+ secretion in Type A intercalated cells that inappropriately enhance absorption of HCO_3^- rather than its excretion. Correction of metabolic alkalosis with volume depletion requires correction of ECF and potassium deficits. When accomplished, the kidney can excrete HCO_3^- efficiently.

tubule is stimulated. The alkalosis is maintained by persistence of contraction of the ECV, secondary hyperaldosteronism, K^+ deficiency, and activation of the H^+,K^+-ATPase, as long as diuretic administration continues. The hypokalemia also enhances ammonium production and excretion. Repair of the alkalosis is achieved by withholding the diuretic, providing isotonic saline to correct the ECV deficit, and repleting the potassium deficit.

BARTTER SYNDROME

Both classic Bartter syndrome and the antenatal type are inherited as autosomal-recessive disorders that impair salt absorption in the thick ascending limb (TAL) of the loop of Henle; this results in salt wasting, volume depletion, and activation of the renin-angiotensin system. These manifestations are the result of loss-of-function mutations of one of the genes that encode three transporters involved in NaCl absorption in the TAL. The most prevalent disorder is a mutation of the gene *NKCC2*, which encodes the Na^+-K^+-$2Cl^-$ cotransporter on the apical membrane. A second mutation has been discovered in the gene *KCNJ1*, which encodes the ATP-sensitive apical K^+ conductance channel (ROMK) that operates in parallel with the Na^+-K^+-$2Cl^-$ cotransporter to recycle K^+. Both defects can be associated with antenatal Bartter syndrome or with classic Bartter syndrome. A mutation of the *CLCNKb* gene encoding the voltage-gated basolateral chloride channel (ClC-Kb) is associated only with classic Bartter syndrome, is milder, and is rarely associated with nephrocalcinosis. All three defects have the same net effect: loss of Cl^- transport in the TAL.

Antenatal Bartter syndrome has been observed in consanguineous families in association with sensorineural deafness, a syndrome linked to chromosome 1p31. The responsible gene, *BSND*, encodes a subunit, barttin, that colocalizes with the ClC-Kb channel in the TAL and K^+-secreting epithelial cells in the inner ear. Barttin appears to be necessary for the function of the voltage-gated chloride channel. Expression of ClC-Kb is lost when coexpressed with mutant barttins. Therefore, mutations in *BSND* define a fourth category of patients with Bartter syndrome.

Such defects predictably lead to ECV contraction, hyperreninemic hyperaldosteronism, and increased delivery of Na^+ to the distal nephron, with consequent alkalosis, renal K^+ wasting, and hypokalemia. Secondary overproduction of prostaglandins, juxtaglomerular apparatus hypertrophy, and vascular pressor unresponsiveness ensue. Most patients have hypercalciuria and normal serum magnesium levels, distinguishing this disorder from Gitelman syndrome.

Bartter syndrome is inherited as an autosomal-recessive defect. Most patients are homozygotes or compound heterozygotes for different mutations in one of these four genes, whereas a few patients with the clinical syndrome have no discernible mutation in any of these genes. Plausible explanations include unrecognized mutations in other genes, a dominant-negative effect of a heterozygous mutation, or other mechanisms. Recently, two groups of investigators reported features of Bartter syndrome in patients with autosomal-dominant hypocalcemia and activating mutations in calcium-sensing receptor, CaSR. Activation of CaSR on the basolateral cell surface of the TAL inhibits the function of ROMK; therefore, mutations in CaSR may represent a fifth gene associated with Bartter syndrome.

For diagnosis, Bartter syndrome must be distinguished from surreptitious vomiting, diuretic administration, and laxative abuse. The finding of a low urinary Cl⁻ concentration is helpful in identifying the vomiting patient (see Table 14.1). The urinary Cl⁻ concentration in a patient with Bartter syndrome would be expected to be normal or increased, rather than depressed.

The therapy for Bartter syndrome focuses on repair of the hypokalemia through inhibition of the renin-angiotensin-aldosterone system or the prostaglandin-kinin system, using propranolol, amiloride, spironolactone, prostaglandin inhibitors, and angiotensin-converting enzyme inhibitors, as well as direct repletion of the deficits with potassium and magnesium.

GITELMAN SYNDROME

Patients with Gitelman syndrome resemble the Bartter syndrome phenotype in that an autosomal-recessive metabolic alkalosis is associated with hypokalemia, a normal-to-low blood pressure, volume depletion with secondary hyperreninemic hyperaldosteronism, and juxtaglomerular hyperplasia. However, the consistent presence of hypocalciuria and the frequent presence of hypomagnesemia are useful in distinguishing Gitelman syndrome from Bartter syndrome on clinical grounds. These unique features mimic the effects of chronic thiazide diuretic administration. A large number of missense mutations in the gene SLC12A3, which encodes the thiazide-sensitive sodium chloride cotransporter in the distal convoluted tubule (NCCT), has been described and accounts for the clinical features, including the classic finding of hypocalciuria. However, it is not clear why these patients have pronounced hypomagnesemia. A study demonstrated that peripheral blood mononuclear cells from patients with Gitelman syndrome express mutated NCCT messenger RNA (mRNA). In a large consanguineous Bedouin family, missense mutations were noted in CLCNKb, but the clinical features overlapped between Gitelman and Bartter syndromes.

Compared to Bartter syndrome, Gitelman syndrome becomes symptomatic later in life and is associated with milder salt wasting. A large study of adults with proven Gitelman syndrome and NCCT mutations showed that salt craving, nocturia, cramps, and fatigue were more common than in sex-matched and age-matched controls. Women experience exacerbation of symptoms during menses, and they may experience complicated pregnancies.

Treatment of Gitelman syndrome consists of a diet high in potassium and potassium salts, typically with the addition of magnesium supplementation. Amiloride is often more helpful than spironolactone or eplerenone, with dose escalation to as much as 10 mg twice daily. Amiloride may be used in combination with spironolactone or eplerenone. Importantly, almost all patients with Gitelman syndrome exhibit some degree of salt craving, some of which may be extreme. To the extent possible, dietary salt should be limited and foods high in salt avoided, because salt loading increases distal delivery of NaCl and greatly amplifies K⁺ secretion by the cortical collecting tubule, a segment not involved in the loss of function mutation of NCCT in the distal tubule. Careful questioning of dietary practices is necessary to expose unusual salt appetites. The author has cared for one patient, for example, who admitted to drinking the liquid from dill pickle jars. Angiotensin-converting enzyme inhibitors have been suggested in selected patients for which frank hypotension is not a complication.

PENDRED SYNDROME

Pendred syndrome consists of sensorineural deafness and goiter caused by impaired iodide uptake, and it is ascribed to a defect in pendrin (encoded by SLC26A4). Pendrin is expressed on the apical membrane of type B intercalated cells of the collecting tubule. Although these patients typically do not have acid-base disorders, two recent reports of severe metabolic alkalosis with hypokalemia (one was a patient prescribed a thiazide diuretic, and another case occurred with alcoholism and severe vomiting after a cochlear implant) suggest that these patients are susceptible because of the inability of type B intercalated cells to secrete bicarbonate. These reports also underscore the importance of bicarbonate secretion during alkalotic challenges. Diuretics should not be prescribed to patients with Pendred syndrome, and clinicians should be aware that protracted vomiting can lead to severe metabolic alkalosis.

NONREABSORBABLE ANIONS AND MAGNESIUM DEFICIENCY

Administration of large quantities of nonreabsorbable anions, such as penicillin or carbenicillin, can enhance distal acidification and K⁺ secretion by increasing the negative transepithelial potential difference. Mg^{2+} deficiency frequently accompanies hypokalemia, and both electrolyte abnormalities must be corrected to ameliorate the metabolic alkalosis.

POTASSIUM DEPLETION

Pure K⁺ depletion causes metabolic alkalosis, although usually of only modest severity. Hypokalemia independently enhances renal ammoniagenesis, which increases net acid excretion and, thereby, the return of "new" bicarbonate to the systemic circulation. When access to salt and K⁺ is restricted, more severe alkalosis develops. Activation of the renal H^+,K^+-ATPase in the collecting duct by chronic hypokalemia probably plays a major role in maintenance of the alkalosis. Specifically, chronic hypokalemia has been shown to increase markedly the abundance of the colonic H^+,K^+-ATPase mRNA and protein in the outer medullary collecting duct. Alkalosis associated with severe K⁺ depletion is resistant to salt administration, with repair of the K⁺ deficiency necessary to correct the alkalosis.

AFTER TREATMENT OF LACTIC ACIDOSIS OR KETOACIDOSIS

When an underlying stimulus for the generation of lactic acid or keto acid is removed rapidly, as with the repair of circulatory insufficiency or administration of insulin therapy, the lactate or ketones are metabolized to yield an equivalent amount of HCO_3^-. Other sources of new HCO_3^- are additive to the original alkali generated by organic anion metabolism to create a surfeit of HCO_3^-. Such sources include new HCO_3^- added to the blood by the kidneys as a result of enhanced acid excretion during the preexisting period of acidosis, and alkali administered during the treatment phase of the acidosis. Acidosis-induced contraction of the ECV and K^+ deficiency act to sustain the alkalosis.

POSTHYPERCAPNIA

Prolonged CO_2 retention with chronic respiratory acidosis enhances renal HCO_3^- absorption and the generation of new HCO_3^- (increased net acid excretion). If the partial pressure of carbon dioxide in arterial blood ($PaCO_2$) is returned to normal by mechanical ventilation or other means, metabolic alkalosis results from the persistently elevated [HCO_3^-]. Associated ECV contraction does not allow complete repair of the alkalosis by correction of the $PaCO_2$ alone, and alkalosis persists until isotonic saline is infused.

METABOLIC ALKALOSIS ASSOCIATED WITH EXTRACELLULAR FLUID VOLUME EXPANSION, HYPERTENSION, AND HYPERALDOSTERONISM

Mineralocorticoid administration or excess production (as a result of primary aldosteronism of Cushing syndrome or adrenal cortical enzyme defects) increases net acid excretion and may result in metabolic alkalosis, which may be worsened by associated K^+ deficiency. ECV expansion from salt retention causes hypertension and antagonizes the reduction in GFR or increases tubule acidification induced by aldosterone and by K^+ deficiency. The kaliuresis worsens K^+ depletion, resulting in a urinary concentrating defect, polyuria, and polydipsia. Increased aldosterone levels may be the result of autonomous primary adrenal overproduction or secondary aldosterone release caused by renal overproduction of renin. In both situations, the normal feedback of ECV on net aldosterone production is disrupted, and hypertension from volume retention can result (see Table 9-2).

LIDDLE SYNDROME

Liddle syndrome is associated with severe hypertension presenting in childhood, accompanied by hypokalemic metabolic alkalosis. These features resemble those of primary hyperaldosteronism, but the renin and aldosterone levels are suppressed (pseudohyperaldosteronism). Liddle originally described patients with low renin and low aldosterone levels that did not respond to spironolactone. The defect is inherited as an autosomal-dominant form of monogenic hypertension, and is attributed to an abnormality in the gene that encodes the β or the γ subunit of the renal epithelial Na^+ channel (ENaC) at the apical membrane of principal cells in the cortical collecting duct. This defect leads to constitutive activation of this channel. Either mutation results in deletion of the cytoplasmic tail (C-terminus) of the affected subunit. The C-termini contain a PY amino acid motif that is highly conserved, and essentially all mutations in Liddle syndrome patients involve disruption or deletion of this motif. Such PY motifs are important in regulating the number of sodium channels in the luminal membrane by binding to the WW domains of the Nedd4-like family of ubiquitin protein ligases. Disruption of the PY motif dramatically increases the surface localization of the ENaC complex by failing to internalize or degrade (Nedd4 pathway)

the channels from the cell surface. Ultimately, persistent Na^+ absorption results in volume expansion, hypertension, hypokalemia, and metabolic alkalosis.

GLUCOCORTICOID-REMEDIABLE HYPERALDOSTERONISM

Glucocorticoid-remediable hyperaldosteronism is an autosomal-dominant form of hypertension, the features of which resemble primary aldosteronism (hypokalemic metabolic alkalosis and volume-dependent hypertension). However, in this disorder glucocorticoid administration corrects the hypertension as well as the excessive excretion of 18-hydroxysteroid in the urine. This disorder results from an unequal crossover between two genes located in close proximity on chromosome 8. This results in the glucocorticoid-responsive promoter region of the gene encoding the 11-β-hydroxylase (*CYP11B1*) attaching to the structural portion of the *CYP11B2* gene encoding aldosterone synthase. The chimeric gene produces excess amounts of aldosterone synthase unresponsive to serum potassium or renin levels, but suppressed by glucocorticoid administration. Although this syndrome is a rare cause of primary aldosteronism, it is important to diagnose, because treatment differs and the syndrome can be associated with severe hypertension and stroke, especially during pregnancy.

CUSHING DISEASE AND CUSHING SYNDROME

Abnormally high glucocorticoid production as a result of adrenal adenoma, carcinoma, or ectopic corticotropin production causes metabolic alkalosis. The alkalosis may be ascribed to coexisting mineralocorticoid (deoxycorticosterone and corticosterone) hypersecretion. Alternatively, glucocorticoids may have the capability of enhancing net acid secretion and NH_4^+ production, which may be caused by cross-reactivity with the mineralocorticoid receptors.

MISCELLANEOUS CONDITIONS

Ingestion of licorice or licorice-containing chewing tobacco can cause a typical pattern of mineralocorticoid excess. The glycyrrhizinic acid contained in genuine licorice inhibits 11β-hydroxysteroid dehydrogenase. This enzyme is responsible for converting cortisol to cortisone, an essential step in protecting the mineralocorticoid receptor from cortisol. When the enzyme is inactivated, cortisol can occupy type I renal mineralocorticoid receptors, mimicking aldosterone. Genetic apparent mineralocorticoid excess (AME) resembles excessive ingestion of licorice, with volume expansion, low renin and aldosterone levels, and a salt-sensitive form of hypertension that may include metabolic alkalosis and hypokalemia. The hypertension responds to thiazides and spironolactone, but without abnormal steroid products in the urine. In genetic AME, 11β-hydroxysteroid dehydrogenase is defective, and monogenic hypertension develops.

SYMPTOMS OF METABOLIC ALKALOSIS

Patients with metabolic alkalosis experience changes in central and peripheral nervous system function similar to those of hypocalcemia. Symptoms may include mental confusion, obtundation, and a predisposition to seizures, paresthesia, muscular cramping, tetany, aggravation of arrhythmias, and hypoxemia in chronic obstructive pulmonary disease. Related electrolyte abnormalities include hypokalemia and hypophosphatemia.

TREATMENT OF METABOLIC ALKALOSIS

The maintenance of metabolic alkalosis represents a failure of the kidney to excrete bicarbonate efficiently because of chloride or potassium deficiency, continuous mineralocorticoid elaboration, or both. Treatment depends on the cause of the metabolic alkalosis, and it is primarily directed at correcting the underlying stimulus for HCO_3^- generation and restoring the ability of the kidney to excrete the excess HCO_3^-. Assistance is gained in the diagnosis and treatment of metabolic alkalosis from the urinary chloride, arterial blood pressure, and volume status of the patient (particularly the presence or absence of orthostasis; see Box 14.1). Helpful in the history is the presence or absence of vomiting, diuretic use, or alkali therapy.

A high urine chloride level and hypertension suggest that primary mineralocorticoid excess is present. If primary aldosteronism is diagnosed, correction of the underlying cause (adenoma, bilateral hyperplasia, Cushing syndrome) will reverse the alkalosis. Patients with bilateral adrenal hyperplasia may respond to spironolactone. Normotensive patients with a high urine chloride level may have Bartter or Gitelman syndrome if diuretic use or vomiting can be excluded. A low urine chloride level and relative hypotension suggest a chloride-responsive metabolic alkalosis such as vomiting or nasogastric suction. Loss of $[H^+]$ by the stomach or kidneys can be mitigated by the use of proton pump inhibitors or the discontinuation of diuretics. The second aspect of treatment is to remove the factors that sustain HCO_3^- reabsorption, such as ECV contraction or K^+ deficiency. Although K^+ deficits should be repleted, NaCl therapy is usually sufficient to reverse the alkalosis if ECV contraction is present, as indicated by a low urine $[Cl^-]$.

Patients with congestive heart failure or unexplained volume expansion represent special challenges in the critical care setting. Patients with a low urine chloride concentration, usually indicative of a "chloride-responsive" form of metabolic alkalosis, may not tolerate normal saline infusion. Renal HCO_3^- loss can be accelerated by administration of the carbonic anhydrase inhibitor acetazolamide (250 mg intravenously) if associated conditions preclude infusion of saline (i.e., elevated pulmonary capillary wedge pressure or evidence of congestive heart failure). Acetazolamide is usually effective in patients with adequate kidney function, but can exacerbate urinary K^+ losses and can cause hypokalemia. Dilute hydrochloric acid (0.1 N HCl) infused into a central vein is also effective, but it can cause hemolysis and may be difficult to titrate. If it is used, the goal should be to restore the pH not to normal, but to a level of approximately 7.50. Alternatively, acidification can also be achieved with oral NH_4Cl, which should be avoided in the presence

of liver disease. Patients receiving continuous renal replacement therapy in the intensive care unit may develop metabolic alkalosis with high-bicarbonate dialysate or if citrate regional anticoagulation is used. Therapy should include reduction of alkali loads via dialysis by reducing the bicarbonate concentration in the dialysate, or, if citrate is being used, by postfiltration infusion of 0.1 N HCl.

BIBLIOGRAPHY

Birkenhager R, Otto E, Schurmann MJ, et al: Mutation of BSND causes bartter syndrome with sensorineural deafness and kidney failure, *Nat Genet* 29:310-314, 2001.

Conn JW, Rovner DR, Cohen EL: Licorice-induced pseudoaldosteronism: hypertension, hypokalemia, aldosteronopenia, and suppressed plasma renin activity, *JAMA* 205:492, 1968.

Cruz DN, Shaer AJ, Bia MJ, et al: Gitelman's syndrome revisited: an evaluation of symptoms and health-related quality of life, *Kidney Int* 59:717-719, 2001.

Diskin CJ, Stokes TJ, Dansby LM, et al: Recurrent metabolic alkalosis and elevated troponins after crack cocaine use in a hemodialysis patient, *Clin Exp Nephrol* 10:156-158, 2006.

DuBose TD Jr: Disorders of acid-base balance. In Brenner BM, editor: *Brenner and Rector's The Kidney*, ed 8. Philadelphia, 2010, Saunders, pp 505-546.

Felsenfeld AJ, Levine BS: Milk alkali syndrome and the dynamics of calcium homeostasis, *Clin J Am Soc Nephrol* 1:641-654, 2006.

Fitzgibbons LJ, Snoey ER: Severe metabolic alkalosis due to baking soda ingestion: case reports of two patients with unsuspected antacid overdose, *J Emerg Med* 17(1):57-61, 1999.

Galla JH: Metabolic alkalosis. In DuBose TD, Hamm L, editors: *Acid-base and electrolyte disorders: a companion to Brenner and Rector's the kidney*, Philadelphia, 2002, Saunders, pp 109-128.

Grotegut CA, Dandolu V, Katari S, et al: Baking soda pica: a case of hypokalemic metabolic alkalosis and rhabdomyolysis in pregnancy, *Obstet Gynecol* 107:484-486, 2006.

Hebert SC, Gullans SR: The molecular basis of inherited hypokalemic alkalosis: bartter's and gitelman's syndromes, *Am J Physiol* 271:F957-F959, 1996.

Hernandez R, Schambelan M, Cogan MG, et al: Dietary NaCl determines severity of potassium depletion-induced metabolic alkalosis, *Kidney Int* 31:1356, 1987.

Hihnala S, Kujala M, Toppari J, et al: Expression of SLC26A3, CFTR and NHE3 in the human male reproductive tract: role in male subfertility caused by congenital chloride diarrhea, *Mol Hum Reprod* 12:107-111, 2006.

Jamison RL, Ross JC, Kempson RL, et al: Surreptitious diuretic ingestion and pseudo-Bartter's syndrome, *Am J Med* 73:142, 1982.

Kamynina E, Staub O: Concerted action of ENaC, Nedd4-2, and Sgk1 in transepithelial Na+ transport, *Am J Physiol Renal Physiol* 283:F377, 2002.

Lifton RP, Dluhy RG, Powers M, et al: Hereditary hypertension caused by chimaeric gene duplications and ectopic expression of aldosterone synthase, *Nat Genet* 2:66-74, 1992.

Morgera S, Haase M, Ruckert M, et al: Regional citrate anticoagulation in continuous hemodialysis: acid-base and electrolyte balance at an increased dose of dialysis, *Nephron Clin Pract* 101(4):c211-c219, 2005.

Sanei-Moghaddam A, Wilson T, Kumar S, et al: An unfortunate case of pendred syndrome, *J Laryngol Otol* 125(9):965-967, 2011 Sep.

Schroeder ET: Alkalosis resulting from combined administration of a "nonsystemic" antacid and a cation-exchange resin, *Gastroenterology* 56:1969, 1969.

Shimkets RA, Warnock DG, Bositis CM, et al: Liddle's syndrome: heritable human hypertension caused by mutations in the beta subunit of the epithelial sodium channel, *Cell* 79:407, 1994.

Yi JH, Han SW, Song JS, et al: Metabolic alkalosis from unsuspected ingestion: use of urine pH and anion gap, *Am J Kidney Dis*, 2012.

Zelikovic I, Szargel R, Hawash A, et al: A novel mutation in the chloride channel gene, CLCNKB, as a cause of gitelman and bartter syndromes, *Kidney Int* 63:24-32, 2003.

15 Respiratory Acidosis and Alkalosis

Nicolaos E. Madias | Horacio J. Adrogué

RESPIRATORY ACIDOSIS

Respiratory acidosis, or primary hypercapnia, is the acid-base disturbance initiated by an increase in carbon dioxide tension of body fluids and in whole-body CO_2 stores. Hypercapnia acidifies body fluids and elicits an adaptive increment in the plasma bicarbonate concentration ($[HCO_3^-]$) that should be viewed as an integral part of the respiratory acidosis. Arterial CO_2 tension (PCO_2), measured at rest and at sea level, is greater than 45 mm Hg in simple respiratory acidosis. Lower values of PCO_2 might still signify the presence of primary hypercapnia in the setting of mixed acid-base disorders (e.g., eucapnia, rather than the expected hypocapnia, in the presence of metabolic acidosis). Another special case of respiratory acidosis is the presence of arterial eucapnia, or even hypocapnia, in association with venous hypercapnia in patients who have an acute severe reduction in cardiac output but relative preservation of respiratory function (i.e., pseudorespiratory alkalosis).

PATHOPHYSIOLOGY

The ventilatory system is responsible for maintaining PCO_2 within normal limits by adjusting minute ventilation ($\dot{V}_E$) to match the rate of CO_2 production. $\dot{V}_E$ consists of two components: ventilation distributed in the gas-exchange units of the lungs (alveolar ventilation, $\dot{V}_A$) and ventilation wasted in dead space ($\dot{V}_D$). Hypercapnia can result from increased CO_2 production, decreased $\dot{V}_A$, or both. Decreased $\dot{V}_A$ can result from a reduction in $\dot{V}_E$, an increase in $\dot{V}_D$, or a combination of the two. The main elements of the ventilatory system are the respiratory pump, which generates a pressure gradient responsible for airflow, and the loads that oppose such action. The respiratory pump comprises the cerebrum, brainstem, spinal cord, phrenic and intercostal nerves, and the muscles of respiration. The respiratory loads include the ventilatory requirement (CO_2 production, O_2 consumption), airway resistance, lung elastic recoil, and chest-wall/abdominal resistance. Most frequently, primary hypercapnia develops from an imbalance between the strength of the respiratory pump and the weight of the respiratory loads, thereby resulting in decreased $\dot{V}_A$. Impairment of the pump can occur because of depressed central drive, abnormal neuromuscular transmission, or muscle dysfunction. Causes of augmented respiratory loads include ventilation/perfusion mismatch (increased $\dot{V}_D$), augmented airway flow resistance, lung/pleural/chest-wall stiffness, and increased ventilatory demand. An increased $\dot{V}_D$ occurs in many clinical conditions, including emphysema, cystic fibrosis, asthma, and other intrinsic lung diseases, as well as chest-wall disorders. A less frequent cause of primary hypercapnia is failure of CO_2 transport caused by decreases in pulmonary perfusion, a condition that occurs in cardiac arrest, circulatory collapse, and pulmonary embolism (thrombus, fat, air).

Overproduction of CO_2 is usually matched by increased excretion, so that hypercapnia is prevented. However, patients with marked limitation in pulmonary reserve and those receiving constant mechanical ventilation might experience respiratory acidosis due to increased CO_2 production caused by increased muscle activity (agitation, myoclonus, shivering, seizures), sepsis, fever, or hyperthyroidism. Increments in CO_2 production might also be imposed by the administration of large carbohydrate loads (>2000 kcal/day) to nutritionally bereft, critically ill patients or during the decomposition of bicarbonate infused in the course of treating metabolic acidosis.

The major threat to life from CO_2 retention in patients who are breathing room air is the associated obligatory hypoxemia. When the arterial oxygen tension (PO_2) falls to less than 40 to 50 mm Hg, harmful effects can occur, especially if the fall is rapid. In the absence of supplemental oxygen, patients in respiratory arrest develop critical hypoxemia within a few minutes, long before extreme hypercapnia ensues. Because of the constraints of the alveolar gas equation, it is not possible for PCO_2 to reach values much higher than 80 mm Hg while the level of PO_2 is still compatible with life. Extreme hypercapnia can be seen only during oxygen administration, and, in fact, it is often the result of uncontrolled oxygen therapy.

SECONDARY PHYSIOLOGIC RESPONSE

An immediate rise in plasma $[HCO_3^-]$ owing to titration of nonbicarbonate body buffers occurs in response to acute hypercapnia. This adaptation is complete within 5 to 10 minutes after the increase in PCO_2. On average, plasma $[HCO_3^-]$ increases by about 0.1 mEq/L for each 1 mm Hg acute increment in PCO_2; as a result, the plasma hydrogen ion concentration ($[H^+]$) increases by about 0.75 nEq/L for each 1 mm Hg acute increment in PCO_2. Therefore, the overall limit of adaptation of plasma $[HCO_3^-]$ in acute respiratory acidosis is quite small; even when PCO_2 increases to levels of 80 to 90 mm Hg, the increment in plasma $[HCO_3^-]$ does not exceed 3 to 4 mEq/L. Moderate hypoxemia does not alter the adaptive response to acute respiratory acidosis. On the other hand, preexisting hypobicarbonatemia (from metabolic acidosis or chronic respiratory alkalosis) enhances the magnitude of the bicarbonate response to acute hypercapnia, whereas this response is diminished in hyperbicarbonatemic states (from metabolic alkalosis or chronic respiratory acidosis). Other electrolyte changes observed in acute respiratory acidosis include mild increases in plasma sodium (1 to 4 mEq/L), potassium (0.1 mEq/L for each 0.1 unit decrease in pH), and phosphorus, as well as small decreases in plasma chloride and lactate concentrations (the latter effect originating from inhibition of the activity of 6-phosphofructokinase and, consequently, glycolysis by intracellular acidosis). A small reduction in the plasma anion gap is also observed, reflecting the decline in plasma lactate and the acidic titration of plasma proteins. Acute respiratory acidosis induces glucose intolerance and insulin resistance that are not prevented by adrenergic blockade. These changes are likely mediated by the direct effects of the low tissue pH on skeletal muscle.

The adaptive increase in plasma $[HCO_3^-]$ observed in the acute phase of hypercapnia is amplified markedly during chronic hypercapnia as a result of the generation of new bicarbonate by the kidneys. Both proximal and distal acidification mechanisms contribute to this adaptation, which requires 3 to 5 days for completion. The renal response to chronic hypercapnia includes chloruresis and the generation of hypochloremia. On average, plasma $[HCO_3^-]$ increases by about 0.35 mEq/L for each 1 mm Hg chronic increment in PCO_2; as a result, the plasma $[H^+]$ increases by about 0.3 nEq/L for each 1 mm Hg chronic increase in PCO_2. More recently, a substantially steeper slope for the change in plasma $[HCO_3^-]$ was reported (0.51 mEq/L for each 1 mm Hg chronic increase in PCO_2), but the small number of blood gas measurements, one for each of 18 patients, calls into question the validity of this conclusion. Empiric observations indicate a limit of adaptation of plasma $[HCO_3^-]$ on the order of 45 mEq/L.

The renal response to chronic hypercapnia is not altered appreciably by dietary sodium or chloride restriction, moderate potassium depletion, alkali loading, or moderate hypoxemia. To what extent chronic kidney disease of variable severity limits the renal response to chronic hypercapnia is currently unknown. Obviously, patients with end-stage kidney disease cannot mount a renal response to chronic hypercapnia, so they are more subject to severe acidemia. The degree of acidemia is more pronounced in patients who are receiving hemodialysis rather than peritoneal dialysis, because the former treatment maintains, on average, a lower plasma level $[HCO_3^-]$. Recovery from chronic hypercapnia is crippled by a chloride-deficient diet. In this circumstance, despite correction of the level of PCO_2, plasma $[HCO_3^-]$ remains elevated as long as the state of chloride deprivation persists, thus creating the entity of "posthypercapnic metabolic alkalosis." Chronic hypercapnia is not associated with appreciable changes in the anion gap or in plasma concentrations of sodium, potassium, or phosphorus.

ETIOLOGY

Respiratory acidosis can develop in patients who have normal or abnormal airways and lungs. Tables 15.1 and 15.2 present, respectively, causes of acute and chronic respiratory acidosis. This classification accounts for the usual mode of onset and duration of the various causes, and it emphasizes the biphasic time course that characterizes the secondary physiologic response to hypercapnia. Primary hypercapnia can result from disease or malfunction within any element of the regulatory system that controls respiration, including the central and peripheral nervous system, respiratory muscles, thoracic cage, pleural space, airways, and lung parenchyma. Not infrequently, more than one cause contributes to the development of respiratory acidosis in a given patient. Chronic obstructive pulmonary disease (COPD) is the most common cause of chronic hypercapnia, a condition that includes emphysema, chronic bronchitis, and small-airway disease.

CLINICAL MANIFESTATIONS

Because hypercapnia almost always occurs with some degree of hypoxemia, it is often difficult to determine whether a specific manifestation is the consequence of the elevated PCO_2 or the reduced PO_2. Clinical manifestations of respiratory acidosis arising from the central nervous system are collectively known as hypercapnic encephalopathy and include irritability, inability to concentrate, headache, anorexia, mental cloudiness, apathy, confusion, incoherence, combativeness, hallucinations, delirium, and transient psychosis. Progressive narcosis or coma might develop in patients receiving oxygen therapy, especially those with an acute exacerbation of chronic respiratory insufficiency in whom PCO_2 levels of ≤100 mm Hg or even higher can occur. In addition, frank papilledema (pseudotumor cerebri) and motor disturbances, including myoclonic jerks, flapping tremor identical to that observed in liver failure, sustained myoclonus, and seizures may develop. Focal neurologic signs (e.g., muscle paresis, abnormal reflexes) might be observed. The neurologic symptom burden depends on the magnitude of hypercapnia, the rapidity with which it develops, the severity of acidemia, and the degree of accompanying hypoxemia. Severe hypercapnia often is misdiagnosed as a cerebral vascular accident or an intracranial tumor.

The hemodynamic consequences of respiratory acidosis include a direct depressing effect on myocardial contractility. An associated sympathetic surge, sometimes intense, leads to increases in plasma catecholamines; however, during severe acidemia (blood pH lower than about 7.20), receptor responsiveness to catecholamines is markedly blunted. Hypercapnia results in systemic vasodilatation via a direct action on vascular smooth muscle; this effect is most obvious in the cerebral circulation, where blood flow increases in direct relation to the level of PCO_2. By contrast, CO_2 retention can produce vasoconstriction in the pulmonary circulation as well as in the kidneys; in the latter case, the hemodynamic response may be mediated via an enhanced sympathetic activity. Mild to moderate hypercapnia is usually associated with an increased cardiac output, normal or increased blood pressure, warm skin, a bounding pulse, and diaphoresis. However, if hypercapnia is severe or considerable hypoxemia is present, decreases in both cardiac output and blood pressure may be observed. Concomitant therapy with vasoactive medications (e.g., β-adrenergic receptor blockers) or the presence of congestive heart failure may further impair the hemodynamic response. Cardiac arrhythmias, particularly supraventricular tachyarrhythmias not associated with major hemodynamic compromise, are common, especially in patients receiving digitalis. They do not result primarily from the hypercapnia, but rather reflect

Table 15.1   Causes of Acute Respiratory Acidosis

Normal Airways and Lungs	Abnormal Airways and Lungs
Central Nervous System Depression General anesthesia Sedative overdosage Head trauma Cerebrovascular accident Central sleep apnea Cerebral edema Brain tumor Encephalitis	**Upper Airway Obstruction** Coma-induced hypopharyngeal obstruction Aspiration of foreign body or vomitus Laryngospasm or angioedema Obstructive sleep apnea Inadequate laryngeal intubation Laryngeal obstruction postintubation
Neuromuscular Impairment High spinal-cord injury Guillain-Barré syndrome Status epilepticus Botulism, tetanus Crisis in myasthenia gravis Hypokalemic myopathy Familial hypokalemic periodic paralysis	**Lower Airway Obstruction** Generalized bronchospasm Severe asthma (status—asthmaticus) Bronchiolitis of infancy and adults Disorders involving pulmonary alveoli Severe bilateral pneumonia Acute respiratory distress syndrome Severe pulmonary edema
Ventilatory Restriction Rib fractures with flail chest Pneumothorax Hemothorax Impaired diaphragmatic function (e.g., peritoneal dialysis, ascites)	**Pulmonary Perfusion Defect** Cardiac arrest* Severe circulatory failure* Massive pulmonary thromboembolism Fat or air embolus
Iatrogenic Events Misplacement or displacement of airway cannula during anesthesia or mechanical ventilation Bronchoscopy-associated hypoventilation or respiratory arrest Increased CO_2 production with constant mechanical ventilation (e.g., due to high-carbohydrate diet or sorbent-regenerative hemodialysis)	

From Madias NE, Adrogué HJ: Respiratory alkalosis and acidosis. In Seldin DW, Giebisch G, editors: The kidney: physiology and pathophysiology. *Philadelphia, 2000, Lippincott Williams & Wilkins, pp 2131-2166.*
*May produce "pseudorespiratory alkalosis."

Table 15.2   Causes of Chronic Respiratory Acidosis

Normal Airways and Lungs	Abnormal Airways and Lungs
Central Nervous System Depression Sedative overdosage Methadone/heroin addiction Primary alveolar hypoventilation (Ondine's curse) Obesity-hypoventilation syndrome (Pickwickian syndrome) Brain tumor Bulbar poliomyelitis	**Upper Airway Obstruction** Tonsillar and peritonsillar hypertrophy Paralysis of vocal cords Tumor of the cords or larynx Airway stenosis after prolonged intubation Thymoma, aortic aneurysm
Neuromuscular Impairment Poliomyelitis Multiple sclerosis Muscular dystrophy Amyotrophic lateral sclerosis Diaphragmatic paralysis Myxedema Myopathic disease	**Lower Airway Obstruction** Chronic obstructive lung disease (bronchitis, bronchiolitis, bronchiectasis, emphysema)
	Disorders Involving Pulmonary Alveoli Severe chronic pneumonitis Diffuse infiltrative disease (e.g., alveolar proteinosis) Interstitial fibrosis
Ventilatory Restriction Kyphoscoliosis, spinal arthritis Obesity Fibrothorax Hydrothorax Impaired diaphragmatic function	

From Madias NE, Adrogué HJ: Respiratory alkalosis and acidosis. In Seldin DW, Giebisch G, editors: The kidney: physiology and pathophysiology. *Philadelphia, 2000, Lippincott Williams & Wilkins, pp 2131-2166.*

the associated hypoxemia and sympathetic discharge, concomitant medications, other electrolyte abnormalities, and underlying cardiac disease. Retention of salt and water is commonly observed in sustained hypercapnia, especially in the presence of cor pulmonale. In addition to the effects of heart failure on the kidney, multiple other factors may be involved, including the prevailing stimulation of the sympathetic nervous system and the renin-angiotensin-aldosterone axis, increased renal vascular resistance, and elevated levels of antidiuretic hormone and cortisol.

DIAGNOSIS

Whenever hypoventilation is suspected, arterial blood gases should be obtained. Alternatively, venous blood gases can be used to assess acid-base status and obtain information about tissue oxygenation. If the acid-base profile of the patient reveals hypercapnia in association with acidemia, at least an element of respiratory acidosis must be present. However, hypercapnia can be associated with a normal or an alkaline pH because of the simultaneous presence of additional acid-base disorders (see Chapter 12). Information from the patient's history, physical examination, and ancillary laboratory data should be used for an accurate assessment of the acid-base status.

THERAPEUTIC PRINCIPLES

Treatment of acute respiratory acidosis should focus on three critical steps: (1) ensuring a patent airway, (2) restoring adequate oxygenation by delivering an oxygen-rich inspired mixture, and (3) securing adequate ventilation to repair the abnormal blood gas composition. Indications for endotracheal intubation/mechanical ventilation include protection of the airway, relief of respiratory distress, improvement of pulmonary gas exchange, assistance with airway and lung healing, and application of appropriate sedation and neuromuscular blockade. As noted, acute respiratory acidosis poses its major threat to survival, not because of hypercapnia or acidemia, but because of the associated hypoxemia. The goal of oxygen therapy is to maintain a PO_2 of at least 60 mm Hg and oxygen saturation of $\geq 90\%$; yet, a PO_2 of 50 to 55 mm Hg might help prevent respiratory depression in patients with hypercapnia and chronic hypoxemia. Supplemental oxygen can be administered to the spontaneously breathing patient with nasal cannulas, Venturi masks, or nonrebreathing masks. Oxygen flow rates ≤ 5 L/min can be used with nasal cannulas, each increment of 1 L/min increasing the FiO_2 by approximately 4%. Venturi masks, calibrated to deliver FiO_2 between 24% and 50%, are most useful in patients with COPD as they allow the PO_2 to be titrated, thus minimizing the risk of CO_2 retention.

If the target PO_2 is not achieved with these measures, and the patient is conscious, cooperative, hemodynamically stable and able to protect the lower airway, a method of noninvasive ventilation through a mask can be used (e.g., bilevel positive airway pressure [BiPAP]). With BiPAP, the inspiratory-pressure support decreases the patient's work of breathing, and the expiratory-pressure support improves gas exchange by preventing alveolar collapse.

Endotracheal intubation with mechanical ventilatory support should be initiated if adequate oxygenation cannot be secured by noninvasive measures, if progressive hypercapnia or obtundation develops, or if the patient is unable to cough and clear secretions. Large tidal volumes during mechanical ventilation often lead to alveolar overdistention, which results in hypotension and barotrauma, two life-threatening complications. To overcome these complications, prescription of tidal volumes of 6 mL/kg body weight (instead of the conventional level of 12 mL/kg body weight) to achieve plateau airway pressures of <30 cm H_2O, has been proposed. Because an increase in PCO_2 develops (but rarely exceeds 80 mm Hg), this approach is termed *permissive hypercapnia* or *controlled mechanical hypoventilation*. If the resultant hypercapnia reduces the blood pH to less than 7.20, many physicians would prescribe bicarbonate; however, this strategy is controversial, and others would intervene only for pH values on the order of 7.00. Several studies indicate that permissive hypercapnia affords improved clinical outcomes. Heavy sedation and neuromuscular blockade are frequently needed with this therapy. After discontinuation of neuromuscular blockade, some patients develop prolonged weakness or paralysis. Contraindications to permissive hypercapnia include cerebrovascular disease, brain edema, increased intracranial pressure, and convulsions; depressed cardiac function and arrhythmias; and severe pulmonary hypertension. Notably, most of these entities can develop as adverse effects of permissive hypercapnia itself, especially if it is associated with substantial acidemia.

The presence of a concurrent *metabolic* acidosis is the primary indication for alkali therapy in patients with acute respiratory acidosis. Administration of sodium bicarbonate to a spontaneously breathing patient with simple respiratory acidosis is not only of questionable efficacy but also involves considerable risk. Concerns include pH-mediated depression of ventilation, enhanced CO_2 production because of bicarbonate decomposition, and volume expansion; however, alkali therapy may have a role in patients with severe bronchospasm by restoring the responsiveness of the bronchial musculature to β-adrenergic agonists. Successful management of intractable asthma in patients with blood pH lower than 7.00 by administering sufficient sodium bicarbonate to raise blood pH to greater than 7.20 has been reported.

Patients with chronic respiratory acidosis frequently develop episodes of acute decompensation that can be serious or life threatening. Common culprits include pulmonary infections, use of narcotics, and uncontrolled oxygen therapy. In contrast to acute hypercapnia, injudicious use of oxygen therapy in patients with chronic respiratory acidosis can produce further reductions in alveolar ventilation. Respiratory decompensation superimposes an acute element of CO_2 retention and acidemia on the chronic baseline. Only rarely can one remove the underlying cause of chronic respiratory acidosis, but maximizing alveolar ventilation with relatively simple maneuvers is often successful in the management of respiratory decompensation. Such maneuvers include treatment with antibiotics, bronchodilators, or diuretics; avoidance of irritant inhalants, tranquilizers, and sedatives; elimination of retained secretions; and gradual reduction of supplemental oxygen, aiming at a PO_2 of about 50 to 55 mm Hg. Administration of adequate quantities of chloride (usually as the potassium salt) prevents or corrects a complicating element of metabolic alkalosis (commonly diuretic-induced) that can further dampen the ventilatory drive. Acetazolamide may be used as an adjunctive measure, but care must be taken to avoid potassium depletion. Potassium and phosphate depletion should be corrected, as they can contribute to the development or maintenance of respiratory failure by impairing the function of skeletal muscles. Restoration of the P_{CO_2} of the patient to near its chronic baseline should proceed gradually, over a period of many hours to a few days. Overly rapid reduction in P_{CO_2} in such patients risks the development of sudden, posthypercapnic alkalemia with potentially serious consequences, including reduction in cardiac output and cerebral blood flow, cardiac arrhythmias (including predisposition to digitalis intoxication), and generalized seizures. In the absence of a complicating element of metabolic acidosis, and with the possible exception of the severely acidemic patient with intense generalized bronchoconstriction who is undergoing mechanical ventilation, there is no role for alkali administration in chronic respiratory acidosis.

RESPIRATORY ALKALOSIS

Respiratory alkalosis, or primary hypocapnia, is the acid-base disturbance initiated by a reduction in carbon dioxide tension of body fluids. Hypocapnia alkalinizes body fluids and elicits an adaptive decrement in plasma $[HCO_3^-]$ that should be viewed as an integral part of the respiratory alkalosis. The level of P_{CO_2} measured at rest and at sea level is lower than 35 mm Hg in simple respiratory alkalosis. Higher values of P_{CO_2} may still indicate the presence of an element of primary hypocapnia in the setting of mixed acid-base disorders (e.g., eucapnia, rather than the anticipated hypercapnia, in the presence of metabolic alkalosis).

PATHOPHYSIOLOGY

Primary hypocapnia most commonly reflects pulmonary hyperventilation caused by increased ventilatory drive. The latter results from signals arising from the lung, from the peripheral (carotid and aortic) or brainstem chemoreceptors, or from influences originating in other centers of the brain. Hypoxemia is a major stimulus of alveolar ventilation, but P_{O_2} values lower than 60 mm Hg are required to elicit this effect consistently. Additional mechanisms for the generation of primary hypocapnia include maladjusted mechanical ventilators, the extrapulmonary elimination of CO_2 by a dialysis device or extracorporeal circulation (e.g., heart-lung machine), and decreased CO_2 production (e.g., sedation, skeletal muscle paralysis, hypothermia, hypothyroidism) in patients receiving constant mechanical ventilation.

A condition termed *pseudorespiratory alkalosis* occurs in patients who have profound depression of cardiac function and pulmonary perfusion but have relative preservation of alveolar ventilation, including patients with advanced circulatory failure and those undergoing cardiopulmonary resuscitation. In such patients, venous (and tissue) hypercapnia is present because of the severely reduced pulmonary blood flow that limits the amount of CO_2 delivered to the lungs for excretion. On the other hand, arterial blood reveals hypocapnia because of the increased ventilation-to-perfusion ratio, which causes a larger than normal removal of CO_2 per unit of blood traversing the pulmonary circulation. However, absolute CO_2 excretion is decreased, and the body CO_2 balance is positive. Therefore, respiratory acidosis, rather than respiratory alkalosis, is present. Such patients may have severe venous acidemia (often resulting from mixed respiratory and metabolic acidosis) accompanied by an arterial pH that ranges from mild acidemia to frank alkalemia. In addition, arterial blood may show normoxia or hyperoxia, despite the presence of severe hypoxemia in venous blood. Therefore, both arterial and mixed (or central) venous blood sampling is needed to assess the acid-base status and oxygenation of patients with critical hemodynamic compromise.

SECONDARY PHYSIOLOGIC RESPONSE

Adaptation to acute hypocapnia is characterized by an immediate drop in plasma $[HCO_3^-]$, principally as a result of titration of nonbicarbonate body buffers. This adaptation is completed within 5 to 10 minutes after the onset of hypocapnia. Plasma $[HCO_3^-]$ declines, on average, by approximately 0.2 mEq/L for each 1 mm Hg acute decrement in P_{CO_2}; consequently, the plasma $[H^+]$ decreases by about 0.75 nEq/L for each 1 mm Hg acute reduction in P_{CO_2}. The limit of this adaptation of plasma $[HCO_3^-]$ is on the order of 17 to 18 mEq/L. Concomitant small increases in plasma chloride, lactate, and other unmeasured anions balance the decline in plasma $[HCO_3^-]$; each of these components accounts for about one third of the bicarbonate decrement. Small decreases in plasma sodium (1 to 3 mEq/L) and potassium (0.2 mEq/L for each 0.1 unit increase in pH) may be observed. Severe hypophosphatemia can occur in acute hypocapnia because of the translocation of phosphorus into the cells.

A larger decrement in plasma $[HCO_3^-]$ occurs in chronic hypocapnia as a result of renal adaptation to the disorder, which involves suppression of both proximal and distal acidification mechanisms. Completion of this adaptation requires 2 to 3 days. Plasma $[HCO_3^-]$ decreases, on average, by about 0.4 mEq/L for each 1 mm Hg chronic decrement in P_{CO_2}; as a consequence, plasma $[H^+]$ decreases by approximately 0.4 nEq/L for each 1 mm Hg chronic reduction in P_{CO_2}. The limit of this adaptation of plasma $[HCO_3^-]$ is on the order of 12 to 15 mEq/L. About two thirds of the decline in plasma $[HCO_3^-]$ is balanced by an increase in plasma chloride concentration, and the remainder reflects an increase in plasma unmeasured anions; part of the remainder results from the alkaline titration of plasma proteins, but most remains undefined. Plasma lactate does not increase in chronic hypocapnia, even in the presence of moderate hypoxemia. Similarly, no appreciable change in the plasma concentration of sodium occurs. In sharp contrast with acute hypocapnia, the plasma concentration of phosphorus remains essentially unchanged in chronic hypocapnia. Although plasma potassium is in the normal range in patients with chronic hypocapnia at sea level, hypokalemia and renal potassium wasting have been described in subjects in whom sustained hypocapnia was induced by exposure to high altitude. Patients with end-stage kidney disease are obviously at risk for development of severe alkalemia in response to chronic hypocapnia, because they cannot mount a renal response. This risk is higher in patients receiving peritoneal dialysis rather than hemodialysis, because the former treatment maintains, on average, a higher plasma level $[HCO_3^-]$.

ETIOLOGY

Primary hypocapnia is the most frequent acid-base disturbance encountered; it occurs in normal pregnancy and with high-altitude residence. Box 15.1 lists the major causes of respiratory alkalosis. Most are associated with the abrupt appearance of hypocapnia, but in many instances the process is sufficiently prolonged to permit full chronic adaptation. Consequently, no attempt has been made to separate these conditions into acute and chronic categories. Some of the major causes of respiratory alkalosis are benign, whereas others are life threatening. Primary hypocapnia is particularly common among the critically ill, occurring either as the simple disorder or as a component of mixed disturbances. Its presence constitutes an ominous prognostic sign, with mortality increasing in direct proportion to the severity of the hypocapnia.

CLINICAL MANIFESTATIONS

Rapid decrements in P_{CO_2} to half the normal values or lower are typically accompanied by paresthesias of the extremities, chest discomfort (especially in patients manifesting increased airway resistance), circumoral numbness, lightheadedness, confusion, and, rarely, tetany or generalized seizures. These manifestations are seldom present in the chronic phase. Acute hypocapnia decreases cerebral blood flow, which in severe cases may reach values <50% of normal, resulting in cerebral hypoxia. This hypoperfusion has been implicated in the pathogenesis of the neurologic manifestations of acute respiratory alkalosis along with other factors, including hypocapnia per se, alkalemia, pH-induced shift of the oxyhemoglobin dissociation curve, and decrements in the levels of ionized calcium and potassium. Some evidence indicates that cerebral blood flow returns to normal in chronic respiratory alkalosis.

Patients who are actively hyperventilating manifest no appreciable changes in cardiac output or systemic blood pressure. By contrast, acute hypocapnia in the course of passive hyperventilation, as typically observed during mechanical ventilation in patients with a depressed central nervous system or receiving general anesthesia, frequently results in a major reduction in cardiac output and systemic blood pressure, increased peripheral resistance, and substantial hyperlactatemia. This discrepant response probably reflects the decline in venous return caused by mechanical ventilation in passive hyperventilation versus the reflex tachycardia consistently observed in active hyperventilation. Although acute

---

Box 15.1   Causes of Respiratory Alkalosis

Hypoxemia or Tissue Hypoxia

Decreased inspired O_2 tension
High altitude
Bacterial or viral pneumonia
Aspiration of food, foreign body,
or vomitus
Laryngospasm
Drowning
Cyanotic heart disease
Severe anemia
Left shift deviation of the HbO_2 curve
Hypotension*
Severe circulatory failure*
Pulmonary edema

Stimulation of Chest Receptors

Pneumonia
Asthma
Pneumothorax
Hemothorax
Flail chest
Acute respiratory distress syndrome
Cardiac failure
Noncardiogenic pulmonary edema
Pulmonary embolism
Interstitial lung disease

Central Nervous System Stimulation

Voluntary
Pain
Anxiety

Psychosis
Fever
Subarachnoid hemorrhage
Cerebrovascular accident
Meningoencephalitis
Tumor
Trauma

Drugs or Hormones

Nikethamide, ethamivan
Doxapram
Xanthines
Salicylates
Catecholamines
Angiotensin II
Vasopressor agents
Progesterone
Medroxyprogesterone
Dinitrophenol
Nicotine

Miscellaneous

Pregnancy
Sepsis
Hepatic failure
Mechanical hyperventilation
Acetate hemodialysis
Heart-lung machine
Extracorporeal membrane oxygenation (ECMO)
Heat exposure
Recovery from metabolic acidosis

From Madias NE, Adrogué HJ: Respiratory alkalosis and acidosis. In Seldin DW, Giebisch G, editors: The kidney: physiology and pathophysiology. Philadelphia, 2000, Lippincott Williams & Wilkins, pp 2131-2166.
HbO_2, Oxyhemoglobin.
*May produce "pseudorespiratory alkalosis."

hypocapnia does not lead to cardiac arrhythmias in normal volunteers, it appears that it contributes to the generation of both atrial and ventricular tachyarrhythmias in patients with ischemic heart disease. Chest pain and ischemic ST-T wave changes have been observed in acutely hyperventilating subjects with or without coronary artery disease. Coronary vasospasm and Prinzmetal angina can be precipitated by acute hypocapnia in susceptible subjects. The pathogenesis of these manifestations has been attributed to the same factors that are incriminated in the neurologic manifestations of acute hypocapnia.

DIAGNOSIS

Careful observation can detect abnormal patterns of breathing in some patients, yet marked hypocapnia may be present without a clinically evident increase in respiratory effort. Therefore, an arterial blood gas analysis should be obtained whenever hyperventilation is suspected. In fact, the diagnosis of respiratory alkalosis, especially the chronic form, is frequently missed; physicians often misinterpret the electrolyte pattern of hyperchloremic hypobicarbonatemia as indicative of a normal anion gap metabolic acidosis. If the acid-base profile of the patient reveals hypocapnia in association with alkalemia, at least an element of respiratory alkalosis must be present; however, primary hypocapnia may be associated with a normal or an acidic pH as a result of the concomitant presence of other acid-base disorders. Notably, mild degrees of chronic hypocapnia commonly leave blood pH within the high-normal range. As always, proper evaluation of the acid-base status of the patient requires careful assessment of the history, physical examination, and ancillary laboratory data (see Chapter 12). After the diagnosis of respiratory alkalosis has been made, a search for its cause should ensue. The diagnosis of respiratory alkalosis can have important clinical implications, often providing a clue to the presence of an unrecognized, serious disorder (e.g., sepsis) or indicating the severity of a known underlying disease.

THERAPEUTIC PRINCIPLES

Management of respiratory alkalosis must be directed whenever possible toward correction of the underlying cause. Respiratory alkalosis resulting from severe hypoxemia requires oxygen therapy. The widely held view that hypocapnia, even if severe, poses little risk to health is inaccurate. In fact, transient or permanent damage to the brain, heart, and lungs can result from substantial hypocapnia. In addition, rapid correction of severe hypocapnia can lead to reperfusion injury in the brain and lung. Therefore, severe hypocapnia in hospitalized patients must be prevented whenever possible, and, if it is present, a slow correction is most appropriate.

Rebreathing into a closed system (e.g., a paper bag) may prove helpful for the patient with the anxiety-hyperventilation syndrome because it interrupts the vicious cycle that can result from the reinforcing effects of the symptoms of hypocapnia. Administration of 250 to 500 mg acetazolamide can be beneficial in the management of signs and symptoms of high-altitude sickness, a syndrome characterized by hypoxemia and respiratory alkalosis. Considering the risks of severe alkalemia, sedation or, in rare cases, skeletal muscle paralysis and mechanical ventilation may be required temporarily to correct marked respiratory alkalosis. Management of pseudorespiratory alkalosis must be directed at optimizing systemic hemodynamics.

BIBLIOGRAPHY

Adrogué HJ, Chap Z, Okuda Y, et al: Acidosis-induced glucose intolerance is not prevented by adrenergic blockade, *Am J Physiol* 255:E812-E823, 1988.

Adrogué HJ, Galla JH, Madias NE, editors: *Acid-base disorders and their treatment*, 2005, Taylor & Francis Group, pp 597-639.

Adrogué HJ, Madias NE: Management of life-threatening acid-base disorders, *N Engl J Med* 338:26-34, 1998.

Adrogué HJ, Madias NE: Respiratory acidosis, respiratory alkalosis, and mixed disorders. In Floege J, Johnson RJ, Feehally J, editors: *Comprehensive clinical nephrology*, ed 4, St. Louis, 2010, Elsevier, pp 176-189.

Adrogué HJ, Madias NE: Secondary responses to altered acid-base status: the rules of engagement, *J Am Soc Nephrol* 21:920-923, 2010.

Adrogué HJ, Rashad MN, Gorin AB, et al: Assessing acid-base status in circulatory failure: differences between arterial and central venous blood, *N Engl J Med* 320:1312-1316, 1989.

Amato MB, Barbas CSV, Medeiros DM, et al: Effect of a protective-ventilation strategy on mortality in the acute respiratory distress syndrome, *N Engl J Med* 338:347-354, 1998.

Arbus GS, Hebert LA, Levesque PR, et al: Characterization and clinical application of the "significance band" for acute respiratory alkalosis, *N Engl J Med* 280:117-123, 1969.

Brackett NC Jr, Cohen JJ, Schwartz WB: Carbon dioxide titration curve of normal man: effect of increasing degrees of acute hypercapnia on acid-base equilibrium, *N Engl J Med* 272:6-12, 1965.

Brackett NC Jr, Wingo CF, Muren O, et al: Acid-base response to chronic hypercapnia in man, *N Engl J Med* 280:124-130, 1969.

Dries DJ: Permissive hypercapnia, *J Trauma* 39:984-989, 1995.

Epstein SK, Singh N: Respiratory acidosis, *Respir Care* 46:366-383, 2001.

Foster GT, Vaziri ND, Sassoon CSH: Respiratory alkalosis, *Respir Care* 46:384-391, 2001.

Grocott MPW, Martin DS, Levett DZH, et al: Arterial blood gases and oxygen content in climbers on mount everest, *N Engl J Med* 360:140-149, 2009.

Jardin F, Fellahi J, Beauchet A, et al: Improved prognosis of acute respiratory distress syndrome 15 years on, *Intensive Care Med* 25:936-941, 1999.

Kollef M: Respiratory failure. In Dale DC, Federman DD, editors: *ACP Medicine*, New York, 2006, WebMD, pp 2791-2804.

Krapf R, Beeler I, Hertner D, et al: Chronic respiratory alkalosis: the effect of sustained hyperventilation on renal regulation of acid-base equilibrium, *N Engl J Med* 324:1394-1401, 1991.

Laffey JG, Kavanagh BP: Hypocapnia. *N Engl J Med* 347:43-53, 2002.

Madias NE, Adrogué HJ: Respiratory acidosis and alkalosis. In Adrogué HJ, editor: *Contemporary management in critical care: acid-base and electrolyte disorders*, New York, 1991, Churchill Livingstone, pp 37-53.

Madias NE, Adrogué HJ: Respiratory alkalosis. In DuBose TD, Hamm LL, editors: *Acid-base and electrolyte disorders*, Philadelphia, 2002, WB Saunders, pp 147-164.

Madias NE, Adrogué HJ: Respiratory alkalosis and acidosis. In Seldin DW, Giebisch G, editors: *The kidney: physiology and pathophysiology*, Philadelphia, 2000, Lippincott Williams & Wilkins, pp 2131-2166.

Madias NE, Wolf CJ, Cohen JJ: Regulation of acid-base equilibrium in chronic hypercapnia, *Kidney Int* 27:538-543, 1985.

Malhotra A: Low-tidal-volume ventilation in the acute respiratory distress syndrome, *N Engl J Med* 357:1113-1120, 2007.

Martinu T, Menzies D, Dial S: Re-evaluation of acid-base prediction rules in patients with chronic respiratory acidosis, *Can Respir J* 10:311-315, 2003.

Tobin MJ: Advances in mechanical ventilation, *N Engl J Med* 344:1986-1996, 2001.

GLOMERULAR DISEASES

16 Glomerular Clinicopathologic Syndromes

J. Charles Jennette | Ronald J. Falk

Injury to glomeruli results in a multiplicity of signs and symptoms of disease, including proteinuria caused by altered permeability of capillary walls, hematuria caused by rupture of capillary walls, azotemia caused by impaired filtration of nitrogenous wastes, oliguria or anuria caused by reduced urine production, edema caused by salt and water retention, and hypertension caused by fluid retention and disturbed renal homeostasis of blood pressure. The nature and severity of disease in a given patient is dictated by the nature and severity of glomerular injury.

Glomerular syndromes include asymptomatic hematuria or proteinuria, nephrotic syndrome, nephritic (glomerulonephritic) syndrome, rapidly progressive glomerulonephritis, and syndromes with concurrent glomerular and extrarenal features, such as pulmonary-renal syndrome. Specific glomerular diseases tend to produce characteristic syndromes of kidney dysfunction (Table 16.1). The diagnosis of a glomerular disease requires recognition of one of these syndromes followed by collection of data to determine which specific glomerular disease is present. Alternatively, if reaching a specific diagnosis is not possible or not necessary, the physician should at least narrow the differential diagnosis to a likely candidate disease.

Evaluation of pathologic features identified in a kidney biopsy specimen is often required for a definitive diagnosis. Figure 16.1 shows the relative frequencies that major categories of glomerular disease are identified in kidney biopsy specimens. These frequencies are different from the overall prevalence of these diseases in patients with these syndromes, because some categories of disease have presentations that are more likely to prompt biopsy (e.g., rapidly progressive glomerulonephritis) than other diseases (e.g., steroid-responsive childhood nephrotic syndrome). Figure 16.2 depicts some of the clinical and pathologic features used to resolve the differential diagnosis in patients with antibody-mediated glomerulonephritis, Figures 16.3 through 16.6 illustrate the distinctive ultrastructural features of some of the major categories of glomerular disease, Figure 16.7 illustrates some of the major patterns of immune deposition identified by immunofluorescence microscopy, and Figure 16.8 illustrates pathologic variants of focal segmental glomerulosclerosis (FSGS).

ASYMPTOMATIC HEMATURIA AND RECURRENT GROSS HEMATURIA

Hematuria is usually defined as greater than three red blood cells per high-power field observed by microscopic examination in a centrifuged urine sediment (see Chapters 4 and 5).

Hematuria is asymptomatic when the patient is unaware of its presence and it is not accompanied by clinical manifestations of nephritis or nephrotic syndrome (i.e., without azotemia, oliguria, edema, or hypertension). Asymptomatic microscopic hematuria occurs in 5% to 10% of the general population. Gross hematuria is characterized by urine discoloration, which often is described as tea-colored or cola-colored. Recurrent gross hematuria may be superimposed on asymptomatic microscopic hematuria, or it may occur in isolation.

Most hematuria is not of glomerular origin. Glomerular diseases cause less than 10% of hematuria in patients who do not have proteinuria; almost 80% is caused by bladder, prostate, or urethral disease. Hypercalciuria and hyperuricosuria also can cause asymptomatic hematuria, especially in children.

Microscopic examination of the urine can help determine whether hematuria is of glomerular or nonglomerular origin. Chemical (e.g., osmotic) and physical damage to red blood cells as they pass through the nephron causes structural changes that are not present in red blood cells that have passed directly into the urine from a gross parenchymal injury in the kidney (e.g., a neoplasm or infection) or from a lesion in the urinary tract (e.g., renal pelvis traumatized by stones or an inflamed bladder). Dysmorphic red blood cells that have transited the urinary tract from the glomeruli usually have lost their biconcave configuration and hemoglobin, and they often have multiple membrane blebs, sometimes producing acanthocytes and "Mickey Mouse" cells. The presence of red blood cell casts and substantial proteinuria (greater than 2 g/24 h) also supports a glomerular origin for hematuria.

Published kidney biopsy series conducted in patients with asymptomatic hematuria show differences in the frequencies of identified underlying glomerular lesions. Differences in the nature of the population analyzed (e.g., military recruits vs. patients undergoing routine physical examination) and differences in pathologic analysis (e.g., failure of earlier studies to recognize thin basement membrane nephropathy) account for the observed disparities. The data presented in Table 16.2 are derived from patients with hematuria who underwent diagnostic kidney biopsy. The data in the first column equate with asymptomatic hematuria and are similar to findings in other published series. In these patients with hematuria, less than 1 g/24 h proteinuria, and serum creatinine less than 1.5 mg/dl, the three major biopsy findings were no pathologic abnormality (30%), thin basement membrane nephropathy (26%), and immunoglobulin A (IgA) nephropathy (28%). Whereas thin basement membrane nephropathy virtually

Table 16.1 Tendencies of Glomerular Diseases to Manifest Nephrotic and Nephritic Features*

Disease	Nephrotic Features	Nephritic Features
Minimal change glomerulopathy	++++	—
Membranous glomerulopathy	++++	+
Diabetic glomerulosclerosis	++++	+
Amyloidosis	++++	+
FSGS	+++	++
Fibrillary glomerulonephritis	+++	++
Mesangioproliferative glomerulopathy†	++	++
MPGN and dense deposit disease‡	++	+++
Proliferative glomerulonephritis†	++	+++
Acute postinfectious glomerulonephritis§	+	++++
Crescentic glomerulonephritisǁ	+	++++

FSGS, Focal segmental glomerulosclerosis; *MPGN*, membranoproliferative glomerulonephritis.

*Most diseases can manifest both nephrotic and nephritic features, but there is usually a tendency for one to predominate. Number of plus signs indicates strength of tendency.

†Mesangioproliferative and proliferative glomerulonephritis (focal or diffuse) are structural manifestations of a number of glomerulonephritides, including IgA nephropathy and lupus nephritis.

‡Both type I (mesangiocapillary) and type II (dense deposit disease).

§Often a structural manifestation of acute poststreptococcal glomerulonephritis.

ǁCan be immune complex mediated, antiglomerular basement membrane antibody mediated, or associated with antineutrophil cytoplasmic antibodies.

always manifests as asymptomatic hematuria or recurrent gross hematuria, IgA nephropathy can manifest as any of the glomerular disease syndromes, because it can cause a variety of glomerular lesions that result in different clinical manifestations (Fig. 16.9).

Alport syndrome is a hereditary disease caused by a defect in the genes that code for basement membrane type IV collagen (see Chapter 43). Approximately 85% of patients have a mutation in the X-chromosomal α5 gene and 15% in the autosomal α3 and α4 genes. In affected men, Alport syndrome initially manifests as asymptomatic microscopic hematuria, sometimes with superimposed episodes of gross hematuria. Although similar within a given kindred, the onset of symptoms varies from childhood to adulthood and typically begins with isolated hematuria. Progressively worsening proteinuria and end-stage renal disease (ESRD) may eventually develop, although the rate of progression is variable. Affected women, who are almost always heterozygous, often have intermittent microscopic hematuria but may have no other manifestations of kidney disease.

Kidney biopsy is not usually performed to evaluate asymptomatic hematuria as the diagnosis will seldom affect treatment in these patients; however, kidney biopsy may be of prognostic value. For example, thin basement membrane nephropathy has a better prognosis and a much greater propensity for familial occurrence than IgA nephropathy. Many patients with asymptomatic hematuria are subjected to repeated invasive

urologic evaluations until a definitive diagnosis can be determined. In these patients, additional urologic evaluation can be avoided if kidney biopsy provides a diagnosis.

In kidney biopsy specimens, thin basement membrane nephropathy is suspected if there is thinning of the glomerular basement membrane (GBM) lamina densa, whereas Alport syndrome is suspected if there is marked lamination of the lamina densa. However, in some patients, especially females with heterozygous X-linked disease, thin basement membrane lesions rather than laminations may be the ultrastructural manifestation of Alport syndrome. In Alport syndrome, the kidney and skin also have diagnostically useful abnormalities in immunohistologic staining for the alpha chains of type IV collagen. The presence of mesangial immune deposits with a dominance or codominance of immunohistologic staining for IgA is diagnostic for IgA nephropathy (see Fig. 16.7).

ACUTE GLOMERULONEPHRITIS AND RAPIDLY PROGRESSIVE GLOMERULONEPHRITIS

Patients with acute glomerulonephritis or rapidly progressive glomerulonephritis often present with acute onset of nephritis with azotemia, oliguria, edema, hypertension, proteinuria, and hematuria along with an "active" urine sediment that often contains red blood cell casts, pigmented casts, and cellular debris. Rapidly progressive glomerulonephritis is defined by a 50% or greater loss of kidney function within weeks to months. If kidney failure ensues, uremia may manifest with symptoms including nausea and vomiting, pruritus, lethargy, and encephalopathy along with signs including volume overload.

The pathologic processes that most often produce the clinical manifestations of acute or rapidly progressive glomerulonephritis are inflammatory glomerular lesions. Lupus glomerulonephritis and IgA nephropathy are the most common causes in children and young adults, whereas antineutrophil cytoplasmic antibody (ANCA) glomerulonephritis is the most common cause in older adults (see Fig. 16.1). The nature and severity of glomerular inflammation correlate with the clinical features of the glomerulonephritis (see Fig. 16.9). Note in Figure 16.9 that the structural stages of glomerular inflammation can change as time passes, and this is reflected by changes in the clinical manifestations of the glomerulonephritis.

The least severe structural injury that can be discerned by light microscopy is mesangial hyperplasia alone, which usually is associated with asymptomatic proteinuria or hematuria, or very mild nephritis. Proliferative glomerulonephritis, which may be focal (affecting less than 50% of glomeruli) or diffuse (affecting more than 50% of glomeruli), is characterized histologically not only by the proliferation of glomerular cells (e.g., mesangial cells, endothelial cells, epithelial cells) but also by the influx of leukocytes, especially neutrophils and mononuclear phagocytes. Necrosis may be present, especially in disease caused by ANCAs or antiglomerular basement membrane (anti-GBM) antibodies. Chronic changes such as glomerular sclerosis, interstitial fibrosis, and tubular atrophy begin to develop within 1 week after the onset of destructive glomerular inflammation and become the dominant features in chronic glomerulonephritis.

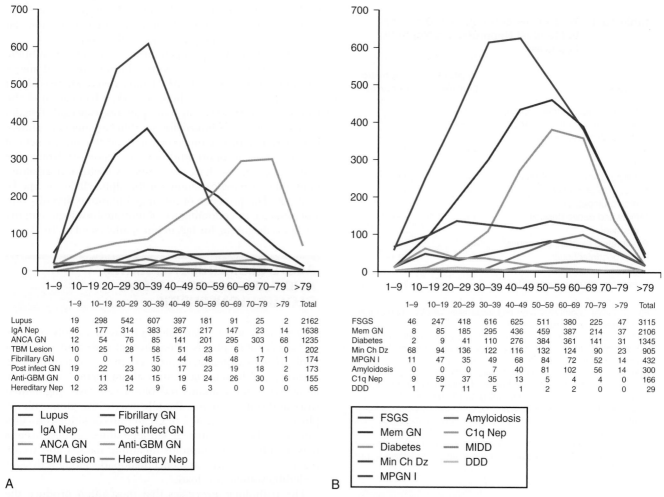

	1–9	10–19	20–29	30–39	40–49	50–59	60–69	70–79	>79	Total
Lupus	19	298	542	607	397	181	91	25	2	2162
IgA Nep	46	177	314	383	267	217	147	23	14	1638
ANCA GN	12	54	76	85	141	201	295	303	68	1235
TBM Lesion	10	25	28	58	51	23	6	1	0	202
Fibrillary GN	0	0	1	15	44	48	48	17	1	174
Post infect GN	19	22	23	30	17	23	19	18	2	173
Anti-GBM GN	0	11	24	15	19	24	26	30	6	155
Hereditary Nep	12	23	12	9	6	3	0	0	0	65

Legend A:
— Lupus   — Fibrillary GN
— IgA Nep   — Post infect GN
— ANCA GN   — Anti-GBM GN
— TBM Lesion   — Hereditary Nep

	1–9	10–19	20–29	30–39	40–49	50–59	60–69	70–79	>79	Total
FSGS	46	247	418	616	625	511	380	225	47	3115
Mem GN	8	85	185	295	436	459	387	214	37	2106
Diabetes	2	9	41	110	276	384	361	141	31	1345
Min Ch Dz	68	94	136	122	116	132	124	90	23	905
MPGN I	11	47	35	49	68	84	72	52	14	432
Amyloidosis	0	0	0	7	40	81	102	56	14	300
C1q Nep	9	59	37	35	13	5	4	4	0	166
DDD	1	7	11	5	1	2	2	0	0	29

Legend B:
— FSGS   — Amyloidosis
— Mem GN   — C1q Nep
— Diabetes   — MIDD
— Min Ch Dz   — DDD
— MPGN I

A   B

Figure 16.1   Frequencies of kidney biopsy diagnoses versus age from 1985-2007 in the UNC Nephropathology Laboratory. The diagnoses are separated into those that usually cause a glomerulonephritic presentation and those that usually cause the nephrotic syndrome. Approximately one third of the patients in this kidney biopsy population from UNC were African Americans, which influences the high frequency of lupus glomerulonephritis and FSGS. **A,** Causes of nephritis. **B,** Causes of nephrotic syndrome. *ANCA,* Antineutrophil cytoplasmic antibody; *DDD,* dense deposit disease; *FSGS,* focal segmental glomerulosclerosis; *GBM,* glomerular basement membrane; *GN,* glomerulonephritis; *IgA,* immunoglobulin A; *Mem,* membranous; *MIDD,* monoclonal immunoglobulin deposition disease; *Min Ch Dz,* minimal change glomerulopathy; *MPGN,* membranoproliferative glomerulonephritis; *Lupus,* systemic lupus erythematosus; *TBM,* thin basement membrane; *UNC,* University of North Carolina.

Lupus glomerulonephritis (Chapter 24) provides a paradigm of the interrelationships among pathogenic mechanisms, pathologic consequences, and clinical manifestations of immune complex glomerular disease (see Fig. 16.5). The mildest expressions of lupus nephritis (International Society of Nephrology/Renal Pathology Society [ISN/RPS] class I minimal mesangial and class II mesangioproliferative lupus glomerulonephritis) are induced by predominantly mesangial localization of immune complexes, which usually causes only mild nephritis or asymptomatic hematuria and proteinuria. Localization of substantial amounts of nephritogenic immune complexes in the subendothelial zones of glomerular capillaries, where they are adjacent to the inflammatory mediator systems in the blood, induces overt glomerular inflammation (focal or diffuse proliferative lupus glomerulonephritis, class III or IV lupus nephritis) and usually causes severe clinical manifestations of nephritis. Qualitative and quantitative characteristics of the pathogenic immune complexes that result in localization, predominantly in subepithelial zones where they are not

in contact with the inflammatory mediator systems in the blood, induce membranous lupus glomerulonephritis (class V lupus glomerulonephritis). This variant usually causes the nephrotic syndrome rather than nephritis. As the nephritogenic immune response in a given patient changes with time, sometimes modified by treatment, transitions may occur among the various lupus nephritis phenotypes.

The structurally most severe form of active glomerulonephritis is crescentic glomerulonephritis, which usually manifests clinically as rapidly progressive glomerulonephritis. In patients with new-onset kidney disease who have a nephritic sediment and serum creatinine greater than 3 mg/dl, glomerulonephritis with crescents is the most common finding in kidney biopsy specimens (see Table 16.2). Crescents are proliferations of cells within Bowman capsule that include both mononuclear phagocytes and glomerular epithelial cells. Crescent formation is a response to glomerular capillary rupture and therefore is a marker of severe glomerular injury. Crescents, however, do not indicate the cause of glomerular injury, because many different pathogenic

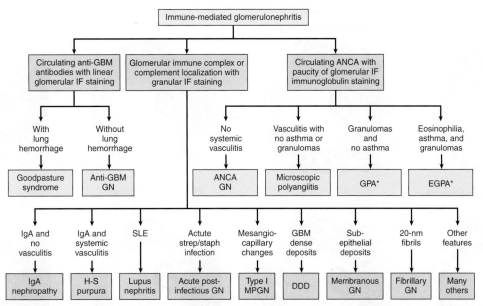

Figure 16.2 **Features that distinguish among different immunopathologic categories of antibody-mediated glomerulonephritis.** *ANCA,* Antineutrophil cytoplasmic antibody; *DDD,* dense deposit disease (which is a C3 glomerulopathy and not an immune complex disease); *EGPA,* eosinophilic granulomatosis with polyangiitis; *GBM,* glomerular basement membrane; *GN,* glomerulonephritis; *GPA,* granulomatosis with poly-angiitis; *IF,* immunofluorescence microscopy; *IgA,* immunoglobulin A; *MPGN,* membranoproliferative glomerulonephritis; *SLE,* systemic lupus erythematosus. *GPA and EGPA were previously known as Wegener granulomatosis and Churg-Strauss syndrome, respectively.

mechanisms can cause crescent formation. There is no consensus on how many glomeruli should have crescents to use the term *crescentic glomerulonephritis* in the diagnosis. Most pathologists use the term if more than 50% of glomeruli include crescents, but the percentage of glomeruli with crescents should be specified in the diagnosis even if it is less than 50% (e.g., IgA nephropathy with focal proliferative glomerulonephritis and 25% crescents). Within a specific pathogenic category of glomerulonephritis (e.g., anti-GBM disease, ANCA disease, lupus glomerulonephritis, IgA nephropathy, poststreptococcal glomerulonephritis), the higher the fraction of glomeruli with crescents, the worse the prognosis; however, among pathogenetically different forms of glomerulonephritis, the pathogenic category may be more important in predicting outcome than the presence of crescents. For example, a patient with poststreptococcal glomerulonephritis with 50% crescents has a much better prognosis for kidney survival, even without immunosuppressive treatment, than a patient with anti-GBM glomerulonephritis or ANCA glomerulonephritis with 25% crescents.

The importance of pathogenic category in predicting the natural history of glomerulonephritis indicates that the pathologic classification of glomerulonephritis by light microscopy into the morphologic categories, shown in Figure 16.9, is not adequate for optimal management. In addition to determining the morphologic severity of glomerular inflammation, the pathogenic or immunopathologic category of disease must be determined. If a kidney biopsy is performed, this is done by immunohistology and electron microscopy (see Figs. 16.2 through 16.7). Immunohistology shows the presence or absence of immunoglobulins and complement components. The distribution (e.g., capillary wall, mesangium), pattern (e.g., granular, linear), and composition (e.g., IgA-dominant, IgG-dominant, IgM-dominant, C3-dominant) of immunoglobulin and complement are

useful for determining specific types of glomerulonephritis; this is discussed in detail in later chapters that address specific types of glomerular disease. Glomerular C3 with little or no immunoglobulin is seen in C3 glomerulopathy, which includes dense deposit disease and C3 glomerulonephritis.

Table 16.3 shows the frequencies of the major pathologic categories of glomerulonephritis in patients with 50% or more crescents who have undergone kidney biopsy. The immune complex category comprises a variety of diseases, including lupus nephritis, IgA nephropathy, and postinfectious glomerulonephritis. Note that most patients with greater than 50% crescents have little or no immunohistologic evidence for immune complex or anti-GBM antibody localization within glomeruli; that is, they have pauci-immune glomerulonephritis. More than 90% of these patients with pauci-immune crescentic glomerulonephritis have circulating ANCAs. Therefore, ANCA glomerulonephritis is the most common form of crescentic glomerulonephritis, especially in older adults.

Because both the structural severity (such as the morphologic stages shown in Fig. 16.9) and the immunopathologic and ultrastructural category of disease (such as the categories presented in Figs. 16.2 through 16.7) are important for predicting the course of disease in a patient with glomerulonephritis, the most useful diagnostic terms should include information about both the morphologic appearance and pathogenic category of injury. Examples are "focal proliferative IgA nephropathy," "diffuse proliferative lupus glomerulonephritis," and "crescentic anti-GBM glomerulonephritis."

Many types of glomerulonephritis are immune-mediated inflammatory diseases and are treated with corticosteroids, cytotoxic drugs, or other antiinflammatory and immunosuppressive agents. The aggressiveness of the treatment, of course, should match the aggressiveness of the disease. For example, active class IV lupus nephritis warrants

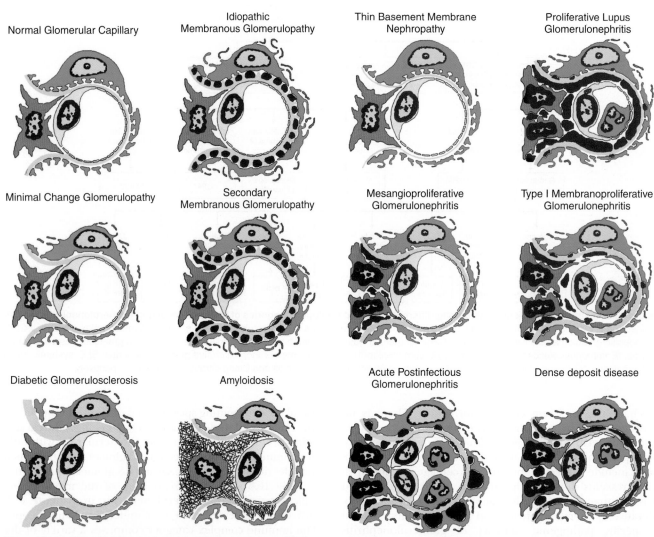

Figure 16.3 Ultrastructural changes in glomerular capillaries caused by glomerular diseases that typically result in the nephrotic syndrome. In the normal glomerular capillary, note the visceral epithelial cell with intact foot processes *(green)*, endothelial cell with fenestrations *(tan)*, mesangial cell *(brown)* with adjacent mesangial matrix *(light gray)*, and basement membrane with lamina densa *(light blue)* that does not completely surround the capillary lumen but splays out as the paramesangial basement membrane. In minimal change glomerulopathy, note the effacement of foot processes and microvillus transformation. In diabetic glomerulosclerosis, note the thickening of the lamina densa and expansion of mesangial matrix. In idiopathic membranous glomerulopathy, note the subepithelial dense deposits with adjacent projections of basement membrane (see also Fig. 16.6). In secondary membranous glomerulopathy, note the mesangial and small subendothelial deposits in addition to the requisite subepithelial deposits. In amyloidosis, note the fibrils within the mesangium and capillary wall. (Courtesy J. Charles Jennette, M.D.)

Figure 16.4 Ultrastructural changes in glomerular capillaries caused by glomerular diseases that typically result in hematuria and the nephritic syndrome. In thin basement membrane nephropathy, note the thin lamina densa of the basement membrane. In mesangioproliferative glomerulonephritis (e.g., mild lupus nephritis, immunoglobulin A nephropathy), note the mesangial dense deposits and mesangial hypercellularity. In acute diffuse proliferative glomerulonephritis (e.g., poststreptococcal glomerulonephritis), note the endocapillary hypercellularity contributed to by leukocytes, endothelial cells, and mesangial cells and the dense deposits, which include not only conspicuous subepithelial "humps" but also inconspicuous subendothelial and mesangial deposits. In proliferative lupus glomerulonephritis (see also Fig. 16.5), note the extensive subendothelial and mesangial dense deposits. In type I membranoproliferative glomerulonephritis (MPGN) (mesangiocapillary glomerulonephritis), note the subendothelial deposits with associated subendothelial interposition of mesangial cytoplasm and deposition of new matrix material resulting in basement membrane replication. In type II MPGN (dense deposit disease), note the intramembranous and mesangial dense deposits. (Courtesy J. Charles Jennette, M.D.)

immunosuppressive treatment, whereas class I or class II lupus nephritis does not.

The two most aggressive forms of glomerulonephritis are anti-GBM crescentic glomerulonephritis and ANCA crescentic glomerulonephritis, and the most important factor in improving kidney outcomes is early diagnosis and treatment. After extensive sclerosis of glomeruli and advanced chronic tubulointerstitial injury have developed, significant response to treatment is unlikely. Both diseases are treated

with immunosuppressive regimens, such as pulse methylprednisolone and intravenous or oral cyclophosphamide. Plasmapheresis is usually added to the regimen for anti-GBM disease and for ANCA disease with pulmonary hemorrhage or severe kidney failure. Immunosuppressive treatment usually can be terminated after 4 to 5 months in patients with

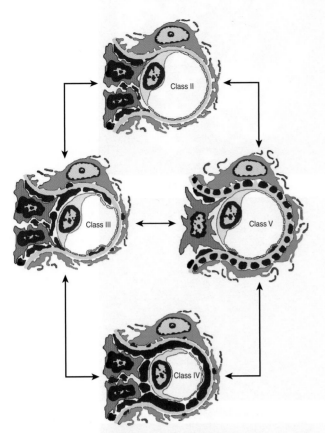

Figure 16.5   Ultrastructural features of the major classes of lupus nephritis. The sequestration of immune deposits within the mesangium in class II (mesangioproliferative) lupus glomerulonephritis causes only mesangial hyperplasia and mild renal dysfunction. Substantial amounts of subendothelial immune deposits, which are adjacent to the inflammatory mediator systems of the blood, cause focal (class III) or diffuse (class IV) proliferative lupus glomerulonephritis with overt nephritic signs and symptoms. Localization of immune deposits predominantly in the subepithelial zone causes membranous (class V) lupus glomerulonephritis, which usually manifests predominantly as the nephrotic syndrome. (Courtesy J. Charles Jennette, M.D.)

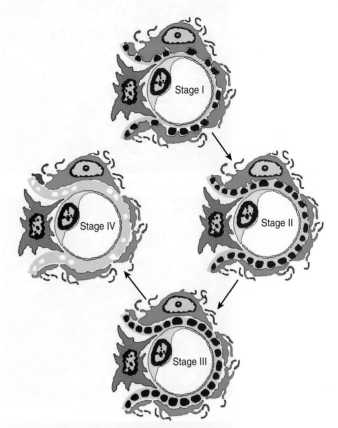

Figure 16.6   Ultrastructural stages in the progression of membranous glomerulopathy. Stage I has subepithelial electron-dense immune complex deposits without adjacent projections of basement membrane material. Stage II has adjacent glomerular basement membrane (GBM) projections that eventually surround the electron-dense immune deposits in stage III. Stage IV has a markedly thickened GBM with electron-lucent zones replacing the electron-dense deposits. (Courtesy J. Charles Jennette, M.D.)

anti-GBM glomerulonephritis with little risk for recurrence (see Chapter 21). The initial induction of remission for ANCA glomerulonephritis often is performed for 6 to 12 months, and even then there is an approximate 25% risk for recurrence that will require additional immunosuppression (Chapter 23).

GLOMERULONEPHRITIS ASSOCIATED WITH SYSTEMIC DISEASES

Some patients with acute or rapidly progressive glomerulonephritis have a pathogenetically related systemic disease. These forms of glomerulonephritis, with known systemic disease causes, may be referred to as *secondary glomerulonephritides.* Immune complex–mediated glomerulonephritis that is induced by infection may involve an antecedent infection, such as streptococcal pharyngitis or pyoderma preceding acute poststreptococcal glomerulonephritis, or a concurrent infection, such as hepatitis C infection concurrent with type I membranoproliferative glomerulonephritis (MPGN). As noted earlier, glomerulonephritis with any of

the morphologic expressions shown in Figure 16.9, as well as membranous glomerulopathy, can be caused by systemic lupus erythematosus (see Fig. 16.6).

Because glomeruli are vessels, glomerulonephritis is a frequent manifestation of systemic small-vessel vasculitides, such as IgA vasculitis (Henoch-Schönlein purpura), cryoglobulinemic vasculitis, microscopic polyangiitis (MPA), granulomatosis with polyangiitis (GPA, formerly Wegener granulomatosis), or eosinophilic granulomatosis with polyangiitis (EGPA, formerly Churg-Strauss syndrome) (see Chapter 23). IgA vasculitis is caused by vascular localization of IgA-dominant immune complexes, which manifests as IgA nephropathy in the glomeruli. Cryoglobulinemic vasculitis is caused by cryoglobulin deposition in vessels and often is associated with hepatitis C infection. In glomeruli, cryoglobulinemia usually causes type I MPGN, but other phenotypes of proliferative and even membranous glomerulonephritis may develop. In MPA, GPA, and EGPA, there is typically a paucity of immune deposits in vessel walls, usually, but not always, accompanied by circulating ANCAs. Glomerulonephritis associated with and probably caused by ANCAs is characterized pathologically by fibrinoid necrosis and crescent formation and often manifests as a rapidly progressive decline in kidney function. Patients with vasculitis-associated glomerulonephritis typically exhibit clinical

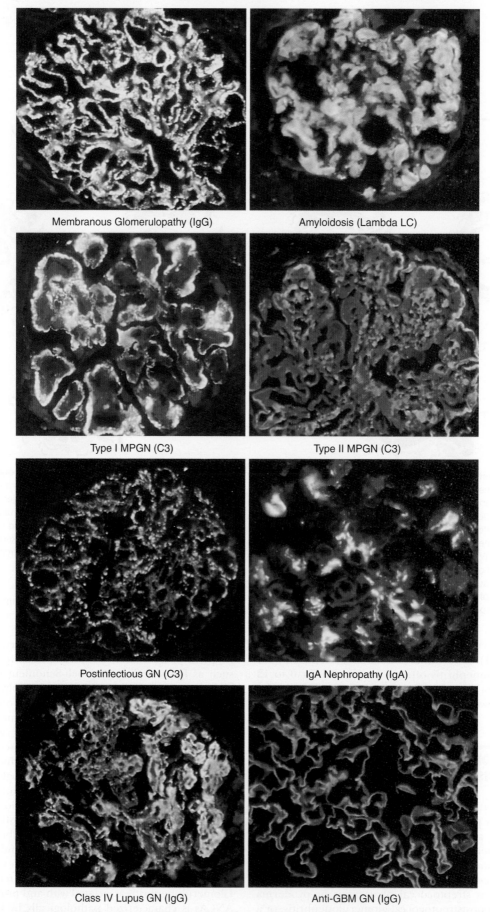

Membranous Glomerulopathy (IgG)

Amyloidosis (Lambda LC)

Type I MPGN (C3)

Type II MPGN (C3)

Postinfectious GN (C3)

IgA Nephropathy (IgA)

Class IV Lupus GN (IgG)

Anti-GBM GN (IgG)

Figure 16.7 **Immunofluorescence microscopy staining patterns for membranous glomerulopathy.** Note the global granular capillary wall staining for IgG. In AL amyloidosis, note the irregular fluffy staining for LCs. In type I MPGN, note the peripheral granular to bandlike staining for C3. In dense deposit disease, note the bandlike capillary wall and coarsely granular mesangial staining for C3. In acute postinfectious GN, note the coarsely granular capillary wall staining for C3. In IgA nephropathy, note the mesangial staining for IgA. In class IV lupus GN, note the segmentally variable capillary wall and mesangial staining for IgG. In anti-GBM GN, note the linear GBM staining for IgG. *anti-GBM,* Antiglomerular basement membrane; *GN,* glomerulonephritis; *IgG,* immunoglobulin G; *LC,* light chain; *MPGN,* membranoproliferative glomerulonephritis.

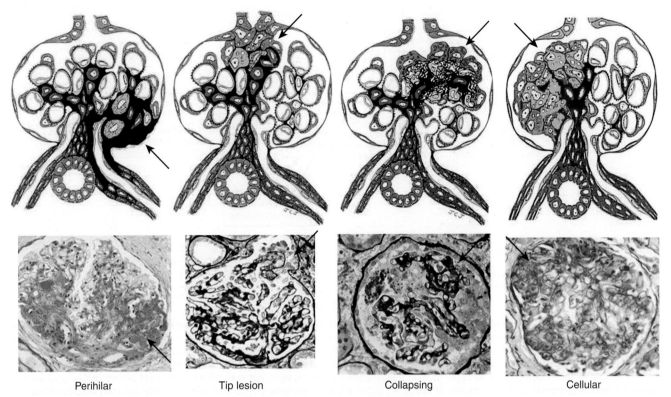

| Perihilar | Tip lesion | Collapsing | Cellular |

Figure 16.8 Pathologic variants of focal segmental glomerulosclerosis (FSGS). Podocytes showing parietal epithelial cells and tubular epithelial cells *(green)*, endothelial cells *(yellow)*, mesangial and arteriolar smooth muscle cells *(red)*, macrophages *(tan)*, and collagenous matrix (black). The photomicrographs of perihilar and cellular FSGS include periodic acid-Schiff (PAS) staining, and the images of tip lesion and collapsing FSGS include Jones silver staining. Perihilar FSGS has perihilar sclerosis and adhesion. Tip lesion FSGS has consolidation of the tuft contiguous with the origin of the proximal tubule. Collapsing FSGS has collapse of capillaries with hypertrophy and hyperplasia of overlying epithelial cells. Cellular FSGS has endocapillary hypercellularity with foam cells.

Table 16.2 Renal Disease in Patients with Hematuria Undergoing Kidney Biopsy*

Disease	Prot <1 g/24 h, Cr <1.5 mg/dl	Prot 1-3 g/24 h	Cr 1.5-3.0 mg/dl	Cr >3 mg/dl
No abnormality	30%	2%	1%	0%
Thin BM nephropathy	26%	4%	3%	0%
IgA nephropathy	28%	24%	14%	8%
GN without crescents[†]	9%	26%	37%	23%
GN with crescents[†]	2%	24%	21%	44%
Other kidney disease[‡]	5%	20%	24%	25%
Total	100% (*n* = 43)	100% (*n* = 123)	100% (*n* = 179)	100% (*n* = 255)

Adapted from Caldas MLR, Jennette JC, Falk RJ, Wilkman AS: NC Glomerular Disease Collaborative Network: what is found by renal biopsy in patients with hematuria? Lab Invest 62:15A, 1990.
BM, Basement membrane; Cr, serum creatinine; GN, glomerulonephritis; IgA, immunoglobulin A; Prot, proteinuria.
*An analysis of kidney biopsy specimens evaluated by the University of North Carolina nephropathology laboratory. Patients with systemic lupus erythematosus were excluded from the analysis.
[†]Proliferative or necrotizing GN other than IgA nephropathy or lupus nephritis.
[‡]Includes causes for the nephrotic syndrome, such as membranous glomerulopathy and focal segmental glomerulosclerosis.

manifestations of vascular inflammation in multiple organs, such as skin purpura caused by dermal venulitis, hemoptysis caused by alveolar capillary hemorrhage, abdominal pain caused by gut vasculitis, and peripheral neuropathy (mononeuritis multiplex) caused by vasculitis in the small epineural arteries of peripheral nerves.

A distinctive and severe clinical presentation for glomerulonephritis is pulmonary-renal vasculitic syndrome, in which rapidly progressive glomerulonephritis is combined with pulmonary hemorrhage. ANCA disease is the most common cause for pulmonary-renal vasculitic syndrome, followed by anti-GBM disease. Histologic and immunohistologic

Light Microscopic Morphology

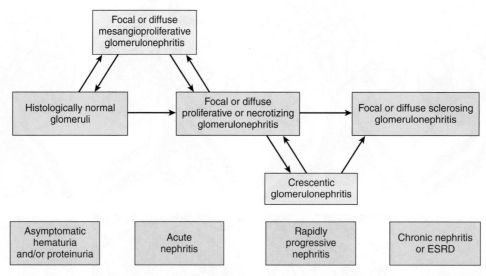

Clinical Manifestations

Figure 16.9   Morphologic stages of glomerulonephritis *(top)* aligned with the usual clinical manifestations *(bottom)*. Certain glomerular diseases, such as antiglomerular basement membrane and antineutrophil cytoplasmic antibody glomerulonephritis, usually exhibit crescentic glomerulonephritis with rapid decline in kidney function if not promptly treated. Others, such as lupus nephritis, have a predilection for causing focal or diffuse proliferative glomerulonephritis with variable rates of progression depending on the activity of the glomerular lesions. Immunoglobulin A nephropathy tends to begin as mild mesangioproliferative lesions but may progress to more severe proliferative lesions. Poststreptococcal glomerulonephritis typically develops an active acute proliferative glomerulonephritis initially but then resolves through a mesangioproliferative phase to normal. Still others, such as immunoglobulin M mesangial nephropathy, rarely progress past the mesangioproliferative phase. *ESRD,* End-stage renal disease. (From Jennette JC, Mandal AK: Syndrome of glomerulonephritis. In Mandal AK, Jennette JC, editors: *Diagnosis and management of renal disease and hypertension*, ed 2, Durham, NC, 1994, Carolina Academic Press, with permission.)

examination of involved vessels, including glomeruli in kidney biopsy specimens, is useful in making a definitive diagnosis (see Fig. 16.2). Serologic analysis for anti-GBM antibodies and ANCA and markers for immune complex disease (e.g., antinuclear antibodies, cryoglobulins, antihepatitis C and B antibodies, complement levels) also may indicate the appropriate diagnosis (see Fig. 16.2).

ASYMPTOMATIC PROTEINURIA AND NEPHROTIC SYNDROME

When proteinuria is severe, it causes the nephrotic syndrome, whereas less severe proteinuria, or severe proteinuria of short duration, may be asymptomatic. The nephrotic syndrome is characterized by massive proteinuria (greater than 3 g/24 h per 1.73 m²), hypoproteinemia (especially hypoalbuminemia), edema, hyperlipidemia, and lipiduria. The most specific microscopic urinalysis finding is the presence of oval fat bodies (Chapter 4). These are sloughed tubular epithelial cells that have reabsorbed some of the excess lipids and lipoproteins in the urine.

Severe nephrotic syndrome predisposes to thrombosis secondary to loss of hemostasis control proteins (e.g., antithrombin III, protein S, protein C), infection secondary to loss of immunoglobulins, and, possibly, accelerated atherosclerosis caused by hyperlipidemia. Volume depletion and inactivity may further increase the risk for venous thrombosis in nephrotic patients. In nephrotic patients with frequent bacterial infections, administration of intravenous gamma globulin may be required.

Any type of glomerular disease can cause proteinuria. In fact, although proteinuria is a sensitive indicator of glomerular damage, not all proteinuria is of glomerular origin. For example, tubular damage can cause proteinuria, but rarely of more than 2 g/24 h.

As noted in Table 16.1, some glomerular diseases are more likely to manifest as nephrotic syndrome than others, although virtually any form of glomerular disease may be the cause. The primary kidney diseases that most often manifest as nephrotic syndrome are minimal change glomerulopathy, FSGS, and membranous glomerulopathy; the secondary forms of kidney disease that most often manifest as nephrotic syndrome are diabetic glomerulosclerosis and amyloidosis.

Age and race may predispose to certain causes of nephrotic syndrome. Among children younger than 10 years, about 80% of nephrotic syndrome is caused by minimal change glomerulopathy, whereas, throughout adulthood, minimal change glomerulopathy accounts for only about 10% to 15% of primary nephrotic syndrome (i.e., nephrotic syndrome not secondary to a systemic disease such as diabetes or amyloidosis). In white adults, membranous glomerulopathy is the most common cause for primary nephrotic syndrome, accounting for approximately 40% of cases, whereas FSGS is the most common cause for primary nephrotic syndrome in African Americans, accounting for more than 50% of cases. Figure 16.1 shows the frequencies of different glomerular disease identified by kidney biopsy specimens across a wide age range. Notably, these biopsy data do not correlate directly with the frequencies of these diseases in all nephrotic patients, because all causes of

Table 16.3 Frequency of Pathologic Categories of Crescentic Glomerulonephritis in Consecutive Native Kidney Biopsy Specimens, by Age of Patient*

Age (yr)	Pauci-immune	Immune Complex	Anti-GBM	Other†
All (n = 632)	60%	24%	15%	1%
1 to 20 (n = 73)	42%	45%	12%	0%
21 to 60 (n = 303)	48%	35%	15%	3%
61 to 100 (n = 256)	79%	6%	15%	0%

Modified from Jennette JC: Rapidly progressive and crescentic glomerulonephritis. Kidney Int 63:1164-1172, 2003.
Anti-GBM, Antiglomerular basement membrane.
*Crescentic glomerulonephritis defined as glomerular disease with 50% or more crescents.
†The "other" category includes all other glomerular diseases, such as thrombotic microangiopathy, diabetic glomerulosclerosis, and monoclonal immunoglobulin deposition disease.

nephrotic syndrome are not biopsied at the same rate. For example, diagnoses of minimal change glomerulopathy in children and diabetic glomerulosclerosis in adults are often made without biopsy.

Membranous glomerulopathy (see Chapter 19) is the most frequent cause of primary nephrotic syndrome in white people during the fifth and sixth decades of life. It is characterized pathologically by numerous subepithelial immune complex deposits (see Figs. 16.3, 16.6, and 16.7). The glomerular lesion evolves through time, with progressive accumulation of basement membrane material around the capillary wall immune complexes (see Fig. 16.6) and eventual development of chronic tubulointerstitial injury in those patients with progressive disease. Most membranous glomerulopathy is caused by autoantibodies specific for an antigen on visceral epithelial cells, M-type phospholipase A_2 receptor (anti-PLA2R). This results in immune complex formation in the subepithelial zone but not in the subendothelial zone or the mesangium of glomeruli. On the other hand, in addition to the numerous subepithelial immune deposits, membranous glomerulopathy secondary to immune complexes composed of antigens and antibodies in the systemic circulation often exhibits immune complex deposits in the mesangium and may include small subendothelial deposits (see Fig. 16.3). Therefore, the ultrastructural identification of mesangial or subendothelial deposits should raise the level of suspicion for secondary membranous glomerulopathy, such as membranous glomerulopathy caused by a systemic autoimmune disease (e.g., lupus, mixed connective tissue disease, autoimmune thyroiditis), infection (e.g., hepatitis B or C, syphilis), or neoplasm (e.g., lung or gut carcinoma). In very young and very old patients, the likelihood of secondary membranous glomerulopathy is greater, although still uncommon. Membranous glomerulopathy occurring in young patients raises the possibility of systemic lupus erythematosus or hepatitis B infection, and in very old patients it raises the possibility of occult carcinoma.

Both type I MPGN and dense deposit disease (DDD, formerly called type II MPGN) typically manifest with mixed nephrotic and nephritic features, sometimes accompanied by hypocomplementemia and C3 nephritic factor, the latter being an autoantibody against the C3 convertase of the alternative complement activation pathway. Both types often exhibit glomerular capillary wall thickening and hypercellularity by light microscopy. Type I MPGN (mesangiocapillary glomerulonephritis) is characterized ultrastructurally by subendothelial immune complex deposits that stimulate subendothelial mesangial interposition and replication of basement membrane material, whereas DDD features pathognomonic intramembranous dense deposits (see Fig. 16.4). This pathognomonic feature, intramembranous dense deposits, is not always accompanied by a MPGN pattern by light microscopy, so *dense deposit disease* (DDD) is the more appropriate diagnostic term. Both MPGN and DDD have extensive glomerular staining for C3 (see Fig. 16.7). Some patients with type I MPGN have prominent immunoglobulin staining, others have exclusively complement staining, whereas DDD has glomerular staining exclusively for complement. Type I MPGN with extensive immunoglobulin deposition is an immune complex disease that may be secondary to cryoglobulinemia, neoplasms, or chronic infections (e.g., hepatitis C or B; infected prostheses, such as a ventriculoatrial shunt; chronic bacterial endocarditis; chronic mastoiditis). Type I MPGN with complement deposition but no immunoglobulin, as well as DDD, are not immune complex diseases but rather are secondary to abnormal activation of the alternative complement pathway by a variety of inherited and acquired abnormalities in complement regulation, such as inherited defects in the complement control protein factor H. The term C3 glomerulopathy refers to DDD and C3-dominant type I MPGN. Less often, C3 glomerulopathy manifests as proliferative or mesangioproliferative glomerulonephritis (C3 glomerulonephritis).

When taken as a group, the various forms of proliferative glomerulonephritis account for a substantial proportion of patients who have nephrotic-range proteinuria. Patients with proliferative glomerulonephritis and marked proteinuria usually also have features of nephritis, especially hematuria. Included in this group are patients with lupus nephritis and IgA nephropathy who have nephrotic-range proteinuria. In the United States, approximately 15% of adults with nephrotic-range proteinuria are found to have IgA nephropathy by kidney biopsy.

FSGS is the most common cause for the nephrotic syndrome in African Americans, but it affects all races. Clinical presentations include asymptomatic proteinuria, indolent nephrotic syndrome, rapid onset nephrotic syndrome, and nephrotic syndrome with rapidly progressive kidney failure. Some forms of FSGS may recur in transplant recipients, suggesting a pathogenic role for a circulating factor (possibly soluble urokinase-type plasminogen activator receptor). The Columbia classification system recognizes five morphologic variants: tip lesion, collapsing, cellular, perihilar, and not otherwise specified (NOS) (see Fig. 16.8). NOS is most common and usually presents as asymptomatic proteinuria or indolent nephrotic syndrome. Although the other variants can have any type of proteinuric presentation, tip lesion FSGS usually presents with rapid onset severe proteinuria resembling minimal change glomerulopathy, collapsing FSGS with severe proteinuria and rapidly progressing kidney failure, and perihilar FSGS with subnephrotic proteinuria. FSGS occurs as a primary (idiopathic) disease or secondary to recognized causes. For example, FSGS NOS may be secondary to mutations in podocyte genes, collapsing FSGS secondary to human immunodeficiency virus infection, and perihilar FSGS secondary to obesity.

Amyloidosis as a cause for the nephrotic syndrome is most frequently seen in older adults. Overall, approximately 10% of adults with unexplained nephrotic syndrome have amyloidosis that appears on kidney biopsy. Currently in the United States, amyloid causing the nephrotic syndrome is approximately 75% AL amyloid rather than AA amyloid, and approximately 75% of AL amyloid is composed of λ rather than κ light chains. Patients with κ light chain paraproteins and the nephrotic syndrome are more likely to experience light chain deposition disease (i.e., nodular sclerosis without amyloid fibrils) rather than amyloidosis (Chapter 26). Amyloid composition can be determined by immunofluorescence microscopy (see Fig. 16.7) or mass spectroscopy. In less developed areas of the world, where chronic infections are more prevalent, AA amyloidosis is more frequent than AL amyloidosis.

CHRONIC GLOMERULONEPHRITIS AND KIDNEY FAILURE

Most glomerular disease, with the possible exceptions of uncomplicated minimal change glomerulopathy and thin basement membrane nephropathy, can progress to chronic glomerular sclerosis with progressively declining kidney function and, eventually, to ESRD. Chronic glomerular disease is the third leading cause of ESRD in the United States after diabetic and hypertensive kidney disease. Clinicopathologic studies of glomerular diseases have shown marked differences in their natural histories. Some diseases, such as anti-GBM and ANCA crescentic glomerulonephritis, result in a high risk for rapid progression to ESRD unless treated. Other diseases, such as IgA nephropathy and FSGS, have more indolent but persistent courses, with ESRD eventually ensuing in a significant number of patients. Some forms of glomerulonephritis, such as acute poststreptococcal glomerulonephritis, may initially manifest with severe nephritis but usually resolve completely with little risk for progression to ESRD, whereas other diseases are unpredictable, such as membranous glomerulopathy, which may remit spontaneously, produce persistent nephrosis for decades without a decline in kidney function, or progress during several years to ESRD.

Chronic glomerulonephritis is characterized pathologically by varying degrees of glomerular scarring that is always accompanied by cortical tubular atrophy, interstitial fibrosis, interstitial infiltration by chronic inflammatory cells, and arteriosclerosis. As the glomerular, interstitial, and vascular sclerosis worsen, they eventually reach a point at which histologic evaluation of the kidney tissue cannot show the initial cause for the kidney injury, and a pathologic diagnosis of ESRD is all that can be concluded.

KIDNEY BIOPSY: INDICATIONS AND METHODS

In a patient with kidney disease, a kidney biopsy provides tissue that can be used to determine the diagnosis, indicate the cause, predict the prognosis, direct treatment, and be used for research, although not all potential applications are accomplished by every kidney biopsy.

Kidney biopsy is indicated in a patient with kidney disease when all three of the following conditions are met: (1) the cause cannot be determined or adequately predicted by less invasive diagnostic procedures; (2) the signs and symptoms suggest parenchymal disease that can be diagnosed by pathologic evaluation; and (3) the differential diagnosis includes diseases that have different treatments, different prognoses, or both.

Situations in which a kidney biopsy serves an important diagnostic function include nephrotic syndrome in adults, steroid-resistant nephrotic syndrome in children, glomerulonephritis in adults other than clear-cut acute poststreptococcal glomerulonephritis, and acute kidney failure of unknown cause. In some kidney diseases for which the diagnosis is relatively certain based on clinical data, a kidney biopsy may be of value not only for confirming the diagnosis but also for assessing the activity, chronicity, and severity of injury (e.g., in patients with suspected lupus glomerulonephritis). Although the diagnosis is strongly supported by positive serologic results in patients with anti-GBM and ANCA glomerulonephritis, the extremely toxic treatment that is used for these diseases warrants the additional level of confirmation that a kidney biopsy provides as well as information about the severity and potential reversibility of the glomerular damage. Figure 16.1 demonstrates the types of native kidney disease that have prompted kidney biopsy among the nephrologists who refer specimens to the University of North Carolina nephropathology laboratory. Nephrologists in community practice performed approximately 80% of these biopsies. Diseases that typically cause nephrotic syndrome (e.g., membranous glomerulopathy, FSGS) were the conditions most often shown by biopsy, followed by diseases that cause nephritis (e.g., lupus nephritis, IgA nephropathy).

Absolute or relative contraindications to percutaneous kidney biopsy include an uncooperative patient, solitary native kidney, hemorrhagic diathesis, uncontrolled severe hypertension, severe anemia or volume depletion, cystic kidney, hydronephrosis, multiple renal arterial aneurysms, acute pyelonephritis or perinephric abscess, kidney neoplasm, and ESRD. Some advocate transjugular kidney biopsy and open kidney biopsy as safer procedures in patients with these risk factors.

Clinically significant complications of kidney biopsy are relatively infrequent but must be kept in mind when determining the risk/benefit ratio of the procedure. Small perirenal hematomas that can be seen on imaging studies (e.g., ultrasonography) are relatively common if observed carefully.

Gross hematuria occurs in fewer than 10% of patients, arteriovenous fistula in less than 1%, hemorrhage requiring surgery in less than 1%, and death in less than 0.1%.

Current percutaneous needle biopsy procedures usually employ real-time ultrasound or computed tomography guidance. Currently, most kidney biopsies are performed with spring-loaded disposable gun devices. Extensive experience and multiple published studies indicate that the use of larger biopsy needles (e.g., 15- and 16-gauge) provides more useful tissue with no more morbidity than smaller needles (e.g., 18-gauge), which are more likely to provide inadequate tissue for diagnosis and especially for prognosis. Therefore, 15- and 16-gauge needles provide a better risk-to-benefit ratio for the patient.

Light microscopy alone is inadequate for the diagnosis of native kidney diseases, although it may be adequate for assessing the basis for kidney allograft dysfunction during the first few weeks after transplantation. All native kidney biopsy samples should be processed for at least light microscopy and immunofluorescence microscopy. Most renal pathologists advocate performing electron microscopy on all native kidney biopsy specimens; however, some fix tissue for electron microscopy but perform the procedure only if the other microscopic findings suggest that it will be useful.

The needle biopsy core sample should be examined with a magnifying glass or a dissecting microscope to confirm that kidney tissue is present and to determine whether it is cortex or medulla. When gently prodded and pulled with forceps, adipose tissue is mushy and strings out, skeletal muscle tissue falls apart into little clumps, and kidney tissue maintains a cylindrical shape. At 15× or higher magnification, adipose tissue looks like clusters of tiny fat droplets (i.e., adipose cells), skeletal muscle is red-brown with irregular bundles of fibers, and kidney tissue is pale pink to tan. Glomeruli in the renal cortex appear as reddish blushes or hemispheres projecting from the surface of the core (Fig. 16.10). Straight red striations produced by the vasa recta are markers for the medulla. If there is extensive glomerular hematuria, the convoluted tubules in the cortex appear as red corkscrews. After the tissue landmarks are identified, portions of tissue should be separated for processing for light, immunofluorescence, and electron microscopy.

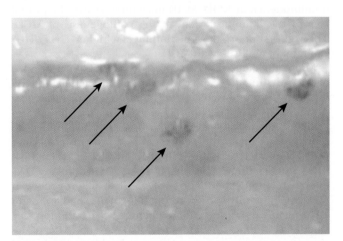

Figure 16.10 Photograph of a fresh 15-gauge needle renal biopsy showing red blushes (*arrows*) corresponding to glomeruli in the renal cortex.

In our experience with kidney biopsy specimens sent to us from more than 200 different nephrologists per year, most of whom are in community practice, approximately 6% of kidney biopsy specimens are inadequate for a definitive diagnosis. The most common cause of this inadequacy is kidney tissue with too little or no cortex. This can be remedied by beginning the sampling procedure with the biopsy needle just barely penetrating the outer cortex. Obviously, if the biopsy needle is inserted too deeply into or through the cortex, the specimen will contain only medulla. However, even specimens that are considered inadequate for a definitive diagnosis may provide useful information. For example, in a patient with nephrotic syndrome, a kidney biopsy specimen that has no glomeruli for light or electron microscopy may have one glomerulus that stains negatively for immunoglobulins, complemented by immunofluorescence microscopy, which rules out any form of immune complex glomerulonephritis (e.g., membranous glomerulopathy) and focuses the differential diagnosis on minimal change glomerulopathy versus FSGS.

BIBLIOGRAPHY

D'Agati VD, Fogo AB, Bruijn JA, et al: Pathologic classification of focal segmental glomerulosclerosis: a working proposal, *Am J Kidney Dis* 43:368-382, 2004.

Eddy AA, Symons JM: Nephrotic syndrome in childhood, *Lancet* 362:629-639, 2003.

Glassock RJ: The pathogenesis of membranous nephropathy: evolution and revolution, *Curr Opin Nephrol Hypertens* 21:235-242, 2012.

Jennette JC: Rapidly progressive and crescentic glomerulonephritis, *Kidney Int* 63:1164-1172, 2003.

Hicks J, Mierau G, Wartchow E, et al: Renal diseases associated with hematuria in children and adolescents: a brief tutorial, *Ultrastruct Pathol* 36:1-18, 2012.

Hudson BG, Tryggvason K, Sundaramoorthy M, et al: Alport's syndrome, Goodpasture's syndrome, and type IV collagen, *N Engl J Med* 348:2543-2556, 2003.

Jennette JC: An approach to the pathologic diagnosis of glomerulonephritis. In D'Agati V, Jennette JC, Silva FG, editors: *Non-neoplastic renal disease*, Washington, D.C, 2005, American Registry of Pathology, pp 239-268, Chapter 10.

Jennette JC: The kidney. In Ruben R, Strayer D, editors: *Rubin's pathology*, ed 6, Philadelphia, 2012, J.B. Lippincott, pp 753-807, Chapter 16.

Jennette JC, Kshirsagar AV: How can the safety and diagnostic yield of percutaneous renal biopsies be optimized? *Nat Clin Pract Nephrol* 4:126-127, 2008.

Jennette JC, Olson JL, Schwartz MM, et al: Primer on the pathologic diagnosis of renal disease. In Jennette JC, Olson JL, Schwartz MM, Silva FG, editors: *Heptinstall's pathology of the kidney*, ed 6, Philadelphia, 2007, Lippincott Williams & Wilkins, pp 100-126.

Kambham N: Crescentic glomerulonephritis: an update on Pauci-immune and Anti-GBM diseases, *Adv Anat Pathol* 19:111-124, 2012.

Reiser J, Wei C, Tumlin J: Soluble urokinase receptor and focal segmental glomerulosclerosis, *Curr Opin Nephrol Hypertens* 21:428-432, 2012.

Sethi S, Nester CM, Smith RJ: Membranoproliferative glomerulonephritis and C3 glomerulopathy: resolving the confusion, *Kidney Int* 81:434-441, 2012.

Smith RJ, Alexander J, Barlow PN, et al: New approaches to the treatment of dense deposit disease, *J Am Soc Nephrol* 18:2447-2456, 2007.

Suzuki H, Kiryluk K, Novak J, et al: The pathophysiology of IgA nephropathy, *J Am Soc Nephrol* 22:1795-1803, 2011.

Walker PD, Cavallo T, Bonsib SM: Ad Hoc committee on renal biopsy guidelines of the renal pathology society: practice guidelines for the renal biopsy, *Mod Pathol* 17:1555-1563, 2004.

Thomas DB, Franceschini N, Hogan SL, et al: Clinical and pathologic characteristics of focal segmental glomerulosclerosis pathologic variants, *Kidney Int* 69:920-926, 2006.

Weening JJ, D'Agati VD, Schwartz MM, et al: The classification of glomerulonephritis in systemic lupus erythematosus revisited, *Kidney Int* 65:521-530, 2004.

17 Minimal Change Disease

Howard Trachtman | Jonathan Hogan | Jai Radhakrishnan

TERMINOLOGY AND HISTOPATHOLOGY

Minimal change disease (MCD) is a common cause of the nephrotic syndrome (NS). Also known as lipoid nephrosis, nil disease, and minimal change nephropathy, the kidney histology on light microscopy in MCD is relatively normal and lacks the significant glomerular cell proliferation, infiltration by circulating immunoeffector cells, immune deposits, tubulointerstitial changes, or alterations in the glomerular basement membrane (GBM) that characterize other glomerular diseases. The defining feature of MCD is diffuse effacement and fusion of podocyte foot processes without electron-dense deposits on electron microscopy. Immunofluorescence is typically negative or may show low-level staining for C3 and IgM.

Although MCD is histologically defined by the previously mentioned criteria, it can also be diagnosed clinically by exhibiting responsiveness to corticosteroid treatment. In children, because MCD is the cause of 90% of cases of idiopathic NS, a kidney biopsy is only warranted if the clinical and laboratory evidence, including disease onset before 6 months of age or following adolescence, unexpected systemic manifestations, or a low serum C3 level, suggests an alternative diagnosis. Children who do not exhibit these characteristics will typically have MCD and will consequently respond to steroids. The nomenclature "steroid-sensitive nephrotic syndrome (SSNS)" is also used to describe such children. Steroid responsiveness is a marker of a favorable long-term prognosis. In contrast, children with steroid-resistant nephrotic syndrome (SRNS) are more likely on subsequent kidney biopsies to show focal segmental glomerulosclerosis (FSGS), a disease that is associated with a worse prognosis. The causes of the NS in adults are more varied and include a higher percentage of cases with membranous nephropathy (MN) and membranoproliferative glomerulonephritis (MPGN). Because MCD only accounts for approximately 10% to 15% of cases, a kidney biopsy is usually warranted to establish the etiology of nephrotic syndrome.

PATHOPHYSIOLOGY

The pathogenesis of MCD is not well understood. The effacement of podocyte foot processes that is a hallmark of MCD may be mediated by various intracellular signaling pathways. For example, it has been demonstrated that markers of focal adhesion complex–mediated Crk-dependent signaling are enhanced in MCD but not FSGS. Moreover, increased production of proteins such as CD80 and angiopoietin-like protein 4 by podocytes in MCD models supports

the central role of podocyte damage in the pathogenesis of MCD. It has been thought that proteinuria occurs solely because of a defect in glomerular permselectivity, although alterations in tubular reabsorption may contribute.

MCD is unique in that it predominantly reflects a decrease in the negative charge present in endothelial cells, the GBM, and podocytes, thereby causing selective proteinuria. The reduction in negative charge appears to be a diffuse abnormality that is manifest in capillaries throughout the body with leakage of albumin in the peripheral circulation and accumulation of interstitial fluid. The cause of the diminished negative charge density probably results from immune-mediated defects that inhibit sulfate incorporation into the GBM rather than a genetic mutation in a podocyte protein. In addition, immunoeffector cells may elaborate soluble molecules, such as vascular endothelial growth factor, that directly increase GBM permeability to protein. It is likely that the molecular identity of circulating permeability factors that cause proteinuria will differ in patients with MCD and FSGS. This is supported by the recent report indicating that circulating levels of soluble urokinase receptor (suPAR) are elevated in nearly 70% of patients with FSGS, but they are undetectable in patients with MCD or MN.

A link between abnormal T-cell function and MCD was initially proposed more than 30 years ago by Shalhoub, and many studies since then have documented altered subtype distribution and activity of lymphocytes in children with MCD. A recent study in which albuminuria and podocyte foot process effacement was induced by injection of CD34+ stem cells isolated from patients with MCD or FSGS into immunodeficient NOD/SCID mice underscores the pivotal role of the immune system in the pathogenesis of MCD. This role is supported by the finding of a higher Th17/Treg cell ratio in children with MCD.

Minimal change disease represents a fascinating instance of organ dysfunction caused by a variable interaction between intrinsic structural defects and immunologic disturbances. Although MCD can occur in a familial pattern with both vertical and horizontal transmission, it has not been linked to mutations in any of the well-recognized proteins associated with FSGS, such as Wilms tumor-1, TRPC6, or α-actinin-4. Interestingly, there have been observations linking frequently relapsing childhood MCD to allelic heterogeneity in the gene for nephrin, a key component of the slit diaphragm and a major genetic locus for congenital NS. In addition, in a study of 214 Chinese patients with MCD, variants in the podocin gene were more common than in healthy controls, and they correlated with the level of urinary protein excretion. Alterations in histone H3 lysine 4 trimethylation in children with MCD raise the possibility that epigenetic changes may contribute to the occurrence of MCD.

MCD also is associated with various "secondary" causes (Box 17.1), including medications, infections, toxins, and malignancies. The pathophysiologic link between these secondary causes and the resulting MCD is not understood.

Minimal change disease can be the cause of significant short-term morbidity and can manifest with a chronic relapsing course with long-term adverse consequences well into adulthood. Both first-line treatment and secondary therapeutic options for more difficult cases can lead to serious toxicity. Therefore, although the long-term prognosis is excellent, optimal management of MCD requires clinical acumen to balance the risks of untreated disease activity against the hazards of available pharmacologic choices. This chapter will review the definition, incidence, presentation, and treatment options for MCD, highlighting key differences between pediatric and adult patients with the goal of providing a rational basis for the management of this disorder.

INCIDENCE

The overall incidence of primary or idiopathic NS comprised of MCD and its variants, FSGS, MN, and MPGN, is approximately three to five cases/100,000 population/yr in children and adults. This rate is fairly constant throughout the world and in most racial and ethnic groups. The contribution of MCD to this general category varies tremendously with the age of the patient. Thus, in prepubertal patients more than 6 months of age, MCD accounts for nearly 90% of all cases of idiopathic NS, whereas in adults the percentage of cases attributable to MCD falls to 10% to 15%. Adolescence represents the transition period between the two ends of the spectrum. In a study of 1523 consecutive Chinese patients who underwent biopsy performed during the evaluation of NS, in those

aged 14 to 24 years, MCD was documented in 33% of the subgroup. Similarly, in a report by Mubarak of biopsy findings in 538 pediatric patients in Pakistan, among whom 365 were younger children (mean age 7.3 years) and 173 were adolescents (mean age 15.1 years), approximately one third of the older group had FSGS and only one fourth had MCD. The incidence of MN and MPGN was significantly higher in the older group than in the younger group. These findings suggest that adolescents correspond more closely to adults than they do to younger children and school-age pediatric patients.

CLINICAL PRESENTATION

Minimal change disease causes the NS with nephrotic range proteinuria, hypoalbuminemia, edema, and hypercholesterolemia. The most common presenting symptom of MCD is edema, and the onset may be acute. There may be an antecedent infection, typically respiratory, that is associated with the onset of MCD. Infections may also trigger subsequent relapses of MCD. The rapidity of the appearance of edema is characteristic of MCD compared to other etiologies of NS. In children, edema can occur anywhere in the body, including the periorbital region, scrotum, or abdomen. Less frequent presenting complaints include infections such as cellulitis secondary to localized accumulation of fluid and skin breakdown, or bacterial peritonitis in patients with ascites. The incidence of thromboembolic events, including renal vein thrombosis and pulmonary emboli, is tenfold higher in adults than in children, and typically these events occur in patients with severe hypoalbuminemia.

Urinalysis reveals microscopic hematuria in 10% to 30% of adults and children with MCD, but gross hematuria is rare. Microscopic examination of the urine may also show waxy casts and oval fat bodies. In one series, acute kidney injury (AKI) occurred in 17.8% of adult patients who presented

---

Box 17.1 Secondary Causes of Minimal Change Disease

Malignancy

Hematologic Tumors

Hodgkin lymphoma
Non-Hodgkin lymphoma
Leukemia

Solid Tumors

Thymoma
Renal cell carcinoma
Lung carcinoma
Mesothelioma

Infection

Syphilis
Mycoplasma
Ehrlichiosis
Strongyloidiasis
Echinococcus
Tuberculosis

HIV
Hepatitis C virus

Drugs

NSAIDs, including COX-2 inhibitors
Antimicrobials (ampicillin, rifampicin, cephalosporins)
Lithium
D-penicillamine
Bisphosphonates (Pamidronate)
Sulfasalazines (mesalazine and salazopyrine)
Trimethadione
Immunizations
Interferon-γ

Other Renal and Systemic Diseases

SLE
Fabry disease
Polycystic kidney disease
IPEX syndrome

HIV, Human immunodeficiency virus; *IPEX,* immune dysregulation polyendocrinopathy, enteropathy, X-linked; *NSAIDs,* nonsteroidal antiinflammatory drugs; *SLE,* systemic lupus erythematosus.

with nephrotic syndrome and were subsequently diagnosed with MCD. These patients tended to be older, male, hypertensive, and had more severe proteinuria and hypoalbuminemia than patients who did not develop AKI. Kidney biopsies of these patients showed a variety of histologic patterns of injury including tubular atropy, interstitial inflammation and fibrosis, and atherosclerotic disease. Serum levels of C3 and C4 are typically normal, and antinuclear antibodies and cryoglobulins are usually absent.

INITIAL TREATMENT

Corticosteroids represent the time-honored initial therapy for presumed and biopsy-confirmed MCD. As mentioned, the sensitivity of MCD to steroid treatment prompts many physicians to empirically treat nephrotic patients with glucocorticoids without a kidney biopsy, particularly children. Prednisone is the usual agent prescribed, and the standard dose in pediatric patients is 60 mg/m^2 or 2 mg/kg daily for 4 to 6 weeks followed by 40 mg/m^2 or 1.5 mg/kg every other day for 4 to 6 weeks. In children, 70% will achieve remission after 10 to 14 days of treatment, and the vast majority will no longer have proteinuria after 4 weeks of therapy. There are conflicting data in the literature as to whether lengthening the course of the initial treatment from 8 to 12 weeks delays the time to first relapse and reduces overall exposure to steroids. Efficacy may vary depending on the patient population, and the precise treatment should be guided by the experience at each center.

Adults are treated with oral prednisone 1 mg/kg/day or alternate-day prednisone at 2 mg/kg/day. However, unlike children, responses in adults may take up to 24 weeks before the patient is designated "steroid responsive" or "steroid resistant." In adults, up to 20% of patients with an initial diagnosis of MCD may be refractory to steroids at the end of 24 weeks.

Relapse therapy involves similar doses, but usually for a shorter period of time. Various modifications in corticosteroid dosing such as extended tapering schedules, avoidance of every other day administration, and prolonged low-dose hydrocortisone to prevent adrenal insufficiency have been tried to prevent relapses and to minimize side effects. Different formulations of steroids such a deflazacort have also been tried with mixed results. Adults do not tolerate relapsing disease as well as children as a consequence of the intrinsic morbidity of MCD and the toxicity related to repeated exposures to corticosteroids. Therefore, these patients are often candidates for prompt implementation of immunosuppressive therapy.

SHORT-TERM COURSE

Minimal change disease is usually a chronic relapsing disease (Fig. 17.1). Less than 10% of cases will remain completely free of relapses after the initial episode. The remaining patients can be divided into three categories. One third will have infrequent relapses that are easily managed by intermittent administration of courses of corticosteroids. Another third will have frequent relapses defined by ≥2 relapses in a 6-month period; however, they, too, are successfully managed with intermittent administration of courses of corticosteroids, and they do not manifest significant steroid-induced side effects. The final third are frequently relapsing patients or those with steroid dependence defined as relapse occurring on alternate-day steroid treatment or within 2 weeks of discontinuing corticosteroids. It has proved difficult to predict the short-term, i.e., ≤2 years after disease onset, prognosis in individual patients. In children, those who go into remission during the first week of corticosteroid treatment and who have no hematuria are more likely to be infrequent relapsers, defined as <2 episodes in 6 months or <3 in 1 year. The presence of small involuted glomeruli, which can be distinguished from other causes of global glomerulosclerosis by the presence of vital podocytes and parietal epithelial cells, may be a marker of frequently relapsing MCD in children.

The last category of patients usually experience steroid toxicity, and they are candidates for the second-line treatments, which will be outlined later. Key steroid-induced side effects in children are impaired linear growth, obesity, behavioral changes, and cosmetic changes. In addition to these clinical effects, children with MCD also experience

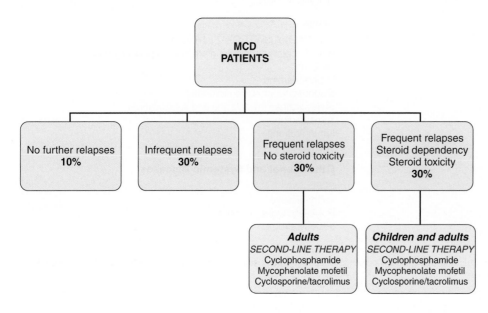

Figure 17.1 Minimal change disease: short-term natural history.

altered quality of life and psychosocial adjustment that is related both to illness-related variables and to alterations in the family climate. In adults, additional evidence of steroid toxicity includes cataracts and altered bone density. Hypertension and hyperlipidemia occur across the age spectrum. It is the last category of patients that most require careful nephrologist attention for ongoing management and care.

LONG-TERM TREATMENT

IMMUNOSUPPRESSIVE THERAPY

Second-line therapy is used in patients who relapse frequently, are steroid dependent, or manifest steroid side effects as a consequence of repeated exposure to the drug (Table 17.1). The first class of drugs that were used under these circumstances was alkylating agents such as cyclophosphamide and chlorambucil. A prolonged remission of at least 1 year was achieved in 70% of patients. With cyclophosphamide, most patients require at least 12 weeks of therapy, and they should be monitored carefully for side effects including leukopenia, infection, hemorrhagic cystitis, gonadal toxicity, and malignancy. However, more than 25% of patients with MCD who were treated with cyclophosphamide were not in sustained remission after puberty, and they required prolonged immunosuppressive treatment. Thus, because of the serious toxicity associated with the alkylating agents, the reluctance to prescribe a second course, and the guarded long-term effect, there has been greater reliance on alternative medications to cyclophosphamide for frequently relapsing or steroid-dependent patients with MCD.

Antimetabolites such as azathioprine and mycophenolate mofetil can reduce the relapse rate by approximately 50%, although they are not as effective as alkylating agents in inducing a permanent remission. They are useful, because they have a more favorable side-effect profile, can be administered for an extended period, and require less intensive monitoring.

A third option is calcineurin inhibitors such as cyclosporine and tacrolimus. These agents induce a prolonged remission in nearly 80% to 90% of patients while the patient is taking the drug; however, relapses frequently occur shortly after stopping the drug. In addition, calcineurin inhibitors can cause undesirable cosmetic changes (hair growth and gingival hyperplasia), hepatoxicity, hypertension, and nephrotoxicity. Therefore, patients taking calcineurin inhibitors for more than 1 year may require periodic blood tests and serial kidney biopsies to insure that irreversible kidney injury does not occur.

Finally, the newest agent used to treat children with frequently relapsing or steroid-dependent MCD and clinical evidence of steroid-induced side effects is rituximab. Administration of this anti-CD20 monoclonal antibody on B cells is likely to achieve remission in up to 80% of steroid sensitive cases when used in combination with calcineurin inhibitors. This was confirmed in a study of 54 children (mean age 11 years) in which rituximab plus low-dose steroids and tacrolimus was as effective as treatment with standard doses of the latter two drugs; however, this therapy is costly, and the long-term risks are unknown. Therefore, it is advisable that randomized clinical trials are performed and ongoing surveillance be maintained to gain perspective on the proper place of this biologic agent in the therapeutic management of children with difficult to treat MCD.

The decision to recommend one of these second-line agents in an effort to alleviate the adverse consequences of steroids must be weighed on an individual basis and must take into account the patient's age, sex, and likely compliance with treatment. Consideration should be given to the severity of the side effect, the likelihood of reversal of the complication, and the odds that the MCD will spontaneously

Table 17.1   Second-Line Treatments of Minimal Change Disease

Drug	Dose	Efficacy	Side Effects
Cyclophosphamide	*Children and adults:* 2-2.5 mg/kg/day × 8-12 wk*	Prolonged remission (>1 yr) in 70%	Leukopenia, hemorrhagic cystitis, alopecia, seizures, gonadal toxicity, malignancy
Chlorambucil	*Children and adults:* 0.15 mg/kg/day × 8-12 wk*		
Mycophenolate mofetil	*Children:* 24-36 mg/kg/day or 600 mg/m²/dose BID *Adults:* 1-1.5 g BID	50% reduction in overall relapse rate	Gastrointestinal complaints, leukopenia, elevated liver enzymes
Cyclosporine	*Children and adults:* 4-5 mg/kg/day in divided doses†	70% to 80% of patients achieve complete remission on treatment	Gingival hyperplasia, tremor, elevated liver enzymes, nephrotoxicity
Tacrolimus	*Children and adults:* 0.05-0.3 mg/kg/day in divided doses†	70%-80%	Tremor, nephrotoxicity
Rituximab	*Children and adults:* 375-1000 mg/m²/dose 2 doses, 2 wk apart	80% in steroid responsive MCD	Infection Malignancy

BID, Twice daily; *SSNS,* steroid-sensitive nephrotic syndrome.
*It is recommended that the duration of therapy be extended to 12 weeks in patients with steroid-dependent disease.
†Target trough levels for cyclosporine and tacrolimus are 100-200 ng/mL and 4-8 ng/mL, respectively. Children may require more frequent dosing to maintain a therapeutic drug level. After achieving remission, reduce doses to the lowest dose compatible with staying in remission.

resolve. Although a number of other immunomodulatory agents have been tried in the past in patients with MCD, the data have been collected in relatively small studies that hinder broad generalizations about efficacy. In addition, drugs such as levamisole are generally not available in the United States for use in patients with MCD. This underscores the need to develop newer agents that can be used to control proteinuria in patients with MCD, especially in children with steroid toxicity and adults with relapsing disease.

SUPPORTIVE CARE

After the initial diagnosis, patients with MCD are usually monitored with daily dipstick testing for proteinuria. In most patients, relapses are detected by the onset of proteinuria 3 to 4 days before edema ensues. In those patients who develop edema before a relapse is recognized or who respond slowly to prednisone, edema can be controlled by prescribing a low-salt (2 g sodium) diet and oral diuretics. Options include loop diuretics, such as furosemide 1 to 2 mg/kg administered once or twice daily or a thiazide diuretic. The duration of action of diuretic agents may be diminished secondary to hypoalbuminemia and enhanced renal clearance, but this is rarely clinically significant because the medications are only needed for 1 to 2 weeks until treatment response occurs and proteinuria resolves. Children who have frequent relapses and persistent edema are at risk for bacterial peritonitis and can be given prophylactic penicillin. Immunization with the pneumococcal vaccine is also helpful under these circumstances. If feasible, the timing of vaccine administration should be delayed for at least 2 weeks after administration of prednisone to ensure maximal immunologic response.

PROGNOSIS

The prognosis for patients with MCD is excellent, and, according to the literature, the disease eventually resolves without further relapses in >95% of patients. However, this presumed benign course is based on scarce data of patients followed into adulthood. A recent study of 42 adult patients, median age 28 years, who were monitored for a median of 22 years after the diagnosis of MCD, demonstrated that 33% were still relapsing in adulthood. Children who had a relapsing course and/or required immunosuppressive medications were more likely to have persistent disease in adulthood. Moreover, although final height was normal, nearly half of adult patients with relapsing MCD have excess weight gain, hypertension, cataracts, osteoporosis, and sperm abnormalities. Whether MCD has any long-term effect on the incidence or age at onset of cardiovascular disease in adults remains unclear. Clinical outcomes in patients enrolled in large health maintenance organizations indicate that persistent NS is associated with an increased incidence of atherosclerotic disease, and the relative risk in patients with MCD versus more refractory forms of idiopathic NS requires further study. Based on the persistence beyond childhood of relapsing disease and the development of serious side effects, transition from a pediatric to an adult nephrologist is warranted in patients with relapsing MCD or a history of prolonged steroid or immunosuppressive drug use for MCD as they reach adulthood.

The overwhelming majority of children with MCD have no evidence of progressive chronic kidney disease. Recognizing that the diagnosis of FSGS can be difficult to establish if a kidney biopsy specimen does not include the few abnormal glomeruli at the corticomedullary junction, it is conceivable that the rare cases of presumed MCD with a poor outcome and progressive GFR loss may represent unidentified FSGS.

CONCLUSION

Although MCD is not a common illness, it causes short-term morbidity related to edema and infection. Initial treatment with corticosteroids results in remission of proteinuria in nearly all patients; however, 90% of patients will manifest a frequently relapsing or steroid-dependent course with steroid toxicity. These patients are candidates for treatment with second-line agents such as cyclophosphamide, mycophenolate mofetil, or tacrolimus. The choice of drug will vary from center to center and reflect local experience and preferences of the individual physician. The disease can persist into adulthood and can lead to chronic sequelae such as bone demineralization, atherosclerosis, and obesity. Therefore, long-term follow-up is warranted in those patients who continue to relapse and require immunosuppressive medication. Further research is needed to define better the cause of MCD, that is, the immunologic basis and/or role of podocyte protein abnormalities, so as to develop more effective treatments that can promote long-term remission without the side effects associated with current therapeutic options.

KEY BIBLIOGRAPHY

Clement LC, Avila-Casado C, Macé C, et al: Podocyte-secreted angiopoietin-like-4 mediates proteinuria in glucocorticoid-sensitive nephrotic syndrome, *Nat Med* 17:117-122, 2011.

Dijkman HBPM, Wetzels JFM, Gemnick JH, et al: Glomerular involution in children with frequently relapsing minimal change nephrotic syndrome: an unrecognized form of glomerulosclerosis? *Kidney Int* 71:44-52, 2007.

Fakhouri F, Bocqueret N, Taupin P, et al: Children with steroid-sensitive nephrotic syndrome come of age: long-term outcome, *J Pediatr* 147:202-207, 2005.

Garin EH, Diaz LN, Mu W, et al: Urinary CD80 excretion increases in idiopathic minimal-change disease, *J Am Soc Nephrol* 20:260-266, 2009.

George B, Verma R, Soofi AA, et al: Crk1/2-dependent signaling is necessary for podocyte foot process spreading in mouse models of glomerular disease, *J Clin Invest* 122:674-692, 2012.

Gulati A, Sinha A, Jordan SC, et al: Efficacy and safety of treatment with rituximab for difficult steroid-resistant and -dependent nephrotic syndrome: multicentric report, *Clin J Am Soc Nephrol* 5:2207-2212, 2010.

Kisner T, Burst V, Teschner S, et al: Rituximab treatment for adults with refractory nephrotic syndrome: a single-center experience and review of the literature, *Nephron Clin Pract* 120:c79-c85, 2012.

Kitamura A, Tsukaguchi H, Hiramoto R, et al: A familial childhood-onset relapsing nephrotic syndrome, *Kidney Int* 71:946-951, 2007.

Kyriels HA, Levtchenko EN, Wetzels JF: Long-term outcome after cyclophosphamide treatment in children with steroid-dependent and frequently relapsing minimal change nephrotic syndrome, *Am J Kidney Dis* 49:592-597, 2007.

McCarthy ET, Sharma M, Savin VJ: Factors in idiopathic nephrotic syndrome and focal segmental glomerulosclerosis, *Clin J Am Soc Nephrol* 5:2115-2121, 2010.

Mubarak M, Kazi JI, Lanewala A, et al: Pathology of idiopathic nephrotic syndrome in children: are the adolescents different from young children? *Nephrol Dial Transplant* 27:722-726, 2012.

Nachman PH, Jennette JC, Falk RJ: Primary glomerular diseases. In Brenner BM, editor: *The kidney*, ed 8, Philadelphia, 2008, W.B. Saunders Company, pp 987-1279.

Palmer SC, Nand K, Strippoli GF: Interventions for minimal change disease in adults with nephrotic syndrome, *Cochrane Database Syst Rev*(1), 2008 Jan 23. CD001537.

Sellier-Leclerc AL, Macher MA, Loirat C, et al: Rituximab efficiency in children with steroid-dependent nephrotic syndrome, *Pediatr Nephrol* 25:1109-1115, 2010.

van Husen M, Kemper MJ: New therapies in steroid-sensitive and steroid-resistant idiopathic nephrotic syndrome, *Pediatr Nephrol* 26:881-892, 2011.

Waldman M, Crew RJ, Valeri A, et al: Adult minimal-change disease: clinical characteristics, treatment, and outcomes, *Clin J Am Soc Nephrol* 2:445-453, 2007.

Wei C, El Hindi S, Li J, et al: Circulating urokinase receptor as a cause of focal segmental glomerulosclerosis, *Nat Med* 17:952-960, 2011.

Zhang L, Dai Y, Peng W, et al: Genome-wide analysis of histone H3 lysine 4 trimethylation in peripheral blood mononuclear cells of minimal change nephrotic syndrome patients, *Am J Nephrol* 30:505-513, 2009.

Zhou FD, Chen M: The renal histopathological spectrum of patients with nephrotic syndrome: an analysis of 1523 patients in a single Chinese center, *Nephrol Dial Transplant* 26:3993-3997, 2011.

Zhu L, Yu L, Wang CD, et al: Genetic effect of the NPHS2 gene variants on proteinuria in minimal change disease and immunoglobulin A nephropathy, *Nephrology* 14:728-734, 2009.

Full bibliography can be found on www.expertconsult.com.

18 Focal Segmental Glomerulosclerosis

Michelle A. Hladunewich | Carmen Avila-Casado | Debbie S. Gipson

Focal segmental glomerulosclerosis (FSGS) is a clinico-pathologic syndrome associated with glomerular injury that may be either idiopathic or secondary to one of a number of other disorders. FSGS accounts for approximately 20% of cases of idiopathic nephrotic syndrome in children and as many as 35% of cases in adults, It is also responsible for clinical cases presenting with isolated and, at times, subnephrotic-range proteinuria. FSGS is the most common pattern of idiopathic nephrotic syndrome among African Americans, and in some published series it is the most common pattern among all races. Studies in North America have documented an increased prevalence of FSGS in biopsy series. Spontaneous remission of FSGS is rare, and both untreated and treatment-resistant idiopathic FSGS frequently progress to kidney failure.

CLINICAL FEATURES AND DIAGNOSIS

FSGS is a pathologic lesion that invariably results in proteinuria ranging from asymptomatic, subnephrotic levels to severe proteinuria with nephrotic syndrome (hypoalbuminemia, hypercholesterolemia, and edema). Proteinuria in FSGS often is nonselective, including both albumin and larger macromolecules. Hypertension is common, and decreased glomerular filtration rate (GFR) is noted in approximately one third of patients at presentation. Although primarily characterized by proteinuria, both microscopic and macroscopic hematuria may be present in FSGS.

FSGS may arise as an idiopathic or primary condition as well as a secondary condition. Across the spectrum of FSGS, there is no absolute confirmatory test that can diagnose FSGS or differentiate idiopathic from secondary FSGS. Consequently, clinicians must carefully assess for potential clinical and pathologic clues with respect to the etiology of this disease. Clinically, idiopathic FSGS typically presents with nephrotic syndrome, whereas secondary FSGS may present with subnephrotic proteinuria. Typically, serum albumin levels are significantly higher, and the edema and dyslipidemia common in nephrotic syndromes less severe in secondary forms of FSGS as compared to idiopathic FSGS.

Causes of secondary FSGS include cancers, drugs, and infections as well as diseases in which prolonged hyperfiltration and intraglomerular hypertension result in glomerular scarring (Box 18.1). Such maladaptive glomerular hemodynamic alterations can arise through: (1) a reduction in the number of functioning nephrons (such as after unilateral renal agenesis, surgical ablation, oligomeganephronia, or any advanced primary kidney disease); or (2) mechanisms that place hemodynamic stress on an initially normal nephron population (as in morbid obesity, cyanotic congenital heart disease, and sickle cell anemia). Finally, both primary and secondary FSGS also must be differentiated from the nonspecific pattern of focal and segmental glomerular scarring that can follow a variety of inflammatory, proliferative, thrombotic, and hereditary conditions. Specific evaluation for cancer, drug exposure, and infections will be guided by the medical history and physical examination, including assessment for human immunodeficiency virus (HIV) infection, which is a routine component in the evaluation of incident nephrotic patients. Evaluation for genetic polymorphisms associated with FSGS will likely prove most beneficial in affected infants, individuals with a family history of FSGS or steroid-resistant nephrotic syndrome, or families with a closely linked ancestry where founder effects may increase the prevalence of autosomal recessive disorders. Notably, for many patients with FSGS who present with nephrotic syndrome, no secondary cause is identified.

PATHOGENESIS

In health, the glomerular filtration barrier functions as a highly organized, semipermeable membrane preventing the passage of the majority of proteins into the urine (Chapter 1). This barrier is composed of the glomerular basement membrane, the podocyte, and the slit diaphragm between the podocytes (Fig. 18.1). Tubular function assists with the recycling of the small amount of proteins that cross the glomerular barrier, maintaining the normal urine protein excretion less than 0.2 g daily. In FSGS, the podocytes lose their cytoarchitecture and, on biopsy specimens, appear with effaced foot processes. With progressive disease, the podocytes die, subsequently separating from the glomerulus followed by excretion in the urine. The degree of podocyte depletion appears to correlate with glomerular sclerosis. When a loss of less than 40% is observed in animal models, limited scarring and mild proteinuria is observed; however, loss of more than 40% of podocytes appears to induce significant scarring and severe proteinuria. In addition, initial podocyte injuries may be followed by a propagation of the injury to adjacent podocytes, which may cumulatively exceed these critical podocyte-loss thresholds.

The pathogenesis of the glomerular sclerosing lesions in FSGS is not completely understood, but, in recent years, the complexity of the podocyte and slit diaphragm has been partially elucidated and specific imperfections in the podocyte architectural and functional components have been identified in children and adults with defined genetic

Box 18.1   Causes of Secondary Focal Segmental Glomerulosclerosis

Genetic Polymorphisms

Nephrin (NPHS1)
Podocin (NPHS2)
α-actinin 4
WT-1
CD2-associated protein
TRPC6
SCARB2
Formin (INF2)
Mitochondrial cytopathies
APOL1

Virus Related

Human immunodeficiency virus (HIV)
Parvovirus B19

Medication or Drug-Related

Heroin
Interferon-α
Lithium
Pamidronate
Anabolic steroids

Malignancy

Hodgkin disease
Non-Hodgkin lymphoma
Plasma cell disorders

Reduced Nephron Mass and/or Hyperfiltration Injury

Oligomeganephronia
Unilateral renal agenesis
Renal dysplasia
Reflux nephropathy
Secondary to surgical or traumatic ablation
Chronic allograft nephropathy
Healed glomerulonephritis
Obesity
Chronic hypertension
Atheroembolic disease
Sickle cell disease

Adapted from the Kidney Disease: Improving Global Outcomes GN Guidelines: http://www.kdigo.org/clinical_practice_guidelines/Glomerulonephritis.php.
APOL1, Apolipoprotein L 1; *CD2*, cluster of differentiation 2; *SCARB2*, scavenger receptor class B, member 2; *TRPC6*, transient receptor potential cation channel, subfamily C; *WT-1*, Wilms tumor.

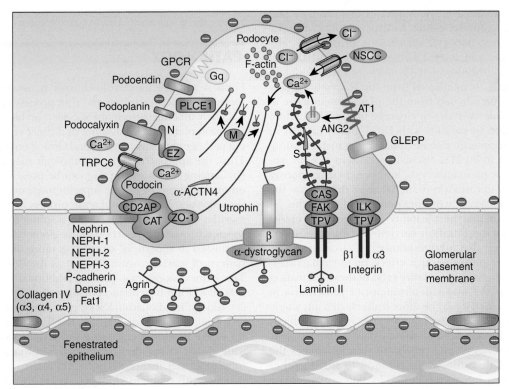

Figure 18.1   Podocyte cytoarchitecture. (Reprinted with permission from Winn MP: 2007 Young Investigator Award: TRP'ing into a new era for glomerular disease, *J Am Soc Nephrol* 19:1071-1075, 2008.)

polymorphisms. Several podocyte-associated genetic polymorphisms affecting the components of the slit diaphragm, actin cytoskeleton, cell membrane, nucleus, lysosome, mitrochronria, and cytosol have been identified (see Fig. 18.1). The frequency of these polymorphisms varies by phenotype and by ancestry. In addition, polymorphisms in the APOL1 gene have been identified as increasing the risk for FSGS in African Americans. The precise role of APOL1 in FSGS remains unknown, but early indicators suggest a role in retarding podocyte senescence.

Another major potential contributor to glomerular disease is the part of the normal circulating proteome that directly or indirectly influences glomerular function in health and disease. In FSGS, the presence of a circulating factor that results in podocyte effacement and disruption of the glomerular filtration barrier has been suggested for decades. Evidence supporting the presence of a circulating factor is derived from clinical cases that have reported virtual immediate recurrence of massive proteinuria following kidney transplantation as well as studies using animal models that have been able to demonstrate that serum from patients with FSGS can increase glomerular permeability to albumin. Using an in vitro assay, Savin and colleagues were the first to demonstrate significantly increased albumin permeability of isolated glomeruli when exposed to plasma from patients with FSGS, yet the specific molecular characteristics and mechanism of action of this permeability factor remained elusive.

Insights into podocyte biology have identified a urokinase receptor (uPAR) integral to the maintenance of the slit diaphragm through its ability to form signaling complexes with other transmembrane proteins, including lipid-dependent activation of $\alpha v \beta 3$ integrin. Activation of this receptor and its downstream pathways results in hypermotility of podocyte foot processes, podocyte effacement, proteinuria, glomerular damage, and loss of kidney function. uPAR is a glycosyl-phosphatidylinisotol (GPI)-anchored three-domain (DI, DII, and DIII, as numbered from the N terminus) protein, which can be released from the plasma membrane as a soluble molecule (suPAR) by cleavage of the GPI anchor. suPAR is elevated in patients with FSGS and is highest in patients with recurrent disease following transplantation. Further, this 20 to 50 kDa circulating protein can be partially removed by plasmapheresis, and beneficial responses can be observed in cases where suPAR levels drop below the threshold of sufficiently activating podocyte $\beta 3$ integrin.

A single circulating permeability factor may be inadequate to disrupt the filtration barrier. Accordingly, others have hypothesized that a large number of circulating proteins have pro- or antiproteinuric effects on normal glomeruli, and that changes in the relative ratio of these circulating proteins may be the major determinant of proteinuria in disease states. In fact, it may be more unlikely that any single protein would cause any specific disease. It is more likely that each specific glomerular disease has a characteristic signature in the circulating proteome that influences the pathogenesis of that disease. In addition to suPAR, other potential soluble proteins implicated in glomerular disease include Angiopoietin-like-4, vascular endothelial growth factor, and hemopexin. All are present in normal circulation and may be components of this signature rather than being individual circulating factors. Research in this area is ongoing.

Box 18.2 Morphologic Classification of Focal Segmental Glomerulosclerosis

Perihilar Variant

Perihilar sclerosis and hyalinosis in more than 50% of segmentally sclerotic glomeruli

Tip Lesion

At least one segmental, either cellular or sclerosing, lesion involving the outer 25% of the glomerulus next to the origin of the proximal tubule

Collapsing Variant

At least one glomerulus with segmental or global collapse and overlying podocyte hyperplasia

Cellular Variant

At least one glomerulus with segmental endocapillary hypercellularity occluding lumina with or without foam cells and karyorrhexis

NOS

At least one glomerulus with segmental increase in matrix obliterating capillary lumina (excludes other variants)

Modified from D'Agati VD, Fogo AB, Bruijn AJ, Jennette JC: Pathologic classification of focal segmental glomerulosclerosis: a working proposal, Am J Kidney Dis 43:368-382, 2004. NOS, Not otherwise specified.

PATHOLOGY

Focal segmental glomerulosclerosis is associated with glomerular podocyte damage and foot process effacement, and it is likely that the pattern of FSGS seen on biopsy represents a common pathway for a number of distinct entities with different pathogenetic mechanisms and clinical courses (Box 18.2). Thus, the approach to a histopathologic diagnosis of FSGS is challenging. Areas of scarring can be present in a variety of other conditions or can be superimposed on other glomerular processes. Early in the disease process, the pattern of glomerular sclerosis is *focal*, involving a subset of glomeruli, and *segmental*, involving a portion of the glomerular tuft, so it may be missed in superficial samples. A more diffuse and global pattern of scarring is usually seen as the disease progresses. The kidney biopsy may provide additional pathologic clues that allow for differentiation of idiopathic FSGS from secondary causes. In idiopathic FSGS, effacement of the podocytes is typically diffuse and extensive. In HIV-associated nephropathy, there is often a collapsing variant of glomerulosclerosis with global rather than segmental involvement along with tubuloreticular inclusions noted on electron microscopy. In patients with remnant kidneys or other forms of hyperfiltration-induced FSGS, enlarged glomeruli with patchy effacement of the foot processes is often noted (Fig. 18.2).

In an effort to classify the glomerular lesions by the location of the scarring, the Columbia classification for FSGS was defined. The five mutually exclusive histologic patterns of

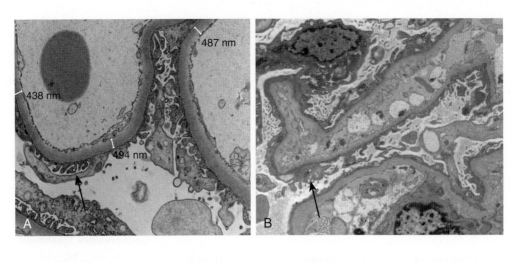

Figure 18.2 Electron microscopy of glomerulus. A, Normal glomerulus with intact foot processes. **B,** Glomerulus with diffuse foot process effacement.

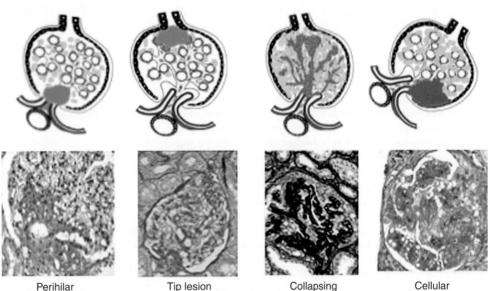

Figure 18.3 Focal segmental glomerulosclerosis histology according to the Columbia classification.

Perihilar   Tip lesion   Collapsing   Cellular

FSGS include the Perihilar Variant, Cellular Variant, Glomerular Tip Lesion, and Collapsing Variant (Fig. 18.3, see Box 18.2). If none of these features is present, the biopsy is classified as FSGS not otherwise specified (NOS). Although the appearance of the glomerular tuft differs in these forms, all share the common feature of podocyte alterations at the ultrastructural level. New insights point toward the conclusion that these morphologic variants may reflect pathogenetic differences and to some degree different causes of podocyte injury.

The morphologic classification of FSGS variants may provide prognostic information. For example, collapsing FSGS exhibits a more aggressive clinical course, with fewer remissions, more frequent kidney failure, and recurrence in the allograft following kidney transplantation, whereas the tip lesion identifies a subset of FSGS that usually responds to steroids and rarely progresses to kidney failure. The cellular lesion is the least common variant of FSGS, identified in only 3% of cases of adult idiopathic FSGS, and the condition is similarly rare in children. The prognostic significance of cellular FSGS is undetermined. The cellular, collapsing, and tip lesions all share clinical presenting features of heavier proteinuria and more frequent nephrotic syndrome compared to FSGS NOS, suggesting that these

three morphologic variants may reflect acute glomerular injury or possibly a response to heavy proteinuria. However, the prognostic value of morphologic classification of FSGS is not universally acknowledged, reflecting the inherent difficulty of accurately classifying focal patterns of injury based on pathologic examination of limited biopsy tissue and the potential for different types of lesions to coexist in individual biopsy samples.

COURSE AND THERAPY

Spontaneous remissions are rare in patients with nephrotic-range proteinuria, occurring in fewer than 5% of patients; if untreated and/or unresponsive, the disease course is typically one of progressive proteinuria and loss of kidney function. FSGS progresses to kidney failure over 6 to 8 years in 50% of patients with no appreciable difference noted in children as compared to adults. Furthermore, FSGS recurs after transplantation in approximately 30% of patients, contributing significantly to loss of graft function. A rapidly progressive course to kidney failure in the native kidneys predicts a greater risk for recurrence following kidney transplant.

Box 18.3   Risk Factors Associated With Worse Kidney Outcomes

Clinical Features
    Male gender
    African ancestry
    Massive proteinuria at presentation
    Elevated serum creatinine at presentation
    Failure to achieve a partial or complete remission
    Relapsing disease
Histopathologic Features
    Collapsing variant
    Tubulointerstitial fibrosis

Box 18.4   Treatment Options for Focal Segmental Glomerulosclerosis

Immunosuppressive Treatment Options

- Oral prednisone: 2 mg/kg/day (max 60 mg) for 6 wk and then 1 mg/kg/alternate days for 6 wk for children; 1 mg/kg/day or 2 mg/kg/alternate days for 3 to 6 mo in adults as tolerated
- Cyclosporine: 3 to 5 mg/kg/day in divided doses for 6 to 12 mo followed by a slow taper as tolerated
- Tacrolimus: 0.2 to 0.3 mg/kg/day in divided doses for 6 to 12 mo followed by a slow taper as tolerated
- MMF: 25 to 35 mg/kg/day in divided doses (max 2 g/day) ± dexamethasone

Conservative Treatment Strategies

- Blockade of the RAAS
- Treatment of hypertension (target BP less than 130/80 mm Hg)
- Statin therapy for hypercholesterolemia
- Diuretics for edema
- Dietary strategies
  - Protein restriction
  - Salt restriction
  - Restricted cholesterol intake
- Anticoagulation in select cases (low serum albumin ± immobilization)

BP, Blood pressure; *MMF*, mycophenolate mofetil; *RAAS*, renin angiotensin aldosterone system.

The presence of genetic polymorphisms is associated with a lower risk for posttransplant recurrence compared with other causes of primary FSGS, but is also suggestive of a lesser opportunity for response to immunomodulating therapy. However partial responses to immunosuppression have been described in children and adults with FSGS-associated genetic polymorphisms.

A number of clinical and histologic features can be informative with respect to predicting disease course (Box 18.3). Female gender appears to be protective, with both slower progression as well as a higher likelihood of a partial or complete remission as compared to men, whereas African ancestry predicts a more aggressive course and, as mentioned previously, recent insights suggest that genetic factors may help explain this predisposition to progressive FSGS (APOL1 gene variants). Severe nephrotic-range proteinuria (greater than 10 g/24 h), impaired kidney function, and increased tubulointerstitial damage on kidney biopsy at the time of presentation all portend a poor prognosis. As mentioned earlier, the collapsing variant is also associated with more rapid progression, whereas the "tip" lesion, which tends to be responsive to immunosuppression, has a better prognosis. During the course of treatment of FSGS, absence of any response to immunosuppressive therapy is the strongest predictor of kidney failure, whereas complete remission of the nephrotic syndrome with normalization of urine protein excretion confers the best prognosis. However, even a partial response to treatment significantly delays progression and is therefore an acceptable treatment goal. Relapse is common (greater than 50%) and is subsequently associated with more rapid progression and poor kidney survival.

The treatment of primary or idiopathic FSGS is controversial because of the paucity of randomized, controlled trials and the lack of effective, well-tolerated treatment options. In patients with nephrotic syndrome, immunosuppression may improve proteinuria and slow progression to kidney failure, but side effects associated with current treatment options, including high doses and prolonged courses of corticosteroids, cytotoxic agents, and calcineurin inhibitors, are significant, and treatment failure and relapses are common. Immunosuppression typically is not used in primary FSGS with subnephrotic-range proteinuria or in FSGS with a suspected secondary cause; conservative management principles, which target symptoms, are preferred (Box 18.4).

Prednisone is the first line of therapy in children and many adults, largely based on data from observational cohorts. The dose and duration of therapy is not clear and therefore has varied widely across clinical centers. Both daily steroid regimens and alternate day regimens have been used. On average, a response in seen within 3 to 4 months, although adults can take much longer to respond. Thus, although the minimum requirement of corticosteroid exposure to define lack of response and resistance remains unclear, many practitioners would define steroid resistance as 3 to 4 months of therapy without significant improvement in urine protein. Among children, 20% to 25% experience a complete remission with corticosteroids. Response rates in adults are lower, and intolerance to steroid therapy tends to be more significant, especially in the presence of advanced age and comorbid conditions such as obesity and diabetes. Steroid resistance, even with prolonged treatment, occurs in more than 50% of adult patients. Prolonged courses of high-dose steroids can result in significant side effects including, but not limited to, cataracts, skin thinning, acne, diabetes, osteoporosis/osteonecrosis, and weight gain regardless of age.

Cytotoxic agents have been used with success in children with relapsing and remitting disease and in adults who have demonstrated at least a partial response to prednisone therapy; however, these agents carry significant immediate and long-term risks including infection, propensity to late onset malignancy, and infertility. Thus, in patients with steroid resistance or intolerance, calcineurin inhibitors have emerged as the therapeutic choice in many centers. In a multicenter, prospective randomized controlled trial, patients with steroid-resistant FSGS were randomized to continue on low-dose prednisone either alone or in combination with cyclosporine. The therapy was continued for 26 weeks and then tapered over 4 weeks. The response rate in the cyclosporine-treated patients exceeded 70%, but relapses after discontinuation of therapy were common, exceeding 50%. In a larger randomized trial conducted over 12 months, only 46% of participants experienced a combined complete and partial remission in response to cyclosporine, and 33% relapsed following discontinuation of cyclosporine. In smaller studies, similar rates of complete and partial remission in patients with steroid-resistant or steroid-dependent nephrotic syndrome are seen for tacrolimus and cyclosporine; accordingly, tacrolimus can be considered an alternative calcineurin inhibitor. Calcineurin inhibitors should be used with caution in patients with significant vascular or interstitial disease noted on kidney biopsy and in patients who have an estimated GFR of less than 40 mL/min/1.73 m^2, because of the potential to cause nephrotoxicity, hyperkalemia, and hypertension.

Other therapeutic options include mycophenolate mofetil (MMF), sirolimus, and rituximab. A randomized controlled trial of children and adults with steroid-resistant FSGS showed that the combination of a 12-month course of MMF with high-dose dexamethasone induced a 33% combined partial and complete remission. Following discontinuation of the MMF and dexamethasone, 18% relapsed, demonstrating only a modest improvement with prolonged dexamethasone exposure and MMF. Case reports noting improvement in FSGS with sirolimus exist, but this drug has been clearly associated with worsening kidney function as well as new-onset de novo FSGS in kidney allografts and therefore may have considerable side effects in patients with preexisting proteinuria. To date, evidence that rituximab might prove effective in patients with FSGS is limited. Although success has been noted in select cases, results have been mixed in patients with either idiopathic FSGS or recurrent FSGS following kidney transplantation. Finally, plasma exchange has been successful in treating some patients with recurrent FSGS in a kidney allograft, and perhaps novel insights into circulating factors might identify patients with native kidney disease wherein this modality may prove particularly useful.

For patients with secondary forms of FSGS, treatment of the primary disorder is the first step in management. Resolution of proteinuria has been documented after discontinuation of culprit drugs or medications as well as after successful treatment of cancer, treatment of HIV with antiretroviral therapy, or cardiac transplant in individuals with FSGS induced by cyanotic heart disease. Some patients with FSGS secondary to obesity have had remissions of proteinuria after weight reduction, including following bariatric surgery. In diseases where there is decreased kidney mass and hyperfiltration, immunosuppression is not indicated; however, in patients with these secondary forms as well is in patients with primary FSGS of any severity, blockers of the renin-angiotensin-aldosterone system should be used to reduce proteinuria, decrease intraglomerular pressure, and prolong kidney survival. Additionally, attention should be paid to controlling hypertension to optimal levels (likely less than 130/80 mm Hg in proteinuric

adults and less than 50% in children) to reduce the rate of progression to kidney failure and to limit the risk for future cardiovascular morbidity. Control of dyslipidemia with diet and pharmacologic therapy is recommended, and fluid retention and edema may be improved with salt restriction and diuretics. Although the risk of venous thromboembolism is highest in patients with membranous nephropathy, patients with FSGS are also at substantially increased risk of venous thromboembolism, such that anticoagulation may be warranted in select patients with low serum albumin levels.

BIBLIOGRAPHY

Barbour SJ, Greenwald A, Djurdjev O, et al: Disease-specific risk of venous thromboembolic events is increased in idiopathic glomerulonephritis, *Kidney Int* 81:190-195, 2012.

Cattran DC, Appel GB, Hebert LA, et al: A randomized trial of cyclosporine in patients with steroid-resistant focal segmental glomerulosclerosis. North America Nephrotic syndrome study group, *Kidney Int* 56:2220-2226, 1999.

Clement LC, Avila-Casado C, Mace C, et al: Podocyte-secreted angiopoietin-like-4 mediates proteinuria in glucocorticoid-sensitive nephrotic syndrome, *Nat Med* 17:117-122, 2011.

Gipson DS, Chin H, Presler TP, et al: Differential risk of remission and ESRD in childhood FSGS, *Pediatr Nephrol* 21:344-349, 2006.

Gipson DS, Trachtman H, Kaskel FJ, et al: Clinical trial of focal segmental glomerulosclerosis in children and young adults, *Kidney Int* 80:868-878, 2011.

Gohh RY, Yango AF, Morrissey PE, et al: Preemptive plasmapheresis and recurrence of FSGS in high-risk renal transplant recipients, *Am J Transplant* 5:2907-2912, 2005.

Haas M, Spargo BH, Coventry S: Increasing incidence of focal-segmental glomerulosclerosis among adult nephropathies: a 20-year renal biopsy study, *Am J Kidney Dis* 26:740-750, 1995.

Kambham N, Markowitz GS, Valeri AM, et al: Obesity-related glomerulopathy: an emerging epidemic, *Kidney Int* 59:1498-1509, 2001.

Kopp JB, Nelson GW, Sampath K, et al: APOL1 genetic variants in focal segmental glomerulosclerosis and HIV-associated nephropathy, *J Am Soc Nephrol* 22:2129-2137, 2011.

Lowik MM, Groenen PJ, Levtchenko EN, et al: Molecular genetic analysis of podocyte genes in focal segmental glomerulosclerosis—a review, *Eur J Pediatr* 168:1291-1304, 2009.

McCarthy ET, Sharma M, Savin VJ: Circulating permeability factors in idiopathic nephrotic syndrome and focal segmental glomerulosclerosis, *Clin J Am Soc Nephrol* 5:2115-2121, 2010.

Ostalska-Nowicka D, Malinska A, Zabel M, et al: Nephrotic syndrome unfavorable course correlates with downregulation of podocyte vascular endothelial growth factor receptor (VEGFR)-2, *Folia histochemica et cytobiologica / Polish Academy of Sciences, Polish Histochemical and Cytochemical Society* 49:472-478, 2011.

Rydel JJ, Korbet SM, Borok RZ, et al: Focal segmental glomerular sclerosis in adults: presentation, course, and response to treatment, *Am J Kidney Dis* 25:534-542, 1995.

Sato Y, Wharram BL, Lee SK, et al: Urine podocyte mRNAs mark progression of renal disease, *J Am Soc Nephrol* 20:1041-1052, 2009.

Sharma M, Sharma R, McCarthy ET, et al: The focal segmental glomerulosclerosis permeability factor: biochemical characteristics and biological effects, *Exp Biol Med* 229:85-98, 2004.

Suthar K, Vanikar AV, Trivedi HL: Renal transplantation in primary focal segmental glomerulosclerosis using a tolerance induction protocol, *Transplant Proc* 40:1108-1110, 2008.

Thomas DB, Franceschini N, Hogan SL, et al: Clinical and pathologic characteristics of focal segmental glomerulosclerosis pathologic variants, *Kidney Int* 69:920-926, 2006.

Troyanov S, Wall CA, Miller JA, et al: Focal and segmental glomerulosclerosis: definition and relevance of a partial remission, *J Am Soc Nephrol* 16:1061-1068, 2005.

Wei C, El Hindi S, Li J, et al: Circulating urokinase receptor as a cause of focal segmental glomerulosclerosis, *Nat Med* 17:952-960, 2011.

Winn MP: 2007 Young Investigator Award: TRP'ing into a new era for glomerular disease, *J Am Soc Nephrol* 19:1071-1075, 2008.

19 Membranous Nephropathy

Daniel C. Cattran | Fernando C. Fervenza

Membranous nephropathy (MN) remains the most common histologic entity associated with adult-onset nephrotic syndrome in Caucasians. This histologic pattern is more properly called nephropathy than nephritis, because there is rarely any inflammatory response in the glomeruli or interstitium (i.e., no nephritis). In the past, the majority of cases were termed idiopathic; however, recent studies have shown that antibodies to the M-type phospholipase–A$_2$-receptor (PLA$_2$R) are present in approximately 70% of patients with MN, and in these cases the nephropathy should be called primary MN. In the other 20% to 30%, when a defined causative agent can be determined, the disease is categorized as secondary (Table 19.1). The idiopathic designation is made by exclusion and should be reserved for patients who are anti-PLA$_2$R negative and for whom a causative agent cannot be determined.

The list of known secondary causes of MN in Table 19.1 is not complete but provides an indication of the variety of disorders that have been seen in association with this histologic pattern. In some, such as hepatitis B or thyroiditis, the specific antigen has been identified as part of the immune complex within the deposits in the glomeruli. In others, the association is less well defined, but the designation remains, because treatment of the underlying condition or removal of the putative agent results in resolution of the clinical and histologic features of the disease.

The clinical manifestations of both primary and secondary MN are similar. Hence a careful history, laboratory evaluation, and review of histologic features must be pursued to rule out potential secondary causes. Ongoing vigilance is also necessary, because the causative agent may not be obvious for months or even years after presentation. MN is rare in children, and, when found, careful screenings for immunologically mediated disorders, especially systemic lupus erythematosus (SLE), are necessary. More recently, high levels of circulating anti-bovine serum albumin (BSA) antibodies, of both IgG1 and IgG4 subclasses, have been reported in children and adults with MN. BSA immunopurified from the serum of children migrated in the basic range of pH, whereas the BSA from adult patients migrated in the neutral region as native BSA. BSA staining colocalized with IgG immune deposits only in four children with circulating cationic BSA, but in none of the adults patients with MN for whom biopsy specimens were available, implying that only cationic BSA can induce MN. Thus, in children, the diagnosis of MN should raise the possibility of BSA-induced MN. In the older patient, neoplasms are the most common cause of secondary MN. There are also marked geographic differences in etiology. In Africa for instance, malaria is a common cause, and, in the Far East, hepatitis B. Universal hepatitis B vaccination has greatly reduced childhood MN associated with hepatitis B.

CLINICAL FEATURES

Membranous nephropathy presents in 60% to 70% of cases with features associated with the nephrotic syndrome, such as edema, proteinuria greater than 3.5 g/day, hypoalbuminemia, and hypercholesterolemia. The other 30% to 40% of cases present with asymptomatic proteinuria, usually in the subnephrotic range (≤3.5 g/day). This variant is commonly found on urine testing performed as part of a routine physical examination. The majority of patients present with normal glomerular filtration rate, specifically a normal serum creatinine and creatinine clearance, but about 10% have diminished kidney function. The urine sediment is often bland, but 30% to 40% have microscopic hematuria and 10% to 20% have granular casts. Hypertension is uncommon at presentation, occurring in only 10% to 20% of cases. The clinical features associated with nephrotic range proteinuria in MN can be severe. Patients with MN almost always have ankle swelling, but ascites, pleural, and rarely pericardial effusions may also be present. This pattern is particularly common in the elderly, and, unless a urinalysis is performed, these symptoms may be incorrectly labeled as signs of primary cardiac failure. Complications of MN include thromboembolic events and hyperlipidemia. A recent study showed that clinically apparent venous thromboembolic events are relatively infrequent, affecting about 8% of patients. In this study, renal vein thrombosis accounted for 30% of the thromboembolic events. This frequency is substantially lower than that previously reported in studies that used systematic screening for thromboembolic events. Secondary hyperlipidemia is also common and is characterized by both an increase in total and low-density lipoprotein (LDL) cholesterol and often a decrease in high-density lipoproteins (HDLs). This is a profile known to be associated with accelerated atherogenesis.

PATHOLOGY

In early MN, the glomeruli appear normal by light microscopy. Increasing size and number of immune complexes in the subepithelial space produce a thickening as well as a rigid appearance of the normally lacy-looking glomerular basement membrane (GBM) on light microscopy (Fig. 19.1). Over time, new basement membrane is formed around the immune complexes (deposits do not stain), producing

Table 19.1   Secondary Causes of Membranous Nephropathy

Etiology	Examples
Neoplasm	Carcinomas, especially solid organ (tumors of the lung, colon, breast, and kidney), leukemia, and non-Hodgkin's lymphoma
Infections	Malaria, hepatitis B and C, secondary or congenital syphilis, leprosy
Drugs	Penicillamine, gold
Immunologic	Systemic lupus erythematosus, mixed connective tissue disease, thyroiditis, dermatitis herpetiformis
Post kidney transplant	Recurrent disease, de novo membranous nephropathy
Miscellaneous	Sickle cell anemia
Bovine serum albumin	In children

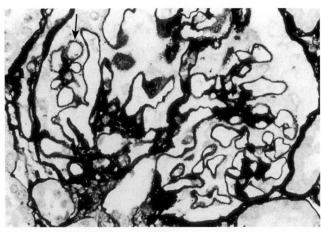

Figure 19.2   Classic spike pattern along glomerular basement membrane as it grows around deposits *(arrow)* (periodic acid-Schiff, original magnification ×400).

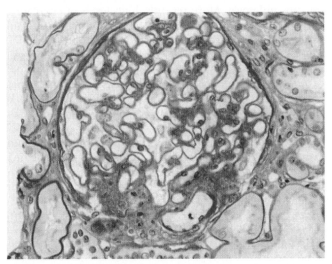

Figure 19.1   Glomerulus from a patient with membranous nephropathy. Capillary walls are diffusely thickened, and there is no increase in mesangial cells or matrix (periodic acid-Schiff, original magnification ×250).

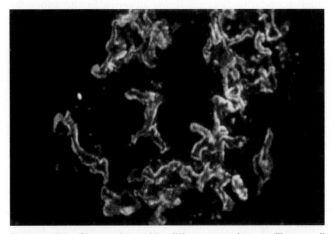

Figure 19.3   Glomerulus with diffuse granular capillary wall staining with anti-IgG antibody (immunofluorescence microscopy, original magnification ×250).

the spikes along the epithelial side of the basement membrane, which are particularly well visualized when using the silver methenamine stains (Fig. 19.2). In contrast, on immunofluorescence microscopy, these immune complexes do stain, most commonly with antihuman immunoglobulin G (IgG) and complement (Fig. 19.3). This produces a beaded appearance along the GBM (capillary wall), a pattern that is pathognomonic of MN on immunofluorescence. In the most extreme cases, this beading can become so dense that careful examination is required to distinguish it from a linear pattern. On electron microscopy, these deposits are initially formed in the subepithelial space (Fig. 19.4). A classification system has been developed based on their specific location on electron microscopic examination. In stage I, the deposits are located only on the surface of the GBM in the subepithelial location without evidence of new basement membrane formation; in stage II, the deposits are partially surrounded by new basement membrane; in stage III, they are surrounded and incorporated into the basement

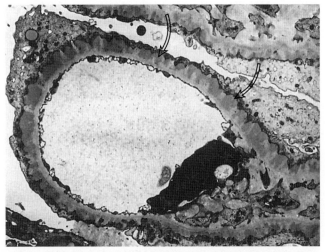

Figure 19.4   Electron photomicrograph of capillary loop with multiple electron-dense deposits along the subepithelial side of the glomerular basement membrane *(arrows)* (original magnification ×7500).

membrane; and in stage IV, the capillary walls are diffusely thickened, but rarefaction (lucent) zones are seen in intramembranous areas previously occupied by the deposits. Unfortunately, the clinical and laboratory correlations with these stages are poor. In some individual cases of MN, the electron microscopic pattern appears as if there had been waves of complex deposition with all of the preceding stages present in the same glomerulus, whereas in others cases the deposits appear as if there had been a continuous production of complexes with the deposit growing in size over time, producing lesions that are all at a similar stage and that can extend from the surface of the subepithelial space and penetrate all the way through the basement membrane.

Although a specific cause cannot usually be determined by standard pathology, there are some features that are helpful in identifying a secondary cause of MN. Features in favor of a secondary cause, in particular an autoimmune disease, include: (1) proliferative features—mesangial or endocapillary, (2) full-house pattern of Ig staining (G, M, and A) including staining for C1q on immunofluorescence microscopy, (3) electron dense deposits in the subendothelial location of the capillary wall and mesangium, or along the tubular basement membrane and vessel walls, and (4) endothelial tubuloreticular inclusions on electron microscopy. Electron microscopy showing only few superficial scattered subepithelial deposits may suggest a drug associated secondary MN. Additional diagnostic value may be obtained by staining renal biopsies for IgG subclasses. IgG1, IgG2, and IgG3 tend to be expressed in lupus MN, whereas IgG1 and IgG4 tend to be more commonly expressed in primary MN.

PATHOGENESIS

Until recently, most of our understanding of the pathogenic mechanisms was derived from experimental models in rats, that is, the Heymann nephritis model. In this model, megalin is the podocyte antigen involved; however, megalin is neither expressed in human podocytes nor detected in the subepithelial deposits in patients with idiopathic/primary MN. Thus, for years the MN target in human podocytes remained elusive. Thanks to modern technology, major advances have occurred in our understanding of the autoimmune processes involved in the development of human MN.

The first breakthrough involved a case report of a patient with neonatal MN caused by the transplacental transfer of circulating antineutral endopeptidase antibodies to the fetus. Neutral endopeptidase (NEP) is a membrane-bound enzyme that is able to digest biologically active peptides and is expressed on the surface of human podocytes, syncytiotrophoblastic cells, lymphoid progenitors, and many other epithelial cells as well as polymorphonuclear leukocytes. Mothers with truncating mutations of the metallomembrane endopeptidase (MME) gene fail to express NEP on cell membranes. NEP-deficient mothers, who were immunized during pregnancy, were able to transplacentally transfer nephritogenic antibodies against NEP to their children, causing MN in the newborns. The fact that rabbits injected with the maternal IgG from these mothers also developed MN was additional proof that the disease was related to circulating

anti-NEP antibodies and was a demonstration of a human counterpart to Heymann nephritis. Subsequent to this discovery, antibodies to the M-type phospholipase–A_2-receptor (PLA$_2$R) were found to be present in approximately 70% of adult patients with MN and a lesser proportion of affected children. These antibodies are not present in the serum of healthy controls, although it remains unclear if these antibodies are specific for primary MN, because low antibody levels have been reported in patients with secondary MN. Levels of anti-PLA$_2$R have more recently been found to correlate with the disease activity: i.e., disappearance of the antibody has been associated with remission of proteinuria whereas reappearance of the antibody has heralded a relapse of nephrotic syndrome. It is hoped that commercially available kits that robustly measure such antibodies will eventually be helpful in distinguishing primary from secondary MN and monitoring response to therapy. This may be especially relevant if these changes in antibody are proven to precede the changes in proteinuria, although how specifically these antibodies lead to the development of proteinuria remains unknown. More recently, high levels of circulating anti-bovine serum albumin antibodies, of both IgG1 and IgG4 subclasses, have been reported in children with MN. The mechanism of BSA-induced MN in these patients is still unclear.

Single-nucleotide polymorphisms (SNPs) in the genes encoding M-type PLA$_2$R and HLA complex class II HLA-DQ alpha chain 1 (HLA-DQA1) have also been reported in Caucasian populations with MN. The risk for primary MN was significantly higher with both the HLA-DQ1 allele and with the PLA$_2$R1 allele, adding a potential pathogenic link between the susceptibility to developing MN in people with these genetic findings and the presence of MN disease in patients with circulating antibodies to anti-PLA$_2$R.

DIAGNOSIS

Membranous nephropathy is a diagnosis based on histology. Primary/idiopathic and secondary forms have similar clinical presentations. As such, secondary MN should be ruled out by careful history, physical, and laboratory examinations, aided by features on pathology. Investigations should include the appropriate screening tests such as a complement profile, assays for antinuclear antibodies, rheumatoid factor, hepatitis B surface antigen and hepatitis C antibody, thyroid antibodies, and cryoglobulins. Malignancy was associated with MN in ≤20% of cases presenting in those older than 60 years. More recent epidemiological data suggest that the standardized incidence ratio of malignancy in MN is in the range of 2 to 3 in all age groups and is independent of the sex of the patient; however, because the absolute incidence of malignancies in younger people is lower, extensive testing for malignancy is not usually performed unless there are clinical clues suggesting malignancy. In contrast, patients who present with MN who are more than 60 years of age should receive a focused history and physical examination, with the clinician looking for an occult tumor. The evaluation should consist of most age-appropriate screening tests, including colon cancer screening, mammography in women, potentially a prostate-specific antigen assay in men, and a chest radiograph (or, in patients with risk factor for lung cancer, chest computed tomography). The precise cost benefit of this additional screening in the absence of symptoms remains unknown.

TREATMENT OF SECONDARY TYPES

In the secondary types of MN, attention should be focused on removing the putative agent or treating the underlying cause. If this can be done successfully, both the histopathology and the clinical manifestations typically resolve with time.

NATURAL HISTORY AND TREATMENT OF PRIMARY/IDIOPATHIC MEMBRANOUS NEPHROPATHY

The natural history of primary/idiopathic MN has been documented in several studies and must be understood before considering specific treatment. Spontaneous complete remissions in proteinuria occur in 20% to 30% of patients with primary/idiopathic MN, whereas progressive kidney failure develops in 20% to 40% of cases after more than 5 to 15 years of observation. In the remaining patients, mild to moderate proteinuria persists. A summary review of 11 large studies demonstrated a 10-year kidney survival rate of 65% to 85%, whereas a more recently pooled analysis of 32 reports indicated a 15-year kidney survival rate of 60%. Complicating the understanding of the natural history is the fact that primary/idiopathic MN often follows a spontaneous remitting and relapsing course. Spontaneous complete remission rates have been reported in 20% to 30% of long-term (greater than 10 years) follow-up studies, with 20% to 50% of these cases exhibiting at least one relapse. A complete remission and a lower relapse rate are more common in patients with persistent low-grade (subnephrotic) proteinuria and in women. In contrast, male gender, age greater than 50 years, high levels of proteinuria (more than 6 g/day), abnormal kidney function at presentation, and tubulointerstitial disease including focal and segmental lesions on biopsy have all been associated with poorer kidney survival rates.

PREDICTING OUTCOME

A semiquantitative method of predicting outcome has been developed and validated. This model takes into consideration the initial creatinine clearance (CrCl), the slope of the CrCl, and the lowest level of proteinuria during a 6-month observation period. This risk score assessment includes good performance characteristics and has been validated in two geographically diverse MN populations, one from Italy and the other from Finland. In its simplest form, the risk score assessment demonstrated that the overall accuracy of predicting patient outcomes was greatly improved compared to nephrotic range proteinuria alone at presentation when proteinuria values during 6-month time frames were monitored. If the proteinuria was consistently ≥4 g/day, its overall accuracy was 71%; if ≥6 g/day, 79%; and when ≥8 g/day, 84%. If the patient had lower than normal estimated

creatinine clearance at the beginning of these periods, or deteriorating kidney function during the 6 months of observation, the odds of progressing were higher. Based on this model, patients who present with a normal CrCl, proteinuria ≤4 g/24 h, and stable kidney function over a 6-month observation period have an excellent long-term prognosis and are classified at low risk of progression. Patients with normal kidney function and whose CrCl remains unchanged during 6 months of observation, but who continue to have proteinuria greater than 4 g but less than 8 g/24 h, have a 55% probability of developing later stage chronic kidney disease and are classified at medium risk of progression, and patients with persistent proteinuria greater than 8 g/24 h, independent of the degree of kidney function impairment, have a 66% to 80% probability of progression to kidney failure within 10 years and are classified in the high risk of progression category (Box 19.1). The advantages of the algorithm are that it only requires standard measurements of kidney function plus its dynamic nature; the risk can be calculated by measuring creatinine clearance and 24-hour urine protein estimates; and the risk can be calculated repeatedly during the period of follow-up of the patient. The issues of age, gender, degree of nephrosclerosis, and hypertension are relevant but are not necessary in this model, because they do not add to its predictive ability. A different approach to outcome prediction also has been developed. It uses urinary excretion rates of large-molecular-weight proteins, such as the urinary excretion of IgG that may reflect glomerular injury, and the approach can be combined with measuring the urinary excretion rates of small-weight proteins such as β2-microglobulin that may reflect damaged tubular cells. The measurements of these protein species excretion rates above certain levels have also predicted both treatment responsiveness and kidney survival. Unfortunately, quantification of urinary α1-microglobulin, β2-microglobulin, IgM, and IgG is not widely available, thus limiting their clinical use, and more recent studies have not supported their advantages over monitoring total proteinuria alone.

It is on this natural history background that our current therapies must be evaluated. One helpful framework is to establish "risk of progression" categories based on the algorithm that relates initial creatinine clearance, as well as quantity of proteinuria and change in function over a 6-month time frame, to outcome. We can then examine the

---

Box 19.1   Risk for Progression Categories

1. Patients with low risks for progression have normal serum creatinine and creatinine clearance estimates and proteinuria of less than 4 g/day during 6 months of observation.
2. Medium-risk patients have normal or near normal creatinine and creatinine clearance estimates and persistent proteinuria during 6 months of between 4 and 8 g/day.
3. High-risk patients include those with high-grade proteinuria (≥8 g/day) persistent during 3 to 6 months and/or creatinine clearance estimates declining during this observation period.
4. In addition, the finding of a urinary IgG excretion rate greater than 250 mg/24 h and/or a urinary β2-microglobulin greater than 0.5 mcg/min is associated with a higher likelihood of progressive MN disease.

laboratory data at entry of the patient into the major clinical trials available and segregate the patients into these risk groups. The treatment benefits in preventing progression compared to the risk associated with treatment are then easier to assess. This is important, because most of our current immunosuppressive routines have potentially significant adverse effects, and these, rather than the symptoms of the disease, are often the overriding concern of both physicians and patients when managing this disease.

RESPONSE GOALS

What the treatment target should be has been debated for some time. Obviously the best target would be a permanent state of complete remission (less than 0.2 g/day of proteinuria), but this only occurs with our current approaches in 30% to 50% of cases, even combining those that occur spontaneously with those that respond to specific drug treatment. However, there is now good evidence that an appropriate and valid target is the achievement of a state of partial remission (less than 3.5 g/day and a 50% reduction from peak proteinuria). Achieving a partial remission is associated with both a very significant slowing in the rate of kidney disease progression as well as a doubling of kidney survival at 10 years when compared to patients who did not experience remission.

TREATMENT

Treatment can be considered in four broad categories:

1. Nonspecific, nonimmunosuppressive therapy focused on reducing proteinuria and perhaps secondarily slowing the progression rate of the kidney disease.
2. Treatment focused on the secondary effects of the disease.
3. Immunosuppressive therapy aimed at slowing or stopping the immune-mediated component of the disease.
4. Treatment prophylaxis aimed at reducing the complications of the immunosuppressive drugs.

Of note, recent preliminary data suggest that the presence of very high levels of the circulating autoantibody to PLA2R is associated with a poor prognosis.

NONSPECIFIC, NONIMMUNOSUPPRESSIVE THERAPY

Nonspecific, nonimmunosuppressive treatment involves restricting dietary sodium to less than 2 g/day, restricting protein intake, and controlling blood pressure, hyperlipidemia, and edema; this treatment is applicable to all patients with MN. Blood pressure reduction has been shown to reduce proteinuria and should be part of the management from the time of diagnosis. Angiotensin-converting enzyme (ACE) inhibitors yield improvement in proteinuria beyond that expected by their antihypertensive action alone, and, unless there is a specific contraindication, they should be the first line of therapy in all cases even when the blood pressure is not significantly elevated. Similar results from angiotensin receptor blockers (ARBs) have been seen in

other proteinuric diseases and should be considered if problems arise with the use of ACE inhibitors. Data on dual ACE inhibitors-ARB therapy in patients with heavy proteinuria, including those with MN, are currently insufficient to draw conclusions. Although dietary protein restriction has never been associated with a complete remission of the nephrotic syndrome, it does result in lower levels of proteinuria; however, this needs to be balanced with the risk for malnutrition.

TREATMENT OF THE SECONDARY EFFECTS OF THE DISEASE

In addition to the efforts to reduce proteinuria and prevent kidney failure, attention must be directed to the associated hyperlipidemia and the increased risks for thromboembolism in patients with primary/idiopathic MN. Patients with nephrotic syndrome have elevated serum cholesterol and triglycerides and normal or low levels of HDL and increased LDL. This hyperlipidemia probably plays a role in the increased risk for cardiovascular disease in patients with prolonged high-grade proteinuria. Although no trial has been conducted to determine if cholesterol lowering reduces the risk for cardiovascular disease in such patients, most clinicians apply evidence from patients without kidney disease to promote the use of HMG CoA (3-hydroxy-3-methylglutaryl coenzyme A) reductase inhibitors in patients with primary/ idiopathic MN and persistent high-grade proteinuria. A recent metaanalysis showed a small benefit on proteinuria reduction, although no beneficial effect on GFR with the use of HMG CoA reductase inhibitors in these proteinuric conditions. Management of dyslipidemia in CKD is more fully discussed in Chapter 56. Studies of the risk for thrombotic disease in primary/idiopathic MN have shown a wide variation in prevalence. This is partly related to the rigor of screening (all patients vs. the selection of high-risk patients) and partly to the detection methods used. A study showed that clinically apparent venous thromboembolic events occurred in approximately 7% of patients with primary/ idiopathic MN. In this study, a serum albumin level less than 2.8 g/dl was the most significant independent predictor of venous thromboembolism. No consensus has emerged as to whether prophylactic anticoagulation should be used in this disease. A majority of physicians use this therapy as primary prevention only in high-risk cases or they reserve its use until after documentation of a thromboembolic event. A positive family history, previous thrombotic event before the patient was known to have MN, prolonged serum albumin levels less than 2 g/dl, bedridden status, or obesity are indicators that should prompt consideration for the earlier use of prophylactic anticoagulation. The precise mechanism of the hypercoagulable state observed in MN is unclear, although a variety of factors do converge that heighten the thrombotic risk, including a local decrease in perfusion pressure in the renal vein from the lowered oncotic pressure, loss of clotting factors in the urine, increased hepatic production of clotting factors, and perhaps even a genetic predisposition to clot.

SPECIFIC IMMUNOSUPPRESSION TREATMENT

LOW RISK FOR PROGRESSION

The prognosis for patients with proteinuria ≤4 g/day and with normal kidney function is excellent. In a series of more than 300 cases from three distinct geographic regions followed for greater than 5 years, fewer than 8% went on to develop a measurable decrease in kidney function. Normalization of blood pressure and reduction of protein excretion through the use of agents such as ACE inhibitors or ARBs should be used. Because some patients do progress, long-term follow-up should include regular measurements of blood pressure, kidney function, and proteinuria. Immunosuppression therapy is not recommended as long as the patient remains in the low-risk for progression category. Approximately 50% of patients who present with nonnephrotic proteinuria in MN will eventually progress to nephrotic range proteinuria. In the great majority of cases (70%), this will occur in the first year after the diagnostic kidney biopsy.

MEDIUM RISK FOR PROGRESSION

There is evidence for a treatment benefit when corticosteroids are combined with a cytotoxic agent. In a series of randomized trials in Italy, a significant increase in both partial and complete remission in proteinuria and long-term improved kidney survival at 10 years were seen after an initial 6-month course of corticosteroids and chlorambucil treatment. Therapy consisted of 1 g of intravenous methylprednisolone on the first 3 days of months 1, 3, and 5, followed by 27 days of oral methylprednisolone at 0.4 mg/kg, alternating in months 2, 4, and 6 with chlorambucil at 0.2 mg/kg/day. This therapeutic routine was compared by the same authors to no specific treatment, to methylprednisolone alone, and to cyclophosphamide substituted for chlorambucil. In their first study that compared the chlorambucil/prednisone regimen to no treatment, 40% of untreated patients reached end-stage renal disease (ESRD) compared to only 8% of treated patients after 10 years. Proteinuria also improved, with the nonnephrotic state maintained during 58% of the follow-up time in the treatment group compared to 22% in the control group. When the chlorambucil/methylprednisolone regimen was compared with methylprednisolone alone, there was a significant initial benefit in the combination-treated patients, but this was not significant by the end of 4 years of follow-up. The original regimen was remarkably safe, with only 4 of 42 treated patients stopping therapy. All adverse events were reversed after stopping the drugs. When 2.5 mg/kg/day oral cyclophosphamide was substituted for chlorambucil and compared with their original regimen, similar complete and partial remission rates of proteinuria were seen. However, a substantial relapse rate of approximately 30% was seen within 2 years in both groups regardless of whether they were treated with chlorambucil or cyclophosphamide. Fewer patients had to discontinue cyclophosphamide (5%) compared to chlorambucil (14%). Kidney function was equally well preserved in both groups for ≤3 years. Similar long-term results using this same regimen recently were reported from a randomized controlled trial from India. Other regimens using longer term cyclophosphamide (1 year) together with lower dose prednisone have also demonstrated an improved outcome, although in these studies the patients were compared to historical controls and were not included in a prospective randomized controlled trial. These results are in contrast to older uncontrolled studies, where cyclophosphamide monotherapy resulted in a frequency of remission similar to that in untreated patients. However, the strength of this evidence is far less than that for randomized clinical trials. Mycophenolate mofetil (MMF), a newer immunosuppressive agent that has proven effective in reducing rejection in the field of solid organ transplantation and is associated with less toxicity than cyclophosphamide, has also been used in treatment trials of patients with MN. Initial results of combined use of MMF with high dose corticosteroids have been similar to cyclophosphamide therapy but with a significantly higher relapse rate after corticosteroids are discontinued (greater than 70% by 3 years posttreatment). Monotherapy with MMF appears ineffective in primary/idiopathic MN.

A different regimen using the immunosuppressive agent cyclosporine has shown results similar to those of the cytotoxic/steroid regimen in terms of improving proteinuria in the medium risk for progression group. Membranous patients who remained nephrotic after a minimum of 6 months of observation, and who were unresponsive to a course of high-dose prednisone, were given 6 months of cyclosporine (3 to 5 mg/kg per day) plus low-dose prednisone (maximum 10 mg/day) and were compared with a prednisone-alone/placebo group. Complete or partial remission in proteinuria was seen in 70% of the cyclosporine group compared to 24% of the control group. There was no difference in kidney survival, but the follow-up period was relatively short at 2 years. Relapses were common within 2 years of discontinuing the drug, with a rate higher than that seen in the Italian cytotoxic trials of approximately 40% to 50%. A study using a longer duration of cyclosporine treatment at a dose of 2 to 4 mg/kg per day for 12 months followed by a 50% reduction in the cyclosporine dosage, and maintaining the cyclosporine therapy in the range of 1.5 mg/kg/day, showed a much lower relapse rate of approximately 20% within the 2-year period. More recently a 12-month randomized controlled trial using tacrolimus monotherapy confirmed the benefit of this class of agent, achieving a partial or complete remission in proteinuria in 75% to 80% of the treated group as well as a significant slowing in the progression rate of the kidney disease compared to a control group; however, nephrotic syndrome reappeared in almost half the patients after tacrolimus withdrawal.

Corticosteroid monotherapy appears ineffective in inducing remission of proteinuria in all controlled trials conducted to date, and in preventing progression in all but one study. Although the follow-up periods were limited to less than 4 years, and the dose and duration of corticosteroid treatment varied, it is generally held that steroid monotherapy should not be used in primary/idiopathic MN treatment. This view is supported by a metaanalysis of studies using corticosteroids alone in MN, although a recent report (albeit not a controlled trial) in patients from Japan did show a benefit to prednisone therapy alone, suggesting that there may be a specific ancestral effect to this class of drugs in the treatment of MN.

Newer therapeutic options include year-long injections of synthetic adrenocorticotrophic hormone. There have been two small but controlled trials with this agent showing short-term benefits similar to the results seen with the cytotoxic/steroid regimen with relatively minor adverse effects. A retrospective case series of 11 patients with nephrotic syndrome resistant to previous immunosuppression treated with a natural, highly purified adrenocorticotrophic hormone (ACTH) gel formulation (H.P. Acthar Gel), currently approved in the United States for remission of proteinuria in the nephrotic syndrome, reported similar encouraging results. The most common treatment regimen used was Acthar Gel 80 units (U) subcutaneous twice weekly for 6 months. Dosing intervals varied from 2 to 3 times weekly. Most patients were treated for a minimum of 6 months, with the longest treatment period being 14 months. Nine of the 11 patients with MN achieved a complete or partial remission. No severe infections were reported in the cohort. These results need to be confirmed but are encouraging. It has been suggested that ACTH mediates its effects via α-melanocyte-stimulating hormone (α-MSH) interaction on melano-corticotropic receptor 1 on podocytes, and this unique interaction may explain why patients who are resistant to previous immunosuppressive therapies respond to ACTH.

Another potential alternative agent is the use of rituximab, a chimeric monoclonal antibody to B cells carrying the CD 20 epitope. Several prospective but nonrandomized pilot studies, using this drug as monotherapy, have resulted in a complete or partial remission in proteinuria in 60% to 80% of the patients by the end of the trial. The great majority of these patients remained in remission at the end of 1 to 2 years of follow up. A B-cell titrated protocol using a single dose of rituximab 1 g has proved to be similarly effective as the 4-doses protocol but at a lower cost. A beneficial effect was also reported in a matched-cohort study comparing 2-year outcomes of 11 consecutive patients with primary MN who received rituximab as second-line therapy for persisting nephrotic syndrome or relapsing disease. Rituximab may also allow successful withdrawal in calcineurin-inhibitor dependent patients. Taken in sum, these results suggest that rituximab is effective for inducing remission of proteinuria in a large number of patients with MN, either as initial treatment or for patients refractory to previous therapeutic attempts. The short-term side-effect profile and compliance issues related to this selective therapy seem preferable to the currently used immunosuppressive regimens, although there are still some concerns about the long-term effects of rare and fatal complications, including reports of progressive multifocal leukoencephalitis potentially related to B-cell depletion therapy. Randomized controlled trials to prove this drug's efficacy and safety are ongoing.

HIGH RISK FOR PROGRESSION

This group includes those with worsening kidney function and/or persistent high-grade proteinuria. The percentage of patients with primary/idiopathic MN in this category is small, and randomized controlled trials focused on this subgroup are rare. In the majority of these cases, if an improvement in proteinuria with conservative therapy is not seen within the first 3 months, an earlier start to immunosuppressive therapy is often warranted. Cyclosporine has been studied in high-risk MN patients in a randomized controlled trial. In this trial, 17 of 64 patients in the conservative, pretreatment phase of the study fulfilled the entry criterion of an absolute reduction in kidney function of 10 mL/min in creatinine clearance. These patients were then randomized to either cyclosporine or placebo for 1 year. The cyclosporine patients showed a substantial improvement in proteinuria compared with placebo, which was sustained for ≤2 years in 50% of cases. The rate of progression as measured by the slope of creatinine clearance was significantly slowed (by greater than 60%) compared with the predrug period during cyclosporine treatment, with no improvement in the placebo group. This drug has substantial nephrotoxic potential, and monitoring for nephrotoxicity and other adverse events must be part of any treatment routine that includes this class of agent.

A recent, randomized, controlled trial at 37 sites in the United Kingdom used an alkalating agent, chlorambucil, in conjunction with steroids in 108 patients with MN who had a greater than 20% decline in GFR within 3 to 24 months of study entry. This combination showed better protection against kidney disease progression than either cyclosporine monotherapy or placebo. Although there was a benefit in preventing a further 20% decline in GFR in the chlorambucil/steroid group, where approximately 60% of participants progressed versus approximately 80% progressing in both the cyclosporine and placebo groups, 117 serious adverse events were reported, with significantly more (particularly hematologic issues) in the chlorambucil group. Accordingly, the inability to avoid serious complications in this rare MN setting should caution against routine application of these therapeutic options. An earlier study reported the treatment of a small group of patients who had progressive deterioration in kidney function with prednisone 1 mg/kg tapering over 6 months to 0.5 mg/kg every other day plus chlorambucil 1.5 mg/kg for 14 weeks, and a significant improvement was found in both their proteinuria and kidney survival at 8 years when compared to an historical control group with similar presenting characteristics. Recent reports have compared more prolonged cytotoxic therapy, that is, 1 year of cyclophosphamide plus prednisone (details outlined in the medium risk patient category mentioned earlier), and these reports show that even repeated courses (≤3) benefited these patients in terms of reducing proteinuria and slowing the rate of kidney disease progression. Obviously the risks associated with prolonged and repeated exposure to potent cytotoxic agents, particularly in relation to the increasing incidence of cancer as drug exposure increases, must be considered. In contrast, in a randomized trial in primary/idiopathic MN patients with documented progression of their disease, treatment with pulse cyclophosphamide combined with pulse methylprednisolone followed by oral prednisone failed to show any significant benefit when compared to prednisone alone.

Although the algorithm for the management of the high-risk patient (Fig. 19.5) lists the option of switching to a cytotoxic agent plus prednisone regimen if there is a failure to respond to the cyclosporine, it must be realized that both options consist of powerful immunosuppressive regimens and carry significant risks. In addition, if kidney function impairment is significant, the dose of cyclophosphamide must be adjusted downward to avoid the risk of significant bone marrow toxicity. Similarly, if the GFR is low (below 30 mL/min per 1.73 m^2) or deteriorating rapidly and/or if the biopsy shows extensive tubular interstitial disease and/or severe vascular changes, the calcineurin inhibitors should either be avoided or approached with great caution. Overall, the decision to treat this group is not to be undertaken without careful consideration of the risks to the patient, and often a second opinion is warranted before initiating these therapies.

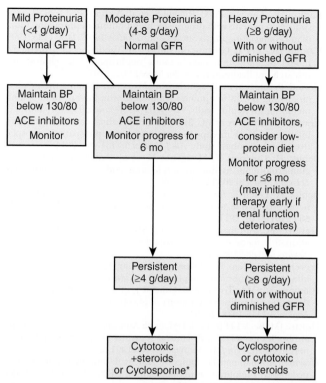

Figure 19.5 Guideline for the treatment of primary/idiopathic membranous nephropathy. Patients may change from one category to another during the course of follow-up. *ACE,* Angiotensin-converting enzyme; *BP,* blood pressure; *GFR,* glomerular filtration rate.

Monotherapy with steroids in this group has not been tested. A subgroup analysis of patients with abnormal kidney function at the time of diagnosis from one of the corticosteroid-alone trials found no differences in the rate of deterioration during 4 years of follow-up between the prednisone-treated group and the control group. One small, uncontrolled trial using pulse methylprednisolone for 5 days followed by a tapering dose of prednisone did show initial stabilization in 15 patients with chronic kidney disease and primary/idiopathic MN. At follow-up, however, two had died and five had developed kidney failure, suggesting at best a transient benefit. These data support the view that corticosteroids alone are not effective in slowing the progression rate in this high risk-of-progression patient.

In sum, specific treatment as well as therapy directed toward secondary effects of the disease may need to be started before the end of the intended conservative monitoring period in these patients especially if there is associated deterioration in glomerular filtration rate.

OTHER TREATMENTS

A large number of other therapies have been tried in MN. These studies have either been small or uncontrolled, or the series have included patients in a variety of risk categories. Some have focused on treating the downstream inflammatory effects of the disease, such as eculizumab a C5b-9 (membrane attack complex) inhibitor, others on the possible benefits of their antioxidant effects, such as probucol, or a potential role as antifibrotic agent, such as pentoxifylline; however, there is insufficient evidence at the

moment to support their general use in this disease. Studies are ongoing, and more are needed.

TREATMENT PROPHYLAXIS

Many large studies in the kidney transplantation field and in postmenopausal women have indicated that agents such as bisphosphonates or supplemental oral calcium and vitamin D reduce bone loss during long-term use of corticosteroids. Certainly the use of such agents in the primary/idiopathic MN patient could be considered when a course of therapy includes prolonged prednisone treatment. Trimethoprim-sulfamethoxazole has reduced the incidence of *Pneumocystis jiroveci* pneumonia infection in patients on prolonged immunosuppressive therapy in both the transplantation field and in certain autoimmune diseases. Its use when the patients with primary/idiopathic MN are exposed to prolonged glucocorticoid treatment, cytotoxic agents, calcineurin inhibitors, or rituximab seems prudent.

MANAGEMENT PLAN

Figure 19.5 shows a treatment framework for patients with primary/idiopathic MN. In addition, the following general rules should be applied:

1. Establish whether the disease is primary or secondary, and take appropriate actions for known causes.
2. For patients with primary/idiopathic MN, monitor kidney function throughout a 6-month period (3 months for the high-risk category patient), and establish a risk-for-progression score.
3. If persistent nephrotic range proteinuria or deterioration in kidney function occurs despite maximum conservative therapy, introduce treatment for the secondary effects of the disease, including a lipid-lowering agent and possibly anticoagulants.
4. Introduce systemic risk-reduction strategies, such as bisphosphonates, when long-term corticosteroids are used, and trimethoprim-sulfamethoxazole if long-term immunosuppressive drugs are used.
5. First choice as specific therapy for patients with a medium risk for progression is chlorambucil or cyclophosphamide cycling monthly with prednisone for 6 months or cyclosporine combined with low-dose prednisone for 6 to 12 months.
6. Specific therapy for high-risk patients (defined by high-grade proteinuria but preserved kidney function) should be cyclosporine for 6 to 12 months. If this fails or if proteinuria is accompanied by low GFR or deteriorating kidney function, a course of chlorambucil or cyclophosphamide combined with ≤6 months of prednisone may be considered if the clinical status of the individual warrants.
7. If both fail, and the clinical status warrants further attempts at treatment, consider one of the newer treatments such as rituximab or ACTH therapy.
8. A significant proportion of the patients who achieve either a partial or complete remission will relapse. Retreatment with the previously successful regimen (or with one of the other proven routines if toxicity is a major

concern) should be undertaken. This should replace labeling the patient as a treatment failure, because even a partial remission is associated with significantly improved kidney survival.

KEY BIBLIOGRAPHY

Adachi JD, Benson WG, Brown J, et al: Intermittent etidronate therapy to prevent corticosteroid induced osteoporosis, *N Engl J Med* 337:382-387, 1997.

Alexopoulos E, Papagianni A, Tsamelashvili M, et al: Induction and long-term treatment with cyclosporine in membranous nephropathy with the nephrotic syndrome, *Nephrol Dial Transplant* 21:3127-3132, 2006.

Beck LH Jr, Bonegio RG, Lambeau G, et al: M-type phospholipase A2 receptor as target antigen in idiopathic membranous nephropathy, *N Engl J Med* 361:11-21, 2009.

Beck LH Jr, Fervenza FC, Beck DM, et al: Rituximab-induced depletion of anti-PLA2R autoantibodies predicts response in membranous nephropathy, *J Am Soc Nephrol: JASN* 22:1543-1550, 2011.

Bjorneklett R, Viksc BE, Svarstad E, et al: Long-term risk of cancer in membranous nephropathy patients, *Am J Kidney Dis* 50:396-403, 2007.

Bomback AS, Tumlin JA, Baranski J, et al: Treatment of nephrotic syndrome with adrenocorticotropic hormone (ACTH) gel, *Drug Des Devel Ther* 5:147-153, 2011.

Branten AJ, du Buf-Vereijken PW, Klasen IS, et al: Urinary excretion of beta 2 microglobulin and IgG predict prognosis in idiopathic membranous nephropathy: a validation study, *J Am Soc Nephrol* 16:169-174, 2005.

Branten AJ, du Buf-Vereijken PW, Vervloet M, et al: Mycofenolate mofetil in idiopathic membranous nephropathy: a clinical trial with comparison to a historical control group treated with cyclophosphamide, *Am J Kidney Dis* 50:248-256, 2007.

Branten AJ, Reichert LJ, Koene RA, et al: Oral cyclophosphamide versus chlorambucil in the treatment of patients with membranous nephropathy and renal insufficiency, *Q J Med* 91:359-366, 1998.

Cattran DC, Appel GB, Hebert LA, et al: Cyclosporine in patients with steroid resistant membranous nephropathy: a randomized trial, *Kidney Int* 59:1484-1490, 2001.

Cattran DC, Greenwood C, Ritchie S, et al: A controlled trial of cyclosporine in patients with progressive membranous nephropathy. Canadian Glomerulonephritis Study Group, *Kidney Int* 47:1130-1135, 1995.

Cattran DC, Pei Y, Greenwood CM, et al: Validation of a predictive model of idiopathic membranous nephropathy: its clinical and research implications, *Kidney Int* 51:901-907, 1997.

Cravedi P, Ruggenenti P, Sghirlanzoni MC, et al: Titrating rituximab to circulating B cells to optimize lymphocytolytic therapy in idiopathic membranous nephropathy, *Clin J Am Soc Nephrol* 2:932-937, 2007.

Cravedi P, Sghirlanzoni MC, Marasa M, et al: Efficacy and safety of rituximab second-line therapy for membranous nephropathy: a prospective, matched-cohort study, *Am J Nephrol* 33:461-468, 2011.

Debiec H, Guigonis V, Mougenot B, et al: Antenatal membranous glomerulonephritis due to anti-neutral endopeptidase antibodies, *N Engl J Med* 346:2053-2060, 2002.

Debiec H, Lefeu F, Kemper MJ, et al: Early-childhood membranous nephropathy due to cationic bovine serum albumin, *N Engl J Med* 364:2101-2110, 2011.

Fervenza FC, Abraham RS, Erickson SB, et al: Rituximab therapy in idiopathic membranous nephropathy: a 2-year study, *Clin J Am Soc Nephrol* 5:2188-2198, 2010.

Fervenza FC, Cosio FG, Ericsson SB, et al: Rituximab treatment of idiopathic membranous nephropathy, *Kidney Int* 73:117-125, 2008.

Hladunewich MA, Troyanov S, Calafati J, et al: The natural history of the non-nephrotic membranous nephropathy patient, *Clin J Am Soc Nephrol* 4:1417-1422, 2009.

Hofstra JM, Beck LH Jr, Beck DM, et al: Anti-phospholipase A receptor antibodies correlate with clinical status in idiopathic membranous nephropathy, *Clin J Am Soc Neph* 6:1286-1291, 2011.

Howman A, Chapman TL, Langdon MM, et al: Immunosuppression for progressive membranous nephropathy: a UK randomised controlled trial. *Lancet* 381(9868):744-751, 2013.

Troyanov S, Wall CA, Miller JA, et al: Idiopathic membranous nephropathy: definition and relevance of a partial remission, *Kidney Int* 66:1199-1205, 2004.

Full bibliography can be found on www.expertconsult.com.

20

Immunoglobulin A Nephropathy and Related Disorders

Jonathan Barratt | John Feehally

Immunoglobulin A nephropathy (IgAN) was first described in 1968 by the Parisian pathologist Jean Berger, and at one time it was known as Berger disease. It is the most common pattern of glomerulonephritis (GN) identified in areas of the world where kidney biopsy is widely practiced. IgAN is defined by mesangial IgA deposition accompanied by a mesangial proliferative GN, and it is an important cause of end-stage renal disease (ESRD). Recurrent gross hematuria is the hallmark of the disease. Closely related to IgAN is Henoch-Schönlein purpura (HSP), and this less common disease is more frequently found in children. HSP is a small vessel systemic vasculitis characterized by IgA deposition in affected blood vessels, with kidney biopsy findings usually indistinguishable from IgAN.

EPIDEMIOLOGY

Immunoglobulin A nephropathy is most common in Caucasian and Asian populations and is relatively rare in people of African decent. The highest worldwide incidence is in Southeast Asia, but this may reflect different approaches to evaluation of kidney disease and different thresholds for kidney biopsy. Peak incidence of IgAN is in the second and third decades of life, and there is a 2:1 male to female predominance in North American and Western European populations. This gender difference is not seen in Asian populations. Subclinical IgAN is estimated to occur in up to 16% of the general population, according to postmortem studies. IgAN is occasionally familial, but the majority of cases are sporadic.

CLINICAL PRESENTATION

EPISODIC GROSS HEMATURIA

Episodic gross hematuria most frequently occurs in the second or third decades of life, and is the presenting complaint in 40% to 50% of patients. The urine is usually brown rather than red and will often be described by the patient as looking like "tea without milk" or "cola-colored." The passage of clots is very unusual. There may be bilateral loin pain accompanying these episodes, which may be attributed to renal capsular swelling. This hematuria usually follows intercurrent mucosal infection, most commonly in the upper respiratory tract, but it is occasionally seen following gastrointestinal infection and also may be provoked by heavy physical exercise. Spontaneous episodes occur as well. The time course is characteristic, with hematuria appearing within 24 hours of the onset of the symptoms of infection. This differentiates it from the 2 to 3 week delay between infection and subsequent hematuria, which is characteristic of postinfectious GN. Visible hematuria resolves spontaneously over a few days in nearly all cases, but microscopic hematuria may persist between attacks. Most patients only experience a few episodes of gross hematuria, and such episodes typically recur for a few years at most. These episodes are infrequently associated with acute kidney injury.

ASYMPTOMATIC MICROSCOPIC HEMATURIA

Asymptomatic microscopic hematuria is usually detected during routine health screening and identifies 30% to 40% of patients with IgAN in most series. Hematuria may occur alone or with proteinuria. It is rare for proteinuria to occur without microscopic hematuria in IgAN.

NEPHROTIC SYNDROME

Nephrotic syndrome is uncommon, occurring in only 5% of all patients with IgAN, but it is more common in children and adolescents. Patients more commonly develop nephrotic-range proteinuria, and this is principally seen in patients with advanced glomerulosclerosis. In those children and adults presenting with concurrent nephrotic syndrome, microscopic hematuria and mesangial IgA deposition, one should always consider the possibility of the coincidence of the two most common glomerular diseases of young adults: minimal change disease and IgAN. A number of case series have reported patients who, on kidney biopsy, have normal light microscopy, foot process effacement on electron microscopy, and electron-dense mesangial IgA deposits and in whom proteinuria resolved completely in response to corticosteroid therapy. Typically in these cases, following resolution of proteinuria, both microscopic hematuria and IgA deposits persist.

ACUTE KIDNEY INJURY

Acute kidney injury is uncommon in IgAN (less than 5% of all cases) and develops by two distinct mechanisms. The first is an acute, severe immune and inflammatory injury resulting in crescent formation—crescentic IgAN. This may be the first presentation of the disease or can occur superimposed on known mild IgAN. Alternatively, acute kidney injury can occur with mild glomerular injury when heavy glomerular hematuria leads to tubular occlusion by red cell casts. This is a reversible phenomenon, and recovery of kidney function occurs with supportive measures.

OTHER PRESENTATIONS

Other presentations of IgAN include hypertension and chronic kidney disease (CKD), where the patient is identified coincidentally, and malignant hypertension.

SECONDARY IMMUNOGLOBULIN A NEPHROPATHY

Mesangial IgA deposition may occur secondary to a number of other diseases, and the kidney biopsy appearances are often indistinguishable from primary IgAN. Although some associations are well established, other anecdotal observations based on single case reports should be interpreted with caution as IgAN is a common disease. The most common form of secondary IgAN is associated with chronic liver disease, particularly with alcoholic cirrhosis. It is usually thought to be a consequence of impaired hepatic clearance of IgA. Mesangial IgA is a common autopsy finding in patients with chronic liver disease; however, few patients have clinical manifestations of kidney disease other than microscopic hematuria. IgAN is also reported in association with HIV infection and AIDS. The polyclonal increase in serum IgA, which is a feature of AIDS, has been cited as a predisposing factor for the disease. The closeness of this association has been controversial however, as autopsy studies have indicated a prevalence of IgAN between zero and 7.75%. Treatment of secondary IgAN should be targeted toward the primary disease.

PATHOLOGY

Elevated serum IgA levels are found in 30% to 50% of adult patients with IgAN. Serum IgA levels do not correlate with disease activity or severity. Likewise, measurement of poorly galactosylated IgA1 O-glycoform levels is neither sensitive nor specific enough to be used as a diagnostic test in IgAN, although there is emerging evidence that high levels of poorly galactosylated IgA1 O-glycoforms may correlate with a worse prognosis. The diagnosis of IgAN requires a kidney biopsy.

LIGHT MICROSCOPY

Light microscopic abnormalities may be minimal, but the most common appearance is mesangial hypercellularity (Fig. 20.1). This is most commonly diffuse and global, but focal segmental hypercellularity is also seen. Focal segmental glomerulosclerosis is also described, and crescentic change may be superimposed on diffuse mesangial proliferation with or without associated segmental necrosis. Crescents are a common finding in biopsies performed during episodes of gross hematuria with reduced GFR.

Tubulointerstitial changes do not differ from those seen in other forms of progressive GN, reflecting the final common pathway of renal parenchymal disease. Mononuclear cell infiltration is associated with tubular atrophy and interstitial fibrosis, ultimately leading to a widening of the cortical interstitium. This finding correlates with a poor prognosis.

IMMUNOHISTOLOGY

The presence of dominant or codominant IgA deposits in the renal mesangium is the defining feature of IgAN. This is detected in kidney biopsy specimens by immunofluorescence or immunohistochemistry (Fig. 20.2). IgA deposition is diffuse and global. In 15% of cases, IgA is the only deposited immunoglobulin. Other immunoglobulins are also frequently detectable (IgG in 50% to 70%, IgM in 31% to 66%), but their presence does not appear to correlate with clinical outcome. The complement component C3 is also commonly present.

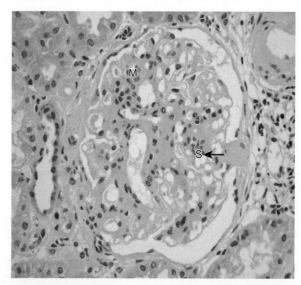

Figure 20.1   Kidney biopsy showing mesangial proliferation (M) and expansion of the mesangial extracellular matrix (S) in a patient with IgA nephropathy. A capsular adhesion can also be seen (arrow).

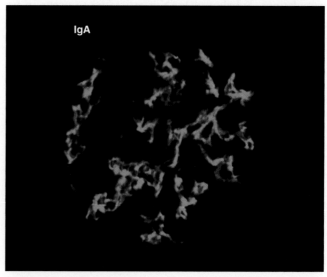

Figure 20.2   Kidney biopsy showing immunofluorescent staining for mesangial immunoglobulin A.

ELECTRON MICROSCOPY

Electron microscopy shows mesangial and paramesangial electron-dense deposits corresponding to IgA immune complexes (Fig. 20.3). The size, shape, quantity, and density of the deposits vary between glomeruli. Glomerular capillary wall deposits may also be seen in the subepithelial, or more commonly, subendothelial space. Capillary loop deposits are associated with disease that is more severe. Glomerular basement membrane abnormalities are seen in 15% to 40% of cases and are associated with heavy proteinuria, more severe glomerular changes, and crescent formation. A group of patients experience thinning of the glomerular basement membrane indistinguishable from thin membrane disease. It remains unclear whether the clinical course of these patients is different.

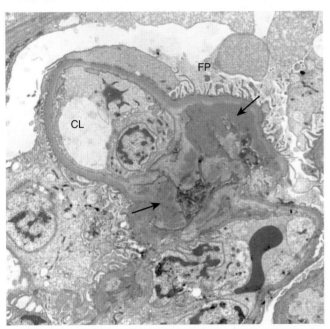

Figure 20.3 Electron micrograph showing immunoglobulin A immune complex deposition within the mesangium and paramesangium (arrows). CL, Capillary loops; **FP,** normal podocyte foot processes.

THE OXFORD CLASSIFICATION OF IMMUNOGLOBULIN A NEPHROPATHY

The Oxford Classification of IgAN, published in 2009, is an international scoring system for evaluating pathological features on kidney biopsy. Four variables were identified that correlated most strongly with clinical outcome, independent of known clinical risk factors including the presence of hypertension, reduced GFR at diagnosis, and degree of proteinuria (Table 20.1). The predictive value of these biopsy features was similar in both adults and children. Studies are ongoing to validate this classification in different patient populations.

PATHOGENESIS

Although considerable progress has been made in characterizing a number of pathogenic pathways operating in IgAN, there remains a great deal we do not understand. In particular, it remains to be established whether IgAN is a single entity or whether mesangial IgA deposition is simply the final common pathway for a number of distinct kidney diseases.

IMMUNOGLOBULIN A IN IMMUNOGLOBULIN A NEPHROPATHY

In humans, IgA is the most abundant antibody. It is predominantly present at mucosal surfaces and in secretions such as saliva and tears, where it protects against mucosal pathogens. The IgA molecule exists as two isoforms, IgA1 and IgA2, with each existing as monomers (single molecules) or polymers (most commonly dimeric IgA). It is predominantly polymeric IgA1 that is found in mesangial IgA deposits in IgAN. The major difference between IgA1 and IgA2 is that IgA1 includes a hinge region that carries a variable complement of O-linked carbohydrates (Fig. 20.4). Changes in the composition of these O-linked sugars is the most consistent finding in patients with IgAN across the world, with identical changes seen in patient cohorts from North America, Europe, and Asia.

The key change is an increase in the serum of IgA1 O-glycoforms that contains less galactose. This increase

Table 20.1 Oxford Classification of Immunoglobulin A Nephropathy

Histologic Variable	Definition	Score	
Mesangial hypercellularity	Mesangial hypercellularity score defined by the proportion of glomeruli with mesangial hypercellularity	M0	≤0.5
		M1	>0.5
Endocapillary hypercellularity	Hypercellularity because of increased number of cells within glomerular capillary lumina, causing narrowing of the lumina	E0	absent
		E1	present
Segmental glomerulosclerosis	Any amount of the tuft involved in sclerosis, but not involving the whole tuft or the presence of an adhesion	S0	absent
		S1	present
Tubular atrophy/interstitial fibrosis	Percentage of cortical area involved by the tubular atrophy or interstitial fibrosis, whichever is greater	T0	0% to 25%
		T1	26% to 50%
		T2	>50%

NOTE: Scoring should be assessed on period acid-Schiff-stained sections.

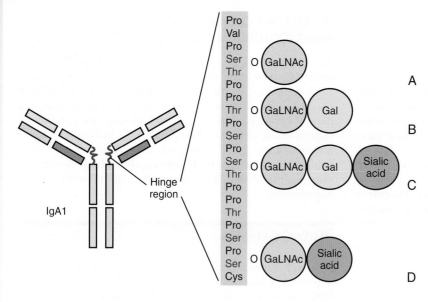

Figure 20.4 *O*-glycosylation of IgA1 hinge region. IgA1 contains a 17 amino-acid hinge region that undergoes co/posttranslational modification by the addition of ≤6 *O*-glycan chains. **A,** These chains comprise N-acetylgalactosamine (GaLNAc) in *O*-linkage with either serine or threonine residues. **B,** Galactose can be β1,3-linked to GaLNAc by the enzyme Core 1 β-3 galactosyltransferase (C1GaLT1) and its molecular chaperone Core 1 β-3 galactosyltransferase molecular chaperone (Cosmc), which ensures its correct folding and stability. **C,** Galactose may also be sialylated. **D,** In addition, sialic acid (N-acetylneuraminic acid, NeuNAc) may be attached directly to GaLNAc by α-2,6 linkage to prevent further addition of galactose. *Cys,* Cysteine; *Pro,* proline; *Ser,* serine; *Thr,* threonine; *Val,* valine.

in poorly galactosylated IgA1 *O*-glycoforms is believed to play a central role in the pathogenesis of IgAN. Poorly galactosylated IgA1 *O*-glycoforms form high molecular weight circulating immune complexes, either through self-aggregation or through the generation of IgG and IgA hinge region specific autoantibodies. These high molecular weight immune complexes are prone to mesangial deposition resulting ultimately in mesangial cell proliferation, release of proinflammatory mediators, and glomerular injury.

ORIGINS OF MESANGIAL IMMUNOGLOBULIN A

Many of the features of mesangial IgA are those typically seen in IgA secreted at mucosal surfaces. Overabundance of this "mucosal-type" IgA in the serum in IgAN might suggest that this IgA originates from mucosal sites. However, mucosal biopsies from patients with IgAN show significantly reduced numbers of polymeric IgA-secreting plasma cells compared to healthy subjects. By comparison, increased numbers of polymeric IgA-secreting plasma cells are seen in bone marrow samples from patients with IgAN, suggesting that mesangial IgA is derived from systemically located plasma cells. This has led to the hypothesis that, in IgAN, mucosally primed IgA-committed B cells relocate to systemic sites such as the bone marrow where they secrete their poorly galactosylated polymeric IgA1 directly into the circulation rather than into the submucosa for passage across the mucosal epithelium. In addition, the systemic microenvironment is likely to be very different from the mucosal sites these plasma cells would normally inhabit, and it is possible that these plasma cells also receive cytokine signals promoting undergalactosylation of IgA1.

It is contended that one of the most likely mechanisms for this displacement is incorrect homing of mucosal lymphocytes to systemic sites. Although there is emerging evidence of altered homing of B and T lymphocyte subsets in IgAN, more work needs to be undertaken to fully evaluate this hypothesis.

KEY EVENTS IN THE DEVELOPMENT OF RENAL SCARRING IN IgA NEPHROPATHY

The Oxford Classification of IgAN publication identified four key pathologic consequences of IgA deposition that independently determine the risk of developing progressive kidney disease: mesangial cell proliferation (M), endocapillary proliferation (E), segmental glomerulosclerosis (S), and tubulointerstitial scarring (T). There is increasing evidence, predominantly from in vitro models, that circulating IgA immune complexes containing poorly galactosylated polymeric IgA1 are key drivers for all of these processes.

Exposure to IgA immune complexes triggers mesangial cell activation, proliferation (M), and release of proinflammatory and profibrotic mediators. These mediators, along with the direct effects of exposure to IgA immune complexes, cause podocyte injury, a process fundamental to segmental glomerular scarring (S), and proximal tubule cell activation, which drives tubulointerstitial scarring (T). Identifying the origins of these IgA immune complexes is therefore key to understanding the pathogenesis of IgAN and is paramount if effective treatments are to be developed.

GENETICS OF IMMUNOGLOBULIN A NEPHROPATHY

Multiple attempts have been made to establish a genetic basis for the IgA nephropathy, both in rare familial cohorts and sporadic IgAN, although, to date, little headway has been made in identifying the genes involved. However, there is now evidence in several ethnic backgrounds to suggest that genetic factors heavily influence the composition of circulating IgA *O*-glycoforms in the serum. From these studies, it is apparent that first-degree unaffected relatives of patients with IgAN often also display high levels of poorly galactosylated IgA1, supporting the hypothesis that changes in the composition of serum IgA1

O-glycoforms is only one part of a "multiple-hit" pathogenic process.

Several susceptibility loci have been identified from genome-wide association studies (GWAS), and one region that has gained particular interest is the major histocompatibility complex (MHC). Polymorphisms within the MHC have been associated with several autoimmune diseases, and an association in IgAN is consistent with an autoimmune component to IgAN. This could be mediated through production of autoantibodies with specificity for the poorly galactosylated IgA1 hinge region.

NATURAL HISTORY AND PROGNOSIS

Fewer than 10% of all patients with IgAN have complete resolution of urinary abnormalities. IgAN has the potential for slowly progressive CKD leading eventually to ESRD. Approximately 25% to 30% of any cohort will require kidney replacement therapy within 20 to 25 years of presentation.

Many studies have identified clinical, laboratory, and histopathologic features at presentation, which mark a poor prognosis (Table 20.2). Although the various prognostic factors listed may be informative for populations of patients, they do not as yet possess the specificity to identify an individual prognosis with complete confidence.

Table 20.2 Prognostic Markers at Presentation in Immunoglobulin A Nephropathy

	Clinical	Histopathologic
Worse prognosis	Increasing age	*Light microscopy*
	Duration of preceding symptoms	Capsular adhesions and crescents
	Severity of proteinuria	Glomerular sclerosis
	Hypertension	Tubular atrophy
	Reduced GFR	Interstitial fibrosis
	Increased body mass index	Vascular wall thickening
	Higher serum uric acid	*Oxford Classification*
		M1 worse than M0
		E1 worse than E0
		S1 worse than S0
		T2 worse than T0
		Immunofluorescence
		Capillary loop IgA deposits
		Ultrastructure
		Capillary wall electron dense deposits
		Mesangiolysis
		GBM abnormalities
Good prognosis	Recurrent gross hematuria (possibly a result of lead time bias)	Minimal light microscopic abnormalities: M0, E0, S0, T0
No effect on prognosis	Gender	Intensity of IgA deposits
	Ethnicity	Co-deposition of mesangial IgG, IgM, or C3
	Serum IgA level	

GBM, Glomerular basement membrane; *GFR,* glomerular filtration rate; *IgA,* immunoglobulin A; *IgG,* immunoglobulin G; *IgM,* immunoglobulin M.

TREATMENT OF IMMUNOGLOBULIN A NEPHROPATHY

Management of patients with IgAN is currently limited to generic strategies applicable to all chronic glomerulonephritides: reduction of proteinuria, use of renin-angiotensin blockade, and control of hypertension (Table 20.3). As with all other causes of CKD, cardiovascular risk factors should be addressed and advice provided regarding smoking cessation, a healthy diet, and exercise.

THE PATIENT WITH MICROSCOPIC HEMATURIA AND LESS THAN 0.5 g/DAY PROTEINURIA

No specific therapy is advised, although long-term follow-up in primary care is recommended to identify development of increasing proteinuria, declining GFR, and hypertension.

THE PATIENT WITH RECURRENT GROSS HEMATURIA

No specific treatment is required for patients with recurrent gross hematuria, and there is no role for prophylactic antibiotics. Tonsillectomy reduces the frequency of acute episodes of gross hematuria when tonsillitis is the provoking factor, and tonsillectomy has its advocates, especially in Japan, as a treatment to reduce progression to ESRD. However, data from clinical trials are conflicting, and larger studies are needed before any conclusion can be drawn regarding the role of tonsillectomy in preserving long-term kidney function in IgAN.

THE PATIENT WITH GREATER THAN 0.5 g/DAY PROTEINURIA AND SLOWLY PROGRESSIVE IgAN

Several randomized controlled trials have shown that renin-angiotensin blockade, with an angiotensin-converting enzyme (ACE) inhibitor or angiotensin II receptor blocker (ARB) to control hypertension and to reduce proteinuria to less than 0.5 g/day, is beneficial in slowing progression of proteinuric IgAN. Therefore an ACE inhibitor or ARB should be introduced and maximized to achieve this threshold. Although the combination of ACE inhibitor and ARB reduces proteinuria in IgAN, long-term beneficial effects on renal survival have not been demonstrated, and the safety of this approach has been questioned in the ONTARGET study.

There are a number of patients who will continue to experience proteinuria in excess of 0.5 g/day and declining kidney function despite maximal doses of ACE inhibitor and/or ARB. In these patients, current evidence regarding additional therapy is controversial.

CORTICOSTEROIDS

The efficacy of corticosteroids in IgAN has been tested in several studies. Overall results have been equivocal, and reports showing positive outcomes have been criticized for inadequate trial design and the presence of multiple confounding factors. The risks of high-dose corticosteroid use must also be considered. A 6-month course of corticosteroids in patients with persistent proteinuria greater than 1 g/day, despite renin-angiotensin blockade and preserved kidney function (eGFR greater than 50 mL/min) may slow progression of GFR loss. The precise utility of corticosteroids should become clear when the STOP-IgAN trial provides a report. In this study, patients with persistent proteinuria greater than 0.75 g/day following optimized supportive therapy for 6 months are randomized to continued supportive therapy or additional immunosuppressive therapy (corticosteroids if eGFR is ≥60 mL/min, corticosteroids plus cyclophosphamide/azathioprine if eGFR is <60 mL/min).

FISH OIL

Fish oil is widely prescribed in IgAN and appears safe, although tolerability is a major issue because of a fishy odor to the breath and perspiration, and increased flatulence. A meta-analysis of available clinical trial data, however, failed to detect a benefit of fish oils on kidney outcomes in IgAN.

OTHER IMMUNOSUPPRESSIVE AGENTS

There is currently insufficient evidence to support the routine use of cyclophosphamide and azathioprine in IgAN. Mycophenolate mofetil (MMF) has been studied in a number of small randomized controlled trials, but results have been inconsistent, and a recent meta-analysis of these trials concluded that there is no significant benefit of MMF in reducing proteinuria in IgAN. In the most recent report providing longer follow-up data, patients with mild histologic lesions did show a benefit in reducing the composite end points of doubling of serum creatinine or ESRD. Further studies of MMF in IgAN are ongoing.

THE PATIENT WITH ACUTE KIDNEY INJURY

In patients known to have IgAN who develop acute kidney injury (AKI) and fail to respond to simple supportive measures, a kidney biopsy is required to differentiate between the two most common causes of AKI in IgAN:

1. *Acute tubular necrosis with intratubular erythrocyte casts.* This requires supportive care only. Recovery to baseline GFR is usual, although some patients may be left with irreversible tubulointerstitial scarring.
2. *Crescentic IgAN.* Patients with rapidly progressive loss of kidney function, active glomerular inflammation and crescents on kidney biopsy, and no significant chronic damage may be treated similarly to other forms of crescentic GN, (i.e., high-dose corticosteroids, cyclophosphamide, and plasma exchange). Evidence for treatment of crescentic IgAN is derived from small case-series and retrospective data. Response to treatment is worse in crescentic IgAN than in other forms of crescentic GN, and renal survival is estimated to be only 50% at 1 year and 20% at 5 years. This may be the consequence of significant preexisting chronic damage at the time of a crescentic transformation, thereby reducing the chances of a response to immunosuppression.

THE PATIENT WITH NEPHROTIC SYNDROME

Nephrotic syndrome in association with mesangial IgA deposition may be a result of advanced glomerular scarring

---

Table 20.3   Treatment Recommendations for Immunoglobulin A Nephropathy According to Clinical Features

Clinical Presentation	Recommended Treatment
Recurrent gross hematuria	No specific treatment—no role for antibiotics or tonsillectomy
Proteinuria <0.5 g/24 h ± microscopic hematuria	No specific treatment—no role for tonsillectomy

Proteinuria >0.5 g/24 h ± microscopic hematuria	Step 1: Maximally tolerated renin-angiotensin blockade with ACE inhibitor and/or ARB
	Step 2: If proteinuria remains >0.5 g/24 h, then consider immunosuppression
	    Little convincing evidence for any particular agent but options include:
	        Fish oil
	        Corticosteroids
	        Mycophenolate mofetil

Acute kidney injury
    Acute tubular necrosis
    Crescentic IgAN (with little or no chronic damage)
	Supportive measures for acute tubular necrosis
	Induction (~8 weeks)
	    Prednisolone 0.5 to 1 mg/kg/day
	    Cyclophosphamide 2 mg/kg/day
	Maintenance
	    Prednisolone in reducing dosage
	    Azathioprine 2.5 mg/kg/day

Nephrotic syndrome
    With minimal change on light microscopy
    With structural glomerular changes
	Prednisolone 0.5 to 1 mg/kg/day for ≤8 weeks
	No specific treatment

Hypertension	Target BP 125/75 if proteinuria >0.5 g/24 h ACE inhibitors/ARB first-choice agents

ACE, Angiotensin converting enzyme; *ARB,* angiotensin receptor blocker; *BP,* blood pressure; *CKD,* chronic kidney disease; *GN,* glomerulonephritis; *IgAN,* immunoglobulin A nephropathy.
NOTE: As with all other causes of CKD, cardiovascular risk factors, including hypertension, should be addressed, and patients should be advised regarding smoking cessation, healthy diet, and exercise. Treatment of crescentic IgAN mirrors that of other systemic vasculitides with rapidly progressive GN (see Chapter 23).

as a consequence of longstanding IgAN, and it therefore may reflect established CKD or an acute podocyte injury indistinguishable from minimal change disease occurring in a patient with coincidental IgAN. A kidney biopsy clearly is the key to distinguishing between these two extremes, and electron microscopy should be performed. Patients with IgAN, nephrotic syndrome, minimal glomerular scarring, and podocyte effacement typical of minimal change disease should be treated as having minimal change disease.

FOLLOW-UP

Patients with IgAN and CKD stages 1 to 3 may be followed up in primary care. On discharge from nephrology services, clear guidance should be provided to the primary-care physician regarding frequency of kidney function, urine dipstick, and blood-pressure monitoring. This will be dictated by local guidelines, although we would suggest this testing be performed at least annually. Patients with CKD 4 to 5 require follow-up in a nephrology clinic.

KIDNEY TRANSPLANTATION AND IMMUNOGLOBULIN A NEPHROPATHY

Recurrence of IgA deposition following kidney transplantation is common, affecting up to 50% of grafts within 5 years. However, graft failure because of recurrence of IgAN is relatively rare, most often occurring in patients who have had a rapidly progressive course in their native kidneys. There is little evidence that the choice of posttransplant immunosuppression protocol modifies the risk of recurrence, and a recently published analysis of the Australia and New Zealand Dialysis and Transplant Registry (ANZDATA) suggests recurrent disease is more common in patients who undergo steroid withdrawal. There is no evidence to support any specific treatment regimen after recurrent IgAN has been diagnosed in a kidney transplant, although a single-center retrospective analysis has suggested that ACE inhibitor/ARB treatment may reduce the rate of decline in allograft function in recurrent IgAN.

HENOCH-SCHÖNLEIN PURPURA

Henoch-Schönlein purpura (HSP) is the most common form of systemic vasculitis in children and is characterized by IgA deposition in affected blood vessels. The renal lesion is a mesangioproliferative GN with mesangial IgA deposition, indistinguishable from IgAN.

EPIDEMIOLOGY

Although HSP may occur at any age, it is most common during childhood between the ages of 3 to 15. There is a slight male predominance. Most cases occur in the winter, spring, and autumn months, which may be because of its association with preceding upper respiratory tract infections.

ETIOLOGY AND PATHOGENESIS

The exact cause of HSP remains unknown. There are, however, many factors that suggest a common pathogenic pathway operating in HSP and IgAN. Identical twins have been reported where one presents with IgAN and the other with HSP. HSP developing on a background of IgAN is described in both adults and children. Both diseases share similar findings on kidney biopsy, and they also share changes in the complement of serum IgA1 O-glycoforms. There is a similar association between mucosal infection and presentation of disease.

NATURAL HISTORY

The kidney disease that accompanies HSP is often transient and self limited in nature, with hematuria or proteinuria typically resolving within weeks of presentation. AKI due to crescentic HSP nephritis is more common than crescentic IgAN (although still uncommon), and AKI tends to occur early in the course of the disease. The prognosis of patients who have transient HSP is generally very good. However, up to 10% of patients with HSP nephritis will develop ESRD.

CLINICAL FEATURES

The classic tetrad of symptoms in HSP is a palpable purpuric rash, arthritis/arthralgia, abdominal pain, and kidney disease. Symptoms appear in any order and can evolve over days to weeks.

The rash is classically distributed on extensor surfaces, with sparing of the trunk and face (Fig. 20.5). It typically appears in crops, and is symmetrically distributed. Polyarthralgia is common, and is usually transient and migratory. There is often swelling and tenderness but no chronic destructive damage. Gastrointestinal symptoms often appear after the rash. Abdominal pain is usually mild and transient, but it may be severe and lead to gastrointestinal hemorrhage, bowel ischemia, intussusception, and perforation. Kidney involvement (HSP nephritis) typically manifests as transient asymptomatic microscopic hematuria and/or

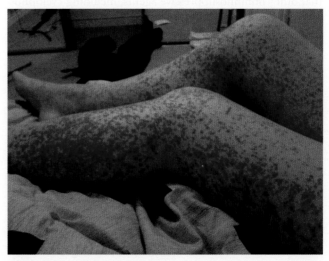

Figure 20.5 Typical appearance of leukocytoclastic vasculitic rash of Henoch-Schönlein purpura.

proteinuria. More severe complications, such as nephrotic syndrome or rapidly progressive deterioration of kidney function, occur less frequently and are more common in adults than in children.

PATHOLOGY

As in IgAN, elevated serum IgA levels are found in 30% to 50% of adult patients with HSP. Serum IgA levels do not correlate with disease activity or severity. Similarly, changes in the levels of undergalactosylated IgA1 *O*-glycoform levels are not sensitive nor specific enough to be used as a diagnostic test in HSP. Confirmation of the clinical diagnosis requires histologic evidence of IgA deposition in affected tissue, often the skin or kidney.

SKIN BIOPSY

Biopsy of the skin rash typically shows a leukocytoclastic vasculitis. IgA immune complex deposition can be seen using immunofluorescent staining, but detection of IgA in the skin is unreliable. If a tissue diagnosis is required, a kidney biopsy should be performed in the presence of nephritis.

KIDNEY BIOPSY

Kidney biopsy is usually reserved for adult cases of diagnostic uncertainty or when a child presents with more severe renal involvement. Histologic features are the same as those in IgAN.

MANAGEMENT

There is little evidence to guide the treatment of HSP nephritis, and that which exists is derived from small retrospective case series. Patients with hematuria, proteinuria, and mildly reduced GFR do not require any specific treatment, and the nephritis usually resolves spontaneously. In patients with crescentic HSP nephritis typified by a rapidly progressive loss of kidney function, there is limited evidence that high-dose corticosteroids are beneficial. Regimens include pulsed methylprednisolone followed by a 3-month course of oral prednisolone. There is currently no conclusive evidence that other immunosuppressive agents, including cyclophosphamide or azathioprine, or other interventions, such as plasmapheresis, have any beneficial effect on outcome.

FOLLOW-UP

Patients should be monitored as for IgAN. As with other forms of glomerular disease, those patients with persistent proteinuria are at highest risk of developing progressive CKD.

TRANSPLANTATION

Kidney transplantation is the treatment of choice in patients with ESRD resulting from HSP nephritis. As with IgAN, recurrence of mesangial IgA deposition may occur, although loss of the graft to HSP nephritis is less common and tends to occur in patients who had an aggressive original disease. Kidney transplantation should be delayed for 12 months from date of presentation.

PREGNANCY

Evidence from cohort studies of children with HSP suggests that all women with a history of HSP should be carefully monitored during pregnancy, even if they had no evidence of kidney disease at the time of diagnosis. These women are at increased risk of developing hypertension and proteinuria during pregnancy.

BIBLIOGRAPHY

IMMUNULOGLOBIN A NEPHROPATHY

Natural History, Epidemiology, and Diagnosis

Berger J, Hinglais N: Les depots intercapillaries d'IgA-IgG, *Journal d Urologie et de Nephrologie* 74:694-695, 1968.

Berthoux FC, Mohey H, Afiani A: Natural history of primary IgA nephropathy, *Semin Nephrol* 28:4-9, 2008.

Cattran DC, Coppo R, Cook HT, et al: The Oxford classification of IgA nephropathy: rationale, clinicopathological correlations, and classification, *Kidney Int* 76:534-545, 2009.

Geddes CC, Rauta V, Gronhagen-Riska C, et al: A tricontinental view of IgA nephropathy, *Nephrol Dial Transplant* 18:1541-1548, 2003.

Mackinnon B, Fraser EP, Cattran DC, et al: Validation of the Toronto formula to predict progression in IgA nephropathy, *Nephron Clin Pract* 109:c148-153, 2008.

Pouria S, Barratt J: Secondary IgA nephropathy, *Semin Nephrol* 28:27-37, 2008.

Pathogenesis

Barratt J, Feehally J: Primary IgA nephropathy: new insights into pathogenesis, *Semin Nephrol* 31:349-360, 2011.

Barratt J, Smith AC, Feehally J: The pathogenic role of IgA1 O-linked glycosylation in the pathogenesis of IgA nephropathy (Review Article), *Nephrology (Carlton)* 12:275-284, 2007.

Moura IC, Benhamou M, Launay P, et al: The glomerular response to IgA deposition in IgA nephropathy, *Semin Nephrol* 28:88-95, 2008.

Novak J, Julian BA, Tomana M, et al: IgA glycosylation and IgA immune complexes in the pathogenesis of IgA nephropathy, *Semin Nephrol* 28:78-87, 2008.

Genetics

Feehally J, Farrall M, Boland A, et al: HLA has strongest association with IgA nephropathy in genome-wide analysis, *J Am Soc Nephrol* 21:1791-1797, 2010.

Gharavi AG, Moldoveanu Z, Wyatt RJ, et al: Aberrant IgA1 glycosylation is inherited in familial and sporadic IgA nephropathy, *J Am Soc Nephrol* 19:1008-1014, 2008.

Treatment

Boyd JK, Cheung CK, Molyneux K, et al: An update on the pathogenesis and treatment of IgA nephropathy, *Kidney Int* 81:833-843, 2012.

Eitner F, Floege J: Glomerular disease: ACEIs with or without corticosteroids in IgA nephropathy? *Nat Rev Nephrol* 6:252-254, 2010.

Strippoli GF, Manno C, Schena FP: An "evidence-based" survey of therapeutic options for IgA nephropathy: assessment and criticism, *Am J Kidney Dis* 41:1129-1139, 2003.

Wang Y, Chen J, Chen Y, et al: A meta-analysis of the clinical remission rate and long-term efficacy of tonsillectomy in patients with IgA nephropathy, *Nephrol Dial Transplant* 26:1923-1931, 2011.

Xu G, Tu W, Jiang D, Xu C: Mycophenolate mofetil treatment for IgA nephropathy: a meta-analysis, *Am J Nephrol* 29:362-367, 2008.

HENOCH-SCHÖNLEIN PURPURA

Kiryluk K, Moldoveanu Z, Sanders J, et al: Aberrant glycosylation of IgA1 is inherited in pediatric IgA nephropathy and Henoch-Schönlein purpura nephritis, *Kidney Int* 80:79-87, 2011.

Ronkainen J, Nuutinen M, Koskimies O: The adult kidney 24 years after childhood Henoch-Schönlein purpura: a retrospective cohort study, *Lancet* 360:666-670, 2002.

Sanders JT, Wyatt RJ: IgA nephropathy and Henoch-Schönlein purpura nephritis, *Curr Opin Pediatr* 20:163-170, 2008.

Goodpasture Syndrome and Other Antiglomerular Basement Membrane Diseases

21

Alan D. Salama | Charles D. Pusey

The term *Goodpasture syndrome* was first used by Stanton and Tange in 1957 in their report of nine patients with pulmonary renal syndrome; it referred back to the original patient described by Goodpasture in 1919. It was not until the 1960s that the development of immunofluorescence techniques led to the detection of immunoglobulin deposited along the glomerular basement membrane (GBM) in this condition. Today the term *Goodpasture syndrome* is often used to describe the combination of rapidly progressive glomerulonephritis (RPGN), pulmonary hemorrhage, and anti-GBM antibodies. However, some researchers use *Goodpasture syndrome* to refer to those patients with the characteristic clinical features from any cause and *Goodpasture disease* to describe those who in addition have anti-GBM antibodies. The term *anti-GBM disease* is also widely used to describe any patient with the typical autoantibodies, regardless of clinical features.

CLINICAL FEATURES

Goodpasture syndrome exhibits a bimodal age distribution, with peak incidences in the third and sixth decades of life, and a slight preponderance toward males. Most patients present with RPGN and lung hemorrhage, although about one third present with isolated glomerulonephritis. Rarely, patients present with isolated lung hemorrhage without kidney failure, although many of these patients will experience hematuria and proteinuria. General malaise, fatigue, and weight loss are the most common systemic features and may relate to anemia.

PULMONARY DISEASE

Pulmonary hemorrhage occurs in about two thirds of patients and is more common in young men. It may precede the development of kidney disease. Patients often complain of breathlessness and cough, which may be accompanied by minor or massive hemoptysis. Cigarette smoking, inhaled toxins, sepsis, or fluid overload can trigger hemoptysis. Clinical signs include tachypnea, respiratory crackles, and eventually cyanosis, but these are often indistinguishable from the signs of pulmonary edema or infection. Radiographic features are nonspecific but usually involve patchy or diffuse alveolar shadowing in the central lung fields (Fig. 21.1). The most sensitive test is an elevation in the carbon monoxide diffusion capacity of the lungs, which is caused by the presence of hemoglobin in the alveolar spaces. Bronchoscopy may reveal diffuse hemorrhage, but it is perhaps of more importance in excluding infection. Despite the common presentation of pulmonary hemorrhage, long-term pulmonary sequelae are uncommon in treated patients.

KIDNEY DISEASE

Although occasional patients may present with isolated hematuria or mildly reduced kidney function, they most commonly present with kidney failure as a result of RPGN. The clinical features are not distinguishable from those of any other cause of RPGN, although, unlike cases of RPGN that are associated with systemic vasculitis, systemic features (other than lung hemorrhage) are uncommon. Urine microscopy typically shows numerous erythrocytes of glomerular origin, red-cell casts, and mild to moderate proteinuria; nephrotic-range proteinuria is rare unless there is a secondary concurrent glomerular disease such as membranous nephropathy. Hypertension and oliguria are late features. Renal ultrasonography usually reveals normal-sized kidneys and is helpful in excluding other kidney disorders.

PATHOLOGY

Light microscopy of the kidney biopsy specimen usually shows diffuse crescentic glomerulonephritis, with most of the crescents at the same stage of evolution (Fig. 21.2). Often, segmental necrosis of glomeruli and some cellular proliferation are present. Blood vessels are usually normal, but vasculitis has been reported. There is usually a prominent interstitial cellular infiltrate. The immunohistology is characteristic, with linear deposits of immunoglobulin G (IgG), sometimes accompanied by IgA or IgM, and complement C3, along the GBM (Fig. 21.3). Less intense linear staining with IgG may occasionally be seen in patients with diabetes, systemic lupus erythematosus, myeloma, or transplanted kidney (termed linear attenuation), but these conditions typically are not associated with crescent formation. Lung histology findings are rarely obtained, because transbronchial biopsy does not provide adequate specimens. Open-lung biopsy can show alveoli full of red cells, hemosiderin-laden macrophages, and fibrin. Immunofluorescence

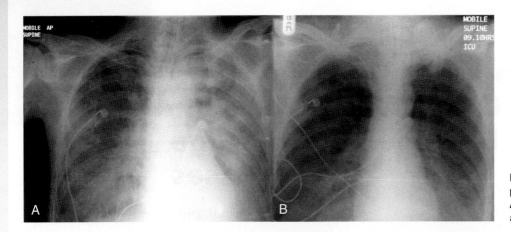

Figure 21.1   Chest radiographs of a patient with Goodpasture disease. **A,** Alveolar hemorrhage. **B,** Resolution after 4 days of treatment.

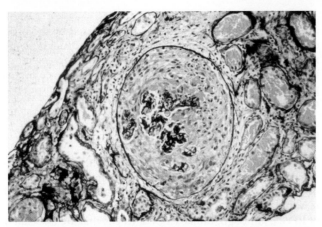

Figure 21.2   Renal biopsy from a patient with Goodpasture disease showing acute crescentic glomerulonephritis *(silver stain).*

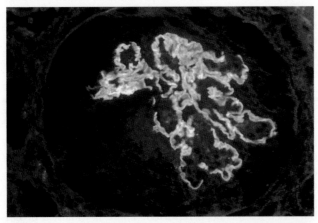

Figure 21.3   Renal biopsy from a patient with Goodpasture disease. Immunofluorescence microscopy shows linear deposition of immunoglobulin G along the glomerular basement membrane.

is technically difficult but may reveal linear deposits of IgG along the alveolar basement membrane.

DIFFERENTIAL DIAGNOSIS

It is important to distinguish anti-GBM disease from other causes of pulmonary renal syndrome and RPGN, because

---

Box 21.1   Causes of Pulmonary Renal Syndrome

More Common Causes

Microscopic polyangiitis
Granulomatosis with polyangiitis
Goodpasture disease
Systemic lupus erythematosus

Less Common Causes

Churg-Strauss syndrome
Henoch-Schönlein purpura
Hemolytic uremic syndrome
Behçet syndrome
Essential mixed cryoglobulinemia
Rheumatoid vasculitis
Penicillamine therapy

---

treatment and prognosis are different. Primary systemic vasculitis associated with antineutrophil cytoplasm antibodies (ANCA) is the most common cause of pulmonary renal syndrome and is the main consideration in the differential diagnosis. Not infrequently, patients have both anti-GBM antibodies and ANCA; this is discussed in more detail later. Other conditions to consider include systemic lupus erythematosus, cryoglobulinemia, Henoch-Schönlein purpura, and various other causes of pulmonary renal syndrome (Box 21.1). The diagnosis of anti-GBM disease can be made by kidney biopsy or by the detection of circulating anti-GBM antibodies. Various enzyme-linked immunosorbent assays (ELISA) are available for serologic testing; although their specificity is generally equivalent, they may vary in their sensitivity. A screen for other relevant antibodies (e.g., ANCA, anti-DNA antibodies) is usually performed at the same time. Rarely, anti-GBM disease can occur in the absence of detectable circulating anti-GBM antibodies but with positive immunohistology on kidney biopsy. These cases have similar antibody properties on biosensor analysis but are not detected on standard ELISA tests. The vast majority of patients' anti-GBM antibodies react with the noncollagenous domain of the α3 chain of type IV collagen and to a lesser extent the α5 chain. Rare reports of reactivity to other collagen chains have been published. Anti-GBM antibodies appear to correlate with disease activity, and their removal via plasmapheresis is associated with clinical improvement.

PATHOGENESIS

There is good evidence that anti-GBM disease is caused by the development of autoimmunity to a component of the GBM known as the Goodpasture antigen. The GBM is formed from a network of type IV collagen molecules, of which the α1 and α2 chains are widespread in vascular basement membranes, whereas the α3, α4, and α5 chains are restricted to the GBM and certain other specialized basement membranes. The Goodpasture antigen is present in the noncollagenous 1 (NC1) domain of the α3 chain of type IV collagen [α3(IV)NC1]. Two main antibody epitopes are closely colocalized in the intact molecule, and these are usually sequestered, suggesting that tolerance is broken after exposure of the cryptic epitopes to the immune system. This hypothesis is further supported by the development of anti-GBM disease after renal insults such as lithotripsy, systemic vasculitis, and membranous glomerulonephritis. Such epitopes may also be generated after the action of reactive oxygen species on GBM. The antigen is also found in basement membranes of the alveoli, choroid plexus, cochlea, and eye, although only lung and renal damage is generally evident.

EPIDEMIOLOGY

Limited epidemiologic studies have suggested that anti-GBM disease has an incidence of 0.5 to 1 case per million population per year. It is found in ≤2% of kidney biopsies and may account for ≤7% of patients with end-stage kidney disease. It is predominantly a disease of whites, but has now been reported in Chinese and Japanese cohorts and is less common in those of African origin.

GENETIC PREDISPOSITION

Goodpasture disease has been reported in siblings and in two sets of identical twins; however, discordant twins have also been documented as having the disease. As in other autoimmune diseases, there are associations with the major histocompatibility complex. There is a strong association with human leukocyte antigen (HLA) DR2, which is carried by approximately 85% of patients with Goodpasture disease. Molecular analysis of HLA class II alleles has confirmed the positive association with DRB1*1501 and DRB1*1502, as well as weaker associations with DRB1*04 and DRB1*03. There are negative associations with DRB1*07 and DRB1*01, suggesting that these are protective alleles. Because of linkage disequilibrium, there are also positive associations with the DQ genes DQA1*01 and DQB1*06. In addition, there are reports of polymorphisms in the inhibitory FcγRIIB and increased copy number of the activatory FcγRIIIA in patients compared to healthy controls.

ENVIRONMENTAL FACTORS

There are several case reports documenting exposure to hydrocarbons before the onset of clinical disease. There are also case-control studies showing a higher incidence of anti-GBM antibodies (usually borderline levels) in those exposed to inhaled industrial hydrocarbons. Cigarette smoking undoubtedly precipitates pulmonary hemorrhage, but it is of uncertain relevance to the etiology. Several clusters of cases have been reported, and there are suggestions of associations with viral infection. However, no clear association with any specific infectious agent has been proved.

ASSOCIATED DISEASES

Antiglomerular basement membrane disease is rarely associated with other autoimmune disorders, except for systemic vasculitis. Up to 30% of patients have been shown to have ANCA, most commonly perinuclear ANCA (P-ANCA) specific for myeloperoxidase. Conversely, relatively few patients with ANCA-associated vasculitis also have anti-GBM antibodies (5% to 10%). A number of recent series have demonstrated that these "double-positive" patients have a kidney prognosis that initially resembles that of patients with isolated anti-GBM disease, in that they are unlikely to recover kidney function after they require dialysis. In contrast to patients with anti-GBM disease, however, relapse in the double-positive group is more common and resembles that in the ANCA-positive patients. Several patients with membranous nephropathy have been reported to develop anti-GBM disease, and conversely patients with anti-GBM disease may go on to develop membranous nephropathy. Anti-GBM disease has also been reported to occur after lithotripsy and after urinary tract obstruction.

AUTOIMMUNITY

In Goodpasture disease, the presence of anti-GBM antibodies is closely linked to the development of clinical features. Titers of anti-GBM antibodies rise rapidly in the months before clinical disease development, but these antibodies often can be found at low titer for some time before. There is a broad correlation between anti-GBM antibody levels at presentation and the severity of disease, and the disease recurs immediately in kidney transplants if the recipient still has circulating antibodies. Importantly, the transfer of anti-GBM antibodies from patients to squirrel monkeys confirmed that the antibodies are directly pathogenic; however, T cells are also involved in pathogenesis, both by providing help for autoreactive B cells and probably by contributing to cell-mediated glomerular injury. In certain rodent models, GBM-specific T cells are capable of mediating disease with minimal antibody responses, demonstrating that either cellular or humoral immunity may predominate in particular individuals and may lead to the same final result. A population of regulatory T cells can be detected in patients who have recovered from the disease, and this regulatory mechanism may account for the rarity of disease recurrence. Recently, low levels of IgG2/IgG4 anti-GBM antibodies have been isolated from healthy individuals. These are not detected on conventional anti-GBM assays but require affinity column isolation. Their clinical relevance is uncertain, but they also suggest that tolerance is actively maintained in healthy subjects.

ANTIGLOMERULAR BASEMENT MEMBRANE DISEASE AND TRANSPLANTATION

Antiglomerular basement membrane disease may develop in the transplanted kidney in patients with Alport syndrome. Patients with X-linked Alport syndrome inherit a defect in the α5 chain of type IV collagen, but they may also lack the α3 chain that contains the Goodpasture antigen. Transplantation of a normal kidney therefore exposes the immune system to an antigen to which tolerance has not developed, and an immune response is provoked. The antibodies may be against either the α5 or the α3 chain. Although many patients show antibody deposition along the GBM of the allograft, only a minority develop severe glomerulonephritis.

TREATMENT

Untreated anti-GBM disease is usually rapidly fatal, and, in the absence of treatment, kidney failure is expected. However, since its introduction in the 1970s, treatment with plasma exchange, cyclophosphamide, and corticosteroids (together with dialysis when required) now allows the great majority of patients to survive. The rationale behind this treatment regimen is that plasma exchange rapidly removes circulating anti-GBM antibodies, whereas cyclophosphamide prevents further antibody synthesis. There has been only one small trial of plasma exchange compared with drug treatment alone, and it suggested a trend toward improved outcome; however, the widely reported improvement in mortality and in kidney function after introduction of the treatment regimen described previously has led to its widespread use. The protocol we currently use is shown in Table 21.1. All patients should be considered for treatment; however, those with limited kidney disease who present dialysis dependent with extensive crescentic glomerulonephritis are least likely to respond, and many practitioners avoid treating them with immunsuppressive therapy. Some patients have been treated with intravenous methylprednisolone, but there is no convincing evidence that it confers a benefit, and it may be associated with a greater risk for infection. Similarly, pulsed intravenous cyclophosphamide has not been formally tested but has been shown to be equivalent to daily oral dosing in ANCA-associated vasculitis with moderate kidney involvement, and it has been used by some practitioners in small cohorts. Cyclosporine, mycophenolate mofetil, and the anti-CD20 monoclonal antibody rituximab have occasionally been used in patients unresponsive to other therapy, but their role is not yet clear, and they cannot be recommended as first-line therapy. In general, long-term treatment is not necessary, and patients can stop cyclophosphamide after 3 months. Some physicians then change to azathioprine, but there is little evidence that this is necessary. Steroids may be tapered off after approximately 6 months.

PROGNOSIS

Most patients now survive the acute disease, although it is important to note that pulmonary hemorrhage and infection remain as causes of death. In recent series, 1-year patient survival was 75% to 90%, but only about 40% of survivors recovered independent kidney function. The serum creatinine concentration usually starts to decrease within 1 or 2 weeks after the initiation of treatment, and most patients with a creatinine level of less than 6.8 mg/dl at presentation recover kidney function. However, it has been reported that those who have a creatinine level greater than 6.8 mg/dl or who are oliguric rarely recover kidney function. A single-center study of 71 treated patients showed that almost all of the patients with a creatinine level of less than 5.7 mg/dl recovered kidney function as did most of those with a level greater than 5.7 mg/dl, but not those requiring dialysis. Crescent scores of greater than 50% are usually, but not always, associated with a poor kidney prognosis. Patients presenting with dialysis-dependent kidney failure may therefore not benefit from immunosuppression unless they also have pulmonary hemorrhage. This is in marked contrast to the outcome in patients with ANCA-associated RPGN, in whom the majority should recover kidney function, even if

---

Table 21.1   Initial Treatment of Goodpasture Disease

Plasma exchange	Daily 4-L exchange for 5% human albumin solution. Use 300-600 mL fresh plasma within 3 days after invasive procedure (e.g., biopsy) or in patients with pulmonary hemorrhage. Continue for 14 days or until antibody levels are fully suppressed.
	Withhold if platelet count is <70,000/μL, fibrinogen <1 g/L or hemoglobin is <9 g/dl. Watch for coagulopathy, hypocalcemia, and hypokalemia.
Cyclophosphamide	Daily oral dosing at 2-3 mg/kg/day (round down to nearest 50 mg; use 2 mg/kg/day in patients >55 years).
	Stop if white cell count is <4 × 10⁹/mL, and restart at lower dose when count increases to >4 × 10⁹/mL.
	Pulsed IV cyclophosphamide has not been tested formally, but is equivalent in ANCA associated vasculitis.
Prednisone	Daily oral dosing at 1 mg/kg/day (maximum, 60 mg). Reduce dose weekly to 20 mg by week 6, and then more slowly.
	There is no evidence of benefit of IV methylprednisolone, and it may increase infection risk (possibly use it if plasma exchange not available).
Prophylactic treatments	Use oral nystatin and amphotericin (or fluconazole) for oropharyngeal fungal infection.
	Use histamine 2 blocker or proton-pump inhibitor for steroid-promoted gastric ulceration.
	Use low-dose cotrimoxazole for PCP.

ANCA, Antineutrophil cytoplasm antibody; *PCP, Pneumocystis jiroveci* pneumonia.

presenting with a creatinine level of greater than 6.8 mg/dl or if dialysis is ongoing. One potential reason for immunosuppression in dialysis-dependent patients is the more rapid elimination of anti-GBM antibodies, which may otherwise persist for years, to enable prompt transplant if a living kidney donor is available.

Exacerbations of pulmonary hemorrhage and worsening kidney function may occur early in the disease in the presence of anti-GBM antibodies, and are often triggered by infection. True late recurrence after anti-GBM antibodies have become undetectable is rare. Kidney transplantation may be performed after anti-GBM antibodies are undetectable, but we usually delay this, on an empiric basis, until at least 6 months after the disappearance of antibodies.

BIBLIOGRAPHY

Borza DB: Autoepitopes and alloepitopes of type IV collagen: role in the molecular pathogenesis of anti-GBM antibody glomerulonephritis, *Nephron Exp Nephrol* 106:e37-e43, 2007.

Cui Z, Zhao MH, Segelmark M, et al: Natural autoantibodies to myeloperoxidase, proteinase 3, and the glomerular basement membrane are present in normal individuals, *Kidney Int* 78:590-597, 2010.

Herody M, Bobrie G, Gouarin C, et al: Anti-GBM disease: predictive value of clinical, histological and serological data, *Clin Nephrol* 40:249-255, 1993.

Johnson JP, Moore JJ, Austin HJ, et al: Therapy of anti-glomerular basement membrane antibody disease: analysis of prognostic significance of clinical, pathological and treatment factors, *Medicine (Baltimore)* 64:219-227, 1985.

Lerner RA, Glassock RJ, Dixon FJ: The role of anti-glomerular basement membrane antibodies in the pathogenesis of human glomerulonephritis, *J Exp Med* 126:989-1004, 1967.

Levy JB, Hammad T, Coulthart A, et al: Clinical features and outcome of patients with both ANCA and anti-GBM antibodies, *Kidney Int* 66:1535-1540, 2004.

Levy JB, Turner AN, Rees AJ, et al: Long-term outcome of anti-glomerular basement membrane antibody disease treated with plasma exchange and immunosuppression, *Ann Intern Med* 134:1033-1942, 2001.

Lockwood CM, Rees AJ, Pearson TA, et al: Immunosuppression and plasma exchange in the treatment of Goodpasture's syndrome, *Lancet* 1:711-715, 1976.

Merkel F, Pullig O, Marx M, et al: Course and prognosis of anti-basement membrane antibody mediated disease: a report of 35 cases, *Nephrol Dial Transplant* 9:372-376, 1994.

Olson SW, Arbogast CB, Baker TP, et al: Asymptomatic autoantibodies associate with future anti-glomerular basement membrane disease, *J Am Soc Nephrol* 22:1946-1952, 2011.

Pedchenko V, Bondar O, Fogo AB, et al: Molecular architecture of the goodpasture autoantigen in anti-GBM nephritis, *N Engl J Med* 363:343-354, 2010.

Phelps RG, Rees AJ: The HLA complex in goodpasture's disease: a model for analyzing susceptibility to autoimmunity, *Kidney Int* 56:1638-1653, 1999.

Pusey CD: Anti-glomerular basement membrane (anti-GBM) disease, *Kidney Int* 64:1535-1550, 2003.

Rutgers A, Slot M, van Paassen P, et al: Coexistence of anti-glomerular basement membrane antibodies and myeloperoxidase-ANCAs in crescentic glomerulonephritis, *Am J Kidney Dis* 46:253-262, 2005.

Salama AD, Chaudhry AN, Holthaus KA, et al: Regulation by CD25+ lymphocytes of autoantigen-specific T-cell responses in Goodpasture's (anti-GBM) disease, *Kidney Int* 64:1685-1694, 2003.

Salama AD, Dougan T, Levy JB, et al: Goodpasture's disease in the absence of circulating anti-glomerular basement membrane antibodies as detected by standard techniques, *Am J Kidney Dis* 39:1162-1167, 2002.

Salama AD, Pusey CD: Immunology of anti-glomerular basement membrane disease, *Curr Opin Nephrol Hypertens* 11:279-286, 2002.

Saus J, Wieslander J, Langeveld JPM, et al: Identification of the Goodpasture antigen as the α3(IV) chain of collagen IV, *J Biol Chem* 263:13374-13380, 1988.

Sinico RA, Radice A, Corace C, et al: Anti-glomerular basement membrane antibodies in the diagnosis of goodpasture syndrome: a comparison of different assays, *Nephrol Dial Transplant* 21:397-401, 2006.

Turner N, Mason PJ, Brown R, et al: Molecular cloning of the human goodpasture antigen demonstrates it to be the alpha 3 chain of type IV collagen, *J Clin Invest* 89:592-601, 1992.

Wilson CB, Dixon FJ: Anti-glomerular basement membrane antibody-induced glomerulonephritis, *Kidney Int* 3:74-89, 1973.

Zhou XJ, Lv JC, Bu DF, et al: Copy number variation of FCGR3A rather than FCGR3B and FCGR2B is associated with susceptibility to anti-GBM disease, *Int Immunol* 22:45-51, 2010.

THE KIDNEY IN SYSTEMIC DISEASE

22

Postinfectious Glomerulonephritis

Alain Meyrier

Infection remains a common cause of proliferative glomerulonephritis (GN). Kidney biopsies demonstrate that the same agent may induce more than one histologic type of GN, and that any given glomerular lesion may be the consequence of a wide array of pathogens. In the early 1970s, this chapter would have been almost entirely devoted to poststreptococcal acute glomerulonephritis (AGN) complicating throat or skin infections and scarlet fever; however, in the ensuing decades, the epidemiology of postinfectious glomerulonephritis (PIGN) has considerably evolved in the Western world. Yet what has now changed in industrialized countries is not entirely applicable to other parts of the world, and poststreptococcal AGN remains a significant public health problem in Latin America, Africa, and most probably Eastern Europe. Any proliferative GN whose etiology is unclear should prompt consideration of an infectious origin, even if this etiology is not readily suggested by the clinical context. In most cases, the diagnosis of PIGN depends on a kidney biopsy evaluated by light microscopy (LM), immunofluorescence (IF), and electron microscopy (EM).

CLINICAL APPROACH

The clinical presentation of PIGN spans a large spectrum. A bacterial cause should be considered in any patient with the acute nephritic syndrome, acute or rapidly progressive GN, or nephrotic syndrome with progressively declining kidney function. An infectious cause is suggested when any of these glomerular syndromes follow or accompany evident bacterial infection; however, the infection may be covert or may be overlooked in the patient's history. These considerations justify wide indications for kidney biopsy, because it may be the pathologist who alerts the clinician to the presence of a possible infectious cause. One such example is a biopsy performed in the course of a febrile episode that discloses glomerular lesions strongly suggestive of infective endocarditis. Along the same line, EM may disclose lesions suggestive of superimposed PIGN on a kidney biopsy performed in a patient with another identified glomerular disease, for instance diabetic glomerulopathy.

ACUTE NEPHRITIC SYNDROME

Acute nephritic syndrome is the common clinical presentation of PIGN, irrespective of the organism. *Streptococcus* and *Staphylococcus* are the most common agents; however, nephritic syndromes are not pathognomonic of PIGN and can be observed in IgA nephropathy, Henoch-Schönlein

purpura, idiopathic membranoproliferative GN (MPGN), and occasionally crescentic pauci-immune GN, among others.

Classically, the illness is characterized by rapid onset of edema, hypertension, oliguria, and concentrated brownish urine with low urinary sodium, heavy proteinuria, and microscopic or often macroscopic hematuria. In contrast to idiopathic nephrotic syndrome (minimal change disease and focal-segmental glomerulosclerosis), volume expansion involves both the interstitial and the intravascular compartments. Thus hypertension, cardiac enlargement, and pulmonary edema may be present along with peripheral pitting edema. Kidney function ranges from normal to oliguric acute kidney injury (AKI). The clinical presentation in children can be fulminant, with abdominal pain, acute cerebral edema, and seizures. In the elderly, volume overload may present with acute pulmonary edema in about 40% of patients versus less than 5% in children. Other features distinguishing AGN in the elderly from the disease in children are, respectively, nephrotic proteinuria in 20% versus less than 5%, AKI in ~75% versus ~35%, and an early mortality in 25% of adults, whereas it is virtually nonexistent in children.

In contrast to IgA nephropathy where macroscopic hematuria shortly follows upper respiratory tract infection (synpharyngitic hematuria) (see Chapter 20), in postpharyngitic forms of PIGN the episode of hematuria typically is delayed by 10 to 20 days after infection.

ACUTE OR RAPIDLY PROGRESSIVE GLOMERULONEPHRITIS

Postinfectious GN can manifest as AKI that is not necessarily correlated with a specific glomerular lesion. Some cases with purely proliferative and exudative GN may be oliguric at presentation, but they resolve completely. However, severely impaired kidney function may also indicate the presence of extracapillary (crescentic) proliferation. A kidney biopsy is almost always required in this setting, both to establish the diagnosis and to guide therapy.

NEPHROTIC SYNDROME AND PROGRESSIVE KIDNEY DISEASE

Hypertension, usually edema, heavy proteinuria (more than 1.5 g/day), and microscopic hematuria point to a more chronic form of glomerular disease. Except when the causative infection is identified, as in shunt nephritis (discussed later) or following a defined illness, the date of onset is generally unknown. The MPGN variant of PIGN often leads to progressive chronic kidney disease (CKD) and eventually end-stage renal disease (ESRD). Chronic GN with nephrotic proteinuria is an indication for kidney biopsy when the kidneys are not atrophic, because atrophy indicates irreversible fibrosis.

PATHOLOGY

The glomerular lesions found in PIGN fall into three light microscopic patterns: acute endocapillary exudative GN, endocapillary plus extracapillary (crescentic) GN, and MPGN.

ACUTE ENDOCAPILLARY EXUDATIVE GLOMERULONEPHRITIS

Acute endocapillary exudative GN is the classic appearance of acute poststreptococcal GN. However, no routine markers are available for histologic identification of the offending microorganism, and the lesions are the same in AGN caused by *Staphylococcus*, other bacteria, and viruses. Many pediatricians defer a biopsy when the clinical picture is typical. This approach is not standard for adults.

CELL PROLIFERATION

By LM, diffuse hypercellularity involves all glomeruli so that the diagnosis can be made on a sample containing just a few or even a single glomerulus. The glomerular tufts are greatly enlarged with few open capillaries and minimal urinary space remaining (Fig. 22.1). Hypercellularity results both from proliferation of resident glomerular cells, mainly mesangial, and the influx of polymorphonuclear leukocytes, monocytes/macrophages, and plasma cells. The old term *exudative* refers to the presence of abundant polymorphonuclear cells, some of which may be eosinophils. It is possible, albeit unusual, to find small focal regions of necrosis with fibrin in some glomeruli. Overall, cell proliferation may range from massive infiltration obstructing virtually all capillary lumina to mild inflammation with a moderate increase in mesangial cellularity and greater than normal numbers of polymorphonuclear leukocytes (normal is fewer than five per glomerulus).

GLOMERULAR BASEMENT MEMBRANE CHANGES

The most characteristic change in acute GN is the postinfectious subepithelial hump. It is usually easily detected on silver staining (Fig. 22.2), and it appears as a triangular or oval structure on the outer aspect of the GBM overlain by a continuous layer of podocyte cytoplasm. The rest of the GBM is normal. Humps are not absolutely pathognomonic of PIGN, but LM and IF easily eliminate other etiologies such as Henoch-Schönlein purpura and idiopathic MPGN. Humps are especially prominent within the first weeks of disease. However, LM findings may be ambiguous. EM is then of diagnostic value, as it demonstrates distinct subepithelial and intramembranous deposits indicative of a postinfectious glomerular injury (Fig. 22.3).

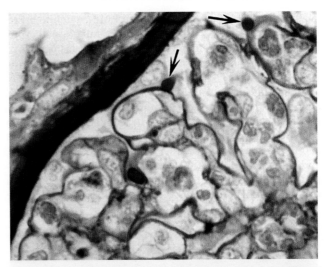

Figure 22.2   Acute poststaphylococcal glomerulonephritis. Typical humps on the outer aspect of the glomerular basement membranes *(arrows)*. Silver methenamine staining was used.

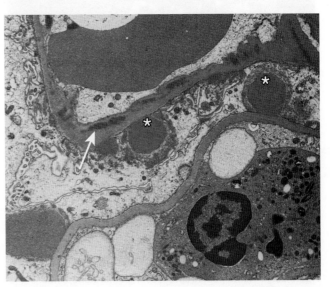

Figure 22.3   Acute poststreptococcal glomerulonephritis. Electron microscopy discloses typical humps *(asterisks)* and intramembranous immune complexes *(arrow)*.

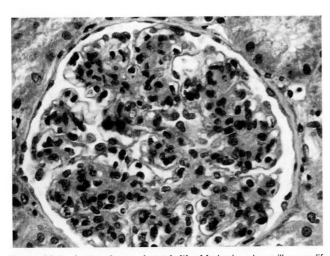

Figure 22.1   Acute glomerulonephritis. Marked endocapillary proliferation. Few capillary lumens remain open. Masson trichrome staining was used.

IMMUNOFLUORESCENCE

Specific antisera disclose granular IgG and C3 deposits along the capillary wall and within the mesangium (Fig. 22.4). Humps appear brightly fluorescent. Two IF patterns have been described. The "garland" type primarily follows the outline of capillary wall. IF shows numerous bright humps. This appearance is often associated with heavy proteinuria. The starry-sky pattern consists of coarser deposits with mesangial predominance and comprises fewer humps. Proteinuria is less abundant than in the garland type. It should be stressed that the absence of complement components on IF preparations casts strong doubt on the infectious origin of a glomerulopathy.

ENDOCAPILLARY PLUS EXTRACAPILLARY (CRESCENTIC) GLOMERULONEPHRITIS

The classical picture of GN associated with systemic bacterial infection consists of focal GN with cellular and necrotic lesions in some of the glomerular tufts. This was described in the early 1900s as "embolic" GN in the course of subacute bacterial endocarditis. However, the most common picture complicating endocarditis and other forms of septicemia, as well as visceral abscesses with negative blood cultures, consists of endocapillary plus extracapillary proliferation (Fig. 22.5). Crescent formation is an ominous finding that is often accompanied by interstitial edema, inflammation, and tubular atrophy. Crescents appear as layers of inflammatory cells comprising parietal epithelial cells (Bowman capsule) and macrophages. Necrosis is characterized by the

presence of fibrin. The size and distribution of crescents may vary from one glomerulus to another. Circumferential crescents anticipate glomerular obsolescence. The spared lobules show the same proliferative changes as described previously. IF shows IgG and C3 deposits as well as fibrin within crescents.

MEMBRANOPROLIFERATIVE GLOMERULONEPHRITIS

That MPGN may be the consequence of infection has been demonstrated in the case of shunt nephritis. The lesions comprise mesangial proliferation, exudative polymorphonuclear cell infiltration, and characteristic GBM changes consisting of double contours caused by interposition of mesangial cells beneath the basement membrane elaborating an additional layer of silver-stained mesangial matrix (Fig. 22.6). Humps and abundant C3 deposits are strongly suggestive of a postinfectious origin of this type of glomerulopathy, and they help to differentiate this type from the "idiopathic" variety.

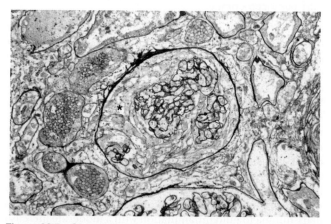

Figure 22.5   Crescentic glomerulonephritis complicating a case of bacterial endocarditis in an elderly patient with urinary tract infection due to *Enterococcus faecalis*. A circumferential crescent *(asterisk)* surrounds the remaining glomerular tuft. Silver methenamine staining was used.

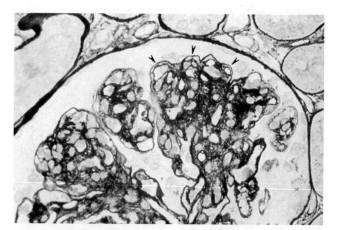

Figure 22.6   Membranoproliferative glomerulonephritis in a 50-year-old man with a lifelong history of acne. Typical glomerular basement membrane double contours *(arrowheads)*. Silver methenamine staining was used.

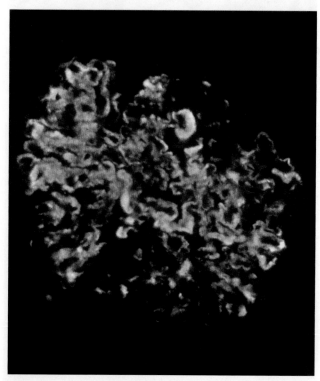

Figure 22.4   Acute poststreptococcal glomerulonephritis. Immunofluorescence with an anti-C3 antiserum discloses widespread "garland-type" C3 labeling, mostly along the glomerular basement membranes.

ETIOLOGY AND EPIDEMIOLOGY

ACUTE POSTINFECTIOUS GLOMERULONEPHRITIS

Acute poststreptococcal GN due to nephritogenic strains of *Streptococcus pyogenes*, group A, remains common in tropical and subtropical regions. It primarily affects children and otherwise healthy adults, including the elderly. The illness is contagious and can be epidemic. The nephropathy is characterized by the rapid onset of acute nephritic syndrome 10 to 20 days after pharyngeal or cutaneous infection. The offending microorganism is not always identified, but serologic markers usually confirm that the etiologic agent is *Streptococcus*. The complement profile is characterized by hypocomplementemia with activation of both the classical and the alternative pathways leading to depressed C3 and C4 levels, followed by normalization within approximately 6 weeks. Spontaneous recovery is the rule. Proteinuria wanes over weeks, but microscopic hematuria can last a few months. Poststreptococcal AGN is most often a benign disease, especially in children. However, in some cases AGN with an initial reassuring histologic appearance of acute exudative GN may progress without remission to crescentic GN. Persistently low complement levels, weeks and months following the initial episode, along with heavy proteinuria, hematuria, and declining kidney function indicate the disease is not following its usual self-limited course and is progressing to chronic GN. Such progression is an indication to perform repeat kidney biopsy.

With regard to long-term prognosis, some publications dating back to the 1970s indicate that, after a protracted period of apparent cure, some patients experience hypertension, renal vascular lesions, and CKD progression even to ESRD. More recent data from Australia also indicate that childhood poststreptococcal GN is a risk factor for CKD in later life.

However, it is difficult to determine the actual long-term outcome of AGN, because kidney biopsies were not performed in these early cohorts. The reported rate of recovery varied from 28% to 100%. The course appears to be more benign in children than in adults. Studies performed during epidemics have determined that, in a substantial number of affected children, kidney disease is clinically silent with GN detected only with proteinuria and microscopic hematuria on screening urinalyses. How many of these clinically silent cases might later eventuate in chronic GN is an unsettled issue. This ascertainment bias may account for the impression that the disease is less severe in children. It has never been clearly established whether cases that are clinically mild and detected only by screening have a better long-term prognosis than the sporadic adult cases that attract attention because kidney involvement is more pronounced and kidney biopsy is almost systematic in adults. In any event, a patient having suffered an episode of AGN should be advised to undergo an annual medical examination incorporating at a minimum assessment of blood pressure, dipstick proteinuria and hematuria, and kidney function. In case of doubt about ongoing glomerular disease, additional clinical and laboratory workup should be pursued. This may include a repeat kidney biopsy.

A retrospective examination of electron microscopic findings in 1012 consecutive kidney biopsies performed at Johns Hopkins in 2003 illustrates the frequency with which infection may be overlooked as the cause of various glomerulopathies. This study showed evidence of resolving or largely healed PIGN in 57 of 543 cases in which a primary diagnosis of an immune complex related glomerular disease had been ruled out by the case history, clinical and laboratory data, and the absence of any specific substructure suggesting a disease other than PIGN (e.g., cryoglobulinemia, fibrillary GN, "fingerprints" suggestive of lupus nephritis). These 57 cases included 26 with an established diagnosis of PIGN. The extant specimens were considered "incidental PIGN" according to EM criteria typical of an infectious etiology. Such findings suggest that clinically silent PIGN is relatively frequent, especially in diabetics who represented 40% of these 57 biopsies.

Acute GN can follow infection with a host of microorganisms. Acute GN complicating staphylococcal infection is virtually indistinguishable from poststreptococcal AGN. This is also true of AGN caused by most of the etiologic agents found in Table 22.1. In the Western world, the incidence of classical poststreptococcal AGN has steadily declined in recent decades, becoming rare in children. On the other hand, microorganisms other than *Streptococcus* are increasingly recognized as etiologic agents for AGN. Thus, the overall incidence of PIGN has remained the same but with a different variety of pathogens. In adults, an immunocompromised background is emerging as a predisposing factor, especially in diabetics, but also in alcoholic and cirrhotic patients. However, individuals with human immunodeficiency virus (HIV) carriage, acquired immunodeficiency syndrome (AIDS), and those receiving immunosuppressive medications do not seem to be at increased risk for AGN.

POSTINFECTIOUS GLOMERULONEPHRITIS WITH RAPID OR SUBACUTE DEVELOPMENT

As noted previously, the typical endocapillary exudative AGN does not always resolve spontaneously. An unfavorable

---

Table 22.1   Infectious Agents Most Frequently Associated With Glomerulonephritis

Bacteria	Viruses
Streptococcus	Hepatitis B
Staphylococcus	Hepatitis C
Pneumococcus	Echovirus
Enterobacteriaceae	Adenovirus
Salmonella typhi	Coxsackievirus
Meningococcus	Cytomegalovirus
Treponema pallidum	Epstein-Barr virus
Brucella	Enteroviruses
Leptospira	Measles
Yersinia	Mumps
Rickettsia	Varicella
Legionella	Rubella

A 2008 American study identified bacteria causing glomerulonephritis were more frequently *Staphylococcus* (46%), *Streptococcus* (16%), and gram-negative organisms. The most common sites of infection were the upper respiratory tract (23%), skin (17%), lung (17%), and heart valves (11.6%). Chronic glomerulonephritis developed in 25% of patients.

course is primarily restricted to patients whose kidney involvement consists of endocapillary plus extracapillary (crescentic) GN. This variety of PIGN is not new. Crescentic GN following septicemia from infectious endocarditis has been known for nearly a century. Nevertheless, its relative frequency, at least in industrialized countries, has grown in inverse proportion to that of acute poststreptococcal GN. Its mode of onset and clinical features are more varied. The onset may be heralded by acute nephritic syndrome or rapidly progressive glomerular filtration rate (GFR) loss. Alternatively, the disorder may not be detected until CKD has developed. The initial focus of infection is not always easy to identify. Most cutaneous, dental, and visceral infections can be complicated by endocapillary and extracapillary GN. Several simultaneous candidate foci may be found in a given patient growing both gram-positive and gram-negative organisms. In contrast to acute poststreptococcal GN, extrarenal manifestations, especially purpura, may be present. In a febrile patient with GN and purpura, especially when purpura is observed on the nape of the neck, a search for endocarditis by transesophageal ultrasound examination and repeated blood cultures is mandatory. In our experience, low serum complement levels were found in only 24% of 25 cases with crescentic GN, likely indicating that the acute initial phase of the disease had occurred in the past.

Risk factors for this form of PIGN include alcoholism, substance abuse, malnutrition, and low socioeconomic level. These factors are associated with poor dental and cutaneous hygiene, and delayed access to medical care. The prognosis depends on the severity of infection, the immunologic status and age of the host, and the findings on kidney biopsy. The extent of crescentic proliferation on a biopsy comprising a sufficient number of glomeruli is the best predictor of progression to ESRD. Early recognition and eradication of the infectious foci with antibiotic treatment and, if necessary, visceral or dental surgery are probably the best means of preventing the progression of kidney disease.

POSTINFECTIOUS MEMBRANOPROLIFERATIVE GLOMERULONEPHRITIS

Membranoproliferative glomerulonephritis (MPGN) was long considered idiopathic in a majority of cases. However, some forms were evidently postinfectious, such as shunt nephritis. Ventriculoatrial shunting (now replaced by ventriculoperitoneal shunting), was devised in the 1950s to relieve hydrocephalus, mostly in children. This procedure consists of a silicon catheter and a valve connecting the cerebral ventricle to the right atrium. The prosthetic material can become colonized with *Staphylococcus epidermidis* or, more rarely, other organisms. Among uncommon strains that may colonize the shunt and induce the MPGN, *Propionibacterium acnes* (a relatively slow growing, typically aerotolerant anaerobic gram-positive bacterium that is linked to acne) deserves mentioning for more general pathophysiologic reasons (see Fig. 22.6).

About 160 cases of "shunt nephritis" have been published. Fever, arthralgias, wasting, purpura, and severe anemia characterize the disease. Laboratory findings suggest an immune complex disease with low serum complement levels, complement-driven hemolytic anemia, antinuclear antibodies, rheumatoid factor, and cryoglobulins. Kidney signs include proteinuria, microscopic hematuria, and GFR loss that can be rapidly progressive.

Kidney biopsy usually discloses type I MPGN, often with numerous endocapillary polymorphonuclear cells and abundant C3 deposits. Endocapillary and extracapillary GN has also been observed. Removal of the shunt (which is a difficult and often complicated neurosurgical procedure) and antibiotic treatment may be followed by stabilization and even regression of the glomerular lesions, a demonstration that type I MPGN is not invariably irreversible. Nevertheless, only half of the patients experience a complete remission.

Several observations are consistent with the theory that other cases of "idiopathic" MPGN are also of infectious origin. These include the presence of C3 made evident by IF, and epidemiologic studies demonstrating the striking simultaneous decrease in the incidence of both AGN and MPGN in Western Europe.

PATHOGENESIS

OFFENDING MICROORGANISMS

A host of microorganisms, including microbes, parasites, and viruses (see Chapter 28 for viral glomerulopathies), can be responsible for PIGN. For historical reasons, the most consistent data are concerned with streptococci. It has been established that only specific strains of group A streptococci can cause acute GN, especially certain strains of Lancefield type 12. The disease is contagious. Some cases are caused by unusual strains with an animal origin, such as strangles in horses (*Streptococcus equi*), mastitis in cows (*Streptococcus zooepidemicus*), and *Streptococcus suis* causing AGN in Asian butchers carving pork. The main sites of human streptococcal infection are the throat, especially in the winter and early spring, and the skin, especially in the late summer and early fall. Tropical or subtropical climates favor skin infection, especially in black children, whereas a pharyngeal origin is more common in temperate climates and in white children. In highly populated areas with low socioeconomic status, poststreptococcal GN is often epidemic. Studies from both the United States and Western Europe have documented a decline in poststreptococcal AGN during recent decades in urban areas, contrasting with a stable incidence in rural areas. In fact, the sharp decline of poststreptococcal AGN and acute rheumatic fever in industrialized countries contrasts with a continuing high incidence in the tropical regions of Africa, Latin America, and the Caribbean. The prevalence remains high in the countries of Mediterranean Africa, which have a dry climate but a low per capita income.

Is this declining incidence just the consequence of better socioeconomic conditions? A French government-sponsored study that focused on eradication of rheumatic heart disease through the systematic free distribution of oral phenoxymethylpenicillin in the French Caribbean was immediately followed by a dramatic decrease in the annual incidence of both rheumatic fever and acute GN, suggesting that early eradication of *Streptococcus pyogenes* group A infection is effective in preventing AGN. The same is likely true for staphylococcal and other etiologic agents.

COMPLEMENT SYSTEM IN POSTINFECTIOUS GLOMERULONEPHRITIS

Low serum complement levels are almost always present during the acute, initial phase of PIGN, indicating the early involvement of the classic pathway. In poststreptococcal GN, low C3 levels characterize this initial phase, with C4 being less depressed than C3. Protein H, a surface protein of *Streptococcus pyogenes*, in association with IgG is also capable of activating the classic complement pathway. Between 15% and 30% of patients with poststreptococcal GN show evidence of reduced C1 and C4 complement component levels. The alternate complement pathway may also be activated, which is mediated by a transient expression of the C3 NeF autoantibody. The lectin pathway of complement activation may be activated in poststreptococcal GN as a result of recognition of the starter molecule mannose-binding lectin by the N-acetyl glucosamine residues of the bacterial wall.

COMPLEX PATHOPHYSIOLOGIC ISSUE OF POSTINFECTIOUS GLOMERULAR INFLAMMATION

Acute PIGN is an immunologic disease. A good clinical argument for this contention is the latent interval between clinical signs of infection and the onset of GN, at least when the onset of infection can be identified. This interval (similar to that of serum sickness) is usually easy to determine in acute GN, but is less readily discerned in endocapillary and extracapillary forms, and rarely is apparent in cases of MPGN. In general, all forms of proliferative GN appear to follow a triphasic course: (1) induction, depending on an antigen, (2) transduction, characterized by immunoglobulin deposits, and (3) mediation. This last phase involves a host of cytokines that originate from monocytes and macrophages, glomerular mesangial cells, platelets, and endothelial cells, including the C5a and C3a complement fractions, and interferon-γ as well as interleukin 2 (IL-2). Activation of these mediators leads to the generation of IL-1, tumor necrosis factor-α, interferon-γ, platelet-derived growth factor, and transforming growth factor-β. The role of C5b-9 in inducing arachidonic acid, free oxygen radicals, and IL-1 release is probably important. The initial event might be the deposition of circulating immune complexes that include a bacterial component, or fixation of bacterial antigens with in situ immune complex formation. In human disease, nephritogenic bacterial antigens are seldom identified within the glomeruli except in some studies evaluating streptococcal or staphylococcal infections. Nephritis-associated plasmin receptor, a group A streptococcal antigen identified as a glyceraldehyde phosphate dehydrogenase (GAPDH), and the cationic cysteine proteinase exotoxin B (SPE B) have been detected in the glomeruli of patients with acute GN following group A streptococcal infection. An antibody response to the latter was present. It is likely that these antigens, especially SPE B, have a pathogenic role in patients with acute poststreptococcal GN. However, considering the diversity of microorganisms and viruses capable of inducing PIGN, identification of specific antigens appears to be a formidable task.

Whatever the triggering mechanism, the usual course of poststreptococcal and poststaphylococcal endocapillary exudative AGN is mostly that of a self-limited disease. This is not the case for crescentic GN. Crescent formation in various conditions seems to be related to segmental destruction of the GBM by polymorphonuclear and macrophagic enzymes. Through these gaps, immune cells, plasma, fibrin, and inflammatory mediators gain access to Bowman space and induce an intense proliferative reaction of the parietal epithelial cells of Bowman capsule. Detached podocytes from the outer aspect of the GBM may participate in crescent formation. The natural history of untreated crescentic GN is evolution to fibrosis and glomerular obsolescence. Why other forms of PIGN produce the chronic form of MPGN is not readily apparent. The fact that the incidence of acute poststreptococcal GN and of MPGN has diminished in parallel suggests that, at least in some cases, the latter might be a mode of progression of an initial occult streptococcal glomerular injury.

POSTSTAPHYLOCOCCAL GLOMERULONEPHRITIS AND ITS IgA-DOMINANT IMMUNOFLUORESCENCE PATTERN

There have been a number of reports of GN with IgA-containing and often IgA-dominant immune complex deposits in association with infections with methicillin-sensitive *S. aureus* (MSSA), methicillin-resistant *S. aureus* (MRSA), and *S. epidermidis*.

CLINICAL CHARACTERISTICS

The typical patient presents with acute GN and massive proteinuria. The kidney biopsy often shows crescent formation. Some patients with MRSA infection may have a less severe clinical picture. The defining characteristic is the IgA dominant or codominant immune deposition in the biopsy. Serum IgA levels are frequently increased. Complement levels may be low or normal. When staphylococcal infection is not proven, these forms may pose a problem of distinguishing poststaphylococcal GN from IgA GN (see Chapter 20).

PATHOLOGY

The histologic features of these cases are variable, including predominantly mesangial proliferative GN, MPGN with or without crescents, and diffuse proliferative and exudative GN closely resembling acute poststreptococcal GN. This was well described in a series of 13 cases of IgA-dominant PIGN. The morphologic features closely resembled those of diffuse proliferative and exudative poststreptococcal GN. Five of the 13 patients were diabetic, and three had coexistent diabetic nephropathy. Six had documented staphylococcal infections before the onset of GN (three MRSA, three MSSA). IgA was the dominant immunoglobulin present in all cases, with five biopsies also staining for IgG and 10 for IgM. C3 was present in all cases with a mean staining intensity equal to that for IgA. Biopsies with histologic changes of acute or subacute PIGN showed a starry-sky pattern of IgA and C3 staining by IF, whereas those with resolving/chronic histology mainly exhibited a mesangial pattern.

PATHOGENESIS

The pathogenesis is poorly elucidated. There is an intense T cell activation resulting in direct binding of staphylococcal superantigens to the major histocompatibility complex class II molecules in antigen presenting cells (APC). The APC engage the Vβ+ T cell receptor region, and T cells activate B cells to produce polyclonal IgA and IgG.

PROGNOSTIC INDICATORS AND OUTCOME OF POSTINFECTIOUS GLOMERULONEPHRITIS

Prognostic indicators stem from both the patient's background and the severity of the infectious focus, as well as features of the glomerulopathy. Patients with poor general health because of malnutrition or cirrhosis are more likely to follow an unfavorable course. Patients with septicemia and those whose sites of infection include visceral abscesses, empyema, meningitis, or endocarditis are more likely to die from the primary disorder than the consequences of their glomerulopathy. Risk of death is significantly higher in older patients and in those with purpura. Initial presentation with nephrotic syndrome, a serum creatinine above ~2.7 mg/dl, and the presence of crescents and interstitial fibrosis on kidney biopsy all usually herald irreversible kidney damage. Two other factors at presentation predict a favorable prognosis: the upper respiratory tract as initial site of infection, and pure endocapillary proliferation with an IF starry-sky pattern. Proteinuria below 1.5 g/day is well correlated with recovery in patients with pure endocapillary proliferation, whereas nephrotic syndrome at presentation is often followed by persistent chronic GN. Persistently low serum complement is associated with worse outcomes.

TREATMENT

In the cases of pure endocapillary GN from three or four decades ago, the course was considered nearly uniformly favorable. More recent experience indicates that the location of the infectious focus is more varied than the throat and the skin, and this focus of infection often is still present at the time of kidney biopsy. Follow-up kidney biopsy months or even years after the initial one may disclose ongoing inflammatory lesions in patients whose infection persists, whereas in those in whom infection had been eradicated the glomerular lesions are mainly inactive and fibrous. This reinforces the need to eradicate any persistent infection with appropriate antibiotic therapy and, if necessary, by a surgical or dental procedure.

Definitive treatment recommendations for the crescentic form of PIGN are unknown. Anecdotal experience with glomerular complications of endocarditis suggests that corticosteroid therapy, cyclophosphamide, or plasmapheresis has a favorable effect on kidney function after infection has been eradicated. Although uncontrolled, these observations suggest that the prognosis of postinfectious crescentic GN is not necessarily disastrous when an aggressive antiinflammatory

and possibly immunosuppressive regimen is used after achieving eradication of infection.

Postinfectious GN is a critical public health problem with significant cost implications. In this respect, early and easy access to medical and dental care, control of drug addiction, and the same prophylactic measures that have proven effective in preventing bacterial endocarditis should also be implemented to reduce the incidence of this kidney disease.

BIBLIOGRAPHY

Bach JF, Chalons S, Forier E, et al: 10-year educational programme aimed at rheumatic fever in two French Caribbean islands, *Lancet* 347:644-648, 1996.

Batsford S, Mezzano S, Mihatsch M, et al: Is the nephritogenic antigen in post-streptococcal glomerulonephritis pyrogenic exotoxin B (SPE B) or GAPDH? *Kidney Int* 68:1120-1129, 2006.

Daimon S, Mizuno Y, Fujii S, et al: Infective endocarditis-induced crescentic glomerulonephritis dramatically improved by plasmapheresis, *Am J Kidney Dis* 32:309-313, 1998.

Frémeaux-Bacchi V, Weiss L, Demouchy C, et al: Hypocomplementaemia of poststreptococcal acute glomerulonephritis is associated with a C3 nephritic factor (C3NeF) IgG autoantibody activity, *Nephrol Dial Transplant* 9:1747-1750, 1994.

Haas M: Incidental healed postinfectious glomerulonephritis: a study of 1012 renal biopsy specimens examined by electron microscopy, *Hum Pathol* 34:3-10, 2003.

Haas M, Racusen LC, Bagnasco SM: IgA-dominant postinfectious glomerulonephritis: a report of 13 cases with common ultrastructural features, *Hum Pathol* 39:1309-1316, 2008.

Haffner D, Schindera F, Aschoff A, et al: The clinical spectrum of shunt nephritis, *Nephrol Dial Transplant* 12:1143-1148, 1997.

Korinek AM, Fulla-Oller L, Boch AL, et al: Morbidity of ventricular cerebrospinal fluid shunt surgery in adults: an 8-year study, *J Neurosurg Sci* 55:161-163, 2011.

Koyama A, Sharmin S, Sakura H, et al: Staphylococcus aureus cell envelope antigen is a new candidate for the induction of IgA nephropathy, *Kidney Int* 66:121-132, 2004.

Montseny JJ, Meyrier A, Kleinknecht D, et al: The current spectrum of infectious glomerulonephritis: experience with 76 patients and review of the literature, *Medicine (Baltimore)* 74:63-73, 1995.

Nasr SH, Fidler ME, Valeri AM, et al: Postinfectious glomerulonephritis in the elderly, *J Am Soc Nephrol* 22:187-195, 2011.

Nasr SH, Markowitz GS, Stokes MB, et al: Acute postinfectious glomerulonephritis in the modern era: experience with 86 adults and review of the literature, *Medicine (Baltimore)* 87:21-32, 2008.

Nasr SH, Markowitz GS, Whelan JD, et al: IgA-dominant acute poststaphylococcal glomerulonephritis complicating diabetic nephropathy, *Hum Pathol* 34:1235-1241, 2003.

Okuyama S, Wakui H, Maki N, et al: Successful treatment of post-MRSA infection glomerulonephritis with steroid therapy, *Clin Nephrol* 70:344-347, 2008.

Roy 3rd S, Stapleton FB: Changing perspectives in children hospitalized with poststreptococcal acute glomerulonephritis, *Pediatr Nephrol* 4:585-589, 1990.

Silva FG: Acute postinfectious glomerulonephritis and glomerulonephritis complicating persistent bacterial infection. In Jennette JC, Olson JL, Schwartz MM, Silva FG, editors: *Heptinstall's pathology of the kidney*, ed 5, Philadelphia, New York, 1998, Lippincott-Raven, pp 389-453.

Wen YK, Chen ML: IgA-dominant postinfectious glomerulonephritis: not peculiar to staphylococcal infection and diabetic patients, *Ren Fail* 33:480-485, 2011.

White AV, Hoy WE, McCredie DA: Childhood post-streptococcal glomerulonephritis as a risk factor for chronic renal disease in later life, *Med J Aust* 174:492-494, 2001.

Kidney Involvement in Systemic Vasculitis

23

J. Charles Jennette | Ronald J. Falk

The kidneys are affected by many forms of system vasculitis (Fig. 23.1), which cause a wide variety of sometimes confusing clinical manifestations. Large-vessel vasculitides, such as giant cell arteritis and Takayasu arteritis, can narrow the abdominal aorta or renal arteries, resulting in renal ischemia and renovascular hypertension. Vasculitides of the medium-sized vessels, such as polyarteritis nodosa and Kawasaki disease, also can reduce flow through the renal artery and may affect intrarenal arteries, resulting in infarction and hemorrhage. Small-vessel vasculitides, such as microscopic polyangiitis (MPA), granulomatosis with polyangiitis (GPA, previously called Wegener granulomatosis), immunoglobulin A (IgA) vasculitis (Henoch-Schönlein purpura), and cryoglobulinemic vasculitis, frequently involve the kidneys and especially the glomerular capillaries, resulting in glomerulonephritis.

PATHOLOGY

As depicted in Figure 23.1 and as described in Table 23.1, different types of systemic vasculitis affect different vessels within the kidney. In addition, each type of vasculitis has different histologic and immunohistologic features.

Giant cell arteritis and Takayasu arteritis predominantly affect the aorta and its major branches. Takayasu arteritis is an important cause of renovascular hypertension, especially in young patients. Giant cell arteritis only rarely causes clinically significant kidney disease, although asymptomatic pathologic involvement is common. Giant cell arteritis often involves the extracranial branches of the carotid arteries, including the temporal artery. Some patients, however, do not have temporal artery involvement, and patients with other types of vasculitis (e.g., MPA, GPA) may have temporal artery involvement. Therefore, temporal artery disease is neither a required nor a sufficient pathologic feature of giant cell arteritis.

Histologically, both giant cell arteritis and Takayasu arteritis are characterized by focal chronic inflammation that frequently has a granulomatous appearance, often, but not always, with multinucleated giant cells. With chronicity, the inflammatory injury evolves into fibrosis and frequently results in vascular narrowing, which is the basis for renovascular hypertension when a renal artery is involved.

Polyarteritis nodosa and Kawasaki disease affect medium-sized arteries (i.e., main visceral arteries) such as the mesenteric, hepatic, coronary, and main renal arteries. These diseases also may involve small arteries, such as arteries within the parenchyma of skeletal muscle, liver, heart,

pancreas, spleen, and kidney (e.g., interlobar and arcuate arteries in the kidney). By the definitions in Table 23.1, polyarteritis nodosa and Kawasaki disease affect arteries exclusively and do not affect capillaries or venules. Therefore, they do not cause glomerulonephritis. The presence of arteritis with glomerulonephritis indicates some form of small-vessel vasculitis rather than a medium-vessel vasculitis.

Histologically, the acute arterial injury of Kawasaki disease and polyarteritis nodosa is characterized by focal artery wall necrosis and infiltration of inflammatory cells. The acute injury of polyarteritis nodosa typically includes conspicuous fibrinoid necrosis, which is absent or less apparent in Kawasaki disease. Fibrinoid necrosis results from plasma coagulation factors spilling into the necrotic areas, where they are activated to form fibrin. Early in the acute injury of polyarteritis nodosa, neutrophils predominate, but within a few days mononuclear leukocytes are most numerous. Thrombosis may occur at the site of inflammation, resulting in infarction. Focal necrotizing injury to vessels erodes into the vessel wall and adjacent tissue, producing an inflammatory aneurysm, which may rupture and cause hemorrhage. Thrombosis of the inflamed arteries causes downstream ischemia and infarction.

Although small-vessel vasculitides may affect medium-sized arteries, these disorders favor small vessels such as arterioles, venules (e.g., in the dermis), and capillaries (e.g., in glomeruli and pulmonary alveoli) (see Fig. 23.1). As described in Table 23.1, there are a variety of clinically and pathogenetically distinct forms of small-vessel vasculitis that have in common focal necrotizing inflammation of small vessels. In the acute phase, this injury is characterized histologically by segmental fibrinoid necrosis and leukocyte infiltration (Fig. 23.2), sometimes with secondary thrombosis. The neutrophils often undergo karyorrhexis (leukocytoclasia). With chronicity, mononuclear leukocytes become predominant and fibrosis develops.

The various forms of small-vessel vasculitis differ from one another with respect to the presence or absence of distinctive features, as summarized in Table 23.1 and Figure 23.1. For example, GPA is characterized by necrotizing granulomatous inflammation, eosinophilic granulomatosis with polyangiitis (EGPA) by blood eosinophilia and asthma, IgA vasculitis (Henoch-Schönlein purpura) by IgA-dominant vascular immune deposits, and cryoglobulinemic vasculitis by circulating cryoglobulins.

The glomerular lesions of MPA, GPA, and EGPA are identical pathologically and are characterized by segmental fibrinoid necrosis, crescent formation (Fig. 23.3), and a paucity

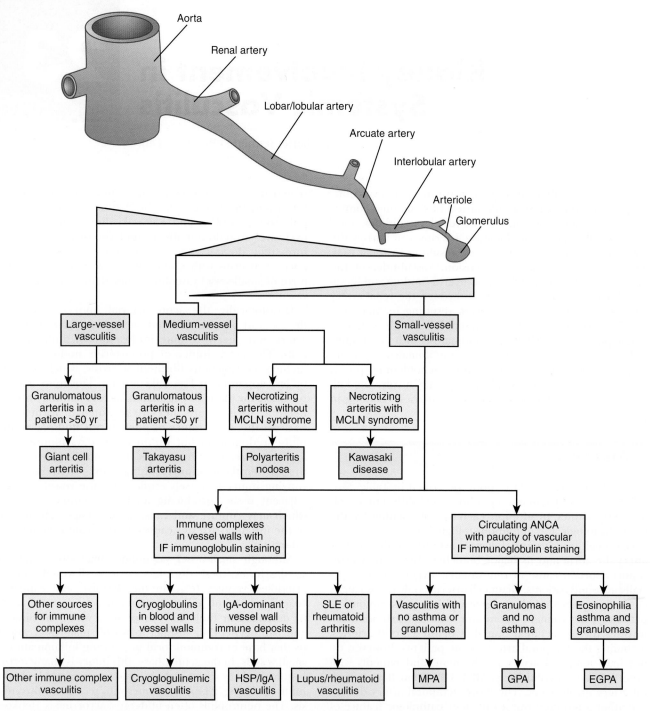

Figure 23.1   Predominant distribution of renal vascular involvement by systemic vasculitides and the diagnostic clinical and pathologic features that distinguish among them. The width of the blue triangles indicates the predilection of small-, medium-, and large-vessel vasculitides for various portions of the renal vasculature. Note that medium-sized renal arteries can be affected by large, medium-, or small-vessel vasculitides, but arterioles and glomeruli are affected by small-vessel vasculitides alone, based on the definitions in Table 23.1. *ANCA,* Antineutrophil cytoplasmic antibodies; *EGPA,* eosinophilic granulomatosis with polyangiitis (previously called Churg-Strauss); *GPA,* granulomatosis with polyangiitis (previously called Wegener granulomatosis); *HSP,* Henoch-Schönlein purpura; *IF,* immunofluorescence; *IgA,* immunoglobulin A; *MCLN,* mucocutaneous lymph node syndrome; *MPA,* microscopic polyangiitis; *SLE,* systemic lupus erythematosus.

of glomerular staining for immunoglobulin (i.e., pauci-immune glomerulonephritis). Leukocytoclastic angiitis of medullary vasa recta (Fig. 23.4) also occurs in the antineutrophil cytoplasmic antibody (ANCA) vasculitides and rarely is severe enough to cause papillary necrosis. More than 90%

of patients with active untreated MPA and GPA have circulating ANCAs. Fewer than half of patients with EGPA have ANCAs; however, the minority of patients with EGPA who have glomerulonephritis and vasculitis as components of the syndrome usually are ANCA-positive.

Table 23.1   Partial Listing of Names and Definitions of Vasculitides Adopted by the 2012 Chapel Hill Consensus Conference on the Nomenclature of Systemic Vasculitis

Name*	Definition
Large-Vessel Vasculitides	
Giant cell arteritis	Arteritis, often granulomatous, usually affecting the aorta and/or its major branches, with a predilection for the branches of the carotid and vertebral arteries. Often involves the temporal artery. Onset usually in patients older than 50 yr and often associated with polymyalgia rheumatica.
Takayasu arteritis	Arteritis, often granulomatous, predominantly affecting the aorta and/or its major branches. Onset usually in patients younger than 50 yr.
Medium-Vessel Vasculitides	
Polyarteritis nodosa	Necrotizing arteritis of medium or small arteries without glomerulonephritis or vasculitis in arterioles, capillaries, or venules, and not associated with ANCA.
Kawasaki disease	Arteritis associated with the mucocutaneous lymph node syndrome and predominantly affecting medium and small arteries. Coronary arteries are often involved. Aorta and large arteries may be involved. Usually occurs in infants and young children.
Small-Vessel Vasculitides	
MPA[†‡]	Necrotizing vasculitis, with few or no immune deposits, predominantly affecting small vessels (i.e., capillaries, venules, or arterioles). Necrotizing arteritis involving small and medium arteries may be present. Necrotizing glomerulonephritis is very common. Pulmonary capillaritis often occurs. Granulomatous inflammation is absent.
GPA (formerly Wegener granulomatosis)[†‡]	Necrotizing granulomatous inflammation usually involving the upper and lower respiratory tract, and necrotizing vasculitis affecting predominantly small to medium vessels (e.g., capillaries, venules, arterioles, arteries, and veins). Necrotizing glomerulonephritis is common.
EGPA (formerly Churg-Strauss syndrome)[†‡]	Eosinophil-rich and necrotizing granulomatous inflammation often involving the respiratory tract, and necrotizing vasculitis predominantly affecting small to medium vessels, and associated with asthma and eosinophilia. ANCA is more frequent when glomerulonephritis is present.
IgA vasculitis (Henoch-Schönlein purpura)[‡]	Vasculitis, with IgA1-dominant immune deposits, affecting small vessels (predominantly capillaries, venules, or arterioles). Often involves skin and gastrointestinal tract, and frequently causes arthritis. Glomerulonephritis indistinguishable from IgA nephropathy may occur.
Cryoglobulinemic vasculitis[‡]	Vasculitis with cryoglobulin immune deposits affecting small vessels (predominantly capillaries, venules, or arterioles) and associated with cryoglobulins in serum. Skin, glomeruli, and peripheral nerves are often involved.
Hypocomplementemic urticarial vasculitis (Anti-C1q Vasculitis)	Vasculitis accompanied by urticaria and hypocomplementemia affecting small vessels (i.e., capillaries, venules, or arterioles), and associated with anti-C1q antibodies. Glomerulonephritis, arthritis, obstructive pulmonary disease, and ocular inflammation are common.
Anti-GBM disease[‡]	Vasculitis affecting glomerular capillaries, pulmonary capillaries, or both, with basement membrane deposition of antibasement membrane autoantibodies. Lung involvement causes pulmonary hemorrhage, and renal involvement causes glomerulonephritis with necrosis and crescents.

Modified from Jennette JC, Falk RJ, Bacon PA, et al: Revised International Chapel Hill Consensus Conference Nomenclature of the Vasculitides. Arthritis Rheum 65:1-11, 2013.
ANCA, Antineutrophil cytoplasmic antibody; EGPA, eosinophilic granulomatosis with polyangiitis; GBM, glomerular basement membrane; GPA, granulomatosis with polyangiitis; MPA, microscopic polyangiitis.
*The term *large vessels* refers to the aorta and the largest branches directed toward major body regions (e.g., extremities, head, and neck); *medium vessels* refers to the main visceral arteries (e.g., renal, hepatic, coronary, mesenteric); and *small vessels* refers to the distal arterial branches that connect with arterioles (e.g., renal arcuate and interlobular arteries), as well as arterioles, capillaries, and venules. Note that some small- and large-vessel vasculitides may involve medium-sized arteries, but large- and medium-vessel vasculitides do not involve vessels other than arteries.
†Strongly associated with ANCAs.
‡May be accompanied by glomerulonephritis and can manifest as nephritis or pulmonary-renal vasculitic syndrome.

The glomerulonephritis of IgA vasculitis (Henoch-Schönlein purpura) is pathologically identical to IgA nephropathy, and these patients have the same abnormal hinge region glycosylation of IgA1. The glomerulonephritis of cryoglobulinemic vasculitis usually manifests as type I membranoproliferative glomerulonephritis (mesangiocapillary glomerulonephritis), although other patterns of proliferative glomerulonephritis occur less often. Cryoglobulinemic vasculitis frequently is associated with hepatitis C infection.

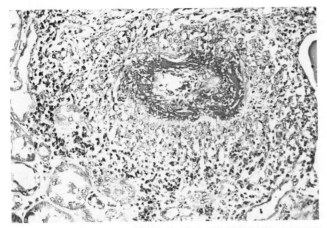

Figure 23.2   Renal interlobular artery with fibrinoid necrosis from a patient with microscopic polyangiitis (Masson trichrome stain).

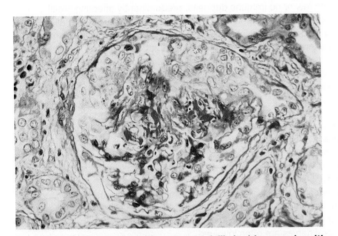

Figure 23.3   Glomerulus with segmental fibrinoid necrosis with red (fuchsinophilic) fibrinous material and an adjacent cellular crescent, from a patient with antineutrophil cytoplasmic antibody small-vessel vasculitis (Masson trichrome stain).

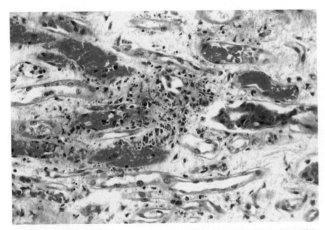

Figure 23.4   Medullary vasa recta with leukocytoclastic angiitis, from a patient with granulomatosis with polyangiitis (hematoxylin and eosin stain).

PATHOGENESIS

Vasculitis is caused by the activation of inflammatory mediator systems in vessel walls. However, the initiating event (cause) is unknown for many forms of vasculitis. An immune response to heterologous antigens (e.g., hepatitis B or C antigens in some forms of immune complex vasculitis) or autoantigens (e.g., proteinase 3 or myeloperoxidase in ANCA vasculitis) is presumed to be the etiologic event in many patients with vasculitis. A number of types of vasculitis are categorized based on the putative immunologic mechanisms listed in Box 23.1.

Primarily because of the pattern of inflammation, T cell–mediated inflammation has been incriminated in the pathogenesis of giant cell arteritis and Takayasu arteritis. Several mechanisms of antibody-mediated injury are thought to be important in the pathogenesis of necrotizing small-vessel vasculitides, but there is evidence that T cells also may play a role.

The vasculitides listed in the immune complex–mediated category in Box 23.1 all produce immunohistologic evidence for vessel wall immune complex localization—that is, granular or linear staining for immunoglobulins and complement. Antibodies bound to antigens in vessel walls activate humoral inflammatory mediator systems (complement, coagulation, plasmin, and kinin systems), which attract and activate neutrophils and monocytes. These activated leukocytes generate toxic oxygen metabolites and release enzymes that cause matrix lysis and cellular apoptosis, resulting in necrotizing inflammatory injury to vessel walls.

This same final pathway of inflammatory injury also can be reached if antibodies bind to antigens that are integral components of vessel walls. The best-documented example is antiglomerular basement membrane (anti-GBM) antibody-mediated glomerulonephritis and Goodpasture

---

Box 23.1   Putative Immunologic Causes of Vasculitis

Immune Complex–Mediated

IgA vasculitis (Henoch-Schönlein purpura)*
Cryoglobulinemic vasculitis*
Lupus vasculitis*
Serum sickness vasculitis*
Hypocomplementemic urticarial vasculitis (Anti-C1q vasculitis)
Anti-GBM disease*

ANCA-Mediated

MPA*
GPA*

Cell-Mediated

Allograft cellular vascular rejection
Giant cell arteritis
Takayasu arteritis

ANCA, Antineutrophil cytoplasmic antibody; *GBM*, glomerular basement membrane; *GPA*, granulomatosis with polyangiitis; *MPA*, microscopic polyangiitis.
*May be accompanied by glomerulonephritis and can manifest as nephritis or pulmonary-renal vasculitic syndrome.

syndrome (see Chapter 21). T cells with specificity for basement membranes or cells also may participate in the mediation or regulation of glomerular injury.

An important group of necrotizing systemic small-vessel vasculitides, which frequently involves the kidneys, occurs without immunohistologic evidence for vascular immune complex localization or direct antibody binding. This paucity of immune deposits is the basis for the designation "pauci-immune" for this group of vasculitides, which includes MPA, GPA, and EGPA. Approximately 90% of patients with pauci-immune glomerulonephritis and vasculitis have circulating ANCAs. In vitro and in vivo experimental evidence indicates that the vascular inflammation is caused by activation of neutrophils and monocytes by ANCAs. T cells also appear to play a role.

ANCAs are specific for proteins within the granules of neutrophils and the peroxidase-positive lysosomes of monocytes. When detected in patient serum by indirect immunofluorescence microscopy using alcohol-fixed normal human neutrophils as substrate, two patterns of neutrophil staining are observed that discriminate between the two major subtypes of ANCAs: cytoplasmic-staining (C-ANCA) and perinuclear-staining (P-ANCA). With the use of specific immunochemical assays such as enzyme-linked immunosorbent assays (ELISAs), most C-ANCAs are found to be specific for a neutrophil and monocyte proteinase called proteinase 3 (PR3-ANCA), and most P-ANCAs are specific for myeloperoxidase (MPO-ANCA).

A leading hypothesis about the pathogenesis of ANCA-associated vasculitides proposes that ANCAs react with cytoplasmic antigens (PR3 and MPO) that are present at the surface of cytokine-stimulated leukocytes, causing the leukocytes to adhere to vessel walls, degranulate, and generate toxic oxygen metabolites. The interaction of ANCAs with neutrophils involves Fc receptor engagement, perhaps by immune complexes formed between ANCAs and ANCA antigens in the microenvironment surrounding the leukocyte. ANCA binding to ANCA antigens on the surface of neutrophils also is involved in neutrophil activation. In vitro and animal model experiments indicate that ANCA-activated neutrophils release factors that activate the alternative complement pathway that initiates an inflammatory amplification loop that is important for tissue injury. ANCA antigens also may become planted in vessel walls, thus providing a nidus for in situ immune complex formation. If such in situ immune complex formation is present, it occurs at a low level, as ANCA vasculitides are characteristically pauci-immune. The most compelling experimental evidence that ANCAs cause vasculitis is the observation that circulating antibodies specific for MPO cause pauci-immune crescentic glomerulonephritis and small-vessel vasculitis in mice and rats. The most convincing clinical observation that supports the pathogenicity of ANCA is a reported occurrence of transplacental transfer of MPO-ANCA IgG that apparently caused glomerulonephritis and pulmonary capillaritis in a newborn, but this result has not been confirmed.

CLINICAL FEATURES

The diagnosis and management of systemic vasculitis can be challenging. The clinical features are extremely varied and are dictated by the category of vasculitis, the type of vessel involved, the organ system distribution of vascular injury, and the stage of disease. Regardless of the type of vasculitis, most patients exhibit accompanying constitutional features of inflammatory disease, such as fever, arthralgias, myalgias, and weight loss. Increased circulating levels of proinflammatory cytokines probably cause these features.

Giant cell arteritis and Takayasu arteritis typically manifest with evidence for ischemia in tissues supplied by involved arteries. Patients with arteritis often develop claudication (especially in the upper extremities), absent pulses, and bruits. Approximately 40% of patients with Takayasu arteritis develop renovascular hypertension, a feature that only rarely complicates giant cell arteritis. Giant cell arteritis can affect virtually any organ in the body, but signs and symptoms of involvement of arteries in the head and neck are the most common clinical manifestations. Superficial arteries (e.g., the temporal artery) may be swollen and tender. Arterial narrowing causes ischemic manifestations in affected tissues (e.g., headache, jaw claudication, loss of vision). About half of the patients with giant cell arteritis have polymyalgia rheumatica, which is characterized by aching and stiffness in the neck, shoulder girdle, or pelvic girdle.

Medium-vessel vasculitides, such as polyarteritis nodosa and Kawasaki disease, often manifest with clinical evidence for infarction in multiple organs, such as abdominal pain with occult blood in the stool and skeletal muscle and cardiac pain with elevated serum muscle enzymes. Laboratory evaluation often demonstrates clinically silent organ damage, such as liver injury with elevated liver function tests and pancreatic injury with elevated serum amylase.

Polyarteritis nodosa frequently causes multiple kidney infarcts and aneurysms. Unlike MPA and GPA, polyarteritis nodosa typically does not cause rapidly progressive loss of kidney function. Rupture of arterial aneurysms with massive retroperitoneal or intraperitoneal hemorrhage is a life-threatening complication of polyarteritis nodosa.

Kawasaki disease almost always occurs in children younger than 6 years of age and has a predilection for coronary, axillary, and iliac arteries. Kawasaki disease is accompanied by the mucocutaneous lymph node syndrome that includes fever, nonpurulent lymphadenopathy, and mucosal and cutaneous inflammation. Although the renal arteries (especially interlobar arteries) frequently are affected pathologically, clinically significant kidney involvement is rare in patients with Kawasaki disease.

Patients with small-vessel vasculitides often present with evidence of inflammation in vessels in multiple organs, but initially there may be involvement of only one organ, followed later by development of disease in other organs. Hematuria, proteinuria, and impaired kidney function caused by glomerulonephritis are frequent clinical features of all forms of small-vessel vasculitis listed in Table 23.1. Other manifestations include purpura caused by leukocytoclastic angiitis in dermal venules and arterioles, abdominal pain and occult blood in the stool from mucosal and bowel wall infarcts, mononeuritis multiplex from arteritis in peripheral nerves, necrotizing sinusitis from upper respiratory tract mucosal angiitis, and pulmonary hemorrhage from alveolar capillaritis.

In addition to these features, which are shared by patients with any type of small vessel vasculitis, patients with GPA and EGPA show distinctive clinical features that set them apart.

Patients with GPA have necrotizing granulomatous inflammation, most often occurring in the upper or lower respiratory tract and rarely in other tissues (e.g., skin, orbit). In the lungs, this inflammation produces irregular nodular lesions that can be observed by radiography. These lesions may cavitate and hemorrhage; however, massive pulmonary hemorrhage in patients with GPA is usually caused by capillaritis rather than granulomatous inflammation. By definition, patients with EGPA have blood eosinophilia and a history of asthma. They also develop eosinophil-rich tissue inflammation, especially in the lungs and gut.

DIAGNOSIS

Multisystem disease in a patient with constitutional signs and symptoms of inflammation, such as fever, arthralgias, myalgias, and weight loss, should raise suspicion of systemic vasculitis. Data to assist in resolving the differential diagnosis include the age of the patient, organ distribution of injury, concurrent syndromes (e.g., mucocutaneous lymph node syndrome in Kawasaki disease, polymyalgia rheumatica in giant cell arteritis, asthma in EGPA), type of vessel involved (e.g., large artery, visceral artery, small vessel other than an artery), lesion histology (e.g., granulomatous, necrotizing), lesion immunohistology (e.g., immune deposits, pauci-immune), and serologic data (e.g., cryoglobulins, hepatitis C antibodies, hypocomplementemia, antinuclear antibodies, ANCAs, cryoglobulins, anti-C1q antibodies, abnormally glycosylated IgA1) (see Fig. 23.1).

Signs and symptoms of tissue ischemia along with angiography demonstrating irregularity, stenosis, occlusion, or, less commonly, aneurysms of large and medium-sized arteries should suggest giant cell arteritis or Takayasu arteritis. A useful discriminator between giant cell arteritis and Takayasu arteritis is age, as the former disorder is rare in individuals younger than 50 years whereas the latter is rare in patients older than 50 years. The presence of polymyalgia rheumatica is a clinical marker for giant cell arteritis.

Polyarteritis nodosa and Kawasaki disease cause visceral ischemia, particularly in the heart, kidneys, liver, spleen, and gut. Arteritis in skeletal muscle and subcutaneous tissues causes tender erythematous nodules that can be identified on physical examination. Angiographic demonstration of aneurysms in medium-sized arteries (e.g., renal arteries) indicates that some type of vasculitis is present, but it is not disease specific, because giant cell arteritis, Takayasu arteritis, polyarteritis nodosa, Kawasaki disease, GPA, MPA, and EGPA all can produce arterial aneurysms. Kawasaki disease almost always occurs in children younger than 6 years and, by definition, is accompanied by the mucocutaneous lymph node syndrome.

A small-vessel vasculitis should be suspected if there is evidence for inflammation of vessels smaller than arteries, such as glomerular capillaries (hematuria and proteinuria), dermal venules (palpable purpura), or alveolar capillaries (hemoptysis). To discriminate among the small-vessel vasculitides, evaluation of serologic data, vessel immunohistology, or concurrent nonvasculitic disease (e.g., asthma, eosinophilia, lupus, hepatitis) is required (see Fig. 23.1).

Evaluation of vessels in biopsy specimens, such as glomerular capillaries in kidney biopsies, alveolar capillaries in lung biopsies, or dermal venules in skin biopsies, can be helpful, especially if immunohistology is performed. The pauci-immune vasculitides lack immune deposits, anti-GBM disease produces linear immunoglobulin deposits, and immune complex vasculitides have granular immune deposits, such as the IgA-dominant deposits of IgA vasculitis.

Serology, especially ANCA analysis, is useful in differentiating among the small-vessel vasculitides. MPA, GPA, and, to a lesser extent, EGPA are associated with ANCAs (Table 23.2). As depicted in Figure 23.5 and listed in Table 23.2, most patients in North America and Europe with active untreated GPA have C-ANCA (PR3-ANCA), whereas a minority have P-ANCA (MPO-ANCA). Therefore, PR3-ANCA is not specific for GPA, because some patients with PR3-ANCA have systemic small-vessel vasculitis without granulomatous inflammation (i.e., MPA) and others have pauci-immune necrotizing and crescentic glomerulonephritis alone. Of note, in Asia, MPO-ANCA is much more common than PR3-ANCA. Patients with EGPA have the lowest frequency of ANCAs and the lowest frequency of kidney involvement by glomerulonephritis. However, EGPA patients with glomerulonephritis have a high frequency of ANCA, usually MPO-ANCA. Some patients with immunopathologic evidence for immune complex–mediated or anti-GBM–mediated vasculitis or glomerulonephritis have concurrent ANCA (see Fig. 23.5). Approximately one fourth to one third of patients with anti-GBM disease are ANCA positive, and these patients experience kidney disease that is intermediate in severity between ANCA disease and anti-GBM disease (which has the worst prognosis), and they may have persistence or recurrence of ANCA disease after the anti-GBM disease remits (Chapter 21). It is important to realize that some patients with MPA, GPA, and especially EGPA are ANCA-negative. In some patients, ANCA titers correlate with disease activity; however, in many patients, especially those with MPO-ANCA, ANCA titers do not mirror disease activity.

Table 23.2   Approximate Frequency of PR3-ANCA or MPO-ANCA in Pauci-Immune Small-Vessel Vasculitis

Antibody	MPA (%)	GPA (%)	EGPA (%)	Renal-Limited Vasculitis (Pauci-Immune Crescentic Glomerulonephritis) (%)
PR3-ANCA	40	75	5	25
MPO-ANCA	50	20	40	65
ANCA-negative	10	5	55	10

EGPA, Eosinophilic granulomatosis with polyangiitis; *GPA,* granulomatosis with polyangiitis; *MPA,* microscopic polyangiitis; *MPO-ANCA,* myeloperoxidase antineutrophil cytoplasmic antibody; *PR3-ANCA,* proteinase 3 antineutrophil cytoplasmic antibody.
Note that more than 75% of patients with EGPA who have glomerulonephritis are ANCA-positive.

Diagnostic serologic tests for immune complex–mediated vasculitides include assays for circulating immune complexes (e.g., cryoglobulins in cryoglobulinemic vasculitis), assays for antibodies known to participate in immune complex formation or to mark the presence of a disease that generates immune complexes (e.g., antibodies to hepatitis B or C, streptococci, DNA), and assays for consumption or activation of humoral inflammatory mediator system components (e.g., assays for reduced complement components or for activated membrane attack complex). Hypocomplementemia is common in patients with cryoglobulinemic vasculitis, lupus vasculitis, and hypocomplementemic urticarial vasculitis. The glomerulonephritis in all three of these vasculitides is characterized by capillary wall and mesangial immune complex deposition and a proliferative or membranoproliferative pattern of injury.

THERAPY AND OUTCOME

All of the vasculitides discussed in this chapter typically respond to antiinflammatory or immunosuppressive therapy. The aggressiveness of treatment should match the aggressiveness of the disease.

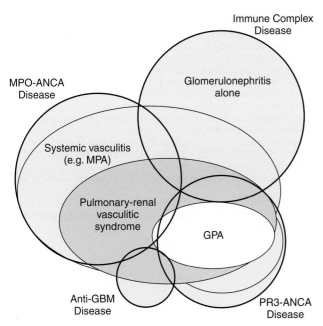

Figure 23.5 Relationship of vasculitic clinicopathologic syndromes to immunopathologic categories of vascular injury in patients with crescentic glomerulonephritis. The circles represent the major immunopathologic categories of vascular inflammation that affect the kidneys, and the shaded ovals represent the clinicopathologic expressions of the vascular inflammation. Note that clinical syndromes can be caused by more than one immunopathologic process; for example, pulmonary-renal vasculitic syndrome can be caused by anti-GBM antibodies (i.e., Goodpasture syndrome), immune complex localization (e.g., lupus erythematosus), or ANCA-associated disease (e.g., MPA, GPA). *GBM,* Glomerular basement membrane; *GPA,* granulomatosis with polyangiitis; *MPA,* microscopic polyangiitis; *MPO-ANCA,* myeloperoxidase antineutrophil cytoplasmic antibody; *PR3-ANCA,* proteinase 3 antineutrophil cytoplasmic antibody. (Modified from Jennette JC: Anti-neutrophil cytoplasmic autoantibody-associated disease: a pathologist's perspective. *Am J Kidney Dis* 18:164-170, 1991, with permission.)

Takayasu arteritis and giant cell arteritis usually respond well to high-dose corticosteroid treatment (e.g., prednisone, 1 mg/kg body weight/day) during the acute phase of the disease, followed by tapering and low-dose maintenance for several months to 1 year depending on disease activity. Patients with severe disease or steroid toxicity benefit from other immunosuppressive agents, including methotrexate, cyclophosphamide, mycophenolate mofetil, or azathioprine. If present, renovascular hypertension should be controlled. After the inflammatory phase has passed and the sclerotic phase has developed, vascular surgery (stent or bypass) may be required to improve flow to ischemic tissues, especially in patients with Takayasu arteritis.

Some patients with polyarteritis nodosa have a persistent viral infection, especially hepatitis B virus infection. These patients are usually ANCA negative. In these cases, antiviral therapy with or without plasma exchange is recommended. In patients with no evidence for infection, management usually consists of corticosteroids with or without cytotoxic drugs.

The preferred treatment for Kawasaki disease is a combination of aspirin (80-100 mg/kg/day) and high-dose intravenous gamma globulins (single 12-hour infusion of 2 g/kg). This controls the inflammatory manifestations of the disease (e.g., the mucocutaneous lymph node syndrome), prevents thrombosis of injured arteries, and retards the frequency of coronary artery involvement. With appropriate treatment, more than 90% of patients with Kawasaki disease have complete resolution of the disease.

Many patients with IgA vasculitis experience mild disease that requires only supportive care (see Chapter 20). IgA vasculitis causes decreased kidney function in approximately 20% of patients 20 years after onset, with a higher rate in patients with later onset disease. Arthralgias can be relieved by nonsteroidal antiinflammatory drugs, whereas corticosteroid treatment is beneficial for patients who experience severe abdominal pain caused by intestinal vasculitis. The treatment of severe glomerulonephritis in patients with IgA vasculitis is controversial. There is anecdotal evidence indicating that aggressive crescent glomerulonephritis should be treated with high-dose corticosteroids, cytotoxic agents, or plasmapheresis, but this has not been documented in controlled trials. Data from a large pediatric population suggest that corticosteroid treatment may decrease the risk for development of kidney involvement in those patients with severe abdominal pain and rash.

Cryoglobulinemic vasculitis caused by hepatitis C infection may respond to pegylated interferon-alfa in combination with antiviral therapy (e.g., ribavirin). As many as 25% to 50% of patients experience either partial or complete response to therapy. In patients with severe vasculitis or glomerulonephritis, an induction phase of immunosuppression (e.g., with rituximab) may be necessary while awaiting the response to antiviral treatments.

The treatments of choice for necrotizing and crescentic glomerulonephritis associated with MPA, GPA, or EGPA or for renal-limited pauci-immune crescentic glomerulonephritis include high-dose corticosteroids (e.g., pulse methylprednisolone) and cytotoxic agents (e.g., cyclophosphamide). Patients with pulmonary-renal vasculitic syndromes in whom hemoptysis is a major clinical feature require emergent therapy with plasma exchange. Plasma exchange also improves kidney survival in patients with severe kidney disease at the time of diagnosis. Induction therapy includes pulse methylprednisolone at a dose of 7 mg/kg/day for 3 days, followed by daily oral prednisone or plasma exchange therapy for 7 to 14 days in addition to daily oral prednisone. Prednisone treatment is typically converted to alternate-day treatment during the second month of therapy. Corticosteroid treatment is terminated by the fourth or fifth month after diagnosis. There are a number of cyclophosphamide protocols, including intravenous or oral cyclophosphamides, that induce remission in almost 90% of patients. Studies suggest that rituximab might be an option for induction therapy in ANCA-associated disease, but it is not clear whether rituximab should be used with glucocorticoids alone or in combination with cyclophosphamide.

After the patient is in remission, treatment may be switched to maintenance therapy that includes azathioprine or mycophenolate mofetil. Some patients may not require any kind of immunosuppressive therapy after they are in remission following 6 to 12 months of overall therapy. As many as 75% to 85% of ANCA-vasculitic patients enter remission with aggressive immunosuppressive therapy, but approximately 20% to 40% experience a relapse within 2 years. Relapses typically occur in the same organ system as the primary disease, although relapses may also occur in other organ systems. Depending on the severity of the relapse, patients may be treated either with another course of corticosteroids and cyclophosphamide or with mycophenolate mofetil, glucocorticoids, azathioprine, or rituximab.

BIBLIOGRAPHY

Alric L, Plaisier E, Thebault S, et al: Influence of antiviral therapy in hepatitis C virus-associated cryoglobulinemic MPGN, *Am J Kidney Dis* 43:617-623, 2004.

Berden AE, Ferrario F, Hagen EH, et al: Histopathological classification of ANCA-associated glomerulonephritis, *Kidney Int* 21:1628-1636, 2010.

Davin JC: Henoch-Schönlein purpura nephritis: pathophysiology, treatment, and future strategy, *Clin J Am Soc Nephrol* 6:679-689, 2011.

de Lind van Wijngaarden RA, Hauer HA, Wolterbeek R, et al: Chances of renal recovery for dialysis-dependent ANCA-associated glomerulonephritis, *J Am Soc Nephrol* 18:2189-2197, 2007.

Falk RJ, Jennette JC: ANCA disease: where is this field going? *J Am Soc Nephrol* 21:745-752, 2010.

Falk RJ, Jennette JC: Rituximab in ANCA-associated disease, *N Engl J Med* 363:285-286, 2010.

Gulati A, Bagga A: Large vessel vasculitis, *Pediatr Nephrol* 25:1037-1048, 2010.

Iannuzzella F, Vaglio A, Garini G: Management of hepatitis C virus-related mixed cryoglobulinemia, *Am J Med* 123:400-408, 2010.

Jayne DR, Gaskin G, Rasmussen N, et al: Randomized trial of plasma exchange or high-dosage methylprednisolone as adjunctive therapy for severe renal vasculitis, *J Am Soc Nephrol* 18:2180-2188, 2007.

Jayne D, Rasmussen N, Andrassy K, et al: A randomized trial of maintenance therapy for vasculitis associated with antineutrophil cytoplasmic autoantibodies, *N Engl J Med* 349:36-44, 2003.

Jennette JC, Falk RJ, Bacon PA, et al: Revised International Chapel Hill Consensus Conference Nomenclature of the Vasculitides, *Arthritis Rheum* 65:1-11, 2013.

Jennette JC, Falk RJ, Gasim AH: Pathogenesis of antineutrophil cytoplasmic autoantibody vasculitis, *Curr Opin Nephrol Hypertens* 20:263-270, 2011.

Jennette JC, Thomas DB: Pauci-immune and antineutrophil cytoplasmic autoantibody glomerulonephritis and vasculitis. In Jennette JC, Olson JL, Schwartz MM, Silva FG, editors: *Heptinstall's pathology of the kidney*, ed 6, Philadelphia, 2007, Lippincott Williams & Wilkins, pp 643-674.

Jennette JC, Thomas DB, Falk RJ: Microscopic polyangiitis (microscopic polyarteritis), *Semin Diagn Pathol* 18:3-13, 2001.

Jennette JC, Xiao H, Falk RJ: The pathogenesis of vascular inflammation by antineutrophil cytoplasmic antibodies, *J Am Soc Nephrol* 17:1235-1242, 2006.

Kamesh L, Harper L, Savage CO: ANCA-positive vasculitis, *J Am Soc Nephrol* 13:1953-1960, 2002.

Koening CL, Langford CA: Novel therapeutic strategies for large vessel vasculitis, *Rheum Dis Clin North Am* 32:173-186, 2006.

Kuo HC, Yang KD, Chang WC, et al: Kawasaki disease: an update on diagnosis and treatment, *Pediatr Neonatol* 53:4-11, 2012.

Morgan MD, Harper L, Williams J, et al: Anti-neutrophil cytoplasm-associated glomerulonephritis, *J Am Soc Nephrol* 17:1224-1234, 2006.

Rossi P, Bertani T, Baio P, et al: Hepatitis C virus-related cryoglobulinemic glomerulonephritis: Long-term remission after antiviral therapy, *Kidney Int* 63:2236-2241, 2003.

Saadoun D, Delluc A, Piette JC, et al: Treatment of hepatitis C-associated mixed cryoglobulinemia vasculitis, *Curr Opin Rheumatol* 20:23-28, 2008.

Seko Y: Giant cell and Takayasu arteritis, *Curr Opin Rheumatol* 19:39-43, 2007.

Vassilopoulos D, Calabrese LH: Hepatitis C virus infection and vasculitis: implications of antiviral and immunosuppressive therapies, *Arthritis Rheum* 46:585-597, 2002.

Kidney Manifestations of Systemic Lupus Erythematosus

24

Andrew S. Bomback | Vivette D. D'Agati

Systemic lupus erythematosus (SLE) is a chronic autoimmune disease that can affect multiple organs, including the skin, joints, brain, peripheral nervous system, heart, gastrointestinal tract, and kidneys. Kidney involvement in SLE, generally termed lupus nephritis, is a major contributor to SLE-associated morbidity and mortality. Up to 50% of SLE patients will have clinically evident kidney disease at presentation, and, during follow-up, kidney involvement occurs in up to 75% of patients, with an even greater representation among children and young adults. Lupus nephritis has been shown to impact clinical outcomes in SLE both directly via target organ damage and indirectly through complications of therapy.

PRESENTATION

Most patients with SLE will have laboratory evidence of kidney involvement at some point in their disease. In about one third of SLE patients, kidney involvement first manifests with proteinuria and/or microhematuria on urinalysis; this eventually progresses to reduction in kidney function. However, early in the course of disease, it is unusual for patients to present with decreased kidney function (i.e., elevated serum creatinine and reduced estimated glomerular filtration rate [GFR]), except for very aggressive cases of lupus nephritis, some of which present as rapidly progressive glomerulonephritis. Instead, patients often present initially with evidence of nonrenal organ involvement, such as malar rash, arthritis, and oral ulcers. After a diagnosis of SLE is confirmed with appropriate laboratory tests, evidence of kidney disease, if present, usually emerges within the first 3 years of diagnosis.

The symptoms of kidney involvement tend to correlate with laboratory abnormalities. For example, patients with nephrotic range proteinuria often present with edema of the lower extremities and, if severe, periorbital edema in the morning. When kidney function is impaired, as is the case with progressive forms of lupus nephritis, elevated blood pressure is a common clinical finding. The rare development of dark or tea-colored urine is a sign of gross hematuria. A number of tools, such as the SLE Disease Activity Index (SLEDAI) and the British Isles Lupus Assessment Group (BILAG) Index, have been developed to assess the systemic severity of lupus symptoms. Although these questionnaires are primarily used to codify symptoms for clinical trial settings, they also can be very helpful to elicit a detailed history from a patient with SLE.

EVALUATION

LABORATORY FINDINGS

The American College of Rheumatology (ACR) has listed 11 diagnostic criteria for SLE: antinuclear antibodies (ANA), arthritis, immunologic disorders (including antidouble-stranded DNA antibody, antiphospholipid antibody, or anti-Smith antibody), malar rash, discoid rash, photosensitivity, oral ulcers, serositis, hematologic disorder, neurologic disorder, and renal disorder (Table 24.1). Ideally, four or more of these criteria should be present to diagnose SLE, including laboratory findings of a positive ANA and/or antidouble-stranded DNA antibody. In addition to the ANA and double-stranded DNA antibody, serum complements (C3, C4, CH50) should be checked whenever kidney involvement is suspected, because these are often low when disease is active, as is usually the case with any severe proliferative lupus nephritis. Antiphospholipid and anticardiolipin antibodies are useful in gauging the risk for clotting abnormalities that can accompany SLE.

Laboratory testing is used both to diagnose kidney involvement and to assess response to therapy in patients with SLE. Traditional parameters, such as serum creatinine and urinary protein excretion (quantified by either 24-hour collection or first morning urine protein:creatinine ratio), are supplemented by serial review of microscopic urinary sediment, changes in serum complement levels, and titers of ANA and double-stranded DNA antibodies. Because cytopenias can often be seen with active SLE, complete blood counts should be checked regularly. A number of urine and serologic tests have been studied as biomarkers for SLE and, specifically, lupus nephritis disease activity. These include molecules specific to lupus (e.g., anti-C1q antibodies), mediators of chronic inflammation (e.g., TNF-like weak inducer of apoptosis [TWEAK]), and generalized markers of kidney injury (urinary neutrophil gelatinase-associated lipocalin [uNGAL]). However, the clinical utility of this approach remains unproven, and no serum or urine disease markers are able to provide as much information as a kidney biopsy. Hence, virtually all patients with SLE with suspected kidney involvement undergo one or more kidney biopsies at some point during their care.

KIDNEY BIOPSY FINDINGS

The classic pattern of lupus nephritis is an immune complex-mediated glomerulonephritis; however, the pathology of lupus nephritis can be varied and at times can cause

215

Table 24.1   American College of Rheumatology Criteria for the Diagnosis of Systemic Lupus Erythematosus

Criteria	Description
Malar rash	Flat or raised erythematous rash over the malar eminences
Discoid rash	Erythematous raised patches, usually circular, with adherent keratotic scaling; atrophic scarring may occur
Photosensitivity	Rash upon exposure to ultraviolet light
Oral ulcers	Oral and/or nasopharyngeal ulcerations
Arthritis	Nonerosive arthritis of at least two peripheral joints, with tenderness and/or swelling
Serositis	Pleuritis or pericarditis
Kidney disorder	Proteinuria, hematuria, and/or elevated creatinine
Neurologic disorder	Seizures or psychosis without other etiologies
Hematologic disorder	Anemia (hemolytic), leukopenia, or thrombocytopenia without other etiologies
Immunologic disorder	Anti-dsDNA, anti-Sm, and/or antiphospholipid antibodies
Antinuclear antibodies	An abnormal ANA titer in the absence of drugs known to induce ANAs

ANA, Antinuclear antibody; *dsDNA,* double-stranded DNA.
Any combination of ≥4 criteria at any time during a patient's course suggests a diagnosis of systemic lupus erythematosus.

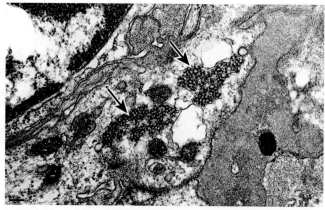

Figure 24.1   Several large endothelial tubuloreticular inclusions (*arrows*) are located in dilated cisternae of the endoplasmic reticulum of this glomerular endothelial cell. These interanastamosing structures, which are commonly identified in systemic lupus erythematosus, are induced in endothelial cells by exposure to ambient interferon, earning them the name "interferon footprints." (Electron micrograph, ×50,000).

confusion with other immune complex-mediated glomerulonephritides. Particular biopsy findings are highly characteristic of lupus nephritis, including: (1) glomerular deposits that stain dominantly for IgG with codeposits of IgA, IgM, C3, and C1q, the so-called "full house" immunofluorescence pattern; (2) extraglomerular immune-type deposits within tubular basement membranes, the interstitium, and blood vessels; (3) the ultrastructural finding of coexistent mesangial, subendothelial, and subepithelial electron-dense deposits; and (4) the ultrastructural finding of tubuloreticular inclusions, which represent "interferon footprints" in the glomerular endothelial cell cytoplasm (Fig. 24.1).

Although lupus may affect all compartments of the kidney, including glomeruli, tubules, interstitium, and blood vessels, disease classification is based largely on the glomerular alterations as assessed by the combined modalities of light microscopy, immunofluorescence, and electron microscopy. Glomerular involvement is the best studied component and correlates well with presentation, course, and treatment response. Over the last four decades, there have been several attempts by different societies, particularly the World Health Organization (WHO), to classify the diverse glomerulopathies associated with SLE. Based on clinicopathologic correlations, a revised classification system of lupus nephritis was developed by a working group of renal pathologists, nephrologists, and rheumatologists under the joint auspices of the International Society of Nephrology (ISN) and the Renal Pathology Society (RPS) and was published in 2004 as the ISN/RPS classification. By refining and clarifying many of the deficiencies of the older WHO classification, this revised schema has eliminated ambiguities and has achieved greater reproducibility. The ISN/RPS classification recognizes six different classes of immune complex-mediated lupus glomerulonephritis based on biopsy findings (Table 24.2). These classes are not static entities, but may transform from one class to another, both spontaneously and after therapy.

ISN/RPS class I represents the mildest possible glomerular lesion—immune deposits limited to the mesangium, without associated mesangial hypercellularity. In class II, the mesangial deposits detected by IF and/or EM are accompanied by mesangial hypercellularity of any degree. In class III, there is focal and predominantly segmental endocapillary proliferation and/or sclerosis affecting less than 50% of glomeruli sampled. The active endocapillary lesions typically include infiltrating monocytes and neutrophils and may exhibit necrotizing features, including fibrinoid necrosis, rupture of glomerular basement membrane, and nuclear apoptosis, forming pyknotic or karyorrhectic debris. These segmental lesions often arise on a background of mesangial proliferation and immune deposits. In class IV, the endocapillary lesions involve ≥50% of glomeruli sampled, typically in a diffuse and global distribution (Fig. 24.2). Subendothelial immune deposits are a feature of the endocapillary lesion in class III and class IV, where they vary from focal and segmental (class III) to more diffuse and global (class IV) (Fig. 24.3). Both class III and class IV may exhibit extracapillary proliferation in the form of cellular crescents, a feature that correlates best with a rapidly progressive clinical course. Subendothelial deposits that are large enough to be visible by light microscopy may form "wire loops," or intracapillary "hyaline thrombi" (Fig. 24.4). A pathognomonic, but uncommon, feature of active lupus nephritis is glomerular "hematoxylin bodies," which consist of extruded nuclei from dying cells that have bound to ambient ANA to form basophilic rounded bodies ("LE bodies") (see Fig. 24.2). Class V denotes membranous lupus nephritis. Subepithelial deposits are the defining feature, usually superimposed on a base of mesangial hypercellularity and/or mesangial immune deposits. Well-developed examples of class V typically

Table 24.2 International Society of Nephrology/Renal Pathology Society 2004 Classification of Lupus Nephritis

Designation	Description	Characteristic Clinical Features
Class I: minimal mesangial lupus nephritis	No LM abnormalities; isolated mesangial IC deposits on IF and/or EM	Normal urine or microscopic hematuria
Class II: mesangial proliferative lupus nephritis	Mesangial hypercellularity or matrix expansion with mesangial IC deposits on IF and/or EM	Microscopic hematuria and/or low-grade proteinuria
Class III: focal lupus nephritis*	<50% of glomeruli on LM display segmental (<50% of glomerular tuft) or global (>50% of glomerular tuft) endocapillary and/or extracapillary proliferation or sclerosis; mesangial and focal subendothelial IC deposits on IF and EM	Nephritic urine sediment and subnephrotic proteinuria
Class IV: diffuse lupus nephritis*	≥50% of glomeruli on LM display endocapillary and/or extracapillary proliferation or sclerosis; class IV-S denotes ≥50% of affected glomeruli have segmental lesions; class IV-G denotes ≥50% of affected glomeruli have global lesions; mesangial and diffuse subendothelial IC deposits on IF and EM	Nephritic and nephrotic syndromes, hypertension, reduced kidney function
Class V: membranous lupus nephritis†	Diffuse thickening of the glomerular capillary walls on LM with subepithelial IC deposits on IF and EM, with or without mesangial IC deposits	Nephrotic syndrome
Class VI: advanced sclerosing lupus nephritis	>90% of glomeruli on LM are globally sclerosed with no residual activity	Markedly reduced kidney function, hypertension

EM, Electron microscopy; *IC,* immune complex; *IF,* immunofluorescence; *LM,* light microscopy.
*Both class III and class IV may have active (proliferative), chronic, inactive (sclerosing), or combined active and chronic lesions subclassified as A, C, or A/C, respectively.
†Class V may coexist with class III or class IV, in which case both classes are diagnosed.

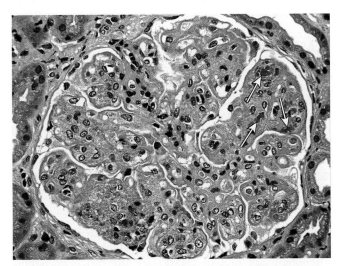

Figure 24.2 **Class IV lupus nephritis: A representative glomerulus shows global narrowing or obliteration of its capillary lumina by endocapillary proliferation, including infiltrating leukocytes.** The glomerular capillary walls are thickened by eosinophilic material, forming wire loops. Rounded basophilic structures ("hematoxylin bodies," *arrows*) represent extruded nuclei altered by binding to antinuclear antibody. (Hematoxylin and eosin, ×400).

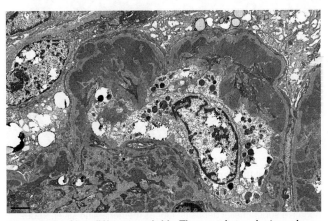

Figure 24.3 **Class IV lupus nephritis: There are large electron-dense deposits within the mesangium and in the subendothelial region.** Podocyte foot processes are effaced. (Electron micrograph, ×6000).

exhibit glomerular basement membrane spikes between the subepithelial deposits (Fig. 24.5). Class V may progress to glomerulosclerosis without the development of a superimposed proliferative lesion. In those patients with combined membranous and endocapillary lesions, a diagnosis of both class V and class III or IV is made. These mixed classes carry a worse prognosis than pure class V lupus nephritis. Class VI

identifies advanced chronic disease exhibiting greater than 90% sclerotic glomeruli, without residual activity.

Unusual kidney biopsy findings in SLE patients include "lupus podocytopathy," presenting as nephrotic syndrome with diffuse foot process effacement in the absence of peripheral capillary wall immune deposits. Such cases resemble minimal change disease or focal segmental glomerulosclerosis in their histopathologic findings and response to glucocorticoids. An altered systemic cytokine milieu, rather than immune complex deposition, is thought to mediate direct podocyte injury. Rare cases of lupus nephritis have predominant tubulointerstitial nephritis with abundant tubulointerstitial immune deposits in the absence of significant glomerular lesions. Some cases with necrotizing and

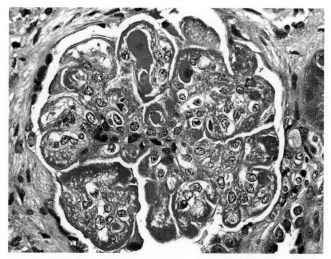

Figure 24.4   Class IV lupus nephritis: Trichrome stain is useful to highlight fuchsinophilic (orange) deposits against the blue-staining glomerular basement membrane and mesangial matrix. In this glomerulus, many subendothelial "wire loops" and intracapillary "hyaline thrombi" are seen. (Masson trichrome, ×600).

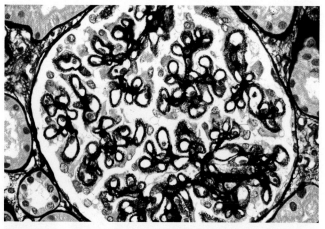

Figure 24.5   Class V lupus nephritis: Membranous lupus nephritis has global thickening of glomerular capillary walls. Silver stain delineates the characteristic silver-positive spikes projecting from the glomerular basement membranes. These spikes form between silver-negative subepithelial deposits. (Jones methenamine silver, ×600).

crescentic features and a paucity of peripheral capillary wall immune deposits are associated with circulating antineutrophil cytoplasmic antibody (ANCA) in addition to ANA. This "pauci-immune" variant is particularly common in lupus nephritis class IV-S, in which there are diffuse but segmental lesions of necrosis and crescent formation. In any patient with SLE who develops thrombotic microangiopathy affecting the glomeruli and/or vessels, the possibility of a circulating lupus anticoagulant or an antiphospholipid antibody should be investigated.

Kidney biopsy evaluation is not complete without an assessment of both histologic activity and chronicity as a guide to therapy. Active lesions include any combination of glomerular endocapillary proliferation, leukocyte infiltration, necrotizing lesions, wire-loop deposits, cellular crescents, and interstitial inflammation, which are graded based on the proportion of glomeruli or cortical area affected. Among features of activity, necrotizing lesions and cellular crescents carry the worst prognosis. Chronic changes include global and segmental glomerular scarring (glomerulosclerosis), fibrous crescents, tubular atrophy, and interstitial fibrosis. Because lesions of activity (A) and chronicity (C) can vary widely in a given biopsy, standard approaches to therapy weigh the extent and severity of active lesions (considered potentially responsive to immunosuppressive therapy) against the extent of chronic, irreversible disease.

TREATMENT

The current approach to treating lupus nephritis, as well as studying new therapeutic modalities in clinical trials, has largely been guided by histologic findings (i.e., ISN/RPS class) with appropriate consideration of presenting clinical parameters and the degree of kidney function impairment (Table 24.3). Class I and class II lupus nephritis, which represent purely mesangial disease, carry a better prognosis and do not require specific therapy directed to the kidney. Rather, conservative, nonimmunomodulatory therapy is appropriate for patients with these findings on kidney biopsy. Optimal control of blood pressure through blockade of the renin-angiotensin-aldosterone system (RAAS) is a cornerstone of conservative therapy in lupus nephritis. Epidemiologic studies have suggested that ACE inhibitor use delays the development of kidney involvement in SLE and reduces overall disease activity.

CLASS III AND IV LUPUS NEPHRITIS

The treatment of active class III and class IV lupus nephritis is generally divided into induction and maintenance phases of immunosuppression. Most patients with active proliferative lupus nephritis are treated initially with corticosteroids, traditionally a "pulse" of intravenous steroids (500-1000 mg/day of methylprednisolone for 3 days), followed by a high-dose oral regimen (usually prednisone at 1 mg/kg/day, not exceeding 60 mg daily) that begins to taper at 8 weeks.

INDUCTION THERAPY

Steroids should be used in conjunction with other immunosuppressive therapy. Currently, cyclophosphamide and mycophenolate mofetil (MMF) are the two main agents used for induction phase immunosuppression. Intravenous, compared to oral, cyclophosphamide therapy involves a lower cumulative exposure to drug, less frequent cytopenias, enhanced bladder protection, and fewer problems with adherence. Several small randomized controlled trials at the National Institutes of Health (NIH) in patients with severe, proliferative lupus nephritis resulted in the induction regimen widely known as the "NIH protocol," which employs six pulses of intravenous cyclophosphamide ($0.5\text{-}1\ g/m^2$) on consecutive months. A trial by the EuroLupus Group aimed to decrease the risk of side effects from cyclophosphamide therapy without sacrificing efficacy; their shorter treatment course (the "EuroLupus protocol") of 500 mg of intravenous cyclophosphamide every 2 weeks for 6 doses (total dose 3 g) was equally effective as the NIH protocol in various

Table 24.3 Treatment Options for Lupus Nephritis, Stratified by International Society of Nephrology Classification and Phase of Therapy

Class	Induction Phase	Maintenance Phase
Class I* Class II	Conservative, nonimmunomodulatory therapy (e.g., RAAS blockade)	Conservative, nonimmunomodulatory therapy (e.g., RAAS blockade)
Class III* Class IV	Pulse IV steroids followed by tapering doses of oral steroids *and* IV cyclophosphamide 0.75-1.0 g/m² IV monthly for 6 doses *or* IV cyclophosphamide 500 mg IV every 2 wk for 6 doses *or* MMF 2000-3000 mg/day for 6 mo	Lowest tolerable amount of oral steroids *and* MMF 2000 mg/day for 6 mo, then 1500 mg/day for 3-6 mo, then 1000 mg/day afterward assuming stable disease *or* Azathioprine 2.0 mg/kg/day for 6 mo, then 1.5 mg/kg/day for 3-6 mo, then 1.0 mg/kg/day afterward assuming stable disease
Class V	Pulse IV steroids followed by tapering doses of oral steroids *and* IV cyclophosphamide 0.75-1.0 g/m² IV monthly for 6 doses *or* Cyclosporine (dose adjusted to goal trough level 125-200 mcg/L) *or* Tacrolimus (dose adjusted to goal trough level 5-10 mcg/L) *or* MMF 2000-3000 mg/day for 6 mo	Lowest tolerable amount of oral steroids *and* MMF 2000 mg/day for 6 mo, then 1500 mg/day for 3-6 mo, then 1000 mg/day afterward assuming stable disease *or* Azathioprine 2.0 mg/kg/day for 6 mo, then 1.5 mg/kg/day for 3-6 mo, then 1.0 mg/kg/day afterward assuming stable disease
Class VI	Conservative, nonimmunomodulatory therapy (e.g., RAAS blockade) with preparation for kidney replacement therapy	Not applicable

IV, Intravenous; *MMF,* mycophenolate mofetil; *RAAS,* renin-angiotensin-aldosterone system.
*Doses listed as mg/day are appropriate for adults. See alternate source for pediatric dosing.

renal and extrarenal outcomes with less toxicity and fewer total infections. Although this trial was largely performed in white subjects and may not be applicable to populations at high risk for poor kidney outcomes, reports from this trial with up to 10 years of follow-up continue to show no differences in outcome between treatment groups.

MMF has emerged as an alternative first choice agent for inducing a remission in severe active proliferative lupus nephritis. An initial report from China compared oral MMF to oral cyclophosphamide and showed similar rates of remission with lower rates of infection and overall mortality in the MMF arm at 1 and 5 years of follow-up. A larger U.S. induction trial in a more diverse population (more than 50% African-Americans) of proliferative or membranous lupus nephritis compared monthly intravenous cyclophosphamide pulses with oral MMF therapy, each in conjunction with a fixed tapering dose of corticosteroids, as induction therapy throughout 6 months. Although the study was powered as a noninferiority trial, complete remissions and complete plus partial remissions at 6 months were significantly more common in the MMF arm (52%) than the cyclophosphamide arm (30%). Most recently, a 370-patient, international multicenter trial of induction therapy with either MMF (3 g/day) or monthly intravenous cyclophosphamide pulses showed, after 6 months of therapy, virtually identical rates of complete and partial remission (56% of patients receiving MMF vs. 53% of patients receiving IV cyclophosphamide). A subgroup analysis of those presenting with significant kidney failure (defined as GFR <30 mL/min) showed no indication that MMF was less effective than cyclophosphamide in this setting.

MAINTENANCE THERAPY

After remission has been achieved, maintenance phase therapy should focus on the long-term management of chronic disease. The goals of continued immunosuppressive therapy are to prevent relapses and flares of disease activity, to eliminate smoldering activity leading to kidney scarring, and to minimize long-term side effects of therapy. Azathioprine and MMF have replaced intravenous cyclophosphamide as the preferred immunosuppressive agents for maintenance therapy. Given the risk for long-term toxicities with all immunosuppressive agents as well as their potential effect on fertility and risk for teratogenicity, the selection and dosage of maintenance therapy are important and modifiable choices that doctors and patients should make together. Although no clinical studies exclude the use of steroids in maintenance therapy, many clinicians will discontinue steroids within the first 1 to 6 months of maintenance therapy to minimize side effects despite a lack of trial data for such a strategy. Until recently, most data suggested equivalence of MMF and azathioprine in sustaining remission during the maintenance phase. For example, in the MAINTAIN Nephritis trial, after standard induction therapy with steroids and cyclophosphamide, 105 subjects with class III (31%), IV (58%), or V (10%) lupus nephritis underwent either azathioprine or MMF maintenance therapy. After at least 3 years of follow-up, both groups showed equal rates of remission, steroid withdrawal, and disease flares. More recently, results from the Aspreva Lupus Management Study maintenance study suggest that MMF may be more effective than azathioprine as maintenance therapy. In this study of 227 patients who had responded to induction therapy with either MMF or intravenous cyclophosphamide, 36 months of maintenance therapy with MMF appeared to be superior to azathioprine with respect to time to treatment failure, time to renal flare, and time to rescue therapy, regardless of induction therapy. Withdrawals resulting from severe adverse events were significantly more common among patients who were administered azathioprine.

CLASS V LUPUS NEPHRITIS

The treatment of class V (membranous) lupus nephritis is also divided into induction and maintenance phases of immunosuppression. As with the proliferative nephritides, induction therapy options include cyclophosphamide and MMF; additionally, in class V, calcineurin inhibitors (cyclosporine or tacrolimus), which have emerged as a first-line therapy for primary membranous nephropathy, are another available treatment. Remission may occur more quickly with a calcineurin inhibitor than with cyclophosphamide or MMF, but these therapies include a higher rate of relapse after withdrawal, similar to the experience of using calcineurin inhibitors in other forms of nephrotic syndrome. One strategy, particularly when a class V lesion is superimposed on a proliferative class III or IV lesion, is to combine a calcineurin inhibitor with MMF. This multitargeted regimen, akin to those used to protect kidney transplants, was tested in a small, randomized trial from China that compared induction therapy with MMF, tacrolimus, and steroids versus intravenous cyclophosphamide and steroids. Intention-to-treat analysis showed a higher rate of complete remission and a lower incidence of adverse events with multitarget therapy at both 6 and 9 months than with cyclophosphamide-based induction therapy.

Because of the unacceptably high rate of treatment failure (30% to 50%) of induction therapies, as well as the high rate of relapsing disease, newer agents and treatment strategies are continuously sought for lupus nephritis. Most of these therapies, when studied in a rigorous manner, are administered in addition to current standard treatment regimens of MMF or cyclophosphamide. Rituximab, an anti-CD20 monoclonal antibody that depletes B cells, was studied in a placebo-controlled trial conducted in 140 patients with severe lupus nephritis, all of whom were receiving concurrent MMF (up to 3 g/day) and tapering dose of corticosteroids. Although more subjects in the rituximab group achieved complete or partial remission, there was no statistically significant difference in the primary clinical endpoint at 1 year. Other agents currently under study for treatment of lupus nephritis include belimumab, a humanized monoclonal antibody that targets the B cell growth factor B lymphocyte stimulator protein; abatacept, a selective T cell costimulation modulator; laquinimod, an oral immunodulatory therapy with an uncertain mechanism of action; and adrenocorticotropic hormone, which has proven effective in some cases of resistant nephrotic syndrome. Plasma exchange has been added to induction therapies in several trials without any demonstrated clear benefit in kidney or patient survival; therefore, the routine use of plasma exchange is not justified in lupus nephritis, although this procedure may be of value in unique individuals, such as those with a refractory antiphospholipid antibody and contraindications to anticoagulation or those with both positive lupus and ANCA serologies.

PROGNOSIS

The proliferative forms of lupus nephritis—class III, class IV, and class V superimposed on class III or IV—are progressive diseases unless a remission is quickly achieved and sustained. In recent decades, the increasing armamentarium of immunosuppressive agents along with an improved knowledge, based on well-performed clinical trials, of how best to dose these agents has led to an improved prognosis for patients with lupus nephritis. Whereas kidney survival at 5 years was as low as 20% before 1980, current treatment strategies have improved this rate to as high as 80% in the past decade. Risk factors for progressive disease include demographic variables, such as male sex, African lineage, Hispanic ethnicity, low socioeconomic status, and young age at presentation, as well as clinical and biopsy features, such as higher serum creatinine at presentation, hypertension, anemia, percentage of glomeruli with necrosis or crescents, and degree of scarring or chronicity in the glomeruli and tubulointerstitium.

When lupus nephritis does progress to end-stage renal disease, most patients experience a gradual complete or partial resolution of their extrarenal manifestations of lupus, including lupus serologies. Furthermore, those patients who continue to experience active disease generally have only mild to moderate symptoms. The mechanisms responsible for this apparent remission of systemic lupus in kidney failure remain unclear. Patients with end-stage renal disease due to lupus nephritis should be dialyzed for at least 3 to 6 months before kidney transplantation is performed; this recommendation holds particular importance for those patients with relatively rapid progression to kidney failure. This period allows for a potential further reduction in lupus activity before transplantation and affords patients with acute kidney injury sufficient time to recover kidney function if therapy is effective. Overall graft survival in patients with lupus who receive a kidney transplant is similar to those in patients with other kidney diseases, despite a recurrence rate of lupus nephritis that ranges from 5% to 30% depending on the indications for kidney allograft biopsy. Recurrence can occur as early as the first week to as late as 10 to 15 years after transplantation. Recurrent lupus nephritis does not necessarily follow the pattern of the native disease but often takes the form of a milder, nonproliferative lesion.

BIBLIOGRAPHY

Appel GB, Contreras G, Dooley MA, et al: Mycophenolate mofetil versus cyclophosphamide for induction treatment of lupus nephritis, *J Am Soc Nephrol* 20:1103-1112, 2009.

Austin 3rd HA, Illei GG, Braun MJ, et al: Randomized, controlled trial of prednisone, cyclophosphamide, and cyclosporine in lupus membranous nephropathy, *J Am Soc Nephrol* 20:901-911, 2009.

Austin HA, Muenz LR, Joyce KM, et al: Diffuse proliferative lupus nephritis: identification of specific pathologic features affecting renal outcome, *Kidney Int* 25:689-695, 1984.

Bao H, Liu ZH, Xie HL, et al: Successful treatment of class V+IV lupus nephritis with multitarget therapy, *J Am Soc Nephrol* 19:2001-2010, 2008.

Bomback AS, Appel GB: Updates on the treatment of lupus nephritis, *J Am Soc Nephrol* 21:2028-2035, 2010.

Chan TM, Li FK, Tang CS, et al: Efficacy of mycophenolate mofetil in patients with diffuse proliferative lupus nephritis. Hong Kong-Guangzhou Nephrology Study Group, *N Engl J Med* 343:1156-1162, 2000.

Dooley MA, Jayne D, Ginzler EM, et al: Mycophenolate versus azathioprine as maintenance therapy for lupus nephritis, *N Engl J Med* 365:1886-1895, 2011.

Duran-Barragan S, McGwin Jr G, Vila LM, et al: Angiotensin-converting enzyme inhibitors delay the occurrence of renal involvement and are associated with a decreased risk of disease activity in patients with systemic lupus erythematosus—results from LUMINA (LIX): a multiethnic US cohort, *Rheumatology (Oxford)* 47:1093-1096, 2008.

Ginzler EM, Dooley MA, Aranow C, et al: Mycophenolate mofetil or intravenous cyclophosphamide for lupus nephritis, *N Engl J Med* 353:2219-2228, 2005.

Gourley MF, Austin 3rd HA, Scott D, et al: Methylprednisolone and cyclophosphamide, alone or in combination, in patients with lupus nephritis. A randomized, controlled trial, *Ann Intern Med* 125:549-557, 1996.

Hill GS, Nochy D: Antiphospholipid syndrome in systemic lupus erythematosus, *J Am Soc Nephrol* 18:2461-2464, 2007.

Houssiau FA, D'Cruz D, Sangle S, et al: Azathioprine versus mycophenolate mofetil for long-term immunosuppression in lupus nephritis: results from the MAINTAIN nephritis trial, *Ann Rheum Dis* 69:2083-2089, 2010.

Houssiau FA, Vasconcelos C, D'Cruz D, et al: The 10-year follow-up data of the euro-lupus nephritis trial comparing low-dose and high-dose intravenous cyclophosphamide, *Ann Rheum Dis* 69:61-64, 2010.

Illei GG, Austin HA, Crane M, et al: Combination therapy with pulse cyclophosphamide plus pulse methylprednisolone improves long-term renal outcome without adding toxicity in patients with lupus nephritis, *Ann Intern Med* 135:248-257, 2001.

Kraft SW, Schwartz MM, Korbet SM, et al: Glomerular podocytopathy in patients with systemic lupus erythematosus, *J Am Soc Nephrol* 16:175-179, 2005.

Markowitz GS, D'Agati VD: Classification of lupus nephritis, *Curr Opin Nephrol Hypertens* 18:220-225, 2009.

Miyasaka N, Kawai S, Hashimoto H: Efficacy and safety of tacrolimus for lupus nephritis: a placebo-controlled double-blind multicenter study, *Mod Rheumatol* 19:606-615, 2009.

Nasr SH, D'Agati VD, Park H-R, et al: Necrotizing and crescentic lupus nephritis with antineutrophil cytoplasmic antibody seropositivity, *Clin J Am Soc Nephrol* 3:682-690, 2008.

Ortega LM, Schultz DR, Lenz O, et al: Lupus nephritis: pathologic features, epidemiology and a guide to therapeutic decisions, *Lupus* 19:557-574, 2010.

Radhakrishnan J, Moutzouris DA, Ginzler EM, et al: Mycophenolate mofetil and intravenous cyclophosphamide are similar as induction therapy for class V lupus nephritis, *Kidney Int* 77:152-160, 2010.

Rovin BH, Zhang X: Biomarkers for lupus nephritis: the quest continues, *Clin J Am Soc Nephrol* 4:1858-1865, 2009.

Weening JJ, D'Agati VD, Schwartz MM, et al: The classification of glomerulonephritis in systemic lupus erythematosus revisited, *J Am Soc Nephrol* 15:241-250, 2004.

25 Pathogenesis, Pathophysiology, and Treatment of Diabetic Nephropathy

Hiddo J. Lambers Heerspink | Paola Fioretto | Dick de Zeeuw

Diabetic nephropathy is the most common cause of end-stage renal disease (ESRD) in adults. In the United States, almost half of patients entering ESRD programs are diabetic, and most of them (≥80%) have type 2 diabetes. The mortality rate of patients with diabetic nephropathy is high, with a marked increase in cardiovascular risk accounting for more than half of the increased mortality risk among these patients. After overt diabetic nephropathy is present, ESRD can often be postponed, but in most instances not prevented, by effective antihypertensive treatment and careful glycemic control. Accordingly, there has been intensive research into early pathophysiologic mechanisms of diabetic kidney injury, predictors of risk for diabetic nephropathy, and early intervention strategies.

PATHOPHYSIOLOGY

Although other important modulating factors may exist, diabetic nephropathy is a result of the long-term metabolic aberrations caused by hyperglycemia. Studies in both type 1 and type 2 diabetes have shown that improved glycemic control can reduce the risk of diabetic nephropathy. Moreover, the development of the earliest diabetic kidney lesions can be slowed or prevented by strict glycemic control, as was demonstrated in a randomized trial in type 1 diabetic kidney transplant recipients. Similarly, intensive insulin treatment decreased the progression rates of glomerular lesions in a controlled trial in microalbuminuric type 1 diabetic patients. Finally, established diabetic glomerular lesions in the native kidneys of type 1 diabetic patients regressed with prolonged normalization of glycemic levels after successful pancreas transplantation. In sum, these studies strongly suggest that hyperglycemia is necessary for the development and maintenance of diabetic nephropathy, as correction of hyperglycemia allows expression of reparative mechanisms that facilitate healing of the original diabetic glomerular injury.

Although hemodynamic mechanisms may be also involved in the pathogenesis of diabetic nephropathy, patients with other causes of hyperfiltration (such as unilateral nephrectomy) do not develop diabetic lesions. Therefore, glomerular hyperfiltration alone cannot fully explain the genesis of the early lesions of diabetic nephropathy; however, clinical observations do suggest that hemodynamic factors may be important in modulating the rate of progression of diabetic lesions that are already well established. It is worth noting that the presence of reduced glomerular filtration rate (GFR) in normoalbuminuric patients with type 1 diabetes has been associated with more severe glomerular lesions, and these patients may be at increased risk of progression to overt diabetic nephropathy. Systemic blood-pressure levels and a lack of normal nocturnal blood-pressure dipping both may be implicated in the progression and genesis of diabetic nephropathy. Supporting this hypothesis is the association between intensive blood-pressure control and decreased rates of progression from normoalbuminuria to microalbuminuria and from microalbuminuria to proteinuria in both normotensive and hypertensive type 2 diabetic patients.

Genetic predisposition to diabetic nephropathy has been strongly suggested in multiple cross-sectional studies in type 1 and type 2 diabetic siblings concordant for diabetes. Importantly, diabetic sibling pairs, known to be concordant for diabetic nephropathy risk, are also highly concordant for diabetic glomerulopathy lesions, and this risk is in part independent of glycemia. Accordingly, there are ongoing searches for genetic loci related to diabetic nephropathy susceptibility through genomic scanning and candidate gene approaches.

The kidney lesions of diabetic nephropathy appear to be mainly related to extracellular matrix (ECM) accumulation in both the glomerular basement membrane (GBM) and the tubular basement membrane (TBM); this ECM accumulation, which reflects an imbalance between ECM synthesis and degradation, is the principal cause of mesangial expansion and a contributor to expansion of the interstitium late in the disease. Many regulatory mechanisms have been proposed to explain the link between a high ambient glucose concentration and ECM accumulation. These include increased levels of TGFβ; activation of protein kinase C, which stimulates ECM production through the cyclic adenosine monophosphate pathway; increased advanced glycation end products; and increased activity of aldose reductase, leading to accumulation of sorbitol. There is also growing evidence that oxidative stress is increased in diabetes and is related to diabetic nephropathy, mediated through altered nitric oxide production and action, and endothelial dysfunction.

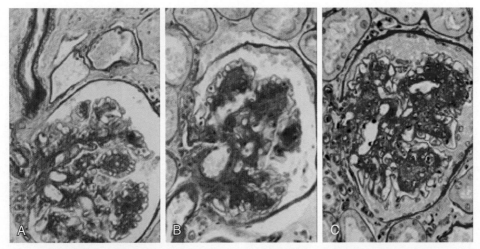

Figure 25.1   Light microscopy photographs of glomeruli in sequential kidney biopsies performed at baseline and after 5 and 10 years of follow-up in a patient with longstanding normoalbuminuric type 1 diabetes with progressive mesangial expansion and kidney function deterioration. A, Diffuse and nodular mesangial expansion and arteriolar hyalinosis in this glomerulus from a patient who was normotensive and normoalbuminuric at the time of this baseline biopsy, 21 years after diabetes onset (periodic acid–Schiff [PAS] stain, original magnification ×400). **B,** Five-year follow-up biopsy showing worsening of the diffuse and nodular mesangial expansion and arteriolar hyalinosis in this now microalbuminuric patient with declining glomerular filtration rate (GFR) (PAS stain, ×400). **C,** Ten-year follow-up biopsy showing more advanced diabetic glomerulopathy in this now proteinuric patient with further reduced GFR. Note also the multiple small glomerular (probably efferent) arterioles in the hilar region of this glomerulus (PAS stain, ×400) and in the glomerulus shown in **A.**

PATHOLOGY

TYPE 1 DIABETES

In patients with type 1 diabetes, glomerular lesions can appear within a few years after diabetes onset. The same time frame is present when a normal kidney is transplanted into a diabetic patient. The changes in kidney structure caused by diabetes are specific, creating a pattern not seen in any other disease, and the severity of these diabetic lesions is related to the functional disturbances of the clinical kidney disease as well as to diabetes duration, glycemic control, and genetic factors. However, the relationship between the duration of type 1 diabetes and extent of glomerular pathology is not precise. This is consistent with the marked variability in susceptibility to this disorder, such that some patients may develop kidney failure after having diabetes for 15 years whereas others escape kidney complications despite having type 1 diabetes for decades.

LIGHT MICROSCOPY

Kidney hypertrophy is the earliest structural change in type 1 diabetes but is not reflected in any specific light microscopic changes. In many patients, glomerular structure remains normal or near normal even after decades of diabetes, whereas others develop progressive diffuse mesangial expansion seen mainly as increased periodic acid–Schiff (PAS)-positive ECM mesangial material. In about 40% to 50% of patients developing proteinuria, there are areas of extreme mesangial expansion called Kimmelstiel-Wilson nodules (nodular mesangial expansion). Mesangial cell nuclei in these nodules are palisaded around masses of mesangial matrix material with compression of surrounding capillary lumina. Nodules are thought to result from earlier glomerular capillary microaneurysm formation. Notably, about half of patients with severe diabetic nephropathy do

not have these nodular lesions; therefore, although Kimmelstiel-Wilson nodules are diagnostic of diabetic nephropathy, they are not necessary for severe kidney disease to develop.

Early changes often include arteriolar hyalinosis lesions involving replacement of the smooth muscle cells of afferent and efferent arterioles with PAS-positive waxy, homogenous material (Fig. 25.1). The severity of these lesions is directly related to the frequency of global glomerulosclerosis, perhaps as the result of glomerular ischemia. GBM and TBM thickening may be seen with light microscopy, although they are more easily seen with electron microscopy. In addition, atubular glomeruli and glomerulotubular junction abnormalities are present in proteinuric type 1 diabetic patients and may be important in the progressive loss of GFR in diabetic nephropathy. Finally, usually quite late in the disease, tubular atrophy and interstitial fibrosis occur.

IMMUNOFLUORESCENCE

Diabetes is characterized by increased linear staining of the GBM, TBM, and Bowman capsule, especially for immunoglobulin G (mainly IgG4) and albumin. Although this staining is removed only by strong acid conditions, consistent with strong ionic binding, the intensity of staining is not related to the severity of the underlying lesions. Care is needed to avoid confusing these findings with anti–basement membrane antibody disorders.

ELECTRON MICROSCOPY

The first measurable change observed in diabetic nephropathy is thickening of the GBM, which can be detected as early as 1.5 to 2.5 years after onset of type 1 diabetes (Fig. 25.2). TBM thickening is also seen and parallels GBM thickening. An increase in the relative area of the mesangium becomes measurable by 4 to 5 years, with the proportion of the volume of the glomerulus that is mesangium increasing from about 20% (normal) to about 40% when proteinuria begins

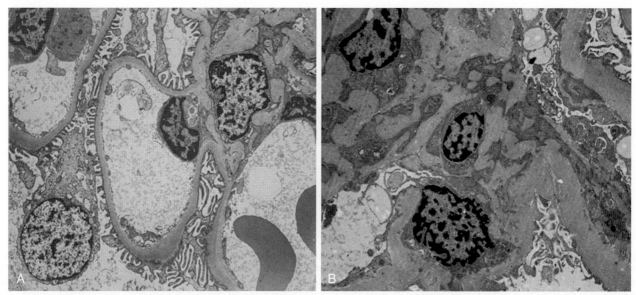

Figure 25.2   Electron microscopy photographs of mesangial area in a normal control subject (A) and in a patient with type 1 diabetes (B) (original magnification ×3900). Note the increase in mesangial matrix and cell content, the glomerular basement membrane thickening, and the decrease in the capillary luminal space in the diabetic patient **(B)**.

and to 60% to 80% in patients with stage 3 chronic kidney disease (CKD). Immunohistochemical studies indicate that these changes in mesangium, GBM, and TBM represent expansion of the intrinsic ECM components at these sites, most likely including types IV and VI collagen, laminin, and fibronectin.

Qualitative and quantitative changes in the renal interstitium are observed in patients with various kidney diseases. Interstitial fibrosis is characterized by an increase in ECM proteins and cellularity. Preliminary studies suggest that the pathogenesis of interstitial changes in diabetic nephropathy is different from the changes that occur in the mesangial matrix, GBM, and TBM in diabetic nephropathy. Whereas, for all but the later stages of diabetic nephropathy, GBM, TBM, and mesangial matrix changes represent the accumulation of basement membrane ECM material, early interstitial expansion is largely a result of cellular alterations and only later, when GFR is already compromised, is interstitial expansion associated with increased interstitium fibrillar collagen and peritubular capillary loss. Consistent with most kidney diseases affecting the glomeruli, the fraction of GBM covered by intact, nondetached foot processes is lower in proteinuric patients with diabetes when compared with either control subjects or individuals with type 1 diabetes with low levels of albuminuria. Moreover, the fraction of the glomerular capillary luminal surface covered by fenestrated endothelium is reduced in all stages of diabetic nephropathy, with increasing severity in normoalbuminuric, microalbuminuric, and overtly proteinuric type 1 diabetics, respectively, as compared with controls.[17]

TYPE 2 DIABETES

Glomerular structure in type 2 diabetes is less well studied but overall seems more heterogeneous than in type 1. Between 30% and 50% of type 2 diabetes patients with clinical features of diabetic nephropathy have typical changes of diabetic nephropathy, including diffuse and nodular

mesangial expansion and arteriolar hyalinosis (Fig. 25.3). Notably, some patients, despite the presence of microalbuminuria or even overt proteinuria, have absent or only mild diabetic glomerulopathy, whereas others have disproportionately severe tubular and interstitial abnormalities and/or vascular lesions and/or an increased number of globally sclerosed glomeruli. Type 2 diabetic patients with microalbuminuria more frequently have morphometric glomerular structural measures in the normal range on electron microscopy and less severe lesions than type 1 diabetic patients with microalbuminuria or overt proteinuria. Interestingly, Pima Indians with type 2 diabetes, a high-risk population for ESRD, have lesions more typical of those seen in type 1 diabetes.

It is currently unclear why some studies show more structural heterogeneity in type 2 than in type 1 diabetes whereas others do not. Regardless, the rate of kidney-disease progression in type 2 diabetes is related, at least in part, to the severity of the classic changes of diabetic glomerulopathy. Although there are reports that patients with type 2 diabetes have an increased incidence of nondiabetic lesions, such as proliferative glomerulonephritis and membranous nephropathy, this likely reflects biopsies more often being performed in patients with atypical clinical features. When biopsies are performed for research purposes, the incidence of other definable kidney diseases is very low (<5%).

STRUCTURAL–FUNCTIONAL RELATIONSHIPS IN DIABETIC NEPHROPATHY

Kidney disease progression rates vary greatly among individuals with diabetes. Patients with type 1 diabetes and patients with proteinuria who are biopsied for research purposes rather than for diagnosis of atypical clinical characteristics always have advanced glomerular lesions and usually have vascular, tubular, and interstitial lesions

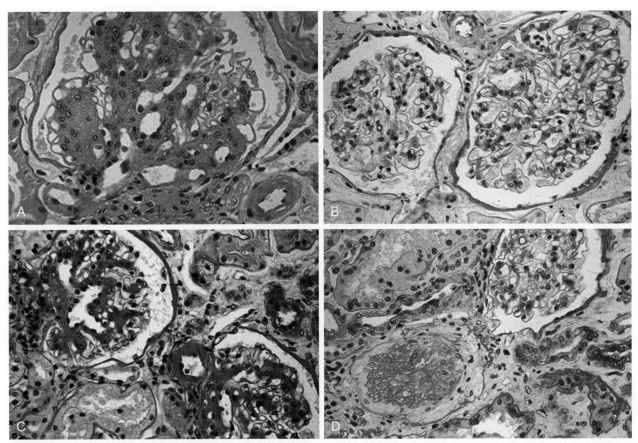

Figure 25.3   Light microscopy photographs of glomeruli from type 1 (A) and type 2 (B through D) diabetic patients. A, Diffuse and nodular mesangial expansion and arteriolar hyalinosis in a glomerulus from a microalbuminuric type 1 diabetic patient (periodic acid–Schiff [PAS] stain, original magnification ×400). **B,** Normal or near-normal kidney structure in a glomerulus from a microalbuminuric type 2 diabetic patient (PAS stain, ×400). **C,** Changes "typical" of diabetic nephropathology (glomerular, tubulointerstitial, and arteriolar changes occurring in parallel) in a kidney biopsy specimen from a microalbuminuric type 2 diabetic patient (PAS stain, ×400). **D,** "Atypical" patterns of injury, with absent or only mild diabetic glomerular changes associated with disproportionately severe tubulointerstitial changes. Note also a glomerulus undergoing glomerular sclerosis (PAS stain, ×400) (**B** through **D**).

as well. Similarly, patients with microalbuminuria biopsied for research purposes usually have well-established lesions, which vary widely in severity. However, there is considerable overlap in glomerular structural changes between long-standing normoalbuminuric and microalbuminuric patients, as some normoalbuminuric patients with long-standing type 1 diabetes can have quite advanced kidney lesions, whereas many patients with longstanding diabetes and normoalbuminuria have structural measurements within the normal range.

Ultimately expansion of the mesangium, mainly resulting from ECM accumulation, reduces or even obliterates the glomerular capillary luminal space, decreasing the glomerular filtration surface and therefore decreasing the GFR. Accordingly, the fraction of the glomerulus occupied by mesangium correlates with both GFR and albuminuria in patients with type 1 diabetes, reflecting in part the inverse relationship between mesangial expansion and total peripheral GBM filtration surface per glomerulus. GBM thickness is also directly related to the albumin excretion rate. Finally, the extent of global glomerulosclerosis and interstitial expansion are correlated with the clinical manifestations of diabetic nephropathy (proteinuria, hypertension, and declining GFR).

In patients with type 1 diabetes, glomerular, tubular, interstitial, and vascular lesions tend to progress more or less in parallel, whereas in type 2 diabetic patients this often is not the case. Current evidence suggests that, among type 2 diabetes patients with microalbuminuria, those patients with typical diabetic glomerulopathy have a higher risk of progressive GFR loss than those with lesser degrees of glomerular changes. A remarkably high frequency of glomerular tubular junction abnormalities can be observed in proteinuric type 1 diabetic patients. Most of these abnormalities are associated with tuft adhesions to Bowman capsule at or near the glomerular tubular junction (tip lesions). The frequency and severity of these lesions (as well as the presence of completely atubular glomeruli) predict GFR loss.

The data on structural–functional relationships in type 2 diabetes based on quantitative morphometric analysis are less abundant. In several small studies, morphometric measures of diabetic glomerulopathy correlated with kidney function parameters similar to those observed in type 1 diabetes, although there seems to be a subset of patients who have normal glomerular structure despite persistent albuminuria. Overall, the relationships between kidney function and glomerular structural variables, although significant, are less precise than in patients with type 1 diabetes. Importantly the rate of GFR decline significantly correlates with the severity of diabetic glomerulopathy lesions. Thus, kidney lesions different from those typical of diabetic glomerulopathy should be considered when investigating the nature of abnormal levels of albuminuria in type 2 diabetes. These lesions include changes in the structure of renal tubules, interstitium, arterioles, and podocytes. For example, Pima Indians with type 2 diabetes and proteinuria have fewer podocytes per glomerulus than those without nephropathy, and, in this population, a lower number of podocytes per glomerulus at baseline was the strongest predictor of greater increases in albuminuria and of progression to overt nephropathy in microalbuminuric patients. Similar findings were noted in another type 2 diabetes cohort, where the density of podocytes per glomerulus was significantly decreased in all diabetic patients compared with controls and was lower in patients with microalbuminuria and overt proteinuria than in patients with normoalbuminuria. In addition, microalbuminuric and proteinuric patients had increased foot process width compared with normoalbuminuric patients, and foot process width was directly related to the level of albuminuria. In sum, these results suggest that changes in podocyte structure and density occur early in diabetic nephropathy and might contribute to increasing albuminuria in these patients.

REVERSAL OF DIABETIC NEPHROPATHY LESIONS

The lesions of diabetic nephropathy have long been considered irreversible. Theoretically, if reversal were possible, this would happen in the setting of long-term normoglycemia. Interestingly, in recipients of successful pancreas transplantation alone, the lesions of diabetic nephropathy were unaffected after 5 years of normoglycemia, whereas, by 10 years after pancreas transplant, reversal of diabetic glomerular and tubular lesions was apparent in all patients, with a remarkable amelioration of glomerular structure abnormalities evident by light microscopy, including total disappearance of Kimmelstiel-Wilson nodular lesions. Although the reasons for the long delay in the reversal of diabetic nephropathy lesions are unknown, the long time necessary for these diabetic lesions to disappear is consistent with their slow rate of development. The understanding of the molecular and cellular mechanisms involved in these repair processes could provide new directions for the treatment of diabetic nephropathy. Other therapeutic approaches, such as antihypertensive agents, have not been described as leading to amelioration or reversal of diabetic kidney lesions.

MEDICAL MANAGEMENT OF DIABETES

Both kidney and cardiovascular morbidity and mortality are increased in patients with type 2 diabetes, particularly in those with nephropathy. Accordingly, treatment goals in these individuals focus on slowing the rate of GFR decline and delaying the onset of kidney failure as well as primary and secondary prevention of cardiovascular disease. This is mainly done by targeting multiple kidney and cardiovascular risk factors, such as hyperglycemia, hypertension, and dyslipidemia. Targeting albuminuria appears of specific interest for kidney protection

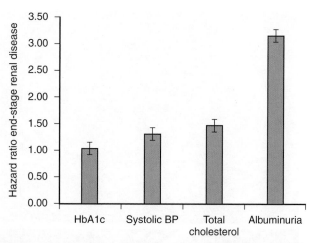

Figure 25.4   Comparison of different risk markers for prediction of end-stage renal disease (ESRD) in patients with type 2 diabetes and nephropathy participating in the Trial to Reduce cardiovascular Events with Aranesp Therapy (TREAT). The risk for ESRD per standard deviation increment in the risk factor is shown. Per standard deviation increment in albuminuria, the risk of ESRD markedly amplifies compared with the other kidney-disease risk factors. (Adapted from Pfeffer MA, Burdmann EA, Chen CY, et al: A trial of darbepoetin alfa in type 2 diabetes and chronic kidney disease, *N Engl J Med* 361:2019-2032, 2009.)

(Fig. 25.4). In the next section, traditional therapeutic options to decrease the risk of kidney and cardiovascular morbidity and mortality are discussed. In addition to traditional risk factors, novel risk factors for diabetic nephropathy are identified, which provide insight into new drug targets and possibilities for new therapeutic interventions. An overview is provided of novel therapeutic avenues that target these novel risk markers.

TRADITIONAL THERAPEUTIC STRATEGIES FOR DIABETIC NEPHROPATHY

GLYCEMIC CONTROL

Rationale

Inadequate glycemic control, as reflected by higher hemoglobin A1c (HbA1c) levels, is associated with markedly worse kidney and cardiovascular outcomes in observational studies of patients with diabetes, and targeting HbA1c values lower than 7% may delay the progression of diabetic kidney disease, including development of microalbuminuria and overt nephropathy. In type 1 diabetics, the benefit of intensive glucose control in the prevention of microvascular complications (i.e., the development of retinopathy or microalbuminuria) was demonstrated in the diabetes control and complications trial (DCCT), where long-term follow-up showed a significant reduction in the risk of developing reduced GFR among individuals who were treated intensively earlier in the course of diabetes. In type 2 diabetes, the United Kingdom prospective diabetes study (UKPDS) documented benefit of intensive glucose targeting on microvascular complications. Of note, although most studies of type 2 diabetes have shown a benefit in kidney outcomes, multiple trials failed to show a benefit of intensive glycemia therapy on mortality and cardiovascular disease, with some trials actually showing increased mortality with intensive control. Accordingly, a careful individualized approach is required when assigning glycemic targets in individuals with diabetes and kidney disease.

Medications of Choice

In principle one uses the same drugs for glycemic control in diabetic patients with and without kidney disease until late stage 3 CKD (Table 25.1). There is some controversy regarding metformin use in advanced CKD, with current suggested use limited to those with serum creatinine ≤1.5 mg/dl (133 µmol/L) in men and 1.4 mg/dl (124 µmol/L) in women because of an increased risk for life-threatening lactic acidosis, although in practice many patients with an estimated glomerular filtration rate (eGFR) of 30 to 60 mL/min/1.73 m^2 receive metformin without any problem. Although it is unlikely to occur, a randomized controlled trial assessing the efficacy and safety of metformin in patients with more advanced CKD is warranted, as metformin is an excellent glucose-lowering agent for many patients. Of note, metformin should be temporarily discontinued before surgery or administration of contrast media.

Reduction in the doses of other oral hypoglycemic agents in later stages of CKD may also be necessary, especially for some sulfonylurea compounds that are metabolized by the kidney. Similarly, as insulin is degraded by the kidney, dose reduction may be needed to prevent hypoglycemia. Finally, thiazolidinediones, such as rosiglitazone or pioglitazone, may affect kidney water and sodium handling, thereby aggravating edema and congestive heart failure. In non-CKD populations, rosiglitazone use is associated with increased risk of heart failure and myocardial infarction compared with placebo, prompting regulatory agencies in Europe to suspend its marketing.

BLOOD-PRESSURE CONTROL

Rationale

Treatment of high blood pressure is of paramount importance for preventing and delaying the progression of diabetic nephropathy. Blood-pressure–lowering therapy is vital during any stage of CKD and is the mainstay of renoprotective therapy in diabetes and nondiabetic kidney diseases. In the UKPDS trial, where average blood-pressure levels of 144/82 mm Hg were achieved, there was no threshold below which further blood-pressure reduction did not reduce risk of progressive diabetic nephropathy and cardiovascular morbidity. However, recent data from the Action to Control Cardiovascular Risk in Diabetes (ACCORD) trial showed that intensive (average 119 mm Hg) versus standard blood pressure (average 134 mm Hg) control conferred no benefit on kidney outcomes in type 2 diabetes patients. Critically, patients with more than 1 g of proteinuria per day were excluded from this trial, leaving the benefits of a lower blood-pressure target (<120 mm Hg systolic) for patients with type 2 diabetes and nephropathy untested. Surprisingly little evidence from randomized controlled trials demonstrates that a lower target blood pressure actually reduces kidney or cardiovascular risk in people with diabetes and CKD. Accordingly, at present, a target of less than 140/90 mm Hg appears to be best supported by evidence.

Drugs of Choice

Any antihypertensive agent can be effectively used in the diabetic population, with agents that block the renin-angiotensin-aldosterone system (RAAS) being the first choice in those with diabetes and hypertension as well as those with (normotensive) diabetes with microalbuminuria or macroalbuminuria. Medication choice is further tailored to the need of the individual patient and the tolerability of the individual drugs. Patients with diabetic nephropathy are often volume overloaded; accordingly diuretic therapy is indicated. Increasing doses of loop diuretics, rather than thiazide diuretics, may become necessary to control fluid retention and accompanying hypertension if GFR declines.

Multiple experimental and clinical studies conclusively demonstrate that RAAS blocking agents lead to additional cardiovascular and renoprotection benefits beyond those expected with blood-pressure reduction alone. This has led many medical societies, such as the National Kidney Foundation and American Diabetes Association, to advocate the use of angiotensin-converting enzyme (ACE) inhibitors or angiotensin receptor blockers (ARB) as first choice antihypertensive therapy to achieve renoprotection. The beneficial effects of ACE inhibitors and ARB appear to be attributable not only to their blood-pressure–lowering effect but also to their antialbuminuric effect, with the degree of the reduction in albuminuria induced by RAAS intervention in the first months of therapy linearly associated with the magnitude of long-term renoprotection both in early and in late stages of diabetic nephropathy.

ACE Inhibitors

The captopril trial by the Collaborative Study Group was the first large trial to show definitively the benefit of ACE inhibitor therapy in delaying progression of overt nephropathy in patients with type 1 diabetes throughout a 4-year period of follow-up, with a nearly 50% reduction in the risk of doubling of serum creatinine concentration or in the combined endpoints of death, dialysis, and kidney transplantation despite similar achieved blood pressure between the captopril and noncaptopril groups. ACE inhibitors should be used in type 1 diabetic patients as soon as persistent microalbuminuria is documented, even if blood pressure is not elevated, to delay and/or prevent the development of overt nephropathy. In type 2 diabetes and normoalbuminuria, ACE inhibitors have consistently reduced the risk of development of microalbuminuria and reduced the rate of kidney function decline. RAAS-blocking drugs can be prescribed for cardioprotective indications in all diabetic patients, regardless of the presence or absence of kidney disease; for example, the subgroup of diabetic patients who received the ramipril in the Heart and Outcome Protection Evaluation (HOPE) trial had significantly fewer cardiovascular events.

Angiotensin Receptor Blockers

The merits of angiotensin receptor blockers (ARB) to protect the kidney and heart beyond blood-pressure control have been demonstrated in numerous randomized placebo-controlled trials, including the Irbesartan in Patients with Type 2 Diabetes and Microalbuminuria (IRMA2) and the Incipient to Overt; Angiotensin II Blocker Telmisartan Investigation on Type 2 Diabetic Nephropathy (INNOVATION) trials, where ARB-based regimens significantly reduced the number of patients with microalbuminuria who progressed to macroalbuminuria. Similarly, large-scale trials in patients with type 2 diabetes and overt nephropathy, including the Reduction in Endpoints in NIDDM with the Angiotensin-II Antagonist Losartan (RENAAL) and Irbesartan Diabetic Nephropathy Trial (IDNT) trials, have shown that ARB-based therapy reduces the risk of a composite endpoint

Table 25.1 Currently Available Oral Hypoglycemic Agents for the Management of Hyperglycemia

Class	Mechanism of Action	Examples of Drugs	Renal Clearance	Hba1c Lowering (%)	Use in Predialysis CKD	Use in Dialysis CKD	Advantage	Disadvantage
Biguanides (European Union 1958; United States 1995*)	Inhibits hepatic glucose production and increases insulin sensitivity	Metformin	Excreted unchanged in urine	1.5	Contraindicated	Contraindicated	Long-term safety; low costs; weight neutral	Risk of lactate acidosis in CKD patients; gastrointestinal side effects
Sulfonylureas (1946*)	Binds to SU receptor in β-cells and increases calcium influx followed by insulin release	Gliclazide Glipizide Glimepiride Glyburide	More than 90% metabolized in liver to weakly active or inactive metabolites and excreted in urine and feces	1.5	May be used	Glipizide may be used; use Glimepiride and glyburide with caution	Long-term safety; low costs	Hypoglycemia; weight gain
Meglitinides (1997*)	Binds to SU receptor (different from SU site) and increases calcium influx followed by insulin release	Nateglinide Repaglinide	Metabolized by liver (100%) and excreted in urine (10%) and feces (90%)	1.0	May be used	No data for patients with renal clearance less than 20 mL/min	Rapid onset of action and short acting	Few long-term safety data; weight gain
Thiazolidinediones (1997*)	Decreases peripheral insulin resistance thus increasing insulin sensitivity	Pioglitazone	Metabolized by liver to weakly active metabolites; excreted in urine (15%) and feces (85%)	0.6 to 1.5	May be used; no dose adjustments necessary	May be used; no dose adjustments necessary	Low-risk hypoglycemia	Pioglitazone is associated with increased risk of bladder cancer; Rosiglitazone withdrawn from the market because of increased cardiovascular risk
Incretin mimetics (2005*)	Binds to the pancreatic GLP-1 receptor and promotes insulin secretion, decreases glucogon secretion, gastric emptying, and appetite	Exenatide Liruglatide	Metabolized by kidney, excreted in urine	0.7 to 1.2 on top of metformin or SU derivatives	Not recommended for patients with moderate or severe renal failure	Not recommended for patients with moderate or severe kidney failure	Seem to have favorable cardiovascular risk profile (blood-pressure lowering/albuminuria lowering)	Long-term safety data not yet known
DPP-4 inhibitors (2006*)	Blocks DPP-4 which inactivates endogenous incretins	Saxagliptin Sitagliptin Linagliptin	Excreted mostly unchanged in urine and feces (Linagliptin metabolized and excreted in feces)	~0.8 (on top of metformin/SU derivatives)	Dose adjustments necessary for saxagliptin and sitagliptin	Dose adjustments necessary for saxagliptin and sitagliptin	Weight neutral; low risk of hypoglycemia	Long-term safety data not yet known
SGLT-2 inhibitors (European Union 2012*)	Inhibits proximal tubular glucose reabsorption	Dapagliflozin	Metabolized by liver to active metabolites; excreted in urine and feces	~0.8 (on top of metformin)	Limited clinical experience	No clinical experience; not recommended	Favorable CV risk profile (blood pressure, body weight lowering)	Long-term safety not yet known; increased risk of urinary or genital tract infections

CKD, Chronic kidney disease; DPP-4, dipeptidylpeptidase 4; GLP-1, glycagon-like peptide-1; SGLT-2, sodium–glucose cotransporter-2; SU, sulphonylurea.
*Year drug became available for clinical use.

consisting of doubling of serum creatinine, ESRD, and all cause mortality. IDNT also established the superiority of irbesartan over the calcium channel blocker (CCB) amlodipine in this setting. Apart from kidney protection, ARBs also afford cardiovascular protection in diabetic patients as demonstrated in the Losartan Intervention for Endpoint Reduction in Hypertension (LIFE) trial.

Comparing ACE Inhibitors to ARBs

Data comparing the benefits of ACE inhibitors and ARB for cardiovascular and/or kidney protection in patients with type 2 diabetic nephropathy are scarce but potentially interesting. One small study directly compared the effects of telmisartan and enalapril on kidney function in type 2 diabetes and reported no difference between the two drugs. Similar results were noted in the Ongoing Telmisartan Alone and in Combination with Ramipril Trial (ONTARGET), where, in people at cardiovascular risk, there was no difference in the incidence of kidney or cardiovascular outcome in subjects treated with ACE inhibitor- or ARB-based regimens in either the overall population or in the third of participants with diabetes. Accordingly, there is no efficacy basis for recommending an ACE inhibitor over an ARB in patients with type 2 diabetes, although the not infrequent occurrence of cough with an ACE inhibitor has increased the popularity of an ARB-based antihypertensive regimen despite the increased cost.

COMBINATIONS OF BLOOD-PRESSURE–LOWERING DRUGS

Rationale

More than one medication is usually required to control blood pressure, with patients with overt diabetic nephropathy usually requiring three or four different antihypertensive drugs, including a diuretic. In addition, synergistic combinations may have the advantage that one can reduce the dose of individual components of the antihypertensive regimen, potentially retaining efficacy while reducing side effects.

Combinations of Choice

Logical combinations can be used just as in uncomplicated hypertensive patients. Since RAAS blockade typically will be the first line agent, clinicians should use other agents, in conjunction with RAAS blockade, that have proven efficacy for preventing both surrogate and hard clinical outcomes.

Diuretic Plus ACE-inhibitor or ARB. This combination effectively reduces both blood pressure and proteinuria in diabetic and non-diabetic patients; however, no studies with hard outcomes have been done to compare this combination with single therapies. The ADVANCE trial showed that the combination of an ACE inhibitor (perindopril) with a diuretic (indapamide) significantly reduces blood pressure and the risk of kidney and cardiovascular complications as compared with placebo therapy in a broad range of patients with type 2 diabetes.

Calcium Channel Blocker Plus ACE Inhibitor or ARB. The combination of a CCB and an ACE inhibitor has been investigated in two large trials. The BENEDICT trial compared the combination of the nondihydropyridine CCB verapamil and the ACE inhibitor trandolapril versus the single use of these

agents in preventing the onset of microalbuminuria in type 2 diabetes, demonstrating that the combination of verapamil and trandolapril provided no advantage over trandolapril alone, whereas trandolapril was superior compared with verapamil. The ACCOMPLISH trial compared benazepril plus hydrochlorothiazide versus benazepril plus amlodipine in high cardiovascular risk patients and reported that the combination of benazepril and amlodipine was superior in preventing cardiovascular and kidney outcomes. Although a prespecified analysis in the diabetic population in ACCOMPLISH (60% of the overall population) showed results similar to the main study, the small number of kidney events in ACCOMPLISH renders the interpretation of this outcome difficult.

COMBINATIONS OF RAAS-INTERVENTIONS

ACE inhibitor+ARB

The recognition of the importance of the RAAS in kidney and cardiovascular health has led to the idea that more stringent RAAS blockade by means of combination of ACE inhibitor and ARB therapy would afford additional protection. Indeed, combination therapy with ACE inhibitors and ARBs does result in additional blood pressure and albuminuria reduction, but the effect of dual therapy on major kidney or cardiovascular events in people with diabetic nephropathy has not been adequately assessed to date. Notably, in early 2013, the VA VA NEPHRON-D trial, which compared ARB alone to combination therapy had medications terminated early per recommendations of the Data Monitoring Committee, based on a greater number of observed acute kidney injury events and hyperkalemia in the combination therapy group. Similarly, the ONTARGET demonstrated that, despite additional blood-pressure reduction and less progression of albuminuria, dual RAAS blockade did not reduce kidney or cardiovascular events in a lower kidney risk population.

ACE inhibitor/ARB and Direct Renin Inhibition

Blockade of the RAAS by renin inhibition was considered an attractive target to prevent kidney and cardiovascular outcomes. The direct renin inhibitor aliskiren is a potent inhibitor of renin, and short-term studies demonstrated its efficacy as well as its safety. However, the large hard outcome ALTITUDE trial, which tested the combination of the direct renin-inhibitor aliskiren plus ACE inhibitor or ARB treatment, demonstrated that aliskiren was associated with adverse kidney and cardiovascular effects in patients with type 2 diabetes at cardiovascular risk, leading to premature termination of the trial and recommendations from drug regulatory agencies that aliskiren is contraindicated in patients with diabetes and moderate or severe CKD who are taking ACE inhibitors or ARBs.

ACE inhibitor/ARB and Mineralocorticoid Receptor Blockers

Adding aldosterone blockers to ACE inhibitors or ARBs is another strategy to block the deleterious effect of the RAAS in diabetic nephropathy. Because aldosterone promotes tissue fibrosis, and to counteract aldosterone breakthrough, a phenomenon defined by elevations of plasma aldosterone levels during chronic ACE inhibitor or ARB treatment that occurs in approximately 40% of patients receiving these agents, mineralocorticoid receptor blocking agents may be beneficial as add-on therapy to ACE inhibitors or ARBs. Targeting aldosterone in these patients is particularly effective on the surrogate marker albuminuria. However, the risk of hyperkalemia and the lack of long-term efficacy and safety data (in particular given the results of ONTARGET and ALTITUDE) warrant caution when combining mineralocorticoid receptor blocking agents with an ACE inhibitor or ARB.

LIPID MANAGEMENT

Rationale

Cholesterol lowering has contributed to improved cardiovascular outcomes in a range of patient populations. However, whether lipid management delays the progression of nephropathy and decreases the risk of ESRD has been subject to debate. Metaanalyses have reported that statin therapy may reduce proteinuria in CKD patients, but the lack of well-designed long-term trials fueled uncertainty as to whether improved lipid management reduces kidney risk. The results of the Study of Heart and Renal Protection (SHARP) trial provided much needed insight into the long-term efficacy and safety of lipid management among kidney disease patients. The SHARP results, which are reviewed in greater detail in Chapter 56, showed that the combination of simvastatin and ezetimibe as compared to placebo treatment reduced the risk of major vascular events by 16% in individuals with advanced CKD. Of note, a recent metaanalysis of all statin trials in CKD, including SHARP, showed that the cardiovascular protective effect of statins is attenuated at lower eGFR levels, and, unfortunately, the combination of simvastatin and ezetimibe in SHARP did not decrease the risk of progression to kidney failure.

Choice of Lipid-Lowering Therapy

Choosing among lipid-lowering strategies in CKD patients is challenging given a lack of adequate data, with most studies focusing on statins. Several studies have assessed the comparative effects of statins on kidney or cardiovascular outcome, with the results of the Prospective Evaluation of Proteinuria and Renal Function in Diabetic Patients with Progressive Renal Disease Trial (PLANET) suggesting a benefit for atorvastatin over rosuvastatin on kidney function. Further studies are needed to evaluate the long-term effects of lipid-lowering therapies on kidney function.

TREATMENT OF TYPE 2 DIABETES IN DIALYSIS PATIENTS

When a diabetic patient approaches kidney failure, the various options for kidney replacement therapies should be offered: peritoneal dialysis, hemodialysis, or kidney transplantation. Survival with any kidney replacement modality is generally worse for patients with diabetes compared with nondiabetic patients, and cardiovascular complications markedly contribute to premature deaths. In fact, more than 70% of deaths in the diabetic ESRD population are attributed to a cardiovascular cause.

Control of Hyperglycemia

Appropriate glycemic control in dialysis patients is important because (severe) hyperglycemia not only increases cardiovascular risk but also causes thirst and high fluid intake. The assessment of glycemic control in dialysis patients is complicated, because interpretation of the commonly used assays for HbA1c is confounded by interference with uremic toxins. In addition, altered red blood cell survival, blood transfusion, and use of erythropoietin all impact the accuracy of HbA1c measurement.

The pharmacologic management of hyperglycemia in dialysis patients must take into account that dialysis reverses insulin resistance so that the insulin requirement is generally lower than before dialysis. The glucose concentration in dialysate typically is 100 mg/dl (6.1 mmol/L) to avoid the risk of hypoglycemic and hypotensive episodes.

Blood-Pressure Control

Previous trials have shown that blood-pressure lowering consistently reduces cardiovascular morbidity and mortality in a broad range of patients, and that the magnitude of blood-pressure reduction is an important driver of protection. However, as most blood-pressure trials have systematically excluded dialysis patients, the benefits and harms of blood-pressure–lowering therapies in this population remains uncertain. Two metaanalyses of small randomized controlled trials suggest that blood-pressure–lowering therapies (including volume control) are associated with a nearly 30% risk reduction for cardiovascular events and 25% risk reduction for cardiovascular death compared with control treatment. Large outcome trials are urgently needed to evaluate this further.

Lipid Control

Based on 4D (Die Deutsche Diabetes Dialysis Study) and the AURORA (A Study to Evaluate the Use of Rosuvastatin in Subjects on Regular Hemodialysis: An Assessment of Survival and Cardiovascular Event) trial, patients treated with hemodialysis should not be started on a statin. Although the SHARP trial noted a benefit in a mixed CKD/ESRD population, metaanalyses of these studies have not demonstrated a substantial benefit in dialysis. Accordingly, we recommend not initiating a statin in patients treated with hemodialysis but often do continue statin treatment in those that are already receiving these agents at dialysis initiation.

NOVEL STRATEGIES AND AGENTS FOR DIABETIC NEPHROPATHY

Optimizing glucose, blood pressure, and lipid control in CKD patients with diabetes has undoubtedly improved their prognosis; however, a considerable proportion of patients continue to develop diabetic nephropathy and progress to kidney failure. An overview of novel agents that target well-established or novel pathophysiologic pathways is provided in the next section. Many of these novel agents not only affect the target for which they are developed (on-target risk factor) but impact multiple other risk markers as well (off-target risk factors) (Table 25.2). Optimizing drug regimens to impact multiple parameters may lead to better drug use in the future.

NEWER GLYCEMIC CONTROL AGENTS

Glycagon-like Peptide-1 and Dipeptidyl Peptidase Inhibitors

Glycagon-like peptide-1 (GLP-1) stimulates insulin secretion and inhibits glucagon secretion in a glucose-dependent manner. Several GLP-1 agonists as well as dipeptidylpeptidase 4 (DPP-4) inhibitors, which block the GLP-1 degrading

Table 25.2   On-Target and Off-Target Effects of Established and Novel Drugs Used in the Management of Diabetic Nephropathy

Drug Class	On-Target Parameter	Off-Target Parameters
Antihyperglycemic Drugs		
Metformin	Glucose ↓	VCAM ↓; ICAM ↓
DPP-4 inhibitors	Glucose ↓	Blood pressure ↓; albuminuria ↓
SGLT-2 inhibitors	Glucose ↓	Blood pressure ↓; body weight ↓; uric acid ↓; albuminuria ↓
Antihypertensive Drugs		
RAAS-intervention	Blood pressure ↓	Albuminuria ↓; K⁺ ↑; Hb ↓; Uric acid ↓ (losartan)
Diuretics	Blood pressure ↓	K⁺ ↓; uric acid ↑
Lipid-Lowering Drugs		
Statins	LDL cholesterol ↓	C-reactive protein ↓; albuminuria ↓
Fibrates	LDL cholesterol ↓ Triglycerides ↓	Uric acid ↓; albuminuria ↓
CETP modulators	HDL cholesterol ↑	Blood pressure ↑ (mainly dalcetrapib)

CETP, Cholesterol ester transfer protein; *DPP-4,* dipeptidylpeptidase 4; *Hb,* hemoglobin; *HDL,* high-density lipoprotein; *ICAM,* intercellular cell adhesion molecule; *K⁺,* potassium; *LDL,* low-density lipoprotein; *SGLT-2,* sodium-glucose cotransporter-2; *VCAM,* vascular cell adhesion molecule.

enzyme DPP-4, have been developed to treat patients with type 2 diabetes (see Table 25.1). DPP-4 inhibitors seem to exert similar effects on HbA1c as alternative agents, with decreases in the range of 0.5% to 1.0%. However, the pharmacokinetic properties vary among the different agents, which could render a specific agent particularly useful for a certain subpopulation. For example, linagliptin is mainly metabolized and eliminated by the liver, making it particularly useful for patients with lower GFR (see Table 25.1). Long-term effects on kidney and cardiovascular outcomes appear promising.

Sodium-Glucose Cotransporter-2 Inhibition

The role of the kidney in maintaining glucose homeostasis has been increasingly appreciated in the last few decades. Plasma glucose is filtered in the glomerulus and reclaimed by tubular reabsorption along with two positively charged sodium ions per glucose molecule. This process involves the sodium-glucose cotransporter-2 (SGLT-2) system, which is located in the proximal tubule. The SGLT-2 transporter accounts for the reabsorption of approximately 90% of all filtered glucose, whereas the SGLT-1 transporter, located in the more distal proximal tubule, reabsorbs the remaining 10%. SGLT-2 inhibitors reversibly inhibit the SGLT-2 transporter, leading to enhanced glucose and sodium excretion and, in turn, to reductions in plasma glucose and HbA1c of up to 0.8% (see Table 25.1). The role of SGLT-2 inhibitors in diabetes management remains uncertain, and their use in patients with lower GFR is likely limited by their mechanism of action.

SGLT-2 inhibitors may have more kidney and cardiovascular protective potential than the protection that is only due to its effects on glucose homeostasis. In addition to the beneficial effects on glycemic control, trends toward increases in sodium excretion and hemoglobin and decreases in body weight and blood pressure have been observed with SGLT-2 inhibition (Fig. 25.5). These blood-pressure–lowering effects could result from enhanced natriuresis and diuresis, whereas the weight loss may reflect

caloric losses. Potential kidney benefits are being evaluated in long-term hard outcome trials.

NOVEL BLOOD-PRESSURE AND LIPID-LOWERING AGENTS

Mineralocorticoid Receptor Blockers

Mineralocorticoid receptor blockers (MRBs) are potent drugs for lowering risk factors such as blood pressure and proteinuria; however, there is concern that these drugs may not improve clinical outcomes in CKD patients because of their tendency to increase serum potassium. To avoid the latter, several new compounds are being tested, including MRBs that may have less effect on potassium homeostasis while retaining the blood-pressure and albuminuria-lowering effect. Today no clinical trials with such drugs are available. Another approach is to use mineralocorticoid synthase inhibitors, which are effective in reducing serum aldosterone and have blood-pressure–lowering capacity. Whether this approach will effectively decrease the incidence of hyperkalemia in patients with diabetes and nephropathy is still unknown. A third approach is using classical MRBs together with agents that prevent or attenuate hyperkalemia. Whether the benefits of this approach will outweigh possible risks of hyperkalemia as well as safety concerns associated with potassium-binding resins remains unknown, although novel potassium-binding resins are in development.

Endothelin Antagonists

Endothelin receptor blockers are promising given potent effects on both blood-pressure and proteinuria reduction; however, the hard outcome study on one of the first agents in this class (avosentan) demonstrated an increased incidence of edema and hospitalization for heart failure with avosentan, leading to the premature discontinuation of the trial. The high risk of heart failure was most likely caused by the drug's sodium retaining effects. Atrasentan, a more specific inhibitor of the endothelin-1A receptor than avosentan, was

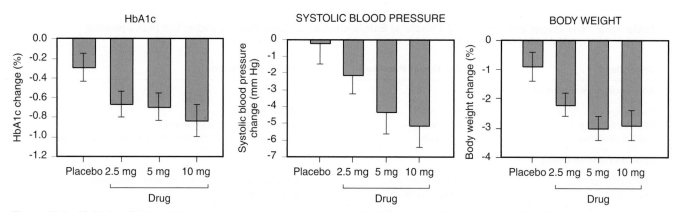

Figure 25.5   Multiple effects of the sodium-glucose cotransporter-2 inhibitor dapagliflozin on renal/cardiovascular risk markers. (Adapted from List JF, et al: Sodium-glucose cotransport inhibition with dapagliflozin in type 2 diabetes, *Diabetes Care* 32:650-657, 2009.)

recently shown to lower albuminuria with fewer side effects (Fig. 25.6). The albuminuria-lowering effects of atrasentan currently are being tested in the Reducing residual Albuminuria in subjects with type 2 Diabetes and nephropathy with AtRasentan (RADAR; NCT01356849) study.

High-Density Lipoprotein-Increasing Drugs

Patients with diabetes are often diagnosed with mixed dyslipidemia, characterized by low levels of high-density lipoprotein (HDL) cholesterol and high levels of triglycerides. Various agents are currently in development for increasing HDL by modulating cholesterol ester transfer protein (CETP), including dalcetrapib; notably, the first-in-class agent, torcetrapib, was abandoned after a hard outcome trial showed an increased risk of cardiovascular events with its use.

LIFESTYLE MODIFICATION

Dietary sodium restriction enhances the blood-pressure and albuminuria-lowering effects of ACE inhibitors and ARBs, with both RENAAL and IDNT showing that the effects of ARBs on hard kidney and cardiovascular outcomes in type 2 diabetic patients are greater in patients with moderately low dietary sodium intake. Prospective studies are needed to definitively confirm or refute these data. Dietary protein restriction has been shown in a metaanalysis of nine randomized controlled trials (seven in type 1 diabetic patients and three in type 2 diabetic patients) to have a small, statistically nonsignificant, long-term beneficial effect in slowing the rate of decline in GFR without demonstrable evidence of malnutrition. Currently, the ADA recommends 0.8 g/kg/day of protein restriction for diabetic patients with increased albuminuria, which is a manageable and safe recommendation for most patients with challenging dietary prescriptions related to their diabetes and CKD. Dietary counseling by a nutritionist may be useful to assist CKD patients in safely implementing dietary changes (Chapter 54).

NOVEL TARGETS

Anemia

A lower hemoglobin level is a risk marker for adverse cardiovascular outcomes, and the interaction between CKD and diabetes amplifies that risk. This observation formed the rationale for the Trial to Reduce cardiovascular Events with Aranesp Therapy (TREAT), which investigated whether

raising hemoglobin targets with darbepoetin-α versus placebo improved kidney and cardiovascular outcomes in patients with diabetic nephropathy. Unfortunately, there was no benefit with darbepoetin, and perhaps a suggestion of increased stroke risk. Accordingly, current erythropoiesis-stimulating agents cannot be recommended for cardiovascular or kidney risk reduction in patients with diabetic nephropathy.

Inflammation

In the past years, increasing evidence has indicated an important role for underlying, low-grade inflammatory processes in the pathogenesis of diabetic nephropathy. Consequently, research in antiinflammatory strategies may open a therapeutic window to halt the progression of disease.

Pyridoxamine Dihydrochloride. Pyridoxamine dihydrochloride (Pyridorin, NephroGenex) inhibits formation of advanced glycation end products and scavenges reactive oxygen species and toxic carbonyls. Whether these effects translate into kidney protection is unknown, although a year-long study of the effects of pyridoxamine dihydrochloride in patients with type 2 diabetes and proteinuria failed to show a difference in kidney function decline with pyridoxamine dihydrochloride in daily doses of 300 or 600 mg versus placebo treatment.

Pentoxifylline. Pentoxifylline is a methylxanthine phosphodiesterase inhibitor with favorable antiinflammatory effects and immunoregulatory properties. Despite this theoretical benefit, pentoxifylline offers at best a small beneficial effect on kidney function and reduction in albuminuria and proteinuria with no apparent serious adverse effects. Importantly, most studies of this agent were poorly reported, small, and methodologically flawed. The results of the PREDIAN study (Pentoxifylline for Renoprotection in Diabetic Nephropathy) will likely shed some further light on the potential use of pentoxifylline for kidney protection in patients with diabetes. Until then, current evidence does not support the use of pentoxifylline in this patient population.

Monocyte Chemoattractant Protein-1 Inhibitors. An increasing body of evidence demonstrates that monocyte chemoattractant protein-1 (MCP-1), a potent cytokine, plays a very important role in initiating and sustaining chronic

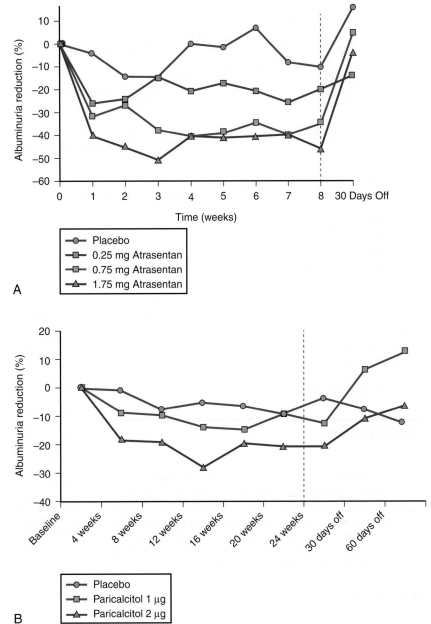

Figure 25.6 Effect of novel drugs on albuminuria. A, Antialbuminuric effect of the endothelin-1 antagonist Atrasentan. **B,** Effect of the vitamin-D receptor activator paricalcitol on albuminuria. (Data are derived from Kohan DE, Pritchett Y, Molitch M, et al: Addition of atrasentan to renin-angiotensin system blockade reduces albuminuria in diabetic nephropathy, *J Am Soc Nephrol* 22:763-772, 2011; and de Zeeuw D, Agarwal R, Amdahl M, et al: Selective vitamin D receptor activation with paricalcitol for reduction of albuminuria in patients with type 2 diabetes (VITAL study): a randomised controlled trial, *Lancet* 376:1543-1551, 2010.)

inflammation in the kidney. MCP-1 is secreted in response to high glucose concentrations. MCP-1 in turn attracts blood monocytes and macrophages and facilitates inflammation. A prospective randomized placebo controlled study showed that inhibition of MCP-1 synthesis further reduced albuminuria when used in addition to ACE inhibitor or ARB therapy in subjects who had macroalbuminuria, although there was no significant effect in individuals with lower levels of albuminuria. To our knowledge there are no hard kidney outcome trials ongoing.

Bardoxolone Methyl. Bardoxolone methyl is an antiinflammatory drug that activates the Nrf2-Keap1 pathway, resulting in inhibition of the proinflammatory cytokine Nf-κB. In a previous nonrandomized 8-week trial, treatment with bardoxolone methyl resulted in a significant increase in estimated GFR. A subsequent 52-week follow-up study showed

that the early bardoxolone-methyl–induced rise in eGFR was sustained throughout the 52-week follow-up period (Fig. 25.7). Unfortunately, a longer-term hard outcome study (Bardoxolone Methyl Evaluation in Patients with Chronic Kidney Disease and Type 2 Diabetes [BEACON], NCT 01351675) was terminated early for safety concerns because of excess serious adverse events and mortality in the bardoxolone methyl arm.

Vitamin Supplements

Vitamin-D Receptor Activation. Emerging data suggest an important role for the vitamin-D axis in kidney and cardiovascular health. The vitamin-D receptor is expressed in numerous tissues, and small studies have shown that activators of this receptor may inhibit the RAAS by suppressing renin synthesis, causing a reduction in albuminuria and inflammatory markers. The Vitamin-D Receptor Activator

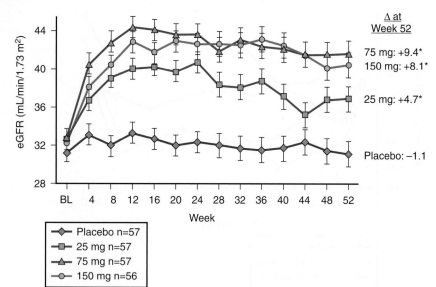

Figure 25.7   Effect of bardoxolone on eGFR.
eGFR, Estimated glomerular filtration rate.

for Albuminuria Lowering (VITAL) study, designed to investigate the antialbuminuric effect of the vitamin-D receptor activator paricalcitol, showed that 24-weeks of treatment with paricalcitol at 2 mcg/day caused a significant fall in albuminuria over time and was well tolerated (see Fig. 25.6). Larger studies with longer follow-up are pending.

CONCLUSION

Despite the successful use of glycemic, lipid, and blood-pressure control, including ACE inhibitor and ARB therapy, kidney risk in patients with diabetes remains very high, leaving the diabetic population with a clear unmet need. As outlined in this section, various novel treatment options are in development that may offer additional renoprotection and have the potential to reduce the high morbidity and mortality rates typically seen in patients with diabetes.

BIBLIOGRAPHY

Barbosa J, Steffes MW, Sutherland DE, et al: Effect of glycemic control on early diabetic renal lesions: a 5-year randomized controlled clinical trial of insulin-dependent diabetic kidney transplant recipients, *JAMA* 272:600-606, 1994.

Brenner BM, Cooper ME, de Zeeuw D, et al: Effects of losartan on renal and cardiovascular outcomes in patients with type 2 diabetes and nephropathy, *N Engl J Med* 345:861-869, 2001.

Cushman WC, Evans GW, Byington RP, et al: Effects of intensive blood-pressure control in type 2 diabetes mellitus, *N Engl J Med* 362:1575-1585, 2010.

de Boer IH, Sun W, Cleary PA, et al: Intensive diabetes therapy and glomerular filtration rate in type 1 diabetes, *N Engl J Med* 365:2366-2376, 2011.

de Zeeuw D, Agarwal R, Amdahl M, et al: Selective vitamin D receptor activation with paricalcitol for reduction of albuminuria in patients with type 2 diabetes (VITAL study): a randomised controlled trial, *Lancet* 376:1543-1551, 2010.

de Zeeuw D, Anzalone D, Cain V, et al: Different renal protective effects of atorvastatin and rosuvastatin in patients with proteinuric diabetic and non-diabetic renal disease; result from the PLANET Trials. 2010.

de Zeeuw D, Remuzzi G, Parving HH, et al: Proteinuria, a target for renoprotection in patients with type 2 diabetic nephropathy: lessons from RENAAL, *Kidney Int* 65:2309-2320, 2004.

Fioretto P, Mauer M: Histopathology of diabetic nephropathy, *Semin Nephrol* 27:195-207, 2007.

Gerstein HC, Miller ME, Byington RP, et al: Effects of intensive glucose lowering in type 2 diabetes, *N Engl J Med* 358:2545-2559, 2008.

Hellemons M, Persson F, Bakker SJ, et al: Initial angiotensin receptor blockade induced decrease in albuminuria predicts long term renal outcome in type 2 diabetic patients with microalbuminuria; a post-hoc analysis of the IRMA-2 trial, *Diabetes Care* 34:2078-2083, 2011.

Kunz R, Friedrich C, Wolbers M, et al: Meta-analysis: effect of monotherapy and combination therapy with inhibitors of the renin angiotensin system on proteinuria in renal disease, *Ann Intern Med* 148:30-48, 2008.

Lewis EJ, Hunsicker LG, Clarke WR, et al: Renoprotective effect of the angiotensin-receptor antagonist irbesartan in patients with nephropathy due to type 2 diabetes, *N Engl J Med* 345:851-860, 2001.

Mehdi UF, Adams-Huet B, Raskin P, et al: Addition of angiotensin receptor blockade or mineralocorticoid antagonism to maximal angiotensin-converting enzyme inhibition in diabetic nephropathy, *J Am Soc Nephrol* 20:2641-2650, 2009.

Parving HH, Lehnert H, Brochner-Mortensen J, et al: The effect of irbesartan on the development of diabetic nephropathy in patients with type 2 diabetes, *N Engl J Med* 345:870-878, 2001.

Patel A, MacMahon S, Chalmers J, et al: Intensive blood glucose control and vascular outcomes in patients with type 2 diabetes, *N Engl J Med* 358:2560-2572, 2008.

Pergola PE, Raskin P, Toto RD, et al: Bardoxolone methyl and kidney function in CKD with type 2 diabetes, *N Engl J Med* 365:327-336, 2011.

Rossing K, Schjoedt KJ, Smidt UM, et al: Beneficial effects of adding spironolactone to recommended antihypertensive treatment in diabetic nephropathy: a randomized, double-masked, cross-over study, *Diabetes Care* 28:2106-2112, 2005.

Shurraw S, Hemmelgarn B, Lin M, et al: Association between glycemic control and adverse outcomes in people with diabetes mellitus and chronic kidney disease: a population-based cohort study. *Arch Intern Med* 171:1920-1927.

The diabetes control and complications trial research group: The effect of intensive treatment of diabetes on the development and progression of long-term complications in insulin-dependent diabetes mellitus, *N Engl J Med* 329:977-986, 1993.

White KE, Bilous RW: Type 2 diabetic patients with nephropathy show structural-functional relationships that are similar to type 1 disease, *J Am Soc Nephrol* 11:1667-1673, 2000.

Dysproteinemias and Amyloidosis

26

Paul W. Sanders

Paraproteinemic kidney diseases are typically the result of deposition of immunoglobulin fragments (heavy chains and light chains) (Fig. 26.1) in specific parts of the nephron, and they can be divided generally into those diseases that manifest primarily as glomerular or tubulointerstitial injury (Box 26.1). Glomerular diseases include AL-type amyloidosis (amyloid composed of light chains), AH-type amyloidosis (amyloid composed of heavy chains), monoclonal light-chain and light- and heavy-chain deposition disease (collectively termed MLCDD in this review), monoclonal heavy-chain deposition disease, immunotactoid glomerulopathy, glomerulonephritis associated with monoclonal immunoglobulin deposition, and glomerulonephritis associated with type I cryoglobulinemia, and, in this review, AL-type amyloidosis, MLCDD, fibrillary glomerulonephritis, and immunotactoid glomerulopathy will be discussed. Patterns of tubular injury include a proximal tubulopathy and cast nephropathy (also known as "myeloma kidney"). In addition to these paraproteinemic kidney lesions, this chapter includes a discussion of Waldenström macroglobulinemia.

Aside from notable exceptions, such as AH-type amyloidosis and heavy-chain deposition disease, immunoglobulin light-chain deposition is directly responsible for most of the various kidney pathologic alterations that occur with paraproteinemia. In one large study of multiple myeloma, kidney dysfunction was present in approximately 2% of patients who did not exhibit significant urinary free light-chain levels, whereas increasing urinary free light-chain levels were strongly associated with kidney failure, with 48% of myeloma patients who had high urinary monoclonal free light chains having kidney failure and associated poor survival. The type of kidney lesion induced by light chains depends on the physicochemical properties of these proteins.

IMMUNOGLOBULIN LIGHT-CHAIN METABOLISM AND CLINICAL DETECTION

The original description of immunoglobulin light chains was attributed to Dr. Henry Bence Jones, who published his findings in 1847. He was the first to report these unique proteins, which now bear his name, and correlate this early urinary biomarker with the disease known as multiple myeloma. More than a century later, Edelman and Gally demonstrated that Bence Jones proteins were immunoglobulin light chains.

Plasma cells synthesize light chains that become part of the immunoglobulin molecule (see Fig. 26.1). In normal states, a slight excess production of light, compared to heavy, chains appears to be required for efficient immunoglobulin synthesis, but this excess results in the release of polyclonal free light chains into the circulation. After entering the bloodstream, light chains are handled similarly to other low-molecular-weight proteins, which are usually removed from the circulation by glomerular filtration. Unlike albumin, these monomers (molecular weight ~22 kDa) and dimers (~44 kDa) are readily filtered through the glomerulus and are reabsorbed by the proximal tubule. Endocytosis of light chains into the proximal tubule occurs through a single class of heterodimeric, multiligand receptor that is composed of megalin and cubilin. After endocytosis, lysosomal enzymes hydrolyze the proteins, and the amino-acid components are returned to the circulation. The uptake and catabolism of these proteins are very efficient, with the kidney readily handling approximately 500 mg of free light chains that are produced daily by the normal lymphoid system. However, in the setting of a monoclonal gammopathy, production of monoclonal light chains increases, and binding of light chains to the megalin-cubilin complex can become saturated, allowing light chains to be delivered to the distal nephron and to appear in the urine as Bence Jones proteins.

Light chains are modular proteins that possess two independent globular regions, termed constant (C_L) and variable (V_L) domains (see Fig. 26.1). Light chains can be isotyped as kappa (κ) or lambda (λ) based on sequence variations in the constant region of the protein. Within the globular V_L domain are four framework regions that consist of β sheets that develop a hydrophobic core. The framework regions separate three hypervariable segments that are known as complementarity determining regions (CDR1, CDR2, and CDR3) (see Fig. 26.1). The CDR domains, which represent those regions of sequence variability among light chains, form loop structures that constitute part of the antigen-binding site of the immunoglobulin. Diversity among the CDR regions occurs because the V_L domain is synthesized through rearrangement of multiple gene segments. Thus, although possessing similar structures and biochemical properties, no two light chains are identical; however, there are enough sequence similarities among light chains to permit categorizing them into subgroups. There are four κ and 10 λ subgroups, although, of the λ subgroups, most patients (94%) with multiple myeloma express λI, λII, λIII, or λV subgroups. Free light chains, particularly the λ isotype, often homodimerize before secretion into the circulation.

The multiple kidney lesions from monoclonal light-chain deposition affect virtually every compartment of the kidney (see Box 26.1) and may be explained by sequence variations particularly in the V_L domain of the offending monoclonal light chain. The light chains that are responsible for

235

monoclonal light-chain deposition disease (MLCDD) are frequently members of the κIV subfamily and appear to possess unusual hydrophobic amino-acid residues in CDR1. In AL-type amyloidosis, sequence variations in the V_L domain of the precursor light chain confer the propensity to polymerize to form amyloid. A classic kidney presentation of multiple myeloma is Fanconi syndrome, which is produced almost exclusively by members of the κI subfamily. Unusual nonpolar residues in the CDR1 region and absence of accessible side chains in the CDR3 loop of the variable domain of κIIlight chains result in homotypic crystallization of the light chain in this syndrome. In cast nephropathy, the secondary

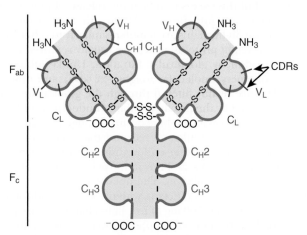

Figure 26.1   Schematic of the immunoglobulin G molecule, which consists of two heavy chains and two light chains that are stabilized by inter- and intramolecular disulfide bonds. Light chains consist of two domains that are termed constant (C_L) and variable (V_L) regions. Within the V_L domain are the complementarity determining regions that are primarily responsible for variations in the amino-acid sequences among light chains. Heavy chains also consist of a variable domain (V_H) and three constant domains (C_H1, C_H2, C_H3). *CDRs,* Complementarity determining regions.

Box 26.1   Monoclonal Light-Chain-Related Renal Lesions

Glomerulopathies

AL-type amyloidosis
MLCDD
Cryoglobulinemia

Tubulointerstitial Lesions

Cast nephropathy ("myeloma kidney")
Fanconi syndrome
Proximal tubulopathy
Tubulointerstitial nephritis (rare)

Vascular Lesions

Asymptomatic Bence Jones Proteinuria

Hyperviscosity Syndrome

Neoplastic Cell Infiltration (Rare)

MLCDD, Monoclonal light-chain and light- and heavy-chain deposition disease.

---

structure of CDR3 is a critical determinant of cast formation. In summary, sequence variations in the V_L domain appear to determine the type of kidney lesion that occurs with monoclonal light-chain deposition.

Free light chains were originally detected using turbidometric and heat tests. Because these tests lack sensitivity, they are no longer in use. The qualitative urine dipstick test for protein also has a low sensitivity for detection of light chains. Although some Bence Jones proteins react with the chemical impregnated onto the strip, other light chains cannot be detected; the net charge of the protein may be an important determinant of this interaction. Because of the relative insensitivity of routine serum protein electrophoresis and urinary protein electrophoresis for free light chains, these tests are not recommended as screening tools in the diagnostic evaluation of the underlying etiology of renal disease. Highly sensitive and reliable immunoassays are available to detect the presence of monoclonal light chains in the urine and serum and are adequate tests for screening when both urine and serum are examined. When a clone of plasma cells exists, significant amounts of monoclonal light chains appear in the circulation and the urine. In healthy adults, the urinary concentration of polyclonal light-chain proteins is about 2.5 mg/L. Causes of monoclonal light-chain proteinuria, a hallmark of plasma cell dyscrasias, are listed (Box 26.2). Urinary light-chain concentration is generally between 0.02 and 0.5 g/L in patients with monoclonal gammopathy of undetermined significance (MGUS) and is often much higher (range 0.02 to 11.8 g/L) in patients with multiple myeloma or Waldenström macroglobulinemia. Immunofixation electrophoresis is sensitive and detects monoclonal light chains and immunoglobulins even in very low concentrations, but it is a qualitative assay that may be limited by interobserver variation. A nephelometric assay that quantifies serum free κ and λ light chains is also useful to nephrologists, because most of the kidney lesions in paraproteinemias are caused by light-chain overproduction and much less commonly heavy chains or intact immunoglobulins. Because an excess of light chains, compared to heavy chains, is synthesized and released into the circulation, this sensitive assay detects small amounts of serum polyclonal free light chains in healthy individuals. This assay can also distinguish polyclonal from monoclonal light chains and further quantifies the free light-chain level in the serum. Quantifying serum

---

Box 26.2   Potential Causes of Monoclonal Light-Chain Proteinuria

Multiple myeloma
AL-type amyloidosis
Monoclonal light-chain deposition disease
Waldenström macroglobulinemia
MGUS
POEMS syndrome (rare)
Heavy-chain (μ) disease (rare)
Lymphoproliferative disease (rare)

MGUS, Monoclonal gammopathy of undetermined significance; *POEMS,* polyneuropathy, organomegaly, endocrinopathy, M protein, and skin changes.

light-chain levels may be of use clinically to monitor chemotherapy as well as to serve as a risk factor for development of kidney failure, because myeloma patients with baseline serum free monoclonal light-chain levels greater than 750 mg/L correlated with depressed kidney function (serum creatinine concentration ≥2 mg/dl) and more aggressive myeloma. In the evaluation of kidney disease, particularly if amyloidosis is suspected, perhaps the ideal screening tests for an associated plasma cell dyscrasia include immunofixation electrophoresis of serum and urine and quantification of serum free κ and λ light chains.

GLOMERULAR LESIONS OF PLASMA CELL DYSCRASIAS

AL-TYPE AMYLOIDOSIS

More than 23 different amyloid proteins have been identified. They are named according to the precursor protein that polymerizes to produce amyloid. AL-type amyloidosis, which is also known as "primary amyloidosis," represents a plasma cell dyscrasia that is characterized by organ dysfunction related to deposition of amyloid and usually only a mild increase in monoclonal plasma cells in the bone marrow. However, about 20% of patients with AL-type amyloidosis exhibit overt multiple myeloma or other lymphoproliferative disorder. In AL-type amyloidosis, the amyloid deposits are composed of immunoglobulin light chains versus AA-type amyloidosis, where the precursor protein (serum amyloid A protein) is an acute phase reactant. The identification of the type of amyloid protein is an essential first step in the management of these patients.

AL-type amyloidosis is a systemic disease that typically involves multiple organs (Table 26.1). Cardiac infiltration frequently produces congestive heart failure and is a common presenting manifestation of primary amyloidosis. Infiltration of the lungs and gastrointestinal tract is also common, but often produces few clinical manifestations. Dysesthesias, orthostatic hypotension, diarrhea, and bladder dysfunction from peripheral and autonomic neuropathies can occur. Amyloid deposition can also produce an arthropathy that resembles rheumatoid arthritis, a bleeding diathesis, and a variety of skin manifestations that include purpura. Kidney involvement is common in primary amyloidosis.

PATHOLOGY

Glomerular lesions are the dominant renal features of AL-type amyloidosis and are characterized by the presence of mesangial nodules and progressive effacement of glomerular capillaries (Fig. 26.2). In the early stage, amyloid deposits are usually found in the mesangium and are not associated with an increase in mesangial cellularity. Deposits may also be seen along the subepithelial space of capillary loops and may penetrate the glomerular basement membrane in more advanced stages. Immunohistochemistry demonstrates that the deposits consist of light chains, although the sensitivity of this test is not high. Amyloid has characteristic tinctorial properties and stains with Congo red, which produces an apple-green birefringence when the tissue section is examined under polarized light and with thioflavins T and S. On electron microscopy, the deposits are characteristic, randomly oriented, nonbranching fibrils 7 to 10 nm in diameter. In some cases of early amyloidosis, glomeruli may appear normal on light microscopy; however, careful examination can identify scattered monotypic light chains on immunofluorescence microscopy. Ultrastructural examination with immunoelectron microscopy to show the fibrils of AL-type amyloid may be required to establish the diagnosis early in the course of renal involvement. Ultrastructural and immunohistochemical examination of biopsies of an affected organ establish the diagnosis, although tissue diagnosis of AL-type amyloidosis can also be difficult, because commercially available antibodies may not detect the presence of the light chain in the tissue. In uncertain cases, the amyloid can be extracted from tissue and examined using tandem mass spectrometry to determine the chemical composition of the

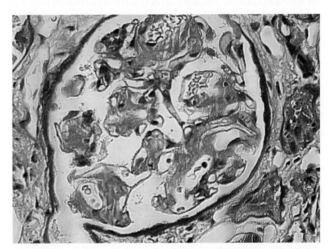

Figure 26.2 Glomerulus from a patient with AL-type amyloidosis showing segmentally variable accumulation of amorphous acidophilic material that is effacing portions of the glomerular architecture (PASH stain, magnification ×40).

Table 26.1 Relative Frequency of Organ Infiltration by Light Chains in AL-Type Amyloidosis and MLCDD

	Isotype	Organ Involvement					
		Renal	Cardiac	Liver	Neurologic	GI	Pulmonary
AL-amyloid	λ > κ	+++	+++	+	+	+++	++++
MLCDD	κ > λ	++++	+++	+++	+	Rare	Rare

GI, Gastrointestinal; *MLCDD,* monoclonal light-chain and light- and heavy-chain deposition disease.
NOTE: From +, uncommon but can occur during the course of the disease, through ++++, extremely common during the course of the disease.

amyloid. As the disease advances, mesangial deposits progressively enlarge to form nodules of amyloid protein that compress the filtering surfaces of the glomeruli and cause renal failure. Epithelial proliferation and crescent formation are rare in AL-type amyloidosis.

CLINICAL FEATURES

Proteinuria and reduced kidney function are the two major kidney manifestations of AL-type amyloidosis. Proteinuria ranges from asymptomatic nonnephrotic proteinuria to nephrotic syndrome. Isolated microscopic hematuria and nephritic syndrome are not common in AL-type amyloidosis. More than 90% of patients have monoclonal light chains either in urine or blood, but occasionally even sensitive assays will not detect a circulating monoclonal light chain in patients with documented kidney involvement from AL-type amyloid. Reduced kidney function is present in 58% to 70% of patients at the time of diagnosis. Scintigraphy using ^{123}I-labeled serum amyloid P component, which binds to amyloid, can assess the degree of organ involvement from amyloid infiltration, but this test is not currently widely available.

PATHOGENESIS

The pathogenesis of AL-type amyloidosis is incompletely understood. Internalization and processing of light chains by mesangial cells produce amyloid in vitro. Presumably, intracellular oxidation or partial proteolysis of light chains allows formation of amyloid, which is then extruded into the extracellular space. With continued production of amyloid, the mesangium expands, compressing the filtering surface of the glomeruli and producing progressive renal failure. There is evidence that amyloidogenic light chains also have intrinsic biological activity that modulates cell function independently of amyloid formation. Not all light chains are amyloidogenic. Members of the λ family are more commonly associated with AL-type amyloidosis, and sequence variations in the V_L domain appear to confer the propensity to polymerize to form amyloid.

TREATMENT AND PROGNOSIS

Patients with both multiple myeloma and AL-type amyloidosis should be managed with treatment regimens that target myeloma. For patients who experience AL-type amyloidosis and lack the criteria for multiple myeloma, the initial approach to management should be to ensure that the patient has AL-type amyloidosis and not amyloidosis related to a nonlymphoid-derived precursor protein, because the approaches to treatment are different. Because a randomized trial suggested improved survival in patients who received chemotherapy, more aggressive antiplasma cell therapies have been undertaken in AL-type amyloidosis, including high-dose chemotherapy with autologous peripheral stem-cell transplantation (HDT/SCT). Although reduced kidney function may not be an exclusion criteria, because of increased treatment-related mortality of HDT/SCT in higher-risk subjects, more conservative approaches should be considered for patients aged ≥80 years, decompensated congestive heart failure, left ventricular ejection fraction less than 0.40, systolic blood pressure less than 90 mm Hg, oxygen saturation less than 95% on room air, or significant overall functional impairment.

Patients who have evidence of multiorgan system dysfunction, particularly cardiac disease, and are considered ineligible for HDT/SCT have an expected median survival of only 4 months, so delays in diagnosis and treatment can be costly. In contrast, one study reported a median survival of 4.6 years in 312 patients who underwent HDT/SCT. Almost half achieved a complete hematologic response, which portended improved long-term survival. Although carefully selected patients with AL-type amyloidosis can respond favorably to HDT/SCT, in a randomized clinical trial comparing HDT/SCT with chemotherapy, which included melphalan and high-dose dexamethasone, the outcome was not superior. Patients with AL-type amyloidosis usually die from organ decompensation from amyloid infiltration and not from tumor burden, and an important observation from these studies is that survival and organ dysfunction can improve with successful reduction in the monoclonal plasma cell population and light-chain production. Other novel chemotherapeutic regimens may be of benefit in AL-type amyloidosis and are being considered, particularly given the potential toxicity of chronic treatment with alkylating agents. The recent success of thalidomide as an alternative treatment of multiple myeloma has prompted treatment of AL-type amyloidosis with this agent in an uncontrolled fashion, although thalidomide is not well tolerated in these patients, and dosage reductions are often required. Lenalidomide, an analog of thalidomide, is another potentially attractive therapy in AL-type amyloidosis. Bortezomib-based regimens have also provided promising results in AL-type amyloidosis. Again, randomized controlled trials are needed to determine efficacy of these pharmacologic agents in AL-type amyloidosis.

MONOCLONAL LIGHT-CHAIN DEPOSITION DISEASE

Monoclonal light-chain deposition disease is a systemic disease that typically presents initially with isolated renal injury related to a glomerular lesion associated with nonamyloid electron-dense granular deposits of monoclonal light chains with or without heavy chains. Isolated deposition of monoclonal heavy chains, termed heavy-chain deposition disease, is extremely rare. MLCDD may accompany other clinical features of multiple myeloma or another lymphoproliferative disorder, or may be the sole manifestation of a plasma cell dyscrasia.

PATHOLOGY

Nodular glomerulopathy with distortion of the glomerular architecture by amorphous, eosinophilic material is the most common pathologic finding observed with light microscopy (Fig. 26.3). These nodules, which are composed of light chains and extracellular matrix proteins, begin in the mesangium. The appearance is reminiscent of diabetic nephropathy. Less commonly, other glomerular morphologic changes in addition to nodular glomerulopathy can be seen in MLCDD. Immunofluorescence microscopy demonstrates the presence of monotypic light chains in the glomeruli. Under electron microscopy, deposits of light-chain proteins are present in a subendothelial position along the glomerular capillary wall, along the outer aspect of tubular basement membranes, and in the mesangium.

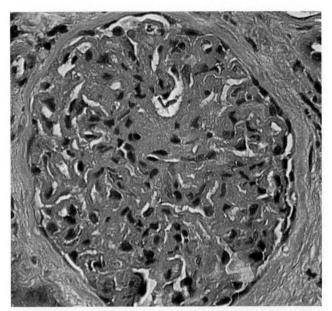

Figure 26.3   Glomerulus from a patient with monoclonal κ light-chain deposition disease showing expansion of the mesangium, related to matrix protein deposition, and associated compression of capillary lumens (hematoxylin-eosin stain, magnification ×40).

There are significant differences between amyloidosis and MLCDD. For amyloid deposition to occur, amyloid P glycoprotein must also be present. The amyloid P component is not part of the amyloid fibrils, but binds them. This glycoprotein is a constituent of normal human glomerular basement membrane and elastic fibrils. In contrast to AL-type amyloid, in MLCDD the light-chain deposits are punctate, granular, and electron-dense and are identified in the mesangium and/or subendothelial space; amyloid P component is absent. Unlike amyloid, the granular light-chain deposits of MLCDD do not stain with Congo red or thioflavin T and S. Another difference between these lesions is the tendency for κ light chains to compose the granular deposits of MLCDD, whereas usually λ light chains constitute AL-amyloid. Both diseases can involve organs other than the kidney (see Table 26.1).

CLINICAL FEATURES

The typical clinical presentation is reminiscent of a rapidly progressive glomerulonephritis. The major symptoms of MLCDD include proteinuria, sometimes in the nephrotic range, microscopic hematuria, and kidney failure. Albumin and monoclonal free light chains are the dominant proteins in the urine. The presence of albuminuria and other findings of nephrotic syndrome are important clues to the presence of glomerular injury and not cast nephropathy. The amount of excreted light chain is usually less than that found in cast nephropathy and can be difficult to detect in some patients. Progressive kidney failure in untreated patients is common. Because kidney manifestations generally predominate and are often the sole presenting features, it is not uncommon for nephrologists to diagnose the plasma cell dyscrasia. Kidney biopsy is necessary to establish the diagnosis. Other organ dysfunction, especially liver and heart, can develop and is related to deposition of light chains in those organs. Although extrarenal manifestations of overt

multiple myeloma can manifest at presentation or over time, a majority (~50% to 60%) of patients with MLCDD will not develop myeloma or other malignant lymphoproliferative disease.

PATHOGENESIS

Monoclonal light-chain deposition disease represents a prototypical model of progressive kidney disease that has a pathogenesis related to glomerulosclerosis from increased production of transforming growth factor-β (TGF-β). The response to monoclonal light-chain deposition includes expansion of the mesangium by extracellular matrix proteins to form nodules and eventually glomerular sclerosis. Experimental studies have shown that mesangial cells exposed to light chains obtained from patients with biopsy-proven MLCDD produce TGF-β, which serves as an autacoid to stimulate these same cells to produce matrix proteins, including type IV collagen, laminin, and fibronectin. Thus, TGF-β plays a central role in glomerular sclerosis from MLCDD. As is true for AL-type amyloidosis, not all light chains can produce MLCDD. Many offending light chains are κ, particularly the κIV subfamily, and appear to possess unusual hydrophobic amino-acid residues in the V_L domain.

Although deposition of light chain is the prominent feature of these glomerular lesions, both heavy chains and light chains can be identified in the deposits. In these specimens, the punctate electron-dense deposits appear larger and more extensive than deposits that contain only light chains, but it is unclear whether the clinical course of these patients differs from the course of isolated light-chain deposition without heavy-chain components, and the management is similar.

TREATMENT AND PROGNOSIS

For patients with both multiple myeloma and MLCDD, therapy is directed toward the myeloma. The treatment of MLCDD without an associated malignant lymphoproliferative disorder is difficult, because guidance from randomized controlled trials is unavailable. However, patients appear to benefit from the same therapeutic approach as that administered for multiple myeloma. The serum creatinine concentration at presentation is an important predictor of subsequent outcome, so intervention should be early in the course of the disease.

Melphalan/prednisone therapy improves kidney prognosis, but the long-term toxicity of melphalan makes this approach less attractive. More aggressive antiplasma cell therapy in the form of HDT/SCT has been used in MLCDD. In the small numbers of patients in which HDT/SCT was performed, the procedure-related death rate was low and, when a complete hematologic response was observed, improvement in affected organ function with histologic evidence of regression of the light-chain deposits occurred. The novel chemotherapeutic agents that include thalidomide- and bortezomib-based regimens also appear to have efficacy in this setting.

The high incidence of progressive kidney disease in MLCDD has prompted treatment with kidney transplantation, but the disease will recur in the allograft if the underlying plasma cell dyscrasia is not addressed. The study with the largest collection of patients (seven) concluded that MCLDD recurred commonly in the renal allograft and significantly reduced long-term graft survival; these findings emphasize the need to control monoclonal light-chain production before kidney transplantation in MLCDD.

FIBRILLARY GLOMERULONEPHRITIS AND IMMUNOTACTOID GLOMERULOPATHY

Fibrillary glomerulonephritis is a rare disorder characterized ultrastructurally by the presence of amyloid-like, randomly arranged fibrillary deposits in the capillary wall (Fig. 26.4). Unlike amyloid, these fibrils are thicker (18 to 22 nm) and Congo red and thioflavin T stains are negative. Immunofluorescence microscopy typically shows IgG (usually IgG4) and C3. Most patients with fibrillary glomerulonephritis do not

have a plasma cell dyscrasia; however, occasionally a plasma cell dyscrasia is present, so screening is advisable. Tests for cryoglobulins and hepatitis C infection should be obtained. Patients typically manifest nephrotic syndrome and varying degrees of renal failure; progression to end-stage renal failure is the rule. Standardized treatment for the idiopathic variety is currently unavailable.

Immunotactoid, or microtubular, glomerulopathy is even more uncommon than fibrillary glomerulonephritis and is usually associated with a plasma cell dyscrasia or other lymphoproliferative disorder. The deposits in this lesion contain thick (greater than 30 nm), organized, microtubular structures that are located in the mesangium and along capillary walls. Cryoglobulinemia, which is discussed in Chapter 28, should be considered in the differential diagnosis and should be ruled out clinically. Treatment of the underlying plasma cell dyscrasia is indicated for this rare disorder.

TUBULOINTERSTITIAL LESIONS OF PLASMA CELL DYSCRASIAS

CAST NEPHROPATHY

PATHOLOGY

Cast nephropathy is an inflammatory tubulointerstitial renal lesion. Characteristically, multiple intraluminal proteinaceous casts are identified mainly in the distal portion of the nephrons (Fig. 26.5). The casts are usually acellular, homogeneous, and eosinophilic with multiple fracture lines. Immunofluorescence and immunoelectron microscopy confirm that the casts contain light chains and Tamm-Horsfall glycoprotein. Persistence of the casts produces giant cell inflammation and tubular atrophy that typify myeloma kidney. Glomeruli are usually normal in appearance.

CLINICAL FEATURES

Kidney failure from this lesion may present acutely or as a chronic progressive disease and may develop at any stage of myeloma. Diagnosis of multiple myeloma is usually evident

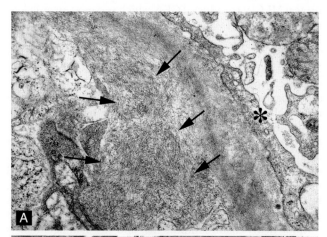

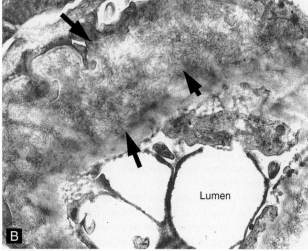

Figure 26.4 Glomeruli. A, Electron micrograph of a glomerulus from a patient with AL-type amyloidosis. Note the randomly arranged relatively straight fibrils with an approximate diameter of 7 to 10 nm *(arrows).* A useful distinction from fibrillary glomerulonephritis **(B)** is that amyloid fibrils will stain with Congo red or thioflavin T. Note fusion of the foot processes *(asterisk)* of the adjacent epithelial cell. **B,** Electron micrograph of a glomerulus from a patient with fibrillary glomerulonephritis. The same random arrangement of nonbranching fibrils *(arrows)* is seen. Careful examination demonstrates that the fibrils are larger (approximately 20 nm in diameter). The overall ultrastructural appearance resembles amyloid except that the fibrils are approximately twice as thick. **(A,** Courtesy Dr. J. Charles Jennette, Department of Pathology, University of North Carolina at Chapel Hill. **B,** Courtesy Dr. William Cook, Department of Pathology, University of Alabama at Birmingham.)

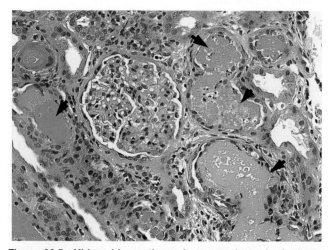

Figure 26.5 Kidney biopsy tissue from a patient who had cast nephropathy. The findings include tubules filled with cast material *(arrows)* and presence of multinucleated giant cells. Glomeruli are typically normal in appearance (hematoxylin-eosin stain, magnification ×20).

when chronic bone pain, pathologic fractures, and hypercalcemia are complicated by proteinuria and renal failure. However, many patients present to nephrologists primarily with symptoms of renal failure or undefined proteinuria; further evaluation then confirms a malignant process. Cast nephropathy should therefore be considered when proteinuria (often more than 3 g/day), particularly without concomitant hypoalbuminemia or albuminuria, is found in a patient who is in the fourth decade of life or older. Hypertension is not a common consequence of cast nephropathy. Diagnosis of myeloma may be confirmed by finding monoclonal immunoglobulins or light chains in the serum and urine and by bone marrow examination, although typical intraluminal cast formation on kidney biopsy is virtually pathognomonic. Nearly all patients with cast nephropathy have detectable monoclonal light chains in the urine or blood.

PATHOGENESIS

Intravenous infusion of nephrotoxic human light chains in rats elevates proximal tubule pressure and simultaneously decreases single nephron glomerular filtration rate; intraluminal protein casts can be identified in these kidneys. Myeloma casts contain Tamm-Horsfall glycoprotein and occur initially in the distal nephron, which provides an optimum environment for precipitation with free light chains. Casts occur primarily because light chains coaggregate with Tamm-Horsfall glycoprotein. Tamm-Horsfall glycoprotein, which is synthesized exclusively by cells of the thick ascending limb of the loop of Henle, comprises the major fraction of total urinary protein in healthy individuals and is the predominant constituent of urinary casts. Cast-forming Bence Jones proteins bind to the same site on the peptide backbone of Tamm-Horsfall glycoprotein; binding results in coaggregation of these proteins and subsequent occlusion of the tubule lumen by the precipitated protein complexes. Intranephronal obstruction and renal failure ensue. Light chains that bind to Tamm-Horsfall glycoprotein are potentially nephrotoxic. The CDR3 domain of the light chain determines binding affinity.

Coaggregation of Tamm-Horsfall glycoprotein with light chains also depends on the ionic environment and the physicochemical properties of the light chain, and not all patients with myeloma develop cast nephropathy, even when the urinary excretion of light chains is high. Increasing concentrations of sodium chloride or calcium, but not magnesium, facilitate coaggregation. The loop diuretic, furosemide, augments coaggregation and accelerates intraluminal obstruction in vivo in the rat. Finally, the lower tubule fluid flow rates of the distal nephron allow more time for light chains to interact with Tamm-Horsfall glycoprotein

and subsequently to obstruct the tubular lumen. Conditions that further reduce flow rates, such as volume depletion, can accelerate tubule obstruction or convert nontoxic light chains into cast-forming proteins. Volume depletion and hypercalcemia are recognized factors that promote acute kidney injury from cast nephropathy.

TREATMENT AND PROGNOSIS

The principles used to guide therapy in cast nephropathy include rapidly decreasing the concentration of circulating light chains and preventing coaggregation of light chains with Tamm-Horsfall glycoprotein (Box 26.3). Prompt and effective chemotherapy should start on diagnosis of multiple myeloma, which is present in virtually all patients with cast nephropathy. The traditional treatment with alkylating agents and steroids has been replaced by HDT/SCT, particularly in younger patients. An advantage with a more aggressive approach is the potential for rapid reductions in the levels of circulating monoclonal light chain. Several randomized trials showed that patients who received HDT/SCT experienced an improvement in overall survival rates than did patients who received conventional chemotherapy. Chemotherapy is usually initiated before HDT/SCT to reduce the plasma cell clone. Chronic treatment with alkylating agents is typically avoided before HDT/SCT, because these drugs may impede peripheral stem cell harvest and are associated with myelodysplasia and acute myelogenous leukemia.

Other therapeutic approaches have been attempted, but they currently lack randomized controlled trials to support their use. For example, patients with advanced kidney failure and refractory myeloma have been treated successfully with bortezomib- and thalidomide-based therapies. These agents are gaining wide acceptance and may ultimately obviate the need for HDT/SCT. Nonmyeloablative allogeneic stem-cell transplantation, so-called mini-allograft therapy, may also provide beneficial results in myeloma without the attendant complications such as severe graft-versus-host disease.

Studies suggest that interstitial fibrosis can develop rapidly in cast nephropathy, promoting persistent and ultimately irreversible kidney failure. Because clinical evidence suggests that prompt reduction in circulating free light chains accelerates renal recovery in cast nephropathy, the delay in reduction of free light-chain levels associated with chemotherapy has provoked exploration of extracorporeal removal of circulating free light chains, with mixed results. Currently, the ancillary role of plasma exchange (PLEX) in acute kidney injury in the setting of multiple myeloma is uncertain. One randomized trial suggested benefit, but two others failed to confirm a survival advantage for patients treated with PLEX along with chemotherapy. The most recent randomized trial suggested no clinical benefit from PLEX for patients with acute kidney injury, although there were limitations to this study. For example, kidney biopsy to document cast nephropathy was not a prerequisite for entry into the study. In addition, the study may have been underpowered to detect differences between the groups. Serum free light chains were not quantified either before or after PLEX. Despite these limitations, a significant theoretical issue related to PLEX is the relatively inefficient removal of light chains, which distribute throughout the extracellular fluid space. Recently, efficient removal of light

---

Box 26.3   Standard Therapy for Cast Nephropathy

Chemotherapy to decrease light-chain production
Increase free water intake to 2 to 3 L/day as tolerated
Treat hypercalcemia aggressively
Avoid exposure to diuretics, radiocontrast agents, and nonsteroidal antiinflammatory agents

chains has been achieved using high-cutoff hemodialysis treatments. Although these early and important studies support this technique for rapid reduction in serum light-chain concentrations, randomized trials, which are ongoing, should inform medical practice. Until additional data are provided, it is probably prudent not to recommend routinely extracorporeal therapies for most patients with acute kidney injury and instead emphasize highly effective chemotherapy, although there may be a subset of patients who have acute kidney injury from cast nephropathy and respond favorably to this additional intervention. If PLEX or high-cutoff hemodialysis is performed, demonstration of the efficacy of treatment by quantifying changes in serum free light-chain levels should be performed. Finally, hyperviscosity syndrome remains an indication for extracorporeal removal of the monoclonal proteins.

Prevention of aggregation of light chains with Tamm-Horsfall glycoprotein is a cornerstone of therapy. Volume repletion, normalization of electrolytes, and avoidance of complicating factors such as loop diuretics and nonsteroidal antiinflammatory agents are helpful in preserving and improving renal function. Although not all patients with light-chain proteinuria develop acute kidney injury following exposure to radiocontrast agents, predicting who is at risk for this complication is difficult, suggesting caution in the use of radiocontrast agents in all patients with multiple myeloma. Daily fluid intake up to 3 L in the form of electrolyte-free fluids should be encouraged, although serum sodium concentration should be monitored periodically. Alkalinization of the urine with oral sodium bicarbonate (or citrate) to keep the urine pH greater than 7 may also be therapeutic, but may be mitigated by the requisite sodium loading, which favors coaggregation of these proteins and also should be avoided in patients who have symptomatic extracellular fluid volume overload.

Hypercalcemia occurs during the course of the disease in more than 25% of patients with multiple myeloma. In addition to being directly nephrotoxic, hypercalcemia enhances the nephrotoxicity of light chains. Treatment of volume contraction with the infusion of saline often corrects mild hypercalcemia. Loop diuretics also increase calcium excretion, but diuretics may also facilitate nephrotoxicity from light chains and should be avoided, if possible. Glucocorticoid therapy (such as methylprednisolone) is helpful for acute management of the multiple myeloma as well as hypercalcemia. Bisphosphonates, such as pamidronate and zoledronic acid, are used to treat moderate hypercalcemia (serum calcium greater than 3.25 mmol/L, or 13 mg/dl) that is unresponsive to other measures. Bisphosphonates lower serum calcium by interfering with osteoclast-mediated bone resorption. Although hypercalcemia of myeloma responds to bisphosphonates, these agents can be nephrotoxic and should be administered only to euvolemic patients. Kidney function should be monitored closely during therapy. Treatment with pamidronate or zoledronic acid allows outpatient management of mild hypercalcemia. In addition to controlling hypercalcemia, bisphosphonates appear to inhibit growth of plasma cells and have been used to treat multiple myeloma, particularly in patients with osseous lesions and bone pain.

Kidney replacement therapy in the form of hemodialysis or peritoneal dialysis is generally recommended in patients with renal failure from monoclonal light-chain-related kidney diseases. Recovery of kidney function sufficient to survive without dialysis occurs in as many as 5% of patients with multiple myeloma, although in some patients this goal requires months to achieve, probably because the traditional chemotherapeutic regimens slowly reduce circulating light-chain levels. Despite the susceptibility to infection in multiple myeloma, the peritonitis rate for continuous ambulatory peritoneal dialysis (one episode every 14.4 months) was not unacceptably high. Neither peritoneal dialysis nor hemodialysis appears to provide a superior survival advantage in patients with myeloma. Kidney transplant also has been performed successfully in selected patients with multiple myeloma in remission. Because the light chain is the underlying cause of cast nephropathy, tests that ensure absence of circulating free light chains are useful in the evaluation of candidacy for kidney transplantation.

OTHER TUBULOINTERSTITIAL KIDNEY LESIONS INCLUDING PROXIMAL TUBULOPATHY

Proximal tubular injury and tubulointerstitial nephritis can occur. A classic kidney presentation of multiple myeloma is Fanconi syndrome, which is characterized by a renal tubular acidosis type II and defective sodium-coupled cotransport processes, producing aminoaciduria, glycosuria, and phosphaturia. Kidney biopsy typically shows crystals of light-chain protein within the epithelium of the proximal tubule. Fanconi syndrome may precede overt multiple myeloma. Plasma cell dyscrasia should therefore be considered in the differential diagnosis when this syndrome occurs in adults.

Unlike most endogenous low-molecular-weight proteins, monoclonal light chains have a propensity to produce tubular injury. Although the more common lesion is cast nephropathy, patients occasionally present with kidney failure from an isolated proximal tubulopathy that is distinct from the pathology associated with Fanconi syndrome. Kidney failure from isolated proximal tubular damage generally improves with effective chemotherapy that reduces the circulating monoclonal free light chain. A major mechanism of damage to the proximal epithelium is related to accumulation of toxic light chains in the endolysosome system. Light chains appear to catalyze sufficient amounts of hydrogen peroxide to generate intracellular oxidative stress to stimulate apoptosis and to activate NF-κB, promoting the production of inflammatory chemokines such as monocyte chemotactic factor-1. Loss of proximal tubular epithelial cells and generation of a proinflammatory milieu may also promote nephron dropout and the tubulointerstitial scarring and inflammation that are prevalent findings in cast nephropathy.

WALDENSTRÖM MACROGLOBULINEMIA

This disorder constitutes about 5% of monoclonal gammopathies and is characterized by the presence of a monoclonal B-cell malignancy consisting of lymphocytoid plasma cells. The origin of these cells is thought to be a postantigen-stimulated memory B cell that has undergone malignant transformation through somatic hypermutation. This condition clinically behaves more like lymphoma, although the malignant cell secretes IgM (macroglobulin), which usually produces most of the clinical symptoms. Lytic bone lesions are uncommon, but hepatosplenomegaly and lymphadenopathy are frequently identified. IgM is a large molecule that is not excreted and accumulates in the plasma to produce hyperviscosity syndrome, which consists of neurological symptoms (headaches, stupor, deafness, dizziness), visual impairment (from hemorrhages and edema), bleeding diathesis (related to IgM complexing clotting factors and to platelet dysfunction), kidney failure, and symptoms of hypervolemia. A reduced glomerular filtration rate occurs in about 30% of patients, and hyperviscosity syndrome and precipitation of IgM in the lumen of glomerular capillaries are the most common causes. About 10% to 15% of patients develop AL-type amyloidosis, but cast nephropathy is rare. Because of the typically advanced age at presentation (sixth to seventh decade) and slowly progressive course, the major therapeutic goal is relief of symptoms. All patients with IgM levels greater than 4 g/dl should have serum viscosity determined. Plasmapheresis is indicated in symptomatic patients and should be continued until symptoms resolve and serum viscosity normalizes. Severe kidney failure requiring kidney replacement therapy is uncommon. The course of the disease can vary, but is often protracted. Factors that portend a worse outcome include age greater than 65 years and organomegaly. Patients lacking these risk factors have a median survival of 10.6 years, whereas patients with either of these risk factors have a reduced chance for survival (median 4.2 years). Symptomatic patients are usually treated with combination chemotherapy that includes an alkylating agent along with rituximab, because these malignant cells express CD20.

BIBLIOGRAPHY

Barlogie B, Shaughnessy J, Tricot G, et al: Treatment of multiple myeloma, *Blood* 103:20-32, 2004.

Clark WF, Stewart AK, Rock GA, et al: Plasma exchange when myeloma presents as acute renal failure: a randomized, controlled trial, *Ann Intern Med* 143:777-784, 2005.

Dember LM, Hawkins PN, Bouke PC, et al: Eprodisate for the treatment of renal disease in AA amyloidosis, *N Engl J Med* 356:2349-2360, 2007.

Deret S, Denoroy L, Lamarine M, et al: Kappa light chain-associated Fanconi's syndrome: molecular analysis of monoclonal immunoglobulin light chains from patients with and without intracellular crystals, *Protein Eng* 12:363-369, 1999.

Drayson M, Begum G, Basu S, et al: Effects of paraprotein heavy and light chain types and free light chain load on survival in myeloma: an analysis of patients receiving conventional-dose chemotherapy in Medical ResearchCouncil UK multiple myeloma trials, *Blood* 108:2013-2019, 2006.

Gertz MA: Immunoglobulin light chain amyloidosis: 2011 update on diagnosis, risk-stratification, and management, *Am J Hematol* 86:181-186, 2011.

Ghobrial IM, Fonseca R, Gertz MA, et al: Prognostic model for disease-specific and overall mortality in newly diagnosed symptomatic patients with Waldenstrom macroglobulinaemia, *Br J Haematol* 133:158-164, 2006.

Hutchison CA, Heyne N, Airia P, et al: Immunoglobulin free light chain levels and recovery from myeloma kidney on treatment with chemotherapy and high cut-off haemodialysis, *Nephrol Dial Transplant* 27:3823-3828, 2012.

Jaccard A, Moreau P, Leblond V, et al: High-dose melphalan versus melphalan plus dexamethasone for AL amyloidosis, *N Engl J Med* 357:1083-1093, 2007.

Lachmann HJ, Booth DR, Booth SE, et al: Misdiagnosis of hereditary amyloidosis as AL (primary) amyloidosis, *N Engl J Med* 346:1786-1791, 2002.

Nasr SH, Valeri AM, Cornell LD, et al: Renal monoclonal immunoglobulin deposition disease: a report of 64 patients from a single institution, *Clin J Am Soc Nephrol* 7:231-239, 2012.

Rosenstock JL, Markowitz GS, Valeri AM, et al: Fibrillary and immunotactoid glomerulonephritis: distinct entities with different clinical and pathologic features, *Kidney Int* 63:1450-1461, 2003.

van Rhee F, Bolejack V, Hollmig K, et al: High serum free-light chain levels and their rapid reduction in response to therapy define an aggressive multiple myeloma subtype with poor prognosis, *Blood* 110:827-832, 2007.

Weichman K, Dember LM, Prokaeva T, et al: Clinical and molecular characteristics of patients with non-amyloid light chain deposition disorders, and outcome following treatment with high-dose melphalan and autologous stem cell transplantation, *Bone Marrow Transplant* 38:339-343, 2006.

Ying WZ, Allen CE, Curtis LM, et al: Mechanism and prevention of acute kidney injury from cast nephropathy in a rodent model, *J Clin Invest* 122:1777-1785, 2012.

Ying WZ, Wang PX, Aaron KJ, et al: Immunoglobulin light chains activate NF-κB in renal epithelial cells through a Src-dependent mechanism, *Blood* 117:1301-1307, 2011.

27 Thrombotic Microangiopathies

Sharon Adler | Cynthia C. Nast

The thrombotic microangiopathies (TMAs) are a group of diverse disorders that have been classified together based on common morphologic features in the kidney. Some of the more common underlying causes of TMA are listed in Table 27.1. Recent advances in the understanding of pathophysiologic mechanisms underlying these disorders have distinguished them substantially from one another, with significant implications for clinical management. This chapter focuses on four of the most common TMAs: thrombotic thrombocytopenic purpura (TTP), hemolytic uremic syndrome (HUS), the antiphospholipid syndrome (APLS), and scleroderma renal crisis.

PATHOLOGY

The characteristic features of the TMAs are shown in Figure 27.1. Histopathologic changes are characterized by fibrin accumulation in the lumina and walls of arteries, arterioles, and glomerular capillaries. By light microscopy, fibrin and platelet thrombi are evident in variable numbers of glomerular capillaries (see Fig. 27.1A). As the disease progresses, glomeruli may develop a lobular appearance with capillary wall double contours, or evidence of ischemia characterized by wrinkled and partially collapsed capillaries (see Fig. 27.1B and C). Arterioles, and to a lesser extent arteries, are thrombosed with fibrin present in the walls. Arterioles also show muscular hypertrophy and mucoid intimal thickening, resulting in luminal narrowing (see Fig. 27.1C and D). Small, and less frequently larger, vessels may have a concentric "onion-skin" appearance because of proliferating intimal cells. Areas of infarcted renal parenchyma are found in patients with cortical necrosis. Immunofluorescence shows fibrin within involved glomerular capillaries, vascular walls, and vascular lumina. Ultrastructurally, the glomerular capillary walls have wide subendothelial zones containing flocculent electron-lucent and electron-dense material representing fibrin with entrapped erythrocytes (see Fig. 27.1E and F). There may be new layers of basement membrane material beneath the widened subendothelial zones accounting for the double-contour appearance of capillaries. Endothelial cells are swollen, capillary lumina are narrowed, and capillaries may contain tactoids of fibrin. There are no electron-dense (immune complex) deposits.

All thrombotic microangiopathic kidney lesions are morphologically similar, although subtle differences have been described. Some have suggested that biopsies from patients with HUS may contain more fibrin and erythrocytes within the thrombi, whereas TTP thrombi are composed predominantly of platelets with little fibrin. TTP thrombi also show entrapped von Willebrand factor (vWF) on immunohistochemical staining. Patients with HUS may be more likely to have cortical necrosis than those with TTP. However, apart from scleroderma, these pathologic findings are not sufficiently distinct to allow a specific diagnosis based on histology. The more distinctive findings seen in scleroderma are described later; however, differentiating among the TMAs always requires clinical assessment.

THROMBOTIC THROMBOCYTOPENIC PURPURA

PATHOGENESIS

Thrombotic thrombocytopenic purpura was once thought to be a disorder pathogenically linked to HUS, but differing somewhat in severity and end-organ involvement. More recently, a more thorough understanding of the pathogenic mechanisms of these entities underscores the notion that TTP and HUS are distinct. TTP is a complex syndrome with most cases characterized by diminished activity of vWF cleaving protein; this disintegrin and metalloprotease with thrombospondin type 1 repeats is referred to as ADAMTS13. In approximately 20% of cases, TTP is caused by an inherited mutation in ADAMTS13; these are more often observed in patients with familial and recurrent forms of TTP. The remaining TTP cases are caused by inactivating autoantibodies. Both mechanisms decrease the functional activity of ADAMTS13, resulting in defective vWF cleavage and abnormally large and numerous circulating vWF multimers. These multimers bind to extracellular matrix (ECM) and platelets, induce platelet aggregation and activation, and lead to intravascular platelet thrombi, organ ischemia, and necrosis. The multimers are found in active TTP but not in cases where TTP is in remission, and the presence of these multimers distinguishes TTP from other causes of hemolysis, thrombosis, or thrombocytopenia. Spacer domains in the ADAMTS13 gene participate in the proteolytic interaction with vWF, and autoantibodies to this motif/region impair ADAMTS13 activity in the majority of the patients with TTP. Severely depressed ADAMTS13 activity distinguishes patients with TTP from those with HUS and other thrombocytopenic conditions, because individuals with TTP tend to have functional ADAMTS13 activity less than 5% to 10% that

Table 27.1   Causes of Thrombotic Microangiopathy

Infectious	Medications
Enteric pathogens	Alpha-interferon
Escherichia coli 0157:H7	Aprotinin
Shigella species	Bevacizumab
Salmonella species	Bleomycin
Campylobacter jejuni	Cisplatinum
Other	Clopidogrel
Mycoplasma pneumoniae	Cocaine
Yersinia	Calcineurin inhibitors
Streptococcus pneumoniae	Cytosine arabinoside
HIV	Doxycycline
Legionella infection	Daunorubicin
Coxsackie A and B virus	Gemcitabine
Histoplasmosis	Interferon
Brucellosis	Mitomycin C
Bartonella	Oral contraceptives
H1N1	Quinine
	Sunitinib
	Ticlopidine
Systemic Diseases	Vinblastine
SLE	
HUS	**Miscellaneous**
Malignant hypertension	Cobalamine deficiency
Neoplasms	Pregnancy
TTP	Vaccinations
APLS	Radiation
Scleroderma	Transplantation

APLS, Antiphospholipid syndrome; *HUS,* hemolytic uremic syndrome; *SLE,* systemic lupus erythematosus; *TTP,* thrombotic thrombocytopenic purpura.

of healthy controls. Less severe inhibition (10% to 30% of normal function) may be seen in other disorders, including HUS and disseminated intravascular coagulation (DIC).

CLINICAL PRESENTATION AND LABORATORY MANIFESTATIONS

Most patients with inherited TTP (known as the Upshaw-Schulman syndrome) are compound heterozygotes and present as neonates or children, although later presentations have been reported. Acquired TTP in patients with autoantibodies tends to present in later life. The classic clinical pentad of TTP consists of fever, microangiopathic hemolytic anemia, thrombocytopenic purpura, kidney disease, and central nervous system symptoms ranging from lethargy, somnolence, and confusion to focal neurologic signs, seizures, and coma. The neurologic symptoms often dominate the overall clinical picture. Rarely, subacute or atypical TTP has been reported; this is characterized by thrombocytopenia or acute neurologic deficits in the absence of hemolytic anemia. Hemolytic anemia in TTP is accompanied by numerous circulating schistocytes and helmet cells, which are likely produced by shear stress injury as erythrocytes flow through vessels narrowed by platelet thrombi. High lactate dehydrogenase (LDH) levels and low platelet counts correlate with the severity and activity of the disease. Kidney involvement may be present in as many as 88% of patients, but often it is mild. Kidney manifestations include microscopic or, rarely, gross hematuria, mild to moderate proteinuria, and reduced

glomerular filtration rate (GFR). Acute kidney injury (AKI) occurs in up to 10% of patients, although it is unusual for individuals with TTP to require acute dialysis.

TTP may present either as an acquired acute disease or in a chronic relapsing form. Certain medications, including quinine, mitomycin-C, calcineurin inhibitors, pamidronate, gemcitabine, bevacizumab, and ticlopidine may trigger the acquired forms. TTP has also rarely been reported in association with statins and clopidogrel therapy. Antibodies to ADAMTS13 have been identified in patients with ticlopidine-associated TTP, HIV infection, and rarely influenza A. However, systematic searches for antibodies related to other conditions and medications associated with TTP have not been reported. Acquired TTP also may complicate collagen-vascular disorders, such as systemic lupus erythematosus (SLE), and neoplasms. For most patients with acquired TTP, no underlying cause is identified. Although the measurement of ADAMTS13 activity now is readily available in commercial clinical laboratories in the United States, there usually is a delay in obtaining the result. Very low levels of activity (e.g., less than 5%) are most consistent with a diagnosis of TTP, but moderately low levels, and occasionally severely low levels, have also been reported in other thrombocytopenic disorders. The need to begin specific therapy urgently, most often before test results are available, represents a continued clinical challenge in the management of this disease. In cases where DIC is a consideration, a prothrombin time within 5 seconds of the upper limit of normal, and a platelet count of less than $20 \times 10^9/L$, may distinguish TTP from DIC in 92% of cases.

THERAPY

Fresh frozen plasma (FFP) or cryosupernatant (cryoprecipitate-poor plasma) infusion is the mainstay of therapy, effectively providing the missing enzyme activity. In the hereditary form, as little as 15 ml/kg of plasma infused every 2 to 3 weeks may be sufficient to prevent episodes of TTP. Particularly in patients with the acquired form, plasma exchange removes circulating ADAMTS13 autoantibody and facilitates the infusion of large amounts of FFP (average course is approximately 21 L). Steroids may be a useful adjunctive therapy by modulating autoantibody production and reducing inflammation in areas of injury. In some cases, rituximab, in conjunction with plasma exchange and steroids, was associated with decreased hospital stay and fewer relapses compared to historical controls. Additionally, in treatment-resistant and frequently relapsing patients, rituximab use was associated with higher ADAMTS13 activity and fewer relapses compared to controls in the first 20 months after treatment. Other therapies are less common, but cyclophosphamide and vincristine continue to be used with some success in refractory patients, and splenectomy may decrease the frequency of relapses potentially by eliminating B-cell clones that produce autoantibodies. Research into novel therapies has been reported. For example, a Phase I/II trial administering an anti-vWF aptamer showed therapeutic promise in patients with congenital TTP, whereas, in a mouse model, N-acetylcysteine reduced intermolecular disulfide bonds in vWF, decreasing its multimolecular size and its aggregability. Platelet inhibitors are of unproven value, and platelet infusions and aspirin are contraindicated. Response to therapy is best monitored by following serial platelet counts and serum LDH levels. In

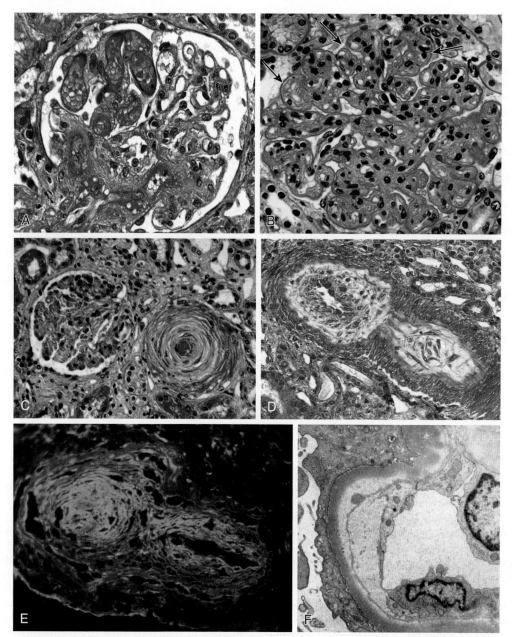

Figure 27.1   Kidney biopsy findings in thrombotic microangiopathy. A, Glomerulus showing many capillary lumina occluded by fibrin thrombi (Masson trichrome, original magnification ×60). **B,** Glomerulus with a lobular membranoproliferative glomerulonephritis type I pattern of injury including many capillary wall double contours *(arrows)* (periodic acid–Schiff, original magnification ×60). **C,** Ischemic glomerulus with wrinkled and partially collapsed capillary walls is adjacent to an arteriole. The arteriole has typical "onion-skin" thickening of the wall and a fibrin thrombus (Masson trichrome, original magnification ×10). **D,** An interlobular artery with mucoid intimal thickening, swollen endothelial cells, and luminal narrowing (Masson trichrome, original magnification ×10). **E,** Immunofluorescence for fibrin showing positive staining in the wall of an artery, corresponding to the mucoid intima in **D** (original magnification ×10). **F,** Electron microscopy of a capillary wall from an involved glomerulus. There is a wide subendothelial lucent zone containing flocculent material, endothelial cell swelling, and podocyte foot process effacement (original magnification ×6000).

those patients whose TTP results from an inherited mutation, long-term treatment with repetitive infusions of plasma or cryosupernatant for acute exacerbations may be required.

COURSE AND PROGNOSIS

Untreated, the mortality of TTP approaches 90%; however, in the era of plasma infusion, with or without plasma exchange, this has fallen to 10%. The long-term prognosis is excellent for those patients in whom an environmental trigger can be identified. When causation is undetermined, recurrence is common, usually within the first year after initial presentation. In most patients, clinical remission is associated with an improvement of ADAMTS13 activity above the 10% level, and relapse is more likely to recur when values drop below this level. However, in some patients, despite clinical remission after treatment, the ADAMTS13 activity levels fail to rise, and autoantibodies continue to be present. In addition, relapse has been reported in patients whose ADAMTS13 activity improves but who retain autoantibodies.

These differing patterns of response indicate a complex relationship between the ADAMTS13 activity level, the presence of autoantibodies, and the underlying inflammatory or environmental triggers of clinical disease.

HEMOLYTIC UREMIC SYNDROME

Hemolytic uremic syndrome includes two major clinical presentations: an atypical form (aHUS, previously referred to as nondiarrheal or D⁻ HUS) and a typical form (previously referred to as diarrheal or D⁺ HUS).

ATYPICAL HUS

PATHOGENESIS

The understanding of the pathogenesis of aHUS has undergone radical revision in recent years, and aHUS is now recognized as a clinical syndrome that occurs because of alternative complement pathway activation in individuals with a limited capacity to regulate this pathway (Table 27.2). In all forms of aHUS, there is dysregulation of complement activation accompanied by complement consumption leading to endothelial injury. Although rare, loss-of-function mutations and polymorphisms of the circulating complement regulatory proteins Factors H (CFH) and I (CFI) are the most common underlying causes of aHUS, and more than 100 CFH mutations have been described. CFH and CFI stabilize the alternative pathway C3 convertase, and, along with tissue-bound membrane cofactor protein (MCP, also known as CD46), cleave and inactivate surface-bound C3b and C4b. Reduced levels of CFH are most commonly associated with an autosomal-recessive mode of inheritance, and clinically manifests with low C3 levels and an earlier onset of disease. Normal levels of dysfunctional CFH are more commonly seen with autosomal-dominant inheritance; these patients present with normal complement levels and later disease onset than autosomal recessive aHUS. The clinical manifestations of autosomal recessive aHUS in patients initially having normal complement levels typically present following a triggering event that initiates complement activation. Other less common mutations of the circulating complement system leading to aHUS include a gain-of-function mutation in complement Factor B (a plasma zymogen that carries the catalytic site of the alternative complement pathway convertase) and mutations in complement C3.

Alternative complement pathway dysregulation may also result from the development of autoantibodies to CFH or CFI, and some patients with CFH mutations also have CFH autoantibodies. Chromosome 1q32 harbors a region rich in complement regulatory proteins, and some individuals express mutations and/or polymorphisms in more than one gene from that region. In patients with chromosomal deletions in this region involving the CFH receptor 1 or 3 genes, autoantibodies to CFH and antinuclear antibodies are often present. This demonstrates that multiple abnormalities may synergistically predispose to aHUS. Deficiency in the antithrombotic prostacyclin prostaglandin I2 has also been implicated in some cases of aHUS.

Table 27.2 Dysregulated Complement Factors in Atypical Hemolytic Uremic Syndrome

Abnormal Factor	Mechanism/ Pathogenesis	Common Presenting Features
Circulating Inhibitors		
Factor H	Autosomal recessive	Younger, low C3
	Autosomal dominant	Older, normal C3
	Autoantibodies	Mildly low C3
	Polymorphisms	HELLP; Calcineurin inhibitor TMAs
Factor H related proteins		
Factor I	Loss of function mutation	Children and adults, normal C3
	Autoantibodies	Associated with CFH mutations
	Polymorphisms	HELLP syndrome
Circulating Activators		
Factor B	Gain of function mutations	Low C3, normal CFB
Factor D	Cleaves, activates CFB	Deficiency predisposes to infections
C3	Gain of function mutations	Childhood presentation, low C3
	Loss of function mutations	Normal factor activities
Membrane Bound		
Factor H	See earlier	
Membrane cofactor protein (CD46)	Loss of function mutations	Young age, best prognosis
Thrombomodulin	Loss of function mutations	Children, young adults variable C3 levels

CFB, Complement factor B; *CFH,* complement factor H; *HELLP,* Hemolysis, elevated liver enzymes, and low platelets; *TMAs,* thrombotic microangiopathies.

Mutations in tissue-bound complement regulatory proteins have also been reported, most commonly in MCP, which accounts for 5% to 12% of aHUS. MCP converts complement C3b on endothelial surfaces to inactive C3bi. The mutant protein binds to C3b poorly, or not at all, limiting C3b inactivation and facilitating endothelial injury and subsequent thrombus formation. Less commonly, other mutations in tissue-bound complement regulators have been reported, including in thrombomodulin, which binds to CFH and C3b and participates in complement regulation by promoting C3b inactivation. Mutations in thrombomodulin likely require additional environmental or genetic factors to induce aHUS.

Mutations in complement regulatory proteins causing aHUS are rare; however, common genetic variations likely contribute to the sporadic cases of aHUS that are more frequently observed than those associated with known genetic mutations. In the genetically predisposed, aHUS may be triggered by environmental factors such as medication use, neoplasms, infections, pregnancy, or collagen-vascular disease (see Table 27.1). For instance, polymorphisms in complement regulatory proteins and CFH or CFI mutations have been reported in a large percentage of women presenting with preeclampsia and the HELLP (hemolysis, elevated liver enzymes, and low platelets) syndrome as well as in kidney transplant recipients with de novo TMA. In these examples, adults without a previous episode of aHUS developed the syndrome in response to exposures, underscoring the concept that environmental stressors may unmask underlying genetic predisposition to aHUS. In this way, complement dysregulation unites a diverse group of rare conditions caused by mutations and single nucleotide polymorphisms.

CLINICAL PRESENTATION AND LABORATORY DIAGNOSIS

Atypical hemolytic uremic syndrome presents with the classic clinical triad of microangiopathic hemolytic anemia, thrombocytopenia, and kidney injury. Many cases of aHUS associated with genetic mutations present in neonates and children, but in up to 30% the initial presentation is in adults. The signs and symptoms of a HUS tend to overlap with those of TTP, but, in a HUS, the hematologic and especially the kidney features predominate.

Most of the reported genetic mutations causing aHUS are autosomal recessive with variable penetrance. Clinical practice guidelines suggest diagnostic evaluation for patients with suspected aHUS that includes measurement of serum C3 and C4; CFH and CFI activity; fluorescent activated cell sorting analysis of MCP on peripheral blood mononuclear cells; molecular genetic analyses for CFH, MCP, CFI, CFB, and C3 including a search for mutations and altered copy number; autoantibody screening for CFH; and ADAMTS13 activity assay. These assays may not be widely available. Some clinical features are common to all genotypes, such as hypertension and AKI. Systemic symptoms, including neurologic complications, do occur, but at a lower frequency than in TTP. Age at presentation and hypocomplementemia are variable (see Table 27.2). Patients with loss-of-function CFH mutations undergo relapses in 60% to 80% of cases, mortality is high, and progression to ESRD is common in survivors. Loss-of-function CFI mutations account for ~10% to 15% of aHUS, and 60% of these individuals progress to ESRD. Patients with gain-of-function mutations in complement C3 progress to ESRD with frequent recurrence in allografts. Mutations in the MCP gene account for 5% to 12% of aHUS, and the majority of patients (60% to 70%) do not progress to ESRD despite multiple relapses. In those who do progress, recurrence in kidney allografts is extremely rare. Thrombomodulin mutations have been identified in less than 5% of patients with aHUS, often with relapsing and severe disease manifestations.

THERAPY

Clinical practice guidelines for the management of aHUS were published in 2009. Eliminating underlying predisposing environmental factors is the most effective therapy, but this is not often feasible, as these factors may be difficult to identify. Plasma exchange with FFP infusion has been advised as primary therapy for all patients with aHUS (weak recommendation). Plasma infusion provides functional protein and is most effective in patients with mutations in circulating complement or complement regulatory proteins. The response is variable, but in ~50%, complete or partial remissions are reported. In patients in whom a circulating autoantibody is present, plasma exchange supplements the efficacy of plasma infusion by also removing the antibody. Plasma therapy is less likely to be effective in patients with aHUS, because of mutations in the tissue-bound complement regulatory proteins, such as MCP or thrombomodulin. However, plasma infusion is reportedly contraindicated for patients with a HUS caused by *Streptococcus pneumoniae*. *S. pneumoniae* produces neuraminidase, which cleaves n-acetyl neuraminic acid on the surfaces of glomerular endothelial cells, platelets, and erythrocytes, thus unmasking the underlying Thomsen-Friedenreich antigen and initiating an inflammatory cascade resulting in thrombosis. Rituximab has been reported to improve outcomes in some patients with resistant or frequently relapsing aHUS. Currently, there are no recommendations regarding complement inhibition or immunosuppression; however, eculizumab, an antibody to the complement C5a protein, has been used for the treatment of aHUS. By inhibiting activation of the complement membrane attack complex and limiting complement-mediated injury, it may confer tissue protection whether the dysregulation is in the circulating or the tissue-bound complement system. Following case reports and small series that demonstrated significant clinical responses in patients with aHUS, the U.S. Food and Drug Administration (FDA) approved the use of eculizumab for aHUS in October 2011.

COURSE AND PROGNOSIS

Poor kidney outcomes have been associated with marked leukocytosis, older age at onset, pregnancy, concurrent pneumococcal infection, anuria, persistent proteinuria, hypertension, and cortical necrosis. TMA occurred in 29% of patients undergoing kidney transplantation for a HUS, compared to 0.8% in patients with kidney failure from other causes. Guidelines suggest that live kidney donor allografts be avoided in aHUS when it is caused by mutations in the circulating complement cascade, because of a high rate of recurrence. However, patients with MCP mutations without additional abnormalities in CFH, CFI, C3, or CFB, or antibodies to these factors have only a low risk of recurrence in allografts.

TYPICAL HEMOLYTIC UREMIC SYNDROME

PATHOGENESIS

In typical HUS, it is postulated that bacteria-derived Shiga-like toxin binds to colonic epithelium and disrupts the barrier function. This permits the Shiga-like toxin to enter the circulation free or bound to PMNs, which then binds to the glycolipid Gb3 membrane receptor on endothelial cells, podocytes, and tubular cells. This binding results in endothelial death by suppression of protein synthesis, which is followed by inflammation, thrombosis, and AKI. In vitro, Shiga toxin activates the fluid-phase complement and reduces the regulatory effect of CFH on cell surfaces, possibly exacerbating thrombosis. Previously, most cases have been attributed to a Shiga toxin produced by *Escherichia coli* (serotype O157:H7) or *Shigella*; however, in a large German outbreak in the spring of 2011, a novel *E. coli* (serotype O104:H4) producing verotoxin, Vtx2a:O104, was responsible.

CLINICAL PRESENTATION AND LABORATORY MANIFESTATIONS

Typical HUS, like aHUS, presents with microangiopathic hemolytic anemia, thrombocytopenia, and kidney disease. Following enteric infection with *E. coli, Shigella, Salmonella, Campylobacter,* or *Yersinia* (see Table 27.1), the incubation period for the development of diarrhea is 2 to 10 days, and the latency period until the development of HUS is an additional 7 days. Most cases are diagnosed clinically, but confirmation can be achieved by obtaining stool culture for enteropathogenic bacteria or by obtaining PCR for Shiga toxin 1 or 2 or verotoxin. HUS caused by *E. coli* O157:H7 disease is often associated with ingestion of undercooked meat or raw vegetables contaminated with *E. coli*, and cases tend to cluster in the summer with children more frequently affected than adults. Diarrhea ranges from watery to hemorrhagic. The classic features of microangiopathic hemolytic anemia and kidney dysfunction frequently manifest as AKI in adults, but less commonly in children where leukocytosis and fever are common. Other systemic manifestations include fluid and electrolyte disturbances, severe hypertension, cerebral edema and seizures, congestive heart failure, pulmonary edema, and cardiac arrhythmias. Hypocomplementemia is occasionally observed during the acute presentation, with normalization on recovery. The clinical manifestations of Shiga-toxin associated HUS are generally less severe than those observed in the massive verotoxin-induced HUS epidemic that occurred in Germany in the spring of 2011. In 2010, the year before the massive epidemic, there were approximately 1000 cases of Shiga-toxin associated diarrhea, 60 cases of HUS, and 2 deaths from HUS reported in Germany. In the 2011 epidemic, atypical features included adults who were more likely to be affected than children, and females more frequently than males. There were approximately 2400 cases of diarrhea, 800 resulting cases of HUS, and 60 attributable deaths.

THERAPY

Therapy has traditionally been supportive, and there is no proven value for treatment with antibiotics, anticoagulants, fibrinolytics, intravenous immunoglobulin, plasma infusion, plasmapheresis, prostacyclin infusion, Shiga-toxin sorbents, or antiplatelet agents. A randomized prospective clinical trial reported in 2003 failed to demonstrate benefit from a Shiga-toxin sorbent. Successful treatment with the complement c5A inhibitor eculizumab was reported in three children with Shiga-toxin associated HUS who were stricken during the 2011 German epidemic. The children had dialysis-dependent kidney failure and severe neurologic disease, and they had failed to respond to plasma therapy. Marked neurologic improvement, kidney recovery, and normalization of LDH and platelet counts occurred after eculizumab treatment.

COURSE AND PROGNOSIS

Once thought to be completely reversible, the AKI of typical HUS may have significant long-term clinical sequelae in a minority of patients, including persistent albuminuria and reduced GFR.

ANTIPHOSPHOLIPID SYNDROME

PATHOGENESIS

The antiphospholipid syndrome (APLS) is a thrombotic microangiopathic disorder caused by antiphospholipid autoantibodies that can induce arterial and venous thrombosis. These antibodies include lupus anticoagulant, anticardiolipin antibody, and antibody against phospholipid-binding protein β_2-glycoprotein I (β_2GPI). Various mechanisms have been proposed to account for the hypercoagulable state, including activation of coagulation in the fluid phase, activation of complement, and activation of the coagulation cascade. The latter likely is a result of autoantibody effects on the endothelium, induction of monocyte tissue factor expression, and platelet activation, and may require a second hit such as an infection or drug exposure to induce thrombosis. Antiphospholipid antibodies can bind to cell membrane phospholipid-binding proteins with subsequent activation of endothelial cells inducing upregulation of adhesion molecules, activation of NFκB, elaboration of cytokines, and alterations in the balance of prothrombotic thromboxane and anticoagulant prostacyclins. Antiphospholipid antibodies may interfere with the function of phospholipid-binding proteins involved in the regulation of coagulation. Candidates for such interference include β_2GPI, prothrombin, protein C, protein S, annexins, and tissue factor. Oxidant-mediated endothelial injury may play a role, with autoantibodies to oxidized low-density lipoprotein (LDL) occurring along with anticardiolipin antibodies. In fact, some anticardiolipin antibodies cross-react with oxidized LDL. Similar to toll-like receptor 4, oxidized β_2GPI can bind to and activate dendritic cells with subsequent upregulation of autoantibody production. Less frequently, there are autoantibodies with specificity to phosphatidyl-serine, phosphatidyl-ethanolamine, phosphatidyl-inositol, or prothrombin. Prothrombin antibodies induce thrombosis by reacting with the prothrombin target molecule on the endothelial cell surface. Genetics likely play a role, with up to 33% of relatives of APLS patients testing positive for antiphospholipid antibodies. There also is an association of anticardiolipin antibodies with specific HLA loci, including DR4 in whites, and DRw53 and DR7 in Hispanics.

CLINICAL AND LABORATORY MANIFESTATIONS

A diagnostic classification was adopted in 1999 and was updated by Miyakis in 2006 requiring at least one laboratory and one clinical criterion to diagnose APLS (Table 27.3). APLS may involve numerous organs including the central nervous system, kidney, endocrine organs, gastrointestinal tract, lungs, skin, and cerebrovascular and cardiovascular systems. Thrombocytopenia is frequent, and there may be additional clinical features associated with APL autoantibodies,

Table 27.3   Criteria for the Antiphospholipid Syndrome*

Clinical Criteria	Laboratory Criteria
Vascular Thrombosis	**Anticardiolipin Abs**
≥1 episode of arterial, venous, or capillary thrombosis in any tissue or organ	IgG or IgM levels (>40 GPL or MPL units or >99 percentile) at least twice, 12 wk apart
Pregnancy Complications	**Lupus Anticoagulant Abs**
≥1 death of a normal fetus at ≥10 wk gestation	Detected at least twice, 12 wk apart
≥1 premature birth of a normal fetus at ≤34 wk	IgG or IgM
≥3 spontaneous abortions at ≤10 wk gestation	**Anti-β_2-glycoprotein I Abs**
	Detected at least twice, 12 wk apart
	IgG or IgM

Based on Miyakis S, Lockshin MD, Atsumi T, et al: International consensus statement on an update of the classification criteria for definite antiphospholipid syndrome (APS). J Thromb Haemost 4:295-306, 2006.
Abs, Antibody; GPL, IgG phospholipid; MPL, IgM phospholipid.
Diagnosis requires ≥1 clinical criterion and ≥1 lab criterion.

including cardiac valve disease, livedo reticularis, thrombocytopenia, kidney disease, and neurologic manifestations, that were recognized by the consensus conference in 2006 as likely consequences of the antibodies but not included in the diagnostic criteria. Approximately 1% to 5% of healthy individuals have circulating anticardiolipin antibodies, and it is unclear how many of these results are false positives versus predating development of the clinical syndrome.

APLS may be present as a primary or as a secondary disorder, with secondary APLS most often seen in association with SLE. In patients with SLE, it has been estimated that 12% to 30% have anticardiolipin antibodies and 15% to 34% have evidence of a lupus anticoagulant; as many as 50% to 70% of these individuals will have an associated clinical event during the course of 20 years of follow-up.

Kidney manifestations in APLS are usually mild, although there are exceptions. Kidney involvement is noted in 8% to 25% of those with APLS, and individuals with lupus anticoagulant more frequently experience concurrent kidney disease. The kidney manifestations are protean and include microscopic hematuria, proteinuria, AKI, mild to malignant hypertension, cortical necrosis, TMA, progressive chronic kidney disease sometimes culminating in end-stage renal disease, and thrombosis of kidney allografts. In one study of 160 patients with primary APLS, membranous glomerulonephritis was identified in four patients and proliferative glomerulonephritis in two. The actual frequencies of these manifestations are not known.

The syndrome may occur in a "catastrophic" form, defined as concurrent involvement of at least three organ systems. The kidney is the most frequently affected organ, involved in 78% of cases of catastrophic APLS. Kidney involvement typically is accompanied by hypertension, which is often malignant, and dialysis is required in 25% of cases.. Other organ systems involved include pulmonary (66%), central nervous system (56%), cardiac (50%), and dermatologic (50%). DIC is uncommon.

THERAPY

The mainstay of therapy is anticoagulation, and warfarin is recommended for both the primary and secondary forms of APLS. In addition to anticoagulation, therapy should include avoidance of prothrombotic drugs such as calcineurin inhibitors, oral contraceptives, hydralazine, procainamide, and chlorpromazine. Aspirin should be prescribed for women with previous pregnancy complications. The role of hydroxychloroquine or chloroquine to prevent thrombosis in patients with SLE is controversial. Although not evidence based, glucocorticosteroids, plasmapheresis, intravenous immunoglobulin, and rituximab have been implemented as salvage therapy in patients with severe or multiple organ involvement.

COURSE AND PROGNOSIS

APLS requires long-term anticoagulation. Low rates of recurrent thrombosis have been reported in patients in whom the INR was kept in the range of 2 to 3. Mortality for patients with the catastrophic syndrome is high, approaching 50%.

SCLERODERMA RENAL CRISIS

PATHOLOGY

The kidney parenchymal changes in scleroderma are similar to those in other forms of TMA, but the changes include subtle features that are more typically associated with scleroderma. The involved vessels more often are the arcuate and interlobular arteries, with less common abnormalities in the arterioles or glomerular capillaries. Arteries are thickened, with wide intimas composed of loose edematous and mucoid fibrosis, embedded fibroblasts, and swollen endothelial cells without inflammation. Intimal proliferation with an "onion-skin" appearance tends to occur in arteries rather than arterioles. Muscular hypertrophy is variable, and there may be fibrosis of the adventitia of arteries. Glomeruli display varying degrees of ischemia with capillary wall wrinkling and other features of TMA, although capillary thrombi are comparatively rare. The juxtaglomerular apparatus often is expanded. The immunofluorescence and electron microscopic changes are similar to those of the other TMAs.

PATHOGENESIS

Scleroderma is a lesion of fibrosis and vascular injury, the pathogenesis of which is complex and not fully understood. It appears to involve a strong genetic component influenced by environmental factors, including exposure to infectious agents, chemicals, and physical substrates such as silica. Exposure to any of these forms of injury on a susceptible genetic background induces dysregulation of the vasculature and innate immunity resulting in fibrosis. Recent results from genome-wide association studies suggest that scleroderma is a polygenic autoimmune disorder with a number of scleroderma susceptibility genes involving immune regulation. These include genes encoding proteins that regulate dendritic and B-cell function, interferon regulators of innate and adaptive immunity, T-cell costimulatory proteins, and proteins involved in Th1 development, among others. In addition, there likely is a role of epigenetic regulation in producing the scleroderma phenotype. The participation of B and T cells, as well as fibroblasts and endothelial cells, implicate the innate immune system acting in concert with adaptive immunity. T cells and macrophages often infiltrate sites of injury in scleroderma, with focal predominance of Th2 factors. T regulatory cells (T_{reg}) have impaired function, although they are increased in number in the peripheral blood. T cells demonstrate antigen-driven immunity to fibroblasts, collagen and other ECM components, and muscle cells, with clonal expansion and production of cytokines. In patients with diffuse systemic sclerosis, monocyte-derived dendritic cells produce increased levels of IL-10 and IL-6, with decreased IL-12. Toll-like receptors also play a role with upregulated expression in fibroblasts from scleroderma patients, and augmented response of immune cells, fibroblasts, and endothelial cells to ligand binding of toll-like receptors. There are increased numbers of activated peripheral B cells, which further activate T cells and also produce scleroderma-associated antibodies such as antitopoisomerase and anticentromere antibodies. Studies have further suggested that reactive oxygen species are involved in autoimmunity in scleroderma.

A plethora of autoantibodies is associated with scleroderma, and there appears to be some specificity linked to the pattern of clinical disease presentation, with anti-RNA polymerase III and anti-Th/To ribonucleoprotein identified frequently in patients who develop scleroderma renal crisis. It is not known whether these phenotype-specific antibodies have a pathogenic role or are merely markers of disease. Antibody binding can change the sites of antigen proteolysis or promote the uptake of complexed proteins, which can spread the immune response to different antigenic components (epitope spreading) and enhance the immune reaction. It is plausible that autoantibodies are directly pathogenic; 25% to 85% of patients with scleroderma have antiendothelial cell antibodies that could induce direct or indirect endothelial injury resulting in vascular damage. This may upregulate growth factors and cytokines including endothelin-1, which is profibrotic, thus providing a link between vascular damage and fibrosis in scleroderma. Endothelial cell damage also causes a decrease in intrinsic complement regulatory proteins, proteolytic activities in serum, and cell-mediated immunity. Vascular dysfunction likely is initiated by endothelial injury, which appears to be the primary process in scleroderma renal crisis. The end results are altered permeability with vascular intimal edema, myointimal proliferation with increased ECM production, platelet activation with aggregation and adhesion, and fibrin deposition. The subsequent vascular narrowing and reduced kidney perfusion increase renin production, exacerbating hypertension. A reduction in the number and differentiation of bone-marrow-derived endothelial progenitor (CD34) cells has also been observed in scleroderma and may impair vascular healing. There is no firm evidence of specific medications inducing scleroderma renal crisis.

In patients with scleroderma, there is aberrant production and accumulation of ECM. Fibroblasts are activated by soluble and ECM-derived factors to overproduce ECM components resulting in accumulation of excess ECM material in the target organs. This process is a result of complex interactions among endothelial cells, lymphocytes, macrophages, and fibroblasts via a number of mediators, including cytokines, chemokines, ECM signaling, and growth factors. Fibroblasts in scleroderma patients express increased levels of TGFβ receptors with enhanced responsiveness to small amounts of TGFβ, whereas TGFβ inhibition via Smad7 is decreased. TGFβ also upregulates PDGFα mRNA and protein levels in scleroderma fibroblasts. Furthermore, scleroderma patients experience increased levels of other proinflammatory and profibrotic cytokines, including IL-4, IL-17, and IL-21 and its receptor. Fibroblast stimulation appears to be a final common pathway, regardless of the upstream pathogenic mechanisms involved.

CLINICAL AND LABORATORY MANIFESTATIONS

Kidney disease was not described as a major cause of morbidity and mortality in systemic sclerosis until 1952. Classic scleroderma renal crisis, defined by the presence of new-onset and often severe hypertension or rapidly progressive AKI occurring in a patient with systemic sclerosis, occurs in approximately 10% of scleroderma patients. However, approximately 10% of patients who develop renal crisis will not be hypertensive, with AKI the only manifestation of their renal crisis. This presentation is more common in patients with cardiac involvement and previous steroid treatment. Patients with diffuse systemic sclerosis carry the greatest risk of renal crisis, with up to 25% of patients developing this complication over a lifetime, although rates of renal crisis appear to be declining to 5% to 10% in more recent reports. In contrast, patients with the CREST syndrome (calcinosis, Raynaud phenomenon, esophagitis, sclerodactyly, and telangiectasias) and limited or localized systemic sclerosis are much less likely to develop renal crisis (approximately 1% to 2%). Increased risk for developing renal crisis is associated with the presence of diffuse disease, especially rapid skin thickening on the trunk or proximal limbs; antitopoisomerase III (Scl-70) as opposed to anticentromere antibodies; onset of scleroderma within the previous 5 years and especially within the previous 1 year; fatigue, weight loss, and polyarthritis; carpal tunnel syndrome; edema; and tendon friction rubs. Seventy-five percent of cases occur within the first 4 years following disease onset. Patients with minimal signs of scleroderma occasionally develop renal crisis. Drugs are another proposed risk factor, including doses of prednisone greater than 15 mg/day, cyclosporine administration within the prior 3 months, and cocaine use. Previously, African-American ethnicity and male gender were considered risks, but prospective studies have not supported this.

The hypertension and increased plasma renin levels characteristic of the disease emerge abruptly, and cases exist where this acute change occurs within days. Striking blood-pressure elevation is the most common presenting manifestation, occurring in 90% of patients. The diastolic blood pressure exceeds 120 mm Hg in 30% of cases. In a minority of patients with normal blood pressures, a significant increment for that individual within the normal range is often observed. In the latter setting, microangiopathic hemolytic anemia and thrombocytopenia are clinical clues to the presence of scleroderma renal crisis. Microscopic hematuria, proteinuria, and AKI frequently accompany accelerated or malignant hypertension at presentation, but they are not helpful in predicting the onset of renal crisis The development of scleroderma, AKI, hemolytic anemia, and thrombocytopenia in the absence of severe hypertension suggests that TMA may occur in scleroderma via a mechanism independent of or in addition to malignant hypertension. Extrarenal manifestations may precede the onset of renal crisis, including pericardial effusions, congestive heart failure, ventricular arrhythmias, microangiopathic hemolytic anemia, thrombocytopenia, and hypertensive encephalopathy. Seizures occur rarely with renal crisis.

Plasma renin levels are invariably high in these patients, but whether this is the cause or a consequence of hypertension and kidney ischemia is uncertain, and following serial renin levels has no clinical utility. Other laboratory features on presentation include nonnephrotic proteinuria, dysmorphic (usually microscopic) hematuria, and an elevated serum creatinine. Microangiopathic hemolytic anemia occurs in 43% of patients. Thrombocytopenia may be seen, but the platelet count rarely falls below 50,000/mm^3. Between 15% and 60% of patients will have anti-RNA-polymerase III antibodies, with most studies showing 30% to 35% of patients affected, but this does not appear to influence survival.

Mild hypertension, proteinuria, microscopic hematuria, and reduced kidney function kidney function may be noted in as many as 50% to 60% of patients with systemic sclerosis who do not have renal crisis, and up to 80% may have kidney disease if abnormalities on kidney biopsy are included in the definition. However, there are many other potential causes of CKD and AKI in people with scleroderma, including medications. Membranous nephropathy and perinuclear-staining antineutrophil cytoplasmic antibody (P-ANCA)-positive pauci-immune crescentic glomerulonephritis have been reported in patients with systemic sclerosis.

THERAPY

The use of ACE inhibitors is the mainstay of treatment for patients with renal crisis. Inasmuch as they are effective in patients with hypertension and in the occasional patient without hypertension, their mechanism of action likely reaches beyond blood pressure control. If ACE inhibitors alone cannot adequately control hypertension, other antihypertensive agents should be prescribed to achieve a blood-pressure target of 125/75 mm Hg. In the treatment of renal crisis, the ACE inhibitor should not be stopped because of concerns that it may be diminishing kidney perfusion pressure and exacerbating the decline in kidney function, although case reports do suggest that combining ACE inhibitors with angiotensin receptor blockers may worsen the kidney outcome.

COURSE AND PROGNOSIS

Once nearly universally fatal at 1 year, patients with renal crisis treated with ACE inhibitors can anticipate 85% survival at 1 year and 65% survival at 5 years. Risk factors for poor outcome in renal crisis include serum creatinine greater than 3 mg/dl at initiation of therapy, delays in initiating antihypertensive treatment or inadequate overall blood-pressure control, older age, male gender, congestive heart failure, arteriolar fibrinoid necrosis, severe glomerular ischemic collapse on kidney biopsy, and renal crisis occurring without hypertension. For those who progress to require dialysis, continued ACE inhibitor therapy is recommended as approximately 50% of patients may recover sufficient kidney function over 3 to 18 months to discontinue dialysis. In those on dialysis, vascular access survival and patient survival were somewhat poorer than in the general dialysis population. Few patients have undergone transplantation, but recurrence in an allograft from an identical twin has been reported.

BIBLIOGRAPHY

Benz K, Amann K: Pathologic aspects of membranoproliferative glomerulonephritis and haemolytic uraemic syndrome/thrombotic thrombocytopenic purpura, *Thromb Haemost* 101:265-270, 2009.

Boyer O, Niaudet P: Hemolytic uremic syndrome: new developments in pathogenesis and treatment, *Int J Nephrol* 2011:908407, 2011,doi:10.4061/2011/908407.

Bussone G, Berezne A, Pestre V, et al: The scleroderma kidney: progress in risk factors, therapy and prevention, *Curr Rheumatol Rep* 13:37-43, 2011.

Crowther MA, Ginsberg JS, Julian J, et al: A comparison of two intensities of warfarin for the prevention of recurrent thrombosis in patients with the antiphospholipid antibody syndrome, *N Engl J Med* 349:1133-1138, 2003.

Galbusera M, Noris M, Remuzzi G: Inherited thrombotic thrombocytopenic purpura, *Haematologica* 94:166-170, 2009.

Gigante A, Gasperini ML, Cianci R, et al: Antiphospholipid antibodies and renal involvement, *Am J Nephrol* 30:405-412, 2009.

Greinacher A, Friesecke S, Abel P, et al: Treatment of severe neurological deficits with IgG depletion through immunoadsorption in patients with Escherichia coli O104:H4-associated haemolytic uraemic syndrome: a prospective trial, *Lancet* 378:1166-1173, 2011.

Kavanagh D, Goodship T: Genetics and complement in atypical HUS, *Pediatr Nephrol* 25:2431-2442, 2010.

Keir L, Coward RJM: Advances in our understanding of the pathogenesis of glomerular thrombotic microangiopathy, *Pediatr Nephrol* 26:423-533, 2011.

Meroni PL, Borghi MO, Raschi E, et al: Pathogenesis of antiphospholipid syndrome: understanding the antibodies, *Nat Rev Rheumatol* 7:330-339, 2011.

Miyakis S, Lockshin MD, Atsumi T, et al: International consensus statement on an update of the classification criteria for definite antiphospholipid syndrome, *J Thromb Haemost* 4:295-306, 2006.

Moake JL: Mechanisms of disease: thrombotic microangiopathies, *N Engl J Med* 347:589-600, 2002.

Moore I, Strain L, Pappworth I, et al: Association of factor H autoantibodies with deletions of *CFHR1, CFHR3, CFHR4*, and with mutations in *CFH, CFI, CD46*, and *C3* in patients with atypical hemolytic uremic syndrome, *Blood* 115:379-387, 2010.

Noris M, Remuzzi G: Atypical hemolytic-uremic syndrome, *N Engl J Med* 361:1676-1687, 2009.

Obrig TG: *Escherichia coli* shiga toxin mechanisms of action in renal disease, *Toxins (Basel)* 2:2769-2794, 2010.

Rock GA, Shumack KH, Buskard NA, et al: the Canadian Apheresis group: comparison of plasma exchange with plasma infusion in the treatment of thrombotic thrombocytopenic purpura, *N Engl J Med* 325:393-397, 1991.

Romano E, Manetti M, Guiducci S, et al: The genetics of systemic sclerosis: an update, *Clin Exp Rheumatol* 29:S75-S86, 2011.

Schmidt CQ, Herbert AP, Hocking HG, et al: Translational mini-review series on complement factor H: structural and functional correlations for factor H, *Clin Exp Immunol* 151:14-24, 2008.

Sinico RA, Cavazzana I, Nuzzo M, et al: Renal involvement in primary antiphospholipid syndrome: retrospective analysis of 160 patients, *Clin J Am Soc Nephrol* 5:1211-1217, 2012.

Tsai HM: Mechanisms of microvascular thrombosis in thrombotic thrombocytopenic purpura, *Kidney Int Suppl* 112:S11-S14, 2009.

Yamamoto T: Autoimmune mechanisms of scleroderma and a role of oxidative stress, *Self/Nonself* 2:4-10, 2011.

Viral Nephropathies 28

Laura H. Mariani | Jeffrey S. Berns

HUMAN IMMUNODEFICIENCY VIRUS, HEPATITIS C VIRUS, AND HEPATITIS B VIRUS

Human immunodeficiency virus (HIV), hepatitis C virus (HCV), and hepatitis B virus (HBV) are among the most important viral-induced causes of kidney disease worldwide. Each can present with glomerular as well as other types of kidney disease, whereas therapy for HIV infection may also be associated with significant nephrotoxicity as well as certain electrolyte and acid-base disorders. Some of the most important features of the kidney diseases associated with these viruses are shown in Table 28.1.

HUMAN IMMUNODEFICIENCY VIRUS

EPIDEMIOLOGY

Kidney disease occurs frequently in the course of HIV disease and has become the fourth leading condition contributing to death in acquired immunodeficiency syndrome (AIDS) patients. Up to 30% of patients with HIV in the United States have chronic kidney disease (CKD) or proteinuria, and HIV is a leading cause of end-stage renal disease (ESRD) among young African-American men; however, the burden of kidney disease resulting from HIV worldwide, especially in sub-Saharan Africa, remains unclear, with estimates of CKD prevalence ranging from 5% to 50% depending on the population studied. Combination antiretroviral therapy (cART) has decreased the incidence of many complications of HIV infection, including HIV-related kidney disease, and has improved life expectancy; as a result of the increased life span of HIV patients, the prevalence of ESRD resulting from HIV has increased. The classic kidney disease related to HIV is a form of collapsing focal segmental glomerulosclerosis (FSGS) referred to as HIV-associated nephropathy (HIVAN), which occurs in 2% to 10% of HIV-infected patients. Other renal complications include fluid and electrolyte disturbances, medication toxicity, acute kidney injury (AKI), and immune-mediated glomerulopathy.

PATHOPHYSIOLOGY OF HUMAN IMMUNODEFICIENCY VIRUS-ASSOCIATED NEPHROPATHY

GENETIC SUSCEPTIBILITY

Human immunodeficiency virus-associated nephropathy (HIVAN) has a strong racial predisposition with nearly 90% of U.S. patients living with ESRD attributed to HIVAN being of African ancestry. Even in transgenic mouse models of HIVAN, only certain genetic backgrounds are susceptible to the disease. International studies have confirmed that a variety of African populations are at much greater risk compared to East Asian and European populations, possibly reflecting polymorphisms in the *APOL1* gene. The gene encodes apolipoprotein L1 (apoL1), a protein that lyses the African parasite *Trypanosome brucei brucei*. The biologic mechanism by which variants in APOL1 and the apoL1 protein lead to HIVAN and whether there is also a contribution of polymorphisms in the *MYH9* gene (which encodes nonmuscle myosin heavy chain IIA and was also associated with FSGS) remain unknown.

DIRECT VIRAL EFFECTS

Evidence from clinical and animal studies supports a direct role for the HIV-1 infection of renal parenchymal cells in the pathogenesis of HIVAN. In humans, HIVAN is typically seen in patients with advanced disease with high viral loads, and the introduction of cART has decreased the incidence of HIVAN. Animal models of HIVAN include a transgenic mouse that expresses a replication-defective HIV-1 construct. These mice develop proteinuria, reduced kidney function, and histologic kidney disease nearly identical to HIVAN. Wild type littermates transplanted with kidneys from the transgenic mice develop nephropathy, but reciprocal transplants from wild type mice into the transgenic mice do not. Similarly, podocyte-specific expression of HIV or HIV genes supports a direct effect of the virus in kidney tissue.

HIV DNA and mRNA have been directly demonstrated in human kidney tissue. A discrepancy between HIV DNA isolated from the kidney and from peripheral mononuclear cells supports local viral replication within kidney tissue and suggests a renal epithelial reservoir for the virus. The mechanism by which HIV enters renal epithelial cells has been unclear, as these cells lack CD4 and other known coreceptors for HIV. Several methods have been proposed for direct infection of epithelial cells and podocytes. For instance, one study of T cells with fluorescently tagged HIV virus cocultured with renal tubular epithelial cells demonstrated direct viral transfer between the cells. The transfer required cell-cell adhesion but did not require CD4. Internalization of the virus resulted in the synthesis of HIV-specific proteins.

Several studies provide better understanding of the particular HIV genes responsible for HIVAN. In vitro studies using transgenic mice have shown that *gag* (which encodes several structural proteins) and *pol* (which encodes several replication machinery proteins) are not necessary; however,

Table 28.1 Important Clinical Features of Viral Nephropathies

	HIV	HCV	HBV
Major Risk Groups	Blacks, individuals of African ancestry	Adults with risk factors for chronic HCV infection	Children of HBV endemic areas
Presentation	Proteinuria, nephrotic syndrome CKD with rapid progression Large, echogenic kidneys CD4 count <200 cells/μL	Hematuria Proteinuria Hypocomplementemia Palpable purpura Systemic vasculitis	Proteinuria Spontaneous remission in children
Primary Renal Pathology	Collapsing FSGS Microcystic dilation of tubules Interstitial inflammation	Membranoproliferative glomerulonephritis	Membranous nephropathy
Pathogenesis	Direct HIV infection of the kidney Host genetic factors	Direct HCV toxicity Cryoglobulinemia	Antigen-antibody complex deposition Vasculitis
Therapy	cART ACE-inhibitors and ARBs	Antiviral therapy Rituximab Cyclophosphamide Plasmapheresis in severe cases	Antiviral therapy

ACE, Angiotensin-converting enzyme; *ARBs,* angiotensin receptor blockers; *cART,* combination antiretroviral therapy; *CKD,* chronic kidney disease; *FSGS,* focal segmental glomerulosclerosis; *HBV,* hepatitis B virus; *HCV,* hepatitis C virus; *HIV,* human immunodeficiency virus.

the *nef* gene, a virulence factor, is necessary and sufficient to produce kidney disease. It appears particularly important in the development of the characteristic glomerular lesion, the proliferation and dedifferentiation of podocytes. Similarly, the *vpr* gene appears to be important in the characteristic tubular pathology.

Multiple cellular pathways are likely responsible for the HIVAN phenotype. The *vpr* gene upregulates the ubiquitin-like protein FAT10, which has a role in apoptosis and cell cycle arrest in the tubular epithelium and may be the cause of the tubular dilation and atrophy seen on biopsy. HIV induces a number of inflammatory mediators in tubular epithelial cells. Activation of the MAPK1,2 and Stat-3 pathways in podocytes has been correlated with the proliferative podocyte phenotype. Transgenic mice and human glomerular tissue have shown downregulation of cyclin-dependent kinase inhibitors. The mammalian target of rapamycin pathway also appears upregulated in a mouse model. Several of these pathways may become possible therapeutic targets.

CLINICAL PRESENTATION

HUMAN IMMUNODEFICIENCY VIRUS-ASSOCIATED NEPHROPATHY

The classic presentation of HIVAN is nephrotic syndrome with moderate or heavy proteinuria, a urinary sediment with relatively few cells or cellular casts, and large, often densely echogenic kidneys on renal ultrasound. Most patients are normotensive and relatively edema-free despite advanced CKD. Untreated, these patients typically experience rapidly progressive kidney failure, often reaching ESRD in a few months. There have been cases of HIVAN occurring at the time of seroconversion, but the majority of cases occur late in the course of HIV disease with high viral loads and low CD4 counts (less than 200 cells/μL).

OTHER GLOMERULAR DISEASES

Although up to 60% of kidney biopsies of HIV-infected patients reveal the typical HIVAN phenotype, several other glomerular diseases have been observed; these include minimal change disease, postinfectious glomerulonephritis, amyloidosis, and IgA nephropathy. Coinfection with hepatitis B and C are common, with membranous nephropathy and membranoproliferative glomerulonephritis (MPGN) somewhat more often observed in such patients.

ACUTE KIDNEY INJURY

The typical causes of AKI that occur in patients without HIV infection are also seen in the HIV population. Prerenal azotemia and acute tubular necrosis can result from volume depletion, sepsis, and hypotension. Nephrotoxic medications used to treat opportunistic infections are also common causes. Interstitial nephritis may result from infections such as cytomegalovirus (CMV), candida, tuberculosis and histoplasmosis, or medications such as antibiotics and nonsteroidal antiinflammatories. CMV-related disease can be associated with nephrocalcinosis. Hemolytic uremic syndrome and thrombotic thrombocytopenic purpura (HUS/TTP) are described and can be the presenting manifestation of HIV disease. The clinical manifestations, pathologic findings, and treatment regimens are similar to the idiopathic form of TTP, although the mechanism by which HIV infection leads to these thrombotic microangiopathies is not well understood. Several medications, specifically acyclovir, sulfadiazine, atazanavir, and indinavir, can result in crystal-induced obstructive AKI, with indinavir causing asymptomatic crystalluria in up to 20% of patients.

ELECTROLYTE AND ACID-BASE DISORDERS

Electrolyte disorders are common in hospitalized HIV-infected patients, particularly hyponatremia, which may affect up to 30% to 50% of hospitalized patients with AIDS. Similarly,

Table 28.2   Common Electrolyte Disorders in Patients With Human Immunodeficiency Virus Infection

Electrolyte Disturbance	Mechanisms in HIV-Positive Patients
Hyponatremia	Volume depletion
	SIADH caused by pulmonary and central nervous system diseases
	Adrenal insufficiency
Hypernatremia	Volume depletion with impaired oral intake
	Acquired nephrogenic diabetes insipidus from medications
Hyperkalemia	Medication effect, especially trimethoprim and pentamadine
	Hyporeninemic hypoaldosteronism
	Adrenal insufficiency
Hypokalemia	Diarrheal losses resulting from GI tract opportunistic infections
	Fanconi syndrome from adefovir, tenofovir, others
Hypocalcemia	Hypoalbuminemia
	Medication effect, especially pentamidine and foscarnet
Hypercalcemia	Granulomatous disease
	Disseminated CMV
Hypomagnesemia	Renal magnesium wasting from amphotericin and pentamidine
Metabolic acidosis	Diarrhea
	Lactic acidosis resulting from NRTIs, especially didanosine and stavudine
Fanconi syndrome	Medication effect, especially cidofovir, adefovir, and tenofovir

CMV, Cytomegalovirus; *GI,* gastrointestinal tract; *HIV,* human immunodeficiency virus; *NRTIs,* nucleoside reverse transcriptase inhibitors; *SIADH,* syndrome of inappropriate antidiuretic hormone.

Table 28.3   Drug-Induced Nephrotoxicity in Patients With Human Immunodeficiency Virus-1 Infection

Drug	Toxicity
cART	
Abacavir	Lactic acidosis
Atazanavir	Nephrolithiasis, acute interstitial nephritis, crystalluria
Didanosine	Lactic acidosis, AKI, Fanconi syndrome, nephrogenic diabetes insipidus
Emtricitabine	Lactic acidosis
Indinavir	Crystalluria, nephrolithiasis, interstitial nephritis
Lamivudine	Lactic acidosis
Rilpivirine	AKI
Ritonavir	AKI, hyperuricemia
Stavudine	Lactic acidosis
Tenofovir	AKI, Fanconi syndrome, lactic acidosis, nephrogenic diabetes insipidus
Zidovudine	Lactic acidosis
Other Antimicrobials	
Acyclovir	AKI, crystalluria, obstructive nephropathy
Adefovir	Fanconi syndrome, AKI
Aminoglycosides	AKI, renal tubular acidosis, Bartter-like syndrome
Amphotericin	AKI, hypokalemia, hypomagnesemia, renal tubular acidosis
Trimethoprim-sulfamethoxazole	Hyperkalemia, acute interstitial nephritis
Cidofovir	Proximal tubular damage, bicarbonate wasting, proteinuria, AKI
Foscarnet	AKI, hypo- and hypercalcemia, hypo- and hyperphosphatemia, hypomagenesemia, nephrogenic diabetes insipidus
Pentamidine	AKI, hyperkalemia, hypocalcemia
Rifampin	Interstitial nephritis
Valacyclovir	Thrombotic microangiopathy

AKI, Acute kidney injury; *cART,* combination antiretroviral therapy.

hyperkalemia has been reported in up to 20% of hospitalized AIDS patients. These and other disturbances are the consequence of direct effects of HIV infection, opportunistic infections, antimicrobial therapy for opportunistic infections, and cART therapy. Some of the more common electrolyte and acid-base disturbances and their mechanisms are listed in Table 28.2.

MEDICATION TOXICITY

Patients with HIV infection are exposed to a variety of medications with potential kidney toxicity (Table 28.3). In particular, nucleoside reverse transcriptase inhibitors (NRTIs) may cause lactic acidosis. Tenofovir, a NRTI, is a well-known cause of AKI, although other drugs in this class may also cause AKI. Tubulopathies such as Fanconi syndrome and nephrogenic diabetes insipidus also occur with tenofovir. It is important to note that NRTIs require dose adjustment in patients with reduced kidney function.

DIAGNOSIS OF HUMAN IMMUNODEFICIENCY VIRUS-ASSOCIATED NEPHROPATHY

PATHOLOGY

Kidney biopsy remains the gold standard for the diagnosis of HIVAN. Light microscopy reveals collapsing FSGS, which typically involves the entire glomerulus (Fig. 28.1). Podocyte proliferation and hypertrophy surround the shrunken glomerulus. Tubular injury is classically marked by microcystic tubular dilation, tubular atrophy, and proteinaceous casts (Fig. 28.2). Tubular cells can contain eosinophilic protein resorption droplets. Many patients have a modest interstitial inflammation with lymphocytes, plasma cells, and monocytes. Immunofluorescence is generally nonspecific. Electron microscopy shows diffuse foot process effacement and tubuloreticular structures in the endothelium without immune complex deposits (Fig. 28.3).

The clinical constellation of proteinuria, azotemia, and low CD4 count is not sufficient for diagnosis without a kidney biopsy; similarly large kidney size and dense kidney echogenicity on ultrasound are also insufficient. Recent small studies suggest that urinary neutrophil gelatinase-associated lipocalin (uNGAL) may be a useful noninvasive

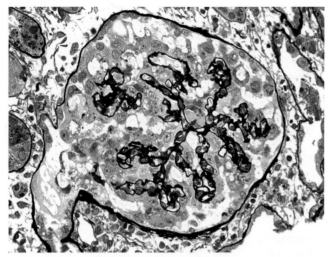

Figure 28.1   Focal segmental glomerulosclerosis of the collapsing variant seen in human immunodeficiency virus-associated nephropathy (HIVAN). (Jones methenamine silver stain, ×400 magnification.) (Courtesy Glen Markowitz, Columbia University.)

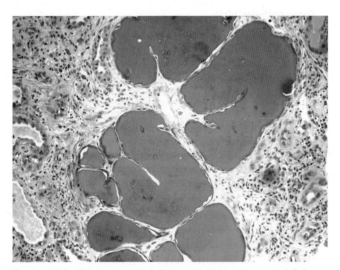

Figure 28.2 Tubulointerstitial disease in human immunodeficiency virus-associated nephropathy (HIVAN), characterized by tubular atrophy, microcystic tubular dilation with proteinaceous casts, and mild interstitial inflammation. (Trichrome stain, ×200 magnification.) (Courtesy Glen Markowitz, Columbia University.)

biomarker for HIVAN, indicating tubular damage. A small series of 25 HIV-positive patients with a variety of glomerular disease showed that elevated uNGAL demonstrated 94% sensitivity and 71% specificity for the diagnosis of HIVAN. Currently, however, if confirmation of HIVAN and exclusion of other kidney lesions is needed for clinical decision making, a kidney biopsy is necessary.

TREATMENT

ANTIRETROVIRAL THERAPY

Although no randomized controlled clinical trials have evaluated the efficacy of cART therapy in the prevention or treatment of HIVAN, multiple observational studies suggest that it is effective. On an epidemiologic basis, a plateau in the incidence of HIVAN coincided with the introduction

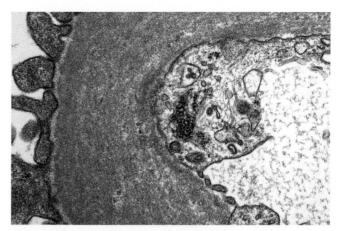

Figure 28.3 Tubuloreticular inclusions in the endothelium classically seen on electron microscopy in human immunodeficiency virus-associated nephropathy (HIVAN). (Electron micrograph, ×50,000 magnification.) (Courtesy Glen Markowitz, Columbia University.)

of cART in the mid-1990s, and several small retrospective studies document patients with biopsy-proven HIVAN, in whom the disease either slowed or even reversed after treatment with cART. Modern cART may also protect against the development of HIVAN; in a retrospective study of 4000 patients with HIV infection, the risk of nephropathy was 60% lower in patients treated with cART, and there were no cases reported among patients who began cART before the development of overt AIDS.

IMMUNOSUPPRESSION

Small, uncontrolled studies demonstrate mixed results regarding the efficacy of corticosteroids, although one small uncontrolled study in children showed an improvement in proteinuria with cyclosporine. In patients with aggressive kidney disease and prominent interstitial inflammation on biopsy, immunosuppressive therapy can be considered, but its use must also be weighed against the potential risk of worsening infections and other toxicities. With the availability of cART, the use of corticosteroids and other immunosuppressive therapies is rarely, if ever, indicated.

ANGIOTENSIN-CONVERTING ENZYME INHIBITORS AND ANGIOTENSIN RECEPTOR BLOCKERS

Several retrospective studies demonstrate that conservative therapy with angiotensin-converting enzyme inhibitors (ACE-inhibitors) and angiotensin receptor blockers may slow progression of kidney disease in HIVAN and improve overall survival; however, these are potentially confounded by concomitant cART therapy, and recommendations for renin-angiotensin-aldosterone system blockade are generally extrapolated from other proteinuric kidney diseases. The specific role of these agents in the era of modern cART is poorly defined, although they are appropriate to use to treat hypertension and for the reduction of proteinuria.

DIALYSIS AND TRANSPLANTATION

Patients with HIV can be successfully treated with peritoneal dialysis or hemodialysis. Although overall survival of these patients was historically much less than other patients with ESRD, it has improved substantially with cART, and survival is now much closer to that of the broader dialysis population. Obviously, careful attention to universal precautions to prevent infection of other patients and dialysis-unit staff is essential.

Safe and effective kidney transplantation in HIV-infected patients was demonstrated in a prospective, nonrandomized trial of 150 patients with CD4 counts greater than 200 cells/µL, undetectable viral loads, and stable antiviral regimens across 19 U.S. transplant centers between 2003 and 2009. Patient survival at 1 and 3 years was 94.6% and 88.2%, respectively, and graft survival at 1 and 3 years was 90.4% and 73.7%, respectively. These survival rates are slightly higher than those seen in ≥65-year-old transplant recipients, another high-risk group. Overall, HIV disease course was stable posttransplant. A variable CD4 drop was seen during the first year, but then recovered and was stable at the end of the study. Interestingly, there was a high rate of acute rejection (31% at 1 year), which may have been a result of difficulty with dosing immunosuppressive agents because of interactions with cART. These results indicate that transplantation is a reasonable option in carefully selected patients with well-controlled HIV.

HEPATITIS C

EPIDEMIOLOGY

The World Health Organization estimates that HCV infection affects 130 to 170 million people worldwide. In the United States, although HCV infection has fallen from a peak of 230,000 new cases per year in the mid-1980s to less than 20,000 new cases per year more recently, 1.6% of the population is HCV-antibody positive, reflecting a high rate of chronic infection.

Large retrospective studies demonstrate an association between HCV infection and the development of CKD and ESRD. The exact incidence of nephropathy caused by HCV is unknown, and a large proportion of HCV-related disease may be undiagnosed. One study of 30 HCV-infected patients undergoing kidney biopsy at the time of liver transplantation showed that 25 had an immune complex glomerulonephritis, with most being unsuspected and asymptomatic. The kidney disease classically associated with HCV infection was cryoglobulinemia with systemic vasculitis and MPGN, but other glomerular diseases have also been observed. Recent advances in therapy for hepatitis C liver disease and associated glomerular disease make accurate identification of HCV-related kidney disease essential.

PATHOPHYSIOLOGY

DIRECT TOXICITY

Direct cytopathic effects of the HCV are thought to play a role in HCV-related kidney disease, but the exact mechanisms by which HCV affects the kidneys are unknown. Kidney tissue expresses many proteins needed for direct viral attachment, endocytosis, and cell entry, but these have not been conclusively demonstrated to occur in renal epithelia or other renal cells; however, several studies have shown HCV-related proteins and RNA in kidney tissue of patients with glomerular disease. In one study, the presence of HCV-related proteins in the mesangium was associated with greater proteinuria. One proposed mechanism involves the upregulation of mesangial toll-like receptor 3 (TLR-3), which has been demonstrated in kidney biopsy tissue of patients with HCV-related MPGN and is associated with chemotactic and inflammatory host responses.

CRYOGLOBULIN-MEDIATED INJURY

Chronic HCV infection causes B cells to overproduce mixed cryoglobulins (type II and III); the cryoglobulins may form with or without viral protein immune complexes. In type II cryoglobulinemia, polyclonal IgG associates with a monoclonal immunoglobulin (typically IgM) to form rheumatoid factor. Type III cryoglobulinemia, composed of polyclonal immunoglobulins, is also seen in HCV infection. Cryoglobulins are deposited in the mesangium and glomerular capillaries. Specifically, the IgM κ component of rheumatoid factor binds fibronectin in the mesangial matrix, leading to complement activation, inflammatory cytokine release, vasculitis, fibrinoid necrosis, and crescent formation.

CLINICAL PRESENTATION

MEMBRANOPROLIFERATIVE GLOMERULONEPHRITIS

Membranoproliferative glomerulonephritis in the setting of cryoglobulinemia is the most common glomerular disease observed with HCV infection. It can develop years or even decades after the initial infection. Cryoglobulinemia often presents with a systemic vasculitis, commonly with palpable purpura that typically involves the lower limbs, arthralgias, neuropathy, and nonspecific symptoms of fever, fatigue, and malaise; however, many patients with cryoglobulinemia are asymptomatic or have mild nonspecific symptoms. Kidney disease presents as hematuria, proteinuria, and acute or chronic reductions in glomerular filtration rate (GFR). Hypertension can be severe, affecting up to 80% of patients, and up to 5% of patients present with severe, oliguric AKI. Laboratory evaluation typically shows marked hypocomplementemia, characterized by a greater reduction in C4 than C3, as well as positive anti-HCV and HCV RNA. Serum aminotransferases are elevated in 70% of patients.

The natural history of this disease can be variable. An Italian series of 146 patients showed that overall survival at 10 years was 80%. Risk factors for ESRD included older age, male gender, and higher serum creatinine and greater proteinuria at the time of diagnosis. Cardiovascular disease was the primary cause of death, but infection, hepatic failure, and malignancy were also seen. At 5 years, 11% of patients reached kidney failure.

MEMBRANOUS NEPHROPATHY

Small case series suggest an association between chronic HCV infection and membranous nephropathy. In one study of HCV-positive transplant patients, 3.6% developed membranous nephropathy within 5 years. A recent biopsy series from Japan indicated that 14% of HCV-positive patients who underwent kidney biopsy had membranous nephropathy; however, HCV overall accounts for a very small fraction of all cases of membranous nephropathy. In most series, patients with membranous nephropathy in the setting of HCV infection have normal or only slightly low complement levels and do not have cryoglulinemia.

POLYARTERITIS NODOSA

Polyarteritis nodosa (PAN), although classically associated with hepatitis B infection, has also been observed in patients with chronic HCV infection. In one series of 161 patients with HCV-related vasculitis, 19% were diagnosed with PAN. Compared to cryoglobulinemic vasculitis, these patients had a more severe presentation but a higher rate of clinical remission. Five-year survival was 86% for all types of vasculitis. Interestingly, cryoglobulin levels did not differ between those patients who presented with PAN versus those with cryoglobulinemic vasculitis.

OTHER GLOMERULAR DISEASES

Several other glomerular diseases have been reported in the setting of HCV infection, including FSGS, IgA nephropathy, postinfectious glomerulonephritis, immunotactoid glomerulopathy, and fibrillary glomerulonephritis. Immunotactoid glomerulopathy and fibrillary glomerulonephritis may share a pathogenesis involving glomerular immunoglobulin deposition. On electron microscopy, random fibrillary deposits are seen in the mesangium and glomerular capillaries, which are larger than those seen with amyloidosis (16 to 24 nm in fibrillary GN, 30 to 50 nm in immunotactoid glomerulopathy, and 10 nm in amyloid). These fibrils do not demonstrate any immunoglobulin light-chain specificity and are Congo-red negative.

DIAGNOSIS

Kidney disease frequently lags many years behind initial infection with HCV and does not appear to correlate well with disease activity in the liver. Cryoglobulin levels are variable and are positive in many patients without kidney disease. As such, kidney biopsy remains the gold standard for diagnosis of HCV-associated glomerular disease.

The classic histologic pattern of MPGN is characterized by an expanded and hypercellular mesangium, endocapillary proliferation, and thickened glomerular capillary loops on light microscopy. There is infiltration of the glomerulus by inflammatory cells, including mononuclear cells. Silver staining shows double contour glomerular basement membranes resulting from immune complex deposition and mesangial cell matrix interposition between the GBM and the endothelial cell, with a new basement membrane forming around these deposits (Fig. 28.4). Immunofluoresence typically shows IgG and C3 granular deposits. Electron microscopy shows subendothelial deposits that can be fibrillary.

TREATMENT

ANTIVIRAL THERAPY

Interferon alpha (IFN-α) has been used with success both as monotherapy as well as in combination therapy. A recent metaanalysis of 11 studies with IFN-α based therapies showed a statistically significant decrease in mean proteinuria of 2.71 g/24 h but a decrease in creatinine by only 0.23 mg/dl with IFN-α treatment. As reported in previous series, those patients with a sustained virologic response to therapy did better than nonresponders. For example, in one trial of 53 patients (40 with kidney involvement) with cryoglobulinemic vasculitis who were randomized to conservative therapy versus IFN-α, 15 of 27 patients in the

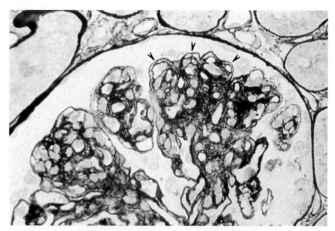

Figure 28.4 Membranoproliferative glomerulonephritis seen in hepatitis C virus infection with typical glomerular basement membrane double contours (arrowheads). (Jones methenamine silver stain.) (Courtesy Glen Markowitz, Columbia University.)

IFN-α arm who had a virologic response showed significant improvement in their clinical symptoms and labs, including serum creatinine level. When the medication was stopped, all 15 patients experienced a recurrence of both cryoglobulinemia and viremia.

Side effects of IFN-α can be severe and include depressive symptoms, malaise, nausea, myalgias, and low-grade fevers. Flulike symptoms are most severe at initiation of therapy and tend to improve over time. Importantly, there have been reports of new onset or worsening of glomerular disease in patients treated with IFN-α for HCV and other conditions.

Pegylated IFN-α (PEG-IFN) is a slow release form of the treatment, which can be dosed weekly and is more commonly used than standard IFN-α. Clearance of PEG-IFN may be reduced in patients with advanced kidney disease; accordingly, guidelines recommend against its use in patients with eGFR less than 15 mL/min/m^2 and in dialysis patients. The most frequent treatment course is 12 months, but longer duration of therapy has been shown in some small series to have higher rates of virologic response, especially in HCV genotype 1, which is generally less responsive to therapy.

Combination therapy with IFN-α and ribavirin leads to improved rates of virologic response and has been shown in several studies to be more effective in treating HCV-related glomerulonephritis than IFN-α monotherapy; however, the kidneys clear ribavirin, and accumulation of the drug in patients with reduced GFR can lead to severe hemolytic anemia. Although there are small case series in which ribavirin has been used safely at reduced dosages, it is generally best avoided in patients with an eGFR less than 50 mL/min/1.73 m^2.

The NS3/4A protease inhibitors, telaprevir and boceprevir, are approved for use in combination with ribavirin and PEG-IFN for treatment of HCV. These agents have been shown as having much higher virologic response rates, especially in genotype 1, but they have not yet been studied for use in HCV-associated glomerular disease.

IMMUNOSUPPRESSIVE THERAPY

In the setting of progressive, severe AKI and nephrotic syndrome, patients are typically treated with aggressive immunosuppressive therapy before antiviral therapy. Plasmapheresis may be used to remove circulating cryoglobulins and steroids are often used to control the acute inflammatory response. Cyclophosphamide has also been used in this setting. However, increased viral replication caused by immunosuppression remains a concern. Rituximab, a monoclonal antibody directed against the B cell antigen CD20 that causes B cell depletion and decreased antibody production, may be useful. In a clinical trial of 59 patients with severe cryoglobulinemic vasculitis randomized to rituximab versus conventional therapy (steroids, cyclophosphamide, azathioprine, and plasmapheresis), treatment with conventional therapy was associated with more treatment failures than rituximab. Serious adverse effects and deaths were similar in both groups.

TRANSPLANTATION

LIVER DISEASE

Patient and graft survival are lower in HCV-positive patients following kidney transplantation compared to HCV-negative patients. The increased risk of death has been attributed to higher rates of infectious complications and liver failure. Importantly, patients with mild and well-compensated liver disease appear to do quite well. A recent study reported on 44 HCV-positive patients who underwent kidney transplantation with pre- and posttransplant liver biopsies, and 77% of patients showed stable or improved liver histology. This report also demonstrated improved patient survival at 6 months compared to those patients who remained on the transplant waiting list.

KIDNEY DISEASE

Recurrence or de novo glomerulonephritis, including MPGN and membranous nephropathy, can occur after kidney transplantation in HCV-infected patients. Additionally, renal thrombotic microangiopathy has been described. Antiviral treatment is challenging in this setting, as IFN is frequently associated with acute kidney transplant rejection. IFN increases expression of HLA antigens on cell surfaces and increases cytokine production. The risk of acute rejection may be greater than 50% and is often refractory to therapy. Monotherapy with ribavirin has been effective in some series, even when levels of viremia did not decrease, but, as in native kidney disease, ribavirin generally must be avoided when eGFR is less than 50 mL/min/1.73 m².

HEPATITIS B

EPIDEMIOLOGY

Hepatitis B virus is a major source of morbidity and mortality worldwide. Affecting more than 2 billion people and resulting in 350 million chronic hepatitis B infections, it is much more infectious than either HIV or HCV. The prevalence of chronic infection varies widely based on geography: in the United States and Western Europe, HBV prevalence is less than 1%, whereas in Southeast Asia, Sub-Saharan Africa, and China prevalence can be as high as 15% to 20%. This disparity reflects highly effective vaccine programs in more developed countries and high rates of perinatal

transmission in endemic areas, with up to 90% of HBV vertical transmissions developing into chronic infections. In the United States, risk factors for infection include intravenous drug use and multiple sexual partners. In contrast to perinatal infections, those infections acquired in adulthood commonly result in recovery, with only 5% to 10% resulting in chronic infection.

Chronic HBV infection is associated with several kidney diseases, including membranous nephropathy, MPGN, and PAN. These disorders, especially membranous nephropathy, most commonly occur in the setting of chronic infection and thus most frequently affect children in endemic areas. The heterogeneity of presentation, pathology, and natural history has made diagnosis and therapeutic trials challenging.

PATHOPHYSIOLOGY

DIRECT TOXICITY

Indirect evidence of HBV as the causal agent for these kidney diseases comes from epidemiologic studies, including demonstration of a decrease in incidence of these diseases following the introduction of vaccine programs. Additionally, other studies have demonstrated viral antigens as well as viral DNA and RNA in glomerular and renal tubular epithelial cells of affected patients, supporting the hypothesis of viral transcription occurring within the kidney and direct toxicity of the virus itself.

IMMUNE MEDIATED

Chronic HBV-associated membranous nephropathy is most commonly seen in children living in endemic areas. It is thought that the subepithelial deposits seen in this form of secondary membranous nephropathy are composed of HBe antigen (HBeAg) and anti-e antibody (anti-HBe) complex. This is supported by the clinical observation that this disease often remits when the patient undergoes clearance of the HBeAg and seroconversion to anti-HBe. Further, it has been reported that children who develop membranous nephropathy in the setting of HBV infection have decreased cellular immune response to the virus, resulting in reduced clearance of the antigen compared to chronic carriers who do not develop membranous nephropathy.

MPGN in the setting of HBV is likely caused by the deposition of circulating antigen-antibody immune complexes in the mesangium and subepithelial space. Deposits containing both HBeAg and hepatitis B surface antigen (HBsAg) have both been reported, along with IgG and C3. A mesangial proliferative lesion has also been reported with prominent IgA mesangial deposition. In some case series, these IgA deposits appear to exhibit a pattern similar to HBsAg and hepatitis B core antigen (HBcAg) deposits; however, it is unclear if this is an incidental finding, as a HBsAg carrier state is less common in IgA nephropathy than in membranous nephropathy or MPGN.

VASCULITIS

There is a known association between PAN and HBV infection. In HBV-associated PAN, antigen-antibody complexes deposit in vessel walls, producing a clinical syndrome that is identical to idiopathic PAN, with vasculitis involving large and medium-sized vessels, leading to glomerular ischemia with hypertension and AKI.

DIAGNOSIS

CLINICAL PRESENTATION

The most common pathologic lesion in HBV-related kidney disease is membranous nephropathy. Patients typically present with a classic nephrotic syndrome, including proteinuria, hyperlipidemia, hypoalbuminemia, and lower extremity edema. In children or adults from endemic areas, the preceding HBV infection is likely to be asymptomatic, whereas adults in low prevalence regions are more likely to have a history of acute hepatitis. There is a male predominance, which is especially strong in children (up to 80%). The natural history of this disease is not well studied. Several small studies in children suggest that spontaneous remission is common, occurring in up to 60% of patients. The long-term prognosis of those who do not undergo remission is not well known. In adults, remission is less common, and CKD and ESRD may develop in a significant proportion of patients.

The clinical presentation of patients with HBV-associated PAN is similar to idiopathic PAN and classically includes hypertension, reduced GFR, and systemic symptoms such as fatigue, malaise, and fever. Other organ system involvement, including the skin, nervous system, and gastrointestinal tract, may be present.

LABORATORY DATA

Laboratory evaluation should include HBV DNA to confirm active replication as well as determination of antigen status, including HBeAg, HBsAg, and HBcAg. Other secondary causes of membranous nephropathy should be excluded, and common coinfections, including hepatitis C and HIV, should also be tested. Unlike idiopathic membranous nephropathy, complement levels may be low. Liver function tests may be normal or only minimally elevated.

PATHOLOGY

Kidney biopsy is the gold standard for diagnosing glomerular disease in the setting of HBV infection. As noted earlier, the most common pathology observed is membranous nephropathy, which is characterized by thickening of the glomerular capillary walls due to immune complex deposition. With silver or trichrome staining, characteristic spikes of the glomerular basement membrane can be seen extending around these deposits (Fig. 28.5). Immunofluorescence demonstrates granular IgG and C3 deposition (Fig. 28.6). Electron microscopy shows classic intramembranous and subepithelial deposits (Fig. 28.7). Some series have reported that membranous nephropathy in the setting of HBV may be differentiated from idiopathic membranous nephropathy by the presence of mesangial proliferation and occasional subendothelial deposits. Other pathologic patterns have been observed in the setting of HBV infection, including MPGN, IgA nephropathy, and a small vessel vasculitis.

TREATMENT

Immunosuppressive therapy has not been shown to be effective for HBV-related kidney disease; in fact, steroid therapy is associated with increased levels of viral DNA, and worsening of liver disease has been reported when steroids are withdrawn. Given these findings, steroid monotherapy is not recommended in HBV-related kidney diseases. The

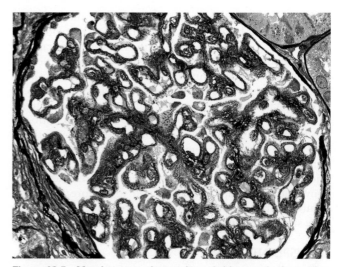

Figure 28.5 Membranous glomerulonephritis seen in the setting of hepatitis B infection. Thickened glomerular basement membrane with spikes extending around immune deposits. (Jones methenamine silver stain, magnification ×400.) (Courtesy Glen Markowitz, Columbia University.)

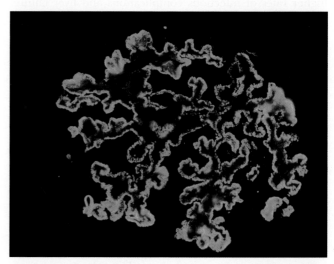

Figure 28.6 Immunofluoresence with granular deposition of IgG in membranous glomerulonephritis resulting from hepatitis B infection. (Magnification ×400.) (Courtesy Glen Markowitz, Columbia University.)

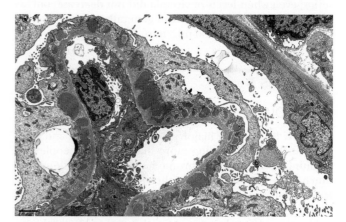

Figure 28.7 Electron microscopy with subepithelial immune deposits in membranous glomerulonephritis resulting from hepatitis B infection. (Magnification ×6000.) (Courtesy Glen Markowitz, Columbia University.)

combination of glucocorticoids with antiviral therapy may be safer than steroids alone and may be reasonable for patients with vasculitis or rapidly progressive glomerulonephritis. Plasmapheresis may also be indicated in the setting of rapidly progressive glomerulonephritis.

Antiviral therapy, with IFN-α and lamivudine therapy, has been studied extensively for treatment of HBV, including in patients with kidney disease, and it is effective at increasing rates of remission of proteinuria and HBV seroconversion. In the landmark study of lamivudine therapy in HBV infection, 10 patients with membranous nephropathy were compared to 12 historic controls from the prelamivudine era. Patients treated with lamivudine showed dramatic reductions in proteinuria, improved liver function tests, and increased clearance of HBV DNA. After 3 years of follow-up, none of those treated with lamivudine were on dialysis as compared with 7 of the historic controls. These findings have been confirmed in subsequent trials. Of note, lamivudine use is associated with a high rate of viral resistance with prolonged use.

Other antiviral agents have not been well studied in this setting. Adefovir and tenofovir are known to be nephrotoxic and are generally avoided, especially in patients with reduced GFR. There are case reports suggesting that entecavir may play a role in treatment of HBV-associated membranous nephropathy.

TRANSPLANTATION

Hepatitis B infection is not a contraindication to kidney transplantation. Although some studies, including a 2005 metaanalysis, report decreased patient survival compared to patients who are not infected, many of these studies were undertaken before modern antiviral therapies. More recent studies including patients treated with lamivudine demonstrate higher patient and graft survival.

Reactivation of viremia after transplant is more common in patients with HBeAg positivity or detectable HBV DNA pretransplant, but this can occur in all patients because of immunosuppression exposure. Although not well studied in kidney transplant patients, a preventative approach is generally recommended to prevent reactivation, and this approach is based on other populations including liver transplant patients and HBV-positive patients undergoing chemotherapy. Entecavir is generally recommended because of its decreased incidence of resistance, especially as several years of therapy may be indicated. As with hepatitis C, interferon therapy should not be used because of the high risk of acute, refractory kidney transplant rejection.

BIBLIOGRAPHY

Chen P, Chen BK, Mosoian A, et al: Virological synapses allow HIV-1 uptake and gene expression in renal tubular epithelial cells, *J Am Soc Nephrol* 22:496-507, 2011.

D'Amico G: Renal involvement in hepatitis C infection: cryoglobulinemic glomerulonephritis, *Kidney Int* 54:650-671, 1998.

De Vita S, Quartuccio L, Isola M, et al: A randomized controlled trial of rituximab for the treatment of severe cryoglobulinemic vasculitis, *Arthritis Rheum* 64:843-853, 2012.

Feng B, Eknoyan G, Guo ZS, et al: Effect of interferon-alpha-based antiviral therapy on hepatitis C virus-associated glomerulonephritis: a meta-analysis, *Nephrol Dial Transplant* 27:640-646, 2012.

Gupta SK, Eustace JA, Winston JA, et al: Guidelines for the management of chronic kidney disease in HIV-infected patients: recommendations of the HIV Medicine Association of the Infectious Diseases Society of America, *Clin Infect Dis* 40:1559-1585, 2005.

Johnson RJ, Gretch DR, Yamabe H, et al: Membranoproliferative glomerulonephritis associated with hepatitis C virus infection, *N Engl J Med* 328:465-470, 1993.

Kamar N, Sandres-Saune K, Selves J, et al: Long-term ribavirin therapy in hepatitis C virus-positive renal transplant patients: effects on renal function and liver histology, *Am J Kidney Dis* 42:184-192, 2003.

Kopp JB, Nelson GW, Sampath K, et al: APOL1 genetic variants in focal segmental glomerulosclerosis and HIV-associated nephropathy, *J Am Soc Nephrol* 22:2129-2137, 2011.

Lucas GM, Eustace JA, Sozio S, et al: Highly active antiretroviral therapy and the incidence of HIV-1-associated nephropathy: a 12-year cohort study, *AIDS* 18:541-546, 2004.

Markowitz GS, Cheng JT, Colvin RB, et al: Hepatitis C viral infection is associated with fibrillary glomerulonephritis and immunotactoid glomerulopathy, *J Am Soc Nephrol* 9:2244-2252, 1998.

Misiani R, Bellavita P, Fenili D, et al: Interferon alfa-2a therapy in cryoglobulinemia associated with hepatitis C virus, *N Engl J Med* 330:751-756, 1994.

Patel HV, Kute VB, Vanikar AV, et al: Clinical outcome of renal transplantation in end-stage renal disease patients with positive pretransplantation hepatitis B surface antigen, *Transplant Proc* 44:72-74, 2012.

Ramos-Casals M, Stone JH, Cid MC, et al: The cryoglobulinaemias, *Lancet* 379:348-360, 2012.

Rosenstiel P, Gharavi A, D'Agati V, et al: Transgenic and infectious animal models of HIV-associated nephropathy, *J Am Soc Nephrol* 20:2296-2304, 2009.

Roth D, Gaynor JJ, Reddy KR, et al: Effect of kidney transplantation on outcomes among patients with hepatitis C, *J Am Soc Nephrol* 22:1152-1160, 2011.

Saadoun D, Terrier B, Semoun O, et al: Hepatitis C virus-associated polyarteritis nodosa, *Arthritis Care Res (Hoboken)* 63:427-435, 2011.

Stock PG, Barin B, Murphy B, et al: Outcomes of kidney transplantation in HIV-infected recipients, *N Engl J Med* 363:2004-2014, 2010.

Trullas JC, Cofan F, Tuset M, et al: Renal transplantation in HIV-infected patients: 2010 update, *Kidney Int* 79:825-842, 2011.

Wyatt CM, Meliambro K, Klotman PE: Recent progress in HIV-associated nephropathy, *Annu Rev Med* 63:147-159, 2012.

Zheng XY, Wei RB, Tang L, et al: Meta-analysis of combined therapy for adult hepatitis B virus-associated glomerulonephritis, *World J Gastroenterol* 18:821-832, 2012.

29 Acute Cardiorenal Syndrome

Andrew A. House | Claudio Ronco

Cardiorenal syndromes (CRSs) are broadly defined as disorders of the heart and kidneys whereby acute or chronic dysfunction in one organ may induce acute or chronic dysfunction of the other. The syndromes represent the intersection and overlap of two very common conditions facing practitioners, and an understanding of the complex bidirectional interactions of these organ systems is paramount for their management.

In this chapter, we focus on the common situation whereby patients with acute decompensated heart failure (ADHF) or acute coronary syndrome (ACS) experience abrupt worsening of kidney function known as acute kidney injury (AKI). This has been termed acute cardiorenal syndrome. Other CRSs include a more indolent form of chronic kidney disease arising in patients with longer term heart failure, termed chronic CRS. This and additional subtypes are highlighted in Box 29.1, but are not discussed in this chapter.

DEFINITION AND EPIDEMIOLOGY OF ACUTE CARDIORENAL SYNDROME

Acute cardiorenal syndrome has been defined as an acute worsening of cardiac function leading to kidney dysfunction. ADHF is typically characterized by rapid worsening of the typical signs and symptoms of heart failure (shortness of breath, pulmonary rales, congestion on chest radiograph, raised jugular venous pressure, and peripheral edema). However, heart failure is a heterogeneous condition with various clinical presentations and multiple contributing factors. Although depressed left ventricular function is an important feature of heart failure, many patients presenting to hospital with ADHF have preserved left ventricular ejection fraction, and, in roughly one third of patients, ACS precipitates the decompensation. Accordingly, the hemodynamic derangements found in patients with ADHF are highly variable and to certain degrees overlapping, potentially including acute pulmonary edema with hypertension, severe peripheral fluid overload, isolated severe right heart failure with hepatic congestion, ascites and edema, cardiogenic shock, and hypotension, as depicted in Figure 29.1. Box 29.2 and Table 29.1 list the European Society of Cardiology diagnostic criteria and presenting clinical phenotypes of the various heart-failure syndromes. Acute CRS patients typically present with hospitalization for one of these heart-failure syndromes and meet criteria for AKI based on acute increase in serum creatinine of at least 0.3 mg/dl (26 μmol/L) and/or oliguria. The ability to detect AKI earlier (with biomarkers such as cystatin c, kidney injury molecule-1, N-acetyl-β-D-glucosaminidase, and neutrophil gelatinase-associated lipocalin) is not part of the current

definition, but may facilitate earlier diagnosis, perhaps affording a better opportunity to reverse or avoid acute CRS.

Heart failure itself is very common, with nearly 7 million Americans estimated to be affected in 2010. In 2004, there were more than 1 million hospitalizations for heart failure, with a total cost of nearly $30 billion. ACS as a primary admitting diagnosis is somewhat less common, although the annual incidence is much higher when secondary diagnoses are included. Of patients admitted with heart failure, acute CRS (defined as an increase in serum creatinine of ≥0.3 mg/dl [26 μmol/L]) may occur in 27% to 40%. Acute CRS in this setting is associated with a nearly 50% increase in mortality, as well as increased length of hospitalization and hospital costs.

PATHOPHYSIOLOGY OF ACUTE CARDIORENAL SYNDROME

HEMODYNAMICS AND THE "TRADITIONAL" CARDIORENAL PARADIGM

One key role of a functioning cardiorenal axis is to maintain appropriate extracellular effective circulating volume, and this homeostasis is achieved through an intricate web of neurohormonal feedback loops, volume and pressure sensors, vasoactive substances, transporters, and other effector mechanisms—including the autonomic nervous system, renin-angiotensin-aldosterone system (RAAS), endothelin, arginine vasopressin, and natriuretic peptides. When these systems are functioning appropriately, they enable rapid response to changing hemodynamics and extracellular fluid volume, allowing for preserved tissue perfusion and oxygen delivery, acid-base and electrolyte homeostasis, and management of nitrogenous and other wastes.

In the past, acute CRS was believed to represent the response to falling cardiac output and renal arterial underfilling with resultant kidney hypoperfusion and diminished glomerular filtration rate (GFR). The exuberant activation of sympathetic nervous system and RAAS then leads to significant increases in systemic angiotensin II and aldosterone, further contributing to the milieu of pressure and volume overload of the failing heart. It has long been recognized that the kidneys of patients with heart failure release substantial amounts of renin into the circulation, and this leads in turn to production of angiotensin II. Angiotensin II has both potent systemic vasoconstrictive effects as well as central effects on thirst and activation of the sympathetic nervous system. The vasoconstrictive effects, coupled with increased sympathetic activity, contribute to increased

Box 29.1   Definition and Classification of the Cardiorenal Syndromes

CRSs General Definition:

Disorders of the heart and kidneys whereby acute or chronic dysfunction in one organ may induce acute or chronic dysfunction in the other

Acute CRS (Type 1)

Acute worsening of cardiac function leading to renal dysfunction

Chronic CRS (Type 2)

Chronic abnormalities in cardiac function leading to renal dysfunction

Acute Renocardiac Syndrome (Type 3)

Acute worsening of renal function causing cardiac dysfunction

Chronic Renocardiac Syndrome (Type 4)

Chronic abnormalities in renal function leading to cardiac disease

Secondary CRSs (Type 5)

Systemic conditions causing simultaneous dysfunction of the heart and kidney

CRS, Cardiorenal syndrome.

Box 29.2   Definition of Heart Failure

Heart failure is a clinical syndrome in which patients have the following features:

- **Symptoms typical of heart failure**
  Breathlessness at rest or on exercise, fatigue, tiredness, ankle swelling
  and
- **Signs typical of heart failure**
  Tachycardia, tachypnea, pulmonary rales, pleural effusion, raised jugular venous pressure, peripheral edema, hepatomegaly
  and
- **Objective evidence of a structural or functional abnormality of the heart at rest**
  Cardiomegaly, third heart sound, cardiac murmurs, abnormality on echocardiogram, raised concentration of natriuretic peptide

Adapted from the 2008 European Society of Cardiology Guidelines for the Diagnosis and Treatment of Acute and Chronic Heart Failure.

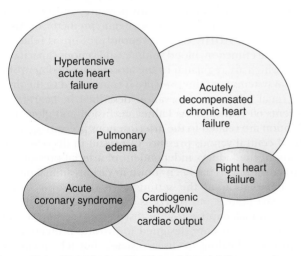

Figure 29.1 Clinical classification of heart-failure syndromes. (Adapted from the 2008 European Society of Cardiology Guidelines for the Diagnosis and Treatment of Acute and Chronic Heart Failure.)

systemic vascular resistance, venous tone and congestion, and increased myocardial contractility, which may cause ventricular demand for oxygen to outstrip its supply. Angiotensin II has potent stimulatory effects on renal sodium reabsorption, and constriction of the efferent arteriole leads to an increase in the filtration fraction, causing an increase in the tubular oncotic pressure, further enhancing proximal tubular sodium and fluid reabsorption. Angiotensin II is also a potent stimulus for aldosterone release from the adrenal gland, leading to even further augmented sodium reabsorption in the distal nephron. Normally, an aldosterone escape phenomenon allows individuals with excess aldosterone to limit this salt-avid state and avoid edema formation; however heart-failure patients lose this escape mechanism because of

the neurohormonal effects that limit distal sodium delivery, hence sodium retention continues, contributing to volume overload and edema formation.

Downstream from the activated RAAS, there is increased synthesis and activity of endothelin-1. Endothelin-1 increases renal vascular resistance and reduces renal blood flow and GFR, and it may cause or amplify ischemic injury to the kidneys. Activation of the endothelin system may also enhance salt and water retention, and it causes systemic vasoconstriction, hence contributing further to volume and pressure overload. Finally, the non-osmotic release of arginine vasopressin in response to decreased effective circulating volume from heart failure leads to further enhanced vasoconstriction through the action of V1a receptors, and to decreased excretion of free water because of enhanced uptake at the level of the collecting ducts mediated through V2 receptors. This in turn contributes to volume and pressure overload and development of hyponatremia (Fig. 29.2).

This traditional "pump and filter" paradigm of cardiorenal pathophysiology is undoubtedly relevant to many patients with decompensated heart failure, but recent observations about the types of patients developing acute CRS require us to expand our thinking. For instance, preserved ejection fraction is found in a growing proportion of patients with heart failure. In one study, almost one half of patients developing acute CRS exhibited preserved left ventricular ejection fraction ≥40%, and a larger proportion of heart-failure patients presented with elevated blood pressure compared to patients without renal complications. The Acute Decompensated Heart Failure Registry (ADHERE) contains information on more than 100,000 heart-failure hospitalizations in the United States, and it provides additional insights into the development of CRS. Using a more conservative definition of AKI (increase of creatinine of 0.5 mg/dl), the investigators categorized patients into four categories, with ejection fraction of less than 25%, 25-40%, 40-55% and ≥55% and they found small but statistically significant incremental increases in incidence of AKI with *increasing* ejection fraction, at 12.1%, 14.7%, 14.9%, and 15.2%, respectively.

Table 29.1   Common Clinical Manifestations of Heart Failure

Dominant Clinical Features	Symptoms	Signs
Peripheral edema/congestion	Breathlessness Tiredness, fatigue Anorexia	Peripheral edema Raised jugular venous pressure Pulmonary edema Hepatomegaly, ascites Fluid overload (congestion) Cachexia
Pulmonary edema	Severe breathlessness at rest	Crackles or rales over lungs, effusion Tachycardia, tachypnea
Cardiogenic shock (low cardiac output state)	Confusion Weakness Cold periphery	Poor peripheral perfusion Systolic blood pressure less than 90 mm Hg Anuria or oliguria
High blood pressure (hypertensive heart failure)	Breathlessness	Usually elevated blood pressure Left ventricular hypertrophy Preserved ejection fraction
Right heart failure	Breathlessness Fatigue	Evidence of right ventricular dysfunction Raised jugular venous pulsation Peripheral edema, hepatomegaly

Adapted from the 2008 European Society of Cardiology Guidelines for the Diagnosis and Treatment of Acute and Chronic Heart Failure.

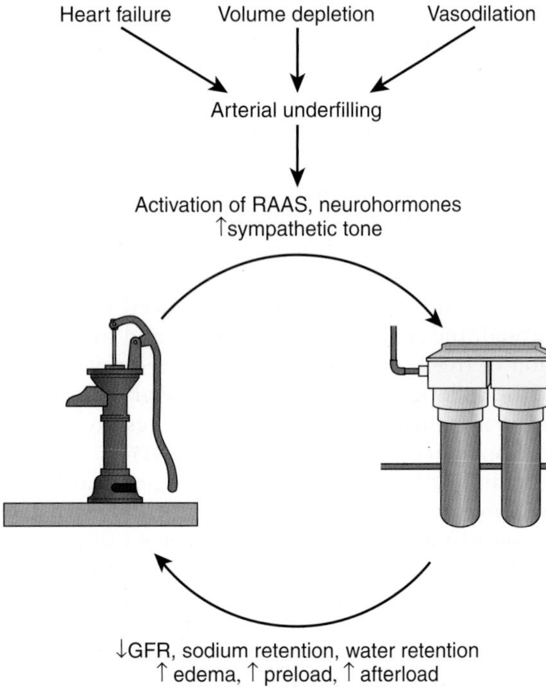

Figure 29.2   Simplistic view of the pump and filter paradigm of the cardiorenal axis. *GFR,* Glomerular filtration rate; *RAAS,* renin-angiotensin-aldosterone system.

Unsurprisingly, the groups with preserved ejection fraction tested with higher blood pressures on average.

ADDITIONAL MECHANISMS

Beyond the traditional pump and filter paradigm, a number of additional mechanisms for acute CRS have been postulated. For instance, observations have implicated high venous pressure and raised intraabdominal pressure leading to renal venous congestion as important contributors to impairment of kidney function. Mullens and colleagues found that raised central venous pressure, and not cardiac index, was the strongest hemodynamic predictor of AKI in the setting of ADHF. Central venous pressure is related to right heart function, blood volume, and venous capacitance, all of which are regulated by the aforementioned neurohormonal systems, and this pressure is transmitted to the draining renal veins, an observation described in heart-failure patients 60 years ago. As kidney perfusion and glomerular filtration are related to the arteriovenous pressure gradient, raised central venous pressure can result in decreased perfusion of the kidneys independent of arterial pressure and cardiac output, as has been shown in various animal models.

Inflammation in the setting of both chronic congestive heart failure and ADHF is increasingly recognized as playing a maladaptive role in disease progression. Inflammatory responses are designed to provide protection and to promote healing in disease states, but left unchecked these responses may in fact promote further tissue damage or may prolong injury. Cardiac myocytes, in response to mechanical stretch or ischemia, are capable of producing a broad array of inflammatory cytokines, and elements of the innate immune response may also be upregulated. Furthermore, venous congestion is postulated to increase gut absorption of endotoxin leading to further augmentation of inflammatory responses—whereas venous congestion itself is a stimulus for peripheral synthesis and release of inflammatory mediators. Clinical evidence for this proinflammatory state is derived from observations that patients with severe heart failure experience markedly elevated levels of tumor necrosis factor-α (TNFα), upregulation of soluble receptors for TNF, and a number of interleukins (IL) including IL-1β, IL-18, and IL-6, as well as several cellular adhesion molecules. It is conceivable that these systemic responses to heart failure could contribute to distant organ damage such as AKI, although direct evidence for this

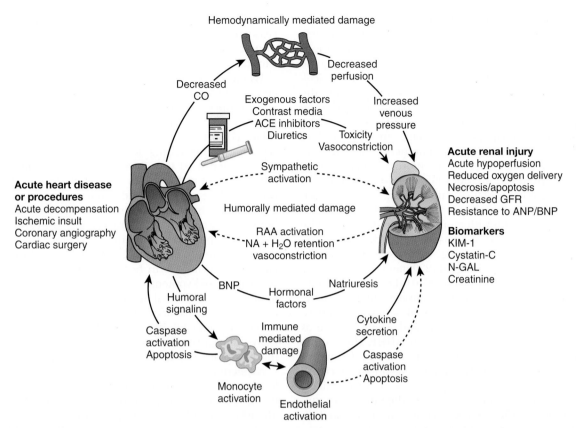

Figure 29.3 Pathophysiologic interactions between the heart and kidney in acute cardiorenal syndrome. *ACE,* Angiotensin-converting enzyme; *ANP,* atrial natriuretic peptide; *BNP,* B-type natriuretic peptide; *CO,* cardiac output; *GFR,* glomerular filtration rate; *KIM,* kidney injury molecule; *N-GAL,* neutrophil gelatinase-associated lipocalin; *RAA,* renin angiotensin aldosterone. (Reproduced from Ronco C, Haapio M, House AA, et al: Cardiorenal syndrome, *J Am Coll Cardiol* 52:1527-1539, 2008, with permission from Elsevier. Original illustration by Rob Flewell.)

cardiorenal link is lacking. The ischemic kidney is capable of producing a postischemic inflammatory state that can induce cardiac apoptosis and in turn contribute to ongoing apoptosis and fibrosis in the kidney. The more indolent response to this heightened proinflammatory state almost certainly contributes to chronic CRS. Furthermore, various inflammatory mediators can contribute to vascular endothelial dysfunction and capillary leak, leading to the movement of fluid into the interstitial compartment. Not only does this add to the signs and symptoms of heart failure through worsening pulmonary and peripheral edema, but movement of fluid into the interstitium further contracts the effective circulating volume, and edema within the peritubular interstitium of the kidneys contributes to tubular dysfunction and impaired GFR.

Additional considerations in the pathophysiology of acute CRS include a failure of counter-regulatory systems such as natriuretic peptides; persistent renal vasoconstriction from tubuloglomerular feedback and various vasoactive substances (adenosine, endothelin); and impaired autoregulation of GFR (particularly in the setting of RAAS blockade). Natriuretic peptides are naturally occurring substances that reduce renal sodium reabsorption, promote diuresis, and work systemically to decrease sympathetic tone, RAAS activity, and to cause vasodilation. Levels of natriuretic peptides are elevated in response to atrial stretch (and are certainly elevated in heart failure), yet heart-failure patients appear to lose responsiveness to these

peptides, providing an additional mechanism for worsening heart and kidney failure.

Diuretics merit special mention in the pathophysiology of acute CRS. Although important for the acute management of dyspnea and pulmonary congestion, they provoke a vigorous activation of both the sympathetic nervous system and RAAS, resulting in the counterproductive and maladaptive responses described earlier. Furthermore, their use is associated with diuretic resistance, requiring higher and higher doses. This resistance is multifactorial and includes decreased solute delivery to tubules because of decreased renal blood flow, decreased GFR, low albumin, and diuretic "braking" as a result of enhanced sodium reabsorption and distal tubular hypertrophy.

A pictorial overview of the complex and multifactorial pathways leading from ADHF to AKI and the acute CRS is presented in Figure 29.3.

TREATMENT OF ACUTE CARDIORENAL SYNDROME

The management and prevention of acute CRS in the hospitalized patient with ADHF or cardiogenic shock is largely empiric, as most treatments aimed at rapid improvement of congestive symptoms or ischemia have not been studied in randomized clinical trials. Diuretics, for instance, would be difficult to withhold (unless tried and found ineffective), but their use is often associated with worsening kidney function. High doses of diuretics have been associated with adverse outcomes, although the severity of heart failure is an obvious source of confounding. Diuretics are used in doses adequate to provide symptom relief through depletion of extracellular fluid volume at a rate that matches refilling from the interstitium to the intravascular space, balanced against the risk of further activation of neurohormonal reflexes.

Loop diuretics including furosemide are preferred to thiazides as the initial choice of diuretic, because the latter produce a smaller effect in the more advanced kidney dysfunction. However, thiazides may need to be added to overcome diuretic resistance. Aldosterone blockade with diuretics such as spironolactone and eplerenone may be problematic in patients with more advanced degrees of kidney insufficiency, who are at high risk of hyperkalemia. Careful introduction and monitoring, while excluding patients with serum creatinine $\geq$2.5 mg/dl (220 µmol/L) or baseline hyperkalemia with potassium level $\geq$5.0 mEq/L, should mitigate this risk. The Diuretic Optimization Strategies Evaluation (DOSE) trial employed a factorial design to compare low-dose with high-dose furosemide and administration as bolus versus infusion in 308 patients with ADHF. The authors reported no differences in their coprimary endpoints of global assessment of symptoms and change in serum creatinine. However, the bolus-group patients were twice as likely to require a dose increase compared to the infusion group, and the low-dose group was less likely to convert to oral therapy at 48 hours and more likely to require a dose increase (24% vs. 9%, $p = 0.003$). There was a nonsignificant trend toward greater improvement in symptoms in the high-dose group, members of which experienced greater net fluid loss, weight loss, and relief from dyspnea, although an acute rise in serum creatinine was more common in the high-dose group. Reassuringly, there were no significant differences between groups in serum creatinine and cystatin C levels at 60 days. A practical approach is to begin therapy for ADHF with bolus intravenous doses of furosemide, but consider rapid conversion to infusion and/or higher doses if diuretic resistance is encountered, while closely monitoring clinical status, electrolytes, and kidney function.

As a nonpharmacologic strategy to treat patients with acute CRS more aggressively, ultrafiltration was shown in one study to be superior to diuretics, with greater fluid loss, less requirement for vasopressors, and fewer rehospitalizations and emergency room visits, although one of the primary efficacy outcomes of dyspnea was not different, and there was not a difference in secondary renal outcomes. The Cardiorenal Rescue Study in Acute Decompensated Heart Failure or CARRESS-HF trial is expected to define further the use of ultrafiltration in acute CRS where change in serum creatinine represents a primary outcome measure.

Blockade of the RAAS is a mainstay of therapy in chronic congestive heart failure, but in acute CRS the ability to autoregulate GFR is highly dependent on angiotensin II and its effects on the efferent arteriole. Therefore, it is prudent to delay introduction of RAAS blockade (or reduce the dose in patients already receiving these drugs), particularly in low cardiac output states and/or hypotension. After kidney function stabilizes, careful introduction and titration of these agents with close monitoring of urine output and kidney function is required. Likewise, blockade

of the sympathetic nervous system with beta blockers is a reasonable goal, but if acute CRS is due to a severe low output state, beta blockers must be used with the utmost caution if at all.

When acute CRS patients present with preserved or elevated blood pressure, vasodilators such as nitroglycerin and nitroprusside are often used to relieve symptoms and to improve hemodynamics, although their use has not been subjected to rigorous controlled study, and their effect on reversing or preventing acute CRS is unknown. Nitroglycerin is often used to relieve symptoms of congestion and ischemia, and at low doses it is a venodilator, decreasing cardiac filling pressures and reducing myocardial oxygen demand. As the dose increases, nitroglycerin can improve both preload and afterload, and can increase cardiac output, although hypotension and nitrate tolerance limit its use. In a similar manner, nitroprusside has been used to dilate vascular smooth muscle in both arterial and venous systems, but because of hypotensive effects its use is generally limited to patients with normal or elevated blood pressure. Because of the potential for accumulation of thiocyanate in patients with decreased GFR, its use in CRS is problematic, although there are reports of its safe use in ADHF patients including those with decreased GFR and hypotension.

As mentioned previously, heart-failure patients become less responsive to endogenous natriuretic peptides. Recombinant human B-type natriuretic peptide (BNP), or nesiritide, when provided in supraphysiologic doses, can reduce levels of catecholamines, angiotension II, and aldosterone and as a result can decrease both preload and afterload, decrease pulmonary vascular resistance, and increase cardiac output. Further, through its effects on the renal tubules nesiritide promotes a prompt diuresis. Hence it provides rapid symptom relief in ADHF. However, studies of exogenous BNP have yielded disappointing results, with some authors suggesting increased risk of acute CRS and greater mortality. To answer adequately questions regarding safety and efficacy, the recently completed Acute Study of Clinical Effectiveness of Nesiritide in Decompensated Heart Failure (ASCEND-HF) enrolled more than 7000 patients and found no significant differences in rates of death or rehospitalization, no increased risk of acute CRS, a small improvement in dyspnea, and a near doubling of hypotension associated with nesiritide. For this reason, nesiritide cannot currently be recommended for routine treatment of patients presenting with ADHF, although studies regarding its role as a renal protective agent are ongoing.

In light of the previously described role of vasoactive substances in the pathogenesis of acute CRS, investigators have reported encouraging results related to a number of novel agents in preclinical and early clinical trials in patients with ADHF. However, as with nesiritide, subsequent larger scale trials have failed to demonstrate any substantive benefit of endothelin antagonists, vasopressin antagonists, or adenosine $\alpha 1$ receptor antagonists.

In cases of low cardiac output causing worsening heart-failure symptoms and threatening renal function, positive inotropes such as dobutamine or phosphodiesterase inhibitors are often used, although there are serious concerns about their capacity to increase myocardial injury and to induce arrhythmias. One randomized trial of milrinone in patients with ADHF showed higher rates of hypotension, arrhythmia, and no benefit related to mortality or hospitalization. Levosimendan is a phosphodiesterase inhibitor that increases myocardial sensitivity to calcium and improves hemodynamics and renal perfusion. Early studies have provided conflicting results in terms of preservation of renal function. Levosimendan appears in the European Society of Cardiology guidelines for management of heart failure, and a recent metaanalysis suggests that it may have some beneficial effects on mortality, but this analysis did not include information on renal outcomes. Levosimendan is not currently available in North America, and its precise role in the management of the prevention of acute CRS remains uncertain.

If, despite a trial of inotropic support, patients with low cardiac output and acute CRS continue to deteriorate, these patients may require more invasive treatments to serve as a bridge to recovery of kidney function, or they may require cardiac transplantation. These therapies include intraaortic balloon pulsation, ventricular assist devices, or artificial hearts; however, limited evidence supports these therapies as means to improve kidney perfusion and GFR.

SUMMARY

Acute CRS is common in patients with ADHF and/or ACS, and its appearance often heralds greater morbidity and mortality. The mechanisms behind acute CRS are complex, multifactorial, and bidirectional. Our current understanding of the pathophysiology has moved beyond the notion of the heart and kidneys operating simply as a pump and a filter, and we increasingly recognize the capacity for inflammation, apoptosis, venous congestion, and other mechanisms to contribute to the downhill spiral in the function of both organ systems. Treatment strategies are for the most part empiric, but recognition of the syndrome has led to the conduct of important, albeit largely disappointing, clinical trials as we continue to search for the optimal management of these complex cases.

BIBLIOGRAPHY

Colombo PC, Ganda A, Lin J, et al: Inflammatory activation: cardiac, renal, and cardio-renal interactions in patients with the cardiorenal syndrome, *Heart Fail Rev* 17:177-190, 2012.

Costanzo MR, Guglin ME, Saltzberg MT, et al: Ultrafiltration versus intravenous diuretics for patients hospitalized for acute decompensated heart failure, *J Am Coll Cardiol* 49:675-683, 2007.

Cuffe MS, Califf RM, Adams KF Jr, et al: Short-term intravenous milrinone for acute exacerbation of chronic heart failure: a randomized controlled trial, *JAMA* 287:1541-1547, 2002.

Damman K, Voors AA, Navis G, et al: The cardiorenal syndrome in heart failure, *Prog Cardiovasc Dis* 54:144-153, 2011.

European Society of Cardiology, Heart Failure Association of the ESC (HFA), European Society of Intensive Care Medicine (ESICM), et al: ESC guidelines for the diagnosis and treatment of acute and chronic heart failure 2008: the task force for the diagnosis and treatment of acute and chronic heart failure 2008 of the European Society of Cardiology. Developed in collaboration with the Heart Failure Association of the ESC (HFA) and endorsed by the European Society of Intensive Care Medicine (ESICM), *Eur J Heart Fail* 10:933-989, 2008.

Felker GM, Lee KL, Bull DA, et al: Diuretic strategies in patients with acute decompensated heart failure, *N Engl J Med* 364:797-805, 2011.

Forman DE, Butler J, Wang Y, et al: Incidence, predictors at admission, and impact of worsening renal function among patients hospitalized with heart failure, *J Am Coll Cardiol* 43:61-67, 2004.

Gottlieb SS, Abraham W, Butler J, et al: The prognostic importance of different definitions of worsening renal function in congestive heart failure, *J Card Fail* 8:136-141, 2002.

House AA, Haapio M, Lassus J, et al: Therapeutic strategies for heart failure in cardiorenal syndromes, *Am J Kidney Dis* 56:759-773, 2010.

Kelly KJ, Burford JL, Dominguez JH: Postischemic inflammatory syndrome: a critical mechanism of progression in diabetic nephropathy, *Am J Physiol Renal Physiol* 297:F923-F931, 2009.

Landoni G, Biondi-Zoccai G, Greco M, et al: Effects of levosimendan on mortality and hospitalization: a meta-analysis of randomized controlled studies, *Crit Care Med* 40:634-646, 2012.

Mullens W, Abrahams Z, Francis GS, et al: Importance of venous congestion for worsening of renal function in advanced decompensated heart failure, *J Am Coll Cardiol* 53:589-596, 2009.

Mullens W, Abrahams Z, Francis GS, et al: Sodium nitroprusside for advanced low-output heart failure, *J Am Coll Cardiol* 52:200-207, 2008.

Neuhofer W, Pittrow D: Role of endothelin and endothelin receptor antagonists in renal disease, *Eur J Clin Invest* 36(Suppl 3):78-88, 2006.

O'Connor CM, Starling RC, Hernandez AF, et al: Effect of nesiritide in patients with acute decompensated heart failure, *N Engl J Med* 365:32-43, 2011.

Roger VL, Go AS, Lloyd-Jones DM, et al: Heart disease and stroke statistics—2012 update: a report from the American Heart Association, *Circulation* 125:e2-e220, 2012.

Ronco C, Haapio M, House AA, et al: Cardiorenal syndrome, *J Am Coll Cardiol* 52:1527-1539, 2008.

Sarraf M, Masoumi A, Schrier RW: Cardiorenal syndrome in acute decompensated heart failure, *Clin J Am Soc Nephrol* 4:2013-2026, 2009.

Smith GL, Lichtman JH, Bracken MB, et al: Renal impairment and outcomes in heart failure: systematic review and meta-analysis, *J Am Coll Cardiol* 47:1987-1996, 2006.

Sweitzer NK, Lopatin M, Yancy CW, et al: Comparison of clinical features and outcomes of patients hospitalized with heart failure and normal ejection fraction (> or = 55%) versus those with mildly reduced (40% to 55%) and moderately to severely reduced (<40%) fractions, *Am J Cardiol* 101:1151-1156, 2008.

30 Hepatorenal Syndrome and Other Liver-Related Kidney Diseases

Vincente Arroyo | Javier Fernández | Wladimiro Jiménez

Patients with cirrhosis frequently develop kidney failure, with causes including hypovolemia, infections, parenchymal kidney diseases, drug toxicity, and hepatorenal syndrome (HRS) (Box 30.1). HRS is the most severe form of kidney failure in cirrhosis. Patients with type 1 and type 2 HRS have a mean survival time of a few weeks and a few months after the onset of kidney failure, respectively. The poor prognosis associated with HRS has led to the incorporation of serum creatinine into algorithms assessing the priority for liver transplantation.

PATHOGENESIS

Current thinking about the basis for kidney dysfunction and ascites in patients with cirrhosis focuses on the peripheral arterial vasodilation hypothesis and the forward theory of ascites formation; accordingly, the mechanisms behind this hypothesis constitute the rationale on which modern treatments of these patients are based.

The peripheral arterial vasodilation hypothesis holds that the primary event leading to renal sodium and water retention in patients with cirrhosis is splanchnic arterial vasodilation caused by a massive release of local vasodilators (i.e., nitric oxide) secondary to portal hypertension. In the initial phases of cirrhosis, compensation occurs through the development of hyperdynamic circulation (high plasma volume, cardiac index, and heart rate); however, as cirrhosis progresses and splanchnic arterial vasodilation increases, this compensatory mechanism is insufficient to maintain circulatory homeostasis. Arterial pressure decreases, leading to stimulation of baroreceptors, homeostatic activation of the sympathetic nervous system (SNS) and the renin-angiotensin-aldosterone system (RAAS), and production of antidiuretic hormone (ADH, or vasopressin), with resultant renal sodium and water retention.

The forward theory of ascites formation follows from the peripheral arterial vasodilation hypothesis and holds that arterial vasodilation in the splanchnic circulation induces the formation of ascites by simultaneously impairing both the systemic circulation (leading to sodium and water retention) and the splanchnic microcirculation (where the forward increase in capillary pressure and permeability from the greatly increased inflow of blood at high pressure into the splanchnic capillaries leads to the leakage of fluid into the abdominal cavity).

More recently, it has been suggested that the pathogenesis of circulatory dysfunction in cirrhosis is even more complex than that just described, such that the primary mechanism behind impaired circulatory function is worsening splanchnic arterial vasodilation that occurs in parallel with the progression of liver disease. It appears that cirrhosis is accompanied by a progressive impairment in both cardiac inotropic and chronotropic functions. The net effect of these abnormalities is a reduction in cardiac output and a decrease or disappearance of the hyperdynamic circulation. The peripheral arterial vasodilation hypothesis has therefore been reformulated, such that progressive circulatory dysfunction, upregulation of the RAAS, the SNS and ADH production, and impairment of kidney function in cirrhosis are caused by both an increase in splanchnic arterial vasodilation and a primary impairment in cardiac function.

The mechanism of cardiac dysfunction in cirrhosis is not well established, but it is probably multifactorial. Whereas cirrhotic cardiomyopathy is characterized by impaired diastolic function, the cardiac output often increases significantly in cirrhosis after volume expansion or following the insertion of a transjugular intrahepatic portosystemic shunt (TIPS), which increases venous return. Together, these findings suggest a role for decreased cardiac preload. Finally, during the course of cirrhosis there is a progressive overactivity of the SNS in the absence of an increase in heart rate, and the acute activation of the SNS during the course of a severe bacterial infection or hypovolemia (i.e., after large volume paracentesis) in cirrhosis is often not associated with normal compensatory tachycardia. All these mechanisms may account for the progressive decrease in cardiac output observed in advanced cirrhosis.

A second major change in our understanding of kidney dysfunction and ascites in cirrhosis relates to the pathogenesis of HRS. Traditionally, type 1 and type 2 HRS were considered to be different expressions of an identical disorder. New evidence suggests that they are completely different syndromes. Type 2 HRS represents genuine functional kidney failure; the extreme expression of impaired circulatory function that slowly and spontaneously develops in patients with decompensated cirrhosis. In contrast, type 1 HRS is acute kidney failure caused by the rapid deterioration of circulatory function that occurs in close temporal association with a precipitating event, commonly severe infection. Acute impairment in the function of other organs, including the

Box 30.1   Causes of Kidney Failure in Patients With Cirrhosis

Bacterial Infections

- The most common precipitant of kidney failure in patients with cirrhosis
- Kidney failure occurring in the absence of septic shock in patients with infections is currently considered a form of HRS

Drug-Induced Kidney Failure

- Current or recent treatment with nephrotoxins, such as nonsteroidal antiinflammatory drugs or aminoglycoside antibiotics

Hypovolemia-Induced Kidney Failure

- Gastrointestinal bleeding or fluid losses (excessive diuretic therapy or diarrhea)

Parenchymal Kidney Disease

- Suspected if proteinuria (greater than 500 mg/day) and/or hematuria are present
- Suspected if kidneys appear abnormal on ultrasound imaging

HRS

- Diagnosis requires the following:
1) Cirrhosis with ascites
2) Serum creatinine greater than 1.5 mg/dL (133 μmol/L)
3) No improvement in serum creatinine after 2 days of diuretic withdrawal and volume expansion with albumin (1 g/kg)
4) Absence of shock
5) No current or recent treatment with nephrotoxic drugs
6) Absence of parenchymal kidney disease

HRS, Hepatorenal syndrome.

Box 30.2   Phases in the Pathogenesis of Kidney Failure in Cirrhosis

Phase 1: Impaired renal sodium metabolism in compensated cirrhosis

Phase 2: Renal sodium retention without activation of the RAAS or the SNSs

Phase 3: Stimulation of the endogenous vasoconstrictor systems with preserved kidney perfusion and GFR

Phase 4: The onset of type 2 HRS, a functional impairment that develops secondary to intense kidney hypoperfusion and is characterized by a moderate and steady decrease in kidney function in the absence of other causes of kidney failure

Phase 5: The onset of type 1 HRS, characterized by a rapid and progressive decline in kidney function with the serum creatinine concentration reaching a level greater than 2.5 mg/dL in less than 2 wk

GFR, Glomerular filtration rate; *HRS,* hepatorenal syndrome; *RAAS,* renin-angiotensin-aldosterone system; *SNSs,* sympathetic nervous systems.

Note that patients can bypass type 2 HRS to develop type 1 HRS, particularly in the setting of precipitating factors, such as spontaneous bacterial peritonitis.

liver, brain, heart, and possibly adrenal glands, is typically also present in type 1 HRS.

NATURAL COURSE OF KIDNEY DYSFUNCTION IN CIRRHOSIS

Reduced ability to excrete sodium and free water and decreased kidney perfusion and glomerular filtration rate (GFR) are the main kidney function abnormalities in cirrhosis. Their course is usually progressive except that, in patients with alcoholic cirrhosis, kidney function may improve after alcohol withdrawal. The main consequence of impaired sodium excretion in cirrhosis is the development of sodium retention and ascites. This occurs when renal sodium excretion decreases to less than the sodium intake and represents a marked impairment in renal sodium handling. The kidney's ability to excrete free water is also reduced in most patients with cirrhosis and ascites, with dilutional hyponatremia (arbitrarily defined as a serum sodium concentration less than 130 mEq/L) developing when electrolyte-free water clearance is severely reduced. Finally, the main consequence of the impaired kidney perfusion is type 2 HRS, which is defined as a GFR of less than 40 mL/min (or a serum creatinine concentration of greater than 1.5 mg/dl) in the absence of any other potential cause of kidney dysfunction.

Sodium retention, dilutional hyponatremia, and HRS tend to appear at different times during the evolution of cirrhosis. Therefore, the clinical course of cirrhosis can be divided into phases according to the onset of each of these complications (Box 30.2).

PHASE 1: IMPAIRED RENAL SODIUM METABOLISM IN COMPENSATED CIRRHOSIS

Chronologically, the first kidney function abnormality that occurs in cirrhosis is impairment of renal sodium handling; this can be detected even before the development of ascites, when cirrhosis is still compensated. During this phase, patients have portal hypertension, increased cardiac output, reduced peripheral vascular resistance, normal or reduced mean arterial pressure, and normal kidney perfusion, GFR, and free water clearance. Although patients remain able to excrete dietary sodium, subtle abnormalities in renal sodium excretion are present. For example, these patients have a reduced natriuretic response to the acute administration of sodium chloride (i.e., infusion of saline solution) and may not be able to escape from the sodium-retaining effect of mineralocorticoids. Abnormal natriuretic responses to changes in posture can also be seen during this phase: urinary sodium excretion is reduced in the upright and increased in the supine posture, compared with normal subjects.

PHASE 2: RENAL SODIUM RETENTION WITHOUT ACTIVATION OF THE RENIN-ANGIOTENSIN-ALDOSTERONE SYSTEM AND SYMPATHETIC NERVOUS SYSTEMS

As cirrhosis progresses, patients become unable to excrete their dietary sodium intake, resulting in retention of sodium together with water, with this excess fluid accumulating in the abdominal cavity as ascites. Urinary sodium excretion, although reduced, is usually greater than 10 mEq/day and in some cases it exceeds 50 to 90 mEq/day; therefore, dietary sodium restriction may be sufficient to effect negative sodium balance and loss of ascites. Kidney perfusion, GFR, the ability to excrete free water, plasma renin activity, and the plasma concentrations of norepinephrine and ADH are normal, indicating that sodium retention therefore is unrelated to any abnormality of the renin-angiotension-aldosterone system (RAAS) or the SNS, the two most important regulators of serum sodium excretion so far identified. Furthermore, plasma levels of atrial natriuretic peptide, brain natriuretic peptide, and natriuretic hormone are increased in these patients, indicating that sodium retention is not caused by a reduced synthesis of endogenous natriuretic peptides. It has been suggested that circulatory dysfunction at this phase (although greater than in compensated cirrhosis without ascites) is not intense enough to stimulate the RAAS and the SNS, but is sufficient to activate an idiopathic, extremely sensitive, sodium-retaining mechanism (renal or extrarenal). No studies have compared the systemic hemodynamics in patients with portal hypertension and compensated cirrhosis with those in patients at this phase of the disease. However, two studies in the latter group of patients clearly showed the presence of hyperdynamic circulation with high cardiac output, low peripheral vascular resistance, and hypervolemia.

PHASE 3: STIMULATION OF THE ENDOGENOUS VASOCONSTRICTOR SYSTEMS WITH PRESERVED KIDNEY PERFUSION AND GLOMERULAR FILTRATION RATE

When sodium retention is intense (urinary sodium excretion less than 10 mEq/day), plasma renin activity and the plasma concentrations of aldosterone and norepinephrine are invariably increased. Aldosterone increases sodium reabsorption in the distal and collecting tubules while renal SNS activity stimulates sodium reabsorption in the proximal tubule and loop of Henle. Therefore, sodium retention in patients at this phase is caused by increased sodium reabsorption throughout the nephron. The plasma volume and peripheral vascular resistance do not differ from those observed in the previous phase. These features are compatible with a progression of splanchnic arterial vasodilation compensated by vasoconstriction in extrasplanchnic organs secondary to an increased activity of the SNS and RAAS. In fact, kidney, cerebral, and muscle blood flow in cirrhosis correlates inversely with plasma renin activity and the concentration of norepinephrine. The most interesting feature is that cardiac output in patients at phase 3 (although higher than in normal subjects) is lower than in patients at phase 2, indicating that progression of circulatory dysfunction is caused not only by an increase in splanchnic arterial vasodilation but also by a decrease in cardiac output. Arterial pressure at this phase of the disease is critically dependent on increased activity of the RAAS and SNS and ADH production, and the administration of drugs that interfere with these systems (angiotensin receptor blockers, angiotensin-converting enzyme inhibitors, clonidine, vasopressin V_{1a} antagonists) may precipitate arterial hypotension. Although angiotensin-II, norepinephrine, and vasopressin are powerful renal vasoconstrictors, kidney perfusion and GFR are normal or only moderately reduced

in this phase, because the vasoconstrictive effects of these hormones on the renal circulation are antagonized by intrarenal vasodilator mechanisms, particularly prostaglandins and nitric oxide. Therefore, severely impaired kidney function may occur at this phase if renal prostaglandins are inhibited with the use of nonsteroidal antiinflammatory drugs. The ability to excrete free water is reduced at this phase of cirrhosis because of the high circulating plasma levels of ADH. However, few patients have significant hyponatremia, because the effect of ADH is partially inhibited by increased renal production of prostaglandin E_2.

PHASE 4: THE ONSET OF TYPE 2 HEPATORENAL SYNDROME

Type 2 HRS is a functional impairment that develops secondary to intense kidney hypoperfusion. Type 2 HRS is characterized by a moderate and steady decrease in kidney function (serum creatinine between 1.5 and 2.5 mg/dl) in the absence of other potential causes of kidney failure. The International Ascites Club considers that serum creatinine concentration should be greater than 1.5 mg/dl or GFR less than 40 mL/min for the diagnosis of HRS to be made; however, many patients with GFR less than 40 mL/min have normal serum creatinine concentration, reflecting loss of muscle mass in patients with advanced liver disease. Therefore the frequency of type 2 HRS is underestimated when serum creatinine alone is used in the clinical evaluation. Type 2 HRS develops in patients with very advanced cirrhosis and significant deterioration of circulatory function. Patients with type 2 HRS have very high plasma levels of renin, norepinephrine, and ADH, as well as significant arterial hypotension. The arterial vascular resistance in these patients is increased not only in the kidneys, but also in the brain, muscle, and skin, indicating generalized arterial vasoconstriction in an attempt to compensate for intense splanchnic arterial vasodilation. Type 2 HRS is probably caused by extreme overactivity of the endogenous vasoconstrictor systems, which overcomes the intrarenal vasodilatory mechanisms. Cardiac output in patients with type 2 HRS is lower than in patients with ascites who have normal serum creatinine concentration, and a significant number of these patients have "normal" cardiac output, indicating the disappearance of the hyperdynamic circulation. The progression of circulatory dysfunction causing type 2 HRS is therefore related to both increased arterial vasodilation and a relative decrease in cardiac output. The degree of sodium retention is very intense in patients with type 2 HRS, caused by a reduction in filtered sodium and a marked increase in sodium reabsorption in the proximal tubule. The delivery of sodium to the distal nephron (where most diuretics act) is very low; therefore, most of these patients do not respond to diuretics and have refractory ascites. Free water clearance is also markedly reduced, and most patients have significant hyponatremia. The prognosis of patients with type 2 HRS is poor with a mortality rate of 50% at 6 months after the onset of impaired kidney function.

PHASE 5: THE ONSET OF TYPE 1 HEPATORENAL SYNDROME

Type 1 HRS is characterized by a rapidly progressive decline in kidney function, defined as a doubling of the serum

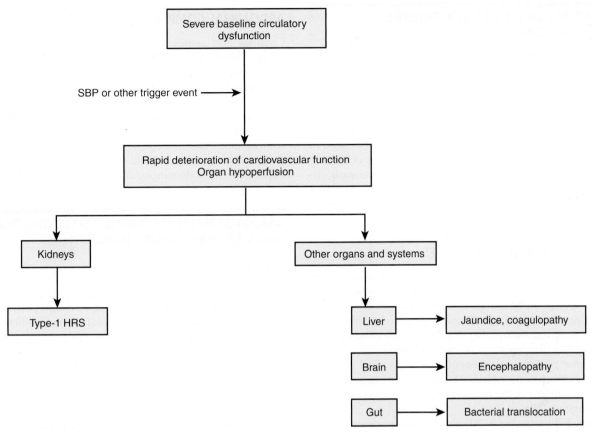

Figure 30.1 Pathogenesis of multiorgan disease in Type 1 hepatorenal syndrome. *HRS,* Hepatorenal syndrome; *SBP,* spontaneous bacterial peritonitis.

creatinine concentration reaching a level greater than 2.5 mg/dl in less than 2 weeks. Although type 1 HRS may arise spontaneously, it frequently occurs in conjunction with a precipitating factor such as severe bacterial infection, acute hepatitis (ischemic, alcoholic, toxic, viral) superimposed on cirrhosis, a major surgical procedure, or massive gastrointestinal hemorrhage. Severe bacterial infections (mainly spontaneous bacterial peritonitis [SBP]) are the most common precipitating event. Patients with type 2 HRS are predisposed to develop type 1 HRS, although the latter may also develop in patients with normal kidney function. Most patients with type 1 HRS have high plasma levels of renin and norepinephrine and, frequently, dilutional hyponatremia, indicating that type 1 HRS has occurred after a precipitating event in patients who already have severe circulatory dysfunction; this event may not be clinically apparent. The prognosis of patients with type 1 HRS is extremely poor, with 80% of patients dying less than 2 weeks after the onset of HRS. Patients succumb from progressive circulatory, hepatic, and kidney failure, along with encephalopathy. Type 1 HRS has been closely investigated in the setting of SBP, as 30% of patients with SBP will develop this type of kidney failure. The two most important predictors of type 1 HRS development in SBP are increased serum creatinine before SBP and an intense intraabdominal inflammatory response, as suggested by high concentrations of polymorphonuclear leukocytes and cytokines (tumor necrosis factor-α and interleukin-6) in ascitic fluid at infection diagnosis. Type 1 HRS after SBP occurs in the setting of an acute and severe deterioration of circulatory function, as indicated by a significant decrease in arterial pressure and a marked increase in the plasma levels of renin and noradrenaline. Two recent studies assessed systemic hemodynamics and kidney function in patients with and without SBP before and after the development of type 1 HRS. These studies suggested that the impairment in circulatory function in patients with HRS is far more complex than initially considered. In addition to accentuated arterial vasodilation, cardiac output significantly decreased during the course of SBP. In some cases, resting cardiac output decreased to values below normal (5 L/min). It is unknown whether this decrease in heart function is caused by cirrhotic or sepsis-related cardiomyopathy, by decreased cardiac preload resulting from central hypovolemia, or by both. The demonstration that using albumin to expand the plasma volume of patients at the diagnosis of SBP reduces the incidence of type 1 HRS by more than 60% and decreases hospital mortality is consistent with the second hypothesis. Cardiac chronotropic function is severely impaired in patients with HRS, because there is no increase in heart rate despite a significant reduction in arterial pressure and a marked increase in plasma norepinephrine concentration and SNS activity. HRS in patients with SBP is associated with impaired circulatory and kidney function and also with reduced hepatic function leading to hepatic encephalopathy. Increased intrahepatic vascular resistance, reduced liver blood flow, and increased portal pressure gradient all correlate closely with an increase in renin and norepinephrine. Type 1 HRS is therefore a complex syndrome of circulatory origin that includes acute deterioration of multiple organs (Fig. 30.1).

OTHER TYPES OF KIDNEY FAILURE IN CIRRHOSIS

DRUG TOXICITY

As stated previously, kidney perfusion and GFR in patients with cirrhosis and ascites are maintained by an increased renal synthesis of vasodilating prostaglandins (PGI2 and PGE2). Nonsteroidal antiinflammatory drugs inhibit prostaglandin synthesis and cause a profound reduction in renal blood flow, with resultant kidney failure occurring in a high proportion of these patients. Patients with cirrhosis and ascites are also susceptible to other nephrotoxins, including aminoglycoside antibiotics and intravenous contrast.

INTRAVASCULAR VOLUME LOSSES

In patients with cirrhosis and upper gastrointestinal bleeding, the incidence of kidney failure is 11%. Risk factors include severity of blood losses and degree of liver failure (prevalence in Child-Pugh C and A-B score patients: 29% vs. 3%). A substantial number of patients with kidney failure following bleeding episodes recover kidney function following volume repletion, consistent with a prerenal state. In other patients, however, kidney failure persists or progresses despite resolution of the bleeding episode, suggesting tubular damage or HRS.

Kidney failure occurs in 30% of cirrhotic patients treated with diuretics. Two scenarios are described. The first occurs in patients continuing diuretic treatment after the complete mobilization of ascites and is caused by volume depletion, whereas the second is observed in patients with ascites, even with tense ascites. The mechanism for both is effective hypovolemia, with compensatory increase in endogenous vasoconstrictor systems and secondary kidney hypoperfusion. Typically, diuretic-induced acute kidney failure does not progress to severe chronic kidney impairment, as the kidney response to diuretics decreases with dropping GFR.

KIDNEY FAILURE ASSOCIATED WITH INFECTION

One third of patients with cirrhosis and SBP develop kidney failure despite rapid resolution of SBP with antibiotic treatment. In 30%, kidney failure is transient, in 25% it persists but does not progress (type 2 HRS), and in 45% rapidly progressive kidney failure develops. The prevalence of steady or progressive kidney failure in other types of infection is significantly lower: 15% in patients with acute pyelonephritis and 13% in those with cellulitis.

PARENCHYMAL KIDNEY DISEASES

Patients with cirrhosis frequently develop parenchymal kidney disease caused by deposition of immunocomplexes related to hepatitis B or C viral antigens or antigens translocated from the intestinal lumen (IgA nephropathy). However, only in a minority of cases are these mechanisms severe enough to cause kidney failure. Kidney diseases associated with hepatitis B and hepatitis C are reviewed in more detail in Chapter 28.

ABDOMINAL COMPARTMENT SYNDROME

Cirrhosis and ascites are classically considered risk factors for the development of abdominal compartment syndrome, an acute and sustained increase in intraabdominal pressure (greater than 20 mm Hg) associated with organ dysfunction, mainly kidney failure and hypotension. This syndrome is infrequent in patients with tense ascites but can be observed in patients with mild or moderate ascites when they develop complications that acutely increase intraabdominal pressure (i.e., massive gastrointestinal bleeding, hemoperitoneum). Rapid abdominal decompression is mandatory for treatment.

MANAGEMENT OF KIDNEY DYSFUNCTION AND ASCITES IN CIRRHOSIS

LOW-SODIUM DIET

Mobilization of ascites occurs when a negative sodium balance is achieved. In the 10% of cirrhotic patients with normal plasma aldosterone, normal norepinephrine concentrations, and relatively high urinary sodium excretion, this can be obtained simply by reducing the sodium intake to 60 to 90 mEq/day. A greater reduction in sodium intake may interfere with nutrition and is not advisable in an already nutritionally vulnerable patient. In most patients with cirrhosis, urinary sodium excretion is very low, and a negative sodium balance cannot be achieved without diuretics. Even in these cases, sodium restriction is important because it reduces diuretic requirements. In fact, a frequent cause of apparently refractory ascites is inadequate sodium restriction, and this should be suspected if ascites does not decrease despite a good natriuretic response to diuretics (see Chapter 9).

DIURETICS

Furosemide and spironolactone are the diuretics most commonly used in the treatment of ascites in cirrhosis. In contrast to healthy subjects (in whom furosemide is more potent than spironolactone), in cirrhotic patients with ascites the reverse is true. Most cirrhotic patients with ascites and marked hyperaldosteronism (comprising 50% of patients with ascites) do not respond to furosemide, whereas most cirrhotic patients with ascites do respond to spironolactone. Patients with normal or slightly increased plasma aldosterone concentration respond to low doses of spironolactone (100 to 150 mg/day), but as much as 300 to 400 mg/day may be required in patients with marked hyperaldosteronism. The mechanism of the resistance to furosemide in patients with hyperaldosteronism is pharmacodynamic. With reduced GFR and avid proximal sodium reabsorption, delivery of sodium to the site of furosemide action (loop of Henle) is reduced. In addition, most of the sodium that is not reabsorbed in the loop because of furosemide's action is subsequently reabsorbed in the distal nephron because of the stimulation by aldosterone. Therefore, spironolactone is the preferred drug for the management of cirrhosis and ascites. The simultaneous administration of furosemide and spironolactone increases the natriuretic effect of both agents and reduces the incidence of hypokalemia or hyperkalemia that may be observed when these drugs are administered alone. There is general agreement that patients not responding to 400 mg/day of spironolactone and 160 mg/day of furosemide will not respond to higher diuretic doses. Diuretic treatment in cirrhosis often leads to complications, particularly in patients requiring high diuretic doses. Approximately 20% of patients develop significant kidney function decline, which is usually moderate and reversible after diuretic withdrawal. Hyponatremia secondary to a decrease in the renal ability to excrete free water occurs in approximately 20% of these patients. The most severe complication related to diuretic treatment is hepatic encephalopathy, which occurs in approximately 25% of patients who are hospitalized with tense ascites and treated with high doses of diuretics. The term *refractory ascites* is applied when ascites cannot be mobilized, when its early recurrence after therapeutic paracentesis cannot be prevented due to lack of response to sodium restriction and maximal diuretic treatment (diuretic-resistant ascites), or when diuretic-induced complications preclude the use of an effective diuretic regimen (diuretic-intractable ascites). Refractory ascites is an infrequent condition, occurring in fewer than 10% of patients hospitalized with tense ascites. Most of these patients have type 2 HRS (serum creatinine concentration greater than 1.5 mg/dl) or less severe but still significantly impaired kidney function (serum creatinine between 1.2 and 1.5 mg/dl). It has been estimated that serum creatinine greater than 1.2 mg/dl reflects a decrease of GFR of more than 50% in patients with cirrhosis, consistent with substantial muscle wasting in this population. Impaired access of diuretics to the renal tubules (because of reduced kidney perfusion) and reduced delivery of sodium to the loop of Henle and distal nephron (secondary to the low GFR and increased sodium reabsorption in the proximal tubule) are the mechanisms of diuretic-resistant ascites. Insufficient sodium restriction or treatment with nonsteroidal antiinflammatory drugs should be excluded before the diagnosis of diuretic-resistant ascites is made.

ARTERIAL VASOCONSTRICTORS

Plasma volume expansion alone (e.g., after the insertion of a peritoneovenous shunt [LeVeen shunt]) does not improve kidney function in patients with HRS, despite a significant suppression of plasma renin activity and norepinephrine concentration. Also, the administration of vasoconstrictors alone does not produce clinically significant increases in GFR in these patients. In contrast, simultaneous treatment of patients with type 1 HRS using intravenous albumin as a plasma expander along with vasoconstrictors for 7 to 14 days is associated with an increase in arterial pressure, a suppression of plasma renin activity and norepinephrine concentration to normal levels, a marked increase in GFR, and a normalization of serum sodium and serum creatinine concentration in a significant number of patients. Type 1 HRS usually does not recur after discontinuation of therapy.

These data are consistent with the hypothesis that type 1 HRS is related to accentuated arterial vasodilation (corrected by the vasoconstrictor) and decreased cardiac output related to central hypovolemia (corrected by the administration of albumin). Very few patients develop side effects related to treatment. The probability of survival after normalization of

serum creatinine increases, and a significant proportion of patients may survive to liver transplantation. Terlipressin, a vasopressin agonist dosed at 0.5 to 2.0 mg every 4 hours, has been the most frequently used vasoconstrictor for the treatment of type 1 HRS. Currently it is not available for use in the United States or Canada. The α-adrenergic agonists noradrenaline and midodrine, at doses that increase arterial pressure by more than 10 mm Hg, also may be effective. Many investigators use an initial dose of albumin of 1 g/kg of body weight, followed by 20 to 40 g/day over 7 to 14 days.

GFR may remain low in many patients with type 1 HRS treated with vasoconstrictors and albumin, suggesting that treatment with vasoconstrictors and albumin is effective for correcting the type 1 HRS component of the syndrome but not the reduced GFR that was present before the development of type 1 HRS in most patients. Two features further support this contention. First, and contrary to what occurs with type 1 HRS, type 2 HRS frequently recurs soon after discontinuation of therapy with vasoconstrictors and albumin. Second, sequential treatment with vasoconstrictors and albumin followed by the insertion of TIPS normalizes serum creatinine and GFR in most patients with type 1 HRS.

V₂ VASOPRESSIN ANTAGONISTS

Dilutional hyponatremia is the most common serum electrolyte abnormality in patients with cirrhosis and ascites. Traditionally, hyponatremia was considered a minor problem in cirrhosis, because it is usually asymptomatic, even in patients with markedly reduced serum sodium concentration. The presence of hyponatremia does not contraindicate diuretic treatment in patients with cirrhosis and ascites; in fact, many cirrhotic patients with ascites and hyponatremia respond to diuretics without a further reduction in serum sodium. However, recent studies suggest that hyponatremia may be more relevant than previously thought, because its presence is associated with a very poor prognosis. The probability of hepatic encephalopathy is significantly higher in patients with hyponatremia than in those with comparable deterioration of hepatic function without hyponatremia. Finally, the incidence of severe neurologic events after liver transplantation is relatively high in patients with dilutional hyponatremia, probably due to the rapid correction of extracellular osmolality during the operation. Therefore, treatment of hyponatremia could be beneficial in patients with decompensated cirrhosis.

Dilutional hyponatremia in cirrhosis is related to severely impaired renal free water excretion, due chiefly to ADH hypersecretion. Other mechanisms involved in the water retention in cirrhosis are impaired renal production of prostaglandin E₂ (a powerful antagonist of the tubular effect of ADH), and reduced sodium and water delivery to the ascending limb of the loop of Henle and the distal convoluted tubule, where urinary dilution occurs. Treatment of dilutional hyponatremia in cirrhosis with ascites should, therefore, be directed toward reducing total body water. The administration of sodium may produce a transient increase in serum sodium, but at the expense of increasing the rate of ascites formation.

Treatment with vasopressin receptor antagonists may be considered in cirrhotic patients with severe hypervolemic hyponatremia (less than 125 mmol/L). The administration of vaptans for a short period of time (1 week to 1 month in most studies) is associated with an increased urine volume and with an improved hyponatremia (45% to 82% of patients) and ascites control. Satavaptan and tolvaptan (oral) and conivaptan (intravenous) are licensed in some countries. Treatment should be started in the hospital and the dose titrated to achieve a slow increase in serum sodium. Rapid increases in serum sodium concentration (greater than 8 to 10 mmol/day) should be avoided to prevent the occurrence of osmotic demyelination syndrome. The duration of treatment with vaptans is not known, and safety has only been established for short-term treatment (approximately 1 month). Recent studies suggest that treatment with vaptans is not clinically beneficial in the long-term management of ascites in cirrhosis and might be associated with an increase in mortality. Further studies are needed to confirm this finding.

THERAPEUTIC PARACENTESIS

Paracentesis is a rapid, effective, and safe treatment of ascites in cirrhosis and is the treatment of choice for tense ascites. The mobilization of ascites by paracentesis is associated with a deterioration of circulatory function, as manifest by a marked increase in plasma renin activity and aldosterone concentration in 60% to 70% of patients following large volume paracentesis. This impairment in circulatory function results from accentuation of arterial vasodilation already present in these patients. The incidence of this complication is reduced to 30% to 40% if paracentesis is followed by plasma volume expansion with synthetic plasma volume expanders (dextran 70 or polygeline), and to 18% if it is accompanied by plasma volume expansion with albumin (8 g/L of ascitic fluid removed).

The occurrence of circulatory dysfunction after paracentesis also depends on the amount of ascitic fluid removed. In patients receiving synthetic plasma expanders, circulatory dysfunction occurred in 18%, 30%, and 54% of patients who had removal of less than 5 L, between 5 and 9 L, and more than 9 L of ascitic fluid, respectively. The corresponding values in patients receiving albumin as plasma expander were 16%, 19%, and 21%, respectively. Therefore, paracentesis-induced circulatory dysfunction is a frequent event in patients with massive ascites that is partially prevented by the use of synthetic plasma expanders and almost totally prevented by the administration of intravenous albumin. Although paracentesis-induced circulatory dysfunction is asymptomatic, it adversely affects the clinical course of the patients and may be associated with shorter survival.

TRANSJUGULAR INTRAHEPATIC PORTOSYSTEMIC SHUNT

Transjugular intrahepatic portosystemic shunt works as a side-to-side portacaval shunt and is extremely effective in improving circulatory and kidney function and reducing ascites. TIPS induces a marked increase in cardiac output, a decrease in systemic vascular resistance, and an elevation in right atrial pressure and pulmonary wedge pressure. These changes are probably caused by increased venous return secondary to the portosystemic shunt. The decrease in systemic vascular resistance is a physiologic response to accommodate the increase in cardiac output and does not represent an impairment in systemic hemodynamics. In fact,

TIPS insertion is associated with a significant reduction in the plasma levels of renin, aldosterone, norepinephrine, and ADH, indicating an improvement in effective arterial blood volume. Suppression of the RAAS is observed within the first week after TIPS treatment and persists during follow-up, whereas suppression of norepinephrine and ADH requires a longer period of time. The improvement in circulatory function induces a rapid increase in urinary sodium excretion, which occurs within the first 1 to 2 weeks and persists during follow-up. Significant increases in serum sodium concentration and GFR are also observed, indicating improved kidney perfusion and free water clearance. However, these latter changes require 1 to 3 months to occur. Of note, TIPS is not curative: TIPS only partially decompresses the portal venous system, and the plasma levels of renin and aldosterone do not decrease to normal levels. Critically, the improvement in systemic and splanchnic hemodynamics associated with TIPS results in either complete disappearance of ascites or a partial response (such that paracentesis is no longer required) in most patients. Only 10% of patients fail to respond to TIPS. Ascites characteristically resolves very slowly (1 to 3 months), but continuous diuretic treatment at lower doses is required in more than 90% of cases, either for the treatment of ascites or to reduce peripheral edema. The persistence of portal hypertension and hyperaldosteronism may account for this feature. Hepatic encephalopathy is the most important complication in cirrhotic patients with refractory ascites treated by TIPS, occurring in more than 40%. Although hepatic encephalopathy before TIPS is a predictor of post-TIPS encephalopathy, new or worsened hepatic encephalopathy develops in approximately 30% of the cases. In most instances, it responds to standard therapy. Shunt dysfunction requiring restenting is also a major problem, occurring in approximately 40% of those receiving uncovered stents. The use of covered stents may reduce this problem.

TREATMENT AT THE DIFFERENT PHASES OF THE DISEASE

The management of ascites and kidney dysfunction in cirrhosis is summarized in Table 30.1.

Table 30.1   Treatment of Ascites and Kidney Dysfunction at Different Phases of the Disease

Phase	Treatment
Moderate ascites	Low-sodium diet and diuretics (spironolactone and furosemide)
Tense ascites	Total paracentesis
Refractory ascites and type 2 HRS	Total paracentesis or TIPS
Type 1 HRS	First option: vasoconstrictors (mainly terlipressin) + intravenous albumin Second option (for patients not responding to pharmacologic treatment): TIPS or albumin dialysis

HRS, Hepatorenal syndrome; *TIPS,* transjugular intrahepatic portosystemic shunt.

PHASE 1: PREASCITIC CIRRHOSIS

At present, specific treatment for the prevention of ascites is not recommended in patients with compensated cirrhosis. These patients should receive a normal sodium diet and should not be treated with diuretics.

PHASES 2 AND 3: MODERATE AND TENSE ASCITES

Patients with moderate ascites respond readily to sodium restriction and low-dose spironolactone with few complications. Therefore, diuretic treatment (spironolactone 100 to 200 mg/day) is the therapy of choice in these patients. In contrast, most patients with tense ascites require higher diuretic doses. Several randomized, controlled trials showed that paracentesis is preferred to diuretic therapy in patients with tense ascites, because it reduces the duration of hospital stays and also is associated with significantly lower incidence of impaired kidney function and hepatic encephalopathy. After ascites has been mobilized, phase 3 patients require dietary sodium restriction and diuretics to prevent recurrence.

PHASE 4: REFRACTORY ASCITES

Five randomized controlled trials in patients with refractory or recurrent ascites clearly showed that TIPS is preferable to therapeutic paracentesis for long-term control of ascites but is inferior if one accounts for the development of severe hepatic encephalopathy. The total time in hospital during follow-up and the probability of survival were similar with the two procedures. Based on these results, the International Ascites Club considers paracentesis to be the first-line treatment of refractory ascites. TIPS may be indicated in those patients who require frequent paracentesis (greater than 3 times per month) if they are without previous episodes of hepatic encephalopathy or cardiac dysfunction, are younger than 70 years of age, and have Child-Pugh scores of less than 12 points.

PHASE 5: TYPE 1 HEPATORENAL SYNDROME

Patients with type 1 HRS must be treated with intravenous albumin and vasoconstrictors drugs for 1 to 2 weeks; with this strategy, reversal of HRS is achieved in 40% to 60% of patients. This is associated with an increase in survival, and a significant proportion of patients may reach liver transplantation. Early morbidity and mortality after liver transplantation are higher, and long-term survival time is shorter in patients with HRS than in those without HRS. These differences were not observed when HRS was reversed preoperatively with intravenous albumin and terlipressin. Therefore, pharmacologic treatment of HRS should also be considered in patients who have HRS before liver transplantation. Two studies have suggested that TIPS could be of value in the management of type 1 HRS in patients with relatively preserved hepatic function. TIPS also could be indicated for those patients not responding to pharmacologic treatment.

Moreover, three large randomized controlled trials suggest that albumin dialysis (MARS or Prometheus systems) may be beneficial for patients with type 1 HRS. In the first study, albumin dialysis with the MARS system was more effective than standard medical therapy for management of patients with grade III-IV hepatic encephalopathy, most of whom had severe HRS. The two other trials compared albumin dialysis with standard medical therapy in patients with type 1 HRS (MARS) or with type 1 and 2 HRS (Prometheus). Significant beneficial effect on hepatic encephalopathy was observed in the MARS study but not in survival. In the Prometheus trial no effect on survival was observed in the whole group, but a significant improvement was observed in type 1 HRS patients. Further studies are needed to ascertain the potential role of albumin dialysis in type 1 HRS.

PREVENTION OF HEPATORENAL SYNDROME

Three randomized controlled studies have shown that HRS can be prevented in specific clinical settings (Table 30.2). Intravenous administration of albumin (1.5 g/kg at infection diagnosis and 1 g/kg on day 3) in patients with cirrhosis and SBP reduced the incidence of type 1 HRS and hospital mortality (10% vs. 29%). Primary prophylaxis of SBP with oral norfloxacin in patients with low ascitic fluid protein concentration (less than 15 g/L) and severe liver or kidney failure (serum creatinine ≥1.2 mg/dl or serum sodium ≤130 mEq/L) led to a significant decrease in 1-year incidence of SBP and type 1 HRS (28% vs. 41%), with a significant increase in survival at 3 months following infection (94% vs. 62%). Finally, the administration of pentoxifylline (400 mg 3 times a day) to patients with severe acute alcoholic hepatitis superimposed on cirrhosis reduced the occurrence of HRS (8% in the pentoxifylline group vs. 35% in the placebo group) and hospital mortality.

CONCLUSIONS

Reduced ability to excrete sodium and free water together with decreased GFR are the main kidney function abnormalities in cirrhosis. Patients with advanced cirrhosis and ascites spontaneously develop a progressive impairment in cardiac and circulatory function. Type 2 HRS is the extreme form of this condition, and it is characterized by slowly progressive functional renal failure and refractory ascites. Type 1 HRS

Table 30.2 Prevention of Hepatorenal Syndrome

Clinical Setting	Prophylactic Measure
Spontaneous bacterial peritonitis	Intravenous albumin administration: 1.5 g/kg body weight at diagnosis and 1.0 g/kg body weight on day 3
Primary prophylaxis of SBP in patients with low protein ascites (less than 15 g/L) and severe liver or kidney failure (serum creatinine ≥1.2 mg/dl)	Oral norfloxacin 400 mg/day
Severe alcoholic hepatitis	Oral pentoxifylline 400 mg every 8 h

is an acute syndrome characterized by rapidly progressive, functional kidney failure, which is usually triggered by a precipitating event and which may be associated with multiorgan failure. Patients with type 2 HRS are usually treated by repeated large-volume paracentesis or TIPS. The treatment of choice for patients with type 1 HRS is intravenous administration of vasoconstrictors and albumin. This treatment reverses HRS in 50% of patients and improves survival. HRS is effectively prevented by the use of intravenous albumin in patients with SBP and by the administration of oral norfloxacin in patients with low protein ascites and poor liver and/or kidney function.

KEY BIBLIOGRAPHY

Angeli P, Volpin R, Gerunda G, et al: Reversal of type 1 hepatorenal syndrome with the administration of midodrine and octreotide, *Hepatology* 29:1690-1697, 1999.

Arroyo V, Ginès P, Gerbes AL, et al: Definition and diagnostic criteria of refractory ascites and hepatorenal syndrome in cirrhosis: International Ascites Club, *Hepatology* 23:164-176, 1996.

Caregaro L, Menon F, Angeli P, et al: Limitations of serum creatinine level and creatinine clearance as filtration markers in cirrhosis, *Arch Intern Med* 154:201-205, 1994.

Epstein M: Renal prostaglandins and the control of renal function in liver disease, *Am J Med* 80:46-55, 1986.

Fernandez J, Navasa M, Planas R, et al: Primary prophylaxis of spontaneous bacterial peritonitis delays hepatorenal syndrome and improves survival in cirrhosis, *Gastroenterology* 133:818-824, 2007.

Ginès A, Fernandez-Esparrach G, Monescillo A, et al: Randomized trial comparing albumin, dextran 70, and polygeline in cirrhotic patients with ascites treated by paracentesis, *Gastroenterology* 111:1002-1010, 1996.

Gines P, Angeli P, Lenz K, et al: EASL clinical practice guidelines on the management of ascites, spontaneous bacterial peritonitis and hepatorenal syndrome in cirrhosis, *J Hepatol* 53:397-417, 2010.

Gines P, Uriz J, Calahorra B, et al: Transjugular intrahepatic portosystemic shunting versus paracentesis plus albumin for refractory ascites in cirrhosis, *Gastroenterology* 123:1839-1847, 2002.

Guevara M, Gines P, Fernandez-Esparrach G, et al: Reversibility of hepatorenal syndrome by prolonged administration of ornipressin and plasma volume expansion, *Hepatology* 27:35-41, 1998.

Hassanein TI, Tofteng F, Brown RS, et al: Randomized controlled study of extracorporeal albumin dialysis for hepatic encephalopathy in advanced cirrhosis, *Hepatology* 46:1853-1862, 2007.

Malbrain ML, Chiumello D, Pelosi P, et al: Incidence and prognosis of intra-abdominal hypertension in a mixed population of critically ill patients: a multiple-center epidemiological study, *Crit Care Med* 33:315-322, 2005.

Martin PY, Ginès P, Schrier RW: Nitric oxide as a mediator of hemodynamic abnormalities and sodium and water retention in cirrhosis, *N Engl J Med* 339:533-541, 1998.

Martin-Llahi M, Pépin MN, Guevara M, et al: Terlipressin and albumin vs albumin in patients with cirrhosis and hepatorenal syndrome: a randomized study, *Gastroenterology* 134:1352-1359, 2008.

Ruiz-del-Arbol L, Urman J, Fernandez J, et al: Systemic, renal, and hepatic hemodynamic derangement in cirrhotic patients with spontaneous bacterial peritonitis, *Hepatology* 38:1210-1218, 2003.

Salerno F, Gerbes A, Gines P, et al: Diagnosis, prevention and treatment of hepatorenal syndrome in cirrhosis, *Gut* 56:1310-1318, 2007.

Schrier RW, Arroyo V, Bernardi M, et al: Peripheral arterial vasodilation hypothesis: a proposal for the initiation of renal sodium and water retention in cirrhosis, *Hepatology* 8:1151-1157, 1988.

Sherman DS, Fish DN, Teitelbaum I: Assessing renal function in cirrhotic patients: problems and pitfalls, *Am J Kidney Dis* 41:269-278, 2003.

Sort P, Navasa M, Arroyo V, et al: Effect of intravenous albumin on renal impairment and mortality in patients with cirrhosis and spontaneous bacterial peritonitis, *N Engl J Med* 341:403-409, 1999.

Trawalé JM, Paradis V, Rautou PE, et al: The spectrum of renal lesions in patients with cirrhosis: a clinicopathological study, *Liver Int* 30:725-732, 2010.

Wong F, Watson H, Gerbes A, et al: Satavaptan for the management of ascites in cirrhosis: efficacy and safety across the spectrum of ascites severity, *Gut* 61:108-116, 2012.

Full bibliography can be found on www.expertconsult.com.

The Kidney in Cancers

31

Colm Magee | Lynn Redahan

Kidney disease frequently complicates cancer and its treatment. The spectrum of disease in this setting includes acute kidney injury (AKI), chronic kidney disease (CKD), and disorders of electrolyte and water balance. Fortunately, these complications are often preventable or reversible with early diagnosis and treatment. Although the causes and management of AKI and CKD in cancer patients overlap significantly with causes in non-cancer patients, certain conditions are either unique to or more common in cancer patients.

This chapter provides a general overview of kidney diseases in individuals with cancer, focusing on conditions such as tumor lysis syndrome, hemolytic uremic syndrome (HUS)/thrombotic thrombocytopenic purpura (TTP), bisphosphonate nephrotoxicity, and kidney disease following hematopoietic cell transplantation. Myeloma associated kidney disease is discussed in Chapter 26.

ACUTE KIDNEY INJURY IN THE CANCER PATIENT

Acute kidney injury in the cancer patient is often multifactorial, but, as in other clinical settings, it is clinically useful to consider prerenal, intrarenal, and postrenal causes (Box 31.1).

PRERENAL ACUTE KIDNEY INJURY

Anorexia, vomiting, and diarrhea (from the cancer itself or, more commonly, from chemotherapy) may predispose to prerenal injury. Additionally, pain is common in cancer patients, and nonsteroidal antiinflammatory drugs (NSAIDs) may be used as treatment. The diagnosis and management of prerenal AKI is similar to that of the general patient, with several conditions more common. Several less common causes include hypercalcemia, interleukin-2 (IL-2) therapy, and hepatorenal syndrome.

HYPERCALCEMIA

Hypercalcemia is a relatively common complication of malignancy and is most often associated with lung cancer, breast cancer, and multiple myeloma. The various types of hypercalcemia associated with malignancy are summarized in Table 31.1. Humoral hypercalcemia, mediated mainly by parathyroid hormone–related peptide (PTHrp), is the most common form. The effects of PTHrp are similar to those of parathyroid hormone, increasing both bone breakdown and renal tubular calcium reabsorption. AKI associated with hypercalcemia is predominantly due to renal vasoconstriction and hypovolemia. Nephrogenic diabetes insipidus can also occur. Treatment involves administration of large volumes of normal saline (+/− loop diuretics) and

bisphosphonates. Measurement of PTHrp or 1,25 vitamin D_3 is rarely required, because treatment is urgent and test results would not alter management. Early control of hypercalcemia usually restores kidney function.

INTERLEUKIN-2

IL-2 therapy is used for selected patients with metastatic renal cell carcinoma or metastatic malignant melanoma. Its use has been limited by severe toxicity, including capillary leak syndrome, which leads to decreased effective circulating volume and a fall in glomerular filtration rate. Vomiting and diarrhea may exacerbate this prerenal syndrome. The typical presentation is oliguria in the first 24 hours of treatment followed by a rising creatinine. Prevention of AKI involves withholding antihypertensive and nephrotoxic medications, administering intravenous fluids, and closely monitoring vital signs and urine output. Treatment of established AKI involves stopping IL-2 therapy and administering intravenous fluids, with close monitoring for development of pulmonary edema.

HEPATORENAL SYNDROME

Hepatorenal syndrome can occur following certain forms of hematopoietic cell transplantation, discussed later in this chapter. Much less commonly, it is seen with massive infiltration of the liver by neoplastic cells. Acute severe hepatitis and hepatorenal syndrome also have been reported with tyrosine kinase inhibitors such as erlotinib.

INTRARENAL AKI

GLOMERULAR DISEASES

Deposition of monoclonal paraproteins in the glomeruli can cause nephrotic syndrome, kidney failure, and, rarely, nephritic syndrome; these conditions are discussed in Chapter 26. Paraneoplastic glomerular disease is a rare but well-described complication of malignancy (Fig. 31.1), in which glomerular disease likely is caused by factors secreted by tumor cells rather than by direct infiltration of the kidney or by deposition of a paraprotein. The diagnosis should be considered if glomerular disease and cancer present at similar times or if the glomerular lesion remits with successful treatment of the malignancy. Membranous nephropathy is the classic example, although the strength of the association (more with solid organ than hematologic cancers) is disputed. The policy in our center is to perform age- and gender-appropriate standard cancer screening in patients with unexplained membranous nephropathy. A careful history and examination may suggest further testing. An association between minimal change disease and Hodgkin's disease is well established albeit uncommon, with an incidence of about 0.4%. Minimal change disease has also been reported with leukemia, non-Hodgkin's lymphoma, thymoma, and a variety of solid organ tumors. Nephrotic syndrome in such cases often improves with treatment of the underlying malignancy.

Paraneoplastic membranoproliferative glomerulonephritis (MPGN) has been reported in cases of lymphoproliferative disorders and carcinomas. Pankhurst and colleagues

---

Box 31.1   Common Causes of Kidney Injury in Cancer Patients

Prerenal

Hypovolemia (poor fluid intake, vomiting, diarrhea, capillary leak syndrome with IL-2)
NSAIDs
Hypercalcemia
Hepatorenal syndrome (after HCT, massive infiltration by cancer cells)

Intrarenal

Glomerular

Membranous nephropathy
ANCA vasculitis
Amyloidosis
Light chain deposition disease
Collapsing glomerulopathy (pamidronate)

Tubulointerstitial

ATN due to sepsis, hypovolemia, IV contrast
ATN due to drugs (cisplatin, ifosfamide, zoledronate)
Acute cast nephropathy (myeloma)*
Tumor lysis syndrome (uric acid and calcium-phosphate deposition)*
Methotrexate*

Vascular

HUS/TTP (gemcitabine, mitomycin C, and other drugs; conditioning regimen for allogeneic HCT)

Postrenal

Obstruction of both urinary tracts by urological and nonurological cancers
Retroperitoneal fibrosis

Other

Bilateral nephrectomy (renal cancer)
Massive infiltration of kidneys by lymphoma

---

*Associated with both tubular injury and tubular obstruction.

---

performed a case-control study comparing 200 patients with antineutrophil cytoplasmic antibody (ANCA)–associated vasculitis and 129 with Henoch-Schönlein purpura (HSP) to age- and sex-matched controls. Because the rate of malignancy was significantly increased in those with ANCA-associated vasculitis or with HSP (relative risk 6.0 and 5.2, respectively), the authors concluded that malignancy should be considered in the differential diagnosis of patients who present with ANCA vasculitis. Of note, cyclophosphamide therapy (particularly when given in small, daily, oral doses) for ANCA vasculitis can cause bladder cancer, often years after administration. Although paraneoplastic glomerulonephritides are rare, they are important to bear in mind when evaluating a patient with malignancy and features suggestive of a glomerular lesion. Treatment should be directed at the underlying malignancy.

TUMOR INFILTRATION

Although many solid organ and hematologic cancers can involve the kidney parenchyma, clinical sequelae are usually not prominent. Lymphomas and leukemias are the most common such cancers, and kidney involvement has been found in up to 50% of autopsy cases of non-Hodgkin lymphoma far exceeding the numbers with clinically evident kidney disease. Accordingly, although lymphomatous involvement of the kidneys may present with AKI, the diagnosis is usually incidental. Typical findings include enlarged kidneys with bland urinalysis. Although kidney biopsy may yield the diagnosis of lymphoma, in cases of known lymphoma with AKI and enlarged kidneys, a presumptive diagnosis of kidney involvement is reasonable and improvement in kidney function and reduction in kidney size with successful chemotherapy can provide further post hoc support for this diagnosis.

Despite advances in nephron-sparing surgery and ablative therapies, full nephrectomy is sometimes still required for primary kidney cancers, including renal cell carcinomas. Patients with preexisting CKD will have significant worsening of their CKD after radical nephrectomy and should be counseled beforehand about this inevitable complication. Occasionally, patients will have bilateral kidney involvement, requiring simultaneous (or staged) bilateral nephrectomy and precipitating "acute" end-stage renal disease (ESRD). Fortunately, patients without extrarenal metastases may still be candidates for kidney transplantation.

TUMOR LYSIS SYNDROME

Tumor lysis syndrome (TLS) describes the metabolic complications of either spontaneous rapid tumor cell turnover or,

---

Table 31.1   Causes of Hypercalcemia in Individuals With Cancer

Type	Proportion	Bone Metastases	Mediator(s)	Typical Cancers
Humoral hypercalcemia of malignancy	80%	Minimal	PTHrp	Squamous cell (of lung, head/neck, cervix), ovarian cell, renal cell
Local bone breakdown	20%	Common and extensive	Cytokines, chemokines	Multiple myeloma, breast cancer, lymphoma
Excess 1,25 vitamin D_3	<1%	Variable	1,25 vitamin D_3	Lymphomas
Excess (ectopic) PTH	<1%	Variable	PTH	Variable

Modified from Stewart AF: Hypercalcemia associated with cancer, N Engl J Med 352:373, 2005.
PTH, Parathyroid hormone; PTHr, parathyroid hormone–related peptide.

more commonly, chemotherapy-induced tumor cell lysis. It occurs most often with the treatment of leukemias and lymphomas but can occur with any rapidly proliferating malignancy that is highly sensitive to treatment. The syndrome is characterized by hyperuricemia, hyperphosphatemia, hypocalcemia, hyperkalemia, and AKI, often with progressive oliguria. Severe forms of TLS are potentially life threatening. The two major mechanisms causing AKI in TLS are the deposition of urate crystals in the renal tubules and the precipitation of calcium-phosphate in the interstitium (Figure 31.2). Urate crystals are both directly toxic to the tubular epithelial cells and also cause intratubular obstruction. Calcium-phosphate precipitation may be exacerbated by alkalinization of the urine.

TLS usually occurs 24 to 72 hours after initiation of chemotherapy, and the cornerstone of management is prevention. Patients at high risk for developing TLS (high tumor burden, rapid cell turnover, hypovolemia, or preexisting kidney disease) should be identified *before* starting chemotherapy. Preventive measures are shown in Table 31.2. Of note, because alkalinization of the urine exacerbates intrarenal calcium-phosphate precipitation, bicarbonate administration is not recommended. AKI associated with TLS is a medical emergency and management involves immediate treatment of electrolyte abnormalities, administration of rasburicase, and diuresis. Severe cases require immediate, high-dose hemodialysis or hemofiltration. The kidney prognosis is good if the patient survives the immediate complications.

MULTIPLE MYELOMA AND RELATED PLASMA CELL DYSCRASIAS

Multiple myeloma and related plasma cell dyscrasias are the most common oncologic causes of severe acute and chronic kidney injury, including cast nephropathy, amyloidosis, and light-chain deposition disease. Myeloma patients are also at increased risk for hypercalcemia-induced AKI and, in some reports, contrast nephropathy and bisphosphonate nephrotoxicity. Multiple myeloma is discussed in detail in Chapter 26.

BISPHOSPHONATE-INDUCED KIDNEY DISEASE

Intravenous bisphosphonates are antiresorptive agents widely used to treat osteolytic metastases and hypercalcemia of malignancy. Their use is particularly common in breast cancer and myeloma. Both nephrotic syndrome and kidney dysfunction have been reported with use of intravenous bisphosphonates in cancer patients, pamidronate being associated with the former and zoledronate with the latter. Risk factors for kidney complications include myeloma, preexisting kidney disease, and higher bisphosphonate dose. Markowitz and colleagues first reported seven patients who developed nephrotic syndrome and kidney dysfunction while receiving pamidronate; histology showed collapsing glomerulopathy with varying degrees of tubular injury. Five of these patients had received very high-dose pamidronate. Notably, the three patients in whom pamidronate was discontinued had subsequent kidney function improvement, whereas the four who continued to receive pamidronate

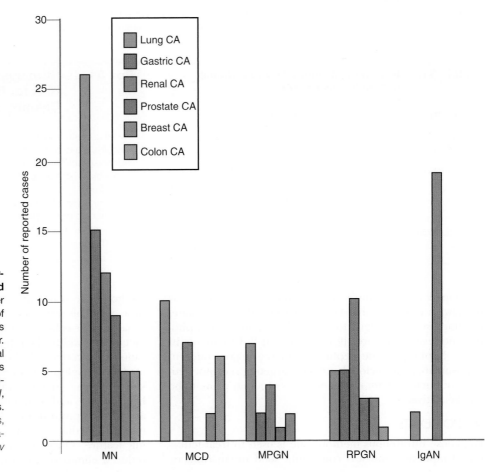

Figure 31.1 Paraneoplastic glomerulonephritis associated with solid tumors. Data are presented as number of reported cases of specific types of paraneoplastic glomerulonephritides associated with each type of cancer. *IgAN*, IgA nephropathy; *MCD*, minimal change disease; *MN*, membranous nephropathy; *MPGN*, membranoproliferative glomerulonephritis; *RPGN*, rapidly progressive glomerulonephritis. (From Lien YH, Lai LW: Pathogenesis, diagnosis and management of paraneoplastic glomerulonephritis, *Nat Rev Nephrol* 7:85-95, 2011.)

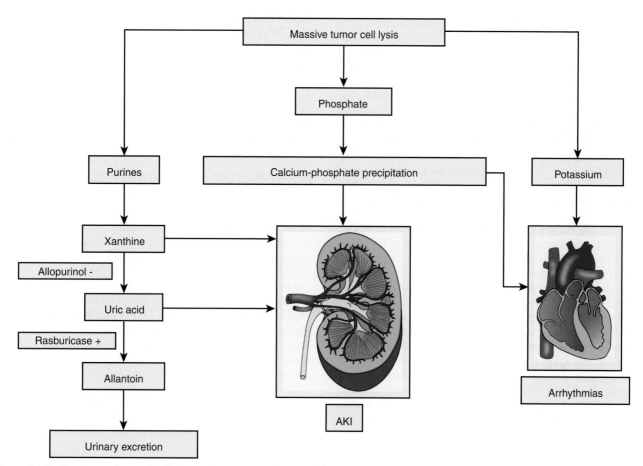

Figure 31.2 The two major mechanisms causing acute kidney injury (AKI) in tumor lysis syndrome are the deposition of urate crystals in the lumina of renal tubules and the precipitation of calcium-phosphate in the interstitium. Hyperkalemia may lead to the development of arrhythmias.

Table 31.2	Prevention of Tumor Lysis Syndrome in a High-Risk Patient
Therapy	**Comment**
Large volume of intravenous saline	Aim to keep urine output >150 mL/hr
Allopurinol	High doses needed Safe and moderately efficacious Inexpensive
Rasburicase	Can be used to treat established cases

Box 31.2   Strategies to Minimize the Risk for Bisphosphonate or Chemotherapy Nephrotoxicity

Avoid supratherapeutic doses
If agents are excreted by the kidneys, adjust dose for lower GFR
Administer high volumes of normal saline or other solution to maintain high urine output before, during, and after infusion of drug
Monitor patient for rising creatinine and proteinuria; consider switching or postponing therapy if these occur
Avoid other nephrotoxins such as NSAIDs and iodinated contrast

developed kidney failure. Severe tubular injury, which is not always reversible, has been reported with zoledronate. Common-sense strategies to reduce the risk for bisphosphonate nephrotoxicity are shown in Box 31.2. In patients in whom bisphosphonate nephrotoxicity is a major concern, denosumab, a monoclonal antibody targeting receptor activator of nuclear factor-κB ligand (RANKL), may prove to be an alternative.

METHOTREXATE

High-dose intravenous methotrexate is used to treat leukemia, lymphoma, and less commonly, solid organ cancers.

Methotrexate is mainly excreted by the kidneys, and high-dose protocols can cause AKI, both by direct toxic effects on renal tubular cells and by precipitation of the drug and its metabolites within the tubular lumen. Intraluminal crystallization is exacerbated by lower urine pH. Other factors associated with development of nephrotoxicity include preexisting kidney disease, concomitant use of other nephrotoxic drugs, hypovolemia, and higher plasma concentrations of the drug at 72 hours postinfusion. An abrupt rise in creatinine during or immediately after the infusion is the typical presenting feature. Once methotrexate nephrotoxicity develops, reduced elimination of the drug results in persistent high plasma levels and an increased risk for severe myelosuppression and hepatitis; thus early recognition and treatment of this complication are vital. The estimated incidence of methotrexate nephrotoxicity is 1.8%. Prevention involves dose adjustment for kidney function, maintenance of both a high urine output and a urine pH higher than 7.0 (by administration of high volumes of sodium bicarbonate fluids before, during, and after methotrexate infusion), and avoidance of other nephrotoxins. Folinic acid (leucovorin) rescue is routinely prescribed. Treatment of established nephrotoxicity involves continued alkalinization of the urine, administration of additional folinic acid, and, in anticipated severe cases, glucarpidase (which rapidly converts methotrexate to nontoxic metabolites). Although hemodialysis is only moderately efficient in removing methotrexate and a rebound in plasma levels may occur upon cessation of dialysis, high-dose hemodialysis may prove useful as a temporizing measure, pending availability of glucarpidase.

CISPLATIN

Cisplatin is commonly used for the treatment of solid organ malignancies, but dose-related nephrotoxicity is a major limiting factor in its use. Tubular injury, which can be permanent, may result in acute and subacute kidney injury, a Fanconi-like syndrome and severe hypomagnesemia. HUS can also occur when the drug is combined with bleomycin or gemcitabine. Strategies to minimize cisplatin nephrotoxicity are summarized in Box 31.2. In some cases, carboplatin can be used as a less nephrotoxic alternative.

IFOSFAMIDE

High cumulative doses of ifosfamide can cause severe tubular damage, manifesting clinically as acute or chronic kidney dysfunction, a Fanconi-like syndrome, or diabetes insipidus. The incidence of AKI in adults treated with various doses of ifosfamide is 4% to 17%. Ifosfamide-associated kidney dysfunction can progress weeks or even months after the drug is stopped, and the Fanconi-like syndrome can be severe and permanent.

OTHER DRUGS

The nitrosoureas (lomustine, carmustine, streptozocin) occasionally cause severe and progressive renal tubular damage. Tyrosine kinase inhibitors such as sunitinib and imatinib have been associated with various forms of kidney injury, including reduced glomerular filtration rate (GFR), proteinuria, and thrombotic microangiopathy.

VASCULAR DISEASES

The most common vascular cause of AKI in patients with cancer is HUS/TTP, which may occur as a complication of cancer itself or, more commonly, as a complication of its treatment (Table 31.3). Carcinomas, particularly gastric, breast, lung, and pancreatic, are the most frequently implicated cancers, whereas mitomycin C, gemcitabine, bleomycin, and cisplatin are the most frequently implicated drugs. HUS/TTP occurs in 0.3% of patients treated with gemcitabine, with median time to diagnosis of 8 months after initiation of gemcitabine. Hypertension is a prominent feature in most cases, with either new or worsened hypertension preceding the diagnosis of HUS/TTP. Patients treated with chemotherapy regimens that are associated with HUS/TTP should be watched

Table 31.3 Settings in Which HUS/TTP May Arise in Individuals With Cancer

Setting	Comment
Spontaneously (before chemotherapy)	Rare
During/after chemotherapy	Gemcitabine, bleomycin + cisplatin, mitomycin C most commonly implicated drugs
During/after VEGF therapy	Uncommon
After HCT	Mainly associated with allogeneic HCT; onset may be delayed

HCT, Hematopoietic cell transplantation; *HUS/TTP,* hemolytic uremic syndrome/thrombotic thrombocytopenic purpura; *VEGF,* vascular endothelial growth factor.

closely for subtle signs of an evolving syndrome, including increasing blood pressure, creatinine and lactate dehydrogenase (LDH), schistocytosis, and falling haptoglobin. Anemia and thrombocytopenia may also occur, but these are difficult to interpret in the setting of chemotherapy. Full-blown HUS/TTP can arise many months after initiation (or completion) of chemotherapy; a similar phenomenon occurs after HCT (see below). Treatment involves cessation of the offending agent, control of hypertension, and other supportive measures. There are few data to support the use of plasma exchange, but some centers use it in severe, resistant cases. Hypertension, proteinuria, and HUS/TTP can also complicate therapy with vascular endothelial growth factor (VEGF) inhibitors, even when these agents are given by the intraocular route alone!

POSTRENAL ACUTE KIDNEY INJURY

Intratubular obstruction due to uric acid (in TLS), methotrexate, or myeloma casts has been discussed earlier. Bilateral urinary tract obstruction, which can occur at any level of the urinary tract, is relatively common in cancer patients and should be considered in the differential diagnosis of AKI. Common obstructing tumors include prostate, bladder, uterus, and cervix cancers (Figure 31.3). Not surprisingly, prognosis is poor, because bilateral obstruction implies high tumor bulk. Nevertheless, nephrostomies and internal ureteric stents can be a good short- and medium-term treatment option. Obstructive uropathy can occur in the absence of hydronephrosis because encasement of the collecting system by retroperitoneal tumor or fibrous tissue may prevent pelviureteric dilation. Retroperitoneal fibrosis can be associated with previous pelvic irradiation or malignancies such as lymphomas and sarcomas.

ELECTROLYTE DISORDERS

Malignancy can be associated with a variety of electrolyte disorders, including hypercalcemia, hypokalemia, hypomagnesemia, hyponatremia, and hypernatremia. Hypercalcemia has been discussed earlier. Hypokalemia can result from gastrointestinal or kidney losses, with the latter most often due to tubular injury from ifosfamide or cisplatin. Tubular injury from these drugs can also cause long-term magnesium wasting and hypomagnesemia.

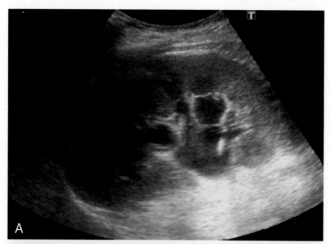

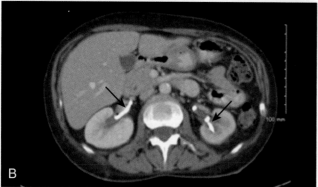

Figure 31.3 A shows hydronephrosis of the right kidney on ultrasonography. This patient was diagnosed with obstructive uropathy secondary to a tumor of the uterine cervix and required insertion of bilateral nephrostomies (indicated by *arrows* on **B**).

Malignancy is a common cause of the syndrome of inappropriate antidiuretic hormone secretion (SIADH; see Chapter 7). Intravenous cyclophosphamide, vincristine, and vinblastine can also cause SIADH, whereas hypovolemic hyponatremia may occur with chemotherapy-related gastrointestinal fluid losses. Hypernatremia is less common, although both primary brain tumors and brain metastases can cause central diabetes insipidus, whereas hypercalcemia can cause nephrogenic diabetes insipidus (Chapter 8).

KIDNEY DISEASE IN HEMATOPOIETIC CELL TRANSPLANTATION

The general purpose of hematopoietic cell transplantation (HCT) is to allow administration of otherwise lethal (and ideally curative) doses of chemoradiotherapy, followed by engraftment of stem or progenitor cells for marrow recovery. Most commonly, HCT is used to treat hematologic cancers, but other indications include genetic disorders (e.g., immunodeficiencies) and severe autoimmune diseases. Conventional myeloablative HCT uses an intensive conditioning regimen (high-dose chemotherapy and radiotherapy) to ablate cancer cells and bone marrow; the hematopoietic system is then reconstituted by infusion and engraftment of stem cells. In allogeneic myeloablative HCT, nonself stem cells are used, whereas in autologous myeloablative HCT, the patient's own cells are used. Nonmyeloablative conditioning regimens have been developed to allow allogeneic HCT in older and sicker patients who would not tolerate standard regimens. In both forms of allogeneic HCT, acute and chronic graft-versus-host disease (GVHD) can be problematic, and calcineurin inhibitors often are used to prevent and treat this complication. The main organs affected by GVHD are the liver, gastrointestinal tract, and skin. Both AKI and CKD are common complications of HCT and are associated with higher early and late mortality. Types and kidney complications of HCT are summarized in Table 31.4.

Table 31.4   Overview of HCT Types and Their Kidney Complications

	Allogeneic Myeloablative	Autologous Myeloablative	Allogeneic Nonmyeloablative
Cancers treated	Many leukemias, lymphomas, myelodysplastic syndromes	Lymphomas, multiple myeloma	As for allogeneic myeloablative
Intensity of conditioning regimen	High	High	Low
GVHD after HCT	Yes (CNIs used as prophylaxis)	No	Yes (CNIs used as prophylaxis)
AKI after HCT	Common; sometimes severe	Rare	Common; rarely severe
Causes of AKI (usually first 3 months)	VOD, shock syndromes, nephrotoxic drugs, CNIs	Shock syndromes, nephrotoxic drugs, occasionally VOD	CNIs
CKD after HCT	Common	Common (but not severe)	Mild forms probably common
Causes of CKD	Irreversible AKI, renal TMA, CNIs; membranous nephropathy	Irreversible AKI; recurrence of original disease (myeloma)	Irreversible AKI, CNIs, membranous nephropathy

AKI, Acute kidney injury; *CKD,* chronic kidney disease; *CNI,* calcineurin inhibitors; *GVHD,* graft-versus-host disease; *HCT,* hematopoietic cell transplantation; *TMA,* thrombotic microangiopathy; *VOD,* venoocclusive disease.

AKI AFTER HCT

CAUSES AND PRESENTATION

AKI is common after HCT (see Table 31.4), most often occurring after myeloablative allogeneic HCT, reflecting the propensity of this regimen to cause profound immunosuppression (with associated risk for severe sepsis) and liver damage (with associated risk for hepatorenal syndrome). Furthermore, calcineurin inhibitors are routinely prescribed for the first 100 days after myeloablative allogeneic HCT, potentially exacerbating the effects of volume depletion and hypoperfusion on the kidney. Myeloablative autologous HCT has an intermediate incidence of AKI, whereas severe AKI is least common after nonmyeloablative HCT, because of the shorter period of pancytopenia and low incidence of hepatorenal syndrome. Regardless of the form of HCT, if dialysis is required for severe AKI, the overall prognosis is very poor (early mortality >70%).

It is useful to consider the causes of AKI according to the time period after HCT. Immediate AKI from TLS or stem cell infusion toxicity is rare; however, during the first few weeks of myeloablative HCT, when the conditioning regimen has caused pancytopenia, mucositis, and liver damage, recipients are at high risk for many forms of AKI. These include prerenal syndromes due to calcineurin inhibitors (CNIs), hypovolemia (caused by vomiting, diarrhea, or bleeding), acute liver disease, and ATN due to septic shock and nephrotoxic drugs (amphotericin, aminoglycosides). Obstructive uropathy is unusual but can be due to severe hemorrhagic cystitis (high-dose cyclophosphamide or viral infection) or fungal infection.

Venoocclusive disease (VOD) of the liver, also known as sinusoidal obstruction syndrome, is one of the more common causes of severe AKI after myeloablative HCT, especially allogeneic HCT. The cause is thought to be radiotherapy- and chemotherapy-induced damage to the endothelium of hepatic venules with subsequent venular thrombosis and sinusoidal and portal hypertension. Risk factors for development of VOD include older age, female sex, preexisting liver disease, use of cyclophosphamide or busulfan in the conditioning regimen, and exposure to methotrexate, progesterone, or antimicrobial drugs. VOD manifests as a form of hepatorenal syndrome, usually within the first 30 days of HCT. The severity of disease varies greatly. Diagnosis is based on typical clinical and laboratory features, including fluid overload, right upper quadrant pain and tenderness, and abnormal LFTs. Occasionally, liver biopsy is performed to exclude other forms of liver disease. Mild to moderate cases often resolve with supportive therapy alone, but severe VOD complicated by liver, kidney, and frequently respiratory failure carries a mortality approaching 100%.

DIAGNOSIS AND MANAGEMENT

The evaluation of AKI following HCT should be similar to that of any patient with hospital-acquired AKI but with particular attention to the possibility of VOD. The patient's cancer diagnosis, conditioning regimen, and type of HCT should be carefully reviewed. Where possible, further exposure to nephrotoxic drugs should be minimized. Reduction in CNI dosage should be considered, particularly if trough concentrations are high. Mild to moderate forms of VOD require supportive therapy, including fluid restriction and cautious diuresis, whereas severe forms of VOD involve multiorgan support, including kidney replacement therapy, often with continuous therapies. Defibrotide, a polynucleotide with antithrombotic and antiischemic properties, may be a promising agent to treat VOD that arises after HCT.

CKD AFTER HCT

CKD is an important long-term complication of HCT, particularly allogeneic HCT. Reported rates vary widely, with one recent review reporting an incidence of 17% in those surviving at least 100 days after HCT. Causes of CKD are summarized in Table 31.4.

RENAL THROMBOTIC MICROANGIOPATHY

Subacute or chronic renal thrombotic microangiopathy (TMA) is an important cause of CKD (particularly severe CKD) after HCT. It typically presents 3 to 12 months after HCT. Characteristic clinical features are slowly rising creatinine, hypertension, and disproportionate anemia. Urine dipstick shows variable proteinuria and hematuria. Some cases have a more fulminant presentation (e.g., nephritic syndrome). Careful review of laboratory data will often show evidence of a low-grade TMA: intermittent or persistent elevation in LDH, low serum haptoglobin, low platelets, low hemoglobin, and sometimes schistocytosis. Kidney imaging is usually unremarkable, and kidney biopsy is rarely required unless the presentation is atypical, because biopsy findings are unlikely to significantly alter management and biopsy carries increased risks in patients with thrombocytopenia and other comorbidities. Histopathology typically shows microthrombi in arterioles and glomerular capillaries, mesangiolysis, glomerular basement membrane duplication, and tubular injury with interstitial fibrosis (Figure 31.4). The main cause of TMA after HCT likely is direct damage to the renal endothelium and tubulointerstitium by the chemoradiotherapy conditioning regimen (particularly the radiotherapy component, Figure 31.5). Kidney tissue has slower turnover than mucosal cells and thus manifests such damage much later. Other factors, such as infection, GVHD, CNIs, and activation of the renin angiotensin system, may play a role. Treatment is mainly supportive, whereas prevention involves shielding the kidneys from radiation and avoidance of nephrotoxic agents at the time of conditioning.

CALCINEURIN INHIBITOR AND SIROLIMUS NEPHROTOXICITY

Calcineurin inhibitors are routinely prescribed after allogeneic HCT to prevent and treat GVHD; however, because CNIs are often stopped 3 to 6 months after HCT (unless there is ongoing GVHD), their contribution to CKD is generally thought to be limited. We have noted a high incidence of TMA when sirolimus is added to CNI therapy, but fortunately this is often reversible.

GLOMERULAR DISEASE

Nephrotic syndrome has been described after both allogeneic and autologous HCT. In allogeneic HCT, it appears to be strongly associated with the presence of GVHD and

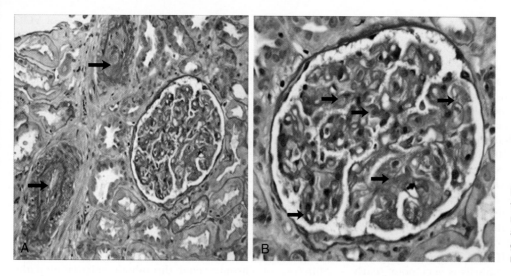

Figure 31.4 Renal biopsy shows typical features of renal TMA with microthrombi in the arterioles (**A**) and glomerular capillaries, mesangiolysis, and duplication of the glomerular basement membrane (**B**).

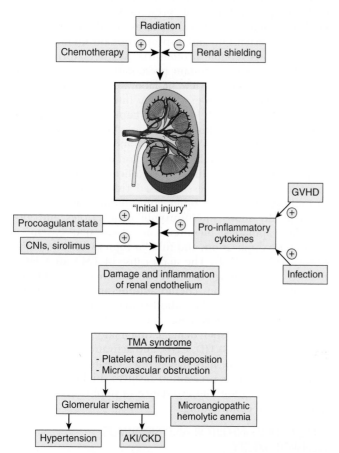

Figure 31.5 Putative pathogenesis of thrombotic microangiopathy after after hematopoietic cell transplantation. *AKI,* Acute kidney injury; *CKD,* chronic kidney disease; *CNI,* calcineurin inhibitors; *GVHD,* graft-versus-host disease; *TMA,* thrombotic microangiopathy.

responds to additional immunosuppression. De novo membranous nephropathy is the most common biopsy finding, although minimal change disease has also been reported. The original hematologic disease (such as myeloma) may also recur with kidney involvement.

DIAGNOSIS AND MANAGEMENT

Careful review of the patient's pre- and post-HCT history is essential. Attention should be paid to the type of HCT and conditioning regimen (in particular, whether total body irradiation was used and at what dose) and degree of exposure to nephrotoxins. Examination frequently shows hypertension and hypervolemia and sometimes skin GVHD. Laboratory results should be reviewed carefully and tests repeated to assess for TMA because the laboratory features of TMA are often intermittent and not florid. Urine dipstick findings of hematuria and moderate proteinuria are suggestive of renal TMA but are not specific to this condition. As with AKI after HCT, kidney ultrasound is often used to exclude postrenal causes, but other imaging studies are usually unnecessary. As discussed earlier, kidney biopsy is rarely indicated. Treatment is similar to that recommended for any patient with CKD, and blood pressure control is warranted. In particular, blockade of the renin-angiotensin system slows progression in animal models of radiation nephropathy and is recommended both for this reason and for its beneficial effects in hypertensive proteinuric CKD. CNI doses should probably be minimized if safe to do so. Plasma exchange does not appear to be beneficial in this setting.

A subset of patients will progress to ESRD, and these patients have worse survival when treated with dialysis than non-HCT controls. Suitability for kidney transplantation should be judged on a case-by-case basis. Occasionally, the allogeneic stem cell donor can donate a kidney; a great benefit of this approach is that a state of tolerance to the allograft should exist, and hence minimal or no immunosuppression is required. If this option is not available and the patient receives a conventional kidney transplant, low-dose immunosuppression should be prescribed because HCT recipients may not have normal immunity and thus remain at higher risk for infection.

CONCLUSION

Acute kidney injury and CKD are important complications of cancer and its treatment. As new chemotherapy regimens are constantly introduced or modified, the spectrum of cancer-associated kidney disease changes. Nevertheless, a simple and systematic approach to assess and treat potential prerenal, intrarenal, and postrenal causes is indicated in all patients. Prompt diagnosis and treatment of kidney disease is vital—both to improve kidney outcomes and to ensure that patients are in optimal condition for further cancer therapy. Close cooperation with oncology colleagues is essential to improve outcomes in these complex patients.

KEY BIBLIOGRAPHY

Ando M, Mori J, Ohashi K, et al: A comparative assessment of the RIFLE, AKIN and conventional criteria for acute kidney injury after hematopoietic SCT, *Bone Marrow Transplant* 45(9):1427-1434, 2010 Sep.

Ando M, Ohashi K, Akiyama H, et al: Chronic kidney disease in long-term survivors of myeloablative allogeneic haematopoietic cell transplantation: prevalence and risk factors, *Nephrol Dial Transplant* 25(1):278-282, 2010 Jan.

Audard V, Larousserie F, Grimbert P, et al: Minimal change nephrotic syndrome and classical Hodgkin's lymphoma: report of 21 cases and review of the literature, *Kidney Int* 69(12):2251-2260, 2006 Jun.

Cairo MS, Coiffier B, Reiter A, et al: TLS Expert Panel. Recommendations for the evaluation of risk and prophylaxis of tumour lysis syndrome (TLS) in adults and children with malignant diseases: an expert TLS panel consensus, *Br J Haematol* 149(4):578-586, 2010 May.

Coppell JA, Richardson PG, Soiffer R, et al: Hepatic veno-occlusive disease following stem cell transplantation: incidence, clinical course, and outcome, *Biol Blood Marrow Transplant* 16(2):157-168, 2010 Feb.

Cutler C, Henry NL, Magee C, et al: Sirolimus and thrombotic microangiopathy after allogeneic hematopoietic stem cell transplantation, *Biol Blood Marrow Transplant* 11(7):551-557, 2005 Jul.

George JN, Li X, McMinn JR, et al: Thrombotic thrombocytopenic purpura-hemolytic uremic syndrome following allogeneic HPC transplantation: a diagnostic dilemma, *Transfusion* 44(2):294-304, 2004 Feb.

Ho VT, Revta C, Richardson PG: Hepatic veno-occlusive disease after hematopoietic stem cell transplantation: update on defibrotide and other current investigational therapies, *Bone Marrow Transplant* 41(3):229-237, 2008 Feb.

Humphreys BD, Sharman JP, Henderson JM, et al: Gemcitabine-associated thrombotic microangiopathy, *Cancer* 100(12):2664-2670, 2004 Jun 15.

Humphreys BD, Soiffer RJ, Magee CC: Renal failure associated with cancer and its treatment: an update, *J Am Soc Nephrol* 16(1):151-161, 2005 Jan.

Jhaveri KD, Flombaum CD, Kroog G, et al: Nephrotoxicities associated with the use of tyrosine kinase inhibitors: a single-center experience and review of the literature, *Nephron Clin Pract* 117(4):c312-c319, 2011.

Markowitz GS, Appel GB, Fine PL, et al: Collapsing focal segmental glomerulosclerosis following treatment with high-dose pamidronate, *J Am Soc Nephrol* 12(6):1164-1172, 2001 Jun.

Markowitz GS, Fine PL, Stack JI, et al: Toxic acute tubular necrosis following treatment with zoledronate (Zometa), *Kidney Int* 64(1):281-289, 2003 Jul.

Pankhurst T, Savage CO, Gordon C, et al: Malignancy is increased in ANCA-associated vasculitis, *Rheumatology (Oxford)* 43(12):1532-1535, 2004 Dec.

Parikh CR, McSweeney PA, Korular D, et al: Renal dysfunction in allogeneic hematopoietic cell transplantation, *Kidney Int* 62(2):566-573, 2002 Aug.

Schlondorff JS, Mendez GP, Rennke HG, et al: Electrolyte abnormalities and progressive renal failure in a cancer patient, *Kidney Int* 71(11):1181-1184, 2007 Jun.

Stewart AF: Clinical practice. Hypercalcemia associated with cancer, *N Engl J Med* 352(4):373-379, 2005 Jan 27.

Troxell ML, Pilapil M, Miklos DB, et al: Renal pathology in hematopoietic cell transplantation recipients, *Mod Pathol* 21(4):396-406, 2008 Apr.

Widemann BC, Adamson PC: Understanding and managing methotrexate nephrotoxicity, *Oncologist* 11(6):694-703, 2006 Jun.

Widemann BC, Balis FM, Kempf-Bielack B, et al: High-dose methotrexate-induced nephrotoxicity in patients with osteosarcoma, *Cancer* 100(10):2222-2232, 2004 May 15.

Full bibliography can be found on www.expertconsult.com.

ACUTE KIDNEY INJURY

32 Pathophysiology of Acute Kidney Injury

Sushrut S. Waikar | Lakshman Gunaratnam | Joseph V. Bonventre

Acute kidney injury (AKI), previously known as acute renal failure (ARF), has been classically defined as the sudden impairment of kidney function resulting in the retention of nitrogenous and other waste products normally cleared by the kidneys. AKI can arise from a heterogeneous group of conditions that lead to a reduction in the glomerular filtration rate (GFR) and, often, the urine volume. The Acute Kidney Injury Network proposed the term AKI to better capture the entire spectrum of ARF that can range in severity from asymptomatic changes in laboratory parameters to life threatening disorders of volume regulation, electrolytes, and acid-base composition of the plasma. The Kidney Disease: Improving Global Outcomes (KDIGO) Clinical Practice Guideline for Acute Kidney Injury proposed the following as the most recent consensus definition of AKI: a rise in serum creatinine concentration of ≥0.3 mg/dl within 48 hours or ≥50% increase within 7 days, or urine output less than 0.5 mL/kg/h for 6 hours. We use the term AKI instead of ARF to describe this syndrome, although many clinicians will continue to use the terms ARF and AKI interchangeably.

In considering the pathophysiology of AKI, it is important to recognize that the serum creatinine level, which is used to estimate GFR, is a very insensitive biomarker for AKI. This is because its rise is delayed after an insult and its level is affected by several factors other than the GFR. Identification of early, sensitive, and specific biomarkers of acute injury, similar to troponin in cardiology, should enable clinicians to recognize kidney injury at earlier time points when the concentration of serum creatinine has not yet been affected. Studies are underway to determine whether assessing kidney function by using creatinine or injury biomarkers can better predict outcome or the need for therapeutic intervention in human AKI.

Historically, AKI has been classified based on its causes—prerenal, intrinsic renal, or postrenal—to simplify the approach to a differential diagnosis. Prerenal AKI, which is common, is a physiologic response to renal hypoperfusion without tubular injury (Fig. 32.1). A functional change in the GFR results from depletion of the intravascular volume resulting from bleeding, low serum protein levels and oncotic pressure, or capillary leak. Congestive heart failure and liver disease can result in reduced cardiac output, splanchnic vasodilation, third spacing of total body water, adverse neurohormonal adaptation, and increased renal venous and intraabdominal pressures, which can all contribute to reduced renal perfusion. Diseases of the large and intermediately sized renal vessels can also interfere with perfusion. The integrity of the renal parenchyma is not disrupted in prerenal AKI, and glomerular filtration is restored on prompt reestablishment of more normal renal perfusion. Postrenal causes of AKI include the various conditions that impede the flow of urine because of urinary tract obstruction (e.g., prostatic hypertrophy). Intrinsic renal or intrarenal AKI is associated with conditions that affect the renal parenchyma (i.e., glomeruli, tubules, interstitium, or vasculature). Ischemia, nephrotoxin exposure, and sepsis are among the most common causes of intrarenal AKI. Other causes of intrinsic AKI are discussed in various chapters in this *Primer*. The clinical approach to differentiating prerenal azotemia, intrinsic causes, and obstruction in AKI is discussed in Chapter 33.

The term *acute tubular necrosis* (ATN) is frequently used to refer to AKI resulting from severe or prolonged hypoperfusion or toxic injury. This is a controversial term, because it is a pathologic description, not a clinical one. The term should not be applied to a patient unless there is documented evidence of tubular cell necrosis such as granular casts or tubular cells in the urine sediment, or biopsy evidence. Prerenal AKI and ATN are at opposite ends of the spectrum of manifestations of renal hypoperfusion, but the most common cause of ATN is progressive prerenal AKI with impaired oxygen delivery to the tubules of the kidney. Ischemic or toxic AKI often follows predictable stages: an initiation phase, characterized by steady increments in serum creatinine levels and reduced urinary volumes; a maintenance phase, in which the GFR is stable at a reduced level and the urinary volume may vary; and a recovery phase, in which the serum creatinine level falls as tubular function is restored. The initiation phase can be further subdivided into initiation and extension periods, as the injury may not occur all at once but instead may be stuttering. All cases of AKI, however, do not follow such a well-defined sequence of events, nor do they all result in oliguria.

This chapter focuses on ischemic and toxic AKI, because our understanding of the pathophysiologic mechanisms of AKI is largely derived from animal models and human studies of these disease entities. In the following sections, we discuss five characteristics of the pathophysiology of AKI: (1) imbalance between vasoconstrictive and vasodilatory factors, (2) inflammation, (3) tubular dysfunction and intratubular obstruction, (4) cell death by necrosis or apoptosis, and (5) adaptive and maladaptive repair

PATHOGENESIS

The pathogenesis of AKI can often be traced to a mismatch at the level of the nephron between oxygen and nutrient delivery and energy demand, or to the direct injury of the tubular cell or vascular endothelium. Relative oxygen deprivation is often not generalized, because certain regions of

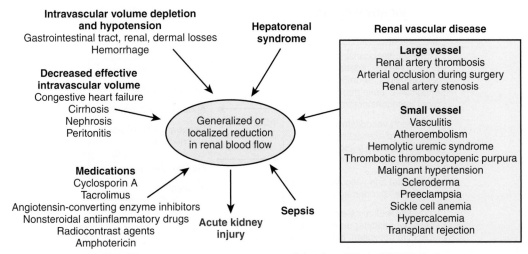

Figure 32.1   Causes of reduced generalized or regional renal blood flow (RBF). Various pathophysiologic states and medications can contribute to the reduction of RBF, causing generalized or localized ischemia to the kidney leading to acute kidney injury. A partial list of contributors is shown here, pointing to ischemia as a common pathway in a variety of clinical states affecting the kidney. (Adapted from Bonventre JV, Yang L: Cellular pathophysiology of ischemic acute kidney injury, *J Clin Invest* 121:4210, 2011.)

the kidney are differentially susceptible to injury because of variations in blood flow or oxygen demand. Because of the complex relationship between the vascular and tubular compartments in the kidney, localized tubular injury can have amplified functional consequences. Figure 32.2 summarizes the complex interplay of vascular and tubular processes that ultimately lead to organ dysfunction.

VASCULAR FACTORS

Although a transient reduction in renal blood flow (RBF) has been observed on reflow in animals after renal ischemia, many cases of profound changes in the GFR in humans are not believed to be related to large generalized reductions in RBF. In toxic AKI, there is little perturbation of renal hemodynamics, but there can be significant organ dysfunction and pathology. The contributions of intrarenal vasoconstriction and regional alterations in blood flow to the pathophysiology of AKI have become increasingly recognized. Potent vasoconstrictors have been identified in the ischemic kidney, including endothelin 1, angiotensin II, thromboxane A_2, prostaglandin H_2, leukotrienes C_4 and D_4, and adenosine, and there is increased sympathetic nerve stimulation. Results of several studies indicate that blockade of endothelin receptors before an ischemic insult protects the rat kidney from injury. Successful reversal strategies of postinjury vasoconstriction in animal models with improved functional response have not, however, translated into practical therapies for humans. Angiotensin converting enzyme inhibition and angiotensin receptor blockade are widely implicated in the induction of ischemic injury through prevention of constriction of postglomerular arterioles with subsequent adverse effects on the forces for filtration within the glomerulus. Renal vasoconstriction in the face of global vasodilation in sepsis-associated AKI is hypothesized to be a physiologic protective mechanism to maintain perfusion pressure to other vital organs such as the brain and heart.

AKI is also characterized by decreased responsiveness of the resistance vessels to vasodilators such as acetylcholine, bradykinin, and nitric oxide, and decreased production

of certain vasodilators. The postischemic kidney endures further injury from perturbations to blood flow within the renal parenchyma due to intrarenal interstitial edema, vascular congestion, and hypoperfusion to the outer medulla. Intrarenal hypoperfusion often persists even after blood flow improves with reperfusion. During early periods of reduced renal perfusion, there is relative preservation of tubular integrity, but as the reduction in blood flow persists, it exacerbates tissue hypoxia and contributes to cellular injury in the cortical and outer medullary tubules. Reduced blood flow to the outer medulla can have particularly detrimental effects on the tubular cells in that region of the kidney, because the outer medulla is, even under normal circumstances, relatively hypoxic because of the countercurrent exchange properties of the vasa recta.

INFLAMMATION

Inflammation is an important component of human AKI. For instance, ischemia and reperfusion cause renal synthesis of proinflammatory cytokines, infiltration of the kidney by leukocytes (neutrophils, macrophages, B cells, T cells), activation of the complement system, and upregulation of vascular adhesion molecules. Although it is incompletely understood, inflammation contributes in an important way to both the reduction in local blood flow within the kidney and to direct tubular injury that leads to reduced kidney function.

The innate and adaptive immune responses are fundamental contributors to the pathobiology of ischemic injury. The innate component is responsible for the early response to infection or injury, and it is independent of foreign antigens. Toll-like receptors, which are important for the detection of exogenous microbial products and the development of antigen-dependent adaptive immunity, recognize host material released during injury and play a central role in the activation of the innate immune system.

Antiinflammatory influences may be important to reduce the injury associated with ischemia and reperfusion or toxins. Resolvins and protectins are families of naturally occurring omega-3 fatty acid docosahexaenoic acid metabolites.

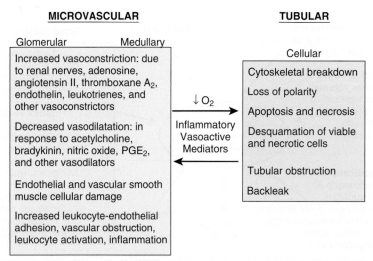

MICROVASCULAR

Glomerular   Medullary

Increased vasoconstriction: due to renal nerves, adenosine, angiotensin II, thromboxane A_2, endothelin, leukotrienes, and other vasoconstrictors

Decreased vasodilatation: in response to acetylcholine, bradykinin, nitric oxide, PGE_2, and other vasodilators

Endothelial and vascular smooth muscle cellular damage

Increased leukocyte-endothelial adhesion, vascular obstruction, leukocyte activation, inflammation

$\downarrow O_2$

Inflammatory Vasoactive Mediators

TUBULAR

Cellular

Cytoskeletal breakdown

Loss of polarity

Apoptosis and necrosis

Desquamation of viable and necrotic cells

Tubular obstruction

Backleak

Figure 32.2   The pathophysiology of acute kidney injury may be divided into a microvascular component and a tubular component. With acute kidney injury, there is enhanced vasoconstriction and decreased vasodilatation in response to agents that are present in the postischemic kidney. With increased endothelial and vascular smooth muscle cellular damage, there is enhanced leukocyte-endothelial adhesion, leading to activation of the coagulation system, vascular obstruction, leukocyte activation, and potentiation of inflammation. At the level of the tubule epithelial cell, there is cytoskeletal breakdown and loss of polarity, followed by apoptosis and necrosis, intratubular obstruction, and backleak of glomerular filtrate through a denuded basement membrane. Tubule cells generate inflammatory vasoactive mediators, which can enhance vascular compromise. In a positive-feedback process, vascular compromise results in decreased oxygen delivery to the tubules, which generates vasoactive inflammatory mediators that enhance the vasoconstriction and the endothelial-leukocyte interactions. *PGE$_2$*, Prostaglandin E$_2$.

They are produced in animals in response to ischemia-reperfusion injury; when administered to animals, these compounds can reduce the severity of AKI caused by ischemia and reperfusion.

LEUKOCYTE-ENDOTHELIAL INTERACTIONS

With ischemia and reperfusion, endothelial cells upregulate integrins, selectins, and members of the immunoglobulin superfamily of adhesion proteins, including intercellular adhesion molecule 1 (ICAM-1) and vascular cell adhesion molecule (VCAM). In animal studies, anti–ICAM-1 antibodies or genetic deletion of ICAM-1 protects the kidney from injury. A number of vasoactive compounds may also affect leukocyte-endothelial interactions. Vasodilators, such as nitric oxide, also can have antiinflammatory effects. Nitric oxide inhibits adhesion of neutrophils to endothelial cells exposed to tumor necrosis factor-α (TNFα). Enhanced leukocyte-endothelial interactions can result in cell–cell adhesion, which can physically impede blood flow. These interactions also activate leukocytes and endothelial cells, and contribute to the generation of local factors that promote vasoconstriction, especially in the presence of other vasoactive mediators. These factors all contribute to compromised local blood flow and impaired tubular cell metabolism, and, if severe enough, cell death. Because of the anatomic relationships of vessels and tubules in the outer medulla, these leukocyte-endothelial interactions compromise blood flow to the outer medulla to a greater extent than to the cortex.

CONTRIBUTION OF TUBULAR CELLS TO INFLAMMATORY INJURY

Both the S3 segment of the proximal tubule and the medullary thick ascending limb of the loop of Henle generate proinflammatory and chemotactic cytokines, such as TNFα

and macrophage chemotactic factors. In addition, inflamed tubular epithelial cells expressing receptors of the innate immune response after ischemia and reperfusion produce complement and express complement receptors. Proximal tubular epithelia are also postulated to acquire the ability to regulate T-lymphocyte activity through expression of costimulatory molecules. Therefore, instead of being a passive victim of injury in AKI, the tubular epithelium is an active participant in the inflammatory response that occurs during the pathogenesis of AKI.

TUBULAR FACTORS

Whether the injury is related to oxygen deprivation, toxin exposure, or a combination of factors, there are many common features of the epithelial cell response. The processes of injury and repair to the kidney epithelium are depicted schematically in Figure 32.3. Injury results in rapid loss of cell polarity and cytoskeletal integrity. With severe injury, cells are desquamated, leaving regions where the basement membrane is the only barrier between the filtrate and the peritubular interstitium. This, together with loss of cell–cell contacts, allows backleak of the filtrate that further contributes to decreased clearance of metabolic waste by the kidney. Backleak is especially prominent when the pressure in the tubule is increased by intratubular obstruction resulting from cellular debris in the lumen that interacts with matrix proteins such as fibronectin.

MECHANISMS OF TUBULAR INJURY

The breakdown in the structural integrity of renal tubular epithelial cells is brought about by one or more specific pathogenic mechanisms of cellular injury that are triggered by relative oxygen deprivation or toxin exposure. A major consequence of acute ischemia and tissue hypoxia is the

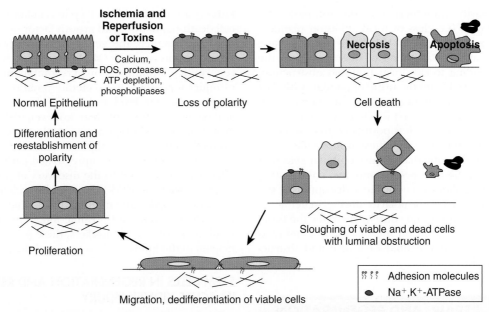

Figure 32.3   With ischemia-reperfusion or toxin-induced injury to the kidney, an early response is loss of the brush border and polarity of the epithelial cell, with mislocation of adhesion molecules, Na⁺,K⁺-ATPase, and other proteins. With increasing injury, cell death occurs by means of necrosis or apoptosis. Some of the necrotic debris is released into the lumen, where it interacts with luminal proteins and can ultimately result in obstruction. Because of the mislocation of adhesion molecules, viable epithelial cells lift off the basement membrane and are found in the urine. The kidney can respond to the injury by initiating a repair process if provided sufficient nutrients and oxygen delivery, and if the basement membrane integrity has not been altered irreparably. Viable epithelial cells migrate and cover denuded areas of the basement membrane. The source of these cells appears to be the kidney itself, not the bone marrow. Bone marrow cells may contribute to the interstitial cellular infiltrate and may produce factors that modulate inflammation and facilitate repair. Cells replacing the epithelium may be derived from dedifferentiated epithelial cells or from a subpopulation of progenitor cells in the tubule. The cells then undergo division and replace lost cells. Ultimately, the cells differentiate and reestablish the normal polarity of the epithelium. *ATP,* Adenosine triphosphate; *ROS,* reactive oxygen species.

depletion of intracellular adenosine triphosphate (ATP) levels because of ATP degradation, and a switch in some epithelia to anaerobic metabolism. Hypoxia and exposure to certain toxins, such as endotoxin or other factors present in sepsis, can also result in mitochondrial dysfunction. The duration of ischemia is a critical determinant of cell survival after reperfusion, because prolonged ischemia can lead to irreversible mitochondrial dysfunction. The major consequences of ATP depletion that lead to cellular injury include the loss of ion gradients, abnormalities of the tight and adherence junctions between epithelial cells, cell swelling, increased intracellular calcium, and activation of intracellular lipases and proteases.

Reactive oxygen species (ROS) that are generated during reperfusion and as a result of the inflammatory response play a major role in cell injury in both ischemic and toxic AKI. ROS are generated by activated, infiltrating leukocytes and by epithelial cells, and the species are directly toxic to tubular cells through the peroxidation of lipids, denaturation of proteins, and damage to DNA.

Activation of phospholipases is a well-documented mode of cellular injury after ischemia in various organs, including the kidney. Increased phospholipase activity leads to marked loss of phospholipid mass and intracellular accumulation of free fatty acids, including arachidonic acid, lysophospholipids, diacylglycerol, and inositol phosphates. Free arachidonic acid leads to the production of eicosanoids, which act as vasoactive and chemotactic mediators that contribute to functional and cytotoxic injury to the kidney during AKI.

FATE OF INDIVIDUAL RENAL TUBULAR CELLS IN ACUTE KIDNEY INJURY

In most cases of AKI, many tubular cells that remain viable or are sublethally injured are able to recover functionally and structurally. The cells within the straight segment (i.e., S3 segment or pars recta) of the proximal tubule and the thick ascending limb in the outer medulla are more susceptible to injury than cells in the cortical region.

The renal tubule consists of highly polarized cells that line the tubular basement membrane. These cells have microvilli that constitute the brush border on their apical side, an array of focal adhesion molecules on the basolateral side that mediate crucial matrix–cell interactions, and tight junctions at cell–cell borders that mediate barrier function. An intricate cytoskeletal network supports the complex cellular architecture and cell polarity of the renal tubular cells. Sublethal damage to tubular cells results in actin cytoskeletal derangements, leading to loss of cell polarity, loss of the brush border, and disruption of cell–cell and cell–substratum adhesion. The actin cytoskeleton is composed of bundles of microfilaments made of G-actin monomers woven into polymers of filamentous actin. ATP depletion induces disassembly of actin bundles and microfilaments. With loss of cell polarity, the expression of Na⁺, K⁺-ATPase channels, normally restricted to the basolateral surface, are rapidly redistributed to the apical membrane during anoxia. Data from ischemia-reperfusion animal models suggest that ischemia causes loss of the junctional complex; this, together with the loss of epithelial cells, explains the backleak of glomerular filtrate and contributes to the functional decline in measured or estimated GFR.

The loss of polarity and tethering of adhesion molecules to the actin network (i.e., loss of focal adhesion plaques) results in detachment of renal epithelial cells from the basement membrane and the shedding of these cells into the tubular lumen, leading to cast formation and obstruction. Tubular cells recovered from the urine of patients with AKI and animals with ischemic injury can be viable, demonstrating that cell death is not required for desquamation of epithelial cells matrix. Moreover, it is postulated that sloughed cells with aberrant expression of adhesion molecules (e.g., integrins) attach to the sublethally injured tubular cells that remain adherent to the basement membrane, contributing further to intraluminal obstruction. Thus, disruption of the actin cytoskeleton and loss of polarity during ischemic or toxic injury may have profound consequences for the tubular cell, and the cells that lift off the basement membrane play a fundamental role in the tubular backleak and obstruction observed in AKI.

CELL DEATH, REPAIR, AND REGENERATION

CELL DEATH BY NECROSIS AND APOPTOSIS IN ACUTE KIDNEY INJURY

Although most cells remain viable after AKI by escapeing injury or recovering from sublethal injury, significant cell death does occur in severe AKI, as evidenced by histologic analysis of biopsy specimens and the presence of cellular debris in the form of casts in the urine. Death can occur by necrosis, which is a chaotic process that can elicit a profound inflammatory response in the organ. An alternative form of cell death, apoptosis, is a highly regulated program that leads to DNA fragmentation and cytoplasmic condensation without triggering an inflammatory response. Inflammation is circumvented by efficient removal of apoptotic cells by phagocytes, which sequester the potentially immunogenic debris. Proteins upregulated during AKI, such as kidney injury molecule 1 (KIM-1), can confer on tubular epithelial cells the ability to phagocytose apoptotic tubular cells. There have been considerable efforts to elucidate the apoptotic mechanisms in AKI in the hope of identifying potential therapeutic strategies to ameliorate injury and enhance recovery.

REPAIR AND REGENERATION

Unlike the brain and the heart, the kidney possesses a remarkable capacity for recovery after acute injury. Some patients who require dialysis and survive their episode of AKI can recover function sufficiently to avoid long-term renal replacement therapy. The efficient reparative process is attributable to the unique capacity of surviving tubular epithelial cells to dedifferentiate, expand rapidly, and redifferentiate to restore the functional integrity of the kidney. Repair of the postnatal kidney parallels organogenesis in the high rate of proliferation and apoptosis, and in patterns of gene expression.

Functional genomics and complementary DNA microarray–based technology have uncovered complex molecular pathways involved in renal injury and repair. Many of the genes identified to be upregulated in the postischemic

kidneys are involved in cell-cycle regulation, inflammation, cell death regulation, and growth factor or cytokine production. For instance, the genes for hepatocyte growth factor (HGF) and its receptor (MET) are rapidly upregulated after renal injury. Administration of recombinant HGF at the time of injury was shown to accelerate renal recovery (based on serum creatinine level and severity of pathologic score) in animal models. It is not clear, however, with HGF and other growth factors, whether accelerated recovery results from a protective effect against injury or from hastening of repair.

Identification of genes upregulated early and specifically after AKI has also led to the discovery of novel protein biomarkers, such as KIM-1, neutrophil gelatinase–associated lipocalin (NGAL), and interleukin 18, which may revolutionize early detection and possible intervention in AKI. Apart from their utility as biomarkers, these proteins may also participate in the injury and/or repair of the kidney after AKI.

STEM CELLS IN REGENERATION AND REPAIR IN ACUTE KIDNEY INJURY

An exciting area of AKI research is identification of the origin of the cells that contribute to repair of the kidney epithelium after injury. Studies support the notion that intrinsic tubular epithelial cell proliferation accounts for replenishment of the tubular epithelium lost after ischemia. There is some evidence that bone marrow derived stromal cells migrate to the injured kidney and likely generate antiinflammatory factors that may influence the proliferative response of the repairing epithelium. Most evidence suggests that intrinsic renal stem cells are not precursors of the cells that repopulate the epithelium after injury; rather, these cells derive from surviving epithelial cells that dedifferentiate.

CHRONIC KIDNEY DISEASE AFTER ACUTE KIDNEY INJURY

Individuals with severe AKI are at increased risk of progressive chronic kidney disease, even after functional recovery of GFR. The pathobiologic underpinning of this phenomenon may be a result of maladaptive repair after injury. AKI can lead to incomplete tubular repair, persistent tubulointerstitial inflammation, fibroblast proliferation, and excessive deposition of extracellular matrix. Postischemic fibrosis may arise from profibrogenic cytokines, such as TGFβ1 and connective tissue growth factor, secreted by surviving tubular epithelial cells that are arrested in the G2/M phase of the cell cycle as a result of severe or sustained tubular cell injury. There is also evidence of proliferation of pericytes and increased numbers of myofibroblasts in the interstitium. Whether there is direct conversion of epithelial cells to fibroblasts remains inconclusive.

THERAPEUTIC CONSIDERATIONS

PRECONDITIONING

An important finding in animal models of ischemic renal injury is that previous ischemic or toxic injury protects from future injury. This preconditioning effect lasts for several weeks. These studies indicate that the kidney can activate endogenous mechanisms, which appear to protect vessels and tubules from injury. Exploiting these mechanisms will likely lead to new therapies.

Although the deliberate induction of sublethal renal ischemia has little practical clinical application, studies of preconditioning in the myocardium have shown that several pharmacologic agents can mediate the same protection as ischemic preconditioning. Cardiac studies have highlighted signaling pathways involving protein kinase A, protein kinase D, and mitogen-activated kinase in preconditioning. Nitric oxide, a pluripotential molecule derived from inducible nitric oxide synthase (iNOS), is a key mediator of protection associated with preconditioning in the kidney. Furthermore, it has been found in a number of systems that remote preconditioning injury to a limb or other organ can confer protection on the kidney or heart.

BENCH TO BEDSIDE

Dialysis and conservative measures remain the foundation of therapy for severe AKI. The unraveling of the novel mechanisms of pathogenesis and repair in AKI has led to the development of novel therapeutic strategies to curb acute injury to the kidney (Table 32.1). Numerous experimental therapies have been explored, but few have been brought to fruition in humans for several reasons. First, the pathogenesis of AKI in animal models is usually less complex than it is in humans, because patients often have many causes of injury and multiorgan dysfunction concurrently. Second, AKI in humans often occurs in the setting of sepsis, and it has been difficult to establish good models of sepsis and AKI in animals. Third, many of the tested strategies in AKI might have been applied too late, because the serum creatinine level was used as the biomarker for the onset of AKI. Trials that take these barriers into consideration are now being conducted to test new compounds and to retest previously studied agents and maneuvers.

BIBLIOGRAPHY

Ali ZA, Callaghan CJ, Lim E, et al: Remote ischemic preconditioning reduces myocardial and renal injury after elective abdominal aortic aneurysm repair: a randomized controlled trial, *Circulation* 116: 105-198, 2007.

Basile DP: The endothelial cell in ischemic acute kidney injury: implications for acute and chronic function, *Kidney Int* 72:151-156, 2007.

Bonventre JV: Dedifferentiation and proliferation of surviving epithelial cells in acute renal failure, *J Am Soc Nephrol* 14(Suppl 1):S55-S61, 2003.

Bonventre JV, Weinberg JM: Recent advances in the pathophysiology of ischemic acute renal failure, *J Am Soc Nephrol* 14:2199-2210, 2003.

Bonventre JV, Yang L: Cellular pathophysiology of ischemic acute kidney injury, *J Clin Invest* 121:4210-4212, 2011.

Bonventre JV, Zuk A: Ischemic acute renal failure: an inflammatory disease, *Kidney Int* 66:480-485, 2004.

Chertow GM, Burdick E, Honour M, et al: Acute kidney injury, mortality, length of stay, and costs in hospitalized patients, *J Am Soc Nephrol* 16:3365-3370, 2005.

Devarajan P: Update on mechanisms of ischemic acute kidney injury, *J Am Soc Nephrol* 17:1503-1520, 2006.

Duffield JS, Bonventre JV: Kidney tubular epithelium is restored without replacement with bone marrow-derived cells during repair after ischemic injury, *Kidney Int* 68:1956-1961, 2005.

Humphreys BD, Bonventre JV: Mesenchymal stem cells in acute kidney injury, *Annu Rev Med* 59:311-325, 2008.

Humphreys BD, Valerius MT, Kobayashi A, et al: Intrinsic epithelial cells repair the kidney after injury, *Cell Stem Cell* 2:284-291, 2008.

Ishani A, Xue JL, Himmelfarb J, et al: Acute kidney injury increases risk of ESRD among elderly, *J Am Soc Nephrol* 20:223-228, 2009.

Jang HR, Ko GJ, Wasowska BA, et al: The interaction between ischemia-reperfusion and immune responses in the kidney, *J Mol Med* 87: 859-864, 2009.

Jo SK, Rosner MH, Okusa MD: Pharmacologic treatment of acute kidney injury: why drugs haven't worked and what is on the horizon, *Clin J Am Soc Nephrol* 2:356-365, 2007.

Johnson GB, Brunn GJ, Platt JL: Activation of mammalian Toll-like receptors by endogenous agonists, *Crit Rev Immunol* 23:15-44, 2003.

Kelly KJ, Williams WW Jr, Colvin RB, et al: Intercellular adhesion molecule-1–deficient mice are protected against ischemic renal injury, *J Clin Invest* 97:1056-1063, 1996.

Le Dorze M, Legrand M, Payen D, et al: The role of the microcirculation in acute kidney injury, *Curr Opin Crit Care* 15:503-508, 2009.

Leemans JC, Stokman G, Claessen N, et al: Renal-associated TLR2 mediates ischemia/reperfusion injury in the kidney, *J Clin Invest* 115:2894-2903, 2005.

Thurman JM: Triggers of inflammation after renal ischemia/reperfusion, *Clin Immunol* 123:7-13, 2007.

Togel F, Hu Z, Weiss K, et al: Administered mesenchymal stem cells protect against ischemic acute renal failure through differentiation-independent mechanisms, *Am J Physiol Renal Physiol* 289:F31-F42, 2005.

Yang L, Besschetnova TY, Brooks CR, et al: Epithelial cell cycle arrest in G2/M mediates kidney fibrosis after injury, *Nat Med* 16:535-543, 2010.

Zuk A, Bonventre JV, Brown D, et al: Polarity, integrin, and extracellular matrix dynamics in the postischemic rat kidney, *Am J Physiol* 275:C711-C731, 1998.

Table 32.1 Examples of Potential Therapies Based on Pathophysiologic Mechanisms

Vascular	Tubular
Vasodilation	**Cell Death/Inflammation**
CO-releasing compounds	Erythropoietin
Natriuretic peptides	Statins
Calcium channel blockers	PPAR agonists
Endothelin receptor antagonists	Caspase inhibitors
Adenosine antagonists	Iron chelators
Growth factors	Acetylcysteine
Nitric oxide	Fibrate
Fenoldopam	Sphingosine-1-phosphate– analogues
Bicarbonate	Klotho
	IL-10, IL-6 antagonists
Leukocyte-Endothelial Interactions	Minocycline
Anti–ICAM-1, CD11a antibody	Edaravone
α-MSH	Levosimendan
PAF antagonists	
A$_{2A}$ adenosine receptor agonists	**Repair**
C5a receptor antagonist	Growth factors
	EGF
Iron Chelation	Heparin-binding EGF
NGAL	IGF-1
Apotransferrin	
	HGF
	Resolvins, protectins
	Mesenchymal stem cells

CO, Carbon monoxide; *EGF,* epidermal growth factor; *HGF,* hepatocyte growth factor; *ICAM,* intercellular adhesion molecule; *IGF,* insulin-like growth factor; *IL,* interleukin; *MSH,* melanocyte-stimulating hormone; *NGAL,* neutrophil gelatinase–associated lipocalin; *PAF,* platelet activating factor; *PPAR,* peroxisome proliferator-activated receptor.

33 Clinical Approach to the Diagnosis of Acute Kidney Injury

Etienne Macedo | Ravindra L. Mehta

Acute kidney injury (AKI) is a complex syndrome associated with several etiologic factors, including specific kidney diseases (e.g., acute interstitial nephritis [AIN], acute glomerular and vasculitic kidney diseases) and nonspecific conditions (e.g., ischemia, toxic injury). AKI occurs in a variety of settings with clinical manifestations ranging from a small elevation in serum creatinine to anuric kidney failure. More than one etiologic factor may coexist in the same patient, and the manifestations and clinical consequences of different causes of AKI can be indistinguishable. However, treatment of AKI is largely dependent on the clinical presentation and the underlying etiology.

The incidence of AKI with and without the need for dialysis has been progressively increasing since the mid-1990s, and it is more pronounced in older hospitalized patients. The first step for the nephrology community to understand AKI better was to develop a uniform definition. Before 2004, acute renal failure (ARF) had more than 30 different definitions reported in the literature. Consequently, epidemiologic studies used different clinical and physiologic endpoints, making it difficult to compare the results between studies. This yielded discrepancies in AKI incidence and prevalence in various clinical settings, ranging from 1% to 31%, and differences in mortality from 28% to 82%. In 2004, the Acute Dialysis Quality Initiative (ADQI) developed the consensus Risk, Injury, Failure, Loss, and End-stage Kidney (RIFLE) classification of ARF. The RIFLE classification system provides three grades of severity for AKI based on changes in either serum creatinine, estimated glomerular filtration rate (eGFR), or urine output from the baseline condition: risk (class R), injury (class I) and failure (class F). Also included were two outcome classes: loss (class L) and end-stage kidney disease (class E) (Fig. 33.1A). In 2007, based on evidence suggesting that small changes in creatinine (≥0.3 mg/dl) were associated with adverse outcomes, the Acute Kidney Injury Network (AKIN) introduced the term *AKI* to more accurately the wider spectrum of the disease than the term *ARF* had suggested. The RIFLE classification was modified to develop the AKIN criteria by introducing a lower threshold for an absolute change in serum creatinine (≥0.3 mg/dl), eliminating the eGFR criteria, and adding a time element of 48 hours for the diagnosis in contrast to the 1-week interval in RIFLE. The terms *Risk, Injury,* and *Failure* were replaced by stages 1, 2, and 3, respectively (Fig. 33.1B). In addition, recognizing that loss and end-stage kidney disease were outcomes of AKI, the categories *Loss* and *End-stage kidney disease* were eliminated. In both

systems, the urine output criteria were unchanged, and it was emphasized that the criteria must follow adequate fluid resuscitation and exclusion of urinary tract obstruction. These criteria were designed to establish a severity stage on diagnosis, with staging determined by the highest creatinine or lowest urine output criteria at the time of evaluation. Sequential assessment of the stage could thus provide information on changes in the patient's course.

Since the mid-2000s, multiple studies in diverse patient populations have validated the concepts proposed in the RIFLE and AKIN systems. Both the serum creatinine and urine output criteria for diagnosis are associated with adverse outcomes, including mortality, morbidity, resource use, and costs. In addition, patient outcome progressively worsens with the severity of AKI. More than 71,000 patients have been included in published studies with the RIFLE classification system; these studies show a stepwise increase in relative risk (RR) for death going from *Risk* (RR: 2.40) to *Injury* (RR: 4.15) to *Failure* (6.37) .

Similarly, studies have validated the AKIN criteria and have shown a higher sensitivity for AKI diagnosis. In a prospective study that evaluated the serum creatinine of 8207 patients using a hospital data survey system, AKI occurred in 1.2% during the study period; 29.2% reached maximum stage 1, 36.5% stage 2, and 34.4% stage 3 AKIN criteria. Mortality for patients with stage 3 AKI (51.5%) was significantly higher than for patients with stages 1 or 2 ($p = 0.013$). Higher rate of renal recovery was observed in patients with lower-stage injuries (71.4%, 60.0%, and 21.2% for stages 1, 2, and 3, respectively). In another study, increased severity of AKI was associated with an increased risk of death independent of comorbidity. Patients with AKIN stages 1, 2, and 3 had odds ratios of 2.2, 6.1, and 8.6, respectively, for hospital mortality.

Although urine output increases the sensitivity of the diagnostic criteria, its specificity has not been defined. The AKIN oliguria criterion has been evaluated in fewer studies than the serum creatinine criterion because of difficulty associated with measuring urine output. Most studies are retrospective and used a modified definition, evaluating urine volume in 2- to 12-hour or 24-hour periods, and shortening the observation time to the first 24 hours of ICU admission or postoperative period. A review of 10 studies showed that patients in the RIFLE *Risk* class defined by the creatinine criterion were more severely ill than those in the same class defined only by the urine output criterion. Although oliguric patients had a higher mortality rate than non-AKI patients, the effect of adding the urine output criterion to

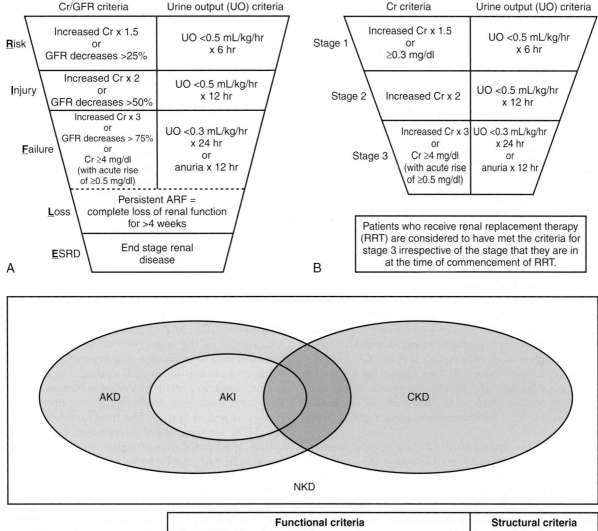

Figure 33.1   A, Risk, Injury, Failure, Loss, and End-stage Kidney (RIFLE), B, Acute Kidney Injury Network (AKIN), and Kidney Disease: Improving Global Outcomes (KDIGO) Classification Systems. The KDIGO definition has modified the serum creatinine criteria for Stage 1 (minimum stage for diagnosis) to include an absolute change in serum creatinine of ≥0.3 mg/dl over 48 hours or a relative change of ≥50% over 7 days. **C,** Definitions of kidney disease and their overlapping relationship. eGFR does not reflect measured GFR as accurately in AKI as in CKD. *AKI,* Acute kidney injury; *AKD,* acute kidney disease; *ARF,* acute renal failure; *CKD,* chronic kidney disease; *Cr,* creatinine; *eGFR,* estimated glomerular filtration rate; *ESRD,* end-stage renal disease; *GFR,* glomerular filtration rate; *mGFR,* measured glomerular filtration rate; *NKD,* no known kidney disease; *RRT,* renal replacement therapy; *SCr,* serum creatinine; *UO,* urine output. (Modified from Barrantes F, Tian J, Vazquez R, et al: Acute kidney injury criteria predict outcomes of critically ill patients, *Crit Care Med* 36:1397-1403, 2004, and Haase M, Bellomo R, Matalanis G, et al: A comparison of the RIFLE and Acute Kidney Injury Network classifications for cardiac surgery-associated acute kidney injury: a prospective cohort study, *J Thorac Cardiovasc Surg* 138:1370-1376, 2009.)

creatinine to predict mortality has shown discordant results. In a systematic review, the RR for death among studies that used both creatinine and urine output criteria was lower than in those studies using only the creatinine criterion. However, these studies used modified urine output criterion or applied it in a shorter period (first 24 or 48 hours).

Patients diagnosed exclusively by AKIN urine output criterion still had more frequent need for dialysis, longer length of ICU stay, and higher mortality rates than patients without AKI. Importantly, the use of the urine output criterion in addition to the creatinine increased the ability of the AKIN classification to predict mortality.

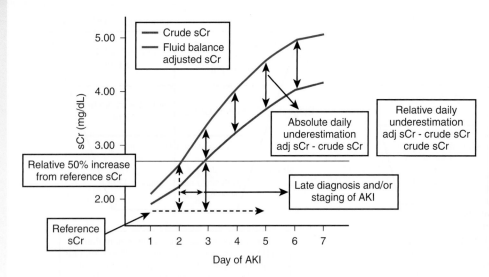

Figure 33.2   Difference between mean crude and adjusted serum creatinine during the follow-up period (late recognition of severity group). *AKI,* Acute kidney injury; *sCr,* serum creatinine. (Modified from Macedo E, Bouchard J, Soroko SH, et al: Fluid accumulation, recognition and staging of acute kidney injury in critically-ill patients, *Crit Care* 14:R82, 2010.)

However, as the RIFLE and AKIN criteria have become more commonly used, their shortcomings have also been recognized. In both systems, the creatinine criterion requires comparison to a "baseline" creatinine that may not always be available. The "baseline" creatinine values should represent the patients' previous chronic kidney disease (CKD) status assessed by creatinine values 90 days before the event. In CKD patients, diagnosis of AKI adds another level of complexity. When relative changes in creatinine are used, the time to achieve a level for diagnosis is greater than for an absolute change.

Recognizing these limitations, the Kidney Disease: Improving Global Outcomes (KDIGO) guidelines for AKI published in 2012 proposed a further modification of the criteria to include a 48-hour interval for absolute changes in creatinine, and a 7-day interval when relative changes in creatinine are considered. Although these enhancements should make the AKIN and RIFLE criteria able to encompass the practical issues for diagnosis, they still need to be validated. The KDIGO group has also proposed a new term, acute kidney disease (AKD), to address the problem in which changes in creatinine may evolve throughout periods longer than 7 days, and thus may not meet the AKI criteria. This term encompasses all conditions affecting kidney structure and function that can be considered acute or chronic, depending on their duration. AKD can occur with or without other acute or chronic kidney diseases and disorders. Future studies will be required to validate these concepts (see Fig. 33.1C).

TOOLS FOR DIAGNOSIS, STAGING, AND EVALUATION OF ACUTE KIDNEY INJURY

STANDARD LABORATORY TESTS

SERUM CREATININE

The current criteria for AKI diagnosis and classification, RIFLE and AKIN, are still based on increases in serum creatinine concentrations and decreases urine output. Many characteristics other than kidney function, such as age, muscle mass, catabolic rate, and race, influence creatinine concentration. In patients with AKI, changes in GFR often correlate poorly with changes in serum creatinine concentration. Three main factors influence the estimation of kidney function: the actual GFR, fluctuations in creatinine production, and fluid balance affecting the volume of distribution (Fig. 33.2). Fluid administration is a common component of the management of critically ill patients. Goal-directed resuscitation has recently focused on early volume expansion in the ICU course. These strategies frequently result in a relative increase in body weight of greater than 10%, sometimes doubling the total body water (TBW) in a short period of time. The fluid accumulation increases the TBW, lowering the concentration of creatinine, and results in potential overestimation of kidney function. The masking of AKI severity by volume expansion may be especially problematic in settings where the creatiniune is rising relatively slowly, owing either to lower creatinine generation (e.g., as might be expected in the elderly or patients with less muscle bulk) or to more modest overall injury. Analysis of the FACTT trial noted that creatinine values corrected for fluid accumulation identified a large number of patients with AKI who had been misclassified. These patients had outcomes similar to those with AKI.

BLOOD UREA NITROGEN

Blood urea nitrogen (BUN) is also used to evaluate kidney function, and elevations in BUN level are often, but not always, a result of a decrease in GFR. Some factors enhance urea production, such as gastrointestinal bleeding, corticosteroid therapy, and high-protein diet, and limit the utility of BUN in assessing kidney function. In the noncatabolic patient with mildly reduced GFR, daily BUN usually increases less than 10 to 15 mg/dl/day and serum creatinine less than 1.5 mg/dl/day. High catabolic states and high protein diets are associated with greater urea nitrogen production, and rises in daily BUN concentration that can exceed 50 mg/dl. In the presence of decreased intravascular effective volume, BUN increase is not proportional to the rise in serum creatinine level and the fall in GFR. Normally, the BUN:serum creatinine ratio is about 15:1, with the BUN and serum creatinine increasing in the absence of GFR by 10 to 15 and 1.0 to 1.5 mg/dl/day, respectively. In situations characterized by decreased glomerular perfusion pressure such as heart failure, BUN can increase independently from serum creatinine. The activation of the renin-angiotensin-aldosterone system

(RAAS) and the sympathetic nervous system are responsible for decreasing the glomerular perfusion pressure and GFR. The increment in vasopressin levels upregulates auqaporin-2 expression and increases water reabsorption. Urea, in contrast to serum creatinine, is not secreted but is reabsorbed by the renal tubules. The increased reabsorption of sodium and water, rather than the reduced GFR, enhances reabsorption of urea and increases BUN levels.

URINE STUDIES

URINE FLOW: OLIGURIA

Although both hydration status and diuretic use influence urine volume, and severe nonoliguric AKI is relatively common, the urinary flow rate often provides helpful information about the cause of AKI. Sustained periods of anuria suggest urinary tract obstruction. Other rare causes of anuria include rapidly progressive glomerulonephritis (GN), mechanical occlusion of renal blood flow, and diffuse renal cortical necrosis. Nonoliguric varieties of AKI are much more common with 33% nonoliguric at AKI diagnosis. Nonoliguric states may be present in all types of AKI, including those following surgery, trauma, hypotension, nephrotoxin exposure, and rhabdomyolysis. Several factors may contribute to the development of nonoliguric AKI, including use of volume expansion, high-dose potent diuretic agents, and renal vasodilators. Another contributory factor is aggressive fluid resuscitation and improved supportive management of critically ill patients. These clinical observations and a large body of experimental data suggest that the residual level of GFR is the primary determinant of urine flow in patients with AKI. The higher level of residual GFR in nonoliguric patients is compatible with improved survival and lower morbidity. Although urine output fluctuations can result from external influences such as diuretic administration, the pattern of change can be detected earlier with more frequent observations. In practice, measuring urine output reliably is often difficult and is usually best done in ICU settings with an indwelling bladder catheter. Dedicated devices for automated recording of urine flow have shown urine output to be a robust parameter for early recognition of AKI. Assessment of urine output over 6- to 12-hour blocks has also been validated as an adequate marker for AKI in epidemiologic studies; however, for prospective diagnostic and intervention studies, urine flow should be measured hourly.

Urine Microscopy

Urinary microscopy is an integral part of the clinical evaluation of patients with kidney disorders and is frequently used to differentiate some clinical conditions (e.g., nephrotic syndrome, urinary tract infection, nephritic syndrome). Drug toxicity has also been assessed by urine microscopy, associated with variable degrees of leukocyturia, crystalluria, and cellular casts.

In AKI, urine microscopy has traditionally been used as a tool to characterize prerenal AKI and acute tubular necrosis (ATN). Sediment containing few formed elements or only hyaline casts strongly suggests prerenal azotemia or obstructive uropathy. With ATN, brownish-pigmented cellular casts and many renal tubular epithelial cells (RTECs) are observed in more than 75% of patients. Sufficient red blood cells to cause microscopic hematuria, especially if

dysmorphic, are traditionally thought to be incompatible with a diagnosis of ATN and usually result from GN or structural kidney disorders (stones, tumor, infection, or trauma). Red blood cell casts suggest the presence of glomerular or vascular inflammatory diseases of the kidney and rarely, if ever, occur with ATN. Red blood cell casts, however, can be seen rarely in AIN. The presence of large numbers of polymorphonuclear leukocytes, singly or in clumps, suggests acute diffuse pyelonephritis or papillary necrosis. In AIN, white blood cell casts or eosinophilic casts on Hansel's stain of urine sediment may be diagnostically helpful. Eosinophiluria may be also present in some forms of GN and in atheroembolic kidney disease. It is rarely encountered in ATN. The combination of brownish-pigmented granular casts and positive occult blood tests on urine in the absence of hematuria indicates either hemoglobinuria or myoglobinuria. In AKI, the finding of large numbers of "football-shaped" uric acid crystals in fresh, warm urine may suggest a diagnosis of acute uric acid nephropathy, whereas the finding of large numbers of "back-of-envelope–shaped" oxalic acid crystals suggests ethylene glycol toxicity. Other agents (e.g., indinavir, atazanavir, sulfadiazine, acyclovir, and methotrexate) also can induce AKI with characteristic crystal appearance in the urine sediment. The clinical value of performing urine microscopy has recently been revised, and an AKI cast-scoring index was developed to standardize urine sediment. The score precision was evaluated in 30 patients with a clinical syndrome compatible, with ATN with renal recovery worse in those patients with a higher cast-scoring index (2.55 ± 0.9 vs. 1.7 ± 0.79; $p = 0.04$). In another study, a different scoring system for differentiating ATN from prerenal AKI was proposed. Using the final AKI diagnosis at discharge as a gold standard, urine microscopy on the day of nephrology consultation was highly predictive of ATN. The odds ratio for ATN incrementally increased with a higher score. The lack of RTECs or granular casts in patients with initial diagnosis of prerenal AKI had a sensitivity of 0.73 and a specificity of 0.75 for excluding the diagnosis of ATN. A scoring point system of urine microscopy findings was also able predict adverse outcomes. Correlation of the urinary-sediment score and AKIN stage at nephrology consultation was demonstrated, and the score was associated with a higher risk of worsening AKI in a dose-dependent manner.

URINARY CHEMICAL INDICES

Fractional excretion of sodium (FE_{Na} = (Urine Na/Plasma Na) ÷ (Urine creatinine/Plasma creatinine) × 100) was initially found to have a high degree of accuracy in differentiating between reversible prerenal azotemia and ATN. However, several caveats in using spot urine chemistries as a diagnostic tool to evaluate the cause of AKI led to a progressive decline in their use. Nevertheless, nearly all studies of spot chemistries were performed at a single time point relatively late in the course of AKI. The lack of serial data is important because AKI is a dynamic process. In the early phases of AKI, renal tubular function is intact. Later, cell injury may result in loss of tubular cell polarity. The resulting urine chemistries, therefore, are dependent on the phase of the course in which they were obtained. This may limit the sensitivity and specificity of urine chemical indices. The fractional excretion of urea nitrogen (FE urea nitrogen = (Urine UN/Plasma UN) ÷ (Urine creatinine/Plasma creatinine) × 100) has been proposed as an alternative marker to evaluate kidney dysfunction. Because intact nephrons reabsorb urea nitrogen from the urine, functional changes without nephron damage should inherently have a low FE_{urea} with a threshold value of less than 35%. With tubular damage, FE_{urea} is expected to parallel changes in FE_{Na}, with the possible advantage of being less affected by diuretic use. However, studies have been conflicting with respect to the value of these parameters for establishing the underlying pathophysiology of AKI. As shown in Table 33.1, the sensitivity, specificity, and predictive value of these tests is variable and influenced by the hydration status and previous use of diuretics. In general, combination of these tests with urinalysis and urine microscopy can help in the differential diagnosis of AKI to determine if structural changes are occurring. Although urine chemical indices are most often used as diagnostic adjuncts in patients with AKI, they

may also provide prognostic information. Some studies suggested that in oliguric patients with AKI, lower values for FE_{Na} and higher values for U/P osmolality are predictive of a diuretic response.

NEW BIOMARKERS

The importance of finding early diagnostic information in AKI has been clarified, and the development of technology has facilitated the search for new biomarkers of kidney injury. Until recently, the importance of the early diagnosis of AKI has been poorly appreciated. In the small number of studies that have been completed, therapeutic interventions have failed to improve outcomes. Since the early 2000s, the concept of interventions based on "windows of opportunity" coupled with targeted therapy became more relevant in other ischemic events, such as acute chest pain syndromes and stroke. Earlier AKI diagnosis provides a wider window to perform supportive and therapeutic interventions. The insensitivity of most commonly used surrogates of kidney function (creatinine and urine output) has led to extensive efforts to identify alternative tools for AKI diagnosis, including urine and serum biomarkers. Compared to the use of more sensitive biomarkers of kidney injury, reliance on serum creatinine may delay the AKI diagnosis by 48 to 72 hours. Most of the studies have focused on the ability of these biomarkers to detect AKI earlier than the classical parameters, but they may be also useful in predicting the course and prognosis of AKI. Several promising candidates have emerged, demonstrating reasonable diagnostic performance for AKI up to 48 hours before a significant change in creatinine.

In addition to facilitating early diagnosis, these biomarkers may also allow for reassessing interventions for AKI that have failed in clinical trials that used serum creatinine as a parameter to guide intervention. Another area of possible application for the new biomarkers is assisting in decisions to initiate renal replacement therapy in patients with AKI.

IMAGING

Ultrasonographic evaluation of the kidney can also help in the diagnosis of AKI. Ultrasound is an excellent modality for structural imaging such as renal parenchymal size, scarring, calcification, and polycystic kidneys. The presence of small kidney size strongly supports a diagnosis of CKD, helping to differentiate acute from chronic kidney injury. The echogenicity of the cortex can be assessed, with a hyperechoic cortex (normal cortex is hypoechoic to liver) present in most cases of CKD, adult polycystic kidney disease being the notable exception. Noncontrast computed tomographic (CT) and magnetic resonance imaging (MRI) scans analyze kidney structure and renal artery calcification. Other functional studies such as mercaptoacetyltriglycine (MAG3) and diethylenetriaminepentaacetic acid (DTPA) show reduced renal uptake and delayed excretion of tracer in AKI.

In ATN, ultrasound usually shows enlarged kidneys with a smooth contour caused by interstitial edema. The cortex demonstrates normal echogenicity with either a normal or hypoechoic medulla. Obstructed kidneys are typically normal sized with dilated ureters, renal pelvis, and calyceal systems. The urine-filled structures appear as anechoic areas

Table 33.1	Fractional Excretion of Sodium and Urea in Clinical Studies	
Performance Measure	FE_{Na} (<1% or >3%)	FE_{urea} (<35%)
Sensitivity		
For prerenal azotemia	78% to 96%	48% to 92%
For prerenal azotemia on diuretic	29% to 63%	79% to 100%
For intrinsic causes	56% to 75%	68% to 75%
Specificity		
For prerenal azotemia	67% to 96%	75% to 100%
For prerenal azotemia on diuretic	81% to 82%	33% to 91%
For intrinsic causes	78% to 100%	48% to 98%
Positive Predictive Value		
For prerenal azotemia	86% to 98%	79% to 100%
For prerenal azotemia on diuretic	86% to 89%	71% to 98%
For intrinsic causes	64% to 100%	43% to 94%
Negative Predictive Value		
For prerenal azotemia	60% to 86%	43% to 83%
For prerenal azotemia on diuretic	18% to 49%	44% to 83%
For intrinsic causes	82% to 86%	79% to 86%

Modified from Himmelfarb J, Joannidis M, Molitoris B, et al: Evaluation and initial management of acute kidney injury, Clin J Am Soc Nephrol 3:962-967, 2008.

FE_{Na}, Fractional excretion of sodium; *FE_{urea},* fractional excretion of urea; *GN,* glomerulonephritis.

Although cutoff values differ among studies, in a patient with acute kidney injury, an FE_{Na} lower than 1% suggests a prerenal cause, whereas a value higher than 3% suggests an intrinsic cause. Similarly, a FE_{urea} less than 35% suggests a functional cause of altered kidney function, whereas a value higher than 50% suggests an intrinsic one. The FE_{Na} can be falsely high in patients taking a diuretic; it can be falsely low in a number of intrinsic kidney conditions, such as contrast-induced nephropathy, rhabdomyolysis, and acute GN.

with posterior acoustic enhancement. The ureter and renal pelvis can be dilated without being obstructed, most commonly after previous obstruction with residual changes, normal pregnancy, or as an anatomical variant (enlarged extrarenal pelvis). False negatives can occur in the hyperacute setting if the renal collecting system has not had time to dilate, or if associated with retroperitoneal fibrosis or ureteral encasement. Noncontrast CT scan is the gold standard for detecting ureteric calculi. The ureters can usually be traced between the kidney and bladder, and a hyperdense stone seen at the site of obstruction. More than 99% of renal calculi are radiopaque on CT scan; however, xanthine and indinavir calculi may be radiolucent. The obstructed kidney is typically edematous with perirenal stranding. A noncontrast study can usually identify bilateral obstruction from extrinsic compression from masses such as retroperitoneal tumors, or cervical or colon carcinomas. Scintigraphic imaging with either Tc-99m-MAG3 or Tc-99m-DTPA can detect ureteric obstruction, and the negative predictive value of nuclear medicine scanning is extremely high.

Doppler ultrasonography is a tool that is emerging to characterize the likelihood of early AKI recovery. The renal arteries can also be evaluated for the resistive index (RI), which is an objective measure of the resistance to renal perfusion. RI is defined as the systolic velocity minus diastolic velocity divided by systolic velocity $(Vs - Vd)/Vs$. Alterations in RI (normal range ≤ 0.70) have been correlated with the severity of AKI. However, these techniques are operator dependent and have not been widely used. Scintigraphic examinations in ATN using Tc-99m-MAG3 nuclear medicine imaging demonstrate relatively well-preserved renal perfusion but delayed tracer uptake, often with a continuing activity accumulation curve. Excretion of tracer into the collecting system is delayed and reduced, but there is no obstruction to drainage of the collecting systems. In CKD, MAG3 studies will show poorly functioning kidneys but no accumulation pattern or obstruction to drainage.

KIDNEY BIOPSY

A kidney biopsy is usually considered in the setting of AKI in the absence of an obvious cause, heavy proteinuria and persistent hematuria, or a prolonged (greater than 2 to 3 weeks) course of AKI. In suspected GN or AIN, the "gold standard" diagnostic test is a kidney biopsy. In clinical practice, most nephrologists choose to biopsy when they are not confident of the cause of the AKI or when kidney injury has an obscure etiology. In a significant proportion of patients with AKI, the clinical context suggests the etiology with a reasonable degree of certainty. In less certain cases, the lack of efficient therapeutic options coupled with the risks of a biopsy decrease the likelihood that the clinician will perform the procedure. However, the development of AKI is often multifactorial, and some other causes of AKI may be misclassified as ATN.

Several studies have examined the clinical utility of kidney biopsy in the setting of AKI. In 9378 cases with biopsy-proven native kidney diseases between 1994 and 2001, AKI was an indication for 12% of kidney biopsies. The majority of the biopsies were in adults and elderly patients, predominantly with the suspicion of vasculitis and crescentic GN. In an Italian survey, 34.1% of 1059 kidney biopsies of patients with AKI demonstrated vasculitis and crescentic GN. In Baltimore, 259 kidney biopsies of adults older than 60 years with AKI showed similar results, with 35.2% of diagnoses being crescentic GN. However, these studies predominantly included patients with active urinary sediment, a selection bias in the indication for biopsy in AKI. In most AKI patients, clinical evaluation can identify functional changes and urinary tract obstruction. However, kidney biopsies should be considered when the underlying clinical diagnosis is not consistent with ATN.

Most important is the necessity of determining the number of patients with unrecognized yet treatable forms of AKI. Several studies have suggested significant discord between prebiopsy and postbiopsy diagnoses in the setting of AKI. In the elderly, the clinical diagnosis was incorrect in 34% of cases biopsied, many of them involving potentially treatable diseases. Among elderly patients with rapidly progressive kidney injury, 71% of the patients were noted to have crescentic GN and 17% interstitial nephritis. Prebiopsy and histopathologic diagnoses differed in 15% of patients, and both groups benefited from therapeutic intervention.

These data emphasize the value of kidney biopsy in the management of AKI of uncertain origin, regardless of the age of the patient. Accurate diagnosis is important to direct appropriate treatment, especially in vasculitis and crescentic GN where delay in diagnosis may affect outcome. Given the safety of the ultrasound or tomographic-guided biopsy, unclear cases of AKI deserve a consideration for kidney biopsy. The transjugular approach has also enhanced our ability to obtain tissue, particularly in patients who are at high risk for bleeding and who cannot be placed in the prone position. The complication rates appear similar to ultrasound-guided biopsies. Major risks for kidney biopsies included bleeding, infection, creation of an intrarenal AV fistula, and injury to adjacent organs. These risks can be mitigated with careful correction of coagulopathy and bleeding times with blood products (fresh frozen plasma and desmopressin [DDAVP]). However, these risks should be weighed in context with developing an effective management strategy and providing prognostic information.

DIFFERENTIAL DIAGNOSIS AND EVALUATION

The definition and classification system of AKI has been standardized. Nevertheless, whether AKI refers only to ATN and other parenchymal diseases or includes reversible functional changes has not been established. Currently, the term "prerenal azotemia" describes reversible forms of kidney dysfunction encompassing different conditions that vary considerably in pathophysiology and course, including intravascular volume depletion, relative hypotension, compromised cardiac output, and hepatorenal syndrome (Fig. 33.3 and Box 33.1). In all these situations, an elevation of serum creatinine or reduction of urine output that resolves with volume resuscitation or improved renal perfusion pressure is the current accepted definition for reversible functional changes. However, there is no agreement on the amount, nature, and duration of fluid resuscitation needed to establish a prerenal state. In most cases, the response to

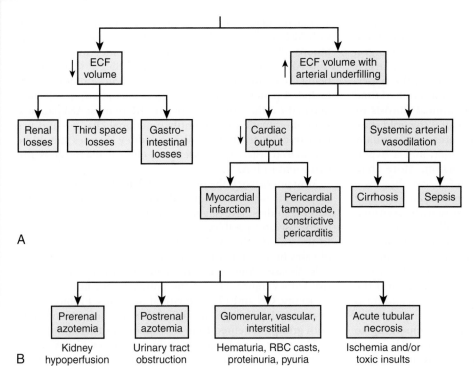

Figure 33.3 A, Causes of prerenal azotemia. B, Acute deterioration in kidney function. (Modified from Schrier RW: Diagnostic value of urinary sodium, chloride, urea, and flow, *J Am Soc Nephrol* 22:1610, 2011.)

fluid expansion or hemodynamic support on kidney function is retrospective and is frequently evaluated by trial and error, and the return of kidney function to the previous baseline within 24 to 72 hours is considered a prerenal or reversible condition. Diagnostic strategies have usually been based on demonstrating a fluid responsive change in kidney function. Unnecessary fluid administration and excessive fluid overload are potential complications of this approach.

Several clinical scenarios are often associated with a potentially reversible or prerenal form of AKI. The use of nonsteroidal antiinflammatory drugs (NSAIDs), volume depletion, hypoalbuminemia, an edematous disorder, advancing age, underlying CKD, or recent diuretic use are all contributing factors for prerenal AKI. A similar reversible form of AKI can complicate angiotensin converting enzyme-inhibitor (ACE-inhibitor) therapy in the presence of decreased renal blood flow from severe bilateral renal artery stenosis, renal artery stenosis in a solitary functioning kidney, and other high-renin, high-angiotensin II states (i.e., edematous states and volume depletion disorders). In these cases, ACE-inhibition with a resultant decrease in both renal perfusion pressure and efferent arteriolar constriction can precipitously decrease GFR. About one third of patients with severe congestive heart failure (CHF) experience an abrupt rise in serum creatinine concentration following ACE-inhibitor therapy. In this setting, the increase in serum creatinine following ACE-inhibition tends to be mild and readily reversible on discontinuation of the drug.

With the availability of new biomarkers of kidney injury, refined paradigms for defining prerenal states are emerging (Fig. 33.4). The diagnosis of reversible functional changes requires a consideration of several factors including preexisting kidney disease, acuity of changes in kidney function, and the response to interventions. There are some promising new biomarkers that may be helpful in distinguishing between reversible and established AKI. During the reversible state,

Box 33.1 Clinical Approach to Acute Kidney Injury

1. Reversible AKI
- Decreased effective renal perfusion
- Extrarenal obstruction to urine flow

2. Self-Limited AKI
- ATN
- AIN
- Intrarenal obstruction, drugs, uric acid
- Acute GN

3. Irreversible AKI
- Cortical necrosis
- Large vessel occlusion
- Certain nephrotoxins: methoxyfluorane
- Microvascular occlusions

AKI, Acute kidney injury; *AIN,* acute interstitial nephritis; *ATN,* acute tubular necrosis; *GN,* glomerulonephritis.

the persistent vasoconstriction associated with metabolic changes and inflammation promotes the release of cell functional markers that can be detected in the blood and urine. However, at the current time, there are no specific markers representing reversible conditions. Urinary neutrophil gelatinase–associated lipocalin (NGAL) levels were evaluated in emergency room patients in whom there was very little overlap in NGAL values in patients with reversible and established AKI, whereas serum creatinine values overlapped significantly.

Some studies have shown a correlation between urinary biomarker concentration and functional severity. Although it is accepted that urinary biomarker concentrations increase

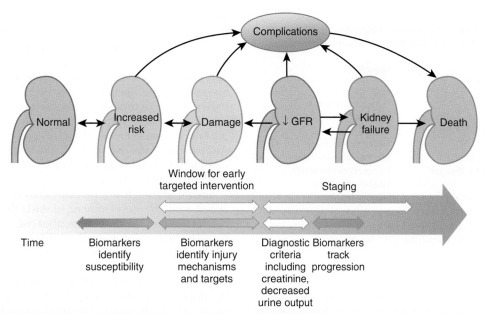

Figure 33.4 Conceptual framework for acute kidney injury. Surveillance could be initiated for high-risk individuals on the basis of clinical and biomarker criteria. Sequential assessment of biomarkers may permit identification of a window of opportunity in which kidney injury has been initiated but has not progressed to kidney functional change. The duration of this window is inherently dependent on the type and site of injury and the nature and specificity of the biomarkers to determine the targets for intervention. Progression of kidney injury would be determined by development of functional changes staged on the basis of the severity of kidney injury. Biomarkers could further define progression, determine need for additional interventions, and predict prognosis. By combining biomarkers, such as urine flow (functional change) and neutrophil gelatinase–associated lipocalin (structural damage), clinicians will have better tools to characterize patients with respect to reversibility and will be able to identify more clearly the phases of the disease. *GFR,* Glomerular filtration rate. (From Mehta RL: Timed and targeted therapy for acute kidney injury: a glimpse of the future. *Kidney Int* 77:947, 2010.)

with reversible functional injury, the rise in these markers differs from patients with established structural damage. It is evident that as biomarkers become available for clinical use, our thresholds for these markers will be defined, and what is currently labeled as prerenal will change.

After reversible and obstructive AKI have been excluded, a variety of kidney disorders can lead to prolonged or sustained AKI. In hospitalized adults, many of these cases are caused by ATN. Three major categories of insults are associated with ATN: prolonged renal ischemia, nephrotoxins, and pigmenturia (myoglobinuria and hemoglobinuria). ATN is often the result of multiple insults. The most common predisposing factor in the development of ATN is renal ischemia from a functional or structural reduction in renal perfusion. Sepsis, and particularly septic shock, has assumed an ever-increasing role as a major predisposing factor in the occurrence of ATN. Nephrotoxins are involved in about 20% of all cases of ATN. Commonly encountered nephrotoxins include aminoglycosides, radiographic contrast materials, NSAIDs, and antineoplasic drugs. A high proportion of patients with AIDS develops nephrotoxicity from drugs used to manage HIV. Several biomarkers have been evaluated in these settings and may have some discriminatory capacity.

DIAGNOSTIC APPROACH

Clinicians currently approach patients with altered kidney function with an aim to classify them as prerenal, intrinsic renal, or postrenal based on the clinical presentation. However, this approach may be somewhat limiting because there is usually no histopathology to confirm the diagnosis. We propose using a revised framework for approaching patients with AKI based on reversibility (see Box 33.1). The first step is to establish a patient's previous level of kidney function to determine whether there is de novo AKI or AKI superimposed on CKD. In most instances, information on previous kidney function based on urine and blood parameters is not available. Nevertheless, a detailed history including comorbidities, medication use, and earlier lab tests should be obtained. Urinary abnormalities such as proteinuria can help establish previous damage. It is preferable to consider creatinine values before 3 months from the episode to determine whether a patient has CKD, because the diagnosis of CKD is based on the presence of abnormalities for greater than 90 days. However, a frequent problem occurs when a baseline serum creatinine is either not available or is unknown. The choice to use a surrogate for baseline creatinine has a marked effect on diagnosing and grading AKI. The most commonly used alternative is the serum creatinine at the time of hospital admission, although this may not reflect the true baseline level of kidney function when the moment of insult is unknown. Misclassification in AKI diagnosis and severity can ultimately lead to different therapeutic approaches and can influence prognosis.

Accurate identification of the AKI risk factors to which the patient has been exposed is fundamental to achieve early diagnosis and accurate assessment of AKI severity. This is essential to developing approaches for earlier intervention, correcting reversible factors, and mitigating the downstream effects of AKI (Table 33.2). In the ICU population, two large prospective observational studies have provided a better understanding of the risk factors associated with

Table 33.2   Nonmodifiable and Modifiable Risk Factors for Acute Kidney Injury

Nonmodifiable	Modifiable
CKD	Hypertension
Diabetes mellitus	Hypoalbuminemia
Older age	Anemia
Chronic liver disease	Sepsis
CHF	Nephrotoxic drugs
Renal artery stenosis	Mechanical ventilation
Peripheral vascular disease	Hypercholesterolemia
AIDS	Rhabdomyolysis
Previous kidney surgery	Hyponatremia

AIDS, Acquired immune deficiency syndrome; *CKD,* chronic kidney disease; *CHF,* congestive heart failure.

AKI: Beginning and Ending Supportive Therapy (BEST) and Program to Improve Care in Acute Renal Disease (PICARD). Both BEST and PICARD found sepsis to be the most common contributing factor to ICU-related AKI. A significant percentage of patients developing severe AKI had baseline CKD. In the BEST study, AKI was associated with septic shock in 47.5% of patients. Thirty-four percent of AKI was associated with major surgery, 27% related to cardiogenic shock, 26% related to hypovolemia, and 19% potentially drug-related. Volume depletion is one of the most common and important risk factors for AKI. In addition to hypovolemia, renal hypoperfusion may be caused by decreased cardiac output, decreased plasma oncotic pressure, hypotension, and decreased renal prostaglandin synthesis. Advanced age, which is often associated with some degree of decreased kidney function and preexisting kidney disease, is another common risk factor associated with AKI. Administration of potentially nephrotoxic agents, or drugs that enhance nephrotoxicity, increase the risk of AKI, as seen with the concurrent use of furosemide and intravenous contrast agents. Sepsis, CHF, nephrotic syndrome, and hepatic disease are common predisposing conditions associated with AKI.

Knowledge of the underlying CKD status and risk factors should prompt a search for specific insults for AKI. Although AKI associated with one specific cause is common outside the ICU, most patients exhibit several etiologic factors contributing to the development of AKI. The most common factors are failure of renal autoregulation, direct nephrotoxicity, ischemia/reperfusion, and inflammatory states. With multiple factors directly influencing kidney function, the nature and timing of the inciting event is often unknown. If a specific etiology can be identified, for example exposure to contrast agents or nephrotoxic antibiotics, the course can be somewhat predictable. However, clinicians should be vigilant in their search for additional factors that may influence the course, such as volume depletion.

Diagnostic strategies using the established parameters of urinalysis, urine microscopy, urine chemistries, and imaging should be combined with newer biomarkers to better differentiate patients with functional reversible changes from those with structural kidney injury. For instance, our current concepts of prerenal AKI represent conditions wherein tubular function is intact, and correction of the underlying condition reverses the kidney dysfunction. Alternatively, structural injury leads to a more protracted course and highlights conditions where biomarkers, such as NGAL and KIM1, are elevated. In the reversible conditions, markers would more likely be below thresholds associated with injury, although there will be some overlap. As we begin to use AKI biomarkers, specific combinations will provide better fingerprints to enable clinicians more optimally to assess AKI patients. After the diagnosis and severity stage have been established, specific interventions can be further designed based on the stage of AKI.

Finally, although several individual risk factors are associated with the development of AKI, the combination of risk factors and the development of risk stratification scores could be better tools to predict AKI in specific patient populations (e.g., after cardiac surgery, contrast exposure, hospitalized patients, general surgery, and high-risk surgery). Few models have examined the clinical risk factors for the development of AKI among the ICU population. Risk profiling can also be used to establish appropriate criteria for surveillance for AKI in hospitalized patients. The use of models to predict the risk of AKI can help clinicians to identify patients at high risk for developing AKI, to make clinical decisions based on this risk, and to provide better patient counseling. A combination of risk assessment, active surveillance, early recognition, rapid response, and targeted intervention can thus be standardized to optimally manage these patients and to improve outcomes.

Thus, because AKI is a common condition that is prevalent in both outpatient and inpatient settings, a practical clinical approach to diagnosis is required. Our understanding of the pathophysiology, mechanism, and pathways has been enhanced in recent years from experimental models and epidemiologic studies. With the availability of new biomarkers, we are now better positioned to approach patients for earlier recognition, active surveillance, and targeted interventions. Strategies for management should focus on identifying reversibility and intervening early to prevent further progression. Several tools are now available to clinicians to manage patients with AKI.

BIBLIOGRAPHY

Anderson GH, Dalakos TG, Elias A, et al: Diuretic therapy and response of essential hypertension to saralasin, *Ann Intern Med* 87:183-187, 1977.

Andreucci VE, Fuiano G, Stanziale P, et al: Role of renal biopsy in the diagnosis and prognosis of acute renal failure, *Kidney Int Suppl* 66:S91-S95, 1998.

Bagshaw SM, George C, Dinu I, et al: A multi-centre evaluation of the RIFLE criteria for early acute kidney injury in critically ill patients, *Nephrol Dial Transplant* 23:1203-1210, 2008.

Bagshaw SM, Uchino S, Bellomo R, et al: Septic acute kidney injury in critically ill patients: clinical characteristics and outcomes, *Clin J Am Soc Nephrol* 2:431-439, 2007.

Barrantes F, Tian J, Vazquez R, et al: Acute kidney injury criteria predict outcomes of critically ill patients, *Crit Care Med* 36:1397-1403, 2008.

Bellomo R, Ronco C, Kellum JA, et al: Acute renal failure—definition, outcome measures, animal models, fluid therapy and information technology needs: the Second International Consensus Conference of the Acute Dialysis Quality Initiative (ADQI) Group, *Crit Care* 8:R204-R212, 2004.

Chawla LS, Dommu A, Berger A, et al: Urinary sediment cast scoring index for acute kidney injury: a pilot study, *Nephron Clin Pract* 110:c145-c150, 2008.

Coca SG, Yalavarthy R, Concato J, et al: Biomarkers for the diagnosis and risk stratification of acute kidney injury: a systematic review, *Kidney Int* 73:1008-1016, 2008.

Collins AJ, Foley RN, Herzog C, et al: Excerpts from the US Renal Data System 2009 Annual Data Report, *Am J Kidney Dis* 55:S1-S420, 2010. A6-A7.

Cruz DN, Bolgan I, Perazella MA, et al: North East Italian Prospective Hospital Renal Outcome Survey on Acute Kidney Injury (NEiPH-ROS-AKI): targeting the problem with the RIFLE Criteria, *Clin J Am Soc Nephrol* 2:418-425, 2007.

Gotfried J, Wiesen J, Raina R, et al: Finding the cause of acute kidney injury: which index of fractional excretion is better? *Cleve Clin J Med* 79:121-126, 2012.

Haase M, Bellomo R, Matalanis G, et al: A Comparison of the RIFLE and Acute Kidney Injury Network classifications for cardiac surgery-associated acute kidney injury: a prospective cohort study, *J Thorac Cardiovasc Surg* 138:1370-1376, 2009.

Himmelfarb J, Joannidis M, Molitoris B, et al: Evaluation and initial management of acute kidney injury, *Clin J Am Soc Nephrol* 3:962-967, 2008.

Joannidis M, Metnitz B, Bauer P, et al: Acute kidney injury in critically ill patients classified by AKIN versus RIFLE using the SAPS 3 database, *Intensive Care Med* 35:1692-1702, 2009.

KDIGO Clinical Practice Guideline for Acute Kidney Injury. *Kidney Int* (Suppl 2):19-68, 2012.

Liaño F, Junco E, Pascual J, et al: The spectrum of acute renal failure in the intensive care unit compared with that seen in other settings. The Madrid Acute Renal Failure Study Group, *Kidney Int Suppl* 66:S16-S24, 1998.

Liaño G, Pascual J: Acute renal failure. Madrid Acute Renal Failure Study Group, *Lancet* 347:479; author reply 479, 1996.

Liu KD, Thompson BT, Ancukiewicz M, et al: Acute kidney injury in patients with acute lung injury: impact of fluid accumulation on classification of acute kidney injury and associated outcomes, *Crit Care Med* 39:2665-2671, 2011.

Macedo E, Bouchard J, Soroko SH, et al: Fluid accumulation, recognition and staging of acute kidney injury in critically-ill patients, *Crit Care* 14:R82, 2010.

Macedo E, Malhotra R, Bouchard J, et al: Oliguria is an early predictor of higher mortality in critically-ill patients, *Kidney Int* 80:760-767, 2011a.

Mehta R, Kellum J, Shah S, et al: Acute Kidney Injury Network: report of an initiative to improve outcomes in acute kidney injury, *Crit Care* 11:R31, 2007.

Mehta RL: Timed and targeted therapy for acute kidney injury: a glimpse of the future, *Kidney Int* 77:947-949, 2012.

Mehta RL, Pascual MT, Soroko S, et al: Spectrum of acute renal failure in the intensive care unit: the PICARD experience, *Kidney Int* 66:1613-1621, 2004.

Nickolas TL, O'Rourke MJ, Yang J, et al: Sensitivity and specificity of a single emergency department measurement of urinary neutrophil gelatinase-associated lipocalin for diagnosing acute kidney injury, *Ann Intern Med* 148:810-819, 2008.

Schrier RW: Diagnostic value of urinary sodium, chloride, urea, and flow, *J Am Soc Nephrol* 22:1610-1613, 2011.

Soni SS, Fahuan Y, Ronco C, et al: Cardiorenal syndrome: biomarkers linking kidney damage with heart failure, *Biomark Med* 3:549-560, 2009.

Stillman IE, Lima EQ, Burdmann EA: Renal biopsies in acute kidney injury: who are we missing? *Clin J Am Soc Nephrol* 3:647-648, 2008.

Uchino S, Kellum JA, Bellomo R, et al: Acute renal failure in critically ill patients: a multinational, multicenter study, *JAMA* 294:813-818, 2005.

34 Acute Tubular Injury and Acute Tubular Necrosis

Jeffrey M. Turner | Steven G. Coca

Traditionally, the term acute tubular necrosis (ATN) defined a sudden decline in kidney function resulting from ischemic or toxin-related damage to the renal tubular epithelial cells (RTECs). In recent years, some have questioned the appropriateness of this nomenclature because of the limited number of frankly necrotic cells found on kidney biopsy. The term acute tubular injury (ATI) has commonly been used in place of ATN as it offers a more inclusive definition that extends beyond just the pathology of necrosis. Being diplomatic, we include both terms in the title of this chapter; however, in the remainder of our narrative, we adopt the sole use of the term *acute tubular injury*. The main focus of this chapter is to discuss etiologies of ATI that occur secondary to ischemic insults and endogenous nephrotoxin exposure.

ISCHEMIC ACUTE TUBULAR INJURY

Acute kidney injury (AKI) commonly occurs as a result of ischemic insult to RTECs. Normal function includes the ability to autoregulate blood flow and perfusion pressure within the renal microvasculature. This allows the kidney to maintain stable hemodynamics despite fluctuations in systemic arterial pressures. In pathologic states, the ability to autoregulate is compromised, and ischemic insults can lead to injury. The clinical manifestations of ischemia-induced insults lie on a continuum, which includes both functional changes in glomerular filtration that are traditionally labeled "prerenal" and direct tubular cell injury that is traditionally labeled "intrarenal." However, the threshold at which prerenal insults result in tubular cell injury is not well understood. Moreover, because of normal variations in regional blood flow and differences in energy and oxygen consumption in different areas of the nephron, tubular injury can be patchy. Thus, ATI is not an "all or none" phenomenon, and many nephrons of the kidney can endure in a prerenal functional state whereas others are injured.

In general, the more severe the renal perfusion defect, the more severe the injury is at the cellular level. However, this association is dynamic depending on the clinical scenario. A number of comorbidities including sepsis, chronic kidney disease, hypertension, and atherosclerosis will lower the threshold at which cellular injury begins to occur. In addition, it has been hypothesized that reduced glomerular filtration rate and the subsequent oliguria that occurs in the setting of AKI are protective mechanisms that attempt to limit mismatches in renal oxygen supply and demand. This creates an interesting dilemma about how we approach the importance of rapidly restoring glomerular filtration and urine output following kidney injury. In this section, we examine some of the common clinical scenarios that lead to ischemic ATI. The causes are divided into those etiologies that result from decreased arterial pressures in the systemic arterial tree and subsequently cause end organ hypoperfusion, and those etiologies that result in localized obstruction or constriction within the renal vasculature causing ischemia in downstream tissues.

CAUSES OF HYPOTENSION-INDUCED ISCHEMIA

In the hospital setting, ATI is the most common cause of AKI, attributable to half of all cases. The typical clinical scenario is a reduction in renal pressure and blood flow in the setting of poor effective arterial perfusion caused by a systemic disorder (Box 34.1). By various mechanisms, shock is a frequent culprit. Septic shock creates a particularly unfriendly environment for the kidney. Not only is oxygen delivery and cellular waste removal impaired because of changes in renal perfusion from systemic vasodilatation and intrarenal vasoconstriction, but the addition of direct tubular damage from endotoxins and inflammatory cytokines also contributes to the pathophysiology. Relatively modest reductions in blood pressure that occur in the setting of sepsis can still result in significant kidney impairment because of this double-hit phenomenon. Like sepsis, distributive shock results in diffuse vasodilatation of the systemic arterial system. Under normal conditions, the kidney receives 20% to 25% of the total cardiac output; however, a significant proportion of blood flow is diverted away from the kidney in this setting.

The cardinal impairment in cardiogenic shock is a reduction in cardiac output. This creates a number of unfavorable conditions for the kidney. In response to underfilling of the systemic arterial vascular bed, compensatory mechanisms lead to increased activity of the sympathetic nervous system and renin–angiotensin-aldosterone system. This in turn causes maladaptive vasoconstriction, particularly within the renal vasculature. The net result is a significant compromise to renal blood flow. In addition, studies have suggested that increased venous congestion and subsequent elevations in intraabdominal pressure are also important contributors to kidney impairment in the setting of reduced systolic function.

Hypovolemic shock commonly occurs secondary to significant volume loss in the setting of diuresis, bleeding, vomiting, or diarrhea. Markedly reduced oncotic pressure from low albumin states such as cirrhosis, nephrotic syndrome, and protein losing enteropathies can also result in severe intravascular volume depletion, despite an excess of total body water. Signs and symptoms of organ dysfunction do not typically occur until approximately 20% to 25% of effective arterial blood volume has been removed.

In addition to shock, a number of other clinical scenarios need to be considered in the etiology of ischemic ATI due to systemic hypotension. Common iatrogenic causes include medications such as antihypertensive agents, alpha antagonists, antiarrhythmics, narcotics, and sedatives. Hypotension related to autonomic dysfunction is most commonly seen in the setting of diabetes mellitus; however, it is also associated with liver disease, Guillain-Barré syndrome, cerebral vascular accidents, dementia, and others. Finally, medications that interfere with the autoregulation of renal blood flow can also contribute or exacerbate ATI from any of the previously mentioned causes. Nonsteroidal antiinflammatory drugs (NSAIDs) can reduce blood flow through the afferent arteriole and can impair medullary blood flow in patients who are prostaglandin-dependent, and angiotensin converting enzyme (ACE) inhibitors and angiotensin receptor blockers (ARBs) may increase the risk for clinical AKI. Whether this effect is purely hemodynamic or results in additional ATI is unclear, because some animal studies demonstrate a protective effect of ACE inhibitors and ARBs against ATI.

DIAGNOSIS

Ischemic ATI is usually suspected based on the clinical setting. Although one expects significant hypotension to have occurred, it is not uncommon for individuals with chronic hypertension and impaired autoregulation to experience normotensive ischemic kidney injury. In such cases, one would see a relative decrease in blood pressure as compared to baseline; however, the nadir pressure may still remain within the normal range. Laboratory data consistent with ischemic ATI include a blood urea nitrogen–to–serum creatinine ratio of less than 20, a fractional excretion of sodium (FE_{Na}) greater than 2%, or a fractional excretion of urea (FE_{Urea}) greater than 50% (FE_{Urea} can be helpful in avoiding a falsely elevated FE_{Na} as a result of diuretic use). It should be noted that sepsis-associated ATI and nonoliguric ATI can present with a FE_{Na} less than 1%. Urine studies usually reflect renal tubule dysfunction. Because of an inability to concentrate or dilute the urine effectively, the specific gravity will be approximately 1.010 (reflecting isosthenuria), and the urine osmolality is typically less than 350 mOsm/kg. Proteinuria can be present, but it is less than 1 g/day. In addition, it is not uncommon to have trace to 1+ heme on urine dipstick. Urine microscopy provides the most useful information to make the diagnosis. The classic finding is dense granular casts or "muddy brown casts," but additional findings include fine granular casts and RTECs. A recently developed scoring system based on the number of granular casts and RTECs seen within a low-power or high-power field, respectively, has been validated as a useful tool in differentiating ATI from prerenal azotemia.

The application of novel biomarkers to predict ATI has been the topic of a number of research articles in recent years. Such markers include neutrophil gelatinase–associated lipocalin (NGAL), interleukin-18, and kidney injury molecule (KIM-1), among others. Their potential application includes diagnosing ATI closer to the time of the actual insult and before the rise in serum creatinine (i.e., the time ATI is typically diagnosed clinically). In addition, biomarkers can be helpful in differentiating acute GFR reductions secondary to functional changes (i.e., prerenal and hepatorenal syndrome) from those caused by true renal tubular injury. Finally, the biomarkers may be able to predict which patients with established clinical AKI will progress to more severe dysfunction, including those who may require acute kidney replacement therapy. These biomarkers are not clinically available currently, but ongoing and future studies will attempt to determine the value of single biomarkers (or biomarker panels) to diagnose accurately and provide the most prognostic information for AKI.

Box 34.1 Causes of Ischemic Acute Tubular Injury/Acute Tubular Necrosis

Decreased Effective Arterial Perfusion

Shock

Septic
Hypovolemic
Cardiogenic
Distributive

Autonomic Dysfunction

Low Oncotic Pressure States

Cirrhosis
Nephrotic syndrome
Protein-losing enteropathies

Adrenal Insufficiency

Iatrogenic

Medication induced
Perioperative

Vasoocclusion Within the Renal Vasculature

Renal Artery Stenosis

Thromboembolism

Atheroembolic Disease

Vasoconstriction Within the Renal Vasculature

Medication Induced

Toxin Induced

CHOLESTEROL ATHEROEMBOLIC KIDNEY DISEASE

Atheromatous plaques form within the walls of arterial beds throughout the body, including in the aorta and renal arteries. These structures are usually composed of smooth muscle and mononuclear cells, calcium deposits, a fibrous cap, and lipids, including cholesterol crystals. Under certain conditions, disrupted plaques can release cholesterol crystals that flow downstream and lodge in small vessels within various organs, including the kidney. As circumstances dictate, isolated kidney involvement can occur or can be a manifestation of multiorgan involvement. Cholesterol atheroembolic kidney disease leads to ischemic kidney injury due to vessel obstruction from cholesterol crystals and the subsequently provoked immune response. Biopsy series have reported incidence rates of 1% among all patients undergoing kidney biopsy, and as high as 6.5% in selected cohorts older than 65. In a chart review of in-patient nephrology consultations, 10% of all cases of AKI were attributed to atheroembolic kidney disease.

CLINICAL PRESENTATION

Cholesterol atheroembolic kidney disease is due to an iatrogenic cause in as many as 77% of cases. The most common etiology is percutaneous coronary interventions, but other procedures include angioplasty for renal artery stenosis, vascular surgery, and coronary artery bypass surgery. These interventions involve vessel cannulation, incision, or clamping that can cause plaque disruption because of mechanical trauma. A small number of case reports have also implicated thrombolytic agents or anticoagulation therapy (unfractionated heparin, low molecular weight [MW] heparin, or coumadin) as the cause of spontaneous atheroemboli. These events occur in the absence of preceding endovascular interventions, and they are thought to occur when the therapeutic agent undermines an overlying stabilizing thrombus. A true cause-and-effect relationship has not been shown in clinical studies, and the absolute risk of an atheroembolic event from thrombolytics and anticoagulation appears to be small.

Patients at high risk for atheroembolic disease have extensive atherosclerosis. Typical patients are men older than 60 years with a history of smoking, diabetes, hyperlipidemia, and hypertension. When plaque disruption occurs and distal tissues are showered with cholesterol emboli, the kidney is the most common organ involved (approximately 75% of all cases). Other frequently affected organs are listed in Table 34.1. After entering the bloodstream, cholesterol crystals typically settle within the arcuate and interlobular arterioles of the kidney, but they can reach the afferent arteriole and glomerular capillary as well. An inflammatory reaction ensues that is characterized initially by granulocyte infiltration and then is followed by mononuclear cell infiltration and giant cell formation. Endothelial proliferation occurs, which leads to intimal thickening and concentric fibrosis. Ultimately this process results in arteriole obstruction and ischemic infarction of downstream tissues including the glomeruli, tubules, and interstitium. Kidney function may decline acutely, subacutely, or slowly over time. Approximately one third of cases will present with fulminant AKI, typically occurring within one week of the triggering event. This scenario is often the result of a large burden of cholesterol emboli, and rarely is the kidney the only organ involved. The more typical presentation is a subacute decline in kidney function, with AKI appearing on average 5.3 weeks after the initial insult. Kidney dysfunction occurs in a stepwise fashion representing ongoing crystal embolization. The least frequently described scenario is a chronic or delayed course, in which significant kidney impairment may not be noted until up to 6 months after the trigger. These cases are likely underrecognized and are typically attributed to other causes of chronic kidney damage, such as nephrosclerosis.

When large burdens of cholesterol crystals are present in the bloodstream, a massive catastrophic syndrome can present with AKI, stroke, gastrointestinal bleeding, necrotic skin ulcerations, and rapid death. In less severe cases,

Table 34.1 Commonly Involved Organs in Cholesterol Atheroembolic Disease

Organ	Percentage (%)
Kidney	75
Spleen	52
Pancreas	52
Gastrointestinal tract	31
Adrenal glands	20
Liver	17
Brain	14
Skin	6

gastrointestinal involvement may be limited to abdominal pain, nausea, or vomiting. Skin manifestations are seen commonly and can be helpful in making the diagnosis. Subjects can present with a classic reticular rash over their lower extremities known as livedo reticularis, as well as blue or purple toes, and purpura. Acalculous cholecystitis can occur with liver involvement, and pancreatitis can also be evident. Funduscopic examination may show Hollenhorst plaques, which are refractive yellow deposits from cholesterol emboli seen within retinal arteries. Central nervous system involvement can lead to transient ischemic events, strokes, amaurosis fugax, or spinal cord infarctions.

DIAGNOSIS

The diagnosis of atheroembolic kidney disease can be elusive and requires a high index of suspicion. In addition to the clinical features described previously, laboratory data can be helpful. Initially, leukocytosis and other inflammatory markers, such as erythrocyte sedimentation rate or C-reactive protein, are commonly elevated in the setting of the provoked immune response. Eosinophilia is present in 25% to 50% of cases, and occasionally hypocomplementemia can be detected. The negative predictive value of these findings is low, and therefore their absence is not helpful in excluding the diagnosis. Additional lab abnormalities can implicate specific organ involvement, including elevated amylase or lipase with pancreatic involvement, increased transaminases with liver involvement, elevated lactate with bowel involvement, and increased creatine kinase concentration with muscle involvement. Urine studies typically show benign sediment without cellular casts and only a minimal amount of proteinuria.

PATHOLOGY

Definitive diagnosis of atheroembolic kidney disease requires a kidney biopsy, but, depending on the clinical circumstances, this may be challenging to perform. A skin or muscle biopsy can also be helpful when these tissues are involved. Often the diagnosis can be made on clinical grounds based on the presenting features, particularly when classic exam findings are present. Kidney lesions found on biopsy include biconvex, needle-shaped clefts within the arcuate and interlobular arterioles (Fig. 34.1). Because the cholesterol crystals dissolve during specimen processing, the clefts are empty and are referred to as "ghost cells." Within

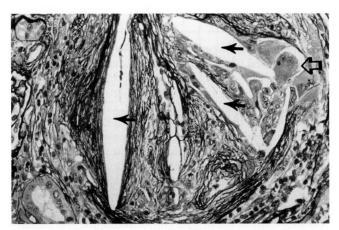

Figure 34.1 Cholesterol atheroembolus occludes the lumen of an interlobular renal artery. Needle-like clefts *(solid arrows)* can be seen, along with a macrophage–multinucleated giant cell reaction *(open arrow)* (methenamine silver–trichrome stain, original magnification ×450). (Courtesy Dr. S.I. Bastacky. From Greenberg A, Bastacky SI, Iqbal A, et al: Focal segmental glomerulosclerosis associated with nephrotic syndrome in cholesterol atheroembolism: clinicopathologic correlations. *Am J Kidney Dis* 29:334-344, 1997, with permission.)

the vessels can be seen intimal thickening and concentric fibrosis; it is not uncommon for giant cells to form in the immediate vicinity of the crystal.

Vascular recanalization, endothelial proliferation, tubulointerstitial fibrosis, glomerular ischemia, and focal segmental glomerulosclerosis also characterize what can be seen on kidney biopsy.

THERAPY AND OUTCOMES

The mainstay of therapy for atheroembolic kidney disease is prevention. Paralleling conventional preventive measures for limiting atherosclerotic disease, patients should avoid smoking, hyperlipidemia, and poorly controlled hypertension or diabetes. The benefits of these modifications are extrapolated from data focusing on risk reduction for cardiovascular events, as there are no controlled trials that specifically address atheroembolic kidney disease prevention. Despite a lack of proven cause and effect, it is advisable to weigh the risks and benefits carefully when planning to initiate or continue anticoagulation or thrombolytic agents in subjects at high risk for cholesterol emboli. The need for elective endovascular procedures should also be critically evaluated, and, when reasonable, medical management should be the preferred option. Alternatively, additional strategies that may reduce atheroembolic events include distal embolic protection devices for renovascular procedures and upper extremity approaches via the radial and brachial arteries for cardiac catheterizations. Data showing a reduction in kidney injury when these practices are implemented are sparse, but suggest that the benefit may be mediated by minimizing the embolization of cholesterol plaques from the renal arteries and abdominal aorta.

After atheroembolic kidney disease has occurred, effective treatment options are limited. To date, there have been no prospective randomized clinical trials evaluating specific agents. The use of steroids has been assessed in observational studies; however, the results have not shown consistent

benefit. The largest prospective study involving 354 patients with atheroembolic kidney disease did not report a benefit in kidney outcomes in those patients treated with steroids. Another study from Spain retrospectively evaluated 45 cases and actually showed worse kidney outcomes in those who received steroids. These findings contradict results from earlier small case series and reports that showed improvement in kidney function with steroid therapy. In summary, data do not support routine use of steroid therapy for atheroembolic kidney disease; however, they may have a role in patients with evidence of a high inflammatory burden and multiorgan involvement.

Statins have also been evaluated for their potential benefit, and it has been hypothesized that they improve kidney outcomes by way of reductions in lipid burden, plaque stabilization, and antiinflammatory effects. Again, the few observational studies involving patients treated with statins have demonstrated conflicting results regarding their effectiveness in limiting kidney injury. However, these agents should routinely be administered to patients with atheroembolic kidney disease because of their well-established ability to reduce the risk of cardiovascular events. Additionally, the routine use of ACE inhibitors or ARBs should also be implemented because of their known benefit to patients with cardiovascular risk factors. Other therapies indicating benefit in isolated reports include pentoxyfylline, iloprost, LDL apheresis, and, in some circumstances, segmental aortic replacement to remove the emboli source.

Overall, renal prognosis is poor in atheroembolic kidney disease with the majority of patients having progressive kidney failure. The number of subjects with severe kidney failure requiring dialysis ranges from 28% to 61% in various studies. In the largest prospective analysis, 33% of patients required dialysis at some point after diagnosis, and 25% remained on chronic dialysis at the end of 2 years. Those treated with statins had more favorable kidney outcomes, irrespective of whether therapy was initiated at the time of diagnosis or was in place before the triggering event. Important predictors of those likely to require dialysis are preexisting chronic kidney disease and longstanding hypertension. However, it has been reported that as many as 39% of those who are started on dialysis recover enough kidney function to be dialysis free at follow-up.

More recent studies have shown decreased mortality with atheroembolic disease as compared to historical case series that documented 1-year survival rates as low as 19%. Belefant et al. implemented an aggressive treatment protocol for 67 consecutive patients diagnosed with atheroembolic kidney disease in an intensive care unit, with a reported 1-year survival rate of 87%. The leading cause of death in atheroembolic kidney failure is from cardiovascular events, and improvement in survival rates in recent studies is a direct result of reducing these risks. Additionally, the widespread use of dialysis has also contributed to reduced mortality rates.

KIDNEY INFARCTION

Abrupt disruption of blood supply to the kidney results in kidney infarction. Overall, this is a relatively rare event. Few studies have been published on this topic, but one retrospective review looking at a 36-month period noted the annual incidence to be 0.007% of all hospital admissions. When kidney infarction occurs, it can involve both kidneys, one entire kidney, or a small subsection depending on the involved vessels. Because of the acute nature of the insult and the lack of collateral blood supply, these events are usually symptomatic. Patients will commonly present with flank or abdominal pain, microscopic hematuria, fever, nausea, and vomiting. When both kidneys, or a single functioning kidney, are involved, oliguric or anuric AKI may occur. Most cases, however, do not present with a rise in creatinine or a change in urine output. Because of the release of renin from the infarcted tissue, an abrupt rise in blood pressure can occur. Laboratory studies show a leukocytosis and a notable rise in lactate dehydrogenase. Given the nonspecific nature of the clinical presentation, imaging is needed to make the diagnosis. A computed tomography (CT) scan with intravenous contrast is often the imaging modality employed, as it allows good delineation of poorly perfused areas in the renal cortex. The classic finding is a wedge-shaped lesion demarcating the area of hypoperfusion (Fig. 34.2). A renal nuclear scan with dimercaptosuccinic acid is a more sensitive study, and it is helpful when a high suspicion remains despite negative findings on CT. Finally, a renal artery angiogram is the gold standard for making the diagnosis, but is rarely needed.

A number of etiologies can lead to kidney infarction (Box 34.2). The most common scenario is a thromboembolism to the renal artery. A thorough investigation for an embolic source should be undertaken. Commonly identified conditions include atrial fibrillation, cardiac thrombus following myocardial infarction, paradoxical emboli from a patent foramen ovale, or thromboemboli from complex atherosclerotic plaques in the aorta. Additional reports have identified acute renal artery thrombosis in the setting of antiphospholipid syndrome and other hypercoagulable states, septic emboli from infective endocarditis, and traumatic injury to the renal artery following a deceleration injury. Aortic or renal artery dissections can create false lumens that obstruct blood flow to the kidney and lead to infarction. Finally, spontaneous renal artery thrombosis can occur in the setting of atherosclerotic disease, aneurysms, or medium and large vessel vasculitidies.

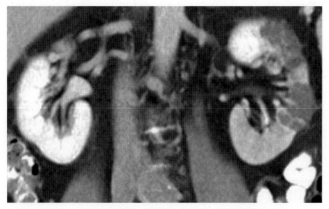

Figure 34.2 Computed tomography with iodinated intravenous contrast demonstrating an infarction in the left kidney. Note the wedge-shaped appearance of the defect, which is typical for this finding.

TREATMENT

Treatment is usually conservative. Antihypertensive therapy should be used to minimize the renin-related hypertension that can occur following infarction; typically ACE inhibitors or ARBs are the agents of choice. Volume overload states should be managed with diuretics and salt restriction. The decision to start anticoagulation is usually dictated by the underlying disorder. When cardiac thrombi or a hypercoagulable state is identified, the initiation of anticoagulation is employed to prevent additional emboli. After infarction has occurred, the tissue is not salvageable. For this reason, revascularization with thrombolysis or angioplasty should only be considered in cases in which the diagnosis is made relatively early in the disease course and under the assumption that restoring perfusion will prevent further tissue involvement. In cases of traumatic renal vascular occlusion, surgical repair of the vessel may provide renal salvage only if the diagnosis is made within the first few hours after occurrence. In patients who develop in situ thrombi in the setting of atherosclerotic kidney disease, previous collateral blood flow has typically developed. These patients often develop ischemic kidney disease without infarction, and it is not unreasonable to use a more liberal revascularization strategy in such cases.

Box 34.2 Causes of Kidney Infarction

Embolism

Cardiac Origin

Atrial fibrillation
Valvular disease
Endocarditis
Ventricular thrombus
Myxoma

Noncardiac Origin

Paradoxical emboli
Fat emboli
Tumor emboli

Thrombosis

Hypercoagulable States

Nephrotic syndrome
Antiphospholipid syndrome
Antithrombin III deficiency
Homocystinuria

Secondary to Structural Changes of the Aorta or Renal Arteries

Atherosclerotic disease
Aneurysms
Dissections

Vasculitis Involving the Renal Artery

Polyarteritis nodosa
Takayasu's arteritis
Kawasaki disease
Thromboangiitis obliterans

Trauma

As a Complication of Endovascular Interventions

ACUTE TUBULAR INJURY FROM ENDOGENOUS NEPHROTOXINS

Endogenous nephrotoxins often cause ATI in specific clinical circumstances. The diagnosis can sometimes be difficult as the toxin exposure will not be readily reported by the patient nor listed in their medical records, as is often the case with exogenous toxins. In addition, preventing further toxin exposure to the kidney is not always readily achieved at the time of diagnosis. Treatment strategies often involve manipulating the biochemical environment in which the kidney and toxin interact to limit injury.

RHABDOMYOLYSIS

The term *rhabdomyolysis* specifically refers to the clinical syndrome associated with muscle necrosis and the release of intracellular contents into the extracellular space. The clinical spectrum can range from a relatively benign course to severe systemic illness with AKI due to heme pigment nephropathy. Bywaters and Bell are credited with the initial description of kidney failure resulting from rhabdomyolysis in four cases involving crush injuries during the bombing of London in World War II. This was a landmark contribution to the understanding of heme pigment nephropathy. The incidence of AKI in rhabdomyolysis has been reported to range from 5% to 51%, and mortality rates are dramatically increased with kidney involvement.

CAUSES AND PATHOPHYSIOLOGY OF RHABDOMYOLYSIS

The etiologies of rhabdomyolysis are listed in Box 34.3. Most notable are crush injuries that accompany natural disasters such as hurricanes and earthquakes. AKI from rhabdomyolysis is one of the most common causes of mortality in these incidents. Immediately following the 2010 earthquake in Haiti, a renal disaster relief task force was dispatched to provide rapid treatment and dialysis support for victims. The goal of this mission was to limit the number of casualties. Compartment syndrome within a limb causes pressure necrosis that leads to tissue damage and rhabdomyolysis. This may require an emergency fasciotomy. Overexertion causes necrosis in otherwise normal muscles because of a mismatch in energy supply and demand. This is most commonly seen in poorly conditioned persons who partake in extreme exercise activities. However, even well-conditioned athletes can manifest rhabdomyolysis and develop AKI. Cases of experienced marathon runners developing kidney failure and requiring dialysis have been reported. The most frequent etiology in a series of 475 patients was from medications and toxin ingestions. Alcohol and cocaine were the two most abused substances associated

---

Box 34.3   Causes of Rhabdomyolysis

Physical Injury

Trauma
Crush injury
Compartment syndrome
Immobilization

Muscle-Fiber Exhaustion

Excessive exercise
Seizures
Heat stroke
Neuroleptic malignant syndrome
Malignant hyperthermia

Medications, Illicit Drugs, and Dietary Supplements

Statins
Fibrates
Zidovudine
Phenytoin
Selective serotonin reuptake inhibitors
Isoniazid
Colchicine
Antipsychotics
Antimilarials
Trimethoprim-sulfamethoxazole in HIV infection
Cocaine
Amphetamines
Heroin
Methadone
Phencyclidine
Creatine
Ephedra

Toxins

Alcohol
Tolulene
Carbon monoxide
Hydrocarbons
Quail poisoning
Mushroom poisoning

Electrolyte Disturbances

Hypokalemia
Hypophosphatemia
Excessive fluid shifts

Inflammatory States

Dermatomysositis and polymyositis
Vasculitis
Systemic inflammatory response
Viral infections (e.g., influenza, parainfluenza, coxsackie, HIV, EBV, CMV, herpes)
Bacterial infection (e.g., Legionnaire's disease, tularemia, toxic shock syndrome, streptococci, staphylococci, *Clostridium, Salmonella*)
Protozoal infections (e.g., *Plasmodium falciparum* malaria)

Deficiencies in Metabolic Enzymes

Muscle phosphorylase deficiency (McArdle's disease)
Carnitine palmotyl transferase deficiency
Phosphofructokinase deficiency in muscle (Tarui disease)

CMV, Cytomegalovirus; *EBV,* Ebstein-Barr virus; *HIV,* human immunodeficiency virus.

with rhabdomyolysis. A number of medications also cause muscle injury; the most frequently implicated agents are antipsychotics, statins, and selective serotonin release inhibitors.

The final common pathologic pathway that leads to the disruption of the muscle-fiber integrity is the increase in the ionized calcium concentration within the cytoplasm (i.e., sarcoplasm). This results in unchecked protease activation and a fatal cascade of cellular events. The elevated intracellular calcium level is a consequence of adenosine triphosphate (ATP) depletion, and Na/K$^+$-ATPase and Ca^{2+}-ATPase failure. This inhibits the normally efficient expulsion of calcium from the cytoplasm.

After muscle-cell necrosis occurs, contents in high concentration within the cell are then expelled into the extracellular fluid, specifically creatine kinase, myoglobin, organic acids, and various electrolytes. Ultimately, it is the pathophysiologic consequences of these substances that lead to morbidity and mortality in rhabdomyolysis. Significant electrolyte imbalances in rhabdomyolysis include hyperkalemia, hyperphosphatemia, and hypocalcemia. Hyperkalemia and hyperphosphatemia reflect their relatively high intracellular concentrations. Ninety-eight percent of total body stores of potassium resides intracellularly, and 70% is within skeletal muscle cells. As opposed to potassium and phosphorous, plasma calcium levels decrease during the acute phase of rhabdomyolysis. This phenomenon occurs because calcium complexes with phosphorous and precipitates within necrotic tissues in the form of calcium-phosphate. As tissue recovery occurs in the following days to weeks, calcium is mobilized from necrotic tissue and can lead to significant rebound hypercalcemia late in the disease course. The release of lactate and other organic acids from muscle cells manifest as an anion gap metabolic acidosis. In addition, elevated uric acid levels may result from purine metabolism after cell injury.

DIAGNOSIS

The most striking clinical feature of patients who present with rhabdomyolysis is typically severe myalgias. However, on occasion patients may have minimal or no symptoms, and in other situations subjects may be incapacitated. A high level of suspicion is needed in these cases. The history often shows circumstances or events that support the diagnosis. Patients should be questioned about vigorous physical activity, medication or toxin ingestion, preceding trauma, or prolonged immobilization on a hard surface.

Urine output may be decreased when AKI is significant and, because of the presence of myoglobin in the urine, will appear reddish-brown in color. Under the microscope, pigmented granular casts will be seen. Urine dipstick shows significant positivity for heme protein with few or no red blood cells seen on microscopy. This apparent discrepancy occurs because the dipstick test is unable to differentiate between myoglobin and hemoglobin. An additional characteristic feature of rhabdomyolysis that is unique from most other forms of ATI is the low fractional excretion of sodium (less than 1%). This is not universal and is typically found early in the disease course. Approximately 50% of cases will have some level of proteinuria detected on urinalysis.

Blood tests show elevations in myoglobin and creatine kinase. Myoglobin levels are not routinely measured, because myoglobin metabolism is rapid and unpredictable,

and therefore unreliable. Creatine kinase, on the other hand, can reach values up to 1000 times the upper limit of normal. The risk of AKI is typically not significant until the creatine kinase levels are greater than 15,000 to 20,000 U/L. Electrolyte and acid-base abnormalities as described earlier are also indicative of the diagnosis.

HEMOGLOBINURIA

Free circulating hemoglobin occurs in the setting of intravascular hemolysis. In small quantities, circulating hemoglobin will be completely bound by plasma haptoglobin to form a hemoglobin-haptoglobin compound that is then cleared by monocytes and macrophages. However, when significant quantities of hemoglobin are present in the plasma, the haptoglobin supply is quickly depleted. Free circulating hemoglobin exists as a tetramer (two α and two β chains; MW 68 kDa), and a dimer (one α and one β chain; MW 32 kDa). Tetrameric hemoglobin and the hemoglobin-haptoglobin complex are not readily filtered because of their large size; however, dimeric hemoglobin can undergo appreciable glomerular filtration. Filtered hemoglobin is taken up by proximal tubule cells, or it contributes to cast formation within the lumen. Hemoglobinuric AKI is included in the spectrum of heme pigment nephropathies. Numerous causes of hemolysis can lead to hemoglobinuria. Common etiologies include transfusion reactions, autoimmune hemolytic anemia, mechanical shearing from prosthetic valves, glucose-6 phosphate dehydrogenase deficiency, paroxysmal nocturnal hemoglobinuria, malaria (blackwater fever), and a number of drugs or toxins.

PATHOGENESIS OF HEME PIGMENT NEPHROPATHY

In addition to the direct tubular toxicity of myoglobin and hemoglobin, additional factors including volume depletion, renal vasoconstriction, acidosis, cytokine release, and tubular cast formation all increase the nephrotoxic potential of heme pigments. Depletion of the intravascular volume is common with rhabdomyolysis because of fluid sequestration into tissues. In addition, the clinical settings that are associated with rhabdomyolysis often result in volume depletion (crush injury in trapped persons, overexertion, drug and alcohol abuse, immobilization). Impaired renal blood flow occurs because of a decrease in the vasodilator nitric oxide, which is avidly scavenged by heme proteins, and an increase in potent vasoconstrictors (i.e., endothelin and isoprostanes). The resultant decrease in renal perfusion results in ischemic injury to renal tubular cells. Cytokine activation also occurs. Heme protein mediated induction of chemokines, such as monocyte chemoattractant-1, results in leukocytic recruitment and additional epithelial cell injury. Acidosis leads to an environment that denatures heme proteins to a confirmation that promotes interaction with Tamm-Horsfall protein and urinary casts formation. Tubular obstruction subsequently occurs, which in turn prolongs the exposure of RTECs to hemoglobin and myoglobin. As a consequence, cellular uptake of heme proteins occurs leading to renal tubular cell injury by way of lipid peroxidation and free radical formation. Ferrihemate, present in muscle injury, is a major cause of tubular injury in this setting. Finally, calcium-phosphate deposition within the kidney also contributes to tubular injury.

TREATMENT

The treatment strategy for heme pigment nephropathy is similar for both rhabdomyolysis and hemoglobinuria. Early aggressive fluid repletion is the most important factor. Not only does this correct volume depletion and subsequent renal ischemia, but it also limits casts formation and excessive heme protein concentrations within the renal tubule. Patients may require 10 L or more of intravenous fluid daily. Although volume repletion is important for treating heme pigment nephropathy, it remains controversial whether saline is the ideal solution to use. Some experts recommend an isotonic sodium bicarbonate solution. The proposed benefits of alkalinizing the urine with sodium bicarbonate include reducing myoglobin binding with Tamm-Horsfall protein, inhibiting the reduction-oxidation (redox) cycling of myoglobin that leads to lipid peroxidation, and preventing metamyoglobin-induced vasoconstriction. These theoretical effects are mainly generated from animal studies, and there are not robust clinical data to show a clear benefit. On the contrary, there is some concern regarding the potential negative effects of sodium bicarbonate administration, as the induced alkalosis may exacerbate the symptoms of hypocalcemia and increase the precipitation of calcium-phosphate in the kidney. The use of mannitol has also been proposed, often in combination with sodium bicarbonate. Mannitol may increase urinary flow and help flush out heme pigment by inducing an osmotic diuresis. In addition, mannitol is a free radical scavenger. Other antioxidant agents that have shown benefit in small case series include pentoxyfylline, vitamin E, and vitamin C. Kidney replacement therapy is mainly supportive when severe kidney failure occurs or rapid correction of electrolyte abnormalities is necessary. Despite the dense ATI that can occur in both settings and the frequent need for kidney replacement therapy, most patients recover enough kidney function to become independent of dialysis, and many regain function back toward their premorbid level.

ACUTE NEPHROPATHY ASSOCIATED WITH TUMOR LYSIS SYNDROME

Tumor lysis syndrome results from the release of a large amount of intracellular contents into the ECF following massive necrosis of tumor cells. This typically occurs after the administration of chemotherapeutic agents for treatment of lymphomas and leukemias, but it can rarely occur spontaneously in rapidly dividing solid tumors that outgrow their blood supply.

Laboratory tests show high serum levels of potassium, phosphate, and uric acid. Acute nephropathy is a common occurrence, and is a direct consequence of uric acid and calcium-phosphate precipitation within the renal tubules. Uric acid crystal formation is enhanced in acidic urine. For this reason, alkalinization of the urine with sodium bicarbonate infusion can be used to prevent or limit urate nephropathy. However, this strategy may in turn lead to more calcium-phosphate deposition and acute nephrocalcinosis. Some experts suggest management with saline alone to induce high urine flow, and only implementing sodium bicarbonate

therapy when the serum uric acid level is greater than 12 mg/dl or uric acid crystals are seen on microscopy. Allopurinol and rasburicase limit the formation of uric acid by either inhibiting its production (allopurinol) or increasing its breakdown (rasburicase). These medications should be considered as prophylaxis in high-risk patients planned for chemotherapy.

OTHER ENDOGENOUS TOXINS

Given the concentrating ability of the kidney, other endogenous substances can accumulate within the renal tubules and cause ATI. Similar to the previous causes, this occurs when pathologic states lead to elevated plasma levels of substances that are relatively benign under normal conditions. In myeloma, free light chains are filtered by the glomerulus in large quantities. After entering the tubule, they cause direct cellular toxicity within the proximal tubule and cast injury in the distal tubule, resulting in myeloma cast nephropathy.

Plasma levels of oxalate can be elevated as a result of either endogenous production or exogenous ingestion. In primary hyperoxaluria, oxalate overproduction occurs as a result of an inborn error in the metabolism of glyoxylate. This leads to urine oxalate concentrations at supersaturated levels. Calcium oxalate precipitation occurs, and results in crystal aggregation and nephrocalcinosis. The resulting tubular injury can lead to significant kidney damage. Hyperoxaluria also occurs following gastric bypass surgery and with other causes of malabsorption (pancreatitis, Crohn's disease). This occurrence is a result of increased gut absorption of oxalate from dietary sources. Exogenous etiologies include ingestion of ethylene glycol (antifreeze), large doses of orlistat, and excessive amounts of vitamin C.

BIBLIOGRAPHY

Abuelo JG: Normotensive ischemic acute renal failure, *N Engl J Med* 357:797-805, 2007.

Belenfant X, Meyrier A, Jacquot C: Supportive treatment improves survival in multivisceral cholesterol crystal embolism, *Am J Kidney Dis* 33:840-850, 1999.

Bywaters EG, Beall D: Crush injuries with impairment of renal function, *Br Med J* 1:427-432, 1941.

Frock J, Bierman M, Hammeke M, et al: Atheroembolic renal disease: experience with 22 patients, *Nebr Med J* 79:317-321, 1994.

Gutierrez Solis E, Morales E, Rodriguez Jornet A, et al: [Atheroembolic renal disease: analysis of clinical and therapeutic factors that influence its progression], *Nefrologia* 30:317-323, 2010.

Howard SC, Jones DP, Pui CH: The tumor lysis syndrome, *N Engl J Med* 364:1844-1854, 2011.

Korzets Z, Plotkin E, Bernheim J, et al: The clinical spectrum of acute renal infarction, *Isr Med Assoc J* 4:781-784, 2002.

Melli G, Chaudhry V, Cornblath DR: Rhabdomyolysis: an evaluation of 475 hospitalized patients, *Medicine (Baltimore)* 84:377-385, 2005.

Meyrier A: Cholesterol crystal embolism: diagnosis and treatment, *Kidney Int* 69:1308-1312, 2006.

Nasr SH, D'Agati VD, Said SM, et al: Oxalate nephropathy complicating Roux-en-Y Gastric Bypass: an underrecognized cause of irreversible renal failure, *Clin J Am Soc Nephrol* 3:1676-1683, 2008.

Perazella MA, Coca SG, Hall IE, et al: Urine microscopy is associated with severity and worsening of acute kidney injury in hospitalized patients, *Clin J Am Soc Nephrol* 5:402-408, 2010.

Scolari F, Ravani P: Atheroembolic renal disease, *Lancet* 375:1650-1660, 2010.

Thurau K, Boylan JW: Acute renal success: the unexpected logic of oliguria in acute renal failure, *Am J Med* 61:308-315, 1976.

Tracz MJ, Alam J, Nath KA: Physiology and pathophysiology of heme: implications for kidney disease, *J Am Soc Nephrol* 18:414-420, 2007.

35 Acute Interstitial Nephritis

Ursula C. Brewster | Asghar Rastegar

In 1898, W.T. Councilman defined acute interstitial nephritis (AIN) as "an acute inflammation of the kidney characterized by cellular and fluid exudation in the interstitial tissue, accompanied by, but not dependent on, degeneration of the epithelium; the exudation is not purulent in character, and the lesions may be both diffuse and focal." This was seen on postmortem examination of patients with scarlet fever and, less commonly, other systemic infectious diseases that had no evidence for direct bacterial invasion of the kidney parenchyma.

More than a century later, definitive diagnosis of AIN requires the pathologic findings of interstitial edema and infiltration with acute inflammatory cells including polymorphonucleocytes (PMNs), eosinophils, and lymphocytes. In the years since Councilman's description, the causes of AIN have changed dramatically with pharmacologic agents the most common etiology (more than 75%). In this chapter we will focus primarily on acute tubulointerstitial inflammation, while briefly covering direct parenchymal invasion by infectious agents.

The incidence of AIN varies greatly depending on the clinical scenario. An incidence of 0.7% is seen in asymptomatic patients with proteinuria or hematuria, whereas hospitalized patients with acute kidney injury (AKI) of unknown etiology experience an incidence of 10% to 15%. Although AIN can occur in all age groups, it is more common in the elderly. In one report, biopsy-proven AIN was seen in 3.0% of the elderly compared to 1.9% of younger subjects. This may reflect greater exposure of elderly patients to drugs and other inciting factors.

CLINICAL PRESENTATION

The presenting symptoms of AIN include an acute or subacute decline in kidney function, often in patients exposed to multiple drugs. Although the "classical" presentation of skin rash, arthralgia, and eosinophilia is occasionally seen, this triad occurs in only 5% to 10% of unselected patients. This presentation is more commonly seen in association with certain drugs, such as penicillin derivatives, in comparison to nonsteroidal antiinflammatory drugs (NSAIDs). Fever, the most common clinical sign, is present in up to 50% of patients with drug-induced AIN but only in 30% of unselected patients. Skin rash is reported in one third of patients and is usually maculopapular. No clinical symptom or sign is sensitive or specific enough to establish a definitive diagnosis. Nonoliguric AKI usually accompanies AIN, but oliguric AKI with rapid rise in creatinine also occurs. Increasingly, AIN develops in patients with underlying chronic kidney disease (CKD) and multiple comorbidities, which makes a diagnosis challenging. AIN should therefore be considered in any patient with acute or subacute decline in kidney function with no clear inciting factor.

LABORATORY FINDINGS

Common laboratory findings in AIN are summarized in Table 35.1. The most common abnormality is a slow and steady rise in blood urea nitrogen and serum creatinine concentration. Rapid and fulminant presentation of AIN occurs less often. Other major laboratory findings include eosinophilia, eosinophiluria, and abnormal urinary sediment. Eosinophilia is common in β-lactam antibiotic associated AIN, reported in up to 80% of cases, where only a third of other drug-induced AIN cases develop eosinophilia. Hyperkalemia, with or without hyperchloremic metabolic acidosis, is occasionally seen.

Urinalysis and examination of the urine sediment are often the most useful laboratory tests. Low-grade proteinuria (1-2+) and positive leukocyte esterase are noted on urine dipstick in most patients. Quantitative proteinuria measurements are usually less than 1 g/day. Macroscopic hematuria is rare, whereas microscopic hematuria is present less than 50% of the time. Leukocytes are present on urine microscopy in virtually all cases of methicillin-induced AIN, but they may be absent in as many as 50% of patients with AIN due to other drugs. The absence of leukocyturia, therefore, should not eliminate this diagnosis from the differential. Classically, urine microscopy will show hematuria, leukocyturia, leukocyte casts, and renal tubular epithelial (RTE) cells (Fig. 35.1). Cellular casts are seen in most cases of methicillin-associated AIN and in up to 50% of patients with AIN resulting from other etiologies.

Eosinophiluria, once thought to be hallmark of this disease, is both insensitive and nonspecific and should not be used to make a diagnosis. This test has a sensitivity of 67% and a specificity of 83% in patients with AKI. The techniques used to stain urine for eosinophils (Wright stain and Hansel stain) have proven unreliable and cumbersome. In addition, other disease states such as cystitis, pyelonephritis, atheroembolic kidney disease, and rapidly progressive glomerulonephritis may present with eosinophiluria, making the test nonspecific in diagnosing AIN.

IMAGING

Kidney ultrasound in the setting of AIN typically shows normal to enlarged kidneys with normal echogenicity. However,

Table 35.1   Laboratory Findings in Acute Interstitial Nephritis

Eosinophilia	Inconsistent finding seen more commonly in drug-induced AIN
Eosinophiluria	Sensitivity 63% to 91%, specificity 52% to 94%
Urinary sediment	Hematuria, leukocyteuria, leukocyte casts, RTE cells, and RTE casts
Protein excretion	Less than 1 g/24 h
Fractional excretion of sodium (FeNa)	Greater than 1%
Proximal tubular defect	Glycosuria, phosphaturia, bicarbonaturia, aminoaciduria
Distal tubular defect	Hyperkalemia, distal RTA, sodium wasting
Medullary defect	Nephrogenic diabetes insipidus

AIN, Acute interstitial nephritis; *RTA,* renal tubular acidosis; *RTE,* renal tubular epithelial.

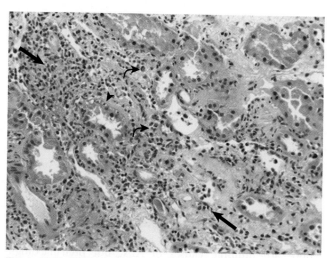

Figure 35.2   Kidney biopsy showing acute interstitial nephritis. A diffuse interstitial infiltrate is present *(arrows)* along with severe tubular injury and tubulitis *(arrowhead)* where lymphocytes have crossed the tubular basement membrane. Also present are eosinophils *(curved arrows).* (Hematoxylin and eosin ×200.)

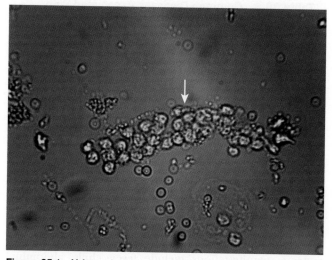

Figure 35.1   Urine microscopy showing a white blood cell cast *(arrow)* and surrounding white blood cells and red blood cells (×60).

these findings are also nonspecific and may be seen with other forms of kidney disease. Although Gallium-67 scan was initially reported as highly sensitive in AIN, this has not been supported over time, and its only role may be to differentiate AIN from acute tubular necrosis (ATN) in those patients who cannot undergo a kidney biopsy. Positron emission tomography has shown diagnostic promise in several AIN cases, but needs further evaluation before widespread use.

PATHOLOGY

Although suspicion of AIN is based on clinical clues, definitive diagnosis often requires a kidney biopsy. Major pathologic findings include interstitial edema, inflammation, and tubulitis without glomerular or vascular involvement (Fig. 35.2). Interstitial infiltration may be diffuse but is often patchy in nature and consists of lymphocytes, mononuclear cells, eosinophils, neutrophils, and plasma

cells. T lymphocytes are primarily composed of CD4 and CD8 cells. The number of eosinophils is highly variable and is more prominent in drug-induced AIN. Granulomas are uncommon but occasionally seen, especially with sarcoidosis and drug-induced AIN. Tubulitis, characterized by the invasion of inflammatory cells though the tubular basement membrane, results in tubular injury and is often seen in association with severe inflammation. Severity of interstitial inflammation, however, does not always correlate with clinical outcome. Poor prognosis is more directly related to the degree of interstitial fibrosis and tubular atrophy. Immunofluorescence and electron microscopic studies are usually unrevealing. NSAID-associated AIN is sometimes associated with glomerular changes of minimal change disease or membranous nephropathy. In contrast to isolated AIN, full-blown nephrotic syndrome accompanies AKI in these cases.

PATHOGENESIS

The clinical and histopathologic findings summarized earlier strongly point to an immune-mediated mechanism initiating and sustaining tubulointerstitial damage. The immunologic basis of injury is supported by the low frequency of AIN in persons exposed to a drug, lack of dose dependency, presence of systemic symptoms in some patients, and recurrence of AIN upon reexposure. The antigens initiating the immune-mediated injury could be of endogenous origin (Tamm-Horsfall protein, megalin, and tubular base membrane components) or exogenous, such as drugs and chemicals. Exogenous antigens may be trapped directly or may circulate as immune complexes that are deposited in the kidney interstitium. They may bind to a tubular antigen acting as a hapten, or mimic a normal tubular or interstitial antigen, thereby triggering an immune reaction. In animal models, both cell-mediated and humoral immunity is involved. The injury is initiated by the presentation of endogenous or exogenous antigens to antigen-presenting lymphocytes resulting in the activation of T cells. These cells induce differentiation and proliferation of other T cells responsible for delayed hypersensitivity and cytotoxicity. The resultant inflammatory infiltrates within the interstitium produce a variety of fibrinogenic cytokines and chemokines, such as transforming growth factor-β (TGF-β), platelet-derived growth factor-BB (PDGF-BB), epidermal growth factor (EGF), and fibroblast growth factor-2 (FGF-2). The fibroblasts invading the interstitium are the product of epithelial-to-mesenchymal transition. Ultimately, this inflammatory process results in the accumulation of extracellular matrix, interstitial fibrosis, and tubular loss.

CAUSES OF ACUTE INTERSTITIAL NEPHRITIS

There are multiple causes of AIN, but pharmacologic agents are the most common (Table 35.2). Diagnosis of AIN should trigger a review of the medication list to identify culpable agents and limit further drug exposure. In addition to various drugs, certain infectious agents may induce AIN. Although less common in the antibiotic era, infectious agents must be considered when the clinical scenario is consistent. Finally, systemic diseases, primarily rheumatologic, are associated with the pathologic finding of AIN. These diseases are usually evident from the clinical presentation (Table 35.3).

DRUG-ASSOCIATED INTERSTITIAL NEPHRITIS

ANTIBIOTICS

β-LACTAM ANTIBIOTICS

Methicillin and other β-lactam antibiotics are the most common agents associated with AIN. Methicillin is immunogenic and leads to a hypersensitivity syndrome more often than other drugs, including those in the β-lactam class. The time course is variable, but AIN usually develops approximately 10 to 14 days following drug exposure, unless the patient was previously sensitized. Patients with β-lactam–induced AIN frequently manifest systemic symptoms of fever, rash, arthralgias, and eosinophilia along with AKI. These symptoms may be fleeting or nonexistent, making them unreliable clinical tools for diagnosing AIN. Urinalysis and urine microscopy demonstrate low-grade proteinuria, hematuria, and leukocyturia in approximately 75% of cases (see Fig. 35.1). Because of its association with AIN, methicillin is rarely used thanks to the availability of other β-lactam agents. Cephalosporins may cause a similar clinical presentation of AIN; however, this is less common than with traditional penicillins. On withdrawal of the drug, kidney function usually recovers, although CKD may persist in some.

NON β-LACTAM ANTIBIOTICS

Rifampin-induced AIN can be severe and appears to occur more frequently with intermittent dosing as compared to continuous dosing regimens. AIN develops in a dose-dependent fashion in most but not all patients, and, at

Table 35.2 Common Drugs Associated With Acute Interstitial Nephritis

Drug Class	Examples
Antibiotics	β-lactams, sulfonamides, fluoroquinolones, rifampin, vancomycin, erythromycin, ethambutol, chloramphenicol
Antivirals	Acyclovir, atazanavir, abacavir, indinavir
Analgesics	NSAIDs, selective COX-2 inhibitors
GI medications	PPIs, H2-receptor blockers, 5-aminosalicylates
Anticonvulsants	Phenytoin, carbamazepine, phenobarbital
Diuretics	Hydrochlorothiazide, furosemide, triamterene, chlorthalidone
Others	Allopurinol, Chinese herbs

COX-2, Cyclooxygenase-2; *GI,* gastrointestinal; *NSAIDs,* nonsteroidal antiinflammatory drugs; *PPIs,* proton pump inhibitors.

Table 35.3 Common Diseases Associated With Acute Interstitial Nephritis

Bacterial infection	Legionella, Staphylococcus, Streptococcus, Yersinia
Viral infection	Hantavirus, CMV, EBV, HIV, herpes simplex, Hep C
Autoimmune	Systemic lupus erythematosis, Sjögren syndrome, sarcoidosis
Neoplastic diseases	Lymphoproliferative disorders, plasma cell dyscrasias

CMV, Cytomegalovirus; *EBV,* Epstein-Barr virus; *Hep C,* hepatitis C virus; *HIV,* human immunodeficiency virus.

times, circulating antibodies to rifampin may be detected. Systemic manifestations include fever, chills, abdominal pain, and myalgia. Laboratory abnormalities include liver function test disturbances, hemolytic anemia, and thrombocytopenia. Renal histopathology demonstrates interstitial inflammation with invasion of mononuclear cells and occasional eosinophils. Tubular epithelial cell injury and tubular necrosis related to vasomotor injury may also occur. Patients with a history of a severe reaction should not be reexposed to the agent because of the potential risk of hemodynamic collapse.

Sulfonamides are widely used antibiotics associated with kidney injury. When these drugs were introduced in the first half of the twentieth century, the most common kidney injury was tubular obstruction from crystalline deposition of insoluble drug and/or metabolite. Currently AIN is the most common cause of kidney injury reported with these agents. Patients exposed to these drugs often present with an acute hypersensitivity syndrome characterized by fever, rash, and eosinophilia. Patients with human immunodeficiency virus (HIV) infection, kidney transplant recipients, or those with underlying CKD appear to be more susceptible to an allergic reaction, but the increased use of agents such as trimethoprim-sulfamethoxazole in these populations may account for this observation. Patients who are slow acetylators of sulfonamides may be at higher risk because of drug accumulation, even with routine dosing schedules.

Fluoroquinolones, particularly ciprofloxacin, may cause kidney injury by several mechanisms; however, AIN is the most common kidney complication. It often presents with a slowly progressive decline in kidney function despite the absence of a hypersensitivity syndrome. Other agents in this class have been associated with AIN, but ciprofloxacin, based on its widespread use, is most commonly described.

Azithromycin, erythromycin, ethambutol, gentamicin, nitrofurantoin, tetracycline, vancomycin, and multiple antiviral agents have all been associated with AIN. No drug is beyond suspicion, and every agent must be considered in the evaluation.

NONSTEROIDAL ANTIINFLAMMATORY AGENTS

Nonsteroidal antiinflammatory agents are widely used by patients including those with chronic illness and chronic pain. Both NSAIDs and the selective cyclooxygenase-2 (COX-2) inhibitors are associated with AIN. Given the high frequency of NSAID use, AIN remains a relatively rare event, supporting an idiosyncratic drug reaction. NSAIDs cause several renal syndromes (see Chapter 37), marked by hemodynamic AKI, electrolyte/acid-base disturbances, and nephrotic syndrome. AIN associated with NSAIDs presents more insidiously than that seen with antibiotics. It often occurs months after starting therapy, with an average onset time of 6 to 18 months. Classically, patients do not develop a hypersensitivity syndrome, and fever, eosinophilia, and rash are rare. An interstitial infiltrate, which is less intense and has fewer eosinophils than seen with other culprit agents, and tubulitis are noted on renal histopathology. Despite multiple classes of NSAIDs with a variety of chemical structures, the pattern of kidney injury is remarkably similar across all agents, arguing against a single epitope-induced immune response. By their mechanism of action, which is inhibition of the conversion of arachidonic acid into its derivatives, NSAIDs may blunt the formation of inflammatory intermediates and the degree of kidney injury. Interestingly, this effect may modulate immune function and alter the clinical presentation, making the diagnosis of AIN more difficult.

GASTROINTESTINAL AGENTS

Proton pump inhibitors (PPIs) have emerged as perhaps the most frequent cause of AIN worldwide. In many countries, these agents are available over the counter, further increasing their use. Since omeprazole became available in the early 1990s, the number of prescriptions for PPIs continues to increase. The mean time to AIN diagnosis from drug initiation is approximately 11 weeks, although it can occur after months of therapy. Only 10% of patients with PPI-induced AIN will present with the classic hypersensitivity syndrome of fever, rash, and eosinophilia, and therefore symptoms are either absent or very mild and nonspecific. Early recognition and treatment of AIN is associated with a relatively good prognosis and rare need

for renal replacement therapy, although CKD does occur in some patients.

5-Aminosalicylates are the mainstay of therapy for patients with inflammatory bowel disease. Most patients require long-term treatment and many years of drug exposure. Kidney impairment is rare with these drugs, occurring in 1 in 200 to 500 patients on therapy. A hypersensitivity reaction can occur and cause AIN. In the absence of early recognition, CKD from chronic interstitial fibrosis may develop. This reaction usually occurs within the first year of therapy, but it can develop at any time in a nondose-dependent fashion.

DIURETICS

Diuretic-induced AKI is almost always related to kidney hypoperfusion from decreased intravascular volume. There are, however, multiple case reports of diuretic-induced AIN from furosemide, hydrochlorothiazide, chlorthalidone, and triamterene. AIN is relatively rare despite widespread use of these drugs. In published reports, most patients experience systemic symptoms including fever, rash, and eosinophilia, suggesting a hypersensitivity syndrome. Drug discontinuation generally leads to renal recovery.

INFECTIONS

INVASIVE INFECTIONS

In the preantibiotic era, streptococcal and diphtheria infections caused inflammatory reactions in the kidney in the absence of direct tissue invasion. However, infection-related AIN diminished in frequency after antibiotics became readily available. Now, when AKI develops in the setting of an infection treated with antibiotics, the drug is assumed to be the culprit. If AKI persists despite antibiotic withdrawal, an acute postinfectious glomerulonephritis or AIN should be considered.

Tubulointerstitial injury can occur either from direct invasion by an organism as in pyelonephritis or indirectly by an immune-mediated mechanism. Unlike AIN, pyelonephritis is usually confined to one pyramid in the kidney. In the setting of urinary obstruction, it becomes more diffuse, resulting in AKI. Although clinical history and symptoms usually differentiate the two conditions readily, CT imaging showing a wedge-shaped area of inflammation supports a diagnosis of pyelonephritis rather than AIN.

A number of infectious agents have been linked with invasive AIN. These include Epstein-Barr virus (EBV), legionella, mycoplasma, cytomegalovirus, adenovirus, and the ricketsial Rocky Mountain spotted fever. Leptospirosis is a classic example of invasive AIN. The spirochete enters the bloodstream through the skin or mucosa, and it transiently invades glomerular capillaries before migrating into the tubulointerstitum. Once in this compartment, the organism induces inflammation and direct tubular injury that, over time, manifests as large, edematous kidneys. In addition, ischemic ATN may coexist with AIN in patients who develop septic shock from overwhelming leptospiral infection. Eradication of infection is associated with recovery of kidney function.

Hantavirus is an RNA virus associated with interstitial edema with infiltration of polymorphonuclear leukocytes, eosinophils, and monocytes. Interstitial hemorrhage accompanies renal inflammation and is associated with gross or microscopic hematuria. Candidemia has been associated with an interstitial inflammatory reaction initially limited to the renal cortex. With time, large fungus balls can form, obstruct the collecting system, and cause AKI as a result of obstructive uropathy.

NONINVASIVE INFECTIONS

Even without direct invasion of the kidney, infectious agents have been associated with AIN. Historically, streptococcal infections were commonly associated with AIN. The clinical syndrome associated with AIN develops early in the course of infection (9 to 12 days). Given the rapidity with which streptococcal infections are treated currently, infection-related AIN has disappeared as a clinical entity.

SYSTEMIC DISEASES

The classic lesions of acute tubulointerstitial inflammation may also complicate a variety of systemic diseases. Whereas rheumatologic diseases primarily cause immune-mediated glomerular disease, they can also induce AIN. Metabolic diseases and malignancy are also associated with interstitial inflammation and AKI.

TUBULOINTERSTITIAL NEPHRITIS WITH UVEITIS

Tubulointerstitial nephritis with uveitis (TINU) is a rare condition of unclear etiology that presents most frequently in adolescent girls, but may appear in adulthood. Weight loss, fever, anemia, and hyperglobulinemia occur before ocular and kidney manifestations. Fanconi syndrome with glucosuria, proteinuria, and aminoaciduria is the initial kidney manifestation, followed by a tubulointerstitial infiltrate, sometimes with granulomas. Certain infections such as toxoplasmosis, Epstein-Barr infection, and giardiasis have been associated with TINU. However, there is no clearly elucidated immune or genetic cause. Steroids are the mainstay of therapy for both the ocular and kidney manifestations of the disease. Fortunately, the prognosis is good in treated patients.

IMMUNOLOGIC DISEASES

The vast majority of rheumatologic diseases complicated by AKI have underlying glomerular disease from anti-glomerular basement membrane (GBM) antibody disease (i.e., Goodpasture disease), immune deposition diseases (lupus or IgA nephropathy among others), or antineutrophil cytoplasmic antibody (ANCA)-related pauci-immune vasculitides. However, there are some rheumatologic ailments, such as Sjögren or sarcoid, which may present with tubulointerstitial inflammation in the absence of glomerular involvement. In the right clinical scenario, these causes of AIN should remain high on the differential diagnosis of kidney injury.

Immune-related injury in a transplanted kidney (cellular rejection) manifests primarily as tubulointerstitial inflammation with or without vascular involvement. The workup and classification of this interstitial disease can be found in Chapter 62.

MALIGNANCY

Patients with underlying cancer are at high risk for AKI because of the malignancy itself or therapies used in its management. Primary lymphoma of the kidney is a rare cause of AKI, whereas non-Hodgkin's lymphoma and acute lymphoblastic leukemias commonly invade the kidney parenchyma. Although it is seen on rare occasions in Hodgkin's lymphoma, infiltrates are usually bilateral and diffuse, and kidneys may appear enlarged on imaging. Multiple myeloma and the plasma cell dyscrasias cause kidney injury when filtered light chains coalesce and obstruct tubular lumens. These obstructive "casts" are accompanied by varying degrees of tubular injury, necrosis, and an interstitial inflammatory reaction on kidney biopsy that resembles classic interstitial nephritis.

TREATMENT

Treatment of AIN depends on the underlying disease that is driving the inflammatory reaction. When the pathologic process is associated with an underlying disease such as a malignancy, therapy is directed at the identified cause. In rheumatologic disease, treatment of the inflammatory condition often improves kidney function as well. In the setting of infection-related interstitial nephritis, eradication of the infection is often associated with kidney recovery.

Treatment of drug-induced AIN is more complicated and controversial. The most important intervention is early recognition of disease and drug discontinuation. This can be a complicated endeavor in patients taking multiple essential medications, making it challenging to identify the culprit drug. Careful scrutiny of the medication record for exposure dates and history of previous drug treatment may point to the offending agent. When a drug is suspected, it should be immediately discontinued and replaced, if necessary, with an agent from a different class. A drug-free trial should be undertaken to determine if kidney function recovers without further intervention. If no improvement is noted after a period of observation (3 to 5 days), or if kidney function is declining rapidly, a trial of corticosteroids is reasonable. Prognosis appears to depend on the timing of diagnosis and drug withdrawal. In general, earlier is better with data supporting a 1- to 2-week time frame. Despite this, a substantial proportion of patients (up to 35%) may develop CKD.

The data published on use of corticosteroids for AIN are incomplete. Assuming the offending drug is withdrawn, steroids improved the rate of kidney recovery in several small studies (fewer than 20 patients). A review of seven nonrandomized retrospective studies including up to 100 patients showed no benefit of steroids in recovery of kidney function or prevention of CKD. However, many of the retrospective studies were biased against steroids as more severely affected patients were treated, confounding the results.

Early steroid therapy, initiated 1 to 2 weeks after diagnosis, is more likely to improve kidney function compared to those started later. In addition, it is reasonable to offer steroids to those with severe AIN where renal replacement therapy is or will likely be required in the absence of rapid kidney recovery. Steroid therapy is recommended for 4 to 6 weeks with a slow taper. If there is no substantial improvement in kidney function after 3 to 4 weeks, response is unlikely, and steroids should be discontinued.

There are limited data available on other forms of immunosuppression. In a small case series of eight patients, mycophenolate mofetil (MMF) improved or stabilized kidney function in patients with steroid-dependent or steroid-resistant AIN. As a result, MMF may offer an alternative therapy to corticosteroids, but more data are required before this agent can be recommended.

BIBLIOGRAPHY

Baldwin DS, Levine BB, McCluskey RT, et al: Renal failure and interstitial nephritis due to penicillin and methicillin, *N Engl J Med* 279:1245-1252, 1968.

Brewster UC, Perazella MA: Proton pump inhibitors and the kidney: critical review, *Clin Nephrol* 68:65-72, 2007.

Clarkson MR, Giblin L, O'Connell FP, et al: Acute interstitial nephritis: clinical features and response to corticosteroid therapy, *Nephrol Dial Transplant* 19:2778-2783, 2004.

Councilman WT: Acute interstitial nephritis, *J Exp Med* 3:393-420, 1898.

González E, Gutiérrez E, Galeano C, et al: Early steroid treatment improves the recovery of renal function in patients with drug-induced acute interstitial nephritis, *Kidney Int* 73:940-946, 2008.

Ivanyi B, Hamilton-Dutoit SJ, Hansen HE, et al: Acute tubulointerstitial nephritis: phenotype of infiltrating cells and prognostic impact of tubulitis, *Virchows Arch* 428:5-12, 1996.

Michel DM, Kelly CJ: Acute interstitial nephritis, *J Am Soc Nephrol* 9:506-515, 1998.

Nielson EG: Pathogenesis and therapy of interstitial nephritis, *Kidney Int* 35:1257-1270, 1989.

Perazella MA, Markowitz GS: Drug-induced acute interstitial nephritis, *Nat Rev Nephrol* 6:461-470, 2010.

Praga M, González E: Acute interstitial nephritis, *Kidney Int* 77:956-961, 2010.

Preddie DC, Markowitz GS, Radhakrishnan J, et al: Mycophenolate mofetil for the treatment of interstitial nephritis, *Clin J Am Soc Nephrol* 1:718-722, 2006.

Rossert J: Drug-induced acute interstitial nephritis, *Kidney Int* 60:804-817, 2001.

Ruffing KA, Hoppes P, Blend D, et al: Eosinophils in urine revisited, *Clin Nephrol* 41:163-166, 1994.

Spanou Z, Keller M, Britschgi M, et al: Involvement of drug-specific T cells in acute drug-induced interstitial nephritis, *J Am Soc Nephrol* 17:2919-2927, 2006.

36 Management of Acute Kidney Injury

Matthew T. James | Neesh Pannu

Acute kidney injury (AKI) is associated with prolonged hospitalization, substantial resource utilization high mortality, and progressive chronic kidney disease (CKD) and end-stage renal disease (ESRD) in survivors. The principles of management of AKI include early recognition of the problem, identification and correction of the underlying cause, and steps to avoid further kidney injury. After AKI is established, the therapeutic options are limited, and mortality remains high despite recent technological advancements. Nonetheless, regional and temporal variations in mortality among hospitalizations for AKI suggest that several elements of management, including supportive care, management of complications, and use of renal replacement therapy (RRT), may influence outcomes. This chapter focuses on the management of early or established AKI resulting from prerenal causes or acute tubular necrosis (ATN). Readers are referred elsewhere in the *Primer* for a review of specific aspects of treatment for acute interstitial nephritis, glomerulonephritis, urinary obstruction, and systemic diseases involving the kidney.

EARLY RECOGNITION AND INITIAL MANAGEMENT

Timely detection and recognition is desirable as it can allow for prompt implementation of interventions to abort early kidney damage and to avoid the development of severe kidney injury and its complications (Box 36.1). AKI is usually identified based on an increase in serum creatinine; however, creatinine is an insensitive early marker of changes in kidney function, and AKI may develop before such changes become apparent. Furthermore, small changes in serum creatinine early in the course of AKI may not be readily appreciated even though they can represent large changes in glomerular filtration rate. Oliguria or anuria is an important sign that can identify AKI before changes in serum creatinine become apparent. Several novel biomarkers for AKI have been identified in recent years including kidney injury molecule-1 (KIM-1), neutrophil gelatinase associated lipocalin (NGAL), interleukin-18 (IL-18), and cystatin C. However, these tests are not yet widely used in clinical practice, and they remain the focus of ongoing studies to determine their appropriate role in guiding management of patients at risk for AKI.

After AKI has been identified, further clinical assessment, investigation, and intervention typically proceed simultaneously. A thorough history and examination are required to identify potential causes of AKI. Ischemia, sepsis, and exposure to nephrotoxic agents are the most common causes of AKI in hospitalized patients. A search for prerenal and postrenal causes should be performed, as their correction can lead to rapid recovery of kidney function. A number of urine studies have been described to distinguish prerenal AKI from ATN, including the urine sodium concentration, fractional excretion of sodium, and fractional excretion of urea. Unfortunately, all of these tests have limitations in their diagnostic performance, and interpretation is dependent on the clinical context. Clinical examination to assess volume status remains an important aspect of early management. AKI due to hypovolemia may be rapidly reversed by the administration of intravenous fluids. Volume status should be frequently reassessed to determine the response to intravenous fluids and to avoid volume overload. Stopping medications that impair glomerular filtration, including nonsteroidal antiinflammatory drugs (NSAIDs) and angiotensin converting enzyme (ACE) inhibitors/angiotensin receptor blockers (ARBs), can help reverse kidney dysfunction, especially in the setting of low effective arterial blood volume. Drugs that cause direct nephrotoxicity, such as aminoglycosides and intravenous radiocontrast, should be avoided. Selected use of renal ultrasound is useful for identifying hydroureter and/or hydronephrosis indicative of a postrenal cause. Lower urinary tract obstruction can be identified and treated by bladder catheterization showing a large postvoid residual urine volume, whereas nephrostomy tubes or ureteric stents can be used to treat upper urinary tract obstruction.

Urinalysis and urine microscopy provide important information about intrinsic renal causes of AKI. Hematuria and proteinuria should prompt further investigations for causes of glomerulonephritis, whereas white bloods cell casts should prompt a careful assessment for causes of interstitial nephritis, including a review of medication exposures. The findings of granular casts and/or renal tubular epithelial cells are associated with an increased likelihood of ATN, and help to predict patients at highest risk for worsening kidney function, the requirement for RRT, or death.

SUPPORTIVE CARE AND MEDICAL MANAGEMENT OF COMPLICATIONS

After AKI is established, management focuses on preventing extension of kidney injury and providing supportive care while awaiting kidney recovery. Attempts are usually made to avoid further exposure to nephrotoxic agents to the greatest extent possible without compromising management of other comorbidities. Doses of medications cleared by the kidney should be adjusted for the level of kidney function. This can be particularly important for antimicrobial agents

---

Box 36.1   Principles of Management of Acute Kidney Injury

- Timely recognition of changes in urine output or kidney function
- Identification and reversal of underlying cause
- Correction of prerenal states and maintenance of hemodynamic stability
- Avoidance of nephrotoxic agents, if possible, and adjustment of medication doses to level of kidney function
- Provision of supportive care, including nutrition and medical interventions to maintain fluid, electrolyte, and acid-base balance
- Initiation of RRT when needed

RRT, Renal replacement therapy.

---

so as to maintain appropriate therapeutic levels in patients with sepsis while avoiding drug toxicity. The involvement of a clinical pharmacist may be helpful.

Supportive care in patients with AKI requires maintenance of fluid, electrolyte, and acid-base balance. Disorders of sodium and water handling, metabolic acidosis, and hyperkalemia are common complications of AKI. Hyponatremia may result from impaired free water excretion, whereas hypernatremia is common in patients with inadequate free water intake, hypotonic fluid losses, or large-volume intravenous saline infusions for resuscitation. These abnormalities may be corrected by modifying free water intake or the composition of intravenous fluids. Acid generation can be reduced by dietary protein restriction, although this may be undesirable in hypercatabolic patients. Alkaline intravenous fluids such as sodium bicarbonate may be provided to correct metabolic acidosis, although volume overload and pulmonary edema may limit this intervention. Hyperkalemia should be treated by discontinuing exogenous sources of potassium. In the presence of ECG changes, calcium gluconate may be administered. Beta-agonists, insulin, and sodium bicarbonate can shift potassium out of the plasma and into cells. Attempts to eliminate potassium through the gastrointestinal tract using ion exchange resins may be used; however, these agents are slow to take effect, have limited efficacy, have been associated with bowl necrosis or perforation, and are unlikely to be adequate in patients with severe hyperkalemia. When medical management of these abnormalities is unsuccessful, or medical interventions cannot be tolerated by the patient, RRT is usually necessary unless recovery of kidney function is imminent.

INTRAVENOUS FLUIDS AND HEMODYNAMIC SUPPORT

Hypotension is a common contributor to AKI, and after AKI is established renal perfusion may be further diminished through disruption of renal autoregulation. Early correction of hypovolemia and hypotension not only reverses most prerenal causes of AKI, but also likely prevents extension and allows recovery from ATN. Strategies to maintain hemodynamic stability include the use of intravenous fluids, vasopressors/inotropic medications, and protocols for

hemodynamic monitoring to guide the use of these therapies. Although more aggressive use of intravenous fluids in the initial phase of illness may be beneficial when AKI is volume responsive, excessive fluid repletion in oliguric patients with established ATN can have adverse effects. A positive fluid balance has been associated with increased mortality in observational studies. Targeting a lower central venous pressure (6 to 8 cm H_2O) may be appropriate in some patients with stable AKI.

Isotonic crystalloids are the principal intravenous fluid for intravascular volume expansion of patients with AKI. Isotonic (0.9%) saline is considered the standard of care for most patients. Colloid solutions such as albumin and starches are theoretically attractive alternatives for intravenous volume expansion given their oncotic properties, but their appropriate use remains controversial. No differences in the incidence or duration of RRT were observed in a randomized trial of critically ill patients comparing treatment with 4% albumin in 0.9% saline with isotonic saline alone. However, a recent systematic review of randomized trials concluded that the use of hyperoncotic albumin solutions reduced the risk of AKI and may be appropriate for some patients, including those with ascites, spontaneous bacterial peritonitis, burns, or following surgery. Hydroxyethyl starch is an alternative colloid solution; however, when compared to crystalloids, hyperoncotic hydroxyethyl starch has been associated with a higher incidence of AKI and features of renal tubular injury (termed *osmotic nephrosis*) on kidney biopsy, suggesting these solutions may be harmful. As colloids have not been shown to consistently reduce mortality when compared with crystalloids across all populations who are at high risk of AKI, these solutions are usually reserved for selected patients, or for those with continuing large fluid requirements.

Distributive shock is a common contributor to AKI in patients with sepsis, anaphylaxis, liver failure, and burns. Aggressive fluid resuscitation remains of paramount importance in these patients; however, after intravascular volume has been repleted, vasopressors such as norepinephrine, dopamine, and vasopressin may be required to maintain hemodynamic stability. Following the publication of several recent randomized trials, management strategies that are focused on achieving specific hemodynamic and oxygenation parameters have gained increasing prominence for the management of patients at risk for AKI from septic shock or in the perioperative period. One randomized trial showed a reduction in in-hospital mortality for patients with septic shock managed according to a protocol for early provision of intravenous fluids, blood transfusion, vasopressors, and inotropes based on specific goals for blood pressure, central venous pressure, serum lactate, central venous oxygen saturation, and urine output. Protocol-based therapies to improve oxygenation and prevent hypotension using intravenous fluids, vasopressors, and blood products also appear to reduce the incidence of perioperative AKI in high-risk surgical patients, although it remains unclear which elements of these protocols are associated with this benefit.

DIURETICS

Fluid overload is one of the major complications of AKI, and diuretics are often prescribed to control fluid balance. The use of loop diuretics may also aid in the management of hyperkalemia and hypercalcemia. It has been proposed that loop diuretics such as furosemide could ameliorate ischemic damage in AKI by reducing the energy requirements of cells within the loop of Henle. However, diuretics can induce hypovolemia leading to prerenal AKI, and their use has been associated with increased mortality and delays in kidney recovery in observational studies. Some small randomized trials of furosemide reported higher risks of AKI when used as a prophylactic agent at the time of imaging and surgical procedures, and systematic reviews of trials that included patients with or at risk for AKI found no significant effects of furosemide on the risks of death, requirement for RRT, or number of dialysis sessions. Furthermore, although furosemide facilitates diuresis, this approach does not appear to improve kidney recovery among patients requiring dialysis for AKI. Nonetheless, diuretics can be used effectively to achieve fluid balance, and may facilitate mechanical ventilation in volume-overloaded patients.

VASODILATORS AND OTHER PHARMACOLOGIC AGENTS

Several pharmacologic agents with renal vasodilatory properties have been studied with the aim of increasing renal blood flow and ameliorating ischemic damage in AKI. However, none of these agents are proven to improve the clinical outcomes of AKI. Low-dose dopamine is associated with increased renal blood flow, increased urine output, and small improvements in creatinine clearance. However, a systematic review of trials including patients with or at risk for AKI showed that low-dose dopamine had no significant effect on survival, need for dialysis, or adverse clinical events. Dopamine is associated with arrhythmias and intestinal ischemia, and is not currently recommended to prevent or treat AKI. Fenoldopam is a dopamine type 1 receptor agonist that also increases renal blood flow, although it decreases systemic vascular resistance. A metaanalysis suggested promising results with the use of fenoldopam in critically ill patients, including reductions in AKI, need for RRT, and in-hospital mortality. However, given its risk of hypotension along with limitations of the existing published trials, further trials are necessary to support the use of fenoldopam for this indication. Atrial natriuretic peptide (ANP) has favorable renovascular effects that increase the glomerular filtration rate in animals. However, large trials of ANP (0.2 μg/kg/min) in critically ill patients with AKI showed no effects on mortality or dialysis-free survival, but did show a higher incidence of hypotension. One systematic review has suggested that low-dose ANP (0.1 μg/kg/min) is not associated with hypotension and may lead to a reduction in the requirement for RRT. Yet again, further large trials of low-dose ANP will be required before this agent can be recommended for AKI prevention or treatment.

There is inadequate efficacy and safety data to support the use of growth factors for AKI. Although insulin-like growth factor-1 showed promising results on recovery of kidney function in animals, small trials have failed to demonstrate beneficial results in humans. A small trial of erythropoietin for the prevention of AKI following cardiac surgery reported a reduction in incidence of AKI in treated patients; however, a subsequent trial in the intensive care unit (ICU) detected no effect.

NUTRITIONAL SUPPORT

Malnutrition is common in patients with AKI, and has been consistently associated with mortality. Although clinical trials assessing the impact of nutrition on clinical endpoints are lacking, it is broadly accepted that appropriate nutritional support should be provided to meet the metabolic requirements of AKI patients. Total energy consumption is not increased in AKI and is only mildly increased above resting energy expenditure in patients with critical illness. A total energy intake of 20 to 30 kcal/kg/day is recommended to maintain nitrogen balance in patients with AKI and to avoid hyperglycemia, hypertriglyceridemia, and fluid accumulation observed with higher caloric provisions.

The optimal protein intake in the setting of AKI is not known. Given the association between protein-calorie malnutrition and mortality in these patients, dietary restriction of protein is not considered appropriate in attempts to delay or prevent the initiation of RRT for azotemia or acidosis. Protein wasting and negative nitrogen balance may occur in patients with AKI because of the inflammatory and physiologic stresses that accompany acute illnesses, particularly in critically ill patients. Nutritional protein administration is therefore usually increased to meet the greater metabolic demands of hypercatabolic patients. Furthermore, losses of amino acids and protein occur in the filtrate on continuous renal replacement therapy (CRRT) and via peritoneal dialysis resulting in additional nutritional requirements for patients receiving these treatments. It is reasonable to aim for a protein intake of 0.8 to 1.0 g/kg/day in noncatabolic patients not requiring RRT, increasing to a maximum of 1.7 g/kg/day for hypercatabolic patients receiving RRT. Consultation with a registered dietician is valuable to estimate the appropriate energy and protein requirements for an individual patient.

Enteral nutrition is the preferred form of support for patients with AKI. If oral feeding is not possible, then enteral (tube) feeding is recommended. Electrolytes (potassium, phosphate) should be monitored following initiation of enteral feeding. Parenteral nutrition may be required in some patients to supplement the enteral route, or in patients without functional gastrointestinal tracts. Potassium, phosphate, and magnesium are usually withheld from parenteral nutrition in patients with AKI.

RENAL REPLACEMENT THERAPY

MODALITIES

Several modalities are currently used for RRT in AKI, including peritoneal dialysis, intermittent hemodialysis (IHD), and CRRTs. Peritoneal dialysis is used for AKI in some pediatric settings and in adults in developing countries where infrastructure for hemodialysis is not available. In industrialized countries, IHD and CRRT are the mainstays of RRT for AKI. Available resources, expertise, hemodynamic stability, and patient comorbidities usually influence the decision of renal replacement modality. In institutions where both modalities are available, it is common for patients to transition between

Table 36.1   Properties of Various Renal Replacement Therapy Modalities Used for Acute Kidney Injury

	Modality	Solute Removal	Blood Flow Rates	Ultrafiltration Rate	Replacement Fluid Rate	Dialysate Flow Rate
Continuous Therapies	CVVHF	Convection (ultrafiltration)	150 to 250 mL/min	1500 to 2000 mL/hr	1500 to 2000 mL/hr for neutral fluid balance. Ultrafiltration in excess of replacement fluid necessary for fluid removal	0
	CVVHD	Diffusion (dialysis)	150 to 250 mL/min	Variable	None	1 to 2 L/hr
	CVVHDF	Diffusion and convection (ultrafiltration and dialysis)	150 to 250 mL/min	1000 to 1500 mL/hr	1000 to 1500 mL/hr for neutral fluid balance. Ultrafiltration in excess of replacement fluid necessary for fluid removal	1 to 2 L/hr
Intermittent Therapies	IHD	Diffusion (dialysis)	200 to 350 mL/min	Variable	None	300 to 500 mL/min
	SLED	Diffusion (dialysis)	100 to 300 mL/min	Variable	None	100 to 300 mL/min
	SCUF	Convection (ultrafiltration)	100 to 200 mL/min	Variable	None	0

CVVHD, Continuous venovenous hemodialysis; *CVVHDF,* continuous venovenous hemodiafiltration; *CVVHF,* continuous venovenous hemofiltration; *IHD,* Intermittent hemodialysis; *SCUF,* sustained continuous ultrafiltration; *SLED,* sustained low-efficiency dialysis.

forms of CRRT and IHD depending on various factors and the setting in which the care is being provided.

CRRT is delivered continuously and uses slower blood flow rates that result in slower fluid and solute removal than IHD. Several forms of CRRT exist, including continuous venovenous hemofiltration (CVVHF), continuous venovenous hemodialysis (CVVHD), and continuous venovenous hemodiafiltration (CVVHDF) (Table 36.1). These modalities are usually only available in ICUs. Although CRRT achieves slower removal of solutes per unit time than IHD, total clearance during a 24-hour period may exceed that provided by IHD. Furthermore, the slower rate of solute clearance may avoid large fluid shifts between intracellular and extracellular fluid compartments. Based on these features, CRRT is often suggested for hemodynamically unstable patients and patients with brain injury at risk of cerebral edema.

IHD is performed for a few hours at a time over spaced intervals. It uses the methods, equipment, and trained nursing staff established for chronic hemodialysis in patients with ESRD. IHD achieves the fastest removal of small solutes and limits the duration a patient is exposed to the extracorporeal circuit. It is a popular therapeutic option for many patients with severe hyperkalemia, poisoning, and tumor lysis syndrome. In recent years, variants of IHD have been implemented using the IHD equipment (see Table 36.1). These hybrid therapies, known as sustained low-efficiency dialysis (SLED), use an extended duration of dialysis with a lower blood flow rate to provide more gradual solute and fluid removal while maintaining hemodynamic tolerability.

Although most patients with AKI are eligible for either modality, it is broadly perceived that CRRT is preferable to IHD for treatment of hemodynamically unstable patients. However, randomized comparisons of CRRT and IHD have shown heterogeneous effects on hemodynamic measurements, with metaanalyses suggesting no significant differences in the risk of hypotension between modalities. Still higher mean arterial blood pressure, and fewer patients

requiring escalation of vasopressor during treatment, were seen with CRRT than with IHD. Experience reported from clinical trials suggests that IHD can be successfully delivered to many patients with hemodynamic instability. Strategies that may help maintain hemodynamic stability during IHD include priming of the dialysis circuit with saline, cooled dialysate, and a high dialysate sodium concentration. Varying the dialysate sodium concentration and ultrafiltration rate during IHD can also improve hemodynamic stability and achieve greater fluid removal.

Several randomized trials and metaanalyses have compared outcomes with CRRT versus IHD in critically ill patients. Data from these trials have demonstrated no significant differences between these modalities in the length of hospitalization, mortality, or the requirement for chronic dialysis in survivors. Although existing data do not provide evidence that either IHD or CRRT results in superior clinical outcomes, further trials remain necessary to compare the hybrid with conventional therapies and to better assess the effect of the major renal replacement modalities on time to kidney recovery.

INITIATION OF RENAL REPLACEMENT THERAPY

Initiating RRT is a clinical decision influenced by several factors, including assessment of fluid, electrolyte, and metabolic status. Little information from clinical trials is available to guide this decision. It is widely accepted that hyperkalemia, metabolic acidosis, and volume overload (refractory to medical management) or overt uremic signs and symptoms constitute traditional indications for RRT. However, it is rare for uremic symptoms to develop in the setting of AKI before initiating dialysis. RRT is usually started after AKI is established and complications are deemed unavoidable. However, in the absence of imminent complications, dialysis may be deferred when there are signs of clinical improvement or kidney recovery. Many patients recover kidney function without the development of absolute indications for RRT,

Table 36.2   Traditional and Early Criteria for Renal Replacement Therapy in Acute Kidney Injury

Criteria	Comment
Traditional Criteria	
Volume overload	Pulmonary edema or respiratory failure that cannot be managed with medical therapy including diuretics
Electrolytes	Hyperkalemia refractory to medical management, severe (K greater than 6.0 mEq/L) or associated with ECG changes
Acidemia	Usually based on severity of metabolic acidosis, but no established threshold
Uremia	Indications include pericarditis, encephalopathy, or uremic bleeding attributed to platelet dysfunction
Early Criteria	
Volume management	To minimize fluid overload, and to facilitate administration of nutritional support and intravenous medication that would otherwise lead to fluid accumulation
Electrolytes	Proactive use to avoid impending electrolyte disorders
Acid-base balance	To maintain arterial pH in the setting of permissive hypercapnea in patients with respiratory failure
Solute control	Severe AKI that is unlikely to recover imminently Remove solutes that are difficult to quantify in the setting of AKI

AKI, Acute kidney injury; *ECG,* electrocardiogram; *K,* serum potassium concentration.

and in some patients complications may be adequately managed medically. Thresholds for starting RRT appear to be lower when AKI is accompanied by multiple organ failure, the rationale being that earlier initiation will facilitate other aspects of management while maintaining fluid, solute, and metabolic control.

There is considerable practice variation for starting renal replacement in the absence of traditional indications (Table 36.2). In theory, earlier initiation may avoid adverse AKI consequences, including metabolic abnormalities and fluid overload, and could improve outcomes. However, earlier initiation can unnecessarily expose some patients to the risk associated with vascular access (infection, thrombosis), anticoagulation (hemorrhage), and RRT itself (hypotension, dialyzer reactions). The majority of studies on the effects of earlier initiation of RRT are observational, and the interpretation of findings is limited by varying definitions of early treatment, comparison with historical cohorts, and possible confounding. However, a small randomized trial that compared early initiation of RRT (oliguria less than 6 hours with creatinine clearance less than 20 mL/min) to conventional

criteria (pulmonary edema, urea greater than 112 mg/dl [40 mmol/L], serum potassium greater than 6.5 mmol/L) did not show an effect of earlier initiation on mortality. Further trials are needed in this area to guide practice.

DOSE OF RENAL REPLACEMENT THERAPY

Several limitations exist regarding the use of urea clearance to quantify the intensity of RRT due to the high catabolic rate and changes in the volume of distribution that commonly accompany AKI. Despite these limitations, urea clearance is often used to prescribe and measure the intensity of RRT in AKI. Urea clearance by hemodialysis is expressed as Kt/V, and may be modified by increasing the surface area of the dialyzer, blood flow rate, dialysate flow rate, treatment duration, or frequency. Urea clearance by CRRT is considered equivalent to the effluent flow rate (ultrafiltrate and/or dialysate) and can be expressed as mL/kg/h of effluent.

One small trial that evaluated the effect of daily versus alternate-day IHD in AKI reported lower mortality and shorter duration of dialysis in the daily IHD group. However, the delivered dose in the alternate-day group was lower than intended with a weekly mean Kt/V of 3.0. More recently, two larger studies of the dose of renal replacement in AKI have provided major advances in our knowledge of this area. The Veterans Affairs ATN study was a randomized trial that evaluated the intensity of RRT while allowing patients to switch between CRRT, IHD, or SLED. In this trial, IHD was prescribed at a Kt/V of 1.4 (mean delivered dose was 1.3) and was performed six times weekly in the intensive arm and three times weekly in the less intensive arm. CRRT was performed using predilution CVVHDF prescribed with effluent flow rate of 35 mL/kg/h in the intensive arm and 20 mL/kg/h in the less intensive arm. Mortality and recovery of kidney function were similar in the intensive and less intensive groups. The RENAL study randomized patients with AKI treated with postdilution CVVHDF to doses of 40 versus 25 mL/kg/h and showed no difference in survival between the two groups.

Based on these results, a delivered dose equivalent to that achieved in the less intensive arm of the ATN study (weekly Kt/V 3.9) appears to be adequate for treatment of patients with IHD. Moreover, a delivered effluent volume consistent with the less intensive arms of the ATN and RENAL studies (20 to 25 mL/kg/h) has been recommended for CRRT. Hemodynamic instability, access failure, technical problems, and time off RRT to perform procedures may reduce the effective time on RRT and result in a lower delivered dose, which may require prescription adjustments. Assessment of the adequacy of renal replacement should also incorporate other factors in addition to small solute (urea) clearance, including fluid management, acid-base status, and electrolyte balance, as these parameters may influence the prescription for RRT. Extracorporeal therapy may be required in some instances for ultrafiltration alone.

VASCULAR ACCESS FOR RENAL REPLACEMENT THERAPY

Venous access is a necessity for CRRT and IHD, and access dysfunction can limit blood flow and the delivery of dialysis.

Because of their large diameter, complications of dialysis catheter insertion (arterial puncture, hematoma, pneumothorax, or hemothorax) can be serious. Indwelling catheters also predispose to bacteremia. Nontunneled catheters are the initial choice for most patients starting RRT. Cuffed, subcutaneous tunneled catheters are more complex to insert; however, they may be less prone to dysfunction, infection, or thrombosis, and thus appropriate if longer (greater than 3 week) durations of RRT are anticipated. Subclavian vein catheters are associated with the highest risk of venous stenosis. As this may compromise future attempts at permanent vascular access, the internal jugular vein is the preferred upper body insertion site for patients at risk for progression to ESRD. Femoral catheters are another reasonable choice, but these restrict mobility and are associated with increased infection in obese patients. Ultrasound guidance is recommended to decrease the risk of insertion complications and to improve the likelihood of successful placement. Insertion should be performed according to infection control protocols, including sterile barrier precautions, skin antisepsis, and catheter use restricted to RRT to minimize the incidence of catheter-related bloodstream infection.

ANTICOAGULATION FOR RENAL REPLACEMENT THERAPY

Clotting of the dialysis filter can lead to extracorporeal blood loss, a reduction in dialysis efficiency, and procedural interruptions. Use of anticoagulation for CRRT and IHD may reduce these problems; however, the benefits of anticoagulation must be balanced against the risk of bleeding complications in acutely ill AKI patients with significant comorbidities. Patients with coagulopathy and thrombocytopenia may not benefit from additional anticoagulation, and CRRT and IHD can often be provided without anticoagulation, aided by intermittent saline flushes of the extracorporeal circuit.

Unfractionated heparin is the most widely used anticoagulant for dialysis. Low molecular weight heparin may also be used, although it has unpredictable clearance in patients with kidney failure. A prolonged half-life requires monitoring of factor Xa levels. Regional citrate anticoagulation has become more common in recent years, especially for anticoagulation on CRRT. Citrate is infused into the prefilter line where it chelates calcium, thereby inhibiting filter coagulation. Some citrate is removed in the extracorporeal circuit, while the citrate returning to the systemic circulation is metabolized to produce bicarbonate and calcium. Additional calcium is infused to replace extracorporeal losses and to maintain normal systemic ionized calcium concentrations. The complexity of this procedure necessitates close monitoring of acid-base status and calcium (total and ionized) levels, and frequent adjustments to infusion rates. Adequately trained staff and adherence to strict protocols are recommended to minimize the complications of metabolic alkalosis, hypocalcemia, and citrate accumulation. Citrate anticoagulation is contraindicated in patients with severely impaired liver function or muscle hypoperfusion who are unable to metabolize citrate. Some small trials suggest that regional citrate anticoagulation reduces the

requirement for transfusion and risk of hemorrhage compared to systematic heparin.

DIALYZER/HEMOFILTER MEMBRANES

Hollow fiber dialyzers used for IHD or CRRT are characterized by their surface area, composition, and flux. Synthetic dialysis membranes are associated with less activation of complement than traditional bioincompatible membranes made of unsubstituted cellulose. Metaanalyses have shown no difference in mortality with biocompatible compared to bioincompatible membranes. However, as a higher risk of death has been suggested with unsubstituted cellulose membranes, these are typically avoided in AKI. Trials to date have shown no difference in outcomes between high-flux and low-flux membranes in AKI, although the increased permeability of high-flux membranes makes them advantageous for hemofiltration.

DIALYSATE AND REPLACEMENT FLUIDS

Dialysate for IHD is produced by the dialysis machine from concentrated electrolyte solutions and treated water from a municipal source. Sterile dialysate and replacement fluid for CRRT may be purchased commercially or produced in local hospital pharmacies. Solutions containing bicarbonate, lactate, and acetate are available for use with CRRT or IHD to correct metabolic acidosis. Bicarbonate-containing solutions have become increasingly available in recent years, and they avoid lactate accumulation in patients with shock or liver failure. When citrate is used for anticoagulation, requirements for additional buffer in dialysate or replacement fluid are limited.

DISCONTINUING RENAL REPLACEMENT THERAPY

Many patients with AKI will experience partial or complete recovery of kidney function, although recovery is less likely in those with severe injury and preexisting CKD. Little is known about the optimal time to stop RRT; however, increasing urine output often identifies patients recovering native kidney function. Changes in interdialytic measurements of serum creatinine, urea, and urinary creatinine clearance can be used to assess native kidney function in patients receiving IHD. For patients receiving a stable prescription of CRRT for several days, urinary creatinine clearance has also been used to measure recovery of native kidney function. Because of the high mortality in patients with AKI accompanying multiorgan failure, some patients will appropriately discontinue RRT as part of withdrawal from life support measures.

LONG-TERM FOLLOW-UP

Acute kidney injury is associated with an increased risk of progressive CKD and ESRD after hospital discharge. Postdischarge follow-up of kidney function is currently recommended for survivors of AKI. Subsequent long-term management of patients with CKD after AKI usually proceeds according to the principles of CKD management.

BIBLIOGRAPHY

Bouman CS, Oudemans-Van Straaten HM, Tijssen JG, et al: Effects of early high-volume continuous venovenous hemofiltration on survival and recovery of renal function in intensive care patients with acute renal failure: a prospective, randomized trial, *Crit Care Med* 30:2205-2211, 2002.

Brienza N, Giglio MT, Marucci M, et al: Does perioperative hemodynamic optimization protect renal function in surgical patients? A meta-analytic study, *Crit Care Med* 37:2079-2090, 2009.

Finfer S, Bellomo R, Boyce N, et al: A comparison of albumin and saline for fluid resuscitation in the intensive care unit, *N Engl J Med* 350:2247-2256, 2004.

Friedrich JO, Adhikari N, Herridge MS, et al: Meta-analysis: low-dose dopamine increases urine output but does not prevent renal dysfunction or death, *Ann Intern Med* 142:510-524, 2005.

Ho KM, Sheridan DJ: Meta-analysis of frusemide to prevent or treat acute renal failure, *BMJ* 333:420-425, 2006.

Klouche K, Amigues L, Deleuze S, et al: Complications, effects on dialysis dose, and survival of tunneled femoral dialysis catheter in acute renal failure, *Am J Kidney Dis* 49:99-108, 2007.

Landoni G, Biondi-Zoccai GG, Tumlin JA, et al: Beneficial impact of fenoldopam in critically ill patients with or at risk for acute renal failure: a meta-analysis of randomized clinical trials, *Am J Kidney Dis* 49:56-58, 2007.

Macias WL, Alaka KJ, Murphy MH, et al: Impact of the nutritional regimen on protein catabolism and nitrogen balance in patients with acute renal failure, *JPEN J Parenter Enteral Nutr* 20:56-62, 1996.

Mehta RL, Pascual MT, Soroko S, et al: Diuretics, mortality, and nonrecovery of renal function in acute renal failure, *JAMA* 288:2547-2553, 2002.

Nigwekar SU, Navaneethan SD, Parikh CR, et al: Atrial natriuretic peptide for management of acute kidney injury: a systematic review and meta-analysis, *Clin J Am Soc Nephrol* 4:261-272, 2008.

Paganini EP, Sandy D, Moreno L, et al: The effect of sodium and ultrafiltration modelling on plasma volume changes and haemodynamic stability in intensive care patients receiving haemodialysis for acute renal failure: a prospective stratified, randomized, cross-over study, *Nephrol Dial Transplant* 11:32-37, 1996.

Pannu N, Klarenbach S, Wiebe N, et al: Renal replacement therapy in patients with acute renal failure: a systematic review, *JAMA* 299:793-805, 2008.

Perel P, Roberts I: Colloids versus crystalloids for fluid resuscitation in critically ill patients, *Cochrane Database Syst Rev* 4, 2007. CD000567.

Rabindranath K, Adams J, Macleod AM, et al: Intermittent versus continuous renal replacement therapy for acute renal failure in adults, *Cochrane Database Syst Rev* 3, 2007. CD003773.

RENAL Replacement Therapy Study Investigators, Bellomo R, Cass A, et al: Intensity of continuous renal-replacement therapy in critically ill patients, *N Engl J Med* 361:1627-1638, 2009.

Schortgen F, Lacherade JC, Bruneel F, et al: Effects of hydroxyethylstarch and gelatin on renal function in severe sepsis: a multicentre randomised study, *Lancet* 357:911-916, 2001.

VA/NIH Acute Renal Failure Trial Network, Palevsky PM, Zhang JH, et al: Intensity of renal support in critically ill patients with acute kidney injury, *N Engl J Med* 359:7-20, 2008.

Wiedermann CJ, Dunzendorfer S, Gaioni LU, et al: Hyperoncotic colloids and acute kidney injury: a meta-analysis of randomized trials, *Crit Care* 14:191, 2010.

DRUGS AND THE KIDNEY

37 Kidney Disease Caused by Therapeutic Agents

Mark A. Perazella | Anushree Shirali

Medications are a mainstay for appropriate patient care, and new agents are being introduced into clinical practice at a rapid pace. Although therapeutic agents are often lifesaving and crucial to the care of many disease states, one unfortunate and relatively frequent adverse consequence is kidney injury. Most drugs are well tolerated; however, a subgroup of individuals may develop nephrotoxicity. This bespeaks the fact that some individuals possess risk factors that predispose to drug-induced renal toxicity.

Kidney injury may result from exposure to the wide array of drugs available in clinical practice. Not unexpectedly, the general population is exposed to various diagnostic and therapeutic agents with nephrotoxic potential on a regular basis. Although most are prescribed, many other preparations are purchased over the counter. Drugs fall into the categories of diagnostic agents, therapeutic medications, alternative or complementary substances, and drugs of abuse, resulting in a variety of renal syndromes (Table 37.1).

RENAL SUSCEPTIBILITY TO NEPHROTOXIC AGENTS

Whereas the kidney performs numerous functions such as clearance of endogenous waste products, excretion of sodium and water, electrolyte and acid-base balance, and endocrine activity, one of its major roles is the metabolism and excretion of exogenously administered drugs. In this role, the kidney is susceptible to various types of injury. There are several factors that increase renal susceptibility to these potential toxins, which can be classified into three simple categories: drug-related factors, kidney-related factors, and host-related factors. One or more of these risk factors often combine to promote nephrotoxicity. As we learn more about drug-induced kidney disease, it appears that these factors explain much of the variability and heterogeneity noted among patients.

Drug-related factors are the critical first step to the development of nephrotoxicity. Innate drug toxicity is important as the drug or its toxic metabolite may cause kidney injury by impairing renal hemodynamics, direct cellular injury, osmotic injury, or intratubular crystal deposition to name a few conditions. Large doses, extended drug exposure, and nephrotoxic drug combinations further enhance nephrotoxicity.

The kidney handling of drugs also determines why certain agents cause nephrotoxicity. As renal blood flow approximates 25% of cardiac output, the kidney is significantly exposed to nephrotoxic drugs. Kidney injury is increased in the loop of Henle where high metabolic rates coexist with a relatively hypoxic environment. Increased drug/metabolite concentrations in the renal medulla also contribute to direct toxicity. Renal drug metabolism from cytochrome P450 (CYP450) and other enzymes increases local toxic metabolite and reactive oxygen species (ROS) formation, which outstrip antioxidants and promote injury via nucleic acid oxidation/alkylation, DNA-strand breaks, lipid peroxidation, and protein damage.

The renal pathway of excretion for many therapeutic agents involves proximal tubular cells. Extensive drug trafficking through the cell via apical and basolateral transporters can lead to cellular injury. Some drugs are endocytosed by the apical membrane of cells, whereas other drugs are transported into the cell via basolateral ion transporters. Such drug transport can be associated with increased cellular concentrations that injure mitochondria, phospholipid membranes, lysosomes, and other organelles.

Host-related factors likely explain the heterogeneity seen in drug-induced kidney injury. Nonmodifiable factors such as older age and female sex increase renal risk through reduced total body water leading to drug overdose. Unrecognized reduced glomerular filtration rate (GFR) and hypoalbuminemia, which result in increased toxic drug concentration, also enhance risk. Pharmacogenetics is important in elucidating individual patient and population risk for drug-related nephrotoxicity. Pharmacogenetic differences likely explain much of the variable response of patients to drugs. Hepatic and renal CYP450 enzyme gene polymorphisms are associated with reduced metabolism and end-organ toxicity. Polymorphisms of genes encoding proteins involved in the metabolism and renal elimination of drugs are correlated with nephrotoxic risk. Another important aspect of genetic makeup is a highly variable host immune response to drugs; one patient reacts with a heightened allergic response, whereas another has a limited reaction with no kidney lesion. Thus, innate host response genes tend to determine the drug reaction.

Renal susceptibility to drug injury is also enhanced by true and effective volume depletion, including nausea/vomiting, diarrhea, and diuretic therapy, as well as heart failure, liver disease with ascites, and sepsis. This physiology enhances the nephrotoxicity of drugs that are excreted primarily by the kidney, drugs reabsorbed/secreted by the proximal tubule, and drugs that are insoluble in the urine. Nephrotoxic risk is also increased in patients with acute kidney injury (AKI) or chronic kidney disease (CKD) because of a lower number of functioning nephrons, reductions in drug clearance, and a robust renal oxidative response to drugs and metabolites. Finally, electrolyte and acid-base disturbances present in some patients also contribute to host susceptibility to drug injury.

Table 37.1   Drug-Induced Clinical Renal Syndromes

Renal Syndrome	Causative Agents
Acute kidney injury	
Prerenal	Cyclosporine, tacrolimus, radiocontrast, AmB, ACE inhibitors, ARBs, NSAIDs, interleukin-2, exenatide
Intrarenal	
Vascular disease	Gemcitabine, anti-VEGF drugs, propylthiouracil, interferon
ATN	Aminoglycosides, AmB, cisplatin, tenofovir, ifosfamide, pemetrexed, polymixins, vancomycin, pentostat, zolendronate, warfarin
AIN	Penicillins, cephalosporins, sulfonamides, rifampin, NSAIDs, interferon, ciprofloxacin, others
Crystal nephropathy	Methotrexate, acyclovir, sulfonamides, indinavir, atazanavir, ciprofloxacin, sodium phosphate
Osmotic nephropathy	IVIG, HES, dextran, mannitol
Postrenal	Methysergide, drug-induced stones, alpha-agonists
Proteinuria	Gold, NSAIDs, anti-VEGF drugs, penicillamine, interferon, pamidronate
Tubulopathies	Aminoglycosides, tenofovir, cisplatin, ifosfamide, AmB, pemetrexed, cetuximab
Nephrolithiasis	Sulfadiazine, atazanavir, indinavir, topiramate, zonisamide
Chronic Kidney Disease	Li$^+$, analgesic abuse, cyclosporine, tacrolimus, cisplatin, nitrosourea

ACE, Angiotensin-converting enzyme; *AIN,* acute interstitial nephritis; *AmB,* amphotericin B; *ARBs,* angiotensin receptor blockers; *ATN,* acute tubular necrosis; *HES,* hydroxyethyl starch; *IVIG,* intravenous immune globulin; *Li$^+$,* lithium; *NSAIDs,* nonsteroidal antiinflammatory drugs; *VEGF,* vascular endothelial growth factor.

KIDNEY INJURY ASSOCIATED WITH MEDICATIONS

Therapeutic agents associated with kidney injury can be classified based on the category of agent or the clinical renal syndrome. Recognizing that all drugs cannot be covered in this chapter, we will describe drug-induced nephrotoxicity by drug category, and within each category highlight the clinical renal syndrome and the segment of nephron injury by the drug. Drug-induced acute interstitial nephritis (AIN) and CKD will be discussed elsewhere.

DIAGNOSTIC AGENTS

RADIOCONTRAST AGENTS

Contrast-induced nephropathy (CIN) is the third most common cause of hospital-acquired AKI and is associated with increased risk of hospital morbidity/mortality and long-term outcomes. It is defined by an absolute or percentage rise in serum creatinine from the baseline within 48 to 72 hours. In general, serum creatinine begins to rise within the first 24 hours after exposure, peaks between 2 and 5 days, and returns to baseline by 7 to 14 days. The course of CIN varies depending on overall patient risk profile.

The incidence of CIN depends on the definition used and the population studied, ranging from 5% to 40%. Two important factors drive this incidence: (1) the increased number of imaging studies and percutaneous procedures using radiocontrast throughout the past decade, and (2) the ever enlarging population of patients with underlying CKD. In the presence of reduced kidney function, the elimination ($T_{1/2}$) of radiocontrast agents is increased. Thus, the kidney undergoes prolonged contrast exposure that increases the likelihood of kidney injury. In CKD stage 3 or greater, the risk of CIN is twofold to fivefold higher compared with normal kidney function, and the risk escalates as the GFR falls.

Radiocontrast media injure the kidney via multiple mechanisms. First, vasoactive substances, such as adenosine and endothelin, mediate vasoconstriction of the afferent arterioles, thereby reducing renal blood flow and promoting renal medullary ischemia. Renal epithelial cell necrosis also occurs with isoosmolar radiocontrast agents as their high viscosity causes sluggish blood flow through the peritubular capillaries and promotes hypoxic renal injury. Lastly, radiocontrast causes direct renal tubular toxicity through hyperosmolar injury, which results in vacuolization of proximal tubular cells, as well as oxidative stress from free oxygen radicals with associated tubular cell apoptosis and necrosis.

The level of kidney function at the time of exposure is one of the most important determinants of risk for CIN. In addition, patient-specific risk factors include older age, volume depletion, congestive heart failure, diabetes mellitus, both hypertension and hypotension, and anemia. The intraaortic balloon pump is associated with increased AKI risk, primarily because it is a surrogate for severe cardiac disease, tenuous cardiac output, and renal hypoperfusion. Emergent procedures increase risk because of reduced use of contrast prophylaxis and increased severity of patient illness. The type, volume, and route of contrast administration also impacts on CIN risk. In regard to radiocontrast type, osmolality and viscosity are the two important characteristics. The osmolality of a solution varies significantly from high-osmolalar contrast media (HOCM) to low-osmolalar media (LOCM) to isoosmolalar media (IOCM). Viscosity, another contrast property, varies from one product to the next, does not correlate with osmolality, and may be associated with CIN. For example, IOCM solutions are about twice as viscous as LOCM products despite having a lower osmolality.

The incidence of CIN is higher with HOCM than with LOCM, and in CKD patients the relative risk is doubled. As a result, LOCM and IOCM agents have replaced HOCM. A metaanalysis of 16 randomized controlled trials suggested a benefit of using IOCM instead of LOCM, with the relative risk reduction of CIN greatest in CKD patients. The maximum increase in serum creatinine was less in CKD patients given ICOM compared with LOCM. However, a randomized trial comparing IOCM with LOCM noted no significant difference in RCIN incidence. Thus, the benefits of low osmolality may be counterbalanced by the detrimental properties of high viscosity, making these agents equal in their risk for CIN. A larger volume of contrast increases CIN, thus a limit of 150 mL for serum creatinine 1.5 to 3.4 mg/dl, and maximum dose of 100 mL for creatinine greater than 3.4 mg/dl, are recommended. The smallest contrast volume required to perform the procedure should be used. Risk of CIN is highest with intraarterial injection, with the intravenous (IV) route presenting a smaller risk. Coronary angiography has an even higher CIN risk than other arterial studies. CKD outpatients have a low CIN risk with nonemergent CT scans.

As radiocontrast exposure is often a predictable occurrence, measures to reduce kidney injury should be undertaken in patients at risk. In addition to limiting volume and using either IOCM or nonionic LOCM, the most important intervention is intravenous fluid (IVF) administration. Studies have uniformly demonstrated the benefit of prophylactic isotonic IVFs administered both before and after radiocontrast administration. Since urinary alkalinization is hypothesized to reduce renal oxidative stress, intravenous sodium bicarbonate has been studied. In an early report, CIN developed in only 2% of CKD patients treated with bicarbonate solution as compared with 14% with IV saline. A later metaanalysis of 23 studies concluded that bicarbonate-containing solutions reduced the risk of RCIN by 38%, but the benefits were noted in small and poor-quality studies. In contrast, larger, better-quality studies did not demonstrate a reduction in CIN. Furthermore, no benefit was demonstrated for AKI requiring dialysis, for heart failure, or for total mortality. Thus, sodium bicarbonate is not superior to isotonic saline, and either solution is acceptable for radiocontrast prophylaxis. For outpatient studies, oral fluids with salt tablets before exposure may provide adequate volume expansion to prevent CIN in CKD.

N-acetylcysteine (NAC) is an antioxidant that is commonly used for CIN prevention. Approximately half of the published randomized controlled trials demonstrate benefit, whereas several metaanalyses suggest either large benefit or no benefit. Beneficial studies are notable for early publication dates, small size, and low quality. Despite the enrollment of nearly 3000 patients, including CKD patients, no beneficial effect of NAC on hard clinical outcomes is noted. The most damning study for NAC as a useful agent to prevent CIN is the Acetylcysteine for Contrast-Induced Nephropathy Trial. This study included 2308 patients and documented no benefit with NAC therapy in the prevention of CIN; the same percentage of NAC- and placebo-treated patients developed CIN (12.7%). Thus, NAC appears to offer no protection against CIN. However, given its favorable safety profile, low cost, easy administration, and wide availability, one could argue for continued use of the drug as prophylaxis. Despite a lack of data, it is reasonable to avoid nonsteroidal antiinflammatory drugs (NSAIDs), calcineurin inhibitors, aminoglycosides, and osmotic agents before radiocontrast exposure. Regarding renin-angiotensin-aldosterone system (RAAS) blockers, some studies note increased CIN risk whereas others show nephroprotection.

Based on its size, lack of protein binding, and small volume of distribution, radiocontrast is efficiently removed with hemodialysis (HD). In fact, approximately 80% is removed over 4 hours with a high-flux dialyzer. HD after radiocontrast exposure to prevent CIN, especially in patients with advanced CKD, has been examined in several studies. Although all HD studies have been negative, one small study demonstrated that

prophylactic HD in stage 5 CKD patients reduced the need for an acute and chronic dialysis requirement after discharge. Hemofiltration (HF) performed 4 to 6 hours before and 18 to 24 hours after contrast reduced the incidence of CIN, in-hospital events, need for acute dialysis, and both in-hospital and 1-year mortality. In contrast, the HF postprocedure alone offered no benefit beyond standard prophylaxis. A systematic review of 11 studies with 1010 patients concluded that one or more sessions of HD, HF, or hemodiafiltration (HDF) performed after contrast did not reduce the incidence of CIN nor the need for acute or chronic dialysis. Examination of HD and HF/HDF separately shows that HD is associated with increased CIN risk, whereas HF/HDF did not affect the occurrence of CIN but did reduce the acute dialysis requirement. Further studies are required to define precisely what cohort of CKD patients, if any, might benefit from this invasive and costly strategy.

GADOLINIUM-BASED CONTRAST AGENTS

Gadolinium-based contrast agents (GBCAs) were considered a safe and effective diagnostic agent, revolutionizing the world of imaging. However, over time, it became clear that GBCAs were not risk free. Rare reports of AKI surfaced, primarily in patients with underlying kidney disease who received large doses via direct arterial injection. Nephrotoxicity may be related to the osmolar or some other effect on tubules. In general, AKI is rare and typically of minor severity in the majority of cases, likely caused by the small volume of contrast required for imaging. A toxicity of greater concern was recognized in 1997—nephrogenic systemic fibrosis (NSF).

GBCAs began to be used widely for imaging patients with kidney disease in the early to mid-1990s, because they offered an outstanding image without the nephrotoxicity of radiocontrast. However, the fibrosing disorder called NSF, first recognized as a skin disease and subsequently as a devastating systemic disorder, was attributed as a complication of GBCAs in 2006. It was reported that two factors were required for NSF to develop: GBCA exposure and underlying kidney disease. Other factors that likely further increased the risk for NSF included infection, inflammation, vascular disease, hypercoaguability, hypercalcemia, hyperphosphatemia, erythropoiesis-stimulating agent (ESA), and iron therapy.

The best approach to NSF is prevention, as therapeutic interventions are at best suboptimal. The high-risk patient should be identified before GBCA exposure, allowing other imaging options to be explored. Such options include non-GBCA MR imaging, CT scan, ultrasonography, and other techniques that can often provide diagnostic results. When a GBCA is necessary to make the diagnosis, the following approach is reasonable: (1) use a macrocyclic GBCA; (2) use the lowest dose required to obtain a diagnostic image; (3) optimize metabolic parameters and restrict ESA and iron use immediately before and after GBCA exposure; (4) wait for kidney recovery or stabilization in AKI; and (5) consider performing HD within hours of GBCA exposure in patients already receiving dialysis. The incidence of NSF has decreased significantly with the implementation of prudent GBCA use in high-risk patients. However, when this disease develops, its consequences are often devastating, and therapeutic options are limited. Although a number of agents have been used, it appears that pain control and physical therapy are most important. Therapies such as extracorporeal photopheresis, sodium thiosulfate, and imitanib show promise; however, only early kidney transplant may offer stabilization or reversal of the fibrosing process.

ORAL SODIUM PHOSPHATE PREPARATION

Although not diagnostic agents in themselves, sodium phosphate preparations are used as purgatives for bowel cleansing before diagnostic colonoscopy and CT virtual colonoscopy. They are administered as a solution or tablets before the procedure, and contain ~38 g of monobasic sodium phosphate and 9 g of dibasic sodium phosphate.

The adverse events associated with phosphate-containing bowel preparations occur with excessive dosing or use in patients with underlying kidney disease. Hypocalcemia and hyperphosphatemia may complicate therapy, but AKI is of greater concern. The pathogenic mechanism was described in 21 patients with AKI after using a phosphate-containing bowel cleansing agent for colonoscopy. Patients were predominantly female, had hypertension, and were on RAAS blockade. AKI was recognized at a median of 3 months after colonoscopy. Minimal proteinuria and bland urine sediment were noted. Tubular injury and atrophy, and abundant calcium phosphate deposits in distal tubules and collecting ducts, were features on kidney biopsy. This entity is coined *acute phosphate nephropathy*.

Two patterns of kidney injury occur with sodium phosphate administration. First, AKI develops within days of exposure and is associated with hyperphosphatemia and hypocalcemia. A second pattern is where AKI is discovered incidentally in patients evaluated weeks or months after exposure. Unfortunately, acute phosphate nephropathy is frequently complicated by CKD. Thus, oral sodium phosphate-based products should not be used in patients with underlying kidney disease, volume depletion, or electrolyte abnormalities. Safe use mandates careful patient selection, appropriate dosing, and maintenance of adequate intravascular volume status. Volume repletion lowers the risk of crystal formation and tubular damage. RAAS blockers, diuretics, and NSAIDs should be discontinued before and immediately after drug exposure. In patients who develop AKI and significant hyperphosphatemia, acute HD should be considered to remove phosphate and enhance kidney recovery.

THERAPEUTIC AGENTS

ANALGESICS

Nonsteroidal antiinflammatory drugs are widely used to treat pain, fever, and inflammation. Numerous NSAIDs are used in clinical practice, and the market flourishes as the pharmaceutical industry designs new drugs with improved efficacy and limited adverse effects. The selective cyclooxygenase-2 (COX-2) inhibitors are the most recent example of creative drug design. More than 20 NSAIDs from seven major classes are approved in the United States, and many are available over the counter. Annually, more than 50 million patients ingest these drugs on an intermittent basis,

> ### Box 37.1 Nonsteroidal Antiinflammatory Drug Clinical Renal Syndromes
>
> Acute kidney injury
>   Prerenal azotemia
>   Acute tubular necrosis
> Glomerular disease
>   Minimal change disease
>   Membranous nephropathy
> Acute interstitial nephritis
> Hyperkalemia/metabolic acidosis (hyporeninemic hypoaldosteronism)
> Hyponatremia
> Hypertension/edema
> Acute papillary necrosis
> Analgesic nephropathy/chronic tubulointerstitial nephritis

whereas 15 to 25 million people in the United States use an NSAID daily.

NSAIDs and selective COX-2 inhibitors are associated with various clinical renal syndromes (Box 37.1). It has been estimated that 1% to 5% of patients who ingest NSAIDs will develop some form of nephrotoxicity, with some calculations based on NSAID use among Americans approximating 500,000 persons likely to develop kidney impairment. These adverse effects are caused primarily by prostaglandin (PG) inhibition; however, other effects are idiosyncratic. PGs are produced by COX enzyme metabolism and are secreted locally in the kidney to modulate the effects of various systemic and local substances. For example, PGs enhance afferent arteriolar vasodilatation in the presence of vasoconstrictors such as angiotensin-II, norepinephrine, vasopressin, and endothelin, thereby providing critical counterbalance to the vasoconstriction that predominates in hypovolemic states. Patients with decreased true or effective circulating volume are at highest risk to develop renal vasoconstriction and reduced GFR. As CKD is a PG-dependent state, these patients are also at higher risk for NSAID-induced kidney injury. In fact, exposure to NSAIDs doubles the risk of hospitalization for AKI in patients with CKD. Similar rates of AKI with NSAID exposure are noted in the elderly, those with cardiac disease, and patients receiving angiotensin-converting enzyme (ACE)-inhibitors. As noted in a nested case-control study, the adjusted relative risk of AKI was 4.1 and 3.2, respectively, in current NSAID users versus nonusers in the general population. Patients with hypertension, heart failure, and diuretic therapy had an adjusted relative risk of 11.6 with NSAIDs.

In addition to increasing arteriolar blood flow, PGs also enhance renal sodium, potassium, and water excretion. PGs modulate renal potassium excretion through stimulation of the RAAS. Inhibition of PGs can result in hyperkalemia when coexistent conditions such as AKI, CKD, diabetes mellitus, and therapy with certain medications (RAAS blockers, potassium-sparing diuretics) are also present. The classic syndrome of hyporeninemic hypoaldosteronism with hyperkalemic metabolic acidosis can be observed with NSAID therapy. Inhibition of PGs is associated with decreased renal sodium excretion, and all NSAIDs cause some degree of sodium retention. Although all patients retain sodium, patients with hypertension, heart disease, and other salt-retentive disease states (cirrhosis, nephrotic syndrome, AKI, CKD) are at highest risk for developing edema, hypertension, or heart failure. Hypertension is a particularly important complication, as small changes in blood pressure are associated with increased cardiovascular events. Hyponatremia from impaired water excretion also complicates therapy as PGs act to antagonize water reabsorption in the distal nephron, an effect that is lost with NSAIDs. Reduced GFR also contributes to water retention and hyponatremia.

Idiosyncratic effects of selective and nonselective NSAIDs include proteinuric glomerular diseases. Minimal change disease is most common, whereas membranous nephropathy is a relatively rare complication of these drugs. Nephrotic-range proteinuria or full-blown nephrotic syndrome is the typical clinical presentation, sometimes accompanied by AKI. NSAID-induced AIN can occur alone or along with these glomerular diseases.

CHEMOTHERAPEUTIC AGENTS

Chemotherapeutic agents are critical to halting or slowing tumor growth, but adverse renal effects often complicate treatment. They are most commonly associated with AKI, but also cause electrolyte and acid-base disturbances, proteinuria, and hypertension.

ANTIANGIOGENESIS DRUGS

Antiangiogenesis drugs target vascular endothelial growth factor (VEGF) or its tyrosine kinase receptor (VEGF-R). VEGF signaling is critical to the tumor angiogenesis, and disruption of the signaling pathways provides novel treatment options for aggressive malignancies. However, VEGF biology is also essential to renal microvasculature and glomerular integrity. Podocytes provide local VEGF to glomerular endothelial cells, allowing maintenance of the integrity of fenestrated endothelium. In animals, pharmacologic reduction in VEGF production or effect causes proteinuria, hypertension, and thrombotic microangiopathy by damaging the renal microvasculature, in particular the glomerular endothelium. A similar clinical syndrome marked by proteinuria (rarely nephrotic) and hypertension occurs in patients treated with antiangiogenesis agents such as bevacizumab and the tyrosine kinase inhibitors. Thrombotic microangiopathy is the most common pathologic lesion noted in patients who undergo kidney biopsy for AKI (Fig 37.1).

INTERFERON

Interferon (α,β,γ) is described as causing glomerular injury and proteinuria. Early reported cases showed minimal change lesions, but more recent reports describe collapsing and noncollapsing focal segmental glomerulosclerosis (FSGS) on biopsy. Patients' presenting symptoms included nephrotic range proteinuria and AKI within weeks of commencing interferon therapy. The time to clinical presentation was shorter for interferon-α as compared to other subtypes. Although proteinuria declined with cessation of interferon therapy, complete reversal

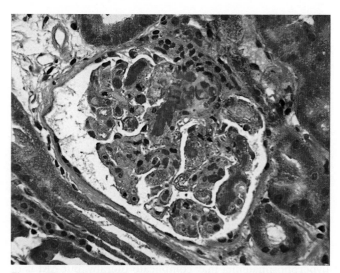

Figure 37.1   Thrombotic microangiopathy as manifested by mesangiolysis, endothelial denudation, red blood cell congestion, and basement membrane duplication in the glomerulus on light microscopy. (Courtesy Michael Kashgarian, Yale University.)

was uncommon. The mechanism underlying interferon-associated glomerular injury is not entirely clear, but it may include direct binding to podocyte receptors and alteration of normal cellular proliferation. Other postulated effects include macrophage activation and skewing of the cytokine profile toward IL-6 and IL-13, which are purported permeability factors in minimal change disease (MCD) and FSGS.

BISPHOSPHONATES

The bisphosphonates are effectively used for malignancy-related bone disorders such as multiple myeloma, hypercalcemia of malignancy, and osteolytic metastases. They are also commonly used in Paget disease and osteoporosis. One of their major adverse effects is nephrotoxicity, seen primarily with pamidronate and zoledronate. Nephrotoxicity is more common with high-dose IV formulations than the oral or low-dose IV preparations used in osteoporosis treatment. Depending on the particular bisphosphonate, glomerular and/or tubular injury may result. Pamidronate-induced kidney injury is dose related, where high dosage and long duration increase risk. Nephrotoxic manifestations include nephrotic-range proteinuria or full-blown nephrotic syndrome associated with collapsing FSGS or MCD, consistent with a toxic podocytopathy. Acute tubular necrosis (ATN) may also accompany collapsing FSGS. Nephrotoxicity is sometimes reversible, but progressive CKD and end-stage renal disease (ESRD) requiring chronic dialysis may develop. IV zoledronate is more commonly associated with AKI from toxic ATN, although rare cases of FSGS are described. Current evidence suggests that ibandronate has the least nephrotoxic potential. As bisphosphonates undergo kidney excretion, prevention of nephrotoxicity hinges on dose reduction in patients with reduced GFR, with clinical guidelines recommending discontinuation of therapy after estimated GFR becomes less than 30 mL/min.

PLATINUM COMPOUNDS

Platinum-based agents are potent antineoplastic drugs that have a high incidence of nephrotoxicity, particularly in patients with CKD. Nonoliguric AKI from toxic ATN is the most common pattern of kidney injury. Cisplatin has the most nephrotoxic potential, although second- and third-generation drugs such as carboplatin and oxaliplatin are also nephrotoxic at high doses. Cisplatin's mechanism of nephrotoxicity is related to its drug characteristics and kidney handling. Chloride at the *cis*-position of the molecule promotes kidney injury, whereas its uptake into proximal tubular cells via OCT-2 also contributes to damage. Other mechanisms of injury are activation of intracellular injury pathways, inflammation, oxidative stress, and vascular injury. The end result is renal tubular cell apoptosis or necrosis, manifesting as clinical AKI and/or a tubulopathy. Platin drugs are also associated with Fanconi syndrome from proximal tubular injury, and sodium-wasting syndrome and hypomagnesemia from cellular injury in the loop of Henle.

In high-risk patients, carboplatin and oxalaplatin are used based on their less nephrotoxic profile. Neither of these molecules is transported by OCT-2, thereby reducing proximal tubular intracellular concentrations. In addition, the chloride at *cis*-position in cisplatin is replaced by carboxylate and cyclobutane in carboplatin and oxalaplatin, respectively, which may further reduce toxicity. Antioxidants such as sodium thiosulfate and amifostine have been proposed as prophylactic measures against platin nephrotoxicity, but concerns of decreased anticancer activity as well as adverse effects limit their utility. Prevention of platin nephrotoxicity focuses on volume repletion with IV saline administration and avoidance of other nephrotoxins.

IFOSFAMIDE

Ifosfamide is an alkylating agent derived from the parent molecule cyclophosphamide. In contrast to cyclophosphamide, ifosfamide causes renal tubular injury primarily through its nephrotoxic metabolite, chloracetaldehyde. Additionally, ifosfamide enters tubular cells via OCT-2, whereas cyclophosphamide does not. Nephrotoxic manifestations include tubulopathies such as isolated proximal tubular injury, Fanconi syndrome, nephrogenic diabetes insipidus (DI), and AKI from ATN, which is often reversible but can be permanent. Tubular cell injury and necrosis with swollen, dysmorphic mitochondria are noted on kidney histopathology. Risk factors for kidney injury include previous cisplatin exposure, cumulative dose greater than 90 g/m², and underlying CKD.

Preventive measures are limited. IV saline and dose reduction are used. As this agent is transported into cells via OCT-2, competitive inhibition of this pathway with cimetidine is being evaluated. Treatment is supportive, addressing electrolyte deficiencies and monitoring for CKD and dialysis-requiring ESRD. Other long-term complications include permanent proximal tubulopathy and isolated renal phosphaturia.

PEMETREXED

Pemetrexed is a methotrexate derivative that inhibits enzymes involved in purine and pyrimidine metabolism, impairing RNA and DNA synthesis in tumors. It is excreted unchanged by the kidneys, although pemetrexed enters proximal tubular cell via apical and basolateral pathways. Apical drug uptake may occur via the folate receptor-α transport pathway, whereas basolateral entry is by the reduced folate carrier. Intracellular pemetrexed is polyglutamylated, which traps the drug within the cell. The higher intracellular drug concentration more fully impairs RNA and DNA synthesis and causes cell injury. Reversible AKI occurs with high-dose therapy, with kidney lesions consisting of ATN and AIN. Tubular dysfunction consisting of nephrogenic DI and distal renal tubular acidosis occur. Most patients present with AKI and minimal proteinuria, which stabilizes with drug discontinuation but can lead to CKD from chronic tubulointerstitial nephritis.

EPIDERMAL GROWTH FACTOR RECEPTOR ANTAGONISTS

Monoclonal antibodies that antagonize epithelial growth factor receptor (EGFR) signaling, including cetuximab and panitumumab, offer promising biologic therapy for colorectal and head and neck tumors. Given the role of EGFR signaling in magnesium homeostasis, these antibodies induce renal magnesium wasting. The EGFR signaling cascade is necessary for activation of transient receptor potential M6 (TRPM6), the epithelial channel in the distal nephron that facilitates magnesium reabsorption. Monoclonal antibodies against EGFR, which have a much higher affinity for EGFR than endogenous EGF, potently inhibit placement of TRPM6 in the apical membrane and prevent luminal magnesium reabsorption. The incidence of hypomagnesemia approaches 43% with cetuximab in clinical trials, whereas nearly all patients develop some reduction in serum magnesium level. Thus, serum magnesium monitoring should be a standard of care with anti-EGFR therapy. Panitumumab causes hypomagnesemia less commonly. The likelihood of hypomagnesemia increases with duration of therapy and may persist for several weeks after drug discontinuation before resolving. Treatment requires IV magnesium repletion, particularly in cancer patients who tend to have diarrhea, vomiting, and decreased oral intake.

ANTIMICROBIAL AGENTS

Several widely prescribed antimicrobial medications to treat infections result in kidney injury, especially in hospitalized patients. Antimicrobial agents are administered to the most severely ill patients who have coexistent processes that can independently affect kidney function and potentiate nephrotoxicity.

ANTIBIOTICS

AMINOGLYCOSIDES

Aminoglycosides (AGs) are frequently associated with kidney injury in hospitalized patients. The reported incidence ranges between 7% and 36% of patients receiving these drugs. This rate increases with the duration of drug administration and may approach 50% with more than 2 weeks of therapy. AGs are freely filtered at the glomerulus and then reabsorbed by proximal tubular cells. Ultimately, renal excretion is the major route of elimination. Their cationic and

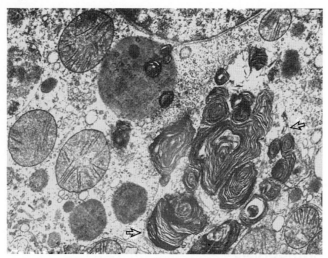

Figure 37.2 Aminoglycoside-induced tubular cell injury manifested by myeloid bodies *(arrows)* **as seen on electron microscopy.** These bodies represent changes in tubular lysosomes caused by the accumulation of polar lipids. (Courtesy Gilbert W. Moeckel, Yale University.)

Box 37.2   Risk Factors for Aminoglycoside Nephrotoxicity

Prolonged course of treatment (>10 days)
Volume depletion
Sepsis
Preexisting kidney disease
Hypokalemia
Advanced age
Combination therapy with certain cephalosporins, particularly cephalothin
Concomitant exposure to other nephrotoxins (e.g., radiocontrast, amphotericin B, cisplatin)
Exposure to gentamicin > amikacin > tobramycin

---

amphophilic properties enhance binding to apical membranes of proximal tubular cells, likely via the megalin receptor, and lead to accumulation of drug within cortical tubular cells. Nephrotoxicity tracks with charge; the more cationic, the more likely the drug will interact with apical membranes, where they undergo endocytosis and accumulate within intracellular lysosomes. Myeloid bodies (Fig. 37.2) visualized on electron microscopy often develop. These structures are membrane fragments and damaged organelles that result from inhibition of lysosomal enzymes. Nephrotoxicity occurs from mechanisms such as disruption of subcellular organelle activity, induction of oxidative stress, and enhanced mitochondrial dysfunction.

AG nephrotoxicity presents clinically as a rising serum creatinine after approximately 5 to 7 days of therapy, but may occur earlier in the presence of risk factors. AKI is often preceded by a concentrating defect. Low-grade proteinuria and urine sediment containing renal tubular epithelial (RTE) cells or granular casts are seen days before clinically obvious AKI, supporting ongoing subclinical kidney injury. Tubular dysfunction is manifested by an elevated fractional excretion of sodium (greater than 1% to 2%), as well as urinary potassium, calcium, and magnesium wasting. Gentamicin has been described as causing a proximal tubulopathy or full-blown Fanconi syndrome in some patients, whereas a Bartter-like syndrome has also been noted. The latter lesion is speculated to occur from the activation of the calcium-sensing receptor by cationic gentamicin, thereby inhibiting the NaK2Cl transporter in the loop of Henle. AKI progressively worsens, but the course may be limited in severity with early drug discontinuation. Nevertheless, a time lag may occur before kidney function improves.

Several risk factors for AG nephrotoxicity have been identified (Box 37.2). This will allow, when alternative antibiotics are unavailable, more intensive monitoring and modification of risk factors, such as volume depletion and electrolyte abnormalities. All members of the AG family can cause nephrotoxicity, but tobramycin exhibits less nephrotoxicity than gentamicin in animal models.

Tailoring AG doses to maintain drug levels within therapeutic range minimizes nephrotoxicity while maintaining bactericidal drug concentrations. When calculating doses, it should be recognized that changes in the serum creatinine often underestimate the true GFR reduction in elderly, cirrhotic, and malnourished patients. In addition to appropriate dose reduction, single daily-dose regimens may reduce AG nephrotoxicity because tubular absorption is saturable, although the data are mixed. Monitoring of peak and trough drug levels, along with serum creatinine concentration, every 2 to 3 days is prudent, but daily monitoring may be required in patients with serious infections and unstable kidney function. Urine microscopic findings will identify kidney injury before serum creatinine changes.

VANCOMYCIN

Vancomycin is a widely prescribed and typically well-tolerated drug. Although AKI rarely occurs as a complication, two lesions have been described. One is an idiosyncratic reaction resulting in AIN, and the other is direct tubular toxicity that occurs with excessive serum concentrations. Kidney biopsies in patients with AKI associated with toxic vancomycin concentrations have demonstrated toxic ATN rather than classic AIN.

POLYMIXINS

The polymixins are a group of antibiotics generally reserved for resistant organisms, primarily because of their high nephrotoxic potential. Colistin and polymyxin B are the two agents that are employed as antimicrobials. Both have a narrow therapeutic window with nephrotoxicity related to their D-amino content and fatty acid component. This increases tubular cell membrane permeability and influx of cations, resulting in tubular cell injury. Patients with underlying risk often develop AKI with increasing duration of therapy.

SULFONAMIDES

Sulfa-based antibiotics are effective antimicrobial agents that can cause three kidney lesions—AIN, crystal nephropathy, and vasculitis. AIN is most common, whereas crystal-induced AKI occurs primarily with high-dose sulfadiazine (other sulfonamides to a lesser degree). Vasculitis is probably the least common sulfonamide-related kidney lesion, typically a hypersensitivity reaction that rarely is associated with development of polyarteritis nodosa. The incidence of AKI ranges from 0.4% to 29%. Crystal-induced kidney injury occurs when insoluble sulfa-drug precipitates within the tubular lumen of the distal nephron. As the drug is a weak acid, this is more likely to happen in an acidic urine (pH less than 6.0), when urine flow rates are low, or with hypoalbuminemia and excessive dose for level of GFR.

Although patients are generally asymptomatic, vague abdominal or flank pain along with an increasing serum creatinine and oliguria occur within 7 days of starting therapy. Urine microscopy reveals strongly birefringent sulfonamide crystals (shocks of wheat, shells), sometimes admixed with white blood cells, RTE cells, and granular casts. Rarely, small radiolucent calculi may also lodge in the kidney parenchyma and/or calyces and appear as layered clusters of echogenic material on kidney ultrasonography. Treatment includes IV fluids, urinary alkalinization, and sulfonamide dose reduction or discontinuation.

CIPROFLOXACIN

The quinolone antibiotic ciprofloxacin is widely used to treat numerous bacterial infections. As noted with other antibiotics, ciprofloxacin causes AKI in patients primarily through the development of AIN. Experimental studies have demonstrated crystalluria following the administration of ciprofloxacin. Less commonly, this drug can be associated with crystal-induced AKI in humans. Ciprofloxacin is insoluble at neutral or alkaline pH, and it crystallizes in alkaline urine (pH greater than 7.3). Intrarenal crystallization may result from excessive drug doses in elderly patients, underlying CKD, volume depletion, and/or alkaline urine. Patients are generally asymptomatic, and the first sign of kidney injury is a rise in serum creatinine after 2 to 14 days of treatment. Urine microscopy shows ciprofloxacin crystals, which appear as strongly birefringent needles, sheaves, stars, fans, butterflies, and other unusual shapes along with other cellular elements and casts. Kidney biopsy reveals crystals within the tubules. To avoid this complication, ciprofloxacin should be dosed appropriately for the level of kidney function. To prevent AKI and crystalluria, patients receiving ciprofloxacin should be volume replete, and alkalinization of the urine should be avoided. Treatment is drug discontinuation or dose reduction and volume repletion with isotonic IV fluids.

ANTIVIRAL DRUGS

ACYCLOVIR

Acyclovir is an effective antiviral agent that is widely used to treat herpes virus infections. Although generally safe, it can cause AKI from intratubular crystal deposition when administered intravenously, particularly at high doses. Acyclovir is excreted in the urine through both glomerular filtration and tubular secretion. Acyclovir is relatively insoluble in the urine, which accounts for its intratubular precipitation at high concentration or with low urine flow rates, resulting in intrarenal urinary obstruction. Isolated crystalluria and asymptomatic AKI are most common, but nausea/vomiting and flank/abdominal pain may occur. Crystal nephropathy typically develops within 24 to 48 hours of acyclovir administration, with an AKI incidence of 12% to 48% when administered as a rapid IV bolus. In contrast, low-dose IV and oral acyclovir therapy rarely cause AKI unless there is severe volume depletion or underlying kidney disease. Urine

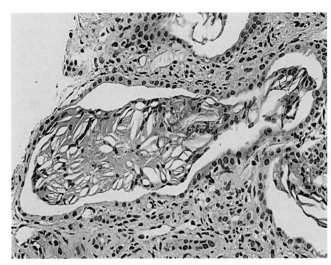

Figure 37.3 Indinavir crystal deposition within renal tubular lumens causes acute and chronic kidney injury, an entity coined *crystal nephropathy*, as seen on light microscopy. (Courtesy Glen S. Markowitz, Columbia University.)

microscopy usually shows both hematuria and pyuria, along with birefringent, needle-shaped crystals. Prevention hinges on avoiding rapid bolus infusion of acyclovir and by repleting intravascular volume before drug exposure. Dose reduction is critical in patients with underlying kidney disease. HD removes significant amounts of acyclovir and is sometimes indicated with severe AKI and concomitant neurotoxicity. Fortunately, most patients recover kidney function with acyclovir discontinuation and volume resuscitation.

INDINAVIR AND ATAZANAVIR

Indinavir and atazanavir are protease inhibitors used in the treatment of human immunodeficiency virus (HIV) infection. Indinavir revolutionized HIV care, but its use was complicated by a number of toxicities including crystal-induced AKI and nephrolithiasis. Atazanavir has gained widespread use, and it is also associated with crystal-related kidney injury and nephrolithiasis.

The kidney clears approximately 20% of indinavir, and intratubular crystal precipitation occurs at urine pH more than 5.5 (Fig. 37.3). Intrarenal tubular obstruction and obstructing calculi can also lead to AKI. Complications include renal colic, dysuria, back/flank pain, or gross hematuria, with an 8% incidence of urologic symptoms. Urine microscopy shows crystals of varying shapes, including platelike rectangles, fan-shaped crystals, and starburst forms. Although most cases of indinavir-associated AKI are mild and reversible, more severe AKI from obstructing calculi and CKD occur. Prevention of intrarenal crystal deposition requires consumption of 2 to 3 liters of fluid per day. Patients with hepatic disease should receive a dose reduction. Discontinuation of indinavir generally reverses nephrotoxicity; however, chronic tubulointerstitial fibrosis has been noted.

Atazanavir also causes kidney disease. It has chemical characteristics and pharmacokinetics similar to indinavir, likely explaining this complication. Crystal nephropathy, nephrolithiasis, and AIN have been described. Thirty cases of atazanavir-associated nephrolithiasis have been reported to the

FDA, whereas another study estimated a 0.97% prevalence of atazanavir stones among those taking the drug. Analysis of kidney stones shows 60% atazanavir metabolite and 40% calcium apatite. Atazanavir-associated crystal nephropathy has also been described, where rodlike atazanavir crystals were noted on urine microscopy as well as within tubular lumens on kidney biopsy. Prevention is best achieved by avoiding intravascular volume depletion. Treatment hinges on IVF therapy and stone removal when indicated. Drug discontinuation is sometimes necessary.

TENOFOVIR

Tenofovir (TF) is an antiviral agent used to treat various viral infections including HIV and hepatitis B virus. Animal models note that TF causes proximal tubular dilatation, abnormalities in mitochondrial ultrastructure, depleted mitochondrial DNA (mtDNA), and depressed respiratory chain enzyme expression. Clinically, patients present with AKI or a proximal tubulopathy, and less commonly with nephrogenic DI. AKI may require temporary dialysis, although a degree of kidney recovery often results in CKD. Kidney histology from patients with clinical nephrotoxicity demonstrates proximal tubular injury and varying degrees of chronic tubulointerstitial scarring. On light microscopy, prominent eosinophilic inclusions within proximal tubular cell cytoplasm represent giant, abnormal mitochondria. On electron microscopy, injured mitochondria vary from small and rounded to swollen with irregular contours.

Host factors that potentiate TF nephrotoxicity include the HIV-infected host's mtDNA depletion, reduced GFR, and genetic defects in drug excretion pathways. TF is eliminated by a combination of glomerular filtration and proximal tubular secretion, which in part explains its compartmental toxicity. It is transported from the basolateral circulation into proximal tubular cells via organic ion transporter-1 (OAT-1), and it is subsequently translocated into the urine through apical efflux transporters such as multidrug resistance proteins (MRP-2/-4). Reduced GFR enhances the amount of drug that is secreted, increasing traffic through proximal tubular cells. Impaired MRP-driven efflux activity can reduce drug secretion and increase intracellular concentrations. A single nucleotide polymorphism (SNP) in the MRP-2 efflux transporter gene (ABCC2) has been documented in HIV-infected patients with TF-induced nephrotoxicity. Excretory pathway defects can lead to increased TF concentrations within tubular cells.

Prevention of and monitoring for TF-related kidney injury is important. Genetic risk factor testing (SNP in ABCC2 gene) to identify high-risk patients, and targeted interventions such as probenicid to reduce OAT-1–mediated drug transport into tubular cells may reduce toxicity. Avoidance of TF in patients with advanced CKD, or at least appropriate dose reduction, will further reduce nephrotoxicity.

ANTIFUNGAL AGENTS

AMPHOTERICIN B

Amphotericin B (AmB) is a polyene antibiotic used in treatment of many serious fungal infections, but it is also associated with nephrotoxicity. The degree of kidney injury is roughly proportional to the total cumulative dose. As this drug is highly bound to cell membranes, it damages membrane integrity and increases permeability. Membrane injury is thought to underlie development of the characteristic clinical syndromes of potassium and magnesium wasting, inability to concentrate urine maximally, and distal tubule acidification defects. These abnormalities, along with urine microscopy findings with RTE cells/casts and granular casts, usually precede the development of clinically apparent AKI. AmB also produces acute afferent arteriolar vasoconstriction, causing a hemodynamic reduction in the GFR. Tubuloglomerular feedback (TGF) triggered by increased sodium permeability has been suggested as playing a role in vasoconstriction.

Reduced kidney function is frequently nonoliguric and progressive, but slowly abates after drug discontinuation. However, high doses and repetitive drug exposure can cause CKD. Volume depletion potentiates nephrotoxicity, whereas sodium loading and volume expansion can ameliorate kidney injury, perhaps by blunting TGF. Risk factors for kidney injury include high dose, prolonged duration of therapy, ICU admission when therapy is initiated, and cyclosporine therapy. Several formulations of AmB in lipid vehicles, including liposomes, have been developed for clinical use and result in fewer constitutional symptoms while retaining antifungal activity. Studies have shown that these formulations are less nephrotoxic, but they can still cause AKI in high-risk patients.

MISCELLANEOUS

EXENATIDE

Exenatide is a synthetic form of endogenous glucagon-like peptide-1, which stimulates insulin secretion, inhibits glucagon release, decreases appetite, and slows gastric emptying. As such, it is used as add-on therapy for diabetes mellitus. This hypoglycemic agent has been associated with several adverse effects, particularly nausea/vomiting and AKI. Exenatide is administered as a subcutaneous injection and is eliminated by glomerular filtration. As a result, the half-life increases from 1.4 hours to 6 hours with underlying kidney disease.

Several adverse drug-event–reporting databases have collected cases of kidney injury associated with exenatide. Many were classified as AKI, and the majority had ≥1 risk factor including stage 4/5 CKD, hypertension, rhabdomyolysis, cardiac disease, and other medications, including diuretics, RAAS blockers, or NSAIDs. Most patients were volume depleted. Limited kidney histology was reported, with five cases demonstrating ATN. Thus, exenatide may cause either prerenal or ischemic ATN in high-risk patients.

WARFARIN-RELATED NEPHROPATHY

A little-known complication of warfarin is AKI from severe glomerular bleeding and obstructing red blood cell casts. This entity has been coined *warfarin nephropathy*, but in actuality it can occur with any form of excessive anticoagulation in at-risk patients. It has been described in patients with and without CKD who are overanticoagulated with warfarin. The mechanism appears to be related to glomerular hemorrhage, often in patients with an underlying glomerulopathy, with subsequent obstruction of tubules by RBC casts. The cause of AKI is not known, although tubular obstruction and/or heme-related tubular injury from lysosmal overload and oxidative damage play a role. Hemoglobin may enter cells via megalin-cubulin receptor-mediated endocytosis, with free hemoglobin promoting lipid peroxidation and heme/iron-generating ROS, mitochondrial damage, and apoptosis. Therapy consists of reversal of anticoagulation initially, followed by more judicious anticoagulation in those who truly require it. Unfortunately, many patients are left with CKD, sometimes requiring chronic dialysis.

OSMOTIC AGENTS

Osmotic nephropathy refers to kidney injury seen when certain macromolecules enter proximal tubular cells through the apical membrane. First described in animal studies, sucrose infusion was associated with tubular cell swelling and kidney dysfunction. Similar histopathology and kidney injury have been described with mannitol, dextran, and, more recently, with intravenous immune globulin (IVIG) and hydroxyethyl starch (HES). Tubular injury begins with drug entry into the tubular cell, followed by accumulation within lysosomes causing tubular epithelia to swell and form vacuoles. This process ultimately disrupts cellular integrity, and if tubular swelling is severe, it obstructs tubular lumens and impedes urine flow causing AKI. Kidney biopsy shows characteristic histopathologic lesions such as swollen, edematous tubules filled with cytoplasmic vacuoles, which represent swollen lysosomes on electron microscopy (Fig. 37.4). With severe injury, tubules may appear degraded, similar to ischemic or toxic ATN.

Osmotic nephropathy is most commonly associated with IVIG, which is stabilized with sucrose, and HES. IVIG-related osmotic nephropathy occurs in patients with underlying kidney disease and the elderly. Nonsucrose formulations of IVIG have not been linked to AKI and thus are preferred for high-risk patients. HES is a potent volume expander that

consists of an amylopectin chain with hydroxyethyl substitutions of varying degrees. Systemic degradation of HES allows glomerular filtration of the smaller HES molecules that enter proximal tubular cells. Similar to sucrose, HES-induced kidney injury has histopathologic features typical of osmotic nephropathy including tubular cell swelling and vacuolization. Clinically, HES is associated with AKI, sometimes requiring dialysis, especially in patients with sepsis and underlying kidney disease. Prevention is based on avoiding these agents in high-risk patients, whereas therapy for osmotic nephropathy is supportive with avoidance of further exposure.

LITHIUM

Lithium (Li^+) is one of the most effective medications used in the treatment of bipolar disorders, making it a cornerstone of therapy despite its various toxicities. Li^+ adversely affects several organ systems, including the kidney, which excretes this cation. Although several renal syndromes occur, the most common complication is nephrogenic DI. This condition develops in as many as 20% to 30% of patients and is a result of induction of renal resistance to the actions of antidiuretic hormone (ADH). ADH resistance reduces water permeability in the distal nephron through inhibition of the generation or action of cyclic-AMP. This decreases expression and attenuates apical targeting of aquaporin-2 water channels in renal epithelial cells. Although polyuria generally improves with Li^+ withdrawal, amiloride therapy can mitigate its effect by antagonizing epithelial sodium channels. This maneuver reduces urine volume in patients who must continue on Li^+ therapy.

Acute Li^+ intoxication can occur with intentional overdose or in patients on stable dose who suffer an acute decline in GFR. It is manifested by symptoms ranging from nausea and tremor to seizures and coma. In addition, AKI can occur. The severity of intoxication generally correlates with serum Li^+ concentrations. Along with gastric lavage and polyethylene glycol, IV saline is used to reverse volume depletion and induce diuresis, thereby facilitating Li^+ excretion. In patients with AKI or CKD, significant neurologic symptoms, and Li^+ levels greater than 4.0 mEq/L, HD should be pursued. HD efficiently clears Li^+, where a 4-hour treatment can reduce plasma levels by about 1 mEq/L.

Long-term Li^+ therapy can cause chronic tubulointerstitial nephritis, characterized by tubular atrophy and interstitial fibrosis, with cortical and medullary tubular microcysts. Rarely, patients develop high-grade proteinuria and FSGS. Although kidney function may improve after drug cessation, irreversible CKD and ESRD may be observed.

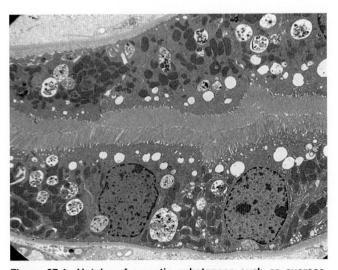

Figure 37.4 Uptake of osmotic substances such as sucrose, hydoxyethyl starch, dextran, and radiocontrast cause acute and chronic tubular injury, an entity known as *osmotic nephropathy*. Electron microscopy demonstrates characteristic cytoplasmic vacuoles. (Courtesy Gilbert W. Moeckel, Yale University.)

BIBLIOGRAPHY

Cruz DN, Goh CY, Marenzi G, et al: Renal replacement therapies for prevention of radiocontrast-induced nephropathy: a systematic review, *Am J Med* 125:66-78, 2012.

Deray G: Amphotericin B nephrotoxicity, *J Antimicrob Chemother* 49:37-41, 2002.

Ermina V, Jefferson A, Kowalewska J, et al: VEGF inhibition and renal thrombotic microangiopathy, *N Engl J Med* 358:1129-1136, 2008.

Gurevich F, Perazella MA: Renal effects of anti-angiogenesis therapy: update for the internist, *Am J Med* 122:322-328, 2009.

Humphreys BD, Soifer RJ, Magee CC: Renal failure associated with cancer and its treatment: an update, *J Am Soc Nephrol* 16:151-161, 2005.

Izzedine H, Harris M, Perazella MA: The nephrotoxic effects of HAART, *Nat Rev Nephrol* 5:563-573, 2009.

Izzedine H, Isnard-Bagnis C, Launay-Vacher V, et al: Gemcitabine-induced thrombotic microangiopathy: a systematic review, *Nephrol Dial Transplant* 21:3038-3045, 2006.

Kintzel PE: Anticancer drug-induced kidney disorders: incidence, prevention and management, *Drug Saf* 24:19-38, 2001.

Markowitz GS, Perazella MA: Acute phosphate nephropathy, *Kidney Int* 76:1027-1034, 2009.

Markowitz GS, Perazella MA: Drug-induced renal failure: a focus on tubulointerstitial disease, *Clin Chim Acta* 351:31-47, 2005.

Perazella MA: Advanced kidney disease, gadolinium and nephrogenic systemic fibrosis: the perfect storm, *Curr Opin Nephrol Hypertens* 18:519-525, 2009.

Perazella MA: Renal vulnerability to drug toxicity, *Clin J Am Soc Nephrol* 4:1275-1283, 2009.

Perazella MA, Markowitz GS: Bisphosphonate nephrotoxicity, *Kidney Int* 74:1385-1393, 2008.

Perazella MA, Moeckel GW: Nephrotoxicity from chemotherapeutic agents: clinical manifestations, pathobiology and prevention/therapy, *Sem Nephrol* 30:570-581, 2010.

Presne C, Fakhouri F, Noel LH, et al: Lithium-induced nephropathy: rate of progression and prognostic factors, *Kidney Int* 64:585-592, 2003.

Weisbord SD, Palevsky PM: Prevention of contrast-induced nephropathy with volume expansion, *Clin J Am Soc Nephrol* 3:273-380, 2008.

Principles of Drug Therapy in Patients with Reduced Kidney Function

38

Gary R. Matzke | Thomas D. Nolin

Reduced kidney function may occur in many situations, including chronic kidney disease (CKD) resulting from such disorders as diabetes mellitus, hypertension, and glomerulonephritis, as well as age-related falls in glomerular filtration rate (GFR). In adults, these conditions are associated with a high use of medications, making these patients particularly susceptible to the accumulation of a drug or its active or toxic metabolites. Clinicians must have a thorough understanding of the impact of reduced kidney function on drug disposition and the appropriate methods by which to individualize drug therapy as they strive to optimize the outcomes of their patients.

Individualization of therapy for those agents that are predominantly (>70%) eliminated unchanged by the kidney can be accomplished with a proportional dose reduction or dosing interval prolongation based on the fractional reduction in GFR or its more commonly evaluated clinical counterparts, creatinine clearance (CL_{Cr}) and estimated GFR. However, because impaired kidney function is associated with progressive alterations in the bioavailability, plasma protein binding, distribution volume, and nonrenal clearance (i.e., metabolism and transport) of many drugs, a more complex adjustment scheme may be required for medications that are extensively metabolized by the liver or for which changes in protein binding and/or distribution volume have been noted. Patients with impaired kidney function may also respond to a given dose or serum concentration of a drug (e.g., phenytoin) differently from those with normal kidney function because of the physiologic and biochemical changes associated with progressive CKD.

Using a sound understanding of basic pharmacokinetic principles, the characteristics of a drug, and the pathophysiologic alterations associated with impaired kidney function, clinicians can design individualized therapeutic regimens. This chapter describes the influence of impaired kidney function resulting from CKD and, when information is available, from acute kidney injury (AKI) on drug absorption, distribution, metabolism, transport, and excretion. The chapter also provides a practical approach to drug dosage individualization for patients with reduced kidney function and those receiving continuous renal replacement therapy (CRRT), peritoneal dialysis, or hemodialysis.

DRUG ABSORPTION

Little quantitative information exists about the influence of reduced kidney function in CKD patients on drug absorption. Several variables, including changes in gastrointestinal transit time, gastric pH, edema of the gastrointestinal tract, vomiting and diarrhea (frequently seen in those with stage 5 CKD), and concomitant administration of phosphate binders, have been associated with alterations in the absorption of some drugs, such as digoxin and many of the fluoroquinolone antibiotics. The fraction of a drug that reaches the systemic circulation after oral versus intravenous administration (termed absolute bioavailability) is rarely altered in CKD patients. However, alterations in the peak concentration (C_{max}) and in the time at which the peak concentration was attained (t_{max}) have been noted for a few drugs, suggesting that the rate, but not the extent of absorption is altered in CKD. Although the bioavailability of some drugs, such as furosemide or pindolol, is reported to be reduced, there are no consistent findings in patients with CKD to indicate that absorption is impaired. However, an increase in bioavailability as the result of a decrease in metabolism during the drug's first pass through the gastrointestinal tract and liver has been noted for some β-blockers, dextropropoxyphene, and dihydrocodeine.

DRUG DISTRIBUTION

The volume of distribution (V_D) of many drugs is significantly altered in patients with stages 4 or 5 CKD (Table 38.1), and changes in patients with oliguric AKI have also been reported. These changes are predominantly the result of altered plasma protein or tissue binding or of volume expansion secondary to reduced renal sodium and water excretion. The plasma protein binding of acidic drugs, such as warfarin and phenytoin, is decreased in patients with CKD, possibly due to changes in the conformation of the binding sites, accumulation of endogenous inhibitors of binding, and decreased concentrations of albumin. In addition, the high concentrations of metabolites of some drugs that accumulate in CKD patients may interfere with the protein binding of the parent compound.

The plasma concentration of the principal binding protein for several basic drug compounds, α1-acid glycoprotein, is increased in kidney transplant patients and in hemodialysis patients. For this reason, the unbound fraction of some basic drugs (e.g., quinidine) may be decreased, and as a result, the V_D in these patients is decreased. The net effect of changes in protein binding is usually an alteration in the relationship between unbound and total drug concentrations, an effect

Table 38.1   Volume of Distribution of Selected Drugs in Patients with Stage 5 CKD

Drug	Normal (L/kg)	Stage 5 CKD (L/kg)	Change from Normal (%)
Amikacin	0.20	0.29	45
Azlocillin	0.21	0.28	33
Cefazolin	0.13	0.17	31
Cefoxitin	0.16	0.26	63
Cefuroxime	0.20	0.26	30
Clofibrate	0.14	0.24	71
Dicloxacillin	0.08	0.18	125
Digoxin	7.3	4.0	-45
Erythromycin	0.57	1.09	91
Gentamicin	0.20	0.32	60
Isoniazid	0.6	0.8	33
Minoxidil	2.6	4.9	88
Phenytoin	0.64	1.4	119
Trimethoprim	1.36	1.83	35
Vancomycin	0.64	0.85	33

CKD, Chronic kidney disease.

frequently encountered with phenytoin. The increase in unbound fraction, to values as high as 20% to 25% from the normal of 10%, results in increased hepatic clearance and decreased total concentrations. Although the unbound concentration therapeutic range is unchanged, the therapeutic range for total phenytoin concentration is reduced to 4 to 10 mcg/mL (normal, 10 to 20 mcg/mL) as GFR falls. Therefore the maintenance of therapeutic unbound concentrations of 1 to 2 mcg/mL provides the best target for individualizing phenytoin therapy in patients with reduced kidney function, and the optimal approach to management relies on the measurement of unbound phenytoin serum concentrations.

Altered tissue binding may also affect the apparent V_D of a drug. For example, the distribution volume of digoxin is reported to be reduced by 30% to 50% in patients with severe CKD. This may be the result of competitive inhibition by endogenous or exogenous digoxin-like immunoreactive substances that bind to and inhibit membrane adenosine triphosphatase (ATPase). The absolute amount of digoxin bound to the tissue digoxin receptor is reduced, and the resultant serum digoxin concentration observed after the administration of any dose is greater than expected.

Therefore in patients with CKD, a normal total drug concentration may be associated with either serious adverse reactions secondary to elevated unbound drug concentrations or subtherapeutic responses because of an increased plasma-to-tissue drug concentration ratio. Monitoring of unbound drug concentrations is suggested for drugs that have a narrow therapeutic range, those that are highly protein bound (>80%), and those with marked variability in the bound fraction (e.g., phenytoin, disopyramide).

DRUG METABOLISM AND TRANSPORT

Nonrenal clearance (CL_{NR}) of drugs includes all routes of drug elimination outside the kidney. Several oxidative and conjugative enzymes and active transporters constitute the primary pathways of CL_{NR}. Alterations in the function of

and interactions between metabolic enzymes and transporters can significantly affect the pharmacokinetic disposition and, correspondingly, patient exposure to drugs that are cleared via nonrenal pathways. The relationship of CKD to cytochrome P450 (CYP)–mediated metabolism (the major oxidative or phase I metabolic pathway) in the liver and other organs has been extensively reviewed and is quite varied. In rat models of end-stage renal disease (ESRD), protein expression in the liver of several CYP enzymes, including CYP3A1 and CYP3A2 (equivalent to human CYP3A4), is reduced by as much as 85%. CYP2C11 and CYP3A2 activity is also significantly reduced, but CYP1A1 activity is unchanged. Hepatic expression of the conjugative enzymes N-acetyltransferases (NATs) are also reduced, whereas uridine diphosphate-glucuronosyltransferases (UGTs) are unchanged. CYP functional expression is also decreased in the intestine; CYP1A1 and CYP3A2 are reduced up to 40% and 70%, respectively. Similarly, functional expression of several intestinal and hepatic transporters is altered in experimental models of kidney disease. The expression and corresponding activities of the efflux transporters P-glycoprotein (P-gp) and multi-drug resistance-associated protein 2 (MRP2) are reduced by as much as 65% in the intestine, but the uptake transporter organic anion transporting polypeptide (OATP) is not affected. Conversely, in the liver, protein expression of P-gp, MRP2, and OATP is increased, unchanged, and decreased, respectively.

In humans with kidney disease, the activities of CYPs appear to be relatively unaffected. It was previously reported that CYP3A4 activity was reduced, but recent data indicate that OATP uptake activity is reduced and thus the perceived changes in CYP3A4 activity were likely due to altered transporter activity, not an alteration in CYP activity. The reduction of CL_{NR} of several drugs that exhibit overlapping CYP and transporter substrate specificity in patients with stages 4 or 5 CKD supports this premise (Table 38.2). These studies must be interpreted with caution, however, because concurrent drug intake, age, smoking status, and alcohol use were often not taken into consideration. Furthermore, pharmacogenetic variations in drug-metabolizing enzymes and transporters that may have been present in the individual before the onset of AKI or progression of CKD must be considered, if known. For these reasons, prediction of the effect of reduced kidney function on the metabolism and/or transport of a particular drug is difficult, and a general quantitative strategy to adjust dosage regimens for drugs that undergo extensive nonrenal clearance has not yet been proposed. However, some qualitative insight may be gained if one knows which enzymes or transporters are involved in the clearance of the drug of interest and how those proteins are affected by a reduction in kidney function.

The effect of CKD on the nonrenal clearance of a particular drug is difficult to predict, even for drugs within the same pharmacologic class. The reductions in CL_{NR} for patients with CKD have frequently been noted to be proportional to the reductions in GFR. In the small number of studies that have evaluated CL_{NR} in critically ill patients with AKI, residual CL_{NR} was higher than in CKD patients with similar levels of CL_{Cr}, whether measured or estimated from the Cockcroft-Gault equation. Because a patient with AKI may have a higher CL_{NR} than does a CKD patient, the resultant plasma concentrations will be lower than expected, and possibly subtherapeutic, if classic CKD-derived dosage guidelines are followed.

Table 38.2   Major Pathways of Nonrenal Drug Clearance and Selected Substrates

CL_{NR} Pathway	Selected Substrates
Oxidative Enzymes	
CYP	
1A2	Polycyclic aromatic hydrocarbons, caffeine, imipramine, theophylline
2A6	Coumarin
2B6	Nicotine, bupropion
2C8	Retinoids, paclitaxel, repaglinide
2C9	Celecoxib, diclofenac, flurbiprofen, indomethacin, ibuprofen, losartan, phenytoin, tolbutamide, S-warfarin
2C19	Diazepam, S-mephenytoin, omeprazole
2D6	Codeine, debrisoquine, desipramine, dextromethorphan, fluoxetine, paroxetine, duloxetine, nortriptyline, haloperidol, metoprolol, propranolol
2E1	Ethanol, acetaminophen, chlorzoxazone, nitrosamines
3A4/5	Alprazolam, midazolam, cyclosporine, tacrolimus, nifedipine, felodipine, diltiazem, verapamil, fluconazole, ketoconazole, itraconazole, erythromycin, lovastatin, simvastatin, cisapride, terfenadine
Conjugative Enzymes	
UGT	Acetaminophen, morphine, lorazepam, oxazepam, naproxen, ketoprofen, irinotecan, bilirubin
NAT	Dapsone, hydralazine, isoniazid, procainamide
Transporters	
OATP	
1A2	Bile salts, statins, fexofenadine, methotrexate, digoxin, levofloxacin
1B1	Bile salts, statins, fexofenadine repaglinide, valsartan, olmesartan, irinotecan, bosentan
1B3	Bile salts, statins, fexofenadine, telmisartan, valsartan, olmesartan, digoxin
2B1	Statins, fexofenadine, glyburide
P-gp	Digoxin, fexofenadine, loperamide, irinotecan, doxorubicin, vinblastine, paclitaxel, erythromycin
MRP	
2	Methotrexate, etoposide, mitoxantrone, valsartan, olmesartan
3	Methotrexate, fexofenadine

Modified from Nolin TD, Unruh ML: Clinical relevance of impaired nonrenal drug clearance in ESRD, Semin Dial *23:482-485, 2010.*
CYP, Cytochrome P450 isozyme; MRP, multidrug resistance-associated protein; NAT, N-acetyltransferase; OATP, organic anion-transporting polypeptide; P-gp, P-glycoprotein; UGT, uridine diphosphate-glucuronosyltransferases.

RENAL EXCRETION OF DRUGS

Renal clearance (CL_R) is the net result of glomerular filtration of unbound drug plus tubular secretion minus tubular reabsorption. An acute or chronic reduction in GFR results in a decrease in CL_R. The degree of change in total body clearance of a drug is dependent on the fraction of the dose that is eliminated unchanged in individuals with normal kidney function, the intrarenal drug transport pathways, and the degree of functional impairment of each of these pathways. The primary renal transport systems of clinical importance with respect to drug excretion include the organic anionic transporters (OATs), organic cationic transporters (OCTs), and P-gp transporters. Diuretics, β-lactam antibiotics, nonsteroidal antiinflammatory drugs, and glucuronide drug metabolites are eliminated by the family of OAT transporters. The OCT transporters contribute to the secretion and excretion of cimetidine, famotidine, and quinidine. And the P-gp transport system in the kidney is involved in the secretion of cationic and hydrophobic drugs (e.g., digoxin, vinca alkaloids). The clearance of drugs that are secreted by the kidney (CL_R >300 mL/min) may be reduced from impairment in one or more of these renal transporters.

Despite the different mechanisms involved in the elimination of drugs by the kidney and the availability of several methods for determining kidney function, the clinical estimation of CL_{Cr} remains the most commonly used index for guiding drug dosage regimen design. The importance of an alteration in kidney function on drug elimination usually depends on two variables: (1) the fraction of drug normally eliminated by the kidney unchanged and (2) the degree of kidney functional impairment. There are a few drugs for which a metabolite is the primary active entity; in that situation, a key variable is the degree of renal clearance of the metabolite. The calculation of CL_{Cr} from a timed urine collection has been the standard clinical measure of kidney function for decades. However, urine is difficult to collect accurately in most clinical settings, and the interference of many commonly used medications with creatinine measurement limits the utility of this approach. Use of radioactive markers ([^{125}I]iothalamate, ^{51}Cr-EDTA, or ^{99}mTc-DTPA) or nonradioactive markers (iohexol, iothalamate, and inulin) of GFR, although scientifically sound, is clinically impractical, because intravenous or subcutaneous marker administration and multiple timed blood and urine collections make the procedures expensive and cumbersome.

ESTIMATION OF KIDNEY FUNCTION FOR DRUG DOSING PURPOSES

The estimation of kidney function by various estimating equations for drug dosing purposes is a critically important issue. In contrast to measured approaches, estimation of CL_{Cr} or GFR requires only routinely collected laboratory and demographic data. The Cockcroft-Gault equation for CL_{Cr} and the equations for estimated GFR (eGFR) from the Modification of Diet in Renal Disease Study (MDRD) and the Chronic Kidney Disease-Epidemiology Collaboration (CKD-EPI) correlate well with CL_{Cr} and GFR measurements in individuals with stable kidney function and average body composition (see Chapter 3). The traditional approach of estimating CL_{Cr} and using it as a continuous variable of kidney function for drug dosing adjustment purposes is now being supplemented—and, in some institutions, replaced—by eGFR. Caution is warranted because the use of eGFR as a guide for drug dosage adjustment has not been systematically validated. Currently, prospective pharmacokinetic data and corresponding dosing recommendations based on GFR estimating equations are limited. Since nearly all of the primary published literature to date has used CL_{Cr} to derive the relationship between kidney function and renal and/or total body clearance of a drug, CL_{Cr} is still the standard metric for drug dosing purposes. Nevertheless, widespread availability of automatically reported eGFR affords clinicians a tool that, if validated for drug dosing, could easily be incorporated into clinical practice. Furthermore, use of eGFR for management of kidney disease and drug dosing, along with harmonization of practice in this regard among physicians, pharmacists, and other clinicians, would be ideal and warrants further evaluation.

Clinicians should consider several issues when assessing CL_{Cr} and eGFR data for drug dosing. First, the MDRD-derived eGFR is currently the most widely reported and provides an estimate that is normalized for body surface area (BSA) in units of mL/min/1.73 m². When used for drug dosing, the eGFR value should be individualized, that is, not normalized for BSA, and converted to units of mL/min, particularly in patients whose BSA is considerably larger or smaller than 1.73 m². The individualized value should be compared with CL_{Cr} estimates (mL/min). Second, when presented with various kidney function estimates that potentially translate into different drug dosing regimens, clinicians should choose the regimen that optimizes the risk-benefit ratio given the patient-specific clinical scenario. For drugs with a narrow therapeutic range, typically more conservative kidney function estimates and corresponding doses should be used, particularly if therapeutic drug monitoring is not readily available. Since CL_{Cr} estimates are more conservative and indicate the need for dose adjustment more often than eGFR, they may be preferred when dosing drugs with narrow therapeutic windows, especially in high-risk subgroups such as older adults. Use of eGFR and a more aggressive dosing strategy may be acceptable for drugs with a wide therapeutic range and a broader margin of safety. Third, when estimating equations are not expected to provide accurate measures of kidney function (i.e., due to altered creatinine generation or unstable serum creatinine concentrations) and therapeutic drug monitoring is not available, it may be reasonable to obtain an accurately timed urine collection to calculate creatinine clearance, particularly for narrow-therapeutic-window drugs with high toxicity. Fourth, before applying data to a specific patient, clinicians must consider the limitations and the study population of the original trials from which the eGFR equations were developed, as well as the subsequent populations in which they have been validated. All of these methods are extremely poor predictors of kidney function in individuals with liver disease, and their use is not recommended for such patients. Finally, although several methods for CL_{Cr} estimation in patients with unstable kidney function (e.g., AKI) have been proposed, the accuracy of these methods has not been rigorously assessed, and at the present time their use cannot be recommended.

STRATEGIES FOR DRUG THERAPY INDIVIDUALIZATION

The design of the optimal dosage regimen for a patient with reduced kidney function depends on the availability of an accurate characterization of the relationship between the pharmacokinetic parameters of the drug and kidney function. Before 1998, there was no consensus regarding the criteria for characterizing the pharmacokinetics of a drug in patients with CKD. An industry report issued by the U.S. Food and Drug Administration in May 1998 provided guidelines regarding when a study should be considered; provided recommendations for study design, data analysis, and assessment of the impact of the study results on drug dosing; and recommended use of renal dose adjustment categories derived from CL_{Cr}. Currently, the FDA is considering including dosing tables based on eGFR and CL_{Cr} in a revised version of the 1998 FDA guideline. In the future, drug dosing recommendations based on eGFR in addition to CL_{Cr}, may be included in FDA-approved drug dosing labels. However, for drugs already approved by the FDA with existing renal dose adjustment recommendations based on CL_{Cr}, it is unlikely drug manufacturers will provide additional eGFR-based dosing recommendations.

Most dosage adjustment references have proposed the use of a fixed dose or interval for patients with a broad range of kidney function. Indeed, "normal" kidney function has often been ascribed to anyone who has a CL_{Cr} greater than 50 mL/min, even though many individuals (e.g., hyperfiltering early diabetics) have values in the range of 120 to 180 mL/min. The "moderate kidney function impairment" category in many guides encompasses a fivefold range of CL_{Cr}, from 10 to 49 mL/min, whereas severe kidney function impairment or ESRD is defined as a CL_{Cr} of less than 10 to 15 mL/min. Each of these categories encompasses a broad range of kidney function, and the calculated drug regimen may not be optimal for all patients within that range.

If specific recommendations or data on the relationship of the pharmacokinetic parameters of a drug to CL_{Cr} are not available, then these parameters can be estimated for a particular patient using the method of Rowland and Tozer, provided that the fraction of drug that is eliminated unchanged by the kidney (f_e) in normal subjects is known. This approach assumes the following: the change in drug clearance is proportional to the change in CL_{Cr}, kidney disease does not alter the drug's metabolism, any metabolites produced are inactive and nontoxic, the drug obeys first-order (linear) kinetic principles, and it is adequately described by a one-compartment model. If these assumptions are true, the kinetic parameter or dosage adjustment factor (Q) can be calculated as follows:

$$Q = 1 - [f_e(1 - KF)]$$

where KF is the ratio of the patient's CL_{Cr} to the assumed normal value of 120 mL/min. As an example, the Q factor for a patient who has a CL_{Cr} of 10 mL/min and a drug that is 85% eliminated unchanged by the kidney would be:

$$Q = 1 - [0.85(1 - 10/120)]$$
$$Q = 1 - [0.85(0.92)]$$
$$Q = 1 - 0.78$$
$$Q = 0.22$$

The estimated clearance rate of the drug in this patient (CL_{PT}) would then be calculated as

$$CL_{PT} = CL_{norm} \times Q$$

where CL_{norm} is the respective value in patients with normal kidney function derived from the literature.

For antihypertensive agents, cephalosporins, and many other drugs for which there are no target values for peak or trough concentrations, attainment of an average steady-state concentration similar to that in normal subjects is appropriate. The principal means to achieve this goal is to decrease the dose or prolong the dosing interval. If the dose is reduced and the dosing interval is unchanged, the desired average steady-state concentration will be near normal; however, the peak will be lower and the trough higher. Alternatively, if the dosing interval is increased and the dose remains unchanged, the peak, trough, and average concentrations will be similar to those in the patients with normal kidney function. This interval adjustment method is often preferred, because it is likely to yield significant cost savings as the result of less frequent drug administration. If a loading dose is not administered, it will take 4 to 5 half-lives for the desired steady-state plasma concentrations to be achieved in any patient; this may require days rather than hours because of the prolonged half-life of many drugs in patients with reduced kidney function (RKF). Therefore to achieve the desired concentration rapidly, a loading dose (D_L) should be administered for most patients with reduced kidney function. D_L can be calculated as follows:

$$D_L = (C_{peak}) \times (V_D) \times (\text{Body weight in kilograms})$$

The loading dose is usually the same for patients with reduced kidney function as it is for those with normal kidney function. However, if the V_D in patients with reduced kidney function is significantly different from that V_D in patients with normal kidney function (see Table 38.1), then the modified value should be used to calculate the D_L.

The adjusted dosing interval (τ_{RKF}) or maintenance dose (D_{RKF}) for the patient can then be calculated from the normal dosing interval (τ_n) and normal dose (D_n), respectively:

$$\tau_{RKF} = \tau_n / Q$$
$$D_{RKF} = D_n \times Q$$

If these approaches yield a time interval or a dose that is impractical, a new dose can be calculated using a fixed, prespecified dose interval (τ_{FPDI}) such as 24 or 48 hours, as follows:

$$D_{RKF} = [D_n \times Q \times \tau_{FPDI}] / \tau_n$$

PATIENTS RECEIVING CONTINUOUS RENAL REPLACEMENT THERAPY

Continuous renal replacement therapy is used primarily in patients with AKI. Drug therapy individualization for the patient receiving CRRT must take into account the fact that patients with AKI may have a higher residual CL_{NR} of a drug than do CKD patients with similar level of kidney function. In addition to patient-specific differences, there are marked differences in the efficiency of drug removal (see Chapter 58) among the three primary types of CRRT: continuous venovenous hemofiltration (CVVH), continuous venovenous hemodialysis (CVVHD), and continuous venovenous hemodiafiltration (CVVHDF). The primary variables that

influence drug clearance during CRRT are the ultrafiltration rate (UFR), the blood flow rate (BFR), and the dialysate flow rate (DFR), as well as the type of hemofilter used. For example, clearance during CVVH is directly proportional to the UFR as a result of convective transport of drug molecules. Drug clearance in this situation is a function of the membrane permeability of the drug, which is called the sieving coefficient (SC), and the UFR. The SC can be approximated by the fraction of drug that is unbound to plasma proteins (f_u), so the clearance can be calculated as follows:

$$CL_{CVVH} = UFR \times SC$$

or

$$CL_{CVVH} = UFR \times f_u$$

Clearance during CVVHD also depends on the DFR and the SC of the drug. If UFR is negligible, CL_{CVVHD} can be estimated to be maximally equal to the product of DFR and f_u or SC. Clearance of a drug by CVVHDF is generally greater than by CVVHD, because drug is removed by diffusion as well as by convection/ultrafiltration. CL_{CVVHDF} in many clinical settings can be mathematically approximated as:

$$CL_{CVVHDF} = (UFR + DFR) \times SC$$

provided that the DFR is less than 33 mL/min and BFR is at least 75 mL/min. Changes in BFR typically have only a minor effect on drug clearance by any mode of CRRT, because BFR is usually much larger than the DFR and is therefore not the limiting factor for drug removal.

Individualization of therapy for CRRT is based on the patient's residual kidney function and the clearance of the drug by the mode of CRRT employed. The patient's residual drug clearance can be predicted as described earlier in this chapter. CRRT clearance can also be approximated from published literature reports, although many of these reports did not specify all the operating conditions, and it may thus be hard to directly apply the findings to a given patient situation. The clearances of several frequently used drugs by CVVH and CVVHDF are summarized in Table 38.3 and Table 38.4, respectively. Whenever feasible, plasma drug concentration monitoring for certain drugs such as aminoglycosides and vancomycin is highly recommended.

PATIENTS RECEIVING CHRONIC HEMODIALYSIS

Drug therapy in hemodialysis patients should be guided by careful evaluation of the patient's residual kidney function, in addition to the added clearance associated with the patient's dialysis prescription. Dosing recommendations are available for many agents, especially those with a wide therapeutic index. However, for those drugs with a narrow therapeutic index, individualization of the drug therapy regimen is highly recommended based on prospective serum concentration monitoring. Although many new hemodialyzers have been introduced in the past 15 years and the average delivered dose of hemodialysis has increased, the effect of hemodialysis on the disposition of a drug is rarely reevaluated after its initial introduction to the market. As a result, most of the published dosing guidelines underestimate the impact of hemodialysis on drug disposition, and clinicians should

Table 38.3   Drug Clearance and Dosing Recommendations for Patients Receiving Continuous Venovenous Hemofiltration (CVVH)

Drug	Hemofilter	CL$_T$ (mL/min, mean or range)	CL$_{CVVH}$ (mL/min, mean or range)	Dosage Recommendation
Acyclovir	PS	0.39	NR	5 mg/kg q12h
Amikacin	PS	10.5	10-16	IND*
Amrinone	PS	40.8	2.4-14.4	None provided
Atracurium	PA	502.5	8.25	None provided
Ceftazidime	AN69, PMMA, PS	NR	7.5-15.6	500 mg q12h
Ceftriaxone	AN69, PMMA, PS	NR	NR	300 mg q12h
	PA	39.3	17	1000 mg q24h
Cefuroxime	PS	32	11	0.75-1.0 g q24h
Ciprofloxacin	AN69	84.4	12.4	400 mg q24h
Fluconazole	AN69	25.3	17.5	400-800 mg q24h
Gentamicin	PS	11.6	3.47	IND*
Imipenem	PS	108.3	13.3	500 mg q6-8h
Levofloxacin	AN69	42.3	11.5	250 mg q24h
Meropenem	PA	76	16-50	0.5-1.0 g q12h
Phenytoin	PS	NR	1.02	IND*
Piperacillin	NR	42	NR	4 g q12h
Ticarcillin	PS	29.7	12.3	2 g q8-12h
Tobramycin	PS	11.7	3.5	IND*
Vancomycin	PA, PMMA,PS	14-29	12-24	750-1250 mg q24h

Modified from Matzke GR, Clermont G: Clinical pharmacology and therapeutics. In Murray P, Brady HR, Hall JB, editors: Intensive Care Nephrology, *London, Taylor and Francis, 2006.*
AN69, Acrylonitrile; *CL$_{CVVH}$,* CVVH clearance; *CL$_T$,* total body clearance; *IND,* individualize; *NR,* not reported; *PA,* polyamide filter; *PMMA,* polymethylmethacrylate filter; *PS,* polysulfone filter.
*Serum concentrations may vary markedly depending on the patient's condition; therefore dose individualization is recommended.

Table 38.4   Drug Clearance and Dosing Recommendations for Patients Receiving Continuous Venovenous Hemodiafiltration (CVVHDF)

Drug	Hemofilter	CL$_T$ (mL/min, mean or range)	CL$_{CVVHDF}$ (mL/min, mean or range)	Dosage Recommendation
Acyclovir	AN69	1.2	NR	5 mg/kg q12h
Ceftazidime	AN69, PMMA, PS	25-31	13-28	0.5-1 g q24h
Ceftriaxone	AN69	—	11.7-13.2	250 mg q12h
	PMMA, PS	—	19.8-30.5	300 mg q12h
Cefuroxime	AN69	22	14-16.2	750 mg q12h
Ciprofloxacin	AN69	264	16-37	300 mg q12h
Fluconazole	AN69	21-38	25-30	400-800 mg q12h
Ganciclovir	AN69	32	13	2.5 mg/kg q24h
Gentamicin	AN69	20	5.2	IND*
Imipenem	AN69, PS	134	16-30	500 mg q6-8h
Levofloxacin	AN69	51	22	250 mg q24h
Meropenem	PAN	55-140	20-39	1000 mg q8-12h
Mezlocillin	AN69, PS	31-253	11-45	2-4 g q24h
Sulbactam	AN69, PS	32-54	10-23	0.5 g q24h
Piperacillin	AN69	47	22	PIP: 4 g q12h PIP/TAZO: 3.375 g q8-12h
Teicoplanin	AN69	9.2	3.6	LD: 800 mg MD: 400 mg q24h × 2, then q48-72h
Vancomycin	AN69	17-39	10-17	7.5 mg/kg q12h
	PMMA	—	15-27.0	1.0-1.5 g q24h
	PS	36	11-22	0.85-1.35 g q24h

Modified from Matzke GR, Clermont G: Clinical pharmacology and therapeutics. In Murray P, Brady HR, Hall JB, editors: Intensive Care Nephrology, *London, Taylor and Francis, 2006.*
AN69, Acrylonitrile; *CL$_{CVVHD}$,* CVVHD clearance; *CL$_T$,* total body clearance; *IND,* individualize; *LD,* loading dose; *MD,* maintenance dose; *NR,* not reported; *PA,* polyamide filter; *PAN,* polyacrylonitrile filter; *PMMA,* polymethylmethacrylate filter; *PS,* polysulfone filter; *TAZO,* tazobactam.
*Serum concentrations may vary markedly depending on the patient's condition; therefore dose individualization is recommended.

Table 38.5   Drug Disposition during Dialysis Depends on Dialyzer Characteristics

| Drug | Hemodialysis Clearance (mL/min) | | Half-Life During Dialysis (hr) | |
	Conventional	High-Flux	Conventional	High-Flux
Ceftazidime	55-60	155 (PA)	3.3	1.2 (PA)
Cefuroxime	NR	103 (PS)	3.8	1.6 (PS)
Foscarnet	183	253 (PS)	NR	NR
Gentamicin	58.2	116 (PS)	3.0	4.3 (PS)
Tobramycin	45	119 (PS)	4.0	NR
Ranitidine	43.1	67.2 (PS)	5.1	2.9 (PS)
Vancomycin	9-21	31-60 (PAN)	35-38	12.0 (PAN)
		40-150 (PS)		4.5-11.8 (PS)
		72-116 (PMMA)		NR

NR, Not reported; *PA*, polyamide filter; *PAN*, polyacrylonitrile filter; *PMMA*, polymethylmethacrylate; *PS*, polysulfone filter.

cautiously consider the prescription of doses that are larger than those conventionally recommended for their critically ill patients. The effect of hemodialysis on a patient's drug therapy depends on the molecular weight, protein binding, and distribution volume of the drug; the composition of the dialyzer membrane and its surface area; BFR and DFR; and whether the dialyzer is reused. Drugs that are small molecules but highly protein-bound are not well dialyzed because the two principal binding proteins (α_1-acid glycoprotein and albumin) are high-molecular-weight entities. Finally, drugs with a large volume of distribution are poorly removed by hemodialysis.

Conventional or low-flux dialyzers are relatively impermeable to drugs with a molecular weight greater than 1000 daltons (Da). High-flux hemodialyzers allow the passage of most drugs that have a molecular weight of 10,000 Da or less.

The determination of drug concentrations at the start and end of dialysis, with subsequent calculation of the half-life during dialysis, has historically been used as an index of drug removal by dialysis. A more accurate means of assessing the effect of hemodialysis is to calculate the dialyzer clearance rate (CL_D) of the drug. Because drug concentrations are generally measured in plasma, the plasma clearance of the drug by hemodialysis (CL_{pD}) can be calculated as follows:

$$CL_{pD} = Q_p([A_p - V_p]/A_p)$$

where A_p is arterial plasma concentration, V_p is venous plasma concentration, and Q_p is the plasma flow rate calculated as:

$$Q_p = BFR \times (1 - Hematocrit)$$

This clearance calculation accurately reflects dialysis drug clearance only if drug does not penetrate or bind to formed blood elements.

For patients receiving hemodialysis, the usual objective is to restore the amount of drug in the body at the end of dialysis to the value that would have been present if the patient had not been dialyzed. The supplementary dose (D_{postHD}) is calculated as follows:

$$D_{postHD} = [V_D \times C] (e^{-k \bullet t} - e^{-k_{HD} \bullet t})$$

where ($V_D \times C$) is the amount of drug in the body at the start of dialysis, $e^{-k \bullet t}$ is the fraction of drug remaining as a result of the patient's residual total body clearance during the dialysis procedure, and $e^{-k_{HD} \bullet t}$ is the fraction of drug remaining as a result of elimination by the dialyzer:

$$k_{HD} = CL_{pD}/V_D$$

Recently, alternative dosing strategies were evaluated for some drugs, such as gentamicin and vancomycin, in which the drug was administered before or during the dialysis procedure. These approaches may save time in the ambulatory dialysis setting but will increase drug cost because more drug will have to be given to compensate for the increased dialysis removal. Values for CL_{pD} of some commonly used drugs are listed in Table 38.5. This information serves only as initial dosing guidance; measurement of predialysis serum concentrations is recommended to guide subsequent drug dosing.

The impact of hemodialysis on drug therapy must not be viewed as a "generic procedure" that will result in removal of a fixed percentage of the drug from the body with each dialysis session; neither should simple "yes/no" answers on the dialyzability of drug compounds be considered sufficient information for therapeutic decisions. Compounds considered nondialyzable with low-flux dialyzers may in fact be significantly removed by high-flux hemodialyzers.

PATIENTS RECEIVING CHRONIC PERITONEAL DIALYSIS

Peritoneal dialysis has the potential to affect drug disposition, but drug therapy individualization is often less complicated in these patients because of the relative inefficiency of the procedure per unit time. Variables that influence drug removal in peritoneal dialysis include drug-specific characteristics such as molecular weight, solubility, degree of ionization, protein binding, and volume of distribution. Patient-specific factors include peritoneal membrane characteristics such as splanchnic blood flow, surface area, and permeability. The contribution of peritoneal dialysis to total body clearance is often low and, for most drugs, markedly less than the contribution of hemodialysis per unit time. Antiinfective agents are the most commonly studied drugs because of their primary role in the treatment of peritonitis, and the dosing recommendations for peritonitis, which are regularly updated, should be consulted as necessary. Most other drugs can generally be dosed according to the residual kidney function of the patient because clearance by peritoneal dialysis is small.

If there is a significant relationship between the desired peak (C_{peak}) or trough (C_{trough}) concentration of a drug for a given patient with reduced kidney function and the potential clinical response (e.g., aminoglycosides) or toxicity (e.g., quinidine, phenobarbital, phenytoin), then attainment of the target plasma concentration value is critical. In these situations, the adjusted dosage interval (τ_{RKF}) and maintenance dose (D_{RKF}) for the patient can be calculated as follows:

$$\tau_{RKF} = ([1/k_{PT}] \times \ln[C_{peak}/C_{trough}]) + t_{inf}$$

$$D_{RKF} = [k_{PT} \times V_D \times C_{peak}] \times [1 - e^{-(k_{PT})(\tau_{RKF})}/1 - e^{-(k_{PT})(t_{inf})}]$$

where t_{inf} is the infusion duration, k_{PT} is the elimination rate constant of the drug for that patient, which can be estimated as:

$$k_{PT} = k_{norm} \times Q$$

and V_D is the volume of distribution of the drug that can be obtained from literature values such as those in Table 38.1. This estimation method assumes that the drug is administered by intermittent intravenous infusion and its disposition is adequately characterized by a one-compartment linear model.

CLINICAL DECISION SUPPORT TOOLS

The availability of health information technology—namely, clinical decision support tools—has increased substantially in recent years, and use of these tools may facilitate renal drug dosing by providing consistent, accurate dosing recommendations in real time. Clinical decision support systems (CDSS) are commonplace in institutional health information computer systems, and their incorporation into computerized provider order entry (CPOE) systems has been shown to improve medication use in CKD and AKI patient populations. In addition, CDSS make individual assessments and comparisons of kidney function estimates feasible. For example, CDSS can easily accommodate new equations (e.g., CKD-EPI) as they become available and facilitate conversion of the MDRD Study equation–derived eGFR to individualized values by modifying units of mL/min/1.73 m^2 to units of mL/min.

Numerous other resources are available for renal drug dosing information, including online sources, as well as portable handheld databases such as Epocrates®, Lexicomp®, and Micromedex®. The *American Hospital Formulary Service Drug Information* text, the *British National Formulary*, *Aronoff's Drug Prescribing in Renal Failure*, and *Martindale's Complete Drug Reference* are excellent resources for drug dosage recommendations for patients with impaired kidney function. All of these are accessible electronically and/or online.

Box 38.1   Key Recommendations for Clinicians

1. Over-the-counter and herbal products, as well as prescription medications, should be assessed to ensure that they are indicated.
2. The least nephrotoxic agent should be used whenever possible.
3. If a drug interaction is suspected and the clinical implication is significant, alternative medications should be used.
4. Although the MDRD eGFR equation may be used for staging CKD, the Cockcroft-Gault equation remains the standard kidney function index for drug dosage adjustment.
5. The dosage of drugs that are more than 30% renally eliminated unchanged should be verified to ensure that appropriate initial dosage adjustments are implemented.
6. Maintenance dosage regimens should be adjusted based on patient response and serum drug concentration determinations when indicated and available.

CKD, Chronic kidney disease; *eGFR*, estimated glomerular filtration rate; *MDRD*, Modification of Diet in Renal Disease.

CONCLUSIONS

The adverse outcomes associated with inappropriate drug use and dosing are largely preventable if the principles illustrated in this chapter are used by the clinician in concert with reliable population pharmacokinetic estimates to design rational initial drug dosage regimens for patients with reduced kidney function and those needing dialysis. Subsequent individualization of therapy should be undertaken whenever clinical therapeutic monitoring tools, such as plasma drug concentrations, are available. These key recommendations for practice are highlighted in Box 38.1.

BIBLIOGRAPHY

Aronoff GR, Bennetl WM, Berns JS, et al: *Drug prescribing in renal failure: dosing guidelines for adults and children,* ed 5, Philadelphia, 2007, American College of Physicians-American Society of Internal Medicine.

Heintz BH, Matzke GR, Dager WE: Antimicrobial dosing concepts and recommendations for critically ill adult patients receiving continuous renal replacement therapy or intermittent hemodialysis, *Pharmacotherapy* 29:562-577, 2009.

Lee W, Kim RB: Transporters and renal drug elimination, *Annu Rev Pharmacol Toxicol* 44:137-166, 2004.

Matzke GR: Status of hemodialysis of drugs in 2002, *J Pharm Practice* 15:405-418, 2002.

Matzke GR, Aronoff GR, Atkinson AJ Jr, et al: Drug dosing consideration in patients with acute and chronic kidney disease-a clinical update from Kidney Disease: Improving Global Outcomes (KDIGO), *Kidney Int* 80:1122-1137, 2011.

Matzke GR, Clermont G: Clinical pharmacology and therapeutics. In Murray PT, Brady HR, Hall JB, editors: *Intensive care in nephrology,* Boca Raton, Fla, 2006, Taylor and Francis, pp 245-265.

Matzke GR, Comstock TJ: Influence of renal disease and dialysis on pharmacokinetics. In Evans WE, Schentag JJ, Burton ME, editors: *Applied pharmacokinetics: principles of therapeutic drug monitoring,* ed 4, Baltimore, 2005, Lippincott Williams and Wilkins.

Mueller BA, Pasko DA, Sowinski KM: Higher renal replacement therapy dose delivery influences on drug therapy, *Artif Organs* 27:808-814, 2003.

Munar MY, Singh H: Drug dosing adjustments in patients with chronic kidney disease, *Am Fam Physician* 75:1487-1496, 2007.

Naud J, Nolin TD, Leblond FA, et al: Current understanding of drug disposition in kidney disease, *J Clin Pharmacol* 52:10S-22S, 2012.

Nolin TD, Frye RF, Le P, et al: ESRD impairs nonrenal clearance of fexofenadine but not midazolam, *J Am Soc Nephrol* 20:2269-2276, 2009.

Nolin TD, Naud J, Leblond FA, et al: Emerging evidence of the impact of kidney disease on drug metabolism and transport, *Clin Pharmacol Ther* 83:898-903, 2008.

Nyman HA, Dowling TC, Hudson JQ, et al: Comparative evaluation of the Cockcroft-Gault Equation and the Modification of Diet in Renal Disease (MDRD) study equation for drug dosing: an opinion of the Nephrology Practice and Research Network of the American College of Clinical Pharmacy, *Pharmacotherapy* 31:1130-1144, 2011.

Piraino B, Bailie GR, Bernardini J, et al: Peritoneal dialysis related infections: 2005 Update, *Perit Dial Int* 25:107-131, 2005.

van dijik EA, Drabbe NRG, Kruijtbosch M, et al: Drug dosage adjustments according to renal function at hospital discharge, *Ann Pharmacother* 40:1254-1260, 2006.

Veltri MA, Neu AM, Fivush BA, et al: Drug dosing during intermittent hemodialysis and continuous renal replacement therapy: special considerations in pediatric patients, *Pediatr Drugs* 6:45-65, 2004.

Verbeeck RK, Musuamba FT: Pharmacokinetics and dosage adjustment in patients with renal dysfunction, *Eur J Clin Pharmacol* 65:757-773, 2009.

Vidal L, Shavit M, Fraser A, et al: Systematic comparison of four sources of drug information regarding adjustment of dose for renal function, *BMJ* 331:263-266, 2005.

HEREDITARY KIDNEY DISORDERS

39

Genetically Based Renal Transport Disorders

Steven J. Scheinman

The coming of age of clinical chemistry in the latter half of the twentieth century, bringing with it the routine measurement of electrolytes and minerals in patient samples, produced descriptions of distinct inherited syndromes of abnormal renal tubular transport. Clinical investigation led to speculation, often ingenious and sometimes controversial, regarding the underlying causes of these syndromes. More recently, the tools of molecular biology made possible the cloning of mutated genes found in patients with monogenic disorders of renal tubular transport. These diseases represent experiments of nature, and for the renal physiologist the insights they have revealed are exciting. Some have provided gratifying confirmation of our existing knowledge of transport mechanisms along the nephron. Examples include mutations in diuretic-sensitive transporters in the Bartter and Gitelman syndromes. In other cases, positional cloning led to the discovery of previously unknown proteins, often surprising ones that appear to play important roles in epithelial transport. For example, the chloride transporter CLC-5 (gene name *CLCN5*), the tight junction claudin 16 (paracellin 1), and the phosphaturic hormone fibroblast growth factor 23 (FGF23) were discovered through positional cloning in the study of Dent disease, inherited hypomagnesemic hypercalciuria, and autosomal dominant hypophosphatemic rickets (ADHR), respectively.

Table 39.1 summarizes genetic diseases of renal tubular transport for which the molecular basis is known. The diseases listed are explained by abnormalities in the corresponding gene product. They are all inherited in Mendelian fashion, either autosomal or X-linked, with the single exception of a syndrome of hypomagnesemia with maternal inheritance that surprisingly results from mutation in a mitochondrial tRNA rather than in the nuclear genome.

DISORDERS OF PROXIMAL TUBULAR TRANSPORT FUNCTION

SELECTIVE PROXIMAL TRANSPORT DEFECTS

Sodium resorption in the proximal tubule occurs through secondary active transport processes in which the entry of sodium is coupled either to the entry of glucose, amino acids, or phosphate or to the exit of protons. Autosomal recessive conditions of impaired transepithelial transport of glucose and dibasic amino acids have been shown to be caused by mutations in sodium-dependent transporters that are expressed in both kidney and intestine, resulting in urinary losses and intestinal malabsorption of these solutes. Other disorders with renal-selective transport defects are thought to result from mutations in transporters expressed specifically in kidney.

IMPAIRED PROXIMAL PHOSPHATE REABSORPTION

X-linked (dominant) hypophosphatemic rickets (XLHR) is characterized by impaired sodium-dependent phosphate reabsorption, in which the maximal transport capacity for phosphate is reduced. This is reflected in fewer units of the sodium-dependent phosphate transporter type 2 (NaPi2) in the apical membrane of proximal tubular cells. XLHR is the most common form of hereditary rickets, and mutations in XLHR involve a phosphate-regulating gene with homologies to a neutral endopeptidase on the X chromosome (PHEX) that is expressed in bone and is thought to be involved in the processing of a circulating phosphate transport-regulating hormone designated *phosphatonin*.

The rare autosomal dominant form of hypophosphatemic rickets (ADHR) is associated with mutations in the gene encoding fibroblast growth factor (FGF23) that protect FGF23 from proteolytic cleavage. It is not clear whether FGF23 is a substrate for the PHEX enzyme or why mutations in PHEX are associated with high FGF23 levels, but the physiologic effects of FGF23 are consistent with its being a phosphatonin, because it inhibits renal phosphate reabsorption by inhibiting expression of two sodium-dependent phosphate transporters in proximal tubule, SLC34A1 (formerly Npt2a) and SLC34A3 (formerly Npt2c). Serum levels of uncleaved FGF23 are excessive in XLHR, ADHR, and tumor-induced hypophosphatemic osteomalacia, all of which are characterized by impaired renal phosphate reabsorption. FGF23 inhibits the 1-hydroxylation of 25-hydroxyvitamin D, likely explaining why hypophosphatemia in these three conditions is not associated with either elevated levels of 1,25-dihydroxyvitamin D or hypercalciuria.

Autosomal recessive inheritance of hypophosphatemic rickets has been reported. Patients with this condition resemble those with autosomal dominant (i.e., FGF23 mutations) and X-linked (PHEX mutations) forms, with renal phosphate wasting, inappropriately normal levels of 1,25-dihydroxyvitamin D, absence of hypercalciuria, and elevated serum levels of FGF23. In this autosomal recessive form, the mutated gene (DMP1) encodes the dentin matrix protein 1 (DMP-1), a bone matrix protein that appears to play a role with PHEX in regulating bone mineralization and FGF23 production.

Hereditary hypophosphatemic rickets with hypercalciuria (HHRH), an autosomal recessive disorder, is different from XLHR and ADHR, both of which are associated with reduced urinary calcium excretion. Unlike XLHR and ADHR, hypophosphatemia in HHRH is associated with appropriate elevations of 1,25-dihydroxyvitamin D levels, and FGF23 levels are normal or reduced. This profile in HHRH is consistent with a primary defect in phosphate transport. The most abundant

Table 39.1 Molecular Bases of Genetic Disorders of Renal Transport

Inherited Disorder	Defective Gene Product
Proximal Tubule	
Glucose-galactose malabsorption syndrome	Sodium-glucose transporter 1
Dibasic aminoaciduria	Basolateral dibasic amino acid transporter (lysinuric protein intolerance)
XLHR	PHEX
ADHR	FGF23 (excess)
Autosomal recessive hypophosphatemic rickets	DMP1
	ENPP1
HHRH	Sodium-phosphate cotransporter Npt2c
Familial hyperostosis-hyperphosphatemia	FGF23 (deficiency)
	GalNac transferase 3
Fanconi syndrome	Aldolase B (hereditary fructose intolerance)
Fanconi-Bickel syndrome	Facilitated GLUT2
Oculocerebrorenal syndrome of Lowe	Inositol polyphosphate-5-phosphatase (OCRL1)
Cystinuria	Apical cystine-dibasic amino acid transporter rBAT
	Light subunit of rBAT
Dent disease (X-linked nephrolithiasis)	Chloride transporter (ClC-5)
	PIP2-5-phosphatase (OCRL1)
Autosomal recessive proximal RTA	Basolateral sodium-bicarbonate cotransporter NBC1
TAL of Loop of Henle	
Bartter syndrome	
Type I	Bumetanide-sensitive Na-K-2Cl cotransporter NKCC2
Type II	Apical potassium channel ROMK
Type III	Basolateral chloride channel ClC-Kb
Type IV, with sensorineural deafness	Barttin (ClC-Kb-associated protein)
Familial hypocalcemia with Bartter features	CaSR (activation)
Familial hypomagnesemia with hypercalciuria and nephrocalcinosis	
Without ocular abnormalities	Claudin-16 (paracellin-1)
With ocular abnormalities	Claudin-19
Familial benign hypercalcemia*	CaSR (inactivation)
Neonatal severe hyperparathyroidism†	CaSR (inactivation)
Familial hypercalciuric hypocalcemia	CaSR (activation)
Familial juvenile hyperuricemic nephropathy	Uromodulin (Tamm-Horsfall protein)
DCT	
Gitelman syndrome	Thiazide-sensitive NaCl cotransporter NCCT
Pseudohypoparathyroidism type Ia‡	Guanine nucleotide-binding protein (Gs)
Familial hypomagnesemia with secondary hypocalcemia	TRPM6 cation channel§
Isolated recessive renal hypomagnesemia	EGF
Isolated renal Mg loss	γ subunit of Na/K-ATPase
SeSAME/EAST syndromes	Kir4.1 potassium channel
Dominant hypomagnesemia with ataxia	Kv1.1 potassium channel
Familial tubulopathy with hypomagnesemia	Mitochondrial tRNA^isoleucine
Dominant hypomagnesemia	CNNM2 (unknown function)
Collecting Duct	
Liddle syndrome	β and γ subunits of epithelial Na channel EnaC
Pseudohypoaldosteronism	
Type 1	
Autosomal recessive	α, β, γ subunits of EnaC
Autosomal dominant	Mineralocorticoid (type I) receptor
Type 2 (Gordon syndrome)	WNK1 and WNK4 kinases
GRA	11β-hydroxylase and aldosterone synthase (chimeric gene)‖
Syndrome of AME	11β-hydroxysteroid dehydrogenase type II
Distal RTA	
Autosomal dominant	Basolateral anion exchanger (AE1) (band 3 protein)
Autosomal recessive, with hemolytic anemia	Basolateral anion exchanger (AE1) (band 3 protein)
Autosomal recessive (with hearing deficit)	β1 subunit of proton ATPase

Continued

Table 39.1   Molecular Bases of Genetic Disorders of Renal Transport (Continued)

Inherited Disorder	Defective Gene Product
Collecting Duct (cont'd)	
Distal RTA (cont'd)	
Autosomal recessive (hearing deficit variable)	α4 isoform of α subunit of proton ATPase
Carbonic anhydrase II deficiency¶	Carbonic anhydrase type II
Nephrogenic diabetes insipidus	
X-linked	AVP 2 (V2) receptor
Autosomal	AQP-2 water channel

ADHR, Autosomal dominant hypophosphatemic rickets; *AME*, apparent mineralocorticoid excess; *AQP-2*, aquaporin 2; *AVP*, arginine vasopressin; *CaSR*, calcium-sensing receptor; *DCT*, distal convoluted tubule; *DMP1*, dentin matrix protein 1; *EAST*, epilepsy, ataxia, sensorineural deafness, and tubulopathy; *EGF*, epidermal growth factor; *ENPP1*, ectonucleotide pyrophosphatase/phosphodiesterase 1; *FGF23*, fibroblast growth factor 23; *GLUT2*, glucose transporter; *GRA*, glucocorticoid-remediable aldosteronism; *HHRH*, hereditary hypophosphatemic rickets with hypercalciuria; *NCCT*, sodium chloride cotransporter; *NKCC2*, Na⁺-K⁺-2Cl⁻ cotransporter; *PHEX*, phosphate regulating gene with homologies to endopeptidases on the X chromosome; *RTA*, renal tubular acidosis; *SeSAME*, seizures, sensorineural deafness, ataxia, mental retardation, and electrolyte imbalance; *TAL*, thick ascending limb; *XLHR*, X-linked hypophosphatemic rickets.
*Results from heterozygous mutation.
†Results from homozygous mutation.
‡Gene also expressed in proximal tubule where functional abnormalities are clinically apparent.
§Gene also expressed in intestine.
ǀGene expressed in adrenal gland.
¶Clinical phenotype can be of proximal RTA, distal RTA, or combined.

phosphate transporter in the proximal tubule, NaPi2a, is encoded by the gene *SLC34A1*, which is not mutated in any of the families with HHRH studied, but several pedigrees have been found to have mutations in *SLC34A3*, encoding another phosphate transporter NaPi2c. Expression of both *SLC34A1* and *SLC34A3* occurs in response to physiologic stimuli such as parathyroid hormone (PTH) and dietary phosphate. Knockout of the mouse homologue of *SLC34A1* reproduces the features of human HHRH except for rickets; a mouse knockout of *SLC34A3* manifests hypercalcemia and hypercalciuria, but not hypophosphatemia, renal calcification, or rickets; and a double knockout of both genes produces mice with the full phenotype of hypophosphatemia, hypercalciuria, nephrocalcinosis, and rickets.

EXCESSIVE PROXIMAL PHOSPHATE REABSORPTION

Inherited hyperphosphatemia in the familial hyperostosis-hyperphosphatemia syndrome represents a mirror image of ADHR and XLHR, with excessive renal phosphate reabsorption, persistent hyperphosphatemia, inappropriately normal levels of 1,25-dihydroxyvitamin D, and low levels of FGF23. This can result from mutations in FGF23 itself or in a Golgi-associated biosynthetic enzyme, *N*-acetylglucosaminyl (GalNac) transferase 3, that is involved in glycosylation of FGF23 and is necessary for its secretion. Together, these discoveries are fleshing out our understanding of the role of bone in the complex regulation of mineral metabolism.

IMPAIRED PROXIMAL BICARBONATE TRANSPORT

Proximal renal tubular acidosis (RTA) is inherited in an autosomal recessive manner and is associated with mutations that inactivate the basolateral sodium bicarbonate cotransporter NBC1, encoded by the gene *SLC4A4*. These patients often suffer blindness from ocular abnormalities, including band keratopathy, cataracts, and glaucoma; these ocular manifestations probably are a consequence of impaired bicarbonate transport in the eye. Mutations in the *SLC4A4* gene result in impaired transporter function or aberrant trafficking of the protein to the basolateral surface. This gene belongs to the same group as the gene encoding the anion exchanger AE1 (now designated *SLC4A1*), which is mutated in distal RTA.

INHERITED FANCONI SYNDROME: HEREDITARY FRUCTOSE INTOLERANCE, LOWE SYNDROME, AND DENT DISEASE

The renal Fanconi syndrome represents a generalized impairment in reabsorptive function of the proximal tubule and comprises proximal RTA with aminoaciduria, renal glycosuria, hypouricemia, and hypophosphatemia. Some or all of these abnormalities are present in individual patients with Fanconi syndrome. Inherited causes of partial or complete Fanconi syndrome include hereditary fructose intolerance, Lowe syndrome, and Dent disease.

Hereditary fructose intolerance is caused by mutations that result in deficiency of the aldolase B enzyme, which cleaves fructose-1-phosphate. Symptoms are precipitated by intake of sweets. Massive accumulation of fructose-1-phosphate occurs, leading to sequestration of inorganic phosphate and deficiency of adenosine triphosphate (ATP). Acute consequences can include hypoglycemic shock, severe abdominal symptoms, and impaired function of the Krebs cycle that produces metabolic acidosis; this is exacerbated by impaired renal bicarbonate reabsorption. ATP deficiency leads to impaired proximal tubular function in general, including the full expression of the Fanconi syndrome with consequent rickets and stunted growth. ATP breakdown can be so dramatic as to produce hyperuricemia, as well as hypermagnesemia from the dissolution of the magnesium-ATP complex. Avoiding dietary sources of fructose can minimize acute symptoms and chronic consequences such as liver disease.

Characteristic features of the oculocerebrorenal syndrome of Lowe include congenital cataracts, mental retardation, muscular hypotonia, and the renal Fanconi syndrome. In contrast, Dent disease is confined to the kidney. In both syndromes, low-molecular-weight (LMW) proteinuria is a prominent feature along with other evidence of proximal tubulopathy such as glycosuria, aminoaciduria, and phosphaturia. One important difference is that proximal RTA with growth retardation can be severe in patients with Lowe syndrome, but it is not a part of Dent disease. Some patients with Lowe syndrome or Dent disease may have rickets, which is thought to be a consequence of hypophosphatemia and, in Lowe syndrome, of acidosis as well. Hypercalciuria is a characteristic feature of Dent disease and is associated with nephrocalcinosis in most and kidney stones in many patients with Dent disease; nephrocalcinosis and nephrolithiasis are less common in Lowe syndrome. Kidney failure is common in both these conditions, typically occurring in young adulthood in Dent disease and even earlier in patients with Lowe syndrome.

Dent disease is caused by mutations that inactivate the chloride transporter CLC-5. This transport protein is expressed in the proximal tubule, the medullary thick ascending limb (MTAL) of the loop of Henle, and the alpha-intercalated cells of the collecting tubule. In the cells of the proximal tubule, CLC-5 colocalizes with the proton-ATPase in subapical endosomes. These endosomes are important in the processing of proteins that are filtered at the glomerulus and taken up by the proximal tubule through adsorptive endocytosis. The activity of the proton-ATPase acidifies the endosomal space, releasing the proteins from membrane-binding sites and making them available for proteolytic degradation. CLC-5 mediates electrogenic exchange of chloride for protons in these endosomes, dissipates the positive charge generated by proton entry, and may provide a brake or set point for endosomal acidification. Mutations that inactivate CLC-5 in patients with Dent's disease interfere with the mechanism for reabsorption of LMW proteins and explain the consistent finding of LMW proteinuria. Glycosuria, aminoaciduria, and phosphaturia are less consistently seen and may be consequences of CLC-5 inactivation, possibly through alterations in membrane trafficking.

Lowe syndrome is associated with mutations in *OCRL1*, which encodes a phosphatidylinositol-4,5-bisphosphate-5-phosphatase. In renal epithelial cells, this phosphatase is localized to the *trans*-Golgi network, which plays an important role in directing proteins to the appropriate membrane. The CLC-5 protein and the OCRL1 phosphatase interact with the actin cytoskeleton and are involved in assembly of the endosomal apparatus. Similarities in the renal features of these two syndromes may be the result of defective membrane trafficking. Still to be explained is why some patients with mutations in *OCRL1* have no cataracts or cerebral dysfunction, and no RTA ("Dent 2" disease).

DISORDERS OF TRANSPORT IN THE MEDULLARY THICK ASCENDING LIMB OF HENLE

BARTTER SYNDROME

Solute transport in the MTAL involves the coordinated functions of a set of transport proteins depicted in Figure 39.1.

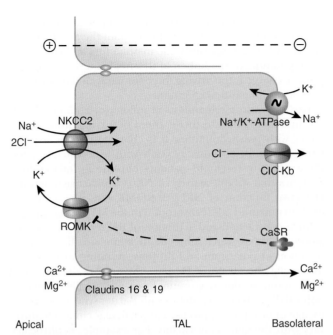

Figure 39.1   Transport mechanisms in the thick ascending limb of loop of Henle transport proteins affected by mutations in genetic diseases. Reabsorption of sodium chloride occurs through the electroneutral activity of the bumetanide-sensitive Na^+-K^+-$2Cl^-$ cotransporter, NKCC2. Activity of the basolateral sodium-potassium adenosine triphosphatase (Na^+,K^+-ATPase) provides the driving force for this transport and also generates a high intracellular concentration of potassium, which exits through the ATP-regulated apical potassium channel, ROMK. This ensures an adequate supply of potassium for the activity of the NKCC2 and also produces a lumen-positive electrical potential, which itself is the driving force for paracellular reabsorption of calcium, magnesium, and sodium ions through the tight junctions, involving the protein paracellin 1. Chloride transported into the cell by NKCC2 exits the basolateral side of the cell through the voltage-gated chloride channel, ClC-Kb. Activation of the extracellular calcium-sensing receptor, CaSR, inhibits solute transport in the TAL by inhibiting activity of the ROMK and possibly by other mechanisms. Mutations that inactivate the CaSR are associated with enhanced calcium transport and hypocalciuria in familial benign hypercalcemia, and mutations that activate the CaSR occur in patients with familial hypercalciuria with hypocalcemia. *ROMK,* Renal outer medullary potassium channel; *TAL,* thick ascending limb.

These proteins are the bumetanide-sensitive Na^+-K^+-$2Cl^-$ cotransporter (NKCC2) and the renal outer medullary potassium channel (ROMK) on the apical surface of cells of the MTAL, and the chloride channel ClC-Kb on the basolateral surface. Optimal function of the ClC-Kb chloride channel requires interaction with a subunit called *barttin*. Mutations in any of the genes encoding these four proteins lead to the phenotype of Bartter syndrome. In addition, activation of the epithelial calcium-sensing receptor (CaSR) inhibits activity of the ROMK potassium channel. Mutations producing constitutive activation of the CaSR cause familial hypocalcemic hypercalciuria. Some patients with hypocalcemic hypercalciuria have the phenotype of Bartter syndrome, and mutations in the CaSR may be considered a fifth molecular cause of this syndrome. Together, these five genes still do not account for all patients with Bartter syndrome.

The ClC-Kb basolateral chloride channel provides the route for chloride exit to the interstitium. Flow of potassium through the ROMK channel ensures that potassium concentrations in the tubular lumen do not limit the activity of the Na⁺-K⁺-2Cl⁻ cotransporter while maintaining a positive electrical potential in the lumen of this nephron segment. This positive charge is the driving force for paracellular reabsorption of calcium and magnesium.

Bartter syndrome manifests in infancy or childhood with polyuria and failure to thrive, often occurring after a pregnancy with polyhydramnios. It is characterized by hypokalemic metabolic alkalosis, typically with hypercalciuria, and these patients resemble patients chronically taking loop diuretics that inhibit activity of NKCC2 pharmacologically. Defective function of NKCC2, ROMK, ClC-Kb, or barttin leads to impaired salt reabsorption in the MTAL, resulting in volume contraction and activation of the renin-angiotensin-aldosterone axis, which subsequently stimulates distal tubular secretion of potassium and protons, resulting in hypokalemic metabolic alkalosis. Despite impaired reabsorption of magnesium, serum magnesium levels are usually normal or only mildly reduced in patients with Bartter syndrome. Severity, age of onset of symptoms, and particular clinical features vary with the gene abnormality. For example, nephrocalcinosis as a consequence of hypercalciuria is most common in individuals with mutations in genes encoding NKCC2 and ROMK. Barttin is expressed in the inner ear, and patients with mutations in its gene have sensorineural deafness. Bartter syndrome is discussed further in Chapter 10.

INHERITED HYPOMAGNESEMIC HYPERCALCIURIA

Reabsorption of calcium and magnesium in the MTAL occurs through the paracellular route, driven by the positive electrical potential in the tubular lumen. The tight junctions between the epithelial cells determine the selective movement of cations (i.e., calcium, magnesium, and sodium). Disturbance of this selective paracellular barrier would be expected to produce parallel disorders in the reabsorption of calcium and magnesium.

Familial hypomagnesemia with substantial renal magnesium losses, hypercalciuria, and nephrocalcinosis (FHHNC) is inherited in an autosomal recessive fashion. These patients develop kidney failure and kidney stones. Investigation of families led to identification by positional cloning of the gene encoding a tight junction protein designated claudin 16 (also called paracellin 1). It is expressed at the tight junction between cells of the MTAL (Fig. 39.2) and in the distal convoluted tubule (DCT). This was the first instance of a disease shown to result from mutations that alter a tight junction protein. Another member of this family, claudin 19, is mutated in other pedigrees in whom FHHNC is associated with ocular abnormalities (e.g., macular colobomas, myopia, horizontal nystagmus) with severe visual impairment. Both claudin 16 and claudin 19 are expressed in the thick ascending limb (TAL), but claudin 19 also is expressed in the retina. These two proteins interact in the tight junction to regulate cation permeability. It is unclear why a defect in tight junctions is associated with hyperuricemia, a consistent finding in this disease.

FAMILIAL HYPOCALCIURIC HYPERCALCEMIA

The extracellular CaSR is expressed in many tissues in which ambient calcium concentrations trigger cellular responses.

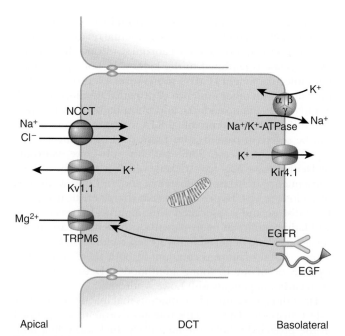

Figure 39.2 Transport mechanisms in the distal convoluted tubule. The basolateral sodium-potassium adenosine triphosphatase (Na⁺,K⁺-ATPase), composed of α, β, and γ subunits, establishes the low intracellular sodium concentration that provides the driving force for coupled sodium and chloride entry across the apical NCCT transporter. It also maintains the high intracellular potassium concentration that drives potassium exit across the apical Kv1.1 potassium channel, which establishes a positive lumen-to-cytosol electrical gradient that drives magnesium entry across the apical TRPM6 cation channel. The basolateral Kir4.1 potassium channel allows potassium exit that may serve to assure an adequate potassium supply for the Na⁺,K⁺-ATPase. The EGF receptor stimulates trafficking of TRPM6 to the apical membrane and stimulates activity of that transporter. Genes encoding these proteins are responsible for inherited electrolyte disturbances discussed in the text. *DCT,* Distal convoluted tubule; *EGF,* epidermal growth factor; *EGFR,* epidermal growth factor receptor; *NCCT,* sodium chloride cotransporter.

In the parathyroid gland, activation of the CaSR suppresses synthesis and release of PTH. In the kidney, the CaSR is expressed on the basolateral surface of cells of the TAL (cortical more than medullary), on the luminal surface of the cells of the papillary collecting duct, and in other portions of the nephron. Activation of the CaSR in the TAL probably mediates the known effects of hypercalcemia to inhibit the transport of calcium, magnesium, and sodium in this nephron segment. For example, CaSR activation inhibits activity of the ROMK potassium channel (see Fig. 39.1). This can be expected to reduce the positive electrical potential in the lumen and thereby suppress the driving force for reabsorption of calcium and magnesium. In the papillary collecting duct, activation of the apical CaSR may explain how hypercalciuria impairs the hydroosmotic response to vasopressin, resulting in nephrogenic diabetes insipidus. Notably, the presence of a large volume of dilute urine produced in this situation is potentially protective against the development of nephrocalcinosis or nephrolithiasis in the setting of hypercalciuria due to hypercalcemia and an increased filtered load.

In familial hypocalciuric hypercalcemia (FHH), loss-of-function mutations of the *CASR* gene increase the set point for calcium sensing, resulting in hypercalcemia with relative elevation of PTH levels. Urinary calcium excretion is low because of enhanced calcium reabsorption in the TAL and PTH-stimulated calcium transport in the DCT. FHH occurs in patients heterozygous for such mutations, and it is benign, because tissues are resistant to the high serum calcium levels. A family history helps to differentiate FHH from primary hyperparathyroidism, and parathyroidectomy should not be performed. Infants of consanguineous parents with FHH can be homozygous for these mutations, resulting in a syndrome of severe hypercalcemia with marked hyperparathyroidism, fractures, and failure to thrive, known as *neonatal severe hyperparathyroidism.*

Other mutations result in constitutive activation of the CaSR, producing hypocalcemia with hypercalciuria without elevated PTH concentrations. As discussed earlier, these circumstances also can produce the phenotype of Bartter syndrome. Polymorphism in the *CASR* gene producing a mild gain-of-function expression of the CaSR without frank hypocalcemia has been associated with idiopathic hypercalciuria.

FAMILIAL JUVENILE HYPERURICEMIC NEPHROPATHY

Mutations in the *UMOD* gene encoding uromodulin (i.e., Tamm-Horsfall protein) occur in families in which children present with hyperuricemia and gout. This syndrome overlaps with medullary cystic kidney disease type 2, which also is associated with *UMOD* mutations. Cytosolic inclusions seen on electron microscopy in the epithelial cells of the MTAL appear to be crystallized uromodulin. A physiologic explanation for the hyperuricemia has not been offered. The occurrence of hyperuricemia in this disease and in the syndrome associated with mutations in paracellin suggests that our understanding of the role of the MTAL in uric acid transport is not fully understood. Families with an indistinguishable phenotype have been identified in whom linkage to the *UMOD* locus is excluded, indicating that genetic heterogeneity is likely (see Chapter 42).

DISORDERS OF TRANSPORT IN THE DISTAL CONVOLUTED TUBULE

GITELMAN SYNDROME

Reabsorption of sodium chloride in the DCT occurs through electroneutral transport mediated by the thiazide-sensitive sodium chloride cotransporter (NCCT). Mutations in the NCCT gene *(SLC12A3)* are associated with Gitelman syndrome, another condition of hypokalemic metabolic alkalosis. Gitelman syndrome once was viewed as a variant of Bartter syndrome; however, an essential distinction between these two conditions is the presence of *hypo*calciuria in Gitelman syndrome, in contrast to the *hyper*calciuria that occurs in Bartter syndrome or in patients taking loop diuretics. Hypocalciuria in Gitelman syndrome resembles the reduction in calcium excretion that occurs in patients taking thiazide diuretics. These findings are satisfying in that they connect the clinical physiology with molecular physiology. However, our understanding of renal transport does not allow us to explain the fact that significant hypomagnesemia with renal magnesium wasting is typical of Gitelman syndrome, whereas in Bartter syndrome it is much less common and, when it does occur, milder.

IMPAIRED DISTAL MAGNESIUM REABSORPTION

Our understanding of the mechanisms involved in distal tubular magnesium transport has been substantially enriched by the identification in recent years of genes responsible for several distinct syndromes of hypomagnesemia. The TRPM6 apical magnesium channel is critical to magnesium transport in the gut as well as in the distal tubule, and mutations in the gene encoding this channel cause a hypomagnesemic syndrome sufficiently severe as to impair PTH release and function, with secondary hypocalcemia. Potassium channels expressed on the apical (Kv1.1) and basolateral (Kir4.1) membranes are also expressed in the brain, and mutations result in hypomagnesemia as well as neurologic dysfunction including ataxia. Hypomagnesemia also results from inherited defects in distal tubule basolateral membrane proteins EGF, the γ subunit of the Na/K ATPase, and a newly discovered protein of unknown function, CNNM2.

FAMILIAL HYPOMAGNESEMIA WITH SECONDARY HYPOCALCEMIA

Patients with this syndrome experience severe hypomagnesemia, often with neonatal seizures and tetany. If not recognized and treated early, the hypomagnesemia can be fatal. Serum magnesium levels fall low enough to impair PTH release or responsiveness, and this is presumed to be the mechanism of the hypocalcemia that commonly accompanies hypomagnesemia in these patients. The primary defect appears to be in intestinal magnesium absorption, although renal magnesium conservation also is deficient. These patients have mutations in a gene *(TRPM6)* encoding the TRPM6 protein. TRPM6 is a member of the long transient receptor potential channel family and is expressed in both the intestine and the DCT. Under experimental conditions, TRPM6 forms functional heteromers with its close homologue TRPM7, which, like TRPM6, has an alpha-kinase domain. Activity of the cation channel formed by these heteromers involves a protein, RACK1, that regulates the alpha-kinase. To date, mutations have not been described in TRPM7 or RACK1.

ISOLATED RECESSIVE RENAL HYPOMAGNESEMIA

This has been described in a single consanguineous Dutch pedigree, in which two sisters presented with hypomagnesemia with renal magnesium wasting, otherwise normal serum and urinary electrolyte metabolism, and associated mental retardation. This disease is linked to the locus encompassing the gene encoding the epidermal growth factor (EGF), and both patients had homozygous mutation in this gene. This mutation leads to abnormal basolateral sorting of pro-EGF. EGF receptors are expressed on DCT cells and elsewhere in the renal epithelium and vasculature, and activation of EGF receptors stimulates activity of TRPM6 magnesium channels whereas blockade of EGF receptors with the monoclonal antibody cetuximab prevents this stimulation. This observation is consistent with the clinical experience with cetuximab used as therapy for colon cancer, because it is associated with hypomagnesemia.

AUTOSOMAL DOMINANT HYPOMAGNESEMIA WITH HYPOCALCIURIA

A syndrome of inherited hypomagnesemia with renal magnesium wasting and hypercalciuria has been described in association with mutation in the *FXYD2* gene encoding the γ subunit of the basolateral Na⁺/K⁺-ATPase. The mechanism is not fully understood. It has been speculated that the mutant subunit results in destabilization of the enzyme complex, leading to a reduced membrane potential in the DCT cells, reducing the driving force for magnesium entry across the apical TRPM6 channel. There is also evidence that the γ subunit can mediate basolateral extrusion of magnesium.

SeSAME/EAST SYNDROMES

The *KCNJ10* gene encoding the Kir4.1 potassium channel is expressed in the brain and distal tubule, and mutations produce an autosomal recessive syndrome that has been labeled "SeSAME syndrome" (for seizures, sensorineural deafness, ataxia, mental retardation, and electrolyte imbalance) and "EAST syndrome" (epilepsy, ataxia, sensorineural deafness, and tubulopathy). In the DCT, the Kir4.1 channel allows potassium recycling from cytosol back to the interstitium. This maintains a negative intracellular potential, and also assures adequate extracellular potassium for optimal functioning of the Na⁺/K⁺-ATPase, which in turn provides the driving force for apical Na⁺ and Cl⁻ influx through NCCT. Loss of function of Kir4.1 therefore results in abnormal electrolyte handling resembling that of NCCT inactivation in Gitelman syndrome, with salt-wasting, secondary activation of renin-angiotensin-aldosterone activity, and hypokalemic metabolic alkalosis, in addition to hypomagnesemia.

ISOLATED HYPOMAGNESEMIA WITH KCNA1 MUTATION

The Kv1.1 apical potassium channel is important in establishing the negative potential across the DCT luminal membrane that provides the driving force for magnesium transport through TRPM6. Mutation is associated with autosomal dominant inheritance of isolated hypomagnesemia, without other electrolyte disturbances. The Kv1.1 channel is also expressed in the cerebellum, and mutations in *KCNA1* are also associated with the rare episodic ataxia type 1, which, however, is not associated with hypomagnesemia. This paradox may relate to tissue-specific splice variants of the gene or differential interactions with tissue-specific Kv1 units.

HYPOMAGNESEMIA WITH MITOCHONDRIAL INHERITANCE

A single but very instructive family has been reported with maternal rather than Mandelian inheritance of symptomatic hypomagnesemia with hypocalciuria and hypokalemia, associated with mutation in a mitochondrial gene encoding a tRNA for isoleucine. The DCT has the highest energy consumption of any nephron segment, and is therefore presumably more susceptible to impairment in energy supply for ATP-dependent sodium transport. Electrolyte abnormalities cluster in this family with hypertension and hypercholesterolemia, suggesting a possible role for mitochondria in the metabolic syndrome.

CNNM2 MUTATIONS IN DOMINANT HYPOMAGNESEMIA

CNNM2 is a protein expressed on the basolateral surface of DCT cells that was identified through studies of families with dominant inheritance of symptomatic hypomagnesemia with renal magnesium wasting. Its expression in cultured DCT cells is increased in magnesium deprivation. Its function is not yet known, but it may represent the postulated basolateral transporter mediating magnesium efflux, or a magnesium sensor.

DISORDERS OF TRANSPORT IN THE COLLECTING TUBULE

LIDDLE SYNDROME

Sodium reabsorption by the principal cells of the cortical collecting duct is physiologically regulated by aldosterone. As in other cells, low intracellular sodium concentrations are maintained by the basolateral Na⁺,K⁺-ATPase, and this drives sodium entry through amiloride-sensitive epithelial sodium channels (ENaC) on the apical surface. Mutations that render the ENaC persistently open produce a syndrome of excessive sodium reabsorption and low-renin hypertension (i.e., Liddle syndrome). This autosomal dominant condition often manifests in children with severe hypertension and hypokalemic alkalosis. It resembles primary hyperaldosteronism, but serum aldosterone levels are quite low, and, for this reason, the disease also has been called *pseudohyperaldosteronism*. In their original description of the syndrome, Liddle and colleagues demonstrated that aldosterone excess was not responsible for this disease and that, although spironolactone had no effect on the hypertension, patients did respond well to triamterene or dietary sodium restriction. They proposed that the primary abnormality was excessive renal salt conservation and potassium secretion independent of mineralocorticoid. This hypothesis proved to be correct, and it is explained by excessive sodium channel activity. Renal transplantation in Liddle's original proband led to resolution of the hypertension, consistent with correction of the defect intrinsic to the kidneys.

In Liddle syndrome, gain-of-function mutations in the ENaC produce channels that are resistant to downregulation by physiologic stimuli such as volume expansion. Three homologous subunits, designated αENaC, βENaC, and γENaC, form the ENaC. Missense or truncating mutations in patients with Liddle syndrome alter the carboxyl-terminal cytoplasmic tail of the β or γ subunit in a domain that is important for interactions with the cytoskeletal protein that regulates activity of the ENaC. In addition to the severe phenotype of Liddle syndrome resulting from these mutations, it has been speculated that polymorphisms in the ENaC sequence that have less dramatic effects on sodium channel function may contribute to the much more common low-renin variant of essential hypertension.

PSEUDOHYPOALDOSTERONISM TYPES 1 AND 2

Pseudohypoaldosteronism types 1 and 2 are referred to as *pseudohypoaldosteronism*, because they feature hyperkalemia and metabolic acidosis without aldosterone deficiency. Type 1 disease is associated with salt wasting and results from mutations that inactivate either the mineralocorticoid receptor (autosomal recessive) or the ENaC (autosomal dominant). The autosomal recessive form is milder and resolves with time, but the autosomal dominant form is more severe and persistent. Type 2 disease differs from hypoaldosteronism in that it is a hypertensive condition. Type 2 pseudohypoaldosteronism is also known as Gordon syndrome or familial hyperkalemic hypertension. It is a mirror image of Gitelman syndrome, with hyperkalemia, metabolic acidosis, and hypercalciuria, although serum magnesium levels are normal.

Gordon syndrome is caused by mutations in two kinases known as WNK1 and WNK4 (with no lysine [K]). Both are expressed in the DCT and collecting duct. WNK4 downregulates the activity of both the NCCT sodium chloride cotransporter and the ENaC. Inactivating mutations in *WNK4* result in increased activity of both pathways for sodium reabsorption. WNK4 also regulates the ROMK potassium channel, but mutations that relieve WNK4's inhibition of sodium transport enhance its inhibition of ROMK, contributing to the hyperkalemia in Gordon syndrome. WNK1 is a negative regulator of WNK4, and gain-of-function *WNK1* mutations indirectly increase NCCT activity. Coordinated regulation of distal ion transport by these WNK kinases may explain how the kidney balances the two effects of aldosterone on sodium reabsorption and potassium secretion, and polymorphisms in this pathway may be relevant to the mechanisms of essential hypertension.

OTHER DISORDERS RESEMBLING PRIMARY HYPERALDOSTERONISM

Two other hereditary conditions produce hypertension in children with clinical features resembling primary hyperaldosteronism. The syndrome of apparent mineralocorticoid excess (AME) is an autosomal recessive disease in which the renal isoform of the 11β-hydroxysteroid dehydrogenase enzyme is inactivated by mutation. In a sense, this is a genetic analogue of the ingestion of black licorice, which contains glycyrrhizic acid that inhibits this enzyme. Inactivation of the enzyme results in failure to convert cortisol to cortisone locally in the collecting duct, allowing cortisol to activate mineralocorticoid receptors and produce a syndrome resembling primary hyperaldosteronism but, like Liddle syndrome, with low circulating levels of aldosterone. As in Liddle syndrome, kidney transplantation has resulted in resolution of hypertension in patients with AME syndrome.

The autosomal dominant condition known as glucocorticoid-remediable aldosteronism (GRA) is caused by a chromosomal rearrangement that produces a chimeric gene in which the regulatory region of the gene encoding the steroid 11β-hydroxylase (which is part of the cortisol biosynthetic pathway and normally is regulated by adrenocorticotropic hormone [ACTH]) is fused to distal sequences of the aldosterone synthase gene. This results in production of aldosterone that responds to ACTH rather than normal regulatory stimuli. Patients with GRA may have variable elevations in plasma aldosterone levels and are often normokalemic. Aldosterone levels are suppressed by glucocorticoid therapy.

Elevated urinary levels of 18-oxacortisol and 18-hydroxycortisol are characteristic of GRA.

HEREDITARY RENAL TUBULAR ACIDOSIS

Secretion of acid by the alpha-intercalated cells of the collecting duct is accomplished by the apical proton-ATPase. Cytosolic carbonic anhydrase catalyzes the formation of bicarbonate from hydroxyl ions, and the bicarbonate then exits the cell in exchange for chloride through the basolateral anion exchanger, AE1 (encoded by the gene *SLC4A1*). Mutations affecting each of these proteins have been documented in patients with hereditary forms of RTA. Autosomal recessive distal RTA is associated with mutations in the β_1 subunit of the proton-ATPase. This form of RTA is often severe, manifesting in young children, and typically is accompanied by hearing loss, consistent with the fact that this ATPase is expressed in the cochlea, endolymphatic sac of the inner ear, and kidney. Other patients with autosomal recessive distal RTA have mutations in the gene encoding a noncatalytic α_4 isoform of the α accessory subunit of the ATPase, and these patients have less severe or no hearing deficit. Autosomal dominant RTA, a more mild disease that often is undetected until adulthood, is associated with mutations in the AE1, which is also the band 3 erythrocyte membrane protein. In Asian patients, mutations in the AE1 occur with recessive inheritance of distal RTA and hemolytic anemia.

Other genetic loci appear to be responsible for additional familial cases of distal RTA. Familial deficiency of carbonic anhydrase II is also characterized by cerebral calcification and osteopetrosis, and the latter condition reflects the important role of carbonic anhydrase in osteoclast function. The acidification defect in carbonic anhydrase II deficiency affects bicarbonate reabsorption in the proximal tubule and the collecting duct.

NEPHROGENIC DIABETES INSIPIDUS

Reabsorption of water across the cells of the collecting duct occurs only when arginine vasopressin (AVP) is present. AVP activates V_2 receptors on the principal cells and cells of the inner medullary collecting duct, initiating a cascade that results in fusion of vesicles containing aquaporin 2 (AQP-2) water channel pores into the apical membranes of these cells (Chapter 8). A gene on the X chromosome encodes the V2 receptor, and inactivating mutations in the V2 receptor gene cause the most common form of inherited nephrogenic diabetes insipidus. This results in vasopressin-resistant polyuria that typically is more severe in male patients and is associated with impaired responses to the effects of AVP that are mediated by extrarenal V_2 receptors, specifically vasodilatation and endothelial release of von Willebrand factor. Less commonly, families have been described with autosomal recessive inheritance of nephrogenic diabetes insipidus, and these patients have mutations in the gene encoding AQP-2 that result in either impaired trafficking of water channels to the plasma membrane or defective pore function. Rare autosomal dominant occurrence of nephrogenic diabetes insipidus with a mutation in AQP-2 has also been reported.

KEY BIBLIOGRAPHY

Bichet DG: Hereditary polyuric disorders: New concepts and differential diagnosis, *Semin Nephrol* 26:224-233, 2006.

Bockenhauer D, Feather S, Stanescu HC, et al: Epilepsy, ataxia, sensorineural deafness, tubulopathy, and KCNJ10 mutations, *N Engl J Med* 360:1960-1970, 2009.

Fry AC, Karet FE: Inherited renal acidoses, *Physiology (Bethesda)* 22:202-211, 2007.

Groenestege WM, Thebault S, van der Wijst J, et al: Impaired basolateral sorting of pro-EGF causes isolated recessive renal hypomagnesemia, *J Clin Invest* 117:2260-2267, 2007.

Hou J, Renigunta A, Konrad M, et al: Claudin-16 and claudin-19 interact and form a cation-selective tight junction complex. *J Clin Invest* 118:619–628.

Jonsson KB, Zahradnik R, Larsson T, et al: Fibroblast growth factor 23 in oncogenic osteomalacia and X-linked hypophosphatemia, *N Engl J Med* 348:1656-1663, 2003.

Kahle KT, Ring AM, Lifton RP: Molecular physiology of the WNK kinases, *Annu Rev Physiol* 70:329-355, 2007.

Kleta R, Bockenhauer D: Bartter syndromes and other salt-losing tubulopathies, *Nephron Physiol* 104:73-80, 2006.

Konrad M, Weber S: Recent advances in molecular genetics of hereditary magnesium-losing disorders, *J Am Soc Nephrol* 14:249-260, 2003.

Scheinman SJ: Dent's disease. In Lifton R, Somlo S, Giebisch G, Seldin D, editors: *Genetic diseases of the kidney*, San Diego, 2008, Elsevier.

Scheinman SJ, Guay-Woodford LM, Thakker RV, et al: Genetic disorders of renal electrolyte transport, *N Engl J Med* 340:1177-1187, 1999.

Sha Q, Pearson W, Burcea LC, et al: Human FXYD2 G41R mutation responsible for renal hypomagnesemia behaves as an inward-rectifying cation channel, *Am J Physiol Renal Physiol* 295:F91-F99, 2008.

Simon DB, Lu Y, Choate KA, et al: Paracellin-1, a renal tight junction protein required for paracellular Mg resorption, *Science* 285:103-106, 1999.

Stuiver M, Lainez S, Will C, et al: CNNM2, encoding a basolateral protein required for renal Mg2+ handling, is mutated in dominant hypomagnesemia, *Am J Hum Genet* 88:333-343, 2011.

Tenenhouse HS: Phosphate transport: molecular basis, regulation and pathophysiology, *J Steroid Biochem Mol Biol* 103:572-577, 2007.

Thakker RV: Diseases associated with the extracellular calcium-sensing receptor, *Cell Calcium* 35:275-282, 2004.

Torres VE, Scheinman SJ: Genetic diseases of the kidney, *NephSAP* 3(1), January 2004. Available at http://www.asn-online.org/education/nephsap/volumes/volume3.aspx. (Accessed May 24, 2013.)

Walder RY, Landau D, Meyer P, et al: Mutation of TRPM6 causes familial hypomagnesemia with secondary hypocalcemia, *Nat Genet* 31:171-174, 2002.

Warnock DG: Liddle syndrome: genetics and mechanisms of Na+ channel defects, *Am J Med Sci* 322:302-307, 2001.

Wilson FH, Hariri A, Farhi A, et al: A cluster of metabolic defects caused by mutation in a mitochondrial tRNA, *Science* 306:1190-1194, 2004.

Full bibliography can be found on www.expertconsult.com.

Sickle Cell Nephropathy

40

Vimal K. Derebail

Sickle cell anemia is caused by the homozygous inheritance (HbSS) of the sickle β-globin gene, produced by a single point mutation in chromosome 11. The resultant β chain of the hemoglobin molecule possesses a substitution of valine for glutamic acid at position 6, leading to an unstable form of hemoglobin (hemoglobin S). Under conditions of low oxygen tension, acidity, extreme temperatures, and other stressors, the altered hemoglobin undergoes polymerization, leading to "sickling" of red blood cells (Figure 40.1). These red cells are rigid, leading to both microvascular obstruction and activation of inflammation and coagulation. Sickle cell disease (SCD) is also seen in the presence of double heterozygous inheritance of hemoglobin mutations (HbS gene and another mutation), such as hemoglobin SCD and sickle β-thalassemia.

The prevalence of sickle cell trait (HbAS) in the United States is between 6% and 9% among African Americans, with sickle cell anemia occurring in approximately 1 of 500 African American live births. Worldwide, the prevalence of the hemoglobin S mutation varies greatly and is often highest in areas where malaria is endemic, related to the protection it affords against malarial infection.

Although SCD affects multiple systems throughout the body and is characterized by acute pain crises and progressive multiorgan damage, the kidney is a particularly susceptible organ. The renal medulla, with its lower oxygen tension, high osmolarity, lower pH, and relatively sluggish blood flow, is an ideal environment for "sickling" and microvascular obstruction. As a result, kidney manifestations are common in SCD (Table 40.1).

PATHOPHYSIOLOGY

Although the classic understanding of SCD is based on microvascular obstruction, its pathophysiology is better understood in the context of vasoocclusion with ischemia-reperfusion injury and hemolytic anemia. In addition to triggering hemoglobin polymerization, inflammation and other stressors also trigger erythrocyte adhesion to endothelium and leukocytes, beginning the process of microvascular obstruction. These processes are dynamic, resulting in ischemia, followed by restoration of blood flow and subsequent reperfusion injury, with resultant oxidative stress and inflammatory cytokine production.

The process of intravascular hemolysis is another contributor to disease burden, with the release of free hemoglobin into the plasma, generating reactive oxygen species and depleting nitric oxide. These processes produce endothelial dysfunction and activate the coagulation system.

Disease severity in SCD appears to be modulated by the relative concentration of sickle hemoglobin (HbS). The presence of fetal hemoglobin (HbF), which can be increased with therapy, reduces the relative content of hemoglobin S; accordingly, haplotypes of the mutation that correlate with lower HbF production, most notably the Central African Republic (CAR) haplotype, typically have the most severe disease manifestations. Similarly, co-inheritance of α-thalassemia mutations reduces intracellular HbS concentration and leads to reduced hemolysis and fewer complications.

Within the kidney, these pathologic mechanisms result in clinical manifestations that lead to changes in kidney hemodynamics, tubulointerstitial damage, and in some patients, glomerular disease.

KIDNEY HEMODYNAMICS

Glomerular hyperfiltration is extraordinarily common among patients with SCD, and can be detected as early as 13 months of age. Glomerulomegaly is evident even in patients without clinical disease and contributes to the hyperfiltration. Glomerular hyperfiltration likely is driven by vasodilatation of the afferent arteriole, which is thought to occur as a compensatory response to chronic tissue hypoxia. The exact mechanisms behind this response are not fully known, but it may be mediated by upregulation of prostaglandins and the nitric oxide systems. Indomethacin and other prostaglandin inhibitors, administered at doses that would not affect glomerular filtration rate (GFR) in normal individuals, can reduce GFR to more normal values in patients with SCD.

TUBULOINTERSTITIAL DISEASE

IMPAIRED URINARY CONCENTRATION

The most commonly reported kidney manifestation in patients with SCD is the loss of complete urinary concentrating ability. Typically, generation of concentrated urine requires an intact collecting duct and a medullary concentration gradient. The juxtamedullary nephrons, which extend deepest into the medulla and are most capable producing a high concentration gradient, are also those most likely to be affected by sickling in the medullary vasa recta. Microangiographic studies demonstrate obliteration of the vasa recta in these patients, with subsequent fibrosis and shortening of the renal papilla. The functional result of these anatomic changes ultimately can

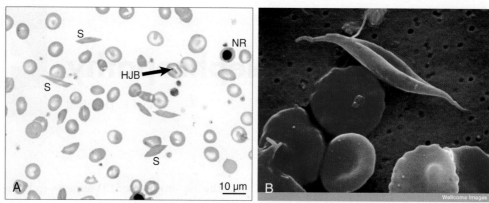

Figure 40.1 **A,** Peripheral blood smear of a patient with sickle cell anemia. This blood film shows irreversibly sickled cells (S), a nucleated red blood cell (NR), and a Howell-Jolly Body (HJB); these last two features are mainly associated with hyposplenism (stained with May-Grunwald-Giemsa). (Reprinted from Rees DC, Williams TN, Gladwin MT: Sickle cell disease, *Lancet* 376:2018-2031, 2010, with permission from Elsevier.) **B,** Scanning electron microscopic image of sickled and other red blood cells, false-colored red. Photographed using Philips 501 SEM. (With permission from EM Unit, UCL Medical School, Royal Free Campus, Wellcome Images.)

Table 40.1   Kidney Pathology in Sickle Cell Disease

Kidney Abnormality	Clinical Consequence
Glomerular	
Hyperfiltration	Increased GFR (early), albuminuria/ proteinuria, sickle glomerulopathy, CKD (late)
Proximal Tubule	
Enhanced proximal tubule activity	Increased creatinine secretion, increased phosphate resorption (hyperphosphatemia)
Depressed renin	Hyporeninemic hypoaldosteronism (hyperkalemia)
Distal Tubule/Cortical Collection Duct	
Impaired hydrogen ion secretion	Metabolic acidosis (type 4 RTA)
Impaired potassium secretion	Hyperkalemia
Impaired urinary concentration	Hyposthenuria
Interstitial	
Chronic "sickling" in vasa recta	Hematuria, renal papillary necrosis (due to ischemia), renal medullary carcinoma

CKD, Chronic kidney disease; *GFR,* glomerular filtration rate; *RTA,* renal tubular acidosis.

manifest by an inability to achieve urinary osmolality greater than 400 mOsm/kg. Early in life, this defect is partially reversible following blood transfusions that rapidly increase normal hemoglobin A (HbA) and reduce sickling in the vasa recta. However, impaired urinary concentration becomes fixed later in life (as early as age 15) and no longer improves with transfusion. As a result, depending on water and solute intake, patients with SCD may have obligatory water losses of up to 2.0 L/day, predisposing them to volume depletion and thereby potentially exacerbating sickle crises. The ability to produce a maximally dilute urine and excrete free water remains intact.

HEMATURIA

Hematuria can be one of the most dramatic kidney presentations in patients with SCD, and may range from microscopic hematuria to gross hematuria. Gross hematuria may occur in patients of any age, including young children. Although the etiology of hematuria remains unclear, the vasoocclusion occurring in the acidic, hyperosmolar, low oxygen tension environment of the medulla is thought to play a central role. Studies of kidneys removed from sickle cell patients with severe hematuria demonstrate severe stasis of peritubular capillaries, particularly those in the medulla, as well as erythrocytes extravasated into the collecting tubules. In addition to the aforementioned vascular occlusion–mediated ischemia and oxidative/reperfusion injury, sickling in these vessels also may lead to vessel wall injury and necrosis, which could cause the structural changes leading to hematuria.

Typically, hematuria is unilateral and occurs nearly four times more often from the left kidney. The longer course and higher venous pressures of the left renal vein as it traverses between the aorta and superior mesenteric artery likely lead to this phenomenon.

Although bleeding is typically benign and self-limited, massive hemorrhage can occur and potentially be life threatening. Treatment consists of conservative management with bed rest and maintenance of high urine output to prevent clots. Alkalinization of the urine may help by raising medullary pH, thereby reducing sickling; however, no proven benefit has been shown in studies. Intravenous fluids may be employed to ensure high urine flow, but must be used with caution in patients at risk for congestive heart failure or acute chest syndrome. Diuretics can also be used to increase urine flow rates, but care must be taken to avoid volume depletion.

For those patients with massive and persistent hematuria despite conservative therapy, ε-aminocaproic acid (EACA) can be beneficial. This agent inhibits fibrinolysis and can induce clotting to halt hematuria. Prior reports have demonstrated improvement with EACA, although no standard dose regimen or length of therapy has been defined. However, EACA can be prothrombotic; accordingly, it must be used with caution

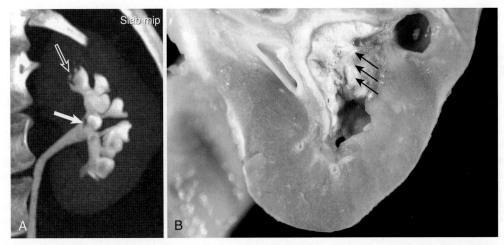

Figure 40.2 **A,** Maximum-intensity-projection (MIP) images from CT urography in a 23-year-old woman with sickle cell trait presenting with intermittent gross hematuria for 5 days. Pooling of contrast material within multiple papillae bilaterally *(open arrow)* is consistent with papillary necrosis. Filling defect within left renal pelvis *(solid arrow)* was shown to represent blood clot at ureteroscopy. (From Chow LC, Kwan SW, Olcott EW et al: Split-Bolus MDCT urography with synchronous nephrographic and excretory phase enhancement, *Am J Roentgenol* 189:314-322, 2007. Reprinted with permission from the American Journal of Roentgenology.) **B,** Gross photomicrograph of a bivalved kidney demonstrating necrosis of a renal papilla *(arrows).* Over time, this area will form a scar with cystic dilation of the calices. (Image courtesy Vincent Moylan.)

in SCD patients who are already at risk for thrombotic events. Currently, EACA use is recommended only for a limited period and at the lowest dose necessary to achieve inhibition of urinary fibrinolytic activity. In addition to EACA, intravenous vasopressin to limit hematuria has been successful in case reports.

In patients who are refractory to medical therapy, invasive intervention may be necessary. If a source of bleeding can be localized via imaging, attempts at percutaneous embolization have been attempted. In rare cases, unilateral nephrectomy of the affected kidney may be required. In all patients presenting with hematuria, and particularly in those with persistent or massive hematuria, alternative causes should be considered, including acquired or hereditary bleeding disorders or abnormalities such as nephrolithiasis, polycystic kidney disease, or renal medullary carcinoma (see next sections).

RENAL PAPILLARY NECROSIS

Renal papillary necrosis (RPN) is fairly common in SCD, occurring in more than 60% of patients in some series. Although often accompanied by hematuria, a similar proportion of patients may be asymptomatic. With severe sickling in the vasa recta, the renal papillae that depend on these vessels can undergo focal, repetitive infarcts leading to necrosis (Figure 40.2). If hematuria is present, as described earlier, patients should undergo an evaluation for other potential causes, including kidney masses or nephrolithiasis. This imaging can be performed with ultrasonography, although helical computed tomography (CT) scan may detect RPN earlier. In many patients, RPN ultimately results in calcification around the renal pelvis. Treatment, as with hematuria, is generally supportive, employing similar measures. If significant sloughing occurs, necrotic and thrombotic material may lead to ureteral obstruction, which can be diagnosed by urography and relieved by stenting.

RENAL MEDULLARY CARCINOMA

Renal medullary carcinoma is an extremely rare occurrence seen almost exclusively in patients with sickle cell trait, although there are a few reports in patients with SCD. Repetitive ischemic injuries to the tubules are postulated to drive the development of this lesion. Most patients present before the age of 20 and are more often male. The typical presentation is gross hematuria accompanied by lumbar pain or abdominal masses, although malignant constitutional symptoms of weight loss, fevers, and fatigue may be present. Regrettably, this malignancy is usually metastatic at diagnosis, with survival of only 6 to 12 months. For these reasons, presentation of gross hematuria in patients with SCD should prompt imaging via ultrasonography or preferably CT scan.

ACIDIFICATION, POTASSIUM EXCRETION, AND OTHER TUBULAR ABNORMALITIES

Acidosis is fairly uncommon in patients with SCD in the absence of kidney failure, although some patients may manifest an incomplete distal renal tubular acidosis (RTA). Hyperkalemia may accompany this; however, this is rare without significant potassium ingestion or medications that interfere with potassium handling. The inability of the damaged distal nephron to excrete ammonium and titratable acids, as well as an inability to respond to aldosterone, lead to these findings. If necessary, treatment with potassium restriction, sodium bicarbonate, and loop diuretics can be effective.

The aforementioned abnormalities generally indicate impaired distal tubule secretory function. The proximal tubule, to the contrary, demonstrates enhanced activity. Sodium reabsorption is increased, leading to less urinary excretion, as well as a relative resistance to loop diuretics. Accompanying this increase in sodium reabsorption is an enhancement of proximal phosphate reabsorption that may cause hyperphosphatemia in settings of increased phosphorus loads (hemolysis, rhabdomyolysis). Additionally, uric acid secretion is increased, perhaps as an adaptive mechanism to the increased uric acid load from chronic hemolysis. Finally, secretion of creatinine in the proximal tubule is also heightened, diminishing the usefulness of creatinine clearance and creatinine-based equations to estimate GFR.

SICKLE CELL GLOMERULOPATHY

The presence of glomerular involvement has long been noted in SCD, with levels of proteinuria ranging from micro-albuminuria to overt nephrotic syndrome. Initial reports of glomerular lesions were those of immune complex deposition and pathology consistent with membranoproliferative glomerulonephritis (MPGN). However, more recent studies have demonstrated glomerulomegaly and development of focal segmental glomerulosclerosis (FSGS) in the majority of patients with sickle cell nephropathy. As in other forms of FSGS, immunofluorescence of biopsy samples may demonstrate minimal staining with immunoglobulin M (IgM), C1q, and C3, but electron microscopy usually fails to identify any electron dense deposits. The clinical sequelae of these lesions are thought to begin with microalbuminuria and evolve into overt proteinuria, loss of kidney function, and advanced chronic kidney disease (CKD).

ALBUMINURIA AND PROTEINURIA

The development of albuminuria and overt proteinuria clearly increases as patients with SCD age, with more than 60% of adults over the age of 35 exhibiting microalbuminuria. However, children below the age of 10 rarely demonstrate this finding. Over 20% of adults with microalbuminuria will progress to overt proteinuria and progressive GFR decline. The nephrotic syndrome itself is fairly rare, but it portends a poor kidney prognosis. An uncommon but well-recognized cause of acute onset of the nephrotic syndrome is parvovirus B19 infection, often leading to the collapsing variant of FSGS. Abnormalities in albumin excretion are more frequent in sickle cell anemia (HbSS disease) than in other sickle hemoglobinopathies (HbSC disease, HbS-β-thalassemia).

Severity of SCD in some series does seem to correlate with the development of albuminuria. Lower hemoglobin levels and pulmonary hypertension may be associated with the development of albuminuria. Finally, as with many other manifestations of SCD, co-inheritance of α-thalassemia may attenuate the development of sickle glomerulopathy.

The underlying pathophysiology of albuminuria is multi-factorial and probably related to a variety of pathologic developments in SCD. Persistence of glomerular hyperfiltration, as in other diseases with this feature, results in albuminuria and eventual GFR decline. As repetitive sickling occurs and interstitial fibrosis leads to dropout of affected nephrons, hyperfiltration is further accentuated in the remaining glomeruli. Additionally, evidence suggests endothelial dysfunction from both direct injury related to sickling and the release of free heme during hemolysis. Subsequently, markers of hemolysis such as reticulocyte hemoglobin and LDH may correlate with albuminuria, as do mediators of endothelial dysfunction including soluble fms-like tyrosine kinase-1 (sFLT-1).

TREATMENT

Therapies for reducing albuminuria and proteinuria have been advocated in hope of delaying progression of CKD, although little prospective data exist to determine whether any therapy is truly effective. As with many diseases in which proteinuria is a feature, inhibition of the renin-angiotensin-aldosterone system (RAAS) forms the mainstay of therapy. Several studies have demonstrated a short-term reduction in both proteinuria and hyperfiltration with the use of angiotensin-converting enzyme (ACE) inhibitors. These effects seem to be independent of any blood pressure lowering and are likely related to reduction of glomerular capillary hypertension. Although specific guidelines do not exist, patients should be screened periodically for albuminuria, and renin-angiotensin blockade should be initiated if albuminuria is detected. With the institution and dose titration of these agents, both kidney function and serum potassium must be monitored closely, because SCD patients are prone to the metabolic effects of reduced eGFR and impaired potassium secretion.

Hydroxyurea, or hydroxycarbamide, is indicated in SCD for those patients with acute chest syndrome, frequent pain crises, and vasoocclusive episodes. Its role in the management of albuminuria and CKD is less well defined. The mechanism of action is not completely understood, but it is in part due to the ability of hydroxyurea to induce HbF production and thereby reduce the overall concentration of hemoglobin S. Hydroxyurea may also affect the synthesis of nitric oxide, and has other beneficial effects. Small studies have demonstrated that the addition of hydroxyurea to ACE inhibitors may provide further reduction in proteinuria. However, a recently published large study of its use in infants failed to demonstrate prevention of hyperfiltration, although this study may not have been of long enough duration or utilized a population old enough to demonstrate a potential benefit. At present, albuminuria alone in SCD is not a clear indication for hydroxyurea.

MANAGEMENT OF CHRONIC KIDNEY DISEASE

The management of SCD patients who develop CKD is similar to patients with CKD due to other causes, with a few exceptions. The first relates to the management of anemia. With chronic ischemic kidney insults and ongoing hemolysis, SCD patients typically have a greater stimulus for erythropoietin and exhibit higher endogenous erythropoietin levels. However, with progressive kidney disease, these patients begin to lose the ability to produce adequate endogenous erythropoietin, typically occurring when GFR falls below 60 mL/min. As with other forms of CKD, erythropoiesis-stimulating agents (ESAs) may be employed to maintain hemoglobin levels and reduce the need for transfusion. SCD patients with CKD are likely to require very large doses of ESAs, and the target hemoglobin is different from what is typical in other CKD or ESRD populations. Generally, a maximum achieved hemoglobin level of 10 mg/dL is recommended to avoid precipitation of vasoocclusive crises. Iron stores should be maintained to maximize erythropoiesis in those not receiving chronic transfusions, although care must be taken to avoid iron overload in this susceptible population.

Finally, even though patients with SCD are at greater risk for advanced CKD, hypertension is an uncommon feature in this population. Despite a prevalence of hypertension of 28% of the general African American population, only about 2% to 6% of African Americans with SCD exhibit hypertension. Various explanations for this finding have been posited, including relative volume depletion and reduced systemic vascular resistance. If hypertension is detected in patients with SCD, therapy should be initiated as in any patient with CKD or at risk for CKD. Most would consider a goal blood pressure of 130/80 mm Hg reasonable. Some suggest avoidance of diuretics given their predisposition to volume depletion, which can induce a pain crisis.

END-STAGE RENAL DISEASE

Once patients with SCD reach ESRD, either peritoneal dialysis or hemodialysis present viable options for kidney replacement therapy. Early referral to a nephrologist is particularly important for this population of patients. Notably, mortality after reaching ESRD for those with SCD may approach 40% in the first year alone, and the mean life expectancy, despite the relative youth of SCD patients with kidney failure, is only 4 years.

Although SCD patients are less likely to be listed for kidney transplantation, this kidney replacement therapy option does appear to offer survival benefit similar to other forms of CKD. One-year graft survival of kidney allografts in SCD patients is similar to other African American patients, although 3-year graft survival is somewhat reduced. Notably, though, patient survival at 10 years for those receiving kidney transplants is far greater than those treated with dialysis alone (56% vs. 14%). After transplantation, SCD patients must be monitored for allograft thrombosis, an increase in vasoocclusive crises, and recurrence of sickle glomerulopathy, which has been reported as early as 3 years after transplantation. Hydroxyurea and exchange transfusion have been used in the posttransplant period, and simultaneous bone marrow transplantation could be curative of the disease as a whole.

SICKLE CELL TRAIT

Patients with a single hemoglobin S mutation are deemed to have sickle cell trait (SCT, HbAS). Although generally viewed as a benign condition, SCT does have manifestations more akin to an intermediate phenotype. Kidney manifestations are by far the most commonly reported comorbidities in SCT, and are similar to those seen in SCD.

Impaired urinary concentration is common, albeit not as severe as that seen in SCD. Again, the severity of the concentrating defect seems to be modulated by the co-inheritance of α-thalassemia. Hematuria and renal papillary necrosis also occur in this population. As noted earlier, renal medullary carcinoma, rarely described in SCD, has been nearly exclusively reported in patients with SCT.

Whether the kidney abnormalities of SCT contribute to the development of CKD remains unclear. A single study has demonstrated an acceleration of progression to ESRD among those with concurrent SCT and adult polycystic kidney disease (ADPKD), whereas another study has noted a higher prevalence of SCT in an African American ESRD population; subsequent studies have not borne out this latter finding.

BIBLIOGRAPHY

Abbott KC, Hypolite IO, Agodoa LY: Sickle cell nephropathy at end-stage renal disease in the United States: patient characteristics and survival, *Clin Nephrol* 58:9-15, 2002.

Ataga KI, Brittain JE, Moore D, et al: Urinary albumin excretion is associated with pulmonary hypertension in sickle cell disease: potential role of soluble fms-like tyrosine kinase-1, *Eur J Haematol* 85(3):257-263, 2010.

Ataga KI, Orringer EP: Renal abnormalities in sickle cell disease, *Am J Hematol* 63:205-211, 2000.

Bruno D, Wigfall DR, Zimmerman SA, et al: Genitourinary complications of sickle cell disease, *J Urol* 166:803-811, Sep 2001.

Day TG, Drasar ER, Fulford T, et al: Association between hemolysis and albuminuria in adults with sickle cell anemia, *Haematologica* 97:201-205, 2012.

Derebail VK, Nachman PH, Key NS, et al: High prevalence of sickle cell trait in African Americans with ESRD, *J Am Soc Nephrol* 21:413-417, 2010.

Falk RJ, Scheinman J, Phillips G, et al: Prevalence and pathologic features of sickle cell nephropathy and response to inhibition of angiotensin-converting enzyme, *N Engl J Med* 326:910-915, 1992.

Guasch A, Navarrete J, Nass K, et al: Glomerular involvement in adults with sickle cell hemoglobinopathies: Prevalence and clinical correlates of progressive renal failure, *J Am Soc Nephrol* 17:2228-2235, 2006.

Haymann JP, Stankovic K, Levy P, et al: Glomerular hyperfiltration in adult sickle cell anemia: a frequent hemolysis associated feature, *Clin J Am Soc Nephrol* 5:756-761, 2010.

Hicks PJ, Langefeld CD, Lu L, et al: Sickle cell trait is not independently associated with susceptibility to end-stage renal disease in African Americans, *Kidney Int* 80:1339-1343, 2011.

Key NS, Derebail VK: Sickle-cell trait: novel clinical significance. Hematology / the Education Program of the American Society of Hematology Education Program, *Am Soc Hematol Educ Program* 418-422, 2010.

Maier-Redelsperger M, Lévy P, Lionnet F, et al: Strong association between a new marker of hemolysis and glomerulopathy in sickle cell anemia, *Blood Cells Mol Dis* 45:289-292, 2010.

McClellan AC, Guasch A, Gilbertson D, et al: Characteristics of Pre-ESRD Care and Early Mortality among Incident ESRD Patients with Sickle Cell Disease (SCD) [abstract F-PO1493]. In *Programs and abstracts of the 42nd Annual Meeting of the American Society of Nephrology*, San Diego: 2009, p 7.

Nath KA, Grande JP, Croatt AJ, et al: Transgenic sickle mice are markedly sensitive to renal ischemia-reperfusion injury, *Am J Pathol* 166:963-972, 2005.

Powars DR, Elliott-Mills DD, Chan L, et al: Chronic renal failure in sickle cell disease: risk factors, clinical course, and mortality, *Ann Intern Med* 115:614-620, 1991.

Rees DC, Williams TN, Gladwin MT: Sickle-cell disease, *Lancet* 376: 2018-2031, 2010.

Scheinman JI: Sickle cell disease and the kidney, *Nat Clin Pract Nephrol* 5:78-88, 2009.

Sharpe CC, Thein SL: Sickle cell nephropathy: a practical approach, *Br J Haematol* 155:287-297, 2011.

Statius van Eps LW, Pinedo-Veels C, de Vries GH, et al: Nature of concentrating defect in sickle-cell nephropathy. Microradioangiographic studies, *Lancet* 1:450-452, 1970.

41 Polycystic and Other Cystic Kidney Diseases

Dana V. Rizk | Arlene B. Chapman

Significant advances have been made in understanding the genetics and molecular pathogenesis of inherited cystic disorders of the kidney. Many of the genes and their respective proteins have been identified (Table 41.1). Final common pathways regarding the formation and development of cysts are being elucidated. Most renal cysts develop because of abnormal function of the primary cilium that resides in all epithelial cells. Recently developed molecularly targeted therapies offer hope for improved outcome or cure of these disorders.

AUTOSOMAL DOMINANT POLYCYSTIC KIDNEY DISEASE

Autosomal dominant polycystic kidney disease (ADPKD) is the most common inherited kidney disorder, occurring in 1 of 400 to 1000 live births. ADPKD has equal representation in all ethnic groups and has been reported worldwide. It accounts for about 5% of the end-stage renal disease (ESRD) cases in the United States. ADPKD is a multisystem disorder that affects almost every organ resulting in significant extrarenal manifestations; however, its hallmark is the gradual and massive cystic enlargement of the kidneys, ultimately resulting in kidney failure.

PATHOGENESIS

Two genes have been implicated in the pathogenesis of ADPKD. *PKD1* mutations account for approximately 85% of cases, whereas *PKD2* mutations account for the remaining 15%. Although mutations in *PKD1* and *2* lead to the same phenotype, their prognostic implications are different as *PKD2* mutations impart a milder disease. Patients with *PKD2* mutations develop renal cysts, hypertension, and ESRD at a later age than their counterparts with *PKD1* mutations (median age of onset of ESRD 74 vs. 54 years, respectively). Given the milder phenotype associated with PKD2, when surveillance autopsies are performed, the relative frequency of PKD2 increases, accounting for up to 27% of all ADPKD cases.

PKD1 is located on the short arm of chromosome 16 (16p13.3) and codes for polycystin-1 (PC1), an integral membrane protein made up of 4304 amino acids. PC1 has a large extracellular N-terminal, 11 transmembrane regions, and a short intracellular C-terminal. PC1 function is not completely understood; it interacts with PC2 through its C-terminal, and the PC1-PC2 complex colocalizes to the primary cilium of epithelial cells. The known properties of PC1 are those of a ligand with extracellular interactions and cell-cycle regulation.

PKD2 is located on the long arm of chromosome 4 (4q12.2) and encodes for polycystin-2 (PC2), a 968 amino acid protein with a short cytoplasmic N-terminal, 6 transmembrane regions, and a short cytoplasmic C-terminal. It localizes to the endoplasmic reticulum, plasma membrane, primary cilium, centrosome, and mitotic spindles in dividing cells. Polycystin-2 belongs to the family of voltage-activated calcium channels (e.g., transient receptor potential polycystin-2 [TRPP-2]), and is involved in intracellular calcium regulation through several pathways. Polycystin-1 and 2 are colocalized in the primary cilium of renal epithelial cells, which functions as a mechanical sensor. Primary cilia create transmembrane calcium current in the presence of stretch or luminal flow. Polycystin-1 and 2 contribute to ciliary function, and the physical interaction between polycystin-1 and 2 is required for a membrane calcium channel to operate properly. Normal polycystin function increases intracellular calcium, which initiates a signaling cascade leading to vesicle fusion and a change in gene transcription.

Each polycystin affects cell proliferation, differentiation, and fluid secretion through G protein or JAK-STAT-mediated signaling pathways. The interaction of polycystin-1 ligand on the basolateral surface with adenylate cyclase, and the G protein–coupled response of adenylate cyclase to binding of vasopressin to the vasopressin V_2 receptor, produce similar results. Both result in increased intracellular concentrations of cyclic adenosine monophosphate (cAMP) and ultimately in chloride secretion across the apical membrane. This chloride-rich fluid secretion is a critical component of cystogenesis, enabling expansion of cysts even after they detach from their parent nephron. The accumulation of cyst fluid, rich in chloride and sodium, relies on the active luminal excretion of chloride primarily through the cystic fibrosis transmembrane conductor regulator (CFTR) (Fig. 41.1).

Less than 5% of all nephrons become cystic in ADPKD. It is thought that renal cysts are derived from a single, clonal hyperproliferative epithelial cell that has genetically transformed. The clonal cystic epithelia proliferate because of a second somatic mutation in the *PKD1* or *PKD2* gene, indicating that a "second hit" is involved in cyst growth and development. Epithelial cell proliferation, fluid secretion, and alterations in extracellular matrix ultimately result in focal outpouching from the parent nephron. Most cysts detach from the parent nephron when cyst size exceeds 2 cm, and continue to secrete fluid autonomously, resulting in cyst and kidney enlargement, and ultimately progressive loss of kidney function.

Table 41.1 Genes and Proteins of Inherited Cystic Disorders of the Kidney

Disease	Frequency	Chromosome	Gene Locus	Protein	Function
ADPKD	1:1000	16p13.3	PKD1	Polycystin 1, which colocalizes with polycystin 2 in the primary cilium	Regulates intracellular cAMP, mTOR, planar polarity
	1:15,000	4q21.2	PKD2	Polycystin 2, which colocalizes with polycystin 1 in the primary cilium and ER	Regulates intracellular Ca levels through ER Ca release, activates Ca channels
ARPKD	1:20,000	6q24.2	PKHD	Fibrocystin or polyductin, located throughout the primary cilium	Serves as receptor to maintain intracellular cAMP levels
VHL	1:36,000	3p25	VHL	VHL, located at the base of the primary cilium	Inhibits HIF-1α and cell turnover, maintains planar polarity, allows ciliogenesis
TSC	1:6000	9q34.3	TSC1	Hamartin	Interacts with tuberin to suppress mTOR activity
		16p13.3	TSC2	Tuberin	Interacts with hamartin to suppress mTOR activity

ADPKD, Autosomal dominant polycystic kidney disease; *ARPKD,* autosomal recessive polycystic kidney disease; *cAMP,* cyclic adenosine monophosphate; *ER,* endoplasmic reticulum; *HIF,* hypoxia inducible factors; *mTOR,* mammalian target of rapamycin; *PKHD,* polycystic kidney and hepatic disease; *TSC,* tuberous sclerosis complex; *VHL,* von Hippel-Lindau.

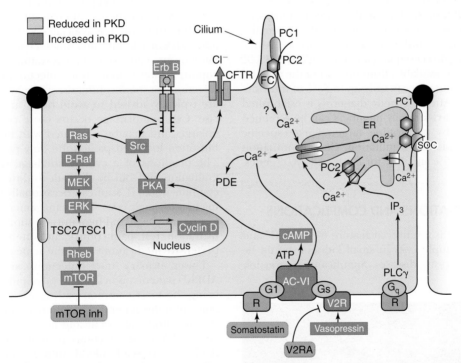

Figure 41.1 Renal tubular epithelial cell showing location and interactions of polycystin 1 (PC1) and polycystin 2 (PC2). *(Top)* The apical surface with a single cilium. *(Both sides and bottom)* The basolateral surfaces. Mutations in PC1 *(gold ovals)* or PC2 *(blue hexagons)* result in changes in the intracellular calcium level or increases in the level of cAMP. A change in the balance of these two critical intracellular components leads to alterations in the Ras pathway, the mTOR pathway, cell turnover, apoptosis, and fluid secretion through the CFTR channel. Mutations in PC1 and PC2 colocalize to the primary cilium and the basolateral membranes. PC2 resides alone in the ER. G-coupled receptor activation increases the concentration of cAMP. Interference with G-coupled receptor processes can return the increased cAMP level seen in ADPKD to normal. Blockade of the vasopressin 2 (V$_2$) receptor by a V$_2$ receptor antagonist is one example. PC1 interacts with the tuberous sclerosis complex proteins (TSC2 and TSC1) regulating the mTOR pathway. Therapies aimed at reducing G-coupled receptor, EGF receptor, CFTR channel, mTOR, and cyclin activity or increasing ER release of calcium may normalize epithelial cell function in ADPKD. *AC-VI,* Adenylate cyclase; *ADPKD,* autosomal dominant polycystic kidney disease; *cAMP,* cyclic adenosine monophosphate; *CFTR,* cystic fibrosis transmembrane conductance regulator; *EGF,* epithelial growth factor; *ER,* endoplasmic reticulum; *ERB,* epidermal growth factor (erythroblastic leukemia, viral); *Inh,* inhibitor; *IP$_3$,* inositol triphosphate; *mTOR,* mammalian target of rapamycin; *PC1,* polycystin 1; *PC2,* polycystin 2; *PDE,* phosphodiesterase; *PKA,* phosphokinase A; *PKD,* polycystic kidney disease; *R,* receptor; *Ras,* renin-angiotensin system; *SRC,* nonreceptor (cytoplasmic) protein tyrosine kinase; *V2R,* vasopressin V$_2$ receptor; *V2RA,* vasopressin V$_2$ receptor antagonist.

DIAGNOSIS

Kidney imaging studies (i.e., ultrasound) remain the mainstay for diagnosing ADPKD. The characteristic findings include enlarged kidneys and the presence of multiple cysts throughout the renal parenchyma (Fig. 41.2). Ravine et al. established age-specific, ultrasound-based diagnostic criteria in the early 1990s. These guidelines were developed focusing on PKD1 related disease. These same criteria are less sensitive in patients with PKD2 mutations whose disease tends to be milder and manifests at a more advanced age, hence leading to a higher rate of false negatives. More recently, unified diagnostic ultrasonographic criteria for at-risk individuals independent of genotype were developed. In individuals ages 15 to 39, the presence of at least three (unilateral or bilateral) renal cysts is sufficient to establish a diagnosis of ADPKD. In those individuals 40 to 59 years of age, two cysts in each kidney are required, and in those older than 60, in whom acquired cystic disease is common, four or more cysts in each kidney are required for diagnosis. For patients with no family history, the diagnostic criteria are more stringent with at least five cysts bilaterally by the age of 30 and a phenotype consistent with ADPKD required (see later).

When disease status must be determined with certainty, for example when an individual is being evaluated as a potential kidney donor or for family-planning purposes, then CT or MRI may be used because they detect smaller cysts. Genetic testing is another diagnostic approach. Mutation screening using direct sequencing of the PKD1 or PKD2 genes is commercially available. Both the cost of the test and its ability to detect mutations in only up to 85% of individuals restricts its use. After a genetic diagnosis is established in a patient, other at-risk family members can be screened at a reduced cost by performing targeted exon-specific sequencing of the identified mutation. Current mutation detection rates are 75% and 95% for PKD1 and PKD2 genes, respectively.

KIDNEY MANIFESTATIONS AND COMPLICATIONS

Kidney enlargement is a universal feature of ADPKD, and individuals with multiple cysts in small kidneys should be screened for other cystic diseases. Significant progression

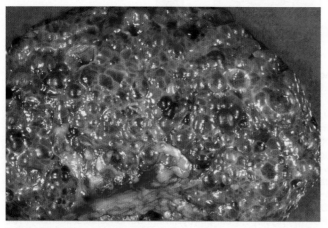

Figure 41.2 Gross pathology of the autosomal dominant polycystic kidney disease kidney.

of cyst growth and kidney enlargement precedes the loss of kidney function by decades in ADPKD. In the Consortium for Radiologic Imaging in the Study of Polycystic Kidney Disease (CRISP), a large multicenter study of 241 ADPKD patients with intact kidney function who were followed prospectively with serial MRI of their kidneys, kidney volumes increased 5.2%/yr. Cysts accounted for more than 95% of total kidney volume, and kidney volume increased approximately 55% after 8 years of follow-up. PKD2 patients have smaller kidney volumes (694 ± 221 vs. 986 ± 204 mL) and lower age-adjusted cyst number per kidney when compared to PKD1 patients, but demonstrated similar rates of growth (4.9 ± 2.3% vs. 5.2 ± 1.6%/yr), indicating that the rate of cyst formation rather than the rate of cyst expansion differs between the two genotypes. More recently, data from the CRISP study showed that height-adjusted total kidney volume of greater than 600 mL/m accurately predicted the development of CKD stage 3 within 8 years. For each 100 mL/m change in height-adjusted total kidney volume, there was a 48% increase in the risk of reaching CKD stage 3. These results suggest that total kidney volume is a good predictive biomarker for the development of future glomerular filtration rate (GFR) loss, with potential application in clinical practice.

Hematuria, whether gross or microscopic, occurs in about 35% to 50% of patients, and typically occurs before the loss of kidney function. It is associated with increased kidney size and with worse kidney outcomes. Hematuria can be precipitated by an acute event such as trauma, heavy exertion, cyst rupture, lower urinary tract infection, pyelonephritis, cyst infection, or nephrolithiasis. Therefore, ADPKD patients are typically advised to avoid heavy and high-impact exercise. Cyst hemorrhage occurs more commonly as kidneys enlarge, and may be associated with hematuria and fever, but often localized pain is the only presenting complaint. The diagnosis of a cyst hemorrhage is based on clinical evaluation and can be difficult to differentiate from renal cyst infection. CT scan can occasionally be helpful in locating hemorrhagic cysts. The management for uncomplicated cyst hemorrhage and hematuria is supportive, and includes hydration, rest, pain control, and often withholding antihypertensive medications until the acute episode has resolved.

Lower urinary tract infections are common among ADPKD patients, as in the general population, with coliforms being the most common pathogens. The treatment is the same as in the general population. Pyelonephritis and renal cyst infections can occur and may be challenging to differentiate. With cyst infections, patients present with fever and flank pain. Typically, blood cultures more often identify the offending pathogen than urine cultures. Most important, treatment of cyst infections requires a prolonged course of 4 weeks with antibiotics that adequately penetrate into the cyst, such as quinolones, vancomycin, chloramphenicol, or trimethoprim-sulfamethoxazole. Recent reports have suggested that Positron Emission Tomography with fluorodeoxyglucose (FDG-PET) may be a promising diagnostic tool for detecting infected cysts in challenging cases.

The incidence of nephrolithiasis is about 5 to 10 times higher among patients with ADPKD compared to the general population. About 25% of those afflicted with kidney stones are symptomatic. Both anatomic deformities and metabolic disturbances including hypocitraturia account for the high incidence of nephrolithiasis. The most common stone type in ADPKD is uric acid, accounting for approximately 50% of all stones, followed by calcium oxalate. Nephrolithiasis should be suspected in any ADPKD patient with acute flank pain. Diagnosis by imaging is difficult given the radiolucent nature of the stones and the presence of calcified cyst walls. Noncontrast CT remains the imaging modality of choice for detecting nephrolithiasis. The medical management of nephrolithiasis in ADPKD is similar to that in non-ADPKD patients. Noninvasive or minimally invasive interventions such as shock-wave lithotripsy and percutaneous nephrolithotomy have been performed on ADPKD patients, however long-term studies regarding safety in this patient population are lacking.

Patients with ADPKD most often complain of increased thirst, polyuria, nocturia, and urinary frequency. A decrease in urinary concentrating ability is one of the earliest manifestations of ADPKD. It is initially mild and worsens with increasing age and declining kidney function. The renal concentrating defect is closely related to the severity of anatomic deformities induced by the cysts, independent of age and GFR. Approximately 60% of affected children demonstrated a decreased response to desmopressin, possibly because of disruption of tubular architecture and alterations in principal cell function.

Pain in ADPKD can be acute or chronic, and is the most common symptom found in ADPKD. Acute episodes are usually related to cyst rupture, cyst or parenchymal infection, and nephrolithiasis. Chronic pain, on the other hand, is typically related to the massive enlargement of the kidneys and liver, and their increased weight. The site of pain can be the lower back, as increased lumbar lordosis has been observed in ADPKD patients. Pain can also be a result of the stretching of the renal capsule or pedicle. Pain management can be challenging, but should include nonpharmacologic as well as pharmacologic interventions.

Hypertension is a common and early manifestation of ADPKD affecting more than 60% of patients before any detectable decline in kidney function. It is the presenting sign of ADPKD in approximately 30% of cases. The average age of onset is 29 years. Studies showed that hypertension occurs earlier and tends to be more severe among *PKD1* versus *PKD2* patients. Hypertension is also associated with a greater rate of kidney enlargement (6.2%/yr vs. 4.5%/yr), suggesting a relationship between cyst expansion and elevations in blood pressure. ADPKD kidneys have an attenuated vasculature with angiographic evidence of intrarenal arteriolar tapering. MRI-based measurements of renal blood flow demonstrate a reduction of blood flow that correlates inversely with kidney volume, and occurs before loss of kidney function. All these findings suggest that renal ischemia induced by cyst expansion plays a role in the etiology of hypertension, and studies have confirmed the intrarenal activation of the renin-angiotensin-aldosterone system. Despite these findings, there is currently no clear evidence that the use of angiotensin converting enzyme (ACE) inhibitors or angiotensin receptor blockers (ARB) is more effective than other antihypertensive agents in delaying the progression of ADPKD to ESRD. Similarly, the optimal blood pressure for ADPKD patients is unknown. The HALT PKD clinical trial that began enrolling patients in 2006 will determine whether rigorous control of blood pressure (≤110/75 vs. ≤130/80)

or maximal inhibition of the renin-angiotensin system (ACE inhibitor + ARB vs. ACE inhibitor + placebo) is effective in slowing progression of ADPKD.

Kidney function among ADPKD patients remains normal for decades despite significant cyst expansion and kidney enlargement. After kidney function becomes impaired, progression is typically universal and rapid, with an average decline in GFR of 4.0 to 5.0 mL/min/yr. There are a number of predictors for progression to ESRD in ADPKD, such as male gender, *PKD1* genotype, early age of onset of hypertension, and the presence of detectable proteinuria. Total kidney volume incorporates all of the aforementioned risk factors, and is the strongest predictor of future GFR loss. Proteinuria is typically mild in ADPKD with an average of 260 mg of protein excretion per day, with only 18% of ADPKD adults having greater than 300 mg/day of protein excretion.

Kidney transplantation remains a viable option for patients approaching ESRD. ADPKD transplant recipients tend to survive longer than those transplanted for other kidney pathologies. Native polycystic kidneys do not have to be removed before transplantation unless chronic infections are present or their large size interferes with nutritional intake or quality of life.

EXTRARENAL MANIFESTATIONS

POLYCYSTIC LIVER DISEASE

Hepatic cysts are the most common extrarenal manifestation in ADPKD. MRI shows presence of hepatic cysts in more than 80% of patients by the age of 30 (Fig. 41.3) with equal gender representation. The hepatic cyst burden, however, is greater in women than in men. Previous estrogen or progesterone exposure either through birth-control pills, hormone replacement therapy, or pregnancy is associated with significant polycystic liver disease. Hepatic function is preserved even in the presence of massive liver cystic disease, and

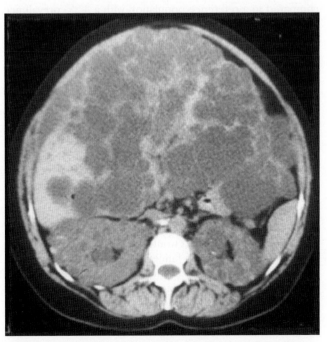

Figure 41.3 CT scan with evidence of kidney and liver cysts in autosomal dominant polycystic kidney disease.

standard biochemical tests are normal except for mild elevation in the serum concentration of alkaline phosphatase. Isolated autosomal dominant polycystic liver disease (ADPLD) without renal cysts exists. ADPLD is a distinct disease, genetically unrelated to ADPKD, instead linked to mutations in two genes: *PRKCSH* (protein kinase C substrate 80K-H) located on chromosome 19, and *SEC 63* located on chromosome 6.

Hepatic enlargement is the predominant complication resulting in symptoms of shortness of breath, pain, early satiety, decreased mobility, ankle swelling, and rarely inferior vena cava compression. This severe form of polycystic liver disease is unusual, occurring in fewer than 10% of all cases. It predominantly affects women and may require surgical cyst deroofing, fenestration, resection, or, in extreme cases, liver transplantation. Recently, the use of somatostatin analogues in the treatment of polycystic liver disease appears to be beneficial. In a small single-center double-blind, placebo-controlled trial of long-acting somatostatin (Octreotide), the investigators showed that over a 12-month period, liver volumes decreased by $4.95 \pm 6.77\%$ in the active drug group compared to placebo. Importantly, somatostatin was well tolerated, and patients experienced an improved perception of bodily pain and physical activity. Mammalian target of rapamycin (mTOR) inhibitors have also generated a lot of interest: an observational study in ADPKD kidney transplant recipients showed that those who were treated with sirolimus had a reduction in polycystic liver volumes by 12% compared to an increase of 14% among patients not receiving sirolimus. The ELATE trial is a randomized, open-label clinical trial that will compare the effect of the mTOR inhibitor everolimus and Octreotide to Octreotide alone on polycystic liver disease during a 12-month period.

CARDIOVASCULAR MANIFESTATIONS

Intracranial aneurysms (ICAs) are the most feared complication of ADPKD. A study showed that ADPKD patients have an adjusted prevalence ratio of 6.9 for unruptured ICAs when compared to a reference population with a 3.2% prevalence of ICAs. ICAs cluster in specific ADPKD families, and occur in 10% of individuals with a family history of a nonruptured ICA and 20% of individuals with a family history of a ruptured ICA. The aneurysms occur most often in the anterior circulation, and multiple ICAs are common in ADPKD patients, similar to what is observed among non-ADPKD familial ICAs. Individuals who underwent screening with magnetic resonance angiography (MRA) and were found to be aneurysm free did not demonstrate a new ICA when screened 7 years later. Ruptured aneurysms contribute to 4% to 7% of deaths among ADPKD patients, and they are associated with an immediate mortality of more than 50% and permanent morbidity of more than 80%. Screening is indicated in asymptomatic patients with a positive family history for ICA or previous history of intracranial hemorrhage, those with high-risk occupations, or before major elective surgery that would affect intracranial hemodynamics. Persons without a family history of ICAs and without these additional concerns do not warrant routine screening. The imaging modality of choice for screening is time-of-flight three-dimensional MRA. Although gadolinium has been used for arteriographic imaging, the occurrence of nephrogenic systemic fibrosis makes routine use of gadolinium particularly complicated in those with impaired kidney function. Moreover, contrast is not needed to visualize accurately the circle of Willis. Although rupture of an ICA is associated with significant morbidity and mortality, only 50% of ADPKD individuals with ICAs have a rupture during their lifetimes. Postoperative complications related to surgical clipping are common, and recovery from elective surgery can be prolonged. For larger aneurysms (greater than 10 mm), the risk of rupture is significantly increased, and the anticipated complications from rupture outweigh the benefits of nonintervention; elective surgical intervention is recommended in these cases. For asymptomatic unruptured ICAs between 5 and 10 mm, the management is controversial and should be individualized in consultation with the treating neurosurgeon and neuroradiologist. Monitoring the rate of growth of these ICAs with periodic imaging is warranted. For those with an ICA smaller than 5 mm, longitudinal studies have not demonstrated significant growth of the ICA, and the risk of rupture is relatively small. Risk factors for aneurysmal growth include smoking and hypertension, and counseling about smoking cessation as well as good blood-pressure control are warranted as part of conservative management of ICA. The current indications for surgical repair of these smaller ICAs are unclear. With the development of less invasive therapies (i.e., coiling or stenting), alternative treatment of small, asymptomatic ICAs may become available.

Left ventricular hypertrophy (LVH) using echocardiographic imaging is common in ADPKD patients, and it has been reported in as many as 48% of hypertensives. More recent data derived from the HALT-PKD study using cardiac MRI in a contemporary cohort of hypertensive ADPKD patients younger than 50 years of age showed a much lower incidence of LVH (less than 4%). However, studies have shown that those with normal blood pressure and preserved kidney function have increased left ventricular mass index (LVMI) and diastolic dysfunction as well. Patients with hypertension who are nondippers (i.e., have elevated nighttime blood pressure) have greater LVMI and total kidney volume than those who are dippers.

Other cardiovascular manifestations of ADPKD include intracoronary aneurysms and mitral valve prolapse and regurgitation occur in 26% of individuals, compared with 3% of the general population. Aortic insufficiency also occurs more frequently (11%) in people with ADPKD.

EFFECTS ON FERTILITY AND PREGNANCY

Overall, fertility rates in ADPKD men and women not yet on dialysis are similar to those in the general population despite a higher incidence of ectopic pregnancies, congenital absence of the seminiferous tubules, and immotile spermatozoa. Affected women with a normal GFR and normal blood pressure experience pregnancy outcomes similar to those of the general population. Hypertensive ADPKD women have a higher incidence of worsening hypertension and preeclampsia during pregnancy, and they have a higher rate of premature delivery. Those with a decreased GFR before pregnancy are at high risk for midgestation fetal loss and progressive loss of kidney function.

AUTOSOMAL DOMINANT POLYCYSTIC KIDNEY DISEASE IN CHILDREN

Children with ADPKD are usually asymptomatic, with only about 1% to 2% of patients presenting with symptoms before the age of 15 years. Longitudinal studies of ADPKD children show a progressive increase in kidney size, which is more significant among those having borderline or overt hypertension. Glomerular hyperfiltration has also been demonstrated in children early in the course of ADPKD, and this has recently been linked to a greater rate of kidney growth and a significantly faster decline in kidney function.

Other kidney manifestations in children include urinary concentrating defects affecting about 60%. Proteinuria is usually low grade and relatively uncommon; however, it is more common in affected children than in adults. Thirty percent of children have microalbuminuria and 23% have overt proteinuria, as compared to 25% and 17% of adults, respectively. Similar to the adult population, proteinuria in children with ADPKD correlates with diastolic hypertension and a more severe cystic kidney disease.

Studies in children with ADPKD show that hypertension is the earliest and most prevalent systemic feature occurring in up to 44% of cases, and it correlates with increased kidney volumes. Moreover, ADPKD children demonstrate abnormal circadian blood pressures with increased nighttime blood pressures. Other cardiovascular abnormalities found in affected children include mitral valve prolapse, increased LVMI, and hyperlipidemia, defined as a fasting cholesterol or triglyceride level above the 95th percentile for age and gender. Although rare among children, cases of ruptured cerebral aneurysms have been reported.

Extrarenal manifestations in children include hepatic cysts, which are typically benign. Rare cases of congenital hepatic fibrosis have been described in children with ADPKD.

At-risk offspring should have regular blood-pressure measurements and urinalyses. However, there are no guidelines for systematic screening of asymptomatic ADPKD children.

THERAPY

Randomized, controlled clinical trials evaluating ACE inhibitors, rigorous blood-pressure control, and dietary protein restriction have failed to demonstrate statistically significant kidney protection in ADPKD when studied late in the course of disease. Other dietary modifications, including abstinence from caffeine and increased water intake, have been suggested but not formally tested in prospective, randomized clinical trials. However, the trials performed have been inadequately designed or powered to definitely determine whether the therapies tested are effective. A metaanalysis of randomized, controlled trials involving at least 142 hypertensive patients with ADPKD showed that ACE inhibitors were associated with significant slowing in GFR loss and decrease in urinary protein excretion in those with greater degrees of proteinuria.

Current recommendations for target blood-pressure level and the initial pharmacologic therapy for ADPKD are based on the Seventh Joint National Committee (JNC7) recommendations for all patients with chronic kidney disease, targeting blood pressure below 130/80 mm Hg using ACE inhibitors or ARB. The HALT PKD clinical trial, which enrolled 1443 hypertensive patients starting in 2006, will determine whether more aggressive control of blood pressure (≤110/75 vs. ≤130/80 mm Hg) or maximal inhibition of the renin-angiotensin system (ACE inhibitor + ARB vs. ACE inhibitor + placebo) is effective in slowing progression of ADPKD.

A promising therapy aimed at reducing intracellular cAMP accumulation by blocking the vasopressin V_2 receptor has successfully retarded renal cyst progression in four distinct genetic forms of cystic disease: the PKD2 WS25 mouse, the Han: SPRD rat, the pcy mouse (a mouse model for familial juvenile nephronophthisis), and the polycystic kidney (pck) rat (a murine model for autosomal recessive polycystic kidney disease). Phase II studies of vasopressin V_2 receptor antagonists in ADPKD subjects demonstrate effective inhibition of the V_2 receptor, resulting in decreased water reabsorption and urinary osmolality over 24 hours. This medication is well tolerated, with patients maintaining serum sodium concentrations and tolerating mild increases in the frequency of nocturia. The Tolvaptan Efficacy and Safety Management of Autosomal Dominant Polycystic Kidney Disease and its Outcomes (TEMPO) 3:4 trial is a phase 3, randomized, double-blind, placebo-controlled trial that was recently completed. Among 1445 participants, and over 3 years of follow-up, the tolvaptan-treated group had a slower rate of kidney volume growth (2.8% vs. 5.5%). The slope of kidney function decline, measured as the reciprocal of the serum creatinine, also favored tolvaptan. It is worth mentioning that aside from expected side effects related to aquaresis in the tolvaptan group, a larger proportion of participants had liver enzyme elevations when compared to the placebo group. These abnormalities were reversed when the drug was discontinued.

Other small, prospective studies evaluating somatostatin (another inhibitor of intracellular cAMP accumulation through inhibition of the G protein and adenylate cyclase pathway) in a randomized, placebo-controlled fashion have demonstrated reduction in the rate of increase in kidney volume in 12 ADPKD patients treated for 6 months compared with controls (2.2 ± 3.7% vs. 5.9 ± 5.4%; P less than 0.05). Recent evidence indicates that normal polycystin 1 interacts with the tuberous sclerosis complex (TSC1/TSC2), and this interaction plays a role in the inhibition of mTOR activity. In support of these findings, the inhibitor of mTOR, sirolimus, has been shown to decrease kidney cyst burden in the Han: SPRD rat. ADPKD patients who received sirolimus for kidney transplantation demonstrate a significant decline in the size of their native kidneys through time.

However, two recent trials of mTOR inhibitor use in ADPKD patients failed to show the anticipated benefit on kidney disease progression. In an 18-month open-label, randomized controlled trial, 100 patients with early polycystic kidney disease were assigned to receive sirolimus versus standard of care. At the conclusion of this study, the investigators found that sirolimus therapy had no effect on kidney volume growth or GFR. However, the sirolimus dose used in this study was extremely low, raising the possibility that the drug dose chosen limited its efficacy.

In another 2-year, double-blind trial, 433 patients with ADPKD were randomly assigned to receive everolimus versus placebo. At the conclusion of this trial, everolimus was found to slow the increase in total kidney volume of ADPKD patients, but not the progression of GFR loss. In fact, the everolimus group experienced a greater decline in the estimated GFR. Additionally, at the end of the 2-year study, proteinuria had significantly increased in the everolimus-treated group when compared to the placebo group. Finally, everolimus use was associated with a high rate of serious adverse events (37.4% of patients who received at least one dose of the drug) and an extremely high rate of study withdrawal (greater than 35%).

AUTOSOMAL RECESSIVE POLYCYSTIC KIDNEY DISEASE

Autosomal recessive polycystic kidney disease (ARPKD) affects 1 in 20,000 live births. Its etiology is linked to mutations in the polycystic kidney and hepatic disease (PKHD) gene located on the short arm of chromosome 6 (6p21.1). The gene encodes for a protein product called fibrocystin (or polyductin), an integral membrane protein of 4074 amino acid with a large extracellular N-terminal and a short cytoplasmic tail. The function of fibrocystin remains to be fully elucidated, but is believed to be a receptor protein involved in the regulation of cellular adhesion, repulsion, proliferation, and/or regulation and maintenance of renal collecting tubules and hepatic biliary ducts. Fibrocystin colocalizes in centrosomes, basal bodies, and primary cilia of epithelial cells.

Mutations have been identified in 42% to 65% of cases. Homozygous mutations that predict immediate stop codons or truncated proteins lead to the most severe phenotype, and are associated with increased perinatal mortality. In a study of 78 ARPKD children with a predominantly mild phenotype, sequence variations confirmed missense mutations in 79% of cases. In the absence of a functional assay or a crystallized structure of fibrocystin, the pathogenicity of such missense mutations remains challenging. Importantly, there is significant variability in the severity of kidney disease among patients carrying the same PKHD1 mutation within the same family, suggesting that modifier genes and environmental factors may play contributory roles. The use of PKHD1 sequencing data for clinical decision making or prenatal counseling is currently limited.

ARPKD is characterized by fibrocystic renal and hepatic involvement of variable severity. The renal cystic disease is a result of fusiform dilatation of renal collecting tubules. Up to 90% of collecting tubules are involved, explaining in part the large variability in the renal phenotype. Unlike ADPKD cysts, the cystic lesions in ARPKD continue to retain their connection to the parent nephron.

In ARPKD, the kidneys are typically enlarged with poor cortical/medullary differentiation. About 50% of ARPKD patients progress to ESRD within the first decade of life. High-resolution ultrasonography is more sensitive in detecting renal pathology limited to the medulla. The presence of imaging anomalies limited to the medulla is associated with a milder kidney disease and predicts preserved kidney function, as opposed to corticomedullary anomalies that tend to present perinatally and are associated with a faster decline in kidney function. In a recent study of 73 patients with ARPKD, a significant but moderate inverse correlation was demonstrated between kidney volume and function.

The liver disease in ARPKD consists of biliary dysgenesis and periportal fibrosis known as congenital hepatic fibrosis, which leads to portal hypertension with subsequent splenomegaly and esophageal varices. Dilation of intrahepatic (Caroli syndrome) and extrahepatic bile ducts can predispose to recurrent ascending cholangitis.

The majority of patients with ARPKD are identified in utero or at birth. Fetuses with severe cases have large echogenic kidneys and oligohydramnios due to poor urinary output, which results in the Potter phenotype with pulmonary hypoplasia and deformed facies, spine, and limbs. In this setting, pulmonary hypoplasia and sepsis are the leading causes of mortality among newborns, with the former accounting for 25% to 30% of deaths. Growth retardation is common among ARPKD children and cannot be solely attributed to chronic kidney disease or lung disease. Hyponatremia has been reported in 26% of neonates diagnosed with ARPKD.

Hypertension is diagnosed in up to 80% of children with ARPKD and is usually associated with reduced GFR. Studies in animal models of ARPKD suggest intrarenal renin and ACE upregulation. The treatment of hypertension includes salt restriction and blockade of the renin-angiotensin-aldosterone system.

The minority of patients are identified with ARPKD later during childhood. Their presenting feature is typically hepatosplenomegaly with predominant liver complications. Hepatic involvement rarely leads to hepatocellular damage with synthetic dysfunction. However, portal hypertension usually develops between the ages of 5 and 10. Therapy includes portosystemic shunts for esophageal varices. Children with advanced liver disease may be eligible for liver or combined kidney-liver transplantation.

TUBEROUS SCLEROSIS COMPLEX

Tuberous sclerosis complex (TSC) is an autosomal dominant disorder that affects approximately 1 in 5800 births. TSC results from either a mutation in the TSC1 gene located on chromosome 9q34 or the TSC2 gene located on chromosome 16p13. Interestingly, TSC2 is adjacent to the PKD1 gene, and a contiguous deletion involving both genes results in a severe, early onset polycystic phenotype.

About 70% to 80% of patients with TSC have no family history of the disorder, suggesting a high rate of spontaneous mutations, most of which involve TSC2 and are associated with a more severe phenotype. TSC1 mutations are twice as likely to occur in familial cases. TSC1 and TSC2 are tumor suppressor genes, and, consistent with the two-hit hypothesis, a mutation in both alleles of either gene is required for characteristic lesions to form. TSC1 encodes TSC1 (or hamartin), a 140 kD protein composed of 1164 amino acids, whereas TSC2 encodes TSC2 (or tuberin), a 200 kD protein composed of 1807 amino acids. TSC1 and TSC2 are coexpressed in the cells of numerous organs including the kidney, brain, lung, and pancreas. Both gene products are tightly bound into a heterodimer with tumor suppressor activity. By 2003, the role of hamartin and tuberin in the inhibitory regulation of the mTOR was elucidated. The mTOR pathway has a key role in regulating protein production, cell growth and proliferation, and angiogenesis. Under normal conditions, protein kinase (Akt)–mediated inactivation of tuberin results in degradation of the tuberin-hamartin complex, allowing mTOR signaling. In TSC cases, allelic mutations in either TSC1 or TSC2 followed by a second hit in the unaffected allele result in disruption of the tuberin-hamartin complex, allowing unregulated mTOR activity.

Clinically, TSC is characterized by the growth of benign tumors in different organ systems that ultimately lead to organ dysfunction. In 1998, the National Institutes of Health sponsored a TSC consensus conference that led to the establishment of clinical diagnostic criteria. For a diagnosis of TSC, a patient should have two major features or one major plus one minor feature. Major features include facial angiofibromas or forehead plaques, nontraumatic ungulas or periungal fibromas, hypomelanotic macules, Shagreen patches, multiple retinal nodular hamartomas, cortical tubers, subependymal nodules, subependymal giant cell astrocytomas, cardiac rhabdomyomas, lymphangiomyomatosis, and renal angiomyolipomas. Minor features include pits in the dental enamel, hamartomatous rectal polyps, bone cysts, cerebral white matter radial migration lines, gingival fibromas, nonrenal hamartomas, retinal achromic patches, confetti-skin lesions, and multiple renal cysts. Most features of the disease become evident only after about 3 years of age. Approximately 85% of TSC patients experience CNS complications that include epilepsy, cognitive impairment, behavioral disorders, or autism. Kidney manifestations are the second most common findings. Fifty percent of patients have renal cystic disease, and 80% have angiomyolipomas. Angiomyolipomas are also thought to underlie the pathogenesis of lymphangioleiomyomatosis (LAM), a devastating pulmonary complication that occurs almost exclusively among women leading to cystic and interstitial lung disease, pneumothoraxes, and chylous pleural effusions.

Hemorrhage from renal angiomyolipomas is the most common cause of death and kidney failure in adults with TSC. After these lesions reach more than 4 cm in size, the risk of bleeding increases significantly. About 20% of patients who present with hemorrhage to the emergency room are in shock. The abundant abnormal vascular structures in these tumors make them prone to aneurysmal formation, and the risk of bleeding increases substantially after aneurysms enlarge beyond 5 mm in diameter. Currently the standard of care to control active bleeding or to prevent bleeding from angiomyolipomas is arterial embolization. Postembolectomy syndrome occurs during the first 48 hours following procedure in most cases, manifests as nausea, pain, fever, and hemodynamic instability, and can be treated with corticosteroids. The aim of any surgical or embolization intervention is to preserve kidney tissue.

Given that disinhibition of the mTOR pathway is central to the pathogenesis of TSC, recent clinical trials have looked at the use of mTOR inhibitors in the treatment of angiomyolipomas as well as other manifestations of TSC. These early trials suggest that the use of mTOR inhibitors is relatively safe and induces a regression in the size of kidney and liver angiomyolipomas, subependymal giant cell astrocytomas, and lymphangioleiomyomas.

VON HIPPEL-LINDAU DISEASE

Von Hippel-Lindau (VHL) disease is a rare autosomal dominant disorder that affects about 1 in 36,000 live births. It is characterized by multiorgan tumors including retinal and central nervous system (CNS) hemangioblastomas, clear cell renal carcinomas, pheochromocytomas, pancreatic islet tumors, and endolymphatic sac tumors. The diagnosis of VHL is based on clinical findings. With a positive family history, the recognition of one of the abovementioned tumors establishes the diagnosis, whereas in the absence of a family history the diagnosis requires the presence of two tumors. About 20% of VHL cases arise from de novo mutations.

The *VHL* gene was mapped to the short arm of chromosome 3 and encodes two proteins: $pVHL_{30}$, a 30kD protein made up of 213 amino acid, and $pVHL_{19}$, a 19 kD protein lacking the first 53 amino acids. Both proteins seem to have similar function. *VHL* is a tumor suppressor gene, and in accordance with the two hit hypothesis, a biallelic mutation is required for tumors to develop. To date, some genotype-phenotype correlations have been established with most renal cell carcinoma (RCC) cases arising from truncating or exon deletion mutations.

The role of pVHL has progressively been elucidated. Under normoxic conditions, pVHL binds to the α subunit of the hypoxia inducible factors (HIF) 1 and 2, and plays an important role in their ubiquitylation and proteosomal degradation. Alternatively, under hypoxic conditions, or when pVHL is inactive or absent (due to a gene mutation), HIF 1 and 2 are stabilized and activate a series of target genes involved in angiogenesis, proliferation, apoptosis, and metabolism such as vascular endothelial growth factor (VEGF), platelet-derived growth factor (PDGF), erythropoietin, etc. This may in part explain the vascular nature of tumors characteristic of VHL disease. More recently, pVHL has been shown to interact with microtubules. This interaction is important for primary cilia maintenance, and it protects from kidney cyst formation by stabilizing microtubules and orienting microtubule growth.

VHL disease is clinically characterized by the development of benign and malignant tumors in many organs. CNS hemangioblastomas occur in 60% to 80% of VHL patients and most commonly occur in the cerebellum, spinal cord, and brain stem. Although benign in nature, hemangioblastomas enlarge with time and cause symptoms related to increased intracranial pressure and mass effect. When symptomatic, they are best treated by surgical removal. Retinal angiomas are identical histopathologically to CNS hemangioblastomas, and are the most common presenting feature of VHL disease. They tend to be bilateral and can lead to vision loss in 35% to 55% of cases. Most lesions respond well to laser photocoagulation. RCCs are an important cause of death in VHL patients. The lifetime risk of RCC varies based on the VHL mutation but can be as high as 70%. Most RCCs are clear cell and tend to be multifocal and bilateral. The best management strategy remains close surveillance for RCCs with serial imaging until the tumor reaches 3 cm in size. Beyond 3 cm, the risk of metastasis increases, and kidney-sparing surgery or ablation is recommended. Pheochromocytomas are seen in 7% to 20% of patients, and the risk varies based on the underlying mutation. They tend to be bilateral, occur at a young age, and can be extraadrenal. Asymptomatic VHL patients scheduled for elective surgery should be screened for pheochromocytomas to prevent hemodynamic and cardiac complications associated with anesthesia and surgery. Endolymphatic sac tumors arise from the membranous labyrinth of the inner ear and when bilateral are pathognomonic of VHL. They can lead to tinnitus, vertigo, and hearing loss. Pancreatic cysts are common but rarely lead to organ dysfunction. Pancreatic tumors occur in 5% to 10% of cases and are usually nonsecretory islet cell tumors. Surgery is indicated when these tumors reach a size greater than 3 cm.

ACQUIRED CYSTIC KIDNEY DISEASE

Acquired cystic kidney disease (ACKD) refers to the development of cysts during a period of chronic kidney disease or ESRD. Its diagnosis requires the presence of at least three cysts in each kidney in a patient with no family history or clinical features of other cystic kidney diseases. Kidneys are usually small or normal in size, and the cysts tend to be of different morphology and size, although classically they are less than 3 cm.

The prevalence of ACKD varies between 8% and 13% among patients initiating renal replacement therapy, increases with the number of years on dialysis, and is higher among males and African Americans. The occurrence of ACKD does not seem to differ based on the dialysis modality.

Most patients with ACKD are asymptomatic, but cysts can rupture causing hematuria or retroperitoneal hemorrhage with flank pain. This later complication occurs mostly in patients on hemodialysis, likely related to the concomitant use of anticoagulation.

RCCs remain the most feared complication affecting about 3% to 6% of patients with ACKD. The tumors tend to occur at a younger age and are more frequently multifocal and bilateral when compared to sporadic RCCs. Papillary cell carcinomas are the most common histologic variant of RCCs in ACKD as compared to clear cell carcinomas in sporadic cases.

More recently, two tumor types exclusive to ACKD patients have been described. Together they represent 60% of ACKD associated RCCs. The first tumor is acquired cystic disease-associated RCC characterized by a well-circumscribed, dense fibrous capsule that separates the tumor from surrounding kidney tissue. The hallmark of this tumor is the presence of oxalate crystals seen under the polarizing microscope. The second type of tumor is the clear cell papillary RCC seen among ESRD patients with or without ACKD. Here again, deposition of oxalate crystals is common. These two types of tumors are distinguished by morphology, cytogenetics, and immunohistochemistry. The theory behind the development of these tumors is that kidney failure leads to cyst and scar formation, and is accompanied by decreased oxalate clearance. The deposition and crystallization of oxalate triggers an oxidative injury leading to genomic damage that in turn stimulates cyst epithelial hyperplasia and tumorigenesis.

To date, there are no clear recommendations regarding the screening of ESRD patients for ACKD and RCC. A decision analysis model showed that screening provides significant benefits only for patients with a life expectancy of at least 25 years. It may, however, be beneficial to screen high-risk individuals (i.e., young, males, African Americans, patients on dialysis for more than 3 years). Ultrasound is a good screening modality, but CT or MRI is more sensitive and recommended for patients that have signs or symptoms suggestive of carcinoma (e.g., hematuria, unexplained anemia, back pain). When detected, tumors larger than 3 cm are treated surgically with total nephrectomy.

Screening guidelines for kidney-transplant candidates or recipients are equally controversial. A study that included 516 patients following kidney transplantation determined a prevalence of RCC of about 5%, and almost all cases were diagnosed in the setting of ACKD of the native kidneys. Risk factors for RCCs in that study included older age, male sex, history of heart disease, larger kidneys, and the presence of renal calcifications. The prevalence of ACKD posttransplant was lower than among ESRD patients, suggesting that better kidney function and/or immunosuppressive therapies may have a negative influence on cyst formation. Given the increasing life expectancy after kidney transplantation and the potential for curative surgical intervention, the screening guidelines may soon be revisited.

BIBLIOGRAPHY

Bonsib S: Renal cystic diseases and renal neoplasms: a mini-review, *CJASN* 4:1998-2007, 2009.

Budde K, Gaedeke J: Tuberous sclerosis complex-associated angiomyolipomas: focus on mTOR inhibition, *AJKD* 59:276-283, 2012.

Chapman AB, Torres VE, Perrone RD, et al: The HALT polycystic kidney disease trials: design and implementation, *CJASN* 5:102-109, 2010.

Dabora SL, Franz DN, Ashwal S, et al: Multicenter phase 2 trial of sirolimus for tuberous sclerosis: kidney angiomyolipomas and other tumors regress and VEGF-D levels decrease, *PLoS One* 6:e23379, 2011.

Fleming S: Renal cell carcinoma in acquired cystic kidney disease, *Histopathology* 56:395-400, 2010.

Goto M, Hoxha N, Osman R, et al: The renin-angiotensin system and hypertension in autosomal recessive polycystic kidney disease, *Pediatr Nephrol* 25:2449-2457, 2010.

Grantham JJ, Torres VE, Chapman AB, et al: CRISP Investigators: volume progression in polycystic kidney disease, *N Engl J Med* 354:2122-2130, 2006.

Guay-Woodford LM, Desmond RA: Autosomal recessive polycystic kidney disease: the clinical experience in North America, *Pediatrics* 111:1072-1080, 2003.

Gunay-Aygun M, Tuchman M, Font-Montgomery E, et al: *PKHD1* sequence variations in 78 children and adults with autosomal recessive polycystic kidney disease and congenital hepatic fibrosis, *Mol Genet Metab* 99:160-173, 2010.

Hyman M, Whittemore VH: National Institutes of Health Consensus Conference: tuberous sclerosis complex, *Arch Neurol* 57:662-665, 2000.

Krueger DA, Care MM, Holland K, et al: Everolimus for subependymal giant-cell astrocytomas in tuberous sclerosis, *N Engl J Med* 363:1801-1811, 2010.

Maher ER, Neumann HPH, Richard S: von Hippel-Lindau disease: a clinical and scientific review, *Eur J Hum Gen* 19:617-623, 2011.

Pei Y, Obaki J, Dupuis A, et al: Unified criteria for ultrasonographic diagnosis of ADPKD, *JASN* 20:205-212, 2009.

Schwarz A, Vatandaslar S, Merkel S, et al: Renal cell carcinoma in transplant recipients with acquired cystic kidney disease, *CJASN* 2:750-756, 2007.

Serra AL, Poster D, Kistler AD, et al: Sirolimus and kidney growth in autosomal dominant polycystic kidney disease, *N Engl J Med* 363:820-829, 2010.

Shneider BL, Magid MS: Liver disease in autosomal recessive polycystic kidney disease, *Pediatr Transplant* 9:634-639, 2005.

Sweeney WE, Avner ED: Molecular and cellular pathophysiology of autosomal recessive polycystic kidney disease (ARPKD), *Cell Tissue Res* 326:671-685, 2006.

Thoma CR, Matov A, Gutbrodt KL, et al: Quantitative image analysis identifies pVHL as a key regulator of microtubule dynamic instability, *J Cell Biol* 190:991-1003, 2010.

Torres VE, Chapman AB, Devuyst O, et al, for the TEMPO 3:4 Trial Investigators: Tolvaptan in patients with autosomal dominant polycystic kidney disease, *N Engl J Med* 367:2407-2418, 2012.

Walz G, Budde K, Mannaa M, et al: Everolimus in patients with autosomal dominant polycystic kidney disease, *N Engl J Med* 363:830-840, 2010.

Yamakado K, Tanaka N, Nakagawa T, et al: Renal angiomyolipoma: relationships between tumor size, aneurysm formation and rupture, *Radiology* 225:78-82S, 2002.

Nephronophthisis and Medullary Cystic Kidney Disease

42

John F. O'Toole | Friedhelm Hildebrandt

Nephronophthisis (NPHP) and medullary cystic kidney disease (MCKD) represent two groups of rare genetic kidney diseases that share similar renal histopathology. NPHP and MCKD can be distinguished by their inheritance pattern and usually by age of onset. NPHP has an autosomal recessive inheritance pattern and results in end-stage renal disease (ESRD) within the first three decades of life. To date, 13 causative genes have been identified. MCKD, on the other hand, has an autosomal dominant inheritance pattern and generally results in ESRD between the fourth to seventh decades of life. There are two known genetic etiologies (Table 42.1).

EPIDEMIOLOGY

Nephronophthisis has long been recognized as a rare cause of ESRD worldwide, but is one of the most common genetic causes of ESRD in the pediatric population. Historically, the incidence of NPHP alone has been quoted as between 1 in 50,000 to 1,000,000 live births. The prevalence of these diseases may be an underestimate, considering that patients often come to clinical attention only after reaching ESRD, and a definitive diagnosis may not be established. In addition, the urinalysis in these disorders is typically bland, without significant proteinuria or hematuria, making aggressive diagnostic procedures such as biopsy less likely to be pursued. Although a presumptive diagnosis of NPHP or MCKD can be made on the basis of clinical features and the renal histopathology seen on biopsy, the only way to definitively diagnose these disorders and ascertain the type (see Table 42.1) is through genetic testing, which until recently, has been unavailable.

PATHOLOGY

The similar appearance of the renal histology in NPHP and MCKD led to the historical association of these two disorders. The classic triad of renal pathology, which is shared by all of the genetic types of NPHP with the exception of NPHP type 2 (NPHP2), includes tubular atrophy with interstitial fibrosis, tubular basement membrane (TBM) disruption, and small corticomedullary cysts. Periglomerular fibrosis and sclerosis has also been noted. Cysts range in size from 1 to 15 mm, and generally arise from the distal convoluted tubule or medullary collecting duct. The kidney size is normal to reduced in these types of NPHP, and the cysts may not be apparent by imaging early in the course of the disease.

In contrast to autosomal dominant polycystic kidney disease (ADPKD), cysts have not been observed in other organs.

NPHP2, infantile nephronophthisis, is caused by mutations in INVS and has kidney pathology and a clinical course that are distinct from the other types of NPHP. NPHP2 results in ESRD in the first decade of life, often within the first 2 years, and is characterized by moderate cystic enlargement of the kidneys bilaterally. Renal pathology is characterized by more prominent cyst formation in the cortex but can also be present in the medulla. Cysts seem to arise from the proximal and distal tubules, and cystic enlargement of the glomerulus has also been noted. Tubulointerstitial nephritis is another prominent finding in NPHP2, one that it shares with the other forms of NPHP. TBM disruption is a less consistent finding in the setting of NPHP2.

The gross appearance of the kidney in MCKD is normal to slightly reduced in size, as in NPHP. The renal histopathology of MCKD is virtually indistinguishable from that of NPHP, which has led to the historic nomenclature of these diseases as the nephronophthisis-medullary cystic kidney disease complex.

PATHOGENESIS

Thirteen causative genes have been identified in NPHP (see Table 42.1). All 13 genes have a broad tissue expression pattern. Two recessive mutations in any one of these genes result in the corresponding NPHP type with complete penetrance, consistent with an autosomal recessive inheritance pattern.

The most common type of NPHP is NPHP type 1 (NPHP1), which accounts for roughly 25% of all cases. Approximately 90% of mutations in NPHP1 consist of large deletions, which typically include the entire gene. The remaining genetic causes of NPHP each account for between 1% and 4% of diagnosed cases of NPHP. The genetic etiology of a majority of NPHP cases has not yet been ascertained.

The study of the products of these 13 genes, the nephrocystins, has provided important insights into the pathogenetic mechanisms underlying NPHP. Many of the nephrocystin proteins have been shown to be present in multiprotein complexes involving other nephrocystins. The interaction among nephrocystin proteins in larger protein complexes suggest that they participate in common functional networks.

Another striking finding has been the common subcellular localization of the nephrocystin proteins to the primary

Table 42.1   Genetic Causes and Extrarenal Manifestations of Nephronophthisis and Medullary Cystic Kidney Disease

Disease	Gene Name	Chromosome	Inheritance	Mean age at kidney failure (range)*	Frequency of Involvement in Extrarenal Organ Systems (%)*				OMIM ID
					Eye	CNS	Liver	Heart	
NPHP1	NPHP1	2q13	AR	13 yr (4-20 yr)†	10	10	1	1	607100
NPHP2	INVS	9q31	AR	2 yr 1 mo (7 mo-5 yr)	17	6		25	243305
NPHP3	NPHP3	3q22	AR	8 yr 5 mo (3-13 yr)		40	20		608002
NPHP4	NPHP4	1p36	AR	17 yr (6-33 yr)	35	10	10		607215
NPHP5	IQCB1	3q21.1	AR	14 yr 10 mo (6-47 yr)	100				609237
NPHP6	CEP290	12q21.3	AR	10 yr 7 mo (2-24 yr)	88	75	6		610142
NPHP7	GLIS2	16p13.3	AR						608539
NPHP8	RPGRIP1L	16q12.2	AR	9 yr 9 mo (4-17 yr)		75	14		610937
NPHP9	NEK8	17q11.1	AR						609799
NPHP10	SDCCAG8	1q43	AR	11yr 3 mo (4-22 yr)	80	20			613524
NPHP11	TMEM67	8q21.13	AR	10 yr 9 mo (2 mo-30 yr)	50	88	78	6	609884
NPHP12	TTC21B	2q24.3	AR						613820
NPHP13	WDR19	4p14	AR						608151
MCKD1	Unknown	1q21	AD	Unknown					174000
MCKD2	UMOD	16p12.3	AD	54 yr (25-70 yr)‡					191845

CNS, Central nervous system; *OMIM*, Online Mendelian Inheritance in Man (http://www.ncbi.nlm.nih.gov/omim); *AR*, autosomal recessive; *AD*, autosomal dominant.

NOTE: NPHP types where fewer than five unique mutations have been identified do not report age at kidney failure or extrarenal organ involvement.

*Unless otherwise indicated, values derived from Hart TC, Gorry MC, Hart PS et al: Mutations of the UMOD gene are responsible for medullary cystic kidney disease 2 and familial juvenile hyperuricaemic nephropathy, J Med Genet 39:882-892, 2002.

†Values derived from Hildebrandt et al: Molecular genetic identification of families with juvenile nephronophthisis type 1: rate of progression to renal failure, Kidney Int 51:261-269, 1997

‡Values derived from Rampoldi L, Caridi G, Santon D et al: Allelism of MCKD, FJHN and GCKD caused by impairment of uromodulin export dynamics, Hum Mol Genet 12:3369-3384, 2003.

cilia/basal body/centrosome complex. The primary cilia are nonmotile and microtubule-based; these arise from the basal body in most polarized cell types and may participate in the sensation of a variety of extracellular cues (e.g., photosensation, mechanosensation, osmosensation, olfactory sensation). Localization to the primary cilia/basal body/centrosome complex is a feature the nephrocystins have in common with other renal cystoproteins, including the mutated gene products in Bardet-Biedl syndrome, autosomal dominant polycystic kidney disease, and autosomal recessive polycystic kidney disease. The common localization of many renal cystoproteins to the primary cilia/basal body/centrosome complex has led to the hypotheses that cilia/basal body/centrosome dysfunction has a central role in the pathogenesis of NPHP.

The ciliary complex transmits extracellular cues through several signaling pathways. Mutations in the NPHP genes likely disrupt effective signaling from the cilia to the cell body, and the nephrocystin proteins have been implicated in several signaling pathways important in the pathogenesis of NPHP. NPHP2/INVS has a role in the regulation of Wnt pathways that contribute to epithelial cell polarization. NPHP7/GLIS2 is a transcription factor that has a role in hedgehog signaling, and animal models of NPHP7/GLIS2 deletion demonstrate increased rates of renal tubular cell apoptosis. Furthermore, genes promoting fibrosis and epithelial-to-mesenchymal transition are upregulated. NPHP9/NEK8 is important for ciliary and centrosomal localization, which is important in cell cycle regulation. The role of nephrocystins in multiple signaling pathways highlights the importance for their coordinate function. When dysregulated, this results in a common renal histopathology of renal fibrosis and tubular atrophy characteristic of the NPHP phenotype.

The phenotype of NPHP can vary with respect to the age of onset of kidney failure, as well as the number and severity of extrarenal manifestations. As an increasing number of causative genes are identified and larger catalogs of gene specific mutations are developed, important relationships are being recognized between the disease phenotype and an individual's genotype, a concept known as genotype-phenotype correlation. Phenotypic variability has been noted with respect to the gene in which mutations are identified (i.e., locus heterogeneity). This is seen in the case of NPHP2/INV mutations, in which the age of onset of kidney failure is less than 4 years of age, or in the case of NPHP5 mutations, which are consistently associated with retinitis pigmentosa. Phenotypic variability may also been be dependent on the severity of the mutations in a given gene (i.e., multiple allelism). This is typified by the observation that two severe mutations within NPHP6 are associated with a greater number of extrarenal organ systems affected with more profound manifestations, but if at least one mutation is less severe, then the number of extrarenal organs affected is reduced and their manifestations tend to be milder. The contribution of multiple allelism to phenotypic variability tends to be less consistent than locus heterogeneity and is likely dependent on the precise location and type of mutation with respect to functional protein domains. A third genetic contribution to phenotypic variability is the concept of disease modifier genes. An example of this is found in a case in which homozygous NPHP1 deletions result in the classic presentation of renal-limited NPHP, but in combination with a single mutation in NPHP6 the disease phenotype is modified and also includes retinitis pigmentosa.

The precise pathogenetic mechanisms by which mutations in the nephrocystin proteins result in kidney disease are not known. However, as noted earlier, recent research has implicated the nephrocystins in the signaling pathways that regulate cell division and the transcriptional pathways that mediate kidney fibrosis. In general, the nephrocystin proteins seem important for the control of fibrosis in the kidney and the maintenance of the tubulointerstitial space.

Two genetic loci have been identified for MCKD, MCKD1 on 1q21 and MCKD2 on 16p12. The causative gene for MCKD1 has not yet been identified. Mutations in uromodulin, the Tamm-Horsfall protein, have been shown to cause MCKD2, familial juvenile hyperuricemic nephropathy (FJHN), and glomerulocystic kidney disease (GCKD). Uromodulin is expressed in the thick ascending limb of the loop of Henle and is the matrix protein for casts. It is the most abundant protein found in the urine. The excretion of uromodulin is reduced in these patients as a result of abnormal intracellular trafficking. Pathologic intracellular accumulation of uromodulin occurs in the tubular epithelial cells of the thick ascending limb.

CLINICAL FEATURES/DIAGNOSIS

NPHP and MCKD differ in the age of onset of kidney disease and the pattern of inheritance in familial cases (see Table 42.1). Kidney disease in NPHP will occur early, resulting in a slow decline in kidney function toward ESRD within the first 3 decades of life. The earliest clinical manifestation of NPHP is a urinary concentrating defect leading to the clinical symptoms of polyuria, polydipsia, and enuresis. These findings may precede the onset of reduced kidney function, anemia, and growth retardation, which occur later

in the course of the disease. A family history demonstrating an autosomal recessive inheritance pattern is strongly suggestive of the diagnosis, but given the rarity of the disease, sporadic cases are more common.

Historically, the age of onset has been felt to be an important clinical distinction between the different types of nephronophthisis leading to the categorization of the disease as infantile (NPHP2), juvenile (NPHP1 and NPHP4), or adolescent (NPHP3). With the exception of NPHP2, which leads to ESRD in the first decade of life, it is not clear that there is truly a predictable difference in the age of onset for the other types of NPHP.

The extrarenal manifestations of NPHP (see Table 42.1) include retinitis pigmentosa, which can be present in most of the NPHP types, but is present in all cases of NPHP5 identified thus far. Many cases of NPHP6 and NPHP8 are identified as a component of Joubert syndrome. Oculomotor apraxia, Cogan type, is associated with mutations in NPHP1 and NPHP4. Situs inversus can occur with NPHP2. Liver fibrosis can occur with NPHP3. A number of additional clinical syndromes have been described with a renal phenotype similar to NPHP, including Jeune, COACH, Arima, Sensenbrenner, and Bardet-Biedl syndromes.

Physical findings related to nephronophthisis include growth retardation from reduced kidney function and high blood pressure, although the latter is less prevalent than would be expected from the degree of functional kidney impairment.

The laboratory evaluation of patients with nephronophthisis includes a urinalysis from first morning void, which is generally normal except for a low specific gravity, reflecting a urinary concentrating defect. The absence of proteinuria or hematuria may serve to distinguish NPHP from other heritable kidney diseases such as focal segmental glomerulosclerosis and Alport syndrome, respectively. Anemia is commonly noted at the time of presentation, which is often related to the severely reduced kidney function. However, in cases in which the diagnosis is made with relatively preserved kidney function, anemia may be due to the significant interstitial infiltration often seen on biopsy with NPHP, resulting in reduced erythropoietin secretion. Other laboratory abnormalities can be seen commensurate with the degree of reduced GFR.

The most relevant diagnostic test is kidney imaging with ultrasound, which demonstrates normal to slightly reduced kidney size with increased echotexture and a loss of the corticomedullary border. Cysts, when present, may be observed at the corticomedullary junction. Many times cysts are not visible on imaging, and their presence is not required for the diagnosis of NPHP. The imaging findings for patients with NPHP2 are substantially different from those of other types of NPHP in that kidney size is often increased and cysts are a prominent finding on imaging studies.

In summary, the diagnosis of NPHP should be entertained when an individual presents in the first three decades of life with reduced kidney function, a bland urine sediment, and normal to small size kidneys on ultrasound with increased echotexture and loss of the corticomedullary junction. The presence of cysts on ultrasound examination of the kidneys is not required for the diagnosis but may be noted. The most common extrarenal manifestation associated with NPHP is retinitis pigmentosa, which often leads to blindness in the first decade of life and occurs in about 10% of cases. The occurrence of similarly affected siblings strongly suggests the diagnosis of NPHP. The parents of affected individuals are not affected, because NPHP is inherited as an autosomal recessive disease.

MCKD is transmitted as an autosomal dominant disease in which one parent of the affected individual is also affected; this distinguishes it from NPHP. MCKD generally presents in the fourth to seventh decades of life. Two exceptions to this are FJHN and GCKD, which are allelic (i.e., caused by mutations in the same gene) to MCKD2 but present within the first three decades of life. MCKD, FJHN, and GCKD all are inherited in an autosomal dominant pattern. The only extrarenal manifestations associated with these diseases, aside from those attributable to declining kidney function, are hyperuricemia and gout, which occur in about 80% of cases.

No other distinctive findings are noted on physical examination associated with MCKD. Laboratory evaluation is notable for a urinary concentrating defect and a reduced fractional excretion of uric acid, but the urinalysis is otherwise unremarkable. Ultrasound examination demonstrates normal to slightly reduced kidney size, increased echogenicity, loss of corticomedullary differentiation, and small cysts that may occur in the cortex and the medulla. Again, these cysts may be too subtle for detection with ultrasound or CT scanning. Ultrasound examination of GCKD patients may reveal normal to small kidney size and cortical cysts.

Although biopsy findings in conjunction with the appropriate clinical and historical presentation can be suggestive of a diagnosis of NPHP or MCKD, the only definitive diagnostic modality is genetic testing. Most genetic testing is done on a research basis, but commercial testing has recently become available.

TREATMENT

No systematic trials have been performed to examine treatment regimens for NPHP or MCKD in human subjects. Some studies have evaluated treatments in a mouse model of NPHP. The pcy mouse is a model of NPHP type 3 (NPHP3). A missense mutation has been identified in the murine homolog of NPHP3, which when present, homozygously results in renal cystic disease and ESRD at around 40 weeks of age. In various studies, these mice have been treated with soy proteins, glucocorticoids, probucol, or vasopressin-2 receptor antagonists. All of these treatments demonstrated a reduction in cyst formation and a slower progression of kidney failure in this mouse model. In the same trial, the vasopressin-2 receptor antagonist was also tested on a rat model of autosomal recessive polycystic kidney disease and demonstrated efficacy. The mechanism by which antagonism of the vasopressin-2 receptor inhibits cystic changes in the renal parenchyma remains incompletely understood, but decreased levels of cyclic adenosine monophosphate (cAMP) were observed in the renal tubules of both animal models, suggesting that cAMP is functioning as a second messenger in the abnormal proliferation of renal epithelial cells in cystic kidney diseases.

Until these therapeutic options are tested in human trials, no disease-specific therapies can be recommended. At present, the standard of care remains conservative therapies known to slow progression of kidney disease and treat the attendant manifestations of reduced kidney function, including anemia, acidosis, and hyperparathyroidism. It is not known whether blockade of the renin-angiotensin-aldosterone axis slows the progression of NPHP, as has been noted in several other kidney diseases. Patients with NPHP and MCKD have successfully undergone kidney transplantation without evidence of recurrent disease.

BIBLIOGRAPHY

Bollee G, Dahan K, Flamant M, et al: Phenotype and outcome in hereditary tubulointerstitial nephritis secondary to UMOD mutations, *Clin J Am Soc Nephrol* 6:2429-2438, 2011.

Chaki M, Hoefele J, Allen SJ, et al: Genotype-phenotype correlation in 440 patients with NPHP-related ciliopathies, *Kidney Int* 80:1239-1245, 2011.

Hart TC, Gorry MC, Hart PS, et al: Mutations of the UMOD gene are responsible for medullary cystic kidney disease 2 and familial juvenile hyperuricaemic nephropathy, *J Med Genet* 39:882-892, 2002.

Hildebrandt F: Nephronophthisis-medullary cystic kidney disease. In Avner ED, Harmon WE, Niaudet P, editors: *Pediatric nephrology*, 5th ed, Philadelphia, Lippincott, 2004, Williams & Wilkins, pp 665-673.

Hildebrandt F, Benzing T, Katsanis N: Ciliopathies, *N Engl J Med* 364:1533-1543, 2011.

Rampoldi L, Caridi G, Santon D, et al: Allelism of MCKD, FJHN and GCKD caused by impairment of uromodulin export dynamics, *Hum Mol Genet* 12:3369-3384, 2003.

43

Alport Syndrome and Related Disorders

Martin C. Gregory

Alport syndrome is a disease of collagen that always affects the kidneys, usually the ears, and often the eyes. Cecil Alport described the association of hereditary hematuric nephritis with hearing loss in a family whose affected male members died in adolescence. Genetic advances have broadened the scope of the condition to include optical defects, platelet abnormalities, late-onset kidney failure, and abnormal hearing in some families. At least 85% of kindreds have X-linked disease, and most or all of those cases result from a mutation of COL4A5, the gene located at Xq22 that codes for the α5 chain of type IV collagen, α5(IV). Autosomal recessive inheritance occurs in perhaps 15% of cases, and autosomal dominant inheritance has been shown in a handful of cases.

JUVENILE AND ADULT FORMS

The distinction between juvenile and adult forms is fundamental to the understanding of Alport syndrome. Kidney failure tends to occur at a broadly similar age in all male members within a family, but this age varies widely among different families, with kidney failure in males occurring in childhood or adolescence in some families and in adulthood in others. Forms with early onset of kidney failure in affected males are called juvenile, and those with kidney failure in middle age are called adult-type. Extrarenal manifestations tend to be more prominent in the juvenile kindreds. Because boys in juvenile kindreds do not commonly survive to reproduce, these kindreds tend to be small and frequently arise from new mutations, whereas adult-type kindreds are typically much larger, and new mutations occur infrequently (Table 43.1).

BIOCHEMISTRY

The open mesh of interlocking type IV collagen molecules that forms the framework of the glomerular basement membrane (GBM) is composed of heterotrimers of α chains. In fetal life, these heterotrimers consist of two α1(IV) chains and one α2(IV) chain, but early in postnatal development, production switches to α3(IV), α4(IV), and α5(IV) chains. The primary chemical defect in Alport syndrome most commonly involves the α5(IV) chain, but faulty assembly of the α3,4,5-heterotrimer produces similar pathology in glomerular, aural, and ocular basement membranes, regardless of which α chain is defective. As an illustration of failure of normal heterotrimer formation, most patients whose genetic defect is in the gene coding for the α5(IV) chain lack demonstrable α3(IV) chains in GBMs.

GENETICS

In most kindreds, inheritance of Alport syndrome is X-linked. This was suggested by classic pedigree analysis, strengthened by tight linkage to restriction-fragment-length polymorphisms, and proved by identification of mutations.

Causative mutations of COL4A5, the gene coding for α5(IV), appear consistently in many kindreds. These mutations include deletions, point mutations, and splicing errors. There is some correlation between the mutation type and the clinical phenotype, but deletions and some splicing errors cause severe kidney disease and early hearing loss. Missense mutations may cause juvenile disease with hearing loss or adult disease with or without hearing loss. Deletions involving the 5′ end of the COL4A5 gene and the 5′ end of the adjacent COL4A6 gene occur consistently in families with esophageal and genital leiomyomatosis.

Homozygotes or mixed heterozygotes for mutations of the COL4A3 or COL4A4 genes (chromosome 2) develop autosomal recessive Alport syndrome. Heterozygotes for these mutations account for many cases of benign familial hematuria (i.e., familial thin basement membrane disease [TBMD]).

Patients with autosomal dominant hematuria and kidney failure with thrombocytopenia, giant platelets (Epstein syndrome), and leukocyte inclusions (Fechtner syndrome) both have mutations of the MYH9 gene on chromosome 22 (vide infra). These patients should no longer be considered to have Alport syndrome but should instead be classified with MYH9-related disorders.

IMMUNOCHEMISTRY

Male patients with X-linked Alport syndrome and patients with autosomal recessive Alport syndrome frequently lack the α3, α4, and α5 chains of type IV collagen in the GBM, and hemizygous males with X-linked Alport syndrome often lack α5(IV) chains in the epidermal basement membrane (EBM). Monoclonal antibodies specific to the α2 and α5 chains of type IV collagen are commercially available and can be used to assist in the diagnosis of Alport syndrome. The GBM and EBM of normal individuals, as well

Table 43.1   Alport Syndrome Types With Chromosomal and Gene Locations and Relative Frequencies

Type	Chromosome	Gene	Relative Frequency*
X-linked	X	COL4A5	85%
Juvenile type			90% of families, 50% of patients
Adult type			8% of families, 25% of patients
Adult type with "normal" hearing			2% of families, 25% of patients
Autosomal recessive	2	COL4A3, COL4A4	15%
Autosomal dominant	2	COL4A3, COL4A4	Less than 1%

*Relative frequencies of the X-linked, autosomal recessive, and autosomal dominant forms are fairly well accepted. The frequencies of "juvenile" (mean age of end-stage renal disease [ESRD] in males less than 30 years), "adult" (mean age of ESRD in males more than 30 years), and adult-type with near-normal hearing are rough estimates from the numbers of patients and families known to the University of Utah Alport Study. In the United States, C1564S is a common mutation causing adult-type Alport syndrome, and L1649R is a common mutation causing adult-type Alport syndrome with near-normal hearing.

as those of all Alport patients, react with the α2 antibody, but most male and female patients with autosomal recessive Alport syndrome and most male patients hemizygous for a COL4A5 mutation show no staining of the GBM with the α5 antibody. Males with X-linked disease commonly show no staining of EBM with antibody to α5, whereas females heterozygous for a COL4A5 mutation show interrupted staining of the GBM and EBM, consistent with mosaicism.

After kidney transplantation, about 10% of male patients with Alport syndrome develop anti-GBM nephritis, presumably because they are exposed for the first time to normal collagen chains including a normal 26-kDa monomer of the α3(IV) chain to which tolerance has never been acquired. Recurrences of anti-GBM nephritis are usual but not inevitable after repeat transplantation. The serum antibodies to GBM developing after transplantation are heterogeneous; all stain normal GBM, and some stain EBM.

PATHOLOGY

In young children, light microscopy of the kidneys may be normal or near normal. Glomeruli with persistent fetal morphology may be seen. As disease progresses, interstitial and tubular foam cells, which arise for reasons that are unclear, may become prominent (Fig. 43.1), although they can also be found in many other conditions. Eventually, progressive glomerulosclerosis and interstitial scarring develop. The results of routine immunofluorescence examination for immunoglobulins and complement components are negative, but staining for the α5(IV) chain may be informative (see "Immunochemistry").

The GBM is up to three times its normal thickness, split into several irregular layers, and frequently interspersed with numerous electron-dense granules about 40 nm in diameter (Fig. 43.2). In florid cases of juvenile types of Alport syndrome, the basement membrane lamellae may branch and rejoin in a complex basket-weave pattern. Early in the development of the lesion, thinning of the GBM may predominate or be the only abnormality visible. The abnormalities in children or adolescents with adult-type Alport syndrome may be unimpressive or indistinguishable from those of TBMD disease (vide infra).

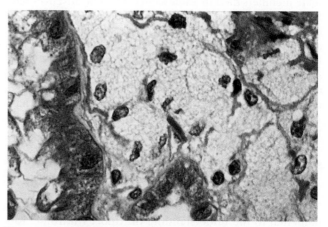

Figure 43.1   High-power photomicrograph shows foam-filled tubular and interstitial cells in a kidney biopsy specimen from a patient with Alport syndrome. Relatively normal proximal tubular cytoplasm stains red in the tubules on the left and at the bottom. The remaining cells appear "foamy" because of the spaces left where lipids have been eluted during processing.

CLINICAL FEATURES

KIDNEY FEATURES

Uninterrupted microscopic hematuria occurs from birth in affected males. Hematuria may become visible after exercise or during fever; this is more common in juvenile kindreds. Microscopic hematuria has a penetrance of approximately 90% in heterozygous females in adult-type kindreds. In juvenile kindreds, the penetrance of hematuria in females has been studied less extensively, but it appears to be common. Urinary erythrocytes are dysmorphic, and red-cell casts usually can be found in affected males. The degree of proteinuria varies, but it occasionally reaches nephrotic levels.

Hemizygous males inevitably progress to end-stage renal disease (ESRD). This occurs at widely different ages, but within each family the age of ESRD is fairly constant. Heterozygous females are usually much less severely affected. About one fourth of them develop ESRD, usually after the age of 50 years, but ESRD can occur in girls in their teens or even younger.

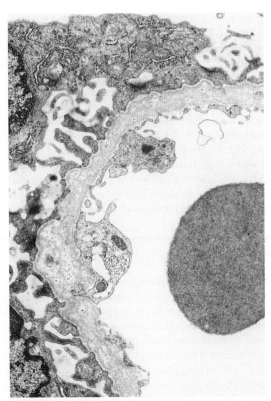

Figure 43.2   High-resolution electron micrograph shows a glomerular basement membrane from a patient with Alport syndrome that varies in thickness. It is split into several layers, which in some areas are separated by lucencies containing small, dense granules. (Courtesy Dr. Theodore J. Pysher.)

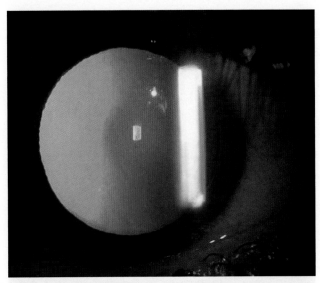

Figure 43.3   Retroilluminated lens photography shows the "oil-drop" appearance of anterior lenticonus, a pathognomonic feature of Alport syndrome. The bulging area of the lens is the dark circular area just to the left of the vertical reflected light artifact from the slit-lamp examination. This is similar to the view obtained through a direct ophthalmoscope using a strong positive lens.

In families with autosomal inheritance, females are affected as severely and as early as males, and kidney failure often occurs before the age of 20 in those who are homozygous for autosomal recessive Alport syndrome.

EXTRARENAL FEATURES

HEARING LOSS

Bilateral, high-frequency cochlear hearing loss occurs in many kindreds, but X-linked disease progressing to ESRD can occur in families without overt hearing loss. It is easy to miss the diagnosis of Alport syndrome if hearing loss is expected as a constant feature (see Table 43.1). In families with juvenile-type disease, hearing loss is almost universal in male hemizygotes and common in severely affected female heterozygotes.

Patterns of hearing loss vary. Often, the most severe loss is at 2 to 6 kHz, but it may occur at a higher frequency if there has been superimposed noise damage. In adult-type Alport syndrome with hearing loss, there is typically no perceptible deficit until 20 years of age, but loss progresses to 60 to 70 dB at 6 to 8 kHz after 40 years of age; hearing loss occurs earlier in juvenile kindreds. The rate at which hearing is lost is not well established in juvenile kindreds, but many children of grade-school age and adolescents require hearing aids.

OCULAR DEFECTS

Ocular defects are common in juvenile kindreds. Myopia, arcus juvenilis, and cataracts occur, but lack diagnostic specificity. Three changes that are present in a minority of kindreds but that are almost diagnostic are anterior lenticonus, posterior polymorphous corneal dystrophy, and retinal flecks. Anterior lenticonus is a forward protrusion of the anterior surface of the ocular lens. It results from a weakness of the type IV collagen forming the anterior lens capsule. The resulting irregularity of the surface of the lens causes an uncorrectable refractive error. The retina cannot be clearly seen by ophthalmoscopy, and with a strong positive lens in the ophthalmoscope the lenticonus often can be seen through a dilated pupil as an "oil drop," or circular smudge on the center of the lens (Fig. 43.3). Retinal flecks are small, yellow or white dots scattered around the macula or in the periphery of the retina (Fig. 43.4). If sparse, they may be difficult to distinguish from small, hard exudates. Macular holes occur rarely but can severely affect sight. Ocular manifestations are often subtle, and consultation with an ophthalmologist familiar with Alport syndrome is invaluable.

Optical coherence tomography is a simple inexpensive test that shows retinal thinning in patients with Alport syndrome. This test appears to have high sensitivity and specificity, but more study is needed.

LEIOMYOMATOSIS

Young members of several families with X-linked Alport syndrome develop striking leiomyomas of the esophagus and female genitalia. Patients frequently have large and multiple tumors, which may bleed or cause obstruction, and their resection can be difficult. All families described have had a deletion at the 5′ ends of the contiguous COL4A5 and COL4A6 genes.

DIAGNOSIS

No single clinical feature is pathognomonic of Alport syndrome. The diagnosis is based on finding hematuria in

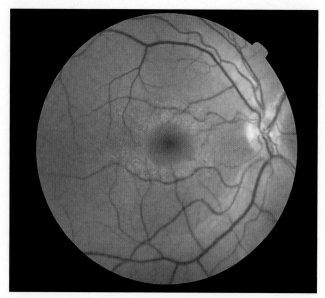

Figure 43.4   Retinal photograph of right fundus from a 14-year-old boy with Alport syndrome shows perimacular dots and flecks that spare the foveola and are more discrete at the outer margin of the ring. Alport retinopathy varies from occasional dots and flecks in the temporal macula to this appearance. (Courtesy Dr. Judith Savige and Dr. Deb Colville.)

many family members, a history of kidney failure in related males, and a kidney biopsy showing characteristic ultrastructural changes in the proband or a relative. Immunofluorescence examination of the biopsy specimen should include staining with antibodies specific to GBM or to α5(IV); the lack of staining in most male patients with Alport syndrome helps to differentiate Alport syndrome from familial TBMD, in which staining is normal. In large families without a known mutation, segregation analysis can help clarify the mode of inheritance and help determine whether a particular individual carries the gene. If the skin of affected family members is known to lack immunofluorescent staining with antibodies to α5(IV), an α5(IV) immunofluorescence examination of a skin biopsy from a suspected case in the family may be diagnostic.

Molecular diagnosis is almost 100% sensitive and specific, but only after a mutation has been found in the family. Sequencing the COL4A5 gene is at least 80% sensitive for mutations, but it is expensive, and sequencing of COL4A3 and COL4A4 may also be required if the COL4A5 test is normal. In families with a previously defined COL4A5 mutation, molecular diagnosis of affected males and gene-carrying females is possible. Specific genetic tests are available for mutations (i.e., C1564S, L1649R, and R1677Q) that commonly cause kidney failure in middle age. These tests are useful in the investigation of potentially affected individuals when a family member is known to carry one of these mutations. It is not clear whether these tests are useful in the investigation of otherwise unexplained hematuria or chronic kidney disease.

The key to diagnosis is clinical suspicion of Alport syndrome in any patient with otherwise unexplained hematuria, glomerulopathy, or kidney failure. In many cases, the familial nature of the condition is not immediately apparent. Inquiry into the family history must be detailed and complete. The patient is usually a boy or young man, and, given the X-linked transmission, may have one or more male

relatives through his mother's family with kidney failure. Urine samples from both of the patient's parents, particularly his mother, should be checked for microscopic hematuria. Although it is a helpful clue, it is crucial to remember that hearing loss is neither a sensitive nor a specific marker of Alport syndrome; it is neither necessary nor sufficient for the diagnosis. Many adults with kidney failure from Alport syndrome do not have conspicuous hearing loss, particularly those with the COL4A5 L1649R mutation. In addition, many patients with hearing loss and kidney disease do not have Alport syndrome, but instead other kidney disorders, most often glomerulonephritis, with a more common cause for hearing loss, such as noise exposure, aminoglycoside therapy, or unrelated inherited hearing loss.

TREATMENT

There is no specific treatment for Alport syndrome. General measures to retard the progression of kidney failure, such as treatment of hypertension, appear warranted, but are unproven. Persuasive observational data from Europe show that angiotensin-converting enzyme inhibition delays onset of kidney failure and prolongs survival, although controlled trials are still lacking. Unconfirmed reports claim benefit from cyclosporine in reducing proteinuria and retarding progression of kidney disease; however, other investigators have found little benefit with risk of cyclosporine nephrotoxicity.

Male patients should wear hearing protection in noisy surroundings. Hearing aids improve but do not completely correct the hearing loss. Tinnitus is usually resistant to all forms of therapy; hearing aids may make it less disruptive by amplifying ambient sounds. Retinal lesions do not commonly affect vision and require no therapy. The serious impairment of vision caused by lenticonus or cataract cannot be corrected with spectacles or contact lenses. Lens removal with reimplantation of an intraocular lens is standard and satisfactory treatment.

RELATED DISORDERS

AUTOSOMAL RECESSIVE ALPORT SYNDROME

A few children have homozygous or compound heterozygous mutations of the genes for the α3(IV) or α4(IV) chains of type IV collagen. Boys and girls are equally affected, and both may develop severe kidney disease before the age of 10 years. The heterozygous parents commonly have TBMD (discussed later), but not all have persistent hematuria.

AUTOSOMAL DOMINANT ALPORT SYNDROME

Families rarely have autosomal dominant Alport syndrome as a consequence of heterozygous mutations of the genes for the α3(IV) or α4(IV) chains of type IV collagen.

ALPORT SYNDROME WITH THROMBOCYTOPATHY: EPSTEIN SYNDROME AND FECHTNER SYNDROME

The Epstein and Fechtner syndromes are uncommon, autosomal dominant syndromes of hematuria and progressive kidney failure associated with moderate thrombocytopenia, severe hearing loss, and kidney failure in males and females. Platelets (about 7 μm in diameter) are much larger than normal (1 to 1.5 μm), and there is a mild or moderate bleeding tendency. In families with Fechtner syndrome, an additional feature is inclusion bodies (Fechtner bodies) in leukocytes. These syndromes are caused by a mutation in the nonmuscle myosin heavy chain 9 gene (MYH9) on chromosome 22q12.3-13.1.

FAMILIAL THIN BASEMENT MEMBRANE DISEASE

Thin basement membrane disease, or benign familial hematuria, is an autosomal dominant basement membrane glomerulopathy. Many cases result from heterozygous mutations of the COL4A3 or COL4A4 gene at chromosome 2q35-2q37; those patients who carry homozygous or compound heterozygous mutations in these same genes develop autosomal recessive Alport syndrome. Ultrastructurally, the GBM is uniformly thinned to about one half its normal thickness. There is no disruption or lamellation of the GBM, nor are any other abnormalities of the glomeruli, tubules, vessels, or interstitium visible by light, immunofluorescence, or electron microscopy. Kidney failure seldom occurs. Longevity is unaffected by this condition, with survivors into the ninth decade documented. Minor degrees of lamellation of the GBM and hearing loss have been described in some families, but these families might have had unrecognized Alport syndrome.

After the precise diagnosis is established, the patient and family can be spared further invasive tests, and an appropriate prognosis can be provided to them and to health insurers. However, the distinction between Alport syndrome and benign familial hematuria is not always easy to make. Being certain of the pattern of inheritance requires a large pedigree with accurate diagnoses for all family members. A single mistaken diagnosis from incidental kidney disease, inaccurate urinalysis, or incomplete penetrance may vitiate conclusions about the pattern of inheritance in the entire pedigree. Even biopsy evidence is fallible. Early cases of Alport syndrome may show ultrastructural changes indistinguishable from those of benign familial hematuria. This is particularly likely if a child from an adult-type Alport kindred is diagnosed based on a biopsy result. Stability of serum creatinine for several years in a child does not exclude adult-type Alport syndrome, and testing for mutations for the common adult types of X-linked Alport syndrome may avoid some diagnostic errors. The situation is further complicated, because cases of autosomal recessive Alport syndrome will occasionally turn up in families with TBMD. In these families, autosomal dominant TBMD and autosomal recessive Alport syndrome are caused by the same mutations.

APPROACH TO THE PATIENT WITH HEREDITARY NEPHRITIS

Although Alport syndrome is less common than polycystic kidney disease, it is probably more common than generally appreciated. Important conditions comprising the differential diagnoses of hematuria in young persons include IgA nephropathy or other glomerulonephritides, renal calculi, and medullary sponge kidney. The differential diagnosis of familial kidney disease with hematuria includes TBMD, familial IgA nephropathy, Fabry disease, and polycystic kidney disease. Familial kidney diseases without hematuria that may be confused with Alport syndrome include polycystic kidney disease, medullary cystic disease, and rare forms of inherited glomerular and tubulointerstitial kidney disease.

If a patient with unexplained hematuria or kidney failure has a family history of hematuria or kidney failure, the family history should be extended, concentrating particularly on the mother's male relatives. Identifying hearing loss strengthens, and finding a specific ocular lesion greatly strengthens, suspicion for Alport syndrome. Kidney biopsy usually is indicated for one family member, but after the diagnosis of a basement membrane nephropathy is established in a family, it is difficult to justify biopsies in other members unless there are features that suggest another diagnosis. The extent of investigation is guided by clinical judgment and relates inversely to the strength of the family history. For example, a young man on the line of descent of a known Alport family whose urine contains dysmorphic erythrocytes needs minimal investigation. He may need no further workup other than an assessment of the glomerular filtration rate and urine protein quantification, unless there are additional clinical features suggesting a systemic disease. A patient with hematuria and an uncertain family history may merit the standard nephrologic workup for hematuria. If suspicion of Alport syndrome is moderate or strong, and the test is available, a skin biopsy with staining for the α5(IV) chain may be considered, particularly if a known affected family member is available as a positive control.

Genetic testing, if undertaken, will generally start with COL4A5 sequencing. If this is normal, sequencing of COL4A3 and COL4A4 can be considered. After a mutation is defined in a family, targeted mutation analysis is an inexpensive way to determine whether other family members carry the mutant gene and may be spared the need for a kidney biopsy. In adults with late-onset kidney failure in the United States, screening with a single assay that is available for the common adult type mutations (C1564S, L1649R, and R1677Q) can be used as an economical first step.

Patients with any hereditary nephropathy should be informed about the nature of the disease, and perhaps be given a copy of the genetic analysis or kidney biopsy report to avoid unnecessary further investigation. Similar recommendations apply to family members who are potential gene carriers. Those with Alport syndrome should be followed regularly for elevation of blood pressure and changes in serum creatinine levels. The frequency of follow-up depends on the anticipated age of onset of kidney functional deterioration in the family. Those with familial TBMD should be checked about every 2 years, because some may ultimately turn out to have Alport syndrome.

BIBLIOGRAPHY

Barker DF, Hostikka SL, Zhou J, et al: Identification of mutations in the COL4A5 collagen gene in Alport's syndrome, Science 248:1224-1227, 1990.

Bekheirnia MR, Reed B, Gregory MC, et al: Genotype-phenotype correlation in X-linked Alport syndrome, J Am Soc Nephrol 21:876-883, 2010.

Gleeson MJ: Alport's syndrome: audiological manifestations and implications, J Laryngol Otol 98:449-465, 1984.

Govan JA: Ocular manifestations of Alport's syndrome: a hereditary disorder of basement membranes? Br J Ophthalmol 67:493-503, 1983.

Gregory MC: Alport's syndrome and thin basement membrane nephropathy: unraveling the tangled strands of type IV collagen, *Kidney Int* 65:1109-1110, 2004.

Gregory MC, Shamshirsam A, Kamgar M, et al: Alport's syndrome, Fabry's disease, and nail-patella syndrome. In Schrier RW, editor: *Diseases of the kidney*, ed 8, Boston, 2007, Little Brown, pp 540-569.

Gross O, Licht C, Anders HJ, et al: Early angiotensin-converting enzyme inhibition in Alport syndrome delays renal failure and improves life expectancy, *Kidney Int* 81:494-501, 2012.

Heath KE, Campos-Barros A, Toren A, et al: Nonmuscle myosin heavy chain IIA mutations define a spectrum of autosomal dominant macrothrombocytopenias: May-Hegglin anomaly and Fechtner, Sebastian, Epstein, and Alport-like syndromes, *Am J Hum Genet* 69:1033-1045, 2001.

Jais JP, Knebelmann B, Giatras I, et al: X-Linked Alport syndrome: natural history in 195 families and genotype-phenotype correlations in males, *J Am Soc Nephrol* 11:649-657, 2000.

Jais JP, Knebelmann B, Giatras I, et al: X-Linked Alport syndrome: natural history and genotype-phenotype correlations in girls and women belonging to 195 families. A "European Community Alport Syndrome Concerted Action" study, *J Am Soc Nephrol* 14:2603-2610, 2003.

Kashtan CE, Ding J, Gregory M, et al: Clinical practice recommendations for the treatment of Alport syndrome: a statement of the Alport Syndrome Research Collaborative, *Pediatr Nephrol*, 2012, Mar 30 Epub.

Kashtan CE, Kleppel MM, Gubler M-C: Immunohistologic findings in Alport's syndrome. In Tryggvason K, editor: *Molecular pathology and genetics of Alport's syndrome*, Basel, 1996, Karger, pp 142-153.

Lemmink HH, Nielsson WN, Mochizuki T, et al: Benign familial hematuria due to mutation of the type 4 collagen gene, *J Clin Invest* 98:1114-1118, 1996.

Tiebosch TA, Frederik PM, van Breda Vriesman PJ, et al: Thin basement membrane nephropathy in adults with persistent hematuria, *N Engl J Med* 320:14-18, 1989.

Fabry Disease
44

Gere Sunder-Plassmann | Manuela Födinger | Renate Kain

Fabry disease (OMIM 301500) is a hereditary lysosomal storage disorder that results from absent or deficient activity of the enzyme α-galactosidase A (αGAL; EC 3.2.1.22). This enzyme is encoded by the *GLA* gene on Xq22 (Fig. 44.1), with more than 600 different mutations so far described (Fig. 44.2). A recent newborn screening study reported the incidence of mutations in *GLA* to be 1:3859 births in Austria. The enzyme defect leads to progressive accumulation of glycosphingolipids, predominantly globotriaoslyceramide (Gb3), in all organs (Fig. 44.3).

Early manifestations during childhood include pain, anhydrosis, and gastrointestinal symptoms among others (Box 44.1). Later, chronic kidney disease (CKD) (Fig. 44.4) leading to end-stage renal disease (ESRD), hypertrophic cardiomyopathy (Fig. 44.5), and cerebral events (Fig. 44.6) are the clinically most important organ manifestations resulting in a reduced life span of hemizygous males and heterozygous females. Most male patients develop the classic phenotype with involvement of all organ systems, whereas alterations in x-inactivation lead to highly variable disease expression in women. Furthermore, renal or cardiac variant phenotypes with later onset of disease, probably linked to some residual enzyme activity, have also been described. Importantly, because of the nonspecific nature of complaints, there is often a delay of more than 10 to 20 years from the earliest symptoms of disease until the correct diagnosis is established. Therefore it is prudent to include Fabry disease in the differential diagnosis if two or more of the clinical problems indicated in Box 44.2 are present in young adults.

Beyond screening individuals with a family history of Fabry disease (Fig. 44.7), many cases are identified by means of kidney biopsy on patients referred to nephrologists for proteinuria or other signs of kidney damage. Other cases are found among high-risk populations such as patients with ESRD, left ventricular hypertrophy, or stroke. A reduced or absent activity of αGAL in leukocytes confirms the diagnosis in male patients. In women genetic testing is mandatory, because αGAL activity may be normal in a significant proportion of women. Urinary excretion of Gb3 is increased in many instances, and lyso-Gb3 in the plasma is a promising marker for diagnosis and treatment monitoring. Proteomics, the large-scale study of the entire complement of proteins, is another valuable research tool directed at finding biomarkers of diagnosis, disease progression, and responsiveness to therapy in the urine or serum of patients with Fabry disease.

KIDNEY MANIFESTATIONS OF FABRY DISEASE

Kidney disease is a major complication of Fabry disease related to glycosphingolipid accumulation throughout the nephron, with interstitial fibrosis and focal or segmental glomerulosclerosis observed early in the course of disease. Progression to ESRD occurs in almost all affected men around the fourth or fifth decade of life, but can also be seen in adolescents. The course of the disease is less severe in women, who also eventually progress to ESRD.

In affected individuals, the urine sediment may show red and white blood cells, hyaline or granular casts, and lipid particles with Maltese cross appearance upon polarization. Early in the course, dysfunction of the proximal and distal tubules includes reduced net acid excretion or a urinary concentrating defect with polyuria, nocturia, and polydypsia. Albuminuria or overt proteinuria sometimes develops during childhood, but by the age of 35 years approximately 50% of men and 20% of women manifest proteinuria. Kidney imaging may show cortical or parapelvic cysts, the cause of which is unknown. Increased blood pressure above 130/80 mm Hg was present in 57% of men and 47% of women in a large analysis of 391 patients presenting with various stages of CKD. A retrospective analysis of 168 female and 279 male patients with Fabry disease from 27 sites in 5 countries showed a more rapid decline of estimated glomerular filtration rate (eGFR) of -6.8 mL/min per 1.73 m^2 in male patients with an eGFR less than 60 mL/min per 1.73 m^2 versus -3.0 mL/min per 1.73 m^2 in patients with eGFR greater than 60 mL/min per 1.73 m^2. The corresponding progression rates for women were -2.1 and -0.9 mL/min per 1.73 m^2, respectively. Similar to other nephropathies, proteinuria and hypertension are also associated with more rapid decline in kidney function. ESRD developed in 49 men and 8 women described in this report. The prevalence of Fabry disease among dialysis patients enrolled in large U.S. and European registries was 1.7% and 1.9%, but most of the case-finding studies during the last decade have shown a prevalence of 0.2% to 0.5% among men with ESRD. In patients with an established diagnosis of Fabry disease, a routine kidney biopsy is not mandatory. Annual monitoring should include measurement of serum creatinine and urinary albumin- or protein-to-creatinine ratio.

PATHOLOGY OF KIDNEY DISEASE IN FABRY DISEASE

GROSS PATHOLOGY

There is a limited number of gross descriptions of the kidneys in Fabry disease, with enlargement caused by both storage and cysts described.

LIGHT MICROSCOPY

Histologic changes show characteristically vacuolated "foamy" podocytes. However, other cell types, including endothelial cells, vascular myocytes, and tubular epithelial cells, may be similarly affected by accumulation of glyco-sphinglolipid. In conventional light microscopy on forma-lin-fixed and paraffin-embedded material, these inclusions appear empty, because their content is removed during pro-cessing. Fixation with osmium and embedding in epoxy res-ins retains the stored material that can easily be visualized by either light microscopy on thin section with Toluidin blue or Methylene blue staining and electron microscopy. The lipid content of the inclusions is sudanophilic and stains with oil red O on frozen section. It may be further charac-terized by immunohistochemistry or lectin binding. Specific histologic changes are usually accompanied by a varying degree of mesangial sclerosis, tubular atrophy, interstitial fibrosis, and sclerosis of arterial blood vessels that correlates with the stage of CKD. Kidney biopsy is therefore consid-ered a valuable instrument in the baseline assessment of Fabry nephropathy, and a validated scoring sheet has been

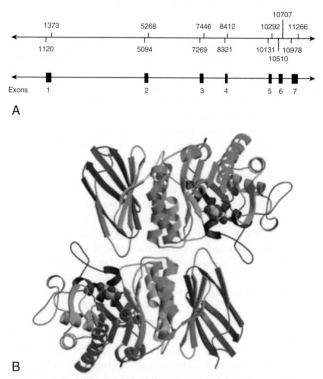

A

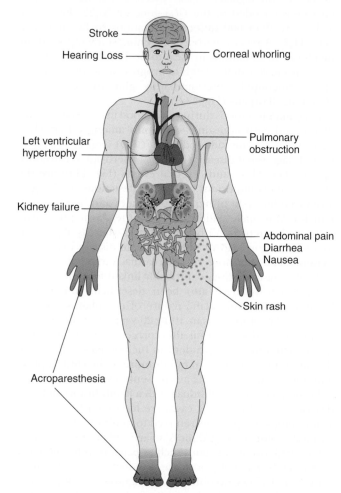

B

Figure 44.1 **A,** Organization of the *GLA* gene on Xq22.1. The whole gene spans 12.4 kb of genomic DNA and contains 7 exons. Black boxes in the lower scheme indicate 7 coding regions (exons) of the *GLA* gene. The upper scheme shows the exon position numbering according to the GenBank database entry X14448.1. **B,** The structure of α-galactosidase A. The structure of the human α-galactosidase A dimer is shown in ribbon representation. The ribbon is colored from blue to red as the polypeptide goes from *N*- to *C*-terminus. The active site is identified by the catalytic product galactose, shown in sphere Corey-Pauling-Koltun (CPK) format. Each monomer in the homodimer contains two domains, a (β/α)8 barrel containing the active site *(blue to yellow)* plus a *C* terminal antiparallel β domain *(yellow to red).* (**A,** From Doctoral thesis, Anita Jallitsch-Halper, Medical University of Vien-na, 2012. **B,** From Garman SC: Structure-function relationships in alpha-galactosidase A, *Acta Paediatr Suppl* 96:6-16, 2007, Fig. 1.)

Figure 44.3 **Organ manifestations in patients with Fabry disease.**

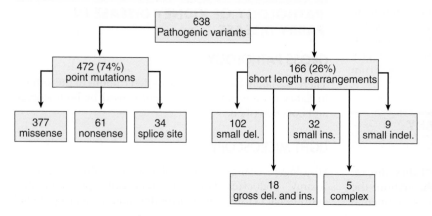

Figure 44.2 **Different types of mutations in *GLA* (as of November 2011).** These mutations include 438 missense and nonsense point mutations, 102 small deletions and 32 small insertions, 9 small indels, 16 gross deletions and 2 gross insertions, as well as 5 complex rearrangements and 34 mutations that affect splice sites. (From Doctoral thesis, Anita Jallitsch-Halper, Medical University of Vienna, 2012.)

Box 44.1   Early Signs and Symptoms of Fabry Disease

Nervous System

Acroparesthesias, nerve deafness, heat intolerance, tinnitus

Gastrointestinal Tract

Nausea, vomiting, diarrhea, postprandial bloating and pain, early satiety, difficulty gaining weight

Skin

Angiokeratoma, hypohidrosis

Eyes

Corneal and lenticular opacities, vasculopathy (retina, conjunctiva)

Kidneys

Albuminuria, proteinuria, impaired concentrating ability, increased urinary Gb3 excretion

Heart

Impaired heart-rate variability, arrhythmias, ECG abnormalities (shortened PR interval), mild valvular insufficiency

Adapted from Germain DP: Fabry disease, Orphanet J Rare Dis 5:30, 2010, p. 30.
ECG, Electrocardiogram; Gb3, globotriaoslyceramide.

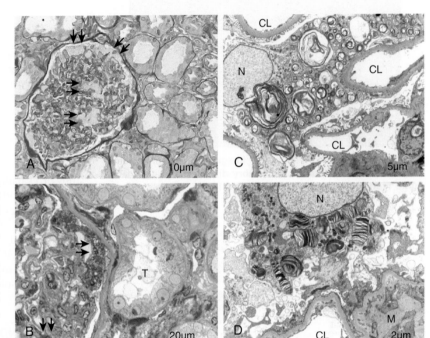

Figure 44.4 Histopathology and electron microscopy of kidney manifestations in Fabry disease. A, Light microsocopy of formalin-fixed and paraffin-embedded material shows "foamy" podocytes *(arrows)* resulting from numerous empty cytoplasmic vacuoles (periodic acid-Schiff). Cytoplasmic inclusions are osmiophilic *(arrows).* **B,** Toluidin blue on Epon-embedded thin section), and they correspond by electron microscopy to lamellated membrane inclusion bodies with either "zebroid" **(C)** or "myelin-like" **(D)** appearance in secondary lysosomes. *CL,* Capillary lumen; *M,* mesangium; *N,* nucleus of podocytes; *T,* proximal tubule.

developed to record progression on serial biopsies by light microscopy (see Fig. 44.4).

ELECTRON MICROSCOPY

Electron microscopy shows podocytes with lamellated membrane inclusion bodies in secondary lysosomes. These consist of concentric "myelin-like" rings, or have a striped "zebroid" appearance (see Fig. 44.4).

TREATMENT ISSUES IN FABRY DISEASE

Fabry disease can affect every organ system. Therefore, various symptoms may require specific therapy (Box 44.3). The most debilitating early symptom, often starting in childhood, is chronic pain; this is typically triggered by vigorous exercise and temperature changes. Pain (and depression) management agents include gabapentin, carbamazepine, phenytoin, amitriptyline, and other antidepressants.

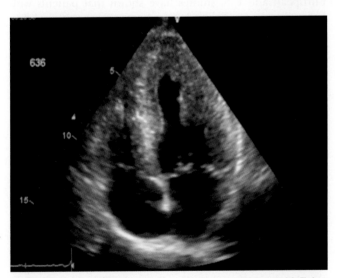

Figure 44.5   Cardiac sonography of a 53-year-old man with Fabry disease showing cardiac hypertrophy. (Courtesy Gerald Mundigler, MD, Medical University of Vienna.)

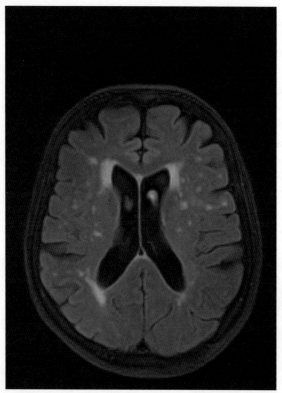

Figure 44.6 Magnetic resonance imaging of the brain of a 63-year-old female patient with Fabry disease showing typical white matter lesions on a T2 weighted image. (Courtesy Paulus Rommer, MD, Medical University of Vienna.)

Box 44.2   Signs and Symptoms Suggestive of Fabry Disease*

1. Acroparesthesia or neuropathic pain in hands or feet beginning in later childhood, precipitated by illness, fever, exercise, emotional stress, or exposure to heat
2. Persistent proteinuria of unknown cause
3. Hypertrophic cardiomyopathy, especially with prominent diastolic dysfunction[†]
4. Progressive CKD[†]
5. Cryptogenic stroke or transient ischemic attack[†]
6. Family history of ESRD, stroke, or hypertrophic cardiomyopathy showing an X-linked pattern of transmission that primarily, but not solely, affects men
7. Vague, persistent, or recurrent abdominal pain associated with nausea, diarrhea, and tenesmus

Adapted from Clarke JT: Narrative review: Fabry disease, Ann Intern Med *146:425-433, 2007.*
CKD, Chronic kidney disease; *ESRD,* end-stage renal disease.
*Any combination of two or more of these problems is highly suggestive of Fabry disease in either gender.
[†]This may be the only clinical manifestation of Fabry disease in patients of either gender with variants of classical Fabry disease.

RENIN-ANGIOTENSIN-ALDOSTERONE SYSTEM BLOCKADE

Blockade of the renin-angiotensin-aldosterone system (RAAS) remains an unresolved issue in Fabry disease. One uncontrolled

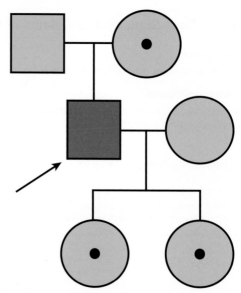

Figure 44.7 Pedigree of a family with Fabry disease. The index case was diagnosed by a nationwide case-finding study among Austrian dialysis patients. His mother and the two daughters carry the same mutation and were asymptomatic at the time of screening. (Case 3 from Kotanko P et al: Results of a nationwide screening for Anderson-Fabry disease among dialysis patients, *J Am Soc Nephrol* 15:1323-1329, 2004.)

study of 11 patients with Fabry disease suggested reduction of proteinuria and stabilization of kidney function with angiotensin converting enzyme (ACE) inhibitors or angiotensin receptor blockers (ARB); however, in the Fabry Outcome Survey (FOS), 208 subjects had a nonstatistically significant reduction in eGFR with ACE inhibitor or ARB use. Furthermore, recombinant αGAL may interact with endogenous ACE and inhibit its activity, resulting in lower blood pressure during enzyme infusion.

DIALYSIS AND TRANSPLANTATION

European and U.S. studies have shown that patients with Fabry disease on dialysis have a poorer 3-year survival rate as compared with nondiabetic controls. The 5-year survival after kidney transplantation is also lower than that of controls. However, Fabry nephropathy does not recur in the allograft, and transplanted Fabry patients appear to have better overall outcomes than those maintained on dialysis. Therefore, kidney transplantation should be recommended as a first choice therapy for patients with Fabry disease.

ENZYME REPLACEMENT THERAPY

Specific enzyme replacement therapy using intravenous recombinant human αGAL has been available for treatment of Fabry disease since 2001. It can be considered for every adult male patient, for symptomatic boys, and for symptomatic women.

Two preparations are currently available, with other products in clinical development. The first, Agalsidase alpha (Replagal, developed by Transkaryotic Therapies, Sweden, now marketed by Shire Human Genetic Therapies, Cambridge, MA), is produced in human skin fibroblasts using

Box 44.3 Concomitant Therapy in Patients with Fabry Disease

Acroparesthesia

Painful crisis: avoiding quick temperature changes, nonsteroidal antiinflammatory drugs
Chronic pain: anticonvulsants

Hypohydrosis

Appropriate temperature and environment

Angiokeratoma

Cosmetic removal with argon laser therapy

Proteinuria

ACE inhibitors or ARB

Kidney failure

Dialysis, transplantation

Gastrointestinal symptoms

Pain relief, H2-blockers, motility agents, pancreatic enzyme supplementation

Hypertension

Regular monitoring and rigorous surveillance following general guidelines (avoid beta-blockers as they can cause sinus bradycardia)

Hyperlipidemia

Regular routine surveillance, statin therapy

Edema

Compression stockings, lymph drainage

Stroke prevention

Address hypertension, diabetes, smoking, dyslipidemia; aspirin, clopidogrel

Depression

Selective serotonin reuptake inhibitors, serotonin norepinephrin reuptake inhibitors

Adapted from Whybra-Trümpler C: Symptomatic and ancillary therapy. In Elstein D, Altarescu G, Beck M, editors: Fabry disease, Dordrecht, Heidelberg, London, New York, 2010, Springer, pp. 481-487.
ACE, Angiotensin converting enzyme; ARB, angiotensin receptor blockers.

gene activation technology. It has been approved at a dose of 0.2 mg/kg every 2 weeks (infusion time: 40 minutes) in the European Union and many other countries, but not in the United States. The other product, Agalsidase beta (Fabrazyme, Genzyme Corporation, Cambridge, MA), is produced in Chinese hamster ovary cells and is registered for use at 1.0 mg/kg every other week (infusion time: several hours). Fabrazyme is the only currently available enzyme replacement in the United States.

Side effects of enzyme replacement therapy include fever, rigors, and chills, typically mild to moderate in nature. These occur in more than half of the patients during the first months of treatment. Infusion related reactions may be due to IgG or IgE antibodies that can be detected in several patients. In case of reactions, the infusion rate should be be decreased or stopped, and the administration of antihistamines and/or corticosteroids should be considered. The infusion can be continued in the case of mild reactions. Some patients need premedication with antihistamines, paracetamol/acetaminophen, or corticosteroids. In patients receiving maintenance dialysis therapy, the infusion can be administered during dialysis treatment.

The clinical effect of both products was examined in two small pivotal trials, a few controlled studies, and numerous uncontrolled studies and registry reports. In a double-blind placebo-controlled trial, Schiffmann et al. randomized 26 adult male patients to receive Agalsidase A (Replagal) at a dosage of 0.2 mg/kg (n = 14; 12 doses total) or placebo (n = 12) every other week. The primary endpoint was neuropathic pain that improved during therapy with Replagal as assessed by a pain questionnaire. Similarly, pain-related quality of life improved during active treatment. Secondary endpoints included kidney function, with no significant difference in the change of measured GFR or renal tissue Gb3 content.

In the other pivotal trial, Eng et al. examined the effect of Agalsidase B (Fabrazyme, 11 infusions total) on 58 adult patients (2 women) with Fabry disease by examining the percentage of patients in whom renal microvascular endothelial Gb3 deposits were cleared. After 20 weeks of treatment, 20 of the 29 patients (69%) in the Agalsidase B group had no microvascular endothelial Gb3 deposits, as compared to no clearance in the placebo group. Among secondary endpoints, there was no difference on pain between active treatment and placebo.

Unfortunately, another important randomized controlled study by Banikazemi et al. was underpowered and failed to show an effect of Agalsidase B on the primary composit endpoint (time to first clinical renal, cardiac, or cerebrovascular event or death) in 82 individuals (10 women and 72 men) with advanced Fabry disease and a mean serum creatinine of 1.6 mg/dl. A per-protocol analysis, adjusted for baseline proteinuria, however, suggested an effect of Agalsidase B as compared to placebo.

Uncontrolled studies suggested stabilization or even improvement of renal and cardiac disease manifestations during enzyme replacement therapy in many patients. Quality of life, gastrointestinal symptoms, hypohydrosis, pulmonary obstruction, and other clinical symptoms also showed improvement. Kidney function, proteinuria, and blood pressure are important predictors of the renal response to enzyme replacement therapy. In a recent analysis of 213 treated patients (Agalsidase B for at least 2 years) enrolled in the Fabry Registry, a higher urinary protein level, poorer initial kidney function, and delayed initiation of enzyme replacement therapy after the onset of symptoms were strong predictors of kidney disease progression in men. A history of cardiac or cerebral events was also associated with a steeper slope of eGFR decline. A total of 75% of the male patients had an eGFR slope of −2.8 to −15.5 mL/min per 1.73 m^2

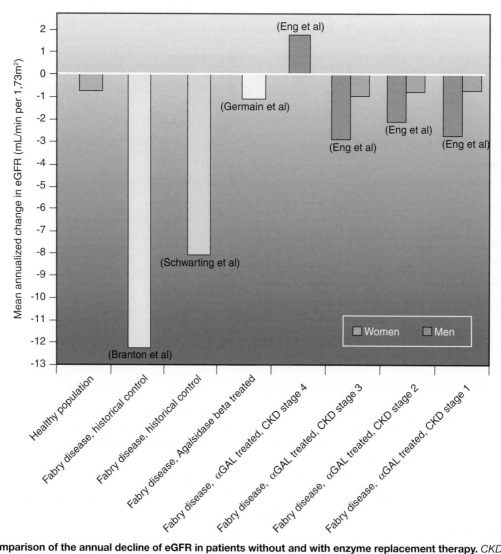

Figure 44.8   Comparison of the annual decline of eGFR in patients without and with enzyme replacement therapy. *CKD,* Chronic kidney disease; *eGFR,* estimated glomerular filtration rate; *ESRD,* end-stage renal disease. (Adapted from Mehta A et al: Enzyme replacement therapy with agalsidase alfa in patients with Fabry's disease: an analysis of registry data. *Lancet* 374:1986-1996, 2009, Fig. 4.)

during enzyme therapy. In a report from the FOS, kidney function was assessed in 208 patients on Agalsidase A treatment for at least 5 years. The mean annual change in eGFR was −2.2 mL/min per 1.73 m² in men and −0.7 mL/min per 1.73 m² in women. Patients with 24-hour protein excretion greater than 1 g/24 h had poorer kidney function at baseline and follow-up compared with patients with protein excretion of 500 to 1000 mg/24 h or less than 500 mg/24 h. Kidney function was worse in patients with baseline hypertension, and there was a more rapid annual decline compared with normotensive patients. Taken together, these data clearly show that Agalsidase A or Agalsidase B cannot halt kidney disease progression in many patients. However, a comparison of treated and untreated patients suggested a somewhat attenuated slope of eGFR decline in treated patients (Fig. 44.8).

Potential reasons for disease progression during enzyme replacement therapy include low physical stability of recombinant αGAL, a short circulating half-life, and variable uptake into different tissues. Thus, novel therapeutic strategies are needed to improve outcomes in patients with Fabry

disease. These include higher frequency and other routes of administration of the enzyme, and the combination or monotherapy with pharmacologic chaperones.

PHARMACOLOGIC CHAPERONES

A pharmacologic chaperone (or pharmacoperone, from "protein chaperone") is a small molecule that causes mutant proteins to fold and route correctly within the cell. Missense mutations in Fabry disease may cause misfolding of αGAL, leading to retention in the endoplasmic reticulum and subsequent degradation. A potent αGAL inhibitor, the iminosugar 1-deoxygalactonojirimycin (migalastat hydrochloride) is an analogon of the terminal galactose of Gb3. It binds to the active site of αGAL, thereby improving stability and trafficking to the lysosomes. It reduces Gb3 storage in vitro and in vivo, and stabilizes wild-type and mutant forms of αGAL. Furthermore, coadministration improves the pharmacologic properties of recombinant human αGAL. It prevents denaturation and activity loss in vitro, and results in substantially higher cellular αGAL and greater Gb3 reduction compared to recombinant human αGAL alone in vivo. Coadministration of 1-deoxygalactono-jirimycin to rats increased the circulating half-life of recombinant human αGAL, and in *GLA* knockout mice resulted in higher αGAL levels and fourfold greater Gb3 reduction than recombinant human αGAL alone. In transgenic mice expressing human mutant αGAL, 1-deoxygalactonojirimycin resulted in significant increases in αGAL activity in various organs, with concomitant reductions in Gb3. Taken together, these data suggest an important clinical potential for this new therapeutic tool, alone or in combination with enzyme replacement therapy.

BIBLIOGRAPHY

Banikazemi M, Bultas J, Waldek S, et al: Agalsidase-beta therapy for advanced Fabry disease: a randomized trial, *Ann Intern Med* 146:77-86, 2007.

Benjamin ER, Khanna R, Schilling A, et al: Co-administration with the pharmacological chaperone AT1001 increases recombinant human alpha-galactosidase A tissue uptake and improves substrate reduction in Fabry mice, *Mol Ther* 20:717-726, 2012.

Branton MH, Schiffmann R, Sabnis SG, et al: Natural history of Fabry renal disease: influence of alpha-galactosidase A activity and genetic mutations on clinical course, *Medicine (Baltimore)* 81:122-138, 2002.

Clarke JT: Narrative review: Fabry disease, *Ann Intern Med* 146:425-433, 2007.

Eng CM, Germain DP, Banikazemi M, et al: Fabry disease: guidelines for the evaluation and management of multi-organ system involvement, *Genet Med* 8:539-548, 2006.

Eng CM, Guffon N, Wilcox WR, et al: Safety and efficacy of recombinant human alpha-galactosidase A replacement therapy in Fabry's disease, *N Engl J Med* 345:9-16, 2001.

Feriozzi S, Torras J, Cybulla M, et al: The effectiveness of long-term agalsidase alfa therapy in the treatment of Fabry nephropathy, *Clin J Am Soc Nephrol* 7:60-69, 2012.

Fogo AB, Bostad L, Svarstad E, et al: Scoring system for renal pathology in Fabry disease: report of the International Study Group of Fabry Nephropathy (ISGFN), *Nephrol Dial Transplant* 25:2168-2177, 2010.

Gal A: Molecular genetics of Fabry disease and genotype-phenotype correlation. In Elstein D, Altarescu G, Beck M, editors: *Fabry disease*. Dordrecht, Heidelberg London New York, 2010, Springer, pp 3-19.

Germain DP, Waldek S, Banikazemi M, et al: Sustained, long-term renal stabilization after 54 months of agalsidase beta therapy in patients with Fabry disease, *J Am Soc Nephrol* 18:1547-1557, 2007.

Linhart A, Kampmann C, Zamorano JL, et al: Cardiac manifestations of Anderson-Fabry disease: results from the international Fabry outcome survey, *Eur Heart J* 28:1228-1235, 2007.

Mechtler TP, Stary S, Metz TF, et al: Neonatal screening for lysosomal storage disorders: feasibility and incidence from a nationwide study in Austria, *Lancet* 379:335-341, 2012.

Mignani R, Feriozzi S, Schaefer RM, et al: Dialysis and transplantation in Fabry disease: indications for enzyme replacement therapy, *Clin J Am Soc Nephrol* 5:379-385, 2010.

Schwarting A, Dehout F, Feriozzi S, et al: Enzyme replacement therapy and renal function in 201 patients with Fabry disease, *Clin Nephrol* 66:77-84, 2006.

Schiffmann R, Kopp JB, Austin HA 3rd, et al: Enzyme replacement therapy in Fabry disease: a randomized controlled trial, *JAMA* 285:2743-2749, 2001.

Schiffmann R, Ries M, Timmons M, et al: Long-term therapy with agalsidase alfa for Fabry disease: safety and effects on renal function in a home infusion setting, *Nephrol Dial Transplant* 21:345-354, 2006.

Schiffmann R, Warnock DG, Banikazemi M, et al: Fabry disease: progression of nephropathy, and prevalence of cardiac and cerebrovascular events before enzyme replacement therapy, *Nephrol Dial Transplant* 24:2102-2111, 2009.

Sunder-Plassmann G: Renal manifestations of Fabry disease. In Mehta A, Beck M, Sunder-Plassmann G, editors: *Fabry disease—perspectives from 5 years of FOS*, Oxford, 2006, Oxford PharmaGenesis, pp 203-214.

Sunder-Plassmann G, Födinger M: Fabry disease case finding studies in high-risk populations. In Elstein D, Altarescu G, Beck M, editors: *Fabry disease*, 2010, Springer, pp 153-162.

Warnock DG, Ortiz A, Mauer M, et al: Renal outcomes of agalsidase beta treatment for Fabry disease: role of proteinuria and timing of treatment initiation, *Nephrol Dial Transplant* 27:1042-1049, 2012.

Warnock DG, Valbuena C, West M, et al: Renal manifestations of Fabry disease. In Elstein D, Altarescu G, Beck M, editors: *Fabry disease. Dordrecht*, Heidelberg London New York, 2010, Springer, pp 211-243.

West M, Nicholls K, Mehta A, et al: Agalsidase alfa and kidney dysfunction in Fabry disease, *J Am Soc Nephrol* 20:1132-1139, 2009.

TUBULOINTERSTITIAL NEPHROPATHIES AND DISORDERS OF THE URINARY TRACT

45 Chronic Tubulointerstitial Disease

Catherine M. Meyers

Primary interstitial nephropathies make up a diverse group of diseases that elicit interstitial inflammation associated with renal tubular cell damage. Traditionally, interstitial nephritis has been classified morphologically and clinically into acute and chronic forms. Acute interstitial nephritis (AIN) generally induces rapid deterioration in kidney function and elicits marked interstitial inflammatory responses characterized by interstitial edema with varying degrees of tubular cell damage. Mononuclear cell infiltrates consist primarily of lymphocytes. This process typically spares both glomerular and vascular structures and is discussed more fully in Chapter 35. By contrast, chronic interstitial nephritis (CIN) follows a more indolent course and is characterized by tubulointerstitial fibrosis and atrophy. It is similarly associated with interstitial mononuclear cell infiltration. Over time, glomerular and vascular structures are involved, with progressive fibrosis and sclerosis within the kidney. Overlap can occur between these two clinical conditions; AIN sometimes presents as a more insidious disease with progression to chronic kidney disease (CKD). Similarly, some forms of CIN are associated with significant cellular.

The U.S. Renal Data System (USRDS) 2011 Annual Data Report indicates that between 2006 and 2010, approximately 4700 (0.9%) incident cases of end-stage renal disease (ESRD) were attributed to primary CIN (including analgesic abuse and lead nephropathy, which are separately reported), with a mean age of 65 years for affected patients. Review of annual incident cases suggests a slight reduction over the last decade, with approximately 1100 cases reported annually in the 1990s, and 850 to 1000 cases reported annually since 2000. In 2009, there were 7000 (1.3%) prevalent cases of ESRD in the United States attributed to primary CIN. The mean age of prevalent cases was 58 years. Since 1990, prevalent cases have slowly increased from approximately 5500 affected patients. Demographic data on patients who develop ESRD as a result of CIN reveal that they are predominantly white (80%).

HISTOPATHOLOGY

Histopathology of CIN is remarkably consistent despite the varied causes (Box 45.1). In addition to tubular cell damage and predominantly mononuclear cell inflammation, CIN is characterized by the development of tubulointerstitial fibrosis and scarring (Figure 45.1). Interstitial granulomatous disease has also been observed in certain forms of CIN (e.g., sarcoidosis). Glomerular and vascular structures may be relatively preserved early in the course of disease, but ultimately become involved in progressive fibrosis and sclerosis. Progressive development of tubulointerstitial fibrosis is a final common pathway to ESRD observed in primary disorders of the tubulointerstitium, as well as in primary glomerular or vascular disorders. All forms of progressive kidney disease eventually result in chronic and progressive interstitial fibrosis.

Similar to AIN, mononuclear cell infiltrates generally accompany CIN, further suggesting a pathogenic immune-mediated mechanism for disease progression. One hypothesis concerning immune recognition of the interstitium suggests that portions of infectious particles or drug molecules may cross-react with or alter endogenous renal antigens. An immune response directed against these inciting agents would therefore also target the interstitium. Intriguing results of a study examining a series of kidney biopsy samples obtained over 8 years at a single center suggest a prominent role of Epstein-Barr virus (EBV) in cases of CIN previously deemed idiopathic. Investigators detected EBV DNA and its receptor, CD21, primarily in proximal tubular cells of all 17 patients with primary idiopathic interstitial nephritis. These findings were not apparent in 10 control kidney biopsy specimens. Such observations imply a more prominent role than previously appreciated for EBV infections in eliciting chronic deleterious immune responses that target the interstitium.

MECHANISMS OF TUBULOINTERSTITIAL FIBROSIS

Observations from the experimental literature suggest that renal tubular epithelial-mesenchymal transition (EMT) may play a role in initiation and progression of tubulointerstitial fibrosis. As the renal epithelium develops from the metanephric mesenchyme via a process of mesenchymal-epithelial transition, observations suggest a unique paradigm of tubulointerstitial response to injury whereby dedifferentiation pathways are activated within the epithelium, resulting in a transition to cells of more mesenchymal characteristics. Dysregulation of such processes in vivo could induce more fibrogenic responses (Figure 45.2). Renal EMT in this setting could thus facilitate accumulation of fibroblasts and myofibroblasts that are characteristic of CIN and other chronic kidney diseases associated with tubulointerstitial fibrosis.

The ability of renal tubular epithelial cells to transform in vitro to fibroblasts and myofibroblasts is well documented. Although the processes relevant for primary CIN in humans have not been elucidated, experimental models of injury and many in vitro studies have implicated a large role for transforming growth factor-β and other fibrogenic

Box 45.1   Chronic Interstitial Nephritis

Drugs/Toxins

Analgesics
Heavy metals (lead, cadmium, mercury)
Lithium
Chinese herbs (aristolochic acid)
Calcineurin inhibitors (cyclosporine, tacrolimus)
Cisplatin
Nitrosoureas

Hereditary Disorders

Polycystic kidney disease
Medullary cystic disease–juvenile nephronophthisis
Hereditary nephritis

Metabolic Disturbances

Hypercalcemia/nephrocalcinosis
Hypokalemia
Hyperuricemia
Hyperoxaluria
Cystinosis

Immune-Mediated Disorders

Kidney allograft rejection
Systemic lupus erythematosus
Sarcoidosis
Granulomatosis with polyangiitis (Wegener granulomatosis)
Vasculitis
Sjögren syndrome

Hematologic Disturbances

Multiple myeloma
Light chain disease
Dysproteinemias
Lymphoproliferative disease
Sickle cell disease

Infections

Kidney
Systemic

Obstruction/Mechanical Disorders

Tumors
Stones
Vesicoureteral reflux

Miscellaneous Disorders

Balkan nephropathy (aristolochic acid)
Radiation nephritis
Aging
Hypertension
Kidney ischemia

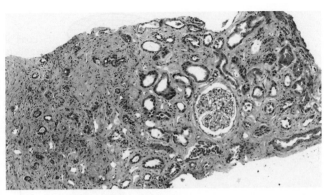

Figure 45.1   Chronic interstitial nephritis. Light microscopy findings demonstrate focal collections of lymphocytes and pronounced loss of normal tubulointerstitial architecture. There is evidence of tubular dilation and atrophy, as well as interstitial fibrosis and relative sparing of glomerular structures. (Hematoxylin-eosin stain, courtesy Dr. James Balow, National Institutes of Health, National Institute of Diabetes, Digestive and Kidney Diseases, Bethesda, Md.)

in vivo in experimental models of disease, have generated apparently conflicting observations regarding the role of EMT in progressive kidney injury. Future studies will likely better characterize pathways that both initiate and propagate renal fibrogenic processes.

CLINICAL FEATURES

As shown in Box 45.1, CIN occurs in a variety of clinical settings, most commonly following exposure to drugs or toxins, or in settings of hereditary disorders, metabolic disorders, immune-mediated diseases, hematologic disturbances, infections, or obstruction. Because CIN tends to occur as a slowly progressive disease, most patients diagnosed with CIN present with systemic complaints of the primary underlying disease, if one exists, or with symptoms of CKD. Laboratory findings in these patients include nonnephrotic-range proteinuria, microscopic hematuria, and sterile pyuria. As listed in Table 45.1, other frequently reported urinary abnormalities such as glucosuria, phosphaturia, and sodium wasting reflect tubular defects. Serologic studies in CIN, such as anti-DNA antibodies, antinuclear antibodies, and complement levels, are typically normal, except when CIN occurs in the setting of a systemic autoimmune disorder.

Affected patients may also have elevated urinary excretion of low-molecular-weight proteins that are commonly associated with tubular injury and damage (e.g., lysozyme, β_2-microglobulin, and retinol-binding protein) and increased enzymuria with N-acetyl-β-D-glucosaminidase, alanine aminopeptidase, and intestinal alkaline phosphatase. However, routine assessment of urinary low-molecular-weight proteins and enzymes is not typically conducted since it is of little diagnostic or prognostic use. Hypertension is another common clinical feature of CIN, although in many forms of CIN it is not apparent until the patient approaches ESRD. With progressive CIN, kidney ultrasonography in patients without significant structural abnormalities (e.g., cystic kidney disease) typically reveals shrunken, echogenic kidneys. Irregular renal contours and renal calcifications are seen in some forms of CIN.

mediators, such as fibroblast growth factor-2, advanced glycation end products, and angiotensin II. These factors regulate the renal fibrogenic responses and renal tubular EMT (see Figure 45.2). In addition, numerous human kidney biopsy studies have demonstrated the colocalization of epithelial and mesenchymal markers on tubular cells in areas of injury, supporting the notion that renal tubular EMT is associated with progressive tubulointerstitial fibrosis in a variety of kidney diseases. However, recent fate-mapping studies, which allow the tagging and tracking of renal epithelial cells

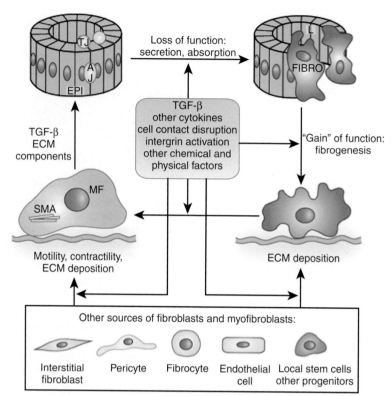

Figure 45.2   The development and progression of renal fibrosis. Fibroblasts and myofibroblasts (MF) originate from other cell types (as noted in the bottom box) and play a significant role in the process of renal fibrosis. The paradigm of tubular epithelial-mesenchymal transition suggests an additional pathway to renal fibrosis, in that tubular epithelium undergoes profound phenotypic changes after exposure to fibrogenic stimuli (center box). This results in loss of epithelial characteristics and gain of mesenchymal characteristics. The transitioning cells might remain in the tubular wall or migrate into the interstitium. Epithelial-derived fibroblasts contribute to the deposition of extracellular matrix (ECM), and a subpopulation may begin expressing α-smooth muscle actin (SMA), a hallmark of the MF phenotype. Activated fibroblasts and MF secrete elevated amounts of transforming growth factor-β (TGF-β), whereas the enhanced contractility of MFs contributes to activation of latent TGF-β through an integrin-mediated mechanochemical pathway. Increasing TGF-β levels along with ECM accumulation might facilitate transformation of previously intact tubules, thereby creating a positive feedback loop of epithelial injury. *AJ*, Adherens junction; *EPI*, epithelium; *FIBRO*, fibroblasts; *L*, lumen; *TJ*, tight junction. (Reprinted by permission from Macmillan Publishers Ltd: Quaggin SE, Kapus A: Scar wars: mapping the fate of epithelial-mesenchymal-myofibroblast transition, *Kidney Int* 80:41-50, 2011.)

Table 45.1   Laboratory Findings in Interstitial Nephritis

Parameter	Finding
Urinary sediment	Erythrocytes, leukocytes (eosinophils), leukocyte casts
Fractional excretion of sodium	Usually >1%
Proximal tubular defects	Glucosuria, bicarbonaturia, phosphaturia, aminoaciduria, proximal RTA
Distal tubular defects	Hyperkalemia, sodium wasting, distal RTA
Medullary defects	Sodium wasting, urine-concentrating defects

RTA, Renal tubular acidosis.

CLINICAL COURSE AND THERAPY

In view of the slowly progressive loss of kidney function observed in most cases of CIN, general therapeutic considerations include treating an underlying systemic disorder (sarcoidosis), avoiding the drug or toxin exposure (analgesics, lead), or eliminating the condition that has induced the chronic interstitial lesion (obstruction). The interstitial fibrosis and scarring, along with the resultant impairment in kidney function, in CIN are not currently amenable to therapeutic intervention. Although definitive diagnosis of CIN requires kidney biopsy, it is probably of limited usefulness in patients with advanced CKD or kidney failure. Therapy for CIN is therefore largely supportive, with renal replacement therapy initiated in patients who develop ESRD. More specific therapies for interstitial lesions associated with lead exposure or sarcoidosis will be discussed in the following section.

DISTINCT CAUSES OF CHRONIC TUBULOINTERSTITIAL NEPHRITIS

Many causes of CIN listed in Box 45.1 are more fully described in other chapters of this text. This section will focus on the common causes of primary CIN. It is also noted that progression to ESRD has been reported with all forms of AIN. The USRDS 2011 Annual Report relates that 1329 (0.2%, 2006-2010 combined) incident cases and 685 (0.1%, 2009) prevalent cases of ESRD in the United States were due to AIN. USRDS data also indicate that both incidence

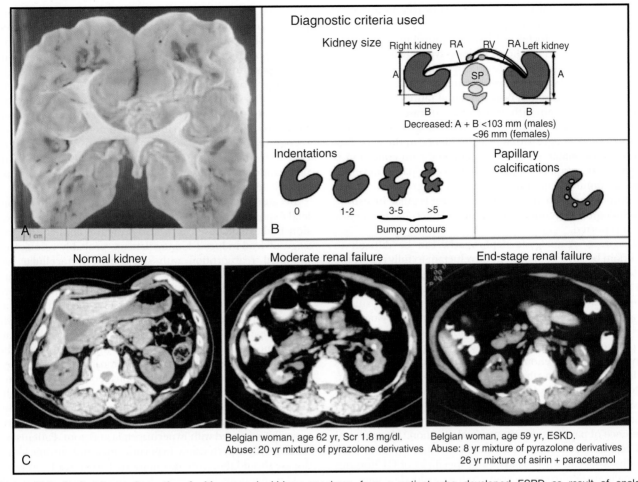

Figure 45.3 Analgesic nephropathy. A, Macroscopic kidney specimen from a patient who developed ESRD as result of analgesic nephropathy. **B,** Characteristic analgesic nephropathy features on CT scanning include reduced kidney size, irregular contours, and papillary calcifications. **C,** Noncontrast CT findings comparing a normal subject with two cases of analgesic nephropathy, with two distinct levels of reduced kidney function. (Reprinted by permission from the *Journal of the American Society of Nephrology*: De Broe ME, Elseviers MM: Over-the-counter analgesic use, *J Am Soc Nephr* 20:2098-2103, 2009.)

and prevalence of ESRD due to AIN have increased steadily since 1990. The mean ages for incident and prevalent ESRD cases were 65 years and 63 years, respectively. Similar to the observations for ESRD assigned to CIN, reported cases are noted predominantly in whites (80%).

ANALGESIC NEPHROPATHY

Analgesic nephropathy has been considered the most common form of drug-induced CIN, particularly in the United States, Europe, and Australia. The condition is associated with chronic excessive consumption of combined analgesic preparations over many years. Affected patients typically have regularly ingested combination analgesic products (e.g., aspirin, phenacetin, paracetamol) that also contain codeine or caffeine. Over the last several decades, however, recognition of the association of analgesic nephropathy with chronic use of over-the-counter combination analgesic products resulted in a marked reduction in availability of these products to the public, as well as a marked reduction in incidence of this disease. Phenacetin-containing combination products were particularly noted for their association with analgesic nephropathy, although the disorder continues to be reported even after these products

were removed from the market. The subsequent removal of other combination analgesic products resulted in a further decrease in the incidence of analgesic nephropathy worldwide. Since 2002, the USRDS Annual Data Report indicates that approximately 180 cases of ESRD due to analgesic nephropathy are reported each year in the United States.

The nephrotoxicity of combination analgesics appears to be dose-dependent, with medullary lesions most prominent early in the disease course. Early medullary capillary and tubular changes then extend to interstitial injury and fibrosis, as well as renal papillary necrosis (RPN) with calcification. RPN is characteristic, but not diagnostic, of analgesic nephropathy, because it occurs in other kidney disorders such as diabetes mellitus, sickle cell disease, renal tuberculosis, and urinary tract obstruction. It has also been reported with use of single reagent analgesic preparations such as nonsteroidal antiinflammatory drugs or aspirin. The mechanism of nephrotoxicity is not completely understood. Ingested compounds and their metabolites are concentrated along the medullary osmotic gradient, likely achieving chronic high levels within the medulla to facilitate the early renal medullary lesions. In addition to high local metabolite concentrations, the relatively vulnerable vascular supply in the medulla could play a major role in initiating and propagating kidney injury.

Similar to many forms of CIN, the clinical manifestations are nonspecific and insidious. Patients typically present with sterile pyuria, mild proteinuria, and slowly progressive disease. As kidney disease progresses, anemia and hypertension develop. The disease has been reported more commonly in women than in men, with 50% to 80% of cases reported in women across several studies. The age range extends from 30 to 70 years of age, with a peak incidence in the early 50s. Daily use of analgesics to treat a chronic pain condition is noted, and estimates suggest that nephropathy develops after a cumulative ingestion of 2 to 3 kilograms of analgesic preparations. In view of the excessive regular ingestion, psychological dependence on these products has frequently been reported.

Diagnosis of analgesic nephropathy can be difficult to ascertain because patients may be reluctant to fully report the extent of chronic analgesic use, and early signs and symptoms are nonspecific. Clinicians frequently rely on a combination of clinical history, urinary findings, and kidney imaging studies to aid in diagnosis of the condition. Intravenous pyelography has not proven useful in view of its low sensitivity and use of nephrotoxic contrast. Computerized tomography (CT) scanning without intravenous contrast is frequently used to assess kidney structures in this setting (Figure 45.3). Several characteristic findings on CT scan support the diagnosis of analgesic nephropathy, including bilateral reduction in kidney volume, cortical scarring with irregular renal contours, and evidence of papillary damage and calcification. These typical CT features are not generally noted in other forms of CIN. Studies assessing the sensitivity and specificity of CT findings in analgesic nephropathy, however, have yielded inconsistent findings. Variability may result from different time frames of study, different geographic regions studied (European and U.S. cohort), and distinct analgesic preparations. The noncontrast CT scan is considered a useful diagnostic test even if performed with patients that do not provide a reliable history of excessive analgesic use.

The clinical course of classic analgesic nephropathy is variable and depends largely on the extent of irreversible renal scarring that has occurred at the time of diagnosis. Like most toxin-induced interstitial diseases, removal of the offending agent before irreversible renal fibrosis is essential for preserving kidney function. Several reports of analgesic nephropathy have described stabilization or mild improvement in kidney function with cessation of analgesic use. In addition to CKD and ESRD, patients with analgesic nephropathy are at increased risk for gastritis and peptic ulcer disease, related to excessive analgesic exposure. This exposure is also associated with development of uroepithelial tumors later in life. Urinary tract malignancies reported are most commonly transitional cell carcinoma, although renal cell carcinoma and sarcoma have also occurred. Excessive analgesic use also appears to confer an increased risk for cardiovascular disease, specifically ischemic heart disease and renal artery stenosis.

CHRONIC LEAD NEPHROPATHY

Exposure to high levels of lead over several years to decades is associated with a progressive CIN referred to as chronic lead nephropathy. Most such exposures are occupational

and seen in the manufacturing or use of lead-containing paints, ammunitions, radiators, batteries, wires, ceramic glazes, solder, and metal cans. In addition, environmental lead exposure can occur in several settings, such as using lead pipes and solder joints in drinking-water lines, consuming crops grown in lead-contaminated soil, or ingesting lead-based paint scraps or "moonshine" generated in lead-lined car radiators. In the developed world, it is rare to see lead exposure high enough to induce lead nephropathy because recognition of its toxicity has resulted in routine removal of lead from sources such as gasoline, paint, and industrial processing. In the absence of such high chronic exposures, chronic lead nephropathy is rarely reported.

Because an early histologic lesion observed with chronic lead exposure consists of proximal tubular intranuclear inclusion bodies composed of a lead-protein complex, the early stage of lead-induced kidney damage probably results from proximal reabsorption with subsequent intracellular lead accumulation. Early clinical manifestations reflect proximal tubular dysfunction with hyperuricemia, aminoaciduria, and glucosuria (see Table 45.1). Because the kidney disease is slowly progressive, affected patients typically present with CKD, hypertension, hyperuricemia, and gout. This symptom complex might, however, suggest the diagnosis of either chronic urate nephropathy or hypertensive nephrosclerosis. Chronic urate nephropathy with tophaceous gout is currently an uncommon condition; moreover, some studies suggest that previously reported cases were actually associated with chronic lead exposure. By contrast, hypertensive nephrosclerosis is not typically associated with hyperuricemia and gout. Patients presenting with hypertension, hyperuricemia, and chronic kidney disease should therefore be questioned about lead exposure.

The diagnosis of chronic lead intoxication is generally established with a lead mobilization test, performed by measuring urinary lead excretion after administering ethylenediaminetetraacetic acid (EDTA). X-ray fluorescence can also be used to determine bone lead levels. The diagnosis of lead nephropathy, however, is frequently made on the basis of a history of lead exposure in the setting of hyperuricemia, hypertension, and slowly progressive kidney disease consistent with CIN. Treatment of lead intoxication consists of chelation therapy with EDTA or oral succimer. In view of the side effects associated with EDTA administration, chelation therapy should be carefully considered, particularly if there is significant preexisting irreversible kidney fibrosis.

It is noted that recent population-based studies have observed a trend of increased blood lead levels in the general population, and a related inverse trend in creatinine clearance. It is unclear, however, whether these population-based observations reflect an increase in chronic lead nephropathy, or an increase in kidney disease that induces lead retention. Such studies suggest, however, that chronic low-level lead exposure in developing countries may confer additional risk for CKD. In addition, some studies have suggested that chelation therapy may slow progression of CKD in patients with excessive total body lead levels.

ARISTOLOCHIC ACID NEPHROPATHY

Rapidly progressive fibrosing interstitial nephritis has been described in clusters of patients in weight loss programs who ingested Chinese herbal preparations tainted with a plant nephrotoxin derived from *Aristolochia fangchi* (aristolochic acid). Kidney lesions are characterized by interstitial fibrosis and tubular atrophy, with a predominance of cortical involvement. Several hundred cases have been reported in the literature thus far, although some cases were observed in patients who ingested herb preparations not containing aristolochic acid. Other reports from Asia suggest that herbal therapy-induced kidney damage is not uncommon. Kidney disease in affected individuals is typically progressive and irreversible despite withdrawal of toxin exposure, with many patients requiring dialysis therapy or transplantation within 1 year of presentation.

The putative nephrotoxin, aristolochic acid, induces tubulointerstitial fibrosis in animal models of disease following chronic daily exposure. The mechanism of aristolochic acid-induced nephrotoxicity, however, has not been delineated. The observation that some patients exposed to toxic herbs do not develop kidney disease further suggests variability in patient susceptibility to kidney injury. Women may be at higher risk for the disorder. In addition, variability in herbal products could significantly alter toxin concentration in batched preparations. Studies in animal models indicate that both toxin exposure and concurrent renal vasoconstriction may be required to precipitate the characteristic progressive kidney disease. A frequent association of cellular atypia and urothelial cell malignancies has also been reported in experimental animals and in many affected patients. Identification of aristolactam-DNA adducts, as well as tumor suppressor *p53* gene mutations, in genitourinary tumors has implicated these factors in malignant urothelial transformation. Because many affected patients have undergone kidney transplantation with immunosuppressive therapy, routine surveillance of urinary cytology is generally recommended in view of this association with urothelial malignancy.

BALKAN NEPHROPATHY

Balkan nephropathy is a form of CIN endemic to the areas of Bulgaria, Romania, Serbia, Croatia, Bosnia, and Herzegovina. It occurs most commonly along the confluence of the Danube River and has been reported almost exclusively in farmers. Although the disease etiology has not been elucidated, several environmental toxins (plant nephrotoxins, mycotoxins, trace metals, and aromatic hydrocarbons) have been explored. The tendency for clustering of cases in families has also suggested that genetic variables may play a role in disease susceptibility, and several recent studies suggest that disease is induced by chronic exposure to aristolochic acid in susceptible individuals. Because *Aristolochia* plants grow abundantly in agricultural areas, harvesting of crops such as wheat from contaminated fields could introduce aristolochic acid into the local food supply, exposing the population to the nephrotoxin. Like many forms of CIN, Balkan nephropathy is a slowly progressive kidney disease, and patients present with blood and urinary evidence of tubular dysfunction. It is typically observed after the fourth decade of life and rarely affects patients younger than 20 years of age. Patients generally present with normal blood pressure and either normal or slightly reduced kidney size on ultrasonography. Renal histologic lesions are characterized by predominant cortical fibrosis and tubular

atrophy. A diagnostic test has not been developed for Balkan nephropathy, and there is not currently a specific treatment or preventive strategy for the disorder.

Although the clinical course and affected populations for Balkan nephropathy and aristolochic acid nephropathy are quite distinct, the two entities share many similarities. Both diseases have been linked to aristolochic acid exposure, have predominant renal cortical pathology, and are associated with urothelial tumors. Studies have reported a wide range of tumor incidence, from 2% to 47%, in patients with Balkan nephropathy. A recent study of renal and urothelial cancer tissue isolated from patients with Balkan nephropathy identified DNA adducts from aristolochic acid as well as *p53* gene mutations—two features that characterize aristolochic acid–induced tumors in experimental models and patients with aristolochic acid nephropathy. These observations have further implicated aristolochic acid in the pathogenesis of Balkan nephropathy.

SARCOIDOSIS

The most common kidney manifestation of sarcoidosis is mediated through disordered calcium metabolism resulting in hypercalcemia and hypercalciuria, occasionally presenting with nephrolithiasis. Although interstitial disease, at times with noncaseating granuloma formation, is relatively common in sarcoidosis (15% to 30%), autopsy series indicate that it is unusual for the interstitial abnormalities to result in clinically significant kidney dysfunction. Moreover, it is unusual to observe interstitial disease in the absence of extrarenal involvement in sarcoidosis. Although most patients with impaired kidney function respond well to corticosteroid therapy, recovery of kidney function is frequently incomplete because of chronic interstitial inflammation and fibrosis. Presentation with hypercalcemia has been associated with more sustained response to corticosteroid therapy 1 year following therapy. Relapse of kidney functional impairment during steroid taper has been reported, but progression to ESRD is rare.

SJÖGREN SYNDROME

Sjögren syndrome, a disorder characterized by lymphocyte and plasma cell infiltration in salivary, parotid, and lacrimal glands, results in progressive organ dysfunction and the sicca syndrome. Involvement of other organs, including the kidney, is frequently reported. Circulating autoantibodies (anti-Ro and anti-La) are associated with Sjögren syndrome, and they support the diagnosis. Kidney involvement has been reported in up to 67% of affected patients in some case series. The kidney lesion noted on biopsy consists predominantly of interstitial cellular infiltrates that invade and destroy renal tubules. Cortical granuloma formation has been reported and may suggest the diagnosis of sarcoidosis or the tubulointerstitial nephritis and uveitis (TINU) syndrome. These other conditions, however, are not associated with sicca syndrome. With disease chronicity in Sjögren syndrome, tubular atrophy and interstitial fibrosis are more apparent, and patients may exhibit biochemical disorders from tubular dysfunction. As with sarcoidosis treatment, patients typically respond to a course of corticosteroids. Although rare, ESRD has been reported.

BIBLIOGRAPHY

Becker JL, Miller F, Nuovo GJ, et al: Epstein-Barr virus infection of renal proximal tubule cells: possible role in chronic interstitial nephritis, *J Clin Invest* 104:1673-1681, 1999.

Brause M, Magnusson K, Degenhardt S, et al: Renal involvement in sarcoidosis—a report of 6 cases, *Clin Nephrol* 57:142-148, 2002.

De Broe ME, Elseviers MM: Over-the-counter analgesic use, *J Am Soc Nephrol* 20:2098-2103, 2009.

Ekong EB, Jaar BG, Weaver VM: Lead-related nephrotoxicity: a review of the epidemiologic evidence, *Kidney Int* 70:2074-2080, 2006.

Evans M, Elinder C- G: Chronic renal failure from lead: myth or evidence-based fact? *Kidney Int* 79:272-279, 2011.

Grollman AP, Shibutani S, Moriya M, et al: Aristolochic acid and the etiology of endemic (Balkan) nephropathy, *Proc Natl Acad Sci USA* 104:12129-12134, 2007.

Henrich WL, Clark RL, Kelly JP, et al: Non-contrast-enhanced computerized tomography and analgesic-related kidney disease: report of the national analgesic nephropathy study, *J Am Soc Nephrol* 17:1472, 2006.

Humphreys BD, Lin SL, Kobayashi A, et al: Fate tracing reveals the pericyte and not epithelial origin of myofibroblasts in kidney fibrosis, *Am J Pathol* 176:85-97, 2010.

Jelaković B, Karanović, Vuković-Lela I, et al: Aristolacam-DNA adducts are a biomarker of environmental exposure to aristolochic acid, *Kidney Int* 81:559-567, 2012.

Kim R, Rotnitsky A, Sparrow D, et al: A longitudinal study of low-level lead exposure and impairment of renal function. The Normative Aging Study, *JAMA* 275:1177-1181, 1996.

Kritz W, Kaissling B, Le Hir M: Epithelial-mesenchymal transition (EMT) is kidney fibrosis: fact or fantasy? *J Clin Invest* 121:468-474, 2011.

Lin JL, Lin-Tan DT, Hsu KU, et al: Environmental lead exposure and progression of chronic renal diseases in patients without diabetes, *N Engl J Med* 348:277-286, 2003.

Mahévas M, Lescure FX, Boffa JJ, et al: Renal sarcoidosis: clinical, laboratory, and histologic presentation and outcome in 47 patients, *Medicine (Baltimore)* 88:98-106, 2009.

Meyers CM: New insights into the pathogenesis of interstitial nephritis, *Curr Opin Nephrol Hypertens* 8:287-292, 1999.

Muntner P, He J, Vupputuri S, et al: Blood lead and chronic kidney disease in the general United States population: Results from NHANES III, *Kidney Int* 63:1044-1050, 2003.

Nortier JL, Martinex M-C, Schmeiser HH, et al: Urothelial carcinoma associated with the use of a Chinese herb (*Aristolochia fangchi*), *N Engl J Med* 342:1686-1692, 2000.

Quaggin SE, Kapus A: Scar wars: mapping the fate of epithelial-mesenchymal-myofibroblast transition, *Kidney Int* 80:41-50, 2011.

Rossert J: Drug-induced interstitial nephritis, *Kidney Int* 60:804-817, 2001.

Strutz F, Okada H, Lo CS, et al: Identification and characterization of a fibroblast marker: FSP1, *J Cell Biol* 130:393-405, 1995.

Obstructive Uropathy

46

Richard W. Sutherland

Obstruction of the urinary tract can occur anywhere from the collecting duct to the urethral meatus. Microcrystals in the collecting duct, urinary calculi, tumors, and luminal strictures can block the normal flow of urine. Regardless of the cause, the ultimate effect is the same, an increase in the hydrostatic pressure of the collecting system, which is transmitted into Bowman space. This reduces the glomerular filtration rate (GFR) and initiates a cascade of events that, if not reversed, will result in kidney scarring and loss of kidney function. The extent of kidney function loss and the damage to the physical structures of the collecting system varies depending on the duration and completeness of the obstruction. The decrease in kidney function is determined by the loss of GFR and the loss of tubular functions. Although both are critical to proper function, GFR is the dominant contributor. In an unobstructed kidney, when glomerular filtration is disrupted tubular functions collapse. The glomerular filtrate is necessary to provide the substrate (i.e., Na^+ ions) for tubular functions. In prolonged obstruction of the kidney, both glomerular and tubular functions are compromised.

UNILATERAL URETERAL OBSTRUCTION

Historically, unilateral and bilateral ureteral obstructions are discussed separately because of the distinct changes in renal physiology that occur after obstruction. In the first hours after obstruction, differences between the two occur in the blood flow to the glomeruli and the ureteral pressure profiles. In unilateral ureteral obstruction (UUO), a triphasic event of vascular blood flow and ureteral pressure is seen. Only two phases are seen in bilateral ureteral obstruction (BUO). In UUO (Fig. 46.1), there is an initial elevation in the luminal hydrostatic pressure. GFR is maintained by a simultaneous increase in the glomerular capillary pressure induced by afferent arteriolar dilation. Prostaglandin E_2 (PGE_2) and nitrous oxide (NO) are considered the initial mediators. Studies using inhibitors of PGE_2 and NO attenuate the increase in renal blood flow and GFR. The exact triggering mechanisms for the production of PGE_2 and NO are less well understood, but may be due to the decreased presentation of Na^+ to the macula densa. These increases in GFR and luminal pressure define the first phase.

The second phase of UUO begins with the decrease of glomerular blood flow. Between 12 and 24 hours after the initial obstruction, there is a switch from afferent arteriolar vasodilation to vasoconstriction. Activation of the renin-angiotensin system occurs during the first phase and becomes the dominant process affecting GFR, whereupon efferent and partial afferent arteriole vasoconstriction overwhelms the PGE_2 and NO vasodilation. Experimental data show that the administration of angiotensin converting enzyme (ACE) inhibitors blunts the vasoconstriction and reduction in GFR. Thromboxane A2 and endothelin reduce glomerular blood flow during UUO. The second phase of UUO is defined by a persistent elevation of hydrostatic pressure from the obstructed lumen even with the reduction of GFR.

The third and last phase of UUO is marked by decreased luminal hydrostatic pressure and renal blood flow. Glomerular capillary blood flow and luminal pressure remain below baseline until the obstruction is relieved. It is during this last phase that the majority of permanent damage is done to the kidney. The return to baseline function is dependent on the overall duration and severity of the initial obstruction. Complete obstruction for 24 hours can produce up to a 50% reduction in GFR in the animal model.

BILATERAL URETERAL OBSTRUCTION

The primary difference between UUO and BUO is persistent postglomerular vasoconstriction of the efferent artery, which maintains GFR. Luminal pressure remains elevated for longer than the 24 hours in BUO, whereas it begins to decrease by 6 hours with UUO. To account for the preglomerular dilation and postglomerular vasoconstriction, it is likely that additional vasoactive substances accumulate in BUO, but not in UUO. Atrial natriuretic peptide (ANP) would be the obvious substance as it is produced in the setting of volume overload and increases diuresis. Increased GFR and associated diuresis occur through vasodilation of the afferent arteriole and vasoconstriction of the efferent arteriole.

There are a number of additional vasoactive substances that affect the kidneys in both UUO and BUO. Vasodilators PGE_2 and NO are likely present because blockade of their production magnifies the already blunted increase in GFR seen in obstruction. This suggests that although ANP produces afferent dilation, PGE_2 and NO enhance this process. Inhibition of TXA-2 and angiotensinogen II production reduces postobstructive diuresis as compared with controls. This minimizes the amount of vasoconstriction that maintains GFR and protects nephron function.

TUBULAR DYSFUNCTION

Loss of tubular function during obstruction occurs primarily from a decrease in GFR rather than direct hydrostatic pressure injury to the tubular cells. Sodium and potassium homeostasis, water handling, and acidification are altered. The decline in GFR initiates a series of compensatory yet maladaptive events

397

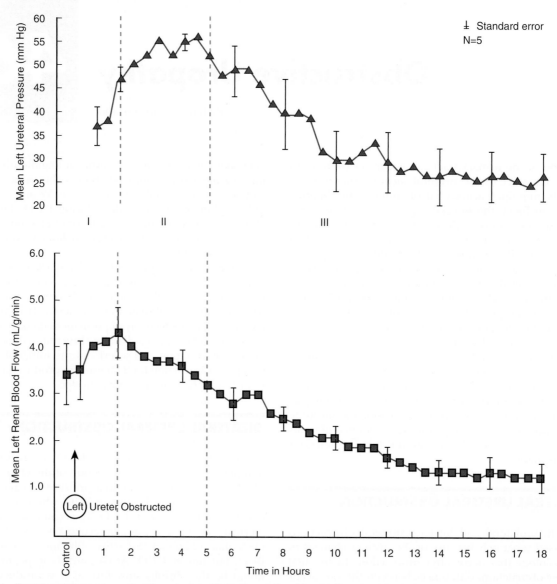

Figure 46.1 Renal resistance in ureteral occlusion. Triphasic relationship of left ureteral luminal pressure and left renal blood flow after occlusion of the left ureter. (Moody TE, Vaughn ED Jr, Gillenwater JY: Relationship between renal blood flow and ureteral pressure during 18 hours of total unilateral urethral occlusion: implications for changing sites of increased renal resistance, *Invest Urol* 13:246-251, 1975.)

that are mediated by vasoactive substances, cytokines, and ischemia. These events alter the amount of filtrate, the composition of the filtrate, tubular transport proteins, and tubular blood flow.

SODIUM REABSORPTION

Obstruction of the kidney impairs Na^+ reabsorption throughout the nephron. Apical Na^+/H^+ exchanger (NHE3), apical $Na^+K^+2Cl^-$ cotransporter (NKCC2), and basolateral Na^+/K^+ ATPase pumps are all thought to be downregulated in obstructed kidneys. Cell suspension studies of distinct nephron segments support this conclusion. In the proximal tubule, reduction of the NHE3 activity is seen. In the loop of Henle, decreased activity of the Na^+K^+ATPase occurs. Diminished activity of the NKCC2 cotransporter is noted in cells studied from the thick ascending limb. Reabsorption of Na^+ also requires apical movement from the lumen

into the cell. This process is similarly affected by furosemide, supporting disruption of the NKCC2 transporter. In the medullary portion of the collecting system, the Na^+/H^+ exchanger has reduced energy consumption and decreased expression of NHE3. Many of these transport processes are energy dependent and require ATP. Although a reduction in the amount of available ATP has been hypothesized due to ischemia, ATP production/supply does not appear to be the rate-limiting step in Na^+ transport.

The actual triggers for the loss of receptor and enzyme activity are still poorly understood. Possible signals include decreased filtrate substrates, natriuretic substances, and direct tubular hydrostatic pressure. Decreased GFR reduces filtrate and Na^+ ion presentation to the cells. Depletion of the Na^+ ion could downregulate its receptor and transport proteins. Additionally, loss of luminal Na^+ reduces the electrochemical gradient, whereas blockade of Na^+ movement into obstructed medullary thick ascending limb cells results in a loss of ouabain-sensitive ATPase. Taken together, decreased Na$^+$ presentation to cells could downregulate Na$^+$-K$^+$-ATPase, which could be at the translational or post-translational level. Ischemia may also play a role.

PGE$_2$ levels change as a result of obstruction, and eventually begin to affect Na$^+$ reabsorption. PGE$_2$ is released during obstruction from increased COX-2 production. COX-2 inhibition reduces the loss of activity of the NKCC2 and Na$^+$-K$^+$-ATPase, implying an effect of PGE$_2$ to impair Na$^+$ reabsorption.

Na$^+$ reabsorption in BUO differs from UUO because of the presence of volume expansion. The addition of ANP and the loss of aldosterone reduces tubular reabsorption of Na$^+$. Much of the impaired Na$^+$ handling in UUO is amplified by the effect of ANP, which blocks release of renin and reduces the ultimate creation of angiotensin II. ANP also directly reduces Na$^+$ reabsorption in the collecting duct and blocks angiotensin II's effect on Na$^+$ reabsorption, the net effect being diuresis and natriuresis.

URINARY CONCENTRATION

Obstruction disrupts normal urinary concentration. With a reduced GFR, less Na$^+$ is available to create the osmolar gradient in the medullary interstitium. As with the defects in Na$^+$ reabsorption, there is loss of the apical and basolateral membrane proteins, NKCC2 cotransporter, and Na$^+$-K$^+$ ATPase. This prevents Na$^+$ transport from the tubular lumen into the medullary interstitium, which is critical to the countercurrent multiplier that creates the medullary gradient. Without the ability to reabsorb Na$^+$ in the ascending limb and dilute the filtrate as it enters the distal convoluted tubule, the solutes required to maintain the gradient are excreted. In the collecting duct of an obstructed kidney, antidiuretic hormone's (ADH) action to increase water permeability is blunted because of decreased AQP-2 in the apical membrane. Several studies have shown this to be a post-cAMP defect. Reduced transcription of the AQP-2 mRNA and a decrease in the phosphorylation necessary to incorporate the AQP-2 vesicles into the apical membrane explain this effect. Finally, a decrease in basolateral membrane AQP-3 and AQP-4 is also noted. After obstruction is removed, overall concentration returns to the kidney paralleling the return of the AQP-2 channel to the apical membrane.

Urea recycling is another process used by the nephron to increase the gradient for urinary concentration. Urea within the filtrate passively exits the collecting duct at its inner medullary segment and enters the interstitium. The vasa recta and the thin portion of the loop of Henle reabsorb it. A maximum medullary interstitial osmotic gradient is created with the recycling of urea. Urea permeability in the collecting duct tubules is controlled by the urea transporter (UT)-A1 and UT-A3 receptors. ADH enhances the permeability of urea, allowing it to flow into the interstitium. Urea reabsorption by the vasa recta is stimulated by UT-B receptors controlled by ADH. In the obstructed kidney, expression of urea transporters UT-A1, UT-A3, and UT-B is reduced. This urea transporter defect reduces the maximal concentrating effect of the gradient by disrupting urea recycling and allowing urea to be excreted.

POTASSIUM

K$^+$ handling in the nephron is not affected directly by obstruction. The initial disturbance in K$^+$ metabolism is explained by defects in Na$^+$ handling, H$^+$ handling, and reduced GFR. With obstruction, there is a decrease in both Na$^+$ reabsorption (reduced Na$^+$ channels) and Na$^+$ presentation to the distal tubule (reduced GFR). Decreased K$^+$ secretion also occurs as a result of increased intraluminal K$^+$. In the low-flow state of obstruction, high urinary potassium concentrations in the collecting duct result in a loss in the gradient between the lumen and the cell's cytoplasm. This results in a reduction in K$^+$ movement into the lumen, and ultimately hyperkalemia.

ACIDIFICATION

Urinary obstruction produces metabolic acidosis best understood as a form of distal (type 1) renal tubular acidosis (RTA) with hyperkalemia, or "voltage dependent" RTA. It is characterized by a failure of distal H$^+$ and K$^+$ secretion. Na$^+$ channel defects play a central role in this acidosis. Loss of Na$^+$ reabsorption from the distal tubule results in impaired urinary acidification in the obstructed kidney. Na$^+$/K$^+$ ATPase dysfunction on the basolateral surface of the cell ultimately disrupts Na$^+$ removal from the lumen of the collecting duct. This decrease in cation reabsorption reduces the opposite passive excretion of H$^+$ into the collecting duct lumen down the electrochemical gradient, and a "voltage-dependent acidosis" occurs. Simultaneous hyperkalemia occurs from failure of Na$^+$-K$^+$-ATPase and Na$^+$ reabsorption. Decreased expression of the H$^+$/ATPase in the collecting duct adds to the metabolic acidosis. Although the defect of the H$^+$/ATPase transporter is critical to classic distal RTA, it cannot account completely for the acidosis in hyperkalemic distal RTA. Urinary acidification occurs in the early phases of obstruction suggesting an intact proton pump. Similarities are noted between voltage dependent RTA and type 4 RTA. In neither of these two processes is H$^+$ secretion felt to be the primary defect. Hypoaldosteronism of type 4 RTA leads to impaired secretion of K$^+$ and hyperkalemia.

FIBROSIS

Persistent obstruction produces tubulointerstitial fibrosis. The activated pathways producing fibrosis do not differ significantly from fibrosis noted with other disease processes. An imbalance in normal kidney homeostasis results in excess accumulation of extracellular matrix (ECM) with the subsequent development of tubulointerstitial fibrosis and, in later stages, glomerular and vascular sclerosis.

Obstructive uropathy produces tissue inhibitors of metalloproteinases (TIMPs), which decrease the activity of the metalloproteinases (MMPs). This decrease in MMPs shifts the normal balance of generation and removal of ECM to one that favors an increase in ECM. At the cellular level, there is an increase in the number of fibroblast and myofibroblasts. Infiltrating macrophages and fibroblasts responding to injury release cytokines and stimulate growth factors such as TGF-β, interleukin (IL)-2, and IL-6. Epithelial tubular cells and endothelial cells transform into mesenchymal cells, losing their epithelial or endothelial phenotype. This epithelial-mesenchymal transition (EMT) and endothelial-mesenchymal transition (EndMT) produce additional fibroblasts necessary for collagen deposition. The presence of angiotensin II, triggered by obstruction, stimulates the expression of TGF-β, a facilitator of fibrosis. Additional growth factors, cytokines, and vasoactive compounds that promote cell growth and fibrosis, such as TNF-α, NF-κB, platelet-derived growth factor (PDGF), vascular cell adhesion molecule-1 (VCAM-1), and basic fibroblast growth factor (bFGF), are upregulated by angiotensin II. Therapeutic strategies, such as ACE-inhibitors to reduce fibrosis, are still hypothetical. There are no good data that support medical intervention to block these pathways in the hope of reducing kidney scarring.

APOPTOSIS

Apoptosis, programmed cell death, is a normal physiologic mechanism that occurs within the kidney and throughout other organ systems of the body. During obstruction, apoptosis is increased through external and internal cellular signals. Extrinsic activation with obstruction occurs from an increase in the tissue levels of TNF-α, which binds its receptor TNFR1. This complex then combines with the cell death domain (TRADD) to activate apoptotic pathways resulting in cell death. Intrinsic activation occurs from oxidative stress, which causes intracellular release of a number of substances from damaged organelle. Mitrochondrial release of cytochrome-c is a known trigger in many organ systems for apoptosis, and this occurs within the kidney. Stress to the endoplasmic reticulum upregulates the apoptotic c-JUN NH2 terminal kinase, resulting in increased inflammation and subsequent fibrosis. The external and internal pathways converge on a single pathway to continue apoptosis through effector caspases, which cleave the nucleus to create apoptotic bodies. There are 12 different caspases, with 3, 8, and 12 identified within the obstructed kidney tissue.

POSTOBSTRUCTIVE DIURESIS

Postobstructive diuresis is a normal physiologic event in patients with prolonged BUO. The rate of diuresis is based on the severity of volume overload, urea accumulation, and electrolyte disturbances that occurred during obstruction. There is no rate of urine output that defines postobstructive diuresis. However, rates of 250 mL/h are common, and 750 mL/h can be seen.

There are several factors that facilitate the physiologic diuresis. Before release of the obstruction, there is a downregulation of the Na^+ transporters, and the inability to reabsorb Na^+ diminishes the osmotic gradient necessary for urinary concentration. In the distal tubule, downregulation and reduced aquaporin activity promote aquaresis. ANP is released because of activation of the cardiac atrial stretch receptors from increased preload, further increasing urine output.

Initial treatment of the postobstructive diuresis is free access to fluids. In the postsurgical patient who is unable to drink, approximately 75% of the urine volume is replaced with 0.45% (½ normal) saline. Intravenous fluids are adjusted based on subsequent urine osmolality, serum osmolality, and

serum electrolyte measurements every 12 hours, depending on the rate of the diuresis and illness of the patient. Aggressive rehydration to "chase" the volume of fluid excreted, rather than kidney pathology, results in "iatrogenic" diuresis after relief of obstruction.

Pathologic postobstructive diuresis does occur. Ongoing excretion of dilute urine can result in severe dehydration. Initial treatment is the same as in physiologic postobstructive diuresis, with resuscitation with water and electrolytes and frequent measurement of serum and electrolytes. In severe cases, laboratory testing every 4 to 6 hours may be required until a stable balance has been created with diet, fluid, and electrolyte therapy.

SPECIFIC CAUSES OF OBSTRUCTIONS

Causes of urinary obstruction are listed in Box 46.1.

NEPHROLITHIASIS

Nephrolithiasis produces an intrinsic obstruction, anywhere from an infundibulum to the urethral meatus. There are three narrow ureteral locations for urinary obstruction to occur from a stone: (1) the ureteropelvic junction (UPJ), (2) the ureter where it crosses the iliac vessels, and (3) the ureterovesicular junction (UVJ). Bladder stones can block the urethra at the trigone. Rarely, urethral stones, generally from prior stricture disease or surgical reconstruction, occlude the urethra or meatus.

Treatment of obstructing stones depends on the location and severity of illness. Stones in the calyces from infundibular stenosis produce pain and infection but do not produce obstructive uropathy. The location of the infundibulum deep within the renal parenchyma makes open surgical management difficult. Endoscopic laser ablation of the calyx may be considered with obliteration of the calyx and resulting loss of function of that portion of the kidney to prevent future obstruction, infection, and pain.

Once within the renal pelvis, a small calcification can form a nidus to create a larger obstructing stone. Renal pelvis stones are excellent candidates for extracorporeal shock wave lithotripsy (ESWL). The retroperitoneal location of the kidney, away from other vital structures and bowel gas, allows for shock waves to penetrate the kidney and fragment the stone. ESWL is an excellent choice for smaller asymptomatic stones. Larger stones require prolonged and repetitive shock-wave treatment, which may damage the surrounding parenchyma. Percutaneous nephrolithotripsy (PCNL) or ureteroscopy may be a better option.

Ureteroscopy is a very effective technique (greater than 85% success) in selected cases. It treats the stone and allows for direct visualization of the ureter and renal pelvis. This ensures there is no structural pathology that may have predisposed the patient to produce the original stone. Abnormal anatomy can make ureteroscopy difficult, requiring direct access through a percutaneous nephrostomy (PCN) tube. With PCN access to the kidney, PCNL can be performed with either laser or ultrasonic probes. Treatment of larger (greater than 2 cm) and harder stones may benefit from PCN because of the ability to use larger and more powerful instruments with better visualization.

Box 46.1   Causes of Urinary Obstruction

Intrinsic Obstruction

Nephron

1. Uric acid crystals/stones
2. Sloughed papillae
3. Gross hematuria with clot

Renal pelvis

1. Malignancy, primary/metastatic
2. Renal cyst
3. Ureteropelvic junction (UPJ) stenosis

Ureteral

1. Ureteral stricture
2. Ureteral stone
3. Aperistaltic ureter (i.e., megaureter or prune belly syndrome)
4. Ureterocele
5. Ectopic ureter

Bladder

1. Neurogenic (i.e., spina bifida, diabetes)
2. Malignancy, transitional cell carcinoma
3. Fibrosis (i.e., radiation, chronic inflammation)

Urethra

1. Posturethral valves
2. Benign prostatic hyperplasia
3. Malignancy
4. Stricture
5. Prostatic abscess
6. Phimosis

Extrinsic Compressions

Renal pelvis

1. Peripelvic cyst
2. Cancer, primary renal or metastatic
3. Trauma

Ureter

1. UPJ crossing vessel
2. Retrocaval ureter
3. Tumor (pelvic malignancy)
4. Retroperitoneal fibrosis
5. Pregnancy
6. Endometriosis
7. Ovarian vein thrombosis

Bladder

1. Bladder neck contraction (previous surgery, malignancy)

While ESWL works well for kidney stones, it has a significantly lower success rate for mid-ureteral stones. ESWL requires focalization of a pressure wave through tissue to fragment the stone. Gas within adjacent bowel impedes shock-wave migration to the stones. Ureteroscopy becomes the treatment of choice for the majority of mid- and lower-ureteral stones. Retrograde access is again the preferred choice, but antegrade access through the renal pelvis and down the ureter can be performed.

STRICTURES

Strictures found within the urinary tract suggest a previous event, such as trauma, infection, or systemic disease. They occur from the UPJ to the urethral meatus. Balloon dilation with a simultaneous full-thickness wall incision of the stricture is a good option. In short isolated strictures, a long-term success rate of 85% to 90% is expected. Postprocedure, temporary stenting facilitates drainage and minimizes extravasation of acidic urine, which can impair healing and result in restenosis. Extensive stricture disease of the ureter or urethra from tuberculosis, infection, or malignancy may require open surgical resection of the diseased portion with reanastomosis.

MALIGNANCY

There are numerous malignancies that can obstruct the urinary tract externally, but few obstruct the system internally. The most common internal malignancy is transitional cell carcinoma (TCC), which is derived from epithelial cells of the urinary mucosa. It is a friable, frondular tumor with a solid stalk found primarily in older patients with a history of tobacco use. Treatment of obstruction is dependent on tumor location; those that fill the renal pelvis can be treated initially with a ureteral stent. TCC can also produce obstruction at the UVJ. Initial treatment includes an attempt with local cystoscopic excision or unroofing the orifice. When unresectable by cystoscopy, a temporizing stent or nephrostomy tube can be placed until surgical reconstruction with ureteral reimplantation and possible cystectomy can be completed.

Extrinsic compression of the ureter from malignancies occurs frequently. The most common are primary pelvic tumors in women. Retroperitoneal adenopathy along the aorta or vena cava adjacent to the ureter can also produce obstruction. Tumors can invade directly into the ureteral wall and occlude the lumen. Initial treatment with a stent is suggested. Large pelvic masses may obliterate the normal anatomy of the bladder and ureteral orifices. This can make ureteral stent placement impossible. In this situation, an initial PCN tube can be placed with subsequent retrograde internalization of the stent at a later date.

BENIGN PROSTATIC HYPERPLASIA/PROSTATE CANCER

An enlarged prostate creates urinary obstruction through bladder decompensation and failure rather than a fixed urethral obstruction. The relatively slow and gradual prostatic enlargement can come from benign or malignant causes. Enlargement of prostate tissue produces a partial obstruction that increases the patient's voiding pressure. The chronic increase in voiding pressure produces a hydrostatic stress to the smooth muscles of the bladder, resulting in bladder muscle hypertrophy. A subsequent increase in fibroblast and smooth muscle results in bladder wall trabeculations and eventual bladder wall deterioration. The loss of muscle tone culminates in bladder dysfunction with the ultimate cause of the uropathy being urinary retention. It is this bladder deterioration that produces the functional obstruction and uropathy. Chronic elevated bladder resting pressures above 40 cm H_2O can also produce obstructive uropathy from disrupted ureteral peristalsis.

Initial treatment of symptomatic benign prostatic hyperplasia (BPH) uses alpha blockers (tamsulosin, terazosin) to reduce prostatic smooth muscle tone. This increases the size of the urethral lumen and allows voiding pressures to decrease. Phosphodiesterase (PD-5) inhibitors are another class of medications that affect smooth muscle and are associated with subjective improvement in voiding symptoms. Combining the PD-5 inhibitor with an alpha blocker improves symptoms better than either medication alone. If medical therapy proves inadequate, transurethral resection of the prostate, open surgical excision, and clean intermittent catheterization (CIC) may be used.

NEUROGENIC BLADDER

Patients with neurogenic bladder must be monitored closely for new onset obstructive uropathy. This was a leading cause of morbidity and uropathy in the adult neurogenic bladder population before the acceptance of CIC in the 1970s. Spinal cord trauma and myelomeningocele are the most common causes of neurogenic bladder in the adult and pediatric population, respectively. The voiding reflex in the normal adult relaxes the urinary sphincter during bladder contraction. Loss of this coordinated reflex in patients with neurogenic bladder results in bladder contraction against a closed sphincter, known as detrusor sphincter dysenergia (DSD). High-pressure voiding puts the patient at risk of bladder deterioration and upper urinary tract damage similar to BPH (Figs. 46.2 and 46.3). Chronic elevated bladder pressure is a more significant risk factor. The bladder fills to a maximum safe volume, but the patient does not recognize the continued urine production. As the volume increases, the constant resting pressure of the bladder rises. In a patient with a small, low volume bladder and tight urethral sphincter, chronically elevated resting pressures above 40 cm H_2O increase the risk of GFR loss. Treatment involves lowering the resting pressure within the bladder. This can be achieved with anticholinergic medication, CIC, urethral dilation, or surgical reconstruction. Incontinent diversions, such as ileal conduits or cutaneous ureterostomies, are other options. Many patients prefer a continent reconstruction with intermittent catheterization through the urethra or cutaneous stoma, such as a Mitrofanoff or Indiana Pouch. Upper urinary tract deterioration with hydroureteronephrosis is generally seen before the irreversible uropathy. A screening renal ultrasound should be performed annually in an

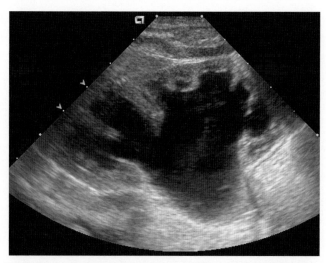

Figure 46.2 Society of Fetal Urology (SFU) grade IV hydronephrosis, which can be seen with or without vesicoureteral reflux, in a patient with a neurogenic bladder and a resting bladder pressure greater than 40 cm H_2O.

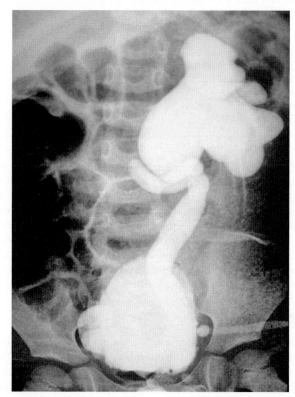

Figure 46.3 Voiding cystourethrogram (VCUG) in a patient with a neurogenic bladder. High resting pressures and dysfunctional voiding result in bladder trabeculations and cellules, with the development of secondary grade 5 reflux.

otherwise healthy urologic patient without urinary tract infections (UTIs) or hydronephrosis.

CONGENITAL DEFECTS IN THE ADULT POPULATION

Congenital defects of the collecting system can present in adults. Defects of the UPJ and UVJ, ectopic ureters, ureteroceles, and even posterior urethral valves can present after childhood. Management depends on the specific signs and symptoms. Patients presenting with pain, infection, or reduced kidney function should be surgically repaired. Intervention can be endoscopic, laparoscopic, or open surgical correction. Asymptomatic abnormalities identified incidentally do not always require treatment. In the adult, there are several anatomic defects that can obstruct the urinary system. UPJ obstruction is identified when stones or infection occur as a result of urinary stasis. Chronic intermittent flank pain previously believed to be of gastrointestinal origin is another common presentation. Treatment of stones and infection will improve the symptoms, but recurrent stone formation or infection is common. Balloon dilation with simultaneous incision of the stricture using the specifically designed Accuise balloon has a success rate approaching 85% in the appropriately selected patient with a UPJ lesion. Long segments of dysplasia at the UPJ have a high failure rate with the Accuise balloon technique. Open surgery or laparoscopic pyeloplasty is an excellent option for reconstruction, approaching a 95% to 97% success rate. In asymptomatic hydronephrotic patients with an UPJ narrowing, intervention should be reserved for those with decreased kidney function. Determination of a functional problem may require a furosemide nuclear scan to examine if kidney dysfunction is caused by obstruction. In a cooperative adult, it is possible to recreate pain during the high urinary flow of the furosemide phase of the study. In the rare equivocal patient with intermittent pain, an indwelling double-J stent can be placed to bypass a possible obstruction to observe if the pain is relieved.

CONGENITAL DEFECTS IN THE PEDIATRIC POPULATION

Congenital obstruction in the pediatric patient occurs throughout the urinary tract. The most common locations are the UPJ, the UVJ, and posterior urethral valves. Prenatal obstruction from a congenital defect can produce dramatic damage to the urinary tract and kidney function. Fortunately, in the majority of children with prenatal hydronephrosis, postnatal development of the urinary tract in the first year results in self-correction of the defect, and a normal unaffected urinary system develops. The goal of managing prenatal congenital defects is to identify the 10% to 30% that will develop progressive disease if left untreated.

Up to 80% of significant partial UPJ obstructions will correct themselves without loss of kidney function. Dramatic hydronephrosis with parenchymal thinning can be monitored if kidney function is comparable to the unaffected contralateral kidney. Megaureters (Fig. 46.4), associated with UVJ obstruction, correct themselves without intervention in 70% of cases. Hydronephrosis does not necessarily mean obstruction.

In the young child with symptomatic UPJ obstruction, pyeloplasty continues to be the best surgical option. A success rate of 95% to 97% should be expected. Laparoscopic pyeloplasty is an excellent technique, except in children less than 1 year old where a slightly higher failure rate is seen.

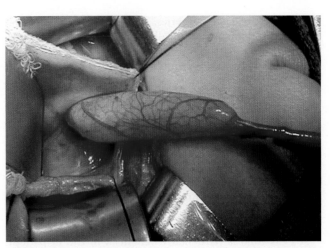

Figure 46.4 Intraoperative megaureter reconstruction. The patient's bladder is open. Initial dissection shows the dilated ureter pulled up into the opened bladder. The distal ureteral narrowing is to the right with proximal healthy, but dilated, vascularized ureter to the left.

PREGNANCY

Hydronephrosis is commonly seen in pregnancy and is rarely pathologic. Hydronephrosis occurs in 40% to 100% of pregnant women depending on the amount of dilation considered abnormal. Postpartum dilation may be seen for up to 6 weeks and is not considered pathologic. Two mechanisms contribute to the hydroureteronephrosis of pregnancy: ureteral compression and hormonal relaxation. By the twentieth week, the gravid uterus achieves adequate size to reach the pelvic rim and extrinsically compress the ureter producing a partial mechanical obstruction. The right kidney is more likely to be dilated because of the position of the uterus. A total of 10% to 15% of women will have hydronephrosis during the first trimester. Hormones present during pregnancy, including estrogen and progesterone that relax the smooth muscle of the ureters, also contribute to hydroureteronephrosis. Identification of hydronephrosis frequently occurs during routine prenatal ultrasound. Follow-up for even moderate hydroureteronephrosis is not needed unless the individual becomes symptomatic.

Treatment of true obstruction from severe extrinsic compression or nephrolithiasis can be performed cystoscopically with ureteral stent placement. Early stent encrustation does occur and will require frequent stent exchange to prevent stent obstruction. PCN can be performed if stent placement is not possible or if the stent is not tolerated.

OBSTRUCTION WITH INFECTION

An obstructed urinary system with an active infection is a medical emergency. Active infection requires close management with early surgical intervention for any systemic progression of illness. Decompression must be accomplished to prevent significant morbidity and mortality. Regardless of the cause of the obstruction, the urgency and means of decompression are dependent on illness severity in the affected patient. Infection is a relative contraindication for many reconstructive surgeries, because the inflammatory process hinders wound healing and promotes fibrosis, scarring, and recurrent obstruction.

Treatment can be as simple as a Foley catheter in an adult male with a urethral stricture, to an open pyelostomy or PCN tube in an infant with a ruptured UPJ. Ureteral obstruction from a stone or a tumor is common, and is best treated early with cystoscopy with stent placement. Definitive reconstruction can be done after the infection and its inflammation resolves. Voiding complaints because of the stent irritating the bladder are common. Anticholinergic medications are indicated for symptomatic patients with bladder hypercontractility. A PCN tube is another excellent option when a previously placed stent is not well tolerated.

A PCN tube is particularly beneficial in the ill patient. The tube can frequently be placed with the patient under sedation rather than using the riskier general anesthesia required for stents. An advantage of a PCN tube is the ability to monitor drainage and to ensure adequate decompression, whereas internalized stents can obstruct asymptomatically. Irrigation of the PCN tube is simple compared to a possible stent exchange. Open surgical drainage is now rarely performed and is reserved for the patient with abnormal anatomy where stenting or PCN is not possible. Patients with severe contractures or ectopic kidneys are in this category. Newborn males with small urethras will not always accept a cystoscope. If the newborn kidney is not significantly hydronephrotic, PCN placement is difficult, and an open decompression procedure may be required. Dilated distal ureters can be brought to the skin as a cutaneous ureterostomy. A pyelostomy can be performed to protect the ureter for future reconstruction.

BIBLIOGRAPHY

Canbay A, Friedman S, Gores GJ: Apoptosis: the nexus of liver injury and fibrosis, *Hepatology* 39:273-278, 2004.

Halachmi S, Pillar G: Congenital urological anomalies diagnosed in adulthood—management considerations, *J Pediatr Urol* 4:2-7, 2008.

Jensen AM, Bae EH, Fenton RA, et al: Angiotensin II regulates V2 receptor and pAQP2 during ureteral obstruction, *Am J Physiol Renal Physiol* 296:F127-F134, 2009.

Jensen AM, Li C, Praetorius HA, et al: Angiotensin II mediates downregulation of aquaporin water channels and key renal sodium transporters in response to urinary tract obstruction, *Am J Physiol Renal Physiol* 291:F1021-F1032, 2006.

Kouba E, Wallen EM, Pruthi RS: Management of ureteral obstruction due to advanced malignancy: optimizing therapeutic and palliative outcomes, *J Urol* 180:444-450, 2008.

Li C, Klein JD, Wang W, et al: Altered expression of urea transporters in response to ureteral obstruction, *Am J Physiol Renal Physiol* 286: F1154-F1162, 2004.

McVary KT, Roehrborn CG, Avins AL, et al: Update on AUA guideline on the management of benign prostatic hyperplasia, *J Urol* 185, 2011. 1793-1780.

Mirone V, Imbimbo C, Longo N, et al: The detrusor muscle: an innocent victim of bladder outlet obstruction, *Eur Urol* 51:57-66, 2007.

Misseri R, Meldrum DR, Dinarello CA, et al: TNF-alpha mediates obstruction-induced renal tubular cell apoptosis and proapoptotic signaling, *Am J Physiol Renal Physiol* 288:F406-F411, 2005.

Sands JM: Critical role of urea in the urine-concentrating mechanism, *J Am Soc Nephrol* 18:670-671, 2007.

Sands JM, Layton HE: The physiology of urinary concentration: an update, *Semin Nephrol* 29:178-195, 2009.

Stødkilde L, Nørregaard R, Fenton RA, et al: Bilateral ureteral obstruction induces early downregulation and redistribution of AQP2 and phosphorylated AQP2, *Am J Physiol Renal Physiol* 301:F226-F235, 2011.

Wang G, Ring T, Li C, et al: Unilateral ureteral obstruction alters expression of acid-base transporters in rat kidney, *J Urol* 182:2964-2973, 2009.

Wolf G: Renal injury due to renin-angiotensin-aldosterone system activation of the transforming growth factor-beta pathway, *Kidney Int* 70:1914-1919, 2006.

Nephrolithiasis

47

Gary Curhan

SCOPE OF THE PROBLEM

Nephrolithiasis is a major cause of morbidity involving the urinary tract. The prevalence of nephrolithiasis in the U.S. population increased from 3.8% in the late 1970s to 8.8% in the late 2000s. The increase in prevalence was observed in both men and women, and both whites and blacks. There were almost 2 million physician office visits for stone disease in 2000. Surprisingly, the estimated annual costs have remained at approximately $2 billion, probably as a result of the shift from inpatient to outpatient procedures.

The lifetime risk of nephrolithiasis is about 19% in men and 9% in women. In men, the first episode of renal colic is most likely to occur after age 30, but it can occur earlier. The incidence for men who have never had a stone is about 0.3% per year between the ages of 30 and 60 years, and it decreases thereafter with age. For women, the rate is about 0.25% per year between the ages of 20 and 30 years, and then declines to 0.15% for the next 4 decades.

The risk of the first recurrent stone after the incident stone in untreated patients remains controversial. Reported frequencies of stone recurrence in uncontrolled studies have ranged from 30% to 50% at 5 years. However, data from the control groups of recent randomized, controlled trials suggest much lower rates of first recurrence after an incident calcium oxalate stone, ranging from 2% to 5% per year. Gender-specific rates are not available from the randomized trials.

ACUTE RENAL COLIC

With the passage of a stone from the renal pelvis into the ureter resulting in partial or complete obstruction, there is sudden onset of unilateral flank pain of sufficient severity that the individual usually seeks medical attention. Despite the use of the misnomer "colic," the pain does not completely remit but rather waxes and wanes. Nausea and vomiting may accompany the pain. The pattern of pain depends on the location of the stone: if it is in the upper ureter, pain may radiate anteriorly to the abdomen; if it is in the lower ureter, pain may radiate to the ipsilateral testicle in men or labium in women; if it is lodged at the ureterovesical junction (UVJ), the primary symptoms may be urinary frequency and urgency. A less common acute presentation is gross hematuria without pain.

The symptoms from a ureteral stone may mimic those of several other acute conditions. A stone lodged in the right ureteropelvic junction can mimic acute cholecystitis.

A stone lodged in the lower right ureter as it crosses the pelvic brim can mimic acute appendicitis. A stone lodged at the UVJ on either side can mimic acute cystitis. A stone lodged in the lower left ureter as it crosses the pelvic brim can mimic diverticulitis. An obstructing stone with proximal infection can mimic acute pyelonephritis. Note that infection in the setting of obstruction is a medical emergency ("pus under pressure") that requires emergent drainage by placement of a ureteral stent or a percutaneous nephrostomy tube. However, because nephrolithiasis is common, the simple presence of a kidney stone does not confirm the diagnosis of renal colic in a patient presenting with acute abdominal pain.

Other conditions to consider in the differential diagnosis of suspected renal colic include muscular or skeletal pain, herpes zoster, duodenal ulcer, abdominal aortic aneurysm, gynecologic causes, ureteral obstruction resulting from other intraluminal factors (e.g., blood clot, sloughed papilla), and ureteral stricture. Extraluminal factors causing compression tend not to result in a presentation with symptoms of renal colic.

The physical examination alone rarely allows for diagnosis, but clues guide the evaluation. The patient typically is in obvious pain and is unable to achieve a comfortable position. There may be ipsilateral costovertebral angle tenderness, or, in cases of obstruction with infection, signs and symptoms of sepsis.

Although blood tests are typically normal, there may be a leukocytosis resulting from stress or infection. The serum creatinine concentration is typically normal, but it may be elevated in the setting of volume depletion, bilateral ureteral obstruction, or unilateral obstruction, particularly in a patient with a solitary functioning kidney. The urinalysis classically shows red blood cells and white blood cells, and it may occasionally show crystals. If ureteral obstruction by the stone is complete, there may be no red blood cells, as urine will not be flowing through that ureter into the bladder.

Because of the often nonspecific physical examination and laboratory findings, imaging studies play a crucial role in making the diagnosis. The imaging modality of choice is helical (spiral) computed tomography (CT), because it does not require a radiocontrast agent and can detect stones as small as 1 mm. Even pure uric acid stones, traditionally considered "radiolucent," are identified. Typically, the study shows a ureteral stone (Fig 47.1) or evidence of recent passage, such as perinephric stranding or hydronephrosis. A plain abdominal radiograph of the kidney, ureter, and bladder (KUB) can miss a stone in the ureter or kidney, even one that is radiopaque, and it provides no information on obstruction. Although KUB is often used to monitor the

405

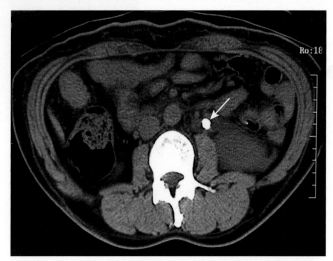

Figure 47.1   Noncontrast-enhanced computed tomography scan shows a radioopaque obstructing stone *(arrow)* in the left ureter.

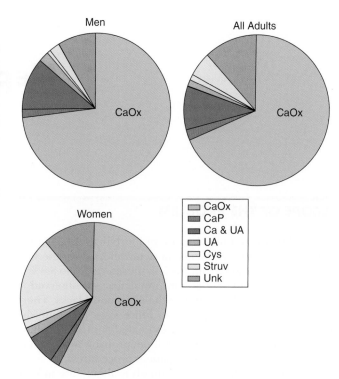

Figure 47.2   Types of stones and their frequency in adults. *Ca,* Calcium; *CaOx,* calcium oxalate; *CaP,* calcium phosphate; *Cys,* cystine; *Struv,* struvite; *UA,* uric acid; *Unk,* unknown. (From Coe F, Parks J, editors: *Nephrolithiasis: pathogenesis and treatment,* Chicago, 1988, Year Book Medical, with permission.)

progress of a ureteral stone or the growth of asymptomatic kidney stones, its sensitivity is limited. An intravenous pyelogram requires contrast and can miss small stones; it should be ordered only rarely for the evaluation and treatment of nephrolithiasis. Although there is a general belief that the osmotic diuresis induced by the radiocontrast agent can facilitate stone passage, there is insufficient confirmatory evidence. Ultrasonography, although avoiding radiation, can image only the kidney and proximal ureter.

Renal colic is one of the most excruciating types of pain, and pain control is essential. Narcotics and parenteral nonsteroidal antiinflammatory drugs are effective, with the latter preferable because they cause fewer side effects. Other treatments that may be effective for promoting stone passage include α-adrenergic blockers and calcium channel blockers. Urinary alkalinization may be effective for dissolving a uric acid stone, but this type is relatively rare and there must be adequate urine flow past the stone.

TYPES OF STONES

Almost 90% of stones in men and 70% of stones in women contain calcium, most commonly as calcium oxalate (Fig. 47.2). Other types of stones, such as cystine, pure uric acid, and struvite, are much less common. However, these types of stone also deserve careful attention, because recurrences are common. No information is available on the frequencies from first-time stone formers, in part because the first stone typically is not retrieved or sent for analysis (although it should be).

PATHOGENESIS

The urinary concentrations of calcium, oxalate, and other solutes that influence stone formation are high enough that they should result in crystal formation in the urine of most individuals, but this is clearly not the case. This condition is termed *supersaturation.* Substances in the urine called *inhibitors* prevent crystal formation. The most clinically important inhibitor is citrate, which works by chelating calcium cations

in the urine and decreasing the free calcium available to bind with oxalate or phosphate anions. If the supersaturation is sufficiently high or there are insufficient inhibitors, precipitation occurs with resulting crystalluria.

The causes of stone formation differ for different stone types. Cystine stones form only in individuals with the autosomal recessive disorder of cystinuria. Uric acid stones form only in those who have persistently acid urine, with or without hyperuricosuria. Struvite stones form only in the setting of an upper urinary tract infection with a urease-producing bacterium. These stones are seen in individuals with recurrent urinary tract infections, particularly those with abnormal urinary tract anatomy, such as patients who have urinary diversions or who require frequent catheterization. Stones may occasionally result from precipitation of medications, such as acyclovir, sulfadiazine, and atazanavir, in the urinary tract.

Calcium-based stones have a multifactorial etiology. Traditionally, stone formation was believed to occur from (1) crystal formation in the renal tubule, followed by (2) attachment of the crystal to the tubular epithelium, usually at the tip of the papilla, and (3) growth of the attached crystal by deposition of additional crystalline material. However, it now appears that the initial event occurs in the medullary interstitium with deposition of calcium phosphate. The calcium phosphate material may then erode through the papillary epithelium, on which calcium oxalate is subsequently deposited. Several medical conditions increase the likelihood of calcium oxalate stone formation. With primary hyperparathyroidism, urinary calcium is increased. Crohn's disease and other malabsorptive states

Table 47.1   Risk Factors for Calcium Oxalate Stone Formation

High Levels	Low Levels
Urinary Risk Factors	
Calcium	Citrate
Oxalate	Total volume
Dietary Risk Factors	
Oxalate	Calcium, dietary
Animal protein	Potassium
Sodium	Phytate
Sucrose	Fluid
Fructose	
Calcium, supplemental	
Vitamin C	
Other Risk Factors	
Obesity	
Gout	
Diabetes	
Anatomic abnormalities	

in which the colon is intact are associated with increased urinary oxalate excretion. With fat malabsorption, calcium is bound in the small bowel to free fatty acids, leaving a smaller amount of free calcium to bind to oxalate. An increased amount of unbound oxalate is then absorbed in the colon. Another possible factor is reduced secretion of oxalate into the intestine, but the contribution of this is uncertain. These patients often lose a fair amount of fluid through the gastrointestinal tract, so the accompanying low urine volume presents an additional risk factor. Citrate reabsorption is increased by metabolic acidosis, leaving less urinary citrate to serve as a calcium chelator. For this reason, distal renal tubular acidosis predisposes to stone formation as well.

Calcium phosphate stones are more likely to form in the presence of high urine calcium, low urine citrate, and alkaline urine. Systemic conditions that are present more frequently in patients with calcium phosphate stones include renal tubular acidosis and primary hyperparathyroidism. The remainder of this chapter focuses on calcium oxalate stones, except where noted.

Urinary variables that increase the risk of calcium oxalate stone formation are higher levels of calcium and oxalate; higher levels of citrate and higher total volume decrease the risk (Table 47.1). Although higher urine uric acid concentration had been thought to increase the risk of calcium oxalate stone formation, results from a recent large study did not support this belief. The traditional approach to urinary abnormalities is based on 24-hour urinary excretion. The normal ranges for urinary factors vary by laboratory; this is because there are no universally agreed-on normal ranges. The following are examples of commonly used definitions of "abnormal" values: hypercalciuria (≥250 mg/day for women, ≥300 mg/day for men), hyperoxaluria (≥45 mg/day for both women and men), hyperuricosuria (≥750 mg/day for women, ≥800 mg/day for men), and hypocitraturia (≤320 mg/day for both women and men). After being evaluated, patients have typically been classified into categories according to their urinary abnormalities, and treatment directed at correcting the abnormalities.

Although this approach has been used for decades, it has several limitations. Stone formation is a disease of concentration. Therefore, it is not just the absolute amount of substances that determines the likelihood of stone formation. The traditional definitions of "abnormal" excretion must be applied cautiously for several reasons. First, there are insufficient data supporting the cutoff points used regarding the risk of actual stone formation. For example, the traditional definition of hypercalciuria is 50 mg/day greater in men than in women, but there is no justification with respect to stone formation for having a higher upper limit of normal in men, particularly because the mean 24-hour urine volume is lower in men than in women. Similarly, another common definition of hypercalciuria is urinary calcium excretion in excess of 4 mg/kg of body weight per day. However, by this definition, an individual who is heavier or gains weight is "allowed" to excrete more calcium than someone who is thinner but still below the cutoff point. Second, an individual could have "normal" absolute excretion of calcium but still have a high urinary calcium concentration because of low urine volume. This situation has therapeutic implications, because the goal is to modify the concentration of the lithogenic factors. Finally, the risk of stone formation is a continuum, so the use of a specific cutoff point may give the false impression that a patient with "high-normal" urinary calcium excretion is not at risk for stone recurrence. Just as cardiovascular risk increases with increasing blood pressure (even in the "normal" range), the risk of stone formation increases with increasing urine calcium levels.

Some investigators have advocated subdividing cases of elevated urinary calcium into three categories: (1) absorptive (caused by increased gastrointestinal absorption of ingested calcium), (2) resorptive (caused by increased bone resorption), and (3) renal (caused by increased urinary excretion of filtered calcium). However, the clinical importance of this approach is uncertain. A substantial proportion of cases cannot be classified, and there is evidence that individuals may change categories when studied years later. Therefore, most clinicians do measure 24-hour urine chemistries as part of the metabolic evaluation, but do not subclassify patients. The underlying mechanisms for idiopathic hypercalciuria remain unknown, although hormones and their receptors involved in calcium metabolism, such as 1,25-dihydroxyvitamin D and the vitamin D receptor, probably play contributing roles.

Higher urinary oxalate concentrations may result from increased gastrointestinal absorption (high dietary oxalate intake or increased fractional dietary oxalate absorption), increased endogenous production, or decreased gastrointestinal secretion. The relative contribution of exogenous and endogenous oxalate sources to urinary oxalate remains controversial. Dietary oxalate most likely contributes 30% to 50%, but other dietary factors (e.g., ascorbic acid) are also important.

Purines are metabolized to uric acid. Increased urinary uric acid is the result of higher purine intake and higher endogenous production from purine turnover. In the steady state, urine uric acid excretion is dependent on generation; the serum uric acid level does not provide any information about 24-hour urine uric acid excretion.

Low urine citrate levels are typically seen in the setting of a systemic metabolic acidosis such as in renal tubular acidosis or excessive gastrointestinal bicarbonate losses from diarrhea. Because citrate is a potential source of bicarbonate, it is actively reclaimed in the proximal tubule after being filtered by the glomerulus.

Dietary variables associated with decreased risk of incident stone formation include higher dietary intakes of calcium, potassium, and fluid; those associated with increased risk include higher intakes of supplemental calcium, oxalate, animal protein, sodium, and sucrose (Table 47.1). Although dietary oxalate intake has been generally believed to be important for stone formation, the magnitude of the risk is not high. Many foods contain small amounts of oxalate, but foods that are high in oxalate are less common. Recently, measurements of the oxalate content of foods have become more reliable.

Data from observational and randomized, controlled studies support the concept that dietary calcium intake is *inversely* associated with risk of stone formation. The mechanism by which dietary calcium may reduce the risk of stone formation is unknown, but it may involve calcium binding to oxalate in the intestine, reducing oxalate absorption. It is also possible that there is some other protective substance in dairy products, the major source of dietary calcium.

Differences in timing of ingestion may explain the apparent contradiction between the protective effect of dietary calcium and the detrimental effect of supplemental calcium. A protective effect would not be expected unless the calcium supplement was ingested with meals containing oxalate; in this case of calcium supplementation, the observed increase in risk might rather be a result of increased urinary calcium excretion without any change in urinary oxalate excretion.

Nondietary factors that increase the risk for kidney stone formation include genitourinary anatomic abnormalities; medical conditions such as medullary sponge kidney, primary hyperparathyroidism, gout, and diabetes mellitus; and larger body size.

CLINICAL EVALUATION

Evaluation after the first kidney stone appears to be cost effective, although there is some disagreement on how much should be done. The decision to proceed depends on several variables. First, what is the stone burden? Even though the episode that brought the patient to medical attention may have been the first symptomatic event, an appreciable proportion of patients has remaining kidney stones and could be considered "recurrent" stone formers. If such a patient had only a KUB or a kidney ultrasonogram during the acute evaluation, either of which could miss small stones, it would seem prudent to obtain a CT scan (preferably a helical CT) to determine whether there are any residual kidney stones. Second, if the initial stone was large (e.g., ≥10 mm) or required an invasive procedure to remove, an evaluation would be indicated. Finally, the patient's preferences are most important, because the recommendations often involve lifelong changes.

A detailed history provides information crucial for treatment recommendations. The following points should be covered: total number of stones, evidence of residual stones, number and types of procedures, types and success

of previous preventive treatments, family history of stone disease, and dietary intake and medication use before the stone event. After having experienced acute renal colic, a patient may attribute a variety of types of chronic back or flank pain to the kidney or to a residual stone. Further questioning often uncovers other causes, particularly musculoskeletal. The physical examination may show findings of systemic conditions associated with stone formation, but these signs are uncommon.

LABORATORY (METABOLIC) EVALUATION

Retrieval of the stone for chemical analysis is an often overlooked but essential part of the evaluation, because treatment recommendations vary by stone type. The stone composition cannot be predicted with certainty from imaging or other laboratory studies. The decision to begin a metabolic evaluation should be guided by the patient's willingness to make lifestyle changes to prevent recurrent stone formation. Some experts advocate proceeding with an evaluation only after the second stone. However, safe and inexpensive interventions (e.g., modifying fluid intake) can be prescribed based on results of the relatively inexpensive 24-hour urine collection. If a metabolic evaluation is pursued, it is identical for first-time and recurrent stone formers. Serum chemistry values that should be measured include electrolytes, kidney function markers, and calcium and phosphorus concentrations. The decision to measure parathyroid hormone or vitamin D concentrations is based on results of the serum and urine chemistries. If the patient has high serum calcium, low serum phosphorus, or high urine calcium, then a parathyroid hormone level should be measured. The cornerstone of the evaluation is the 24-hour urine collection. Two 24-hour urine collections should be performed while the patient is consuming his or her usual diet. Because individuals often change their dietary habits soon after an episode of renal colic, a patient should wait at least 6 weeks before carrying out the collections. Two collections are needed because there is substantial day-to-day variability in the values.

The critical variables that should be measured in the 24-hour urine collections are total volume, calcium, oxalate, citrate, uric acid, sodium, potassium, phosphorus, pH, and creatinine. Some laboratories calculate the relative supersaturation from measurements of the urine factors, which can be used to gauge the impact of therapy.

MEDICAL TREATMENTS

Because stones can remain asymptomatic for years, the actual time of formation of the stone that brought the patient to medical attention is usually unknown. The current metabolic evaluation may, in fact, be completely normal with no changes to lifestyle needed. Whether the patient is an active stone former influences the decision to treat. The likelihood of recurrence can be estimated but not definitely predicted from the urine chemistry results; a repeat imaging study 1 year later helps determine whether the patient is an active stone former. For patients who are at risk for stone recurrence, lifestyle modification should be attempted first, tailoring the recommendation according to stone type and urine chemistry findings. Lifelong changes are needed to prevent recurrence of this chronic condition. Because the supersaturation required for an existing stone to grow is lower than that needed for a new stone to form, recommendations to prevent stone growth may be more aggressive than those to prevent new stone formation.

DIETARY RECOMMENDATIONS

Dietary recommendations that are useful in preventing nephrolithiasis are listed in Table 47.2. There is no evidence that dietary calcium restriction is helpful in preventing stone formation, and there is substantial evidence that it is harmful. Decreasing intake of animal protein (meat, chicken, and seafood) may be helpful. Patients who have low urine citrate concentrations should increase their intake of potential alkali (fruits and vegetables), and decrease intake of acid-producing foods such as animal protein. The role of calcium supplements deserves comment, as use of supplements is common. In someone who has never had a kidney stone, the risk attributable to supplemental calcium is low. For a patient who has had a calcium-containing stone and wishes to continue taking the supplement, 24-hour urine chemistry values should be measured while the patient is taking, and not taking, the supplement; if the urine calcium is higher than desired while taking the supplement, then it should be discontinued. Increased fluid intake decreases the risk of stone formation and recurrence. On the basis of the urine volume, the patient should be instructed how many additional 8-ounce glasses of fluid to drink each day, with the goal of producing approximately 2 L of urine daily.

For patients with high urine oxalate levels, the benefit of a low-oxalate diet is less clear because of the previously addressed issues regarding the oxalate content of food; however, spinach should be avoided and intake of nuts moderated. There is no accepted definition of a low-oxalate diet. An increase in dietary calcium with meals may reduce oxalate absorption and thereby reduce urine oxalate excretion. In addition, vitamin C supplementation should be avoided, because higher vitamin C intake may increase urine oxalate excretion.

PHARMACOLOGIC OPTIONS

The use of medication is indicated if dietary recommendations are unsuccessful in adequately modifying the urine composition. The three most commonly used classes of medications for stone prevention are (1) thiazides (e.g., chlorthalidone, hydrochlorothiazide), which reduce urine calcium excretion; (2) alkali (e.g., potassium citrate), which increase urine citrate excretion; and (3) xanthine oxidase inhibitors (e.g., allopurinol), which reduce urine uric acid excretion.

For patients who have elevated urinary calcium levels but do not have excessive calcium intake (i.e., less than 1500 mg/day), a thiazide diuretic has been demonstrated to reduce the likelihood of stone recurrence and to help maintain bone density. The dosages required to reduce urinary calcium adequately are substantially higher than those typically used for treatment of hypertension (at least 25 mg/day, and often 50 to 100 mg/day). Randomized trials of at least 3 years' duration have consistently shown a 50% reduction in the risk of recurrence. Adequate sodium restriction (to less than 3 g/day) is necessary to achieve maximum benefit from the thiazides; a higher sodium intake leads to greater distal sodium delivery and minimizes or negates the beneficial effect of the thiazides. For patients who are unable to increase their fluid intake, a thiazide may be helpful even if the total urine calcium excretion is not high, because it will reduce the urinary calcium excretion and thus the calcium concentration. In addition, a thiazide may be more readily prescribed if there is evidence of low bone density.

For patients with low urine citrate levels, any form of alkali will increase the urine citrate. However, citrate is the base of choice because it is better tolerated than bicarbonate. Potassium salts are preferred more than sodium because of the potential effect on urinary calcium excretion. The alkali preparations must be taken at least twice daily to maintain adequate citrate levels. Randomized trials suggest a greater than 50% reduction in risk of recurrence with alkali supplementation.

Table 47.2   Dietary and Pharmacologic Treatments to Prevent Nephrolithiasis, According to Urinary Abnormality

Urinary Abnormality	Dietary Changes	Medication
High calcium concentration	Avoid excessive intake of calcium supplements Maintain adequate dietary calcium intake Reduce intake of animal protein Reduce sodium intake to less than 3 g/day Reduce sucrose intake	Thiazide
High oxalate concentration	Avoid high-oxalate foods Maintain adequate dietary calcium intake Avoid vitamin C supplements	High-dose pyridoxine?
High uric acid concentration	Reduce purine intake (i.e., meat, chicken, fish)	Xanthine oxidase inhibitor
Low citrate concentration	Increase intake of fruits and vegetables Reduce intake of animal protein	Alkali (e.g., potassium citrate)
Low volume	Increase total fluid intake	Not applicable

In one randomized trial, allopurinol reduced the recurrence rate by 50% among individuals with a history of recurrent calcium oxalate stones and isolated hyperuricosuria. Given the epidemiologic observation that higher urine uric acid levels do not increase a person's likelihood of being a stone former, it is unclear whether the benefit was caused by the reduction in urine uric acid concentration or by some other mechanism.

NONCALCIUM STONES

For the less common types of stones (uric acid, struvite, and cystine), there is little or no information on the influence of dietary factors on actual stone formation, rather than simply changes in urine composition. The following recommendations are based on our current understanding of the pathophysiology of these stone types, but caution is warranted, because they are derived from studies of urine composition rather than actual stone formation.

URIC ACID STONES

A higher intake of nondairy animal protein may increase the risk of uric acid stone formation. Consumption of meat, chicken, and seafood increases uric acid production because of the purine content of animal flesh. Animal protein has a greater content of sulfur-containing amino acids than vegetable protein, and their metabolism leads to increased acid production with a subsequent lowering of the urinary pH. Both increased uric acid excretion and lower urine pH increase the risk of uric acid crystal formation. Higher intake of fruits and vegetables, which are high in potential base, may raise the urine pH, thereby reducing the risk of uric acid crystal formation.

Alkali supplementation is the most effective treatment of existing uric acid stones. If the urine pH is maintained at 6.5 or higher (which often requires 90 to 120 mEq of supplemental alkali per day), pure uric acid stones will dissolve. Slightly lower doses may be used to prevent new uric acid stone formation. A xanthine oxidase inhibitor is the second-line choice if the patient has marked hyperuricosuria or is unable to maintain a urine pH higher than 6.5.

CYSTINE STONES

Higher sodium intake may increase urine cystine excretion. Because the solubility of cystine increases as pH rises, a higher consumption of fruits and vegetables may have a beneficial effect by increasing urine pH. Although restriction of proteins high in cystine (e.g., animal protein) seems advisable, there is little evidence to support this recommendation as a means of directly lowering urinary cystine levels; however, reducing animal protein intake may be beneficial by leading to an increase in the urine pH.

Medications such as tiopronin and penicillamine increase the solubility (not the total amount) of the filtered cystine. The effectiveness of these drugs is limited by the amount of cystine excreted daily and the high side-effect profile. If adequate amounts of the medication enter the urine, cystine stones can be dissolved. Supplemental potassium alkali salts may also provide benefit by increasing the urine pH.

STRUVITE STONES

Because struvite stones form only in the setting of an infection in the upper urinary tract with urease-producing bacteria, it is unlikely that dietary factors can directly influence struvite stone formation. Struvite stones are almost always large and may fill the renal pelvis, referred to as "staghorn calculi"; an experienced urologist should remove these stones. In addition to the complete removal of all residual fragments, prevention of urinary tract infections is the cornerstone for avoiding recurrence. Acetohydroxamic acid is the only drug available that inhibits urease; however, it should be used with extreme caution because of its very common and serious side effects.

CALCIUM PHOSPHATE STONES

Information on dietary issues related to actual calcium phosphate stone formation is limited. However, on the basis of the known physicochemical aspects, nutrients that might stimulate calcium phosphate crystal formation include excessive calcium intake (resulting in higher urinary calcium excretion), higher phosphate intake (resulting in higher urinary phosphate excretion), and higher intake of fruits and vegetables (resulting in a higher urinary pH). Nonetheless, caution is advised, because the "theoretical" benefits of limiting these nutrients may not be realized, and there are, of course, other reasons to maintain an adequate intake of calcium, fruits, and vegetables.

Reduction in urine calcium can be achieved with thiazides using an approach similar to that recommended for calcium oxalate stones. Because patients who form calcium phosphate stones may also have low urine citrate concentrations, alkali supplementation may be used with caution. Alkali supplementation often increases urine pH and therefore could increase the risk of calcium phosphate crystal formation.

SURGICAL MANAGEMENT OF STONES

In the acute setting, the urologist will assist in the management. If the stone does not pass rapidly, the patient can be sent home with appropriate oral analgesics, an α-blocker or calcium channel blocker to increase the likelihood of stone passage, and instructions to return in case of fever or uncontrollable pain. Most urologists wait several days before intervening for a ureteral stone unless one of the following conditions exists: urinary tract infection, stone greater than 6 mm in size, presence of an anatomic abnormality that would prevent passage, or intractable pain. A cystoscopically placed ureteral stent is typically used, but anesthesia is required. The stent can be uncomfortable and not infrequently causes gross hematuria. Although it is debatable whether a stent helps with stone passage, the cystoscopy or stent placement may push the stone back up into the renal pelvis, thus relieving the obstruction and permitting its management on a nonemergent basis.

The method of stone removal is determined by stone size, location, and composition; the urinary tract anatomy; availability of technology; and the experience of the urologist.

Extracorporeal shock wave lithotripsy (ESWL) is the least invasive method. Cystoscopic stone removal, by either basket extraction or fragmentation, is invasive but more effective than ESWL, and newer instruments allow removal of stones even in the kidney. Percutaneous nephrostolithotomy, an approach requiring the placement of a nephrostomy tube, is more invasive but necessary for large stone burdens and for kidney stones that cannot be removed cystoscopically; this is the gold standard for making a patient "stone-free." Open procedures such as ureterolithotomy or nephrolithotomy are rarely needed.

The surgical treatment of asymptomatic stones is controversial. The availability of ESWL has lowered the threshold for treating asymptomatic stones; most urologists consider treating only asymptomatic stones that are at least 1 cm in size.

With the increasing prevalence of obesity in the United States, the treatment of existing stones in morbidly obese individuals deserves mention. The ability to image the urinary tract may be limited if the patient's size prohibits access to scanning by CT. ESWL may not be an option, because morbid obesity can impede stone localization and the ability of the shock waves to reach the calculus; therefore, more invasive approaches, such as ureteroscopy, may be necessary.

LONG-TERM FOLLOW-UP

The nephrologist or primary-care provider should assume responsibility for the long-term prevention program, and should consult with the urologist as needed for further surgical interventions. The plan should include recommendations for prevention based on the evaluation; interventions should be followed by repeat metabolic measurements to assess their success, adjustment of recommendations, and follow-up imaging.

Adherence to recommendations frequently declines with time. In addition, the long-term sequelae of the treatments and the underlying abnormalities may have other implications for the health of the patient. For example, individuals with higher urine calcium excretion typically have lower bone density and are at increased risk for osteoporosis. With appropriate attention and evaluation, the morbidity and cost of recurrent stone disease can be dramatically reduced.

BIBLIOGRAPHY

Borghi L, Schianchi T, Meschi T, et al: Comparison of two diets for the prevention of recurrent stones in idiopathic hypercalciuria, *N Engl J Med* 346:77-84, 2002.

Coe FL, Evan A, Worcester E: Pathophysiology-based treatment of idiopathic calcium kidney stones, *Clin J Am Soc Nephrol* 6:2083-2092, 2011.

Curhan GC, Willett WC, Rimm EB, et al: A prospective study of dietary calcium and other nutrients and the risk of symptomatic kidney stones, *N Engl J Med* 328:833-838, 1993.

Evan AP, Lingeman JE, Coe FL, et al: Randall's plaque of patients with nephrolithiasis begins in basement membranes of thin loops of Henle, *J Clin Invest* 111:607-616, 2003.

Ferraro PM, Taylor EN, Gambaro G, Curhan GC: Soda and other beverages and the risk of kidney stones. *Clin J Am Soc Nephrol* 2013 (in press).

Mandeville JA, Gnessin E, Lingeman JE: Imaging evaluation in the patient with renal stone disease, *Semin Nephrol* 31:254-258, 2011.

Pearle MS, Calhoun EA, Curhan GC: Urolithiasis. In Litwin MS, Saigal CS, editors: *Urologic diseases in America*, U.S. Department of Health and Human Services, Public Health Service, National Institutes of Health, National Institute of Diabetes and Digestive and Kidney Diseases. Washington, DC, 2004, U.S. Government Publishing Office, pp 3-39.

Taylor EN, Curhan GC: Oxalate intake and the risk for nephrolithiasis, *J Am Soc Nephrol* 18:2198-2204, 2007.

Taylor EN, Stampfer MJ, Curhan GC: Dietary factors and the risk of incident kidney stones in men: new insights after 14 years of follow-up, *J Am Soc Nephrol* 15:3225-3232, 2004.

Taylor EN, Stampfer MJ, Curhan GC: Obesity, weight gain, and the risk of kidney stones, *JAMA* 293:455-462, 2005.

Taylor EN, Stampfer MJ, Mount DB, et al: DASH-style diet and 24-hour urine composition, *Clin J Am Soc Nephrol* 5:2315-2322, 2010.

Teichman JMH: Acute renal colic from ureteral calculus, *N Engl J Med* 350:684-693, 2004.

48 Urinary Tract Infection and Pyelonephritis

Lindsay E. Nicolle

Urinary infection is the presence of microbial pathogens within the normally sterile urinary tract. Infections are overwhelmingly bacterial, although fungi, viruses, and parasites may occasionally be pathogens (Table 48.1). Urinary infection is the most common bacterial infection in humans, and can be either symptomatic or asymptomatic. Symptomatic infection is associated with a wide spectrum of morbidity, from mild irritative voiding symptoms to bacteremia, sepsis, and occasionally, death. Asymptomatic urinary infection is defined as isolation of bacteria from urine in quantitative counts consistent with infection, but without localizing genitourinary or systemic signs or symptoms attributable to the infection.

The term *bacteriuria* simply means bacteria present in the urine, although it is generally used to imply isolation of a significant quantitative count of organisms. This term is often used interchangeably with *asymptomatic urinary infection*. Recurrent urinary infection is common in individuals who experience an initial infection. It may be either relapse (i.e., recurrence subsequent to therapy with the pretherapy isolate) or reinfection (i.e., recurrence with a different organism). An important consideration in the management of urinary infection is whether the patient has a functionally and structurally normal (uncomplicated urinary infection or acute nonobstructive pyelonephritis) or abnormal (complicated urinary infection) genitourinary tract.

The microbiologic diagnosis of urinary infection requires isolation of a pathogenic organism in sufficient quantitative amounts from a urine specimen collected in a manner that minimizes contamination from vaginal or periurethral organisms. A quantitative bacterial count of $\geq 10^5 \text{cfu/mL}$ is the usual standard to discriminate infection from organisms present as contaminants. The use of the quantitative urine culture is essential for the diagnosis of urinary infection and the description of natural history, but the quantitative standard of $\geq 10^5$ cfu/mL must be interpreted in the context of clinical presentations.

ACUTE UNCOMPLICATED URINARY INFECTION

Acute uncomplicated urinary infection, or acute cystitis, is infection occurring in individuals with a normal genitourinary tract and no recent instrumentation. It is a common syndrome that occurs virtually entirely in women; 60% of all women experience at least one infection in their lifetime. From 1% to 2% of women have frequent recurrent infection. The highest incidence is in young, sexually active women. Risk factors for infection in these women are both genetic and behavioral. Women with recurrent acute uncomplicated urinary infection are more likely to have first-degree female relatives with urinary infections and to be nonsecretors of blood group substances. Recent studies have suggested that polymorphisms of genes encoding elements of the innate immune response contribute to the genetic propensity to recurrent infection. Sexual activity is strongly associated with infection, and frequency of infection correlates with frequency of intercourse. The use of spermicides or a diaphragm for birth control also increase the risk for infection; risk is not increased by use of oral contraceptives or condoms without spermicide. For young women, behavioral practices such as postvoid personal hygiene, type of underwear, postcoital voiding, or bathing rather than showering have no association with infection. For postmenopausal women, frequency of sexual intercourse is not a risk factor for infection. The most important predictor of infection in older women is a history of urinary infection at a younger age.

E. coli is isolated from 80% to 85% of episodes. *Staphylococcus saprophyticus*, a coagulase-negative staphylococcus, occurs in 5% to 10% of episodes. This organism is rarely isolated in other clinical syndromes and has a unique seasonal variation with increased frequency in the late summer and early fall. *Klebsiella pneumoniae* and *Proteus mirabilis* are each isolated in 2% to 3% of cases. Organisms that cause infection originate from the normal gut flora, colonize the vagina and periurethral area, and ascend to the bladder. Women who experience this syndrome frequently have alterations in vaginal flora characterized by decreased or absent hydrogen peroxide (H_2O_2) producing lactobacilli, resulting in increased vaginal pH and colonization with *E. coli* and other potential uropathogens.

The clinical presentation, diagnosis, and recommended treatment for acute uncomplicated urinary infection are summarized in Table 48.2. New onset frequency, dysuria, and urgency together with the absence of vaginal discharge or pain are 90% accurate to diagnose infection. From 30% to 50% of women have quantitative counts of less than 10^5 cfu/mL of a uropathogen isolated. Any quantitative count of a potential uropathogen with pyuria is considered sufficient for microbiologic diagnosis when accompanied by consistent clinical symptoms. Because the clinical presentation is characteristic, bacteriology predictable, and quantitative microbiology often not definitive, it is recommended that symptomatic episodes be managed with empiric antimicrobial therapy and routine pretherapy urine culture not be obtained. A urine specimen for culture should be obtained before antimicrobial treatment if there is uncertainty about the diagnosis, failure of an initial therapeutic regimen, or

Table 48.1 Nonbacterial Pathogens Causing Urinary Tract Infection

Fungi	Viruses	Parasites
Candida albicans	JC, BK viruses	Schistosoma
Candida parapsolosis	Adenovirus types	hematobium
Candida glabrata	11, 21	
Candida tropicalis	Mumps	
Blastomyces dermatitidis*	Hantavirus†	
Aspergillus fumigatus*		
Cryptococcus neoformans*		
Histoplasma capsulatum*		

*With disseminated infection.
†Hemorrhagic fever and renal syndrome.

early recurrence after therapy. The differential diagnosis includes urethritis due to sexually transmitted diseases such as *Neisseria gonorrheae* or *Chlamydia trachomatis*, yeast vulvovaginitis, or genital herpes.

Antimicrobial therapy is selected based on consideration of patient tolerance, documented efficacy for treating urinary infection, and local prevalence of resistance in community-acquired *E. coli*. Trimethoprim-sulfamethoxazole (TMP/SMX) has been the recommended empiric therapy for many years. However, if the regional prevalence of resistance of community *E. coli* isolates to this antimicrobial is over 20%, an alternate empiric regimen should be prescribed. Recommended alternates are nitrofurantoin for 5 days, single-dose fosfomycin trometamol, or 5 days of pivmecillinam; all of these have indications virtually limited to treatment of this syndrome. Fluoroquinolones and β-lactam antimicrobials are not considered first-line therapy because of the propensity to induce resistance in gut flora and, for β-lactams, a lower efficacy. The increasing global resistance of community *E. coli*, especially the widespread dissemination of extended-spectrum beta-lactamase (ESBL) or carbapenemase-producing strains, is a concern. These organisms are also usually resistant to TMP/SMX and fluoroquinolones but, to date, most remain susceptible to nitrofurantoin, fosfomycin, and pivmecillinam. A 3-day course of antimicrobial therapy with TMP/SMX or a fluoroquinolone is effective. A longer course of 7 days is recommended when the duration of symptoms is more than 7 days, for women with an early recurrence of symptomatic infection (less than 30 days) following prior antimicrobial therapy, and when treatment is with a β-lactam antimicrobial.

Frequent recurrent acute cystitis is a disruptive and distressing problem for many women. Antimicrobial prophylaxis, given either as a long-term low-dose regimen or after intercourse, will prevent 95% or more of recurrent episodes (Table 48.3). Increasing resistance of *E. coli* strains may limit the effectiveness of TMP/SMX. Continuous low-dose prophylaxis taken at bedtime is recommended, with an initial course of 6 to 12 months. This remains effective when continued for as long as 2 to 5 years. When prophylactic therapy is discontinued, the frequency of urinary infection is similar to that observed before prophylaxis. Approximately 50% of women will have recurrent infection within 3 months.

Postcoital prophylaxis is, obviously, most appropriate for women who identify sexual intercourse as a precipitating factor for recurrent symptomatic episodes. An alternate approach preferred by some women, especially with less frequent recurrences, is self-treatment. This has been shown to be effective with short-course TMP/SMX, ciprofloxacin, or ofloxacin. It is appropriate for women who are compliant with management and reliable in identifying their symptomatic episodes.

The most important nonantimicrobial intervention for prevention of recurrent urinary infection is avoidance of spermicide use. The daily intake of cranberry or lingonberry juice or cranberry tablets was previously reported to decrease the frequency of recurrent infection by 30%, but recent blinded placebo controlled trials have not reported a benefit. Vaccines to prevent recurrent uncomplicated urinary infection and use of probiotics to reestablish normal gut or vaginal flora are being investigated, but studies to date have not shown consistent benefit with either of these approaches.

ACUTE NONOBSTRUCTIVE PYELONEPHRITIS

Acute nonobstructive pyelonephritis is a symptomatic kidney infection occurring in women with a normal genitourinary tract. Women who experience acute uncomplicated urinary infection are also at risk for nonobstructive pyelonephritis, with the frequency of episodes of cystitis relative to pyelonephritis reported to be 18-29 to 1. Risk factors for developing acute pyelonephritis are similar to those for acute cystitis for premenopausal women; frequency of sexual intercourse is the most important. *E. coli* is isolated from 85% of episodes. These strains are characterized by expression of specific virulence factors. The P fimbria, an adhesin that attaches to uroepithelial cells and induces an inflammatory response, is the most important. Additional organism virulence factors include production of hemolysin, which may lyse host cells, and aerobactin, an iron scavenger, which may promote bacterial growth.

Acute pyelonephritis presents classically with fever and costovertebral angle pain and tenderness. There are often associated lower urinary tract symptoms. Fever may be low grade or, occasionally, absent. A urine specimen for culture and susceptibility testing should be obtained before the initiation of antimicrobial therapy from every woman with a suspected diagnosis of pyelonephritis. Growth of $\geq 10^4$ cfu/mL of a uropathogen with pyuria together with consistent clinical findings is sufficient for diagnosis, but $\geq 10^5$ cfu/mL of organisms is isolated from 95% of cases. Bacteremia occurs in about 10% of episodes, and is more frequent in older adult women and women with diabetes. When women with pyelonephritis present with sepsis or shock, urgent imaging should be obtained to exclude obstruction or other lesions requiring immediate intervention for source control, as severe presentations are unusual with acute nonobstructive pyelonephritis.

The majority of women can be treated as outpatients with oral antimicrobial therapy (see Table 48.2). A common approach is to give a single dose of parenteral antibiotic in the emergency department, usually gentamicin 3 to 5 mg/kg

Table 48.2   Diagnosis and Management of Common Symptomatic Syndromes of Urinary Infection

Clinical Presentation	Microbiologic Diagnosis	First-Line Treatment	Second-Line Treatment	Parenteral Treatment
Acute uncomplicated urinary infection (acute cystitis) Lower-tract irritative symptoms: dysuria, frequency, urgency, suprapubic discomfort, hematuria	≥10³ cfu/mL of uropathogen with pyuria	TMP/SMX 160/180 mg bid, 3 days TMP 200 mg bid, 3 days Nitrofurantoin 50-100 mg qid, or monohydrate/macrocrystals 100 mg bid × 5 days Fosfomycin trometamol 3 g, one dose Pivmecillinam 400 mg bid,* 3 or 7 days	Norfloxacin 400 mg bid, 3 days Ciprofloxacin 250 mg bid, 3 days Ciprofloxacin extended-release 500 mg daily, 3 days Ofloxacin 400 mg bid, 3 days Levofloxacin 400 mg daily, 3 days Amoxicillin/clavulanic acid 500 mg bid, 7 days Cephalexin 500 mg qid, 7 days Cefixime 400 mg daily, 7 days Cefpodoxime 100 mg bid, 3 days	
Acute nonobstructive pyelonephritis Costovertebral angle pain and tenderness; ± fever, ±lower-tract symptoms	≥10⁴ cfu/mL	Norfloxacin 400 mg bid Ciprofloxacin 500 mg bid Ofloxacin 400 mg bid Levofloxacin 500-750 mg daily	TMP/SMX 160/800 mg bid† TMP 100 mg bid† Amoxicillin/clavulanic acid 500 mg tid Cephalexin 500 mg qid† Cefixime 400 mg daily	Gentamicin 3-5 mg/kg/24 hr in one or two doses ± ampicillin 1g q4-6h Ceftriaxone 1-2 g q24h Cefotaxime 1g tid Ciprofloxacin 400 mg bid Levofloxacin 500-750 mg daily
Complicated urinary infection Variable symptoms, including lower-tract symptoms; pyelonephritis; systemic symptoms (fever, shock)	≥10⁵ cfu/mL	TMP/SMX 160/800 mg bid Norfloxacin 400 mg bid Ciprofloxacin 250-500 mg bid Ciprofloxacin extended-release, 1 g daily Ofloxacin 400 mg bid Levofloxacin 500 mg daily Amoxicillin/clavulanic acid 500 mg tid Cephalexin 500 mg qid Cefixime 400 mg po daily		Gentamicin or tobramycin 3-5 mg/kg/24 hr in one or two doses ± ampicillin 1 g q4-6h or piperacillin 3 g q4h Amikacin 15 mg/kg in one or two doses Piperacillin/tazobactam 3.375 g q6h Ceftazidime 1 g tid Cefotaxime 1 g tid or ceftriaxone 1-2 g q24h Ertapenem 1 g q24h Meropenem 500 mg q6h Doripenem 500 mg q8h

bid, Twice daily; *tid,* three times daily; *TMP/SMX,* trimethoprim/sulfamethoxazole; *qid,* four times daily.
*Not licensed in the United States.
†If organism is known to be susceptible.

or ceftriaxone, 1 or 2 g, followed by a course of oral therapy. Hospitalization and initial parenteral antimicrobial therapy are recommended for women with hemodynamic instability, for whom oral medication may not be tolerated because of severe gastrointestinal symptoms, or when there are significant systemic signs of illness and concern about compliance with outpatient therapy. The parenteral antimicrobial can usually be replaced by oral therapy once clinical improvement has occurred, usually by 48 to 72 hours. The urine culture results are also available by this time and will direct selection of a specific oral antimicrobial for continuing therapy.

By 48 to 72 hours following initiation of effective antimicrobial therapy, there should be evidence of clinical improvement, including decreased costovertebral angle discomfort and a decrease in or resolution of fever. If there is not substantial clinical improvement by this time or if symptomatic infection recurs soon after an adequate course of therapy, a resistant bacterial strain or abnormality within the genitourinary tract causing urinary obstruction or abscess formation should be excluded. The imaging approach should be individualized depending on presentation, clinical course, and access to diagnostic testing. Computed tomography (CT) scanning with contrast, however, is generally superior

Table 48.3 Prophylactic Antimicrobial Therapy for Women With Frequent Recurrence of Acute Uncomplicated Urinary Infection

	Regimen	
Agent	Long-Term	Postcoital (One Dose)
TMP/SMX*	80/400 mg daily or 3 × weekly	80/400 mg
TMP*	100 mg daily	100 mg
Nitrofurantoin*	50 mg daily	50-100 mg
Cephalexin	125 mg daily	250 mg
Norfloxacin	200 mg every other day	200-400 mg
Ciprofloxacin	–	250 mg

TMP/SMX, Trimethoprim/sulfamethoxazole.
*Recommended first-line agents.

Table 48.4 Abnormalities of the Genitourinary Tract Associated With Complicated Urinary Infection

Abnormality	Examples
Metabolic or structural	Medullary sponge kidney
	Nephrocalcinosis
	Malakoplakia
	Xanthogranulomatous pyelonephritis
Congenital	Cystic disease
	Duplicated drainage system with obstruction
	Urethral valves
Obstruction	Vesicoureteral reflux
	Pelvicalyceal obstruction
	Papillary necrosis
	Urethral fibrosis/stricture
	Bladder diverticulum
	Neurogenic bladder
	Prostatic hypertrophy
	Tumors
	Urolithiasis
Instrumentation	Indwelling catheter
	Intermittent catheterization
	Cystoscopy
	Ureteric stent
	Nephrostomy tube
Other	Immunocompromised
	Subsequent to kidney transplant
	Neutropenic

to ultrasonography or magnetic resonance imaging (MRI) for characterizing potential kidney abnormalities.

COMPLICATED URINARY INFECTION

The most important host defense preventing urinary infection is intermittent, unobstructed voiding of urine. Any abnormality of the genitourinary tract that impairs voiding increases the risk for urinary infection. Urinary infection in individuals with structural or functional abnormalities of the urinary tract, including those who have undergone instrumentation, is considered a *complicated urinary infection* (Table 48.4). The likelihood and frequency of infection is determined by the underlying abnormality, and is independent of gender or age. For some abnormalities, such as an infected cyst with polycystic kidney disease, infection is infrequent but difficult to manage. In other patients, such as those with an indwelling catheter, infection is very frequent, with a rate of 5% per day. For patients with chronic indwelling devices, biofilm formation on the device results in 100% of patients being bacteriuric.

The clinical presentation of symptomatic infection varies along a spectrum from mild lower tract irritative symptoms to systemic manifestations with fever or even septic shock. Individuals with complete obstruction of urine flow or with mucosal bleeding are at greatest risk for the most severe clinical presentations. A quantitative count of organisms in the urine of $\geq 10^5$ cfu/mL remains the standard for the microbiologic diagnosis of complicated urinary infection. Organisms isolated are characterized by a greater diversity of infecting species and an increased prevalence of antimicrobial resistance when compared with uncomplicated infection. They are less likely to express virulence factors because the host abnormality of impaired voiding is itself sufficient for infection. Increased antimicrobial resistance is common because of nosocomial acquisition of infecting organisms or repeated prior courses of antimicrobial therapy for recurrent infection. In cases where broad-spectrum antimicrobial therapy has been given for prolonged periods, reinfection may occur with yeast species or highly resistant bacteria, such as *Pseudomonas aeruginosa* or *Acinetobacter* species.

Antimicrobial treatment is selected based on clinical presentation, patient tolerance, and the known or predicted susceptibilities of the infecting organism. When possible, antimicrobial therapy should be delayed until urine culture results are available. Patients with moderate to severe symptoms should have empiric therapy initiated pending culture results. The recent history of antimicrobial use and prior urine culture results in an individual patient are helpful in directing the choice of empiric therapy. Initial parenteral therapy is required for patients with severe systemic manifestations, where oral therapy is not tolerated, or when the infecting organism is suspected or known to be resistant to any available oral therapy. When the clinical presentation is of lower tract symptoms, 7 days of therapy are generally adequate. In cases with fever or other systemic symptoms, 10 to 14 days of therapy are recommended, although 7 days is effective with some fluoroquinolone antimicrobials.

Complicated urinary infection can be prevented if the underlying abnormality is corrected. There is a high likelihood of recurrent infection when the underlying genitourinary abnormality persists. For instance, 50% of patients with a neurogenic bladder and voiding managed by intermittent catheterization will experience recurrent infection by 4 to 6 weeks after antimicrobial therapy. For hospitalized patients, the most important interventions to limit infection are to avoid indwelling catheter use and, if a catheter is indicated, to minimize the amount of time it remains in situ. Prophylactic antimicrobials are not recommended, because this approach has not been shown to decrease symptomatic infections and it increases reinfection with organisms resistant to the antimicrobial given. In selected patients who experience frequent, severe symptomatic recurrences and have an abnormality that cannot be corrected, such as men with chronic prostatitis or individuals with infection in a nonfunctioning kidney, long-term suppressive therapy may be considered. This approach is individualized in every case. Full therapeutic antimicrobial doses are initiated and may subsequently be decreased to one half the regular dose if the urine culture remains negative and the clinical course is satisfactory.

ASYMPTOMATIC URINARY INFECTION

Asymptomatic bacteriuria is isolation of one or more uropathogens in quantitative counts consistent with urinary infection ($\geq 10^5$cfu/mL) in a patient with no localizing genitourinary signs or symptoms. Pyuria is common, being present in 50% to 90% of patients. Asymptomatic bacteriuria occurs with increased frequency in persons who also experience symptomatic urinary infection, but does not, in itself, cause symptomatic infection. This suggests that the biologic defect promoting symptomatic and asymptomatic infection is similar. Treatment is indicated only for pregnant women and patients who will undergo an invasive genitourinary procedure with a high likelihood of mucosal bleeding. Identification and treatment of asymptomatic bacteriuria in early pregnancy prevents pyelonephritis as well as negative fetal outcomes of premature delivery and low birth weight. For patients undergoing an invasive genitourinary procedure, prophylaxis is initiated immediately before the intervention to prevent perioperative sepsis. For other populations, asymptomatic infection, with or without pyuria, does not require treatment. Long-term cohort studies do not document adverse effects attributable to bacteriuria, and prospective randomized trials have not identified any clinical benefits of antimicrobial treatment. In fact, adverse antibiotic effects and reinfection with organisms of increased resistance occur when treatment is attempted.

SPECIAL POPULATIONS

URINARY INFECTION IN CHILDREN

Urinary infection occurs more frequently in boys than girls in the first year of life. Infection in boys usually occurs within 3 months of birth and is often associated with congenital anomalies of the urinary tract. The clinical presentation is of neonatal sepsis without localizing genitourinary tract signs, and these episodes are treated as neonatal sepsis. Subsequent to the first year of life, urinary infection occurs more frequently in girls than boys, and the clinical presentation is with genitourinary symptoms. Most episodes in girls are acute uncomplicated urinary infection, and these girls will also experience urinary infection more frequently as adults. Vesicoureteral reflux, which may lead to impaired kidney function, must be excluded. Imaging studies including voiding cystourethrogram, ultrasonography, ^{99}Tc-dimercaptosuccinic acid (DMSA), or CT scan are indicated for any child presenting with pyelonephritis, for a first urinary infection in a boy of any age or a girl under 3 years, for a second urinary infection in a girl older than 3 years, and for a first urinary infection at any age with a family history of urinary tract abnormalities. Other indications for imaging include urinary infection accompanied by abnormal voiding, hypertension, or poor growth.

Treatment of acute lower tract infection in young girls is for 3 to 7 days. Pyelonephritis should be treated for 10 to 14 days. Generally, the antimicrobials used are similar to those in adults, with appropriate dose adjustments for weight. The fluoroquinolones are not recommended for children under the age of 16 years because of potential adverse effects on cartilage. Long-term low-dose prophylactic therapy is indicated for young girls with frequent symptomatic recurrences, or with severe vesicoureteral reflux (grades IV or V) and recurrent urinary infection. Asymptomatic urinary infection is common in school-age girls. Treatment of asymptomatic urinary infection does not alter the natural history of kidney disease in young girls or prevent renal scarring. In fact, treatment of asymptomatic bacteriuria with antimicrobials appears to increase the frequency of symptomatic infection. Thus it is not recommended to screen for or treat asymptomatic bacteriuria in girls.

URINARY INFECTION IN PREGNANCY

Hormonal changes in pregnancy produce hypotonicity of the autonomic musculature, leading to urine stasis and ureteric reflux. In addition, obstruction at the pelvic brim—more marked on the right than the left side—occurs with the enlarging fetus. These changes are maximal at the end of the second trimester and beginning of the third trimester, correlating with the highest incidence of pyelonephritis. Acute pyelonephritis may precipitate premature labor and delivery, as may any febrile illness in later pregnancy. About 30% of women identified with asymptomatic bacteriuria in early pregnancy who are not treated with antimicrobials develop acute pyelonephritis later in the pregnancy. From 75% to 90% of these episodes are prevented by early identification and treatment of asymptomatic bacteriuria. Premature delivery and low birth rate are also decreased with treatment.

Because of these benefits in treating asymptomatic bacteriuria, all pregnant women should be screened for bacteriuria by urine culture at 12 to 16 weeks' gestation. If significant bacteriuria is identified, it should be confirmed with a second urine culture, and treated if persistent. Antimicrobial therapy is selected based on the susceptibilities of the infecting organism, patient tolerance, and safety for use in pregnancy. A 3-day course of amoxicillin, nitrofurantoin, or cephalexin is usually sufficient. TMP/SMX has been widely used and is effective, but it may be associated with increased fetal abnormalities when given in the first trimester and should be avoided early in pregnancy. Fluoroquinolones are contraindicated. Women treated for an initial episode of asymptomatic bacteriuria or symptomatic urinary infection in early pregnancy should be followed with monthly urine cultures throughout the remainder of the pregnancy to identify recurrent infection. If a second episode of either symptomatic or asymptomatic infection occurs, low-dose prophylactic therapy should be initiated following treatment of the infection and continued until delivery.

URINARY INFECTION IN MEN

Men rarely present with acute uncomplicated urinary infection or acute nonobstructive pyelonephritis. Lack of circumcision, acquisition of an infecting strain from a new sexual partner, and men who have sex with men are potential risk factors in the few cases that do occur. *E. coli* is the usual infecting organism. Uncomplicated infection, however, is so uncommon in men that any man presenting with urinary infection should be investigated for the possibility of an underlying abnormality.

Older adult men have an increased frequency of urinary infection as prostatic hypertrophy leads to obstruction and turbulent urine flow. These men may also develop chronic bacterial prostatitis. Once bacteria are established in the prostate, poor diffusion of antibiotics into the prostate and formation of prostate stones make the infection very difficult to eradicate. The prostate then serves as a nidus for recurrent symptomatic or asymptomatic bladder infection. If recurrent symptomatic infection occurs and chronic bacterial prostatitis is diagnosed, a more prolonged antimicrobial course of 4 to 6 weeks of therapy may increase the likelihood of long-term cure. Fluoroquinolones are the recommended first-line agents, but TMP/SMX, tetracyclines, and azithromycin may also be used, depending on the susceptibility of the organisms isolated.

URINARY TRACT INFECTIONS IN OLDER ADULTS

Urinary infection is the most common infection occurring in both ambulatory and institutionalized older adult populations. The prevalence of bacteriuria is 5% to 10% for women and 5% in men over 65 years of age living in the community. These rates increase with advancing age. In long-term care facilities, 25% to 50% of all older adult residents have asymptomatic bacteriuria at any time. The prevalence increases with increasing functional impairment, including dementia and bladder and bowel incontinence. Asymptomatic bacteriuria in older adult patients should not be treated with antimicrobials. Antimicrobial treatment does not decrease morbidity or mortality, but is associated with increased adverse drug effects, cost, and antimicrobial resistance. It follows that asymptomatic older adult populations should not be screened for bacteriuria.

Symptomatic infection in older adults usually has clinical presentations similar to those in younger populations. However, particularly in the institutionalized or functionally impaired population, the diagnosis may not be straightforward. Difficulties in communication, comorbid illnesses with chronic symptoms, and the high frequency of asymptomatic bacteriuria all impair diagnostic acumen. A decreased fever response and lower frequency of leukocytosis characterize infection in older adults, and acute confusion may be a prominent presenting symptom. Despite this, a diagnosis of symptomatic urinary infection in an older individual without an indwelling urinary catheter should not be made in the absence of localizing genitourinary symptoms. Foul-smelling or cloudy urine is not, by itself, an indication for antimicrobial treatment.

Antimicrobial regimens for therapy are similar to those in younger populations, including duration of treatment. The dosage should be adjusted for kidney function but not for age. Cure rates with any duration of therapy are lower for older women. Posttreatment urine cultures to document microbiologic cure are not recommended unless symptoms persist or recur. Some women with frequent, recurrent, symptomatic infection may have a decreased number of infections with use of topical intravaginal estradiol, although this is less effective for prevention than prophylactic antimicrobials. Systemic estrogen therapy has been associated with an increased risk for infection.

URINARY INFECTION IN PATIENTS WITH IMPAIRED KIDNEY FUNCTION

Treatment of urinary infection requires adequate concentrations of effective antimicrobials in the kidneys or urine. There is decreased excretion of antimicrobials into the urine when kidney function is impaired, so therapeutic urinary antimicrobial levels may not be achieved. With severe kidney impairment, it is often difficult to cure urinary infection. When kidney function is impaired, antimicrobials such as nitrofurantoin and tetracyclines other than doxycycline may have increased toxicity and should be avoided. Aminoglycosides may not diffuse into nonfunctioning kidneys sufficiently to provide effective therapy. The penicillins and cephalosporins, as well as fluoroquinolones, are effective treatment for most individuals with mild or moderately impaired kidney function. Obviously, dosage adjustments appropriate for the level of kidney function are necessary. In some situations, such as infected native kidneys in transplant recipients, infection cannot be eradicated and long-term suppressive therapy may be necessary to manage frequent symptomatic recurrences.

If impaired kidney function is unilateral, the functioning kidney will preferentially excrete the antimicrobial into the urine. High urinary antimicrobial levels will sterilize bladder urine, but antimicrobial levels in the nonfunctioning kidney may not be therapeutic. If there is infection in the impaired kidney, relapse of infection from this source can occur once antimicrobial therapy is discontinued.

URINARY INFECTION IN PATIENTS WITH CYSTIC KIDNEY DISEASE

Patients with polycystic kidney disease may develop infection of one or more cysts, and the management of these infections frequently presents diagnostic and therapeutic challenges. Symptoms usually include abdominal pain or tenderness, and bacteremia is frequent. Recurrent bacteremia is common if initial therapy is inadequate. The infected cyst should be identified and, wherever possible, cyst contents aspirated for culture. A wide variety of organisms, including yeast species, may cause infection, so optimal treatment requires knowledge of the infecting organism and susceptibilities. MRI and white cell labeled scans may be useful imaging techniques to identify infected cysts. Treatment includes prolonged antimicrobial therapy with an agent effective against the infecting organism and that has good penetration into the cyst. Potential agents that achieve therapeutic cyst levels include TMP/SMX, fluoroquinolones, or chloramphenicol. At least 4 weeks of antimicrobial therapy is recommended, although clinical trials to define optimal therapy are not available. Surgery may be necessary for selected cases in which antimicrobial therapy, with or without drainage, does not lead to cure.

OTHER PRESENTATIONS OF URINARY INFECTION

FUNGAL URINARY INFECTION

Fungal urinary infection has been increasing in frequency. It is primarily a healthcare-acquired infection that occurs in the setting of diabetes, indwelling urethral catheters, and intense broad-spectrum antimicrobial therapy. *Candida albicans* is most frequently isolated, but other *Candida* species such as *C. glabrata*, *C. krusei*, *C. parapsolosis*, and *C. tropicalis* also occur. The clinical significance of a positive urine culture is often difficult to assess because most of these patients have complex medical or surgical problems. If there are no genitourinary symptoms or evidence of invasive infection, treatment of funguria is not beneficial and should be avoided. If an indwelling urethral catheter is present, it should be discontinued when possible. Fungus balls may develop, leading to obstruction, and should be excluded in individuals with obstruction and persistent candiduria or candidemia. If present, they must be surgically removed.

When symptoms are referable to the genitourinary tract and repeated cultures have grown yeast organisms at $\geq 10^4$cfu/mL without other potential pathogens, treatment of funguria is indicated. Fluconazole 100 to 400 mg/day for 7 to 14 days is recommended, because it is excreted in the urine and may be given as oral therapy. 5-Fluorocytosine (50 to 150 mg/kg/day for 7 days) and amphotericin B are also effective. The echinocandins (caspofungin, micafungin, anidulafungin) and other azoles (voriconazole, posocconazole) are not excreted in the urine and not recommended for therapy. *Candida* species such as *C. krausei* or *C. glabrata*, which are resistant to fluconazole, require treatment with amphotericin B. Amphotericin B bladder irrigation (50 mg/L continuous for 5 days) is no longer considered first-line therapy because it requires urethral catheterization and is no more effective than other therapeutic options. In selected situations, however, particularly in subjects with chronic kidney disease and bladder infection, the washout method may still be useful. The cure rate with any treatment is only about 70%, but assessment of outcome is often limited by serious comorbidities.

XANTHOGRANULOMATOUS PYELONEPHRITIS

Xanthogranulomatous pyelonephritis is an uncommon subacute or chronic suppurative process of the kidney characterized by destruction of the renal parenchyma and replacement by granulomatous tissue containing histiocytes and foamy cells. Perinephric tissues may also be involved. The etiology remains unknown, but potential contributing factors include chronic urinary tract infection, abnormal lipid metabolism, lymphatic obstruction, impaired leukocyte function, and vascular occlusion. Infection is usually present; *Proteus mirabilis* and *E. coli* are the most frequent organisms. *Klebsiella/Enterobacter* species, *Pseudomonas aeruginosa*, and *Staphylococcus aureus* may also be isolated. The usual clinical presentation is with subacute or chronic fever, flank or abdominal pain, weight loss, lower urinary tract symptoms, and gross hematuria. Renal calculi are invariably present, and a history of recurrent urinary tract infections and previous urologic procedures is common. The diagnosis is usually made with a CT scan. The characteristic imaging findings are an enlarged kidney with replacement of renal parenchyma and multiple fluid filled cavities. Urolithiasis is often seen. Management is nephrectomy; antimicrobial therapy has only a secondary role. If the diagnosis is made early when only focal renal involvement is present, partial nephrectomy may be curative.

MALAKOPLAKIA

Malakoplakia is a rare chronic granulomatous inflammatory disorder of the bladder and, occasionally, the ureter or kidneys. It occurs primarily in immunocompromised or debilitated adults, but has been described in normal adults and children. Chronic infection is uniformly present, with *E. coli* isolated from 85% to 90% of cases. The pathophysiology is not fully understood, but defective macrophage lysosomal digestion of phagocytosed bacteria, particularly coliforms, is thought to play a role. The clinical presentation is variable, with chronic or subacute fever, urinary symptoms, and abdominal or pelvic pain the most frequent symptoms. Anemia and leukocytosis are common. The characteristic radiologic feature of bladder involvement is one or more mucosal-based sessile nodular lesions less than 1 cm in diameter. Rarely, the disease presents as a kidney mass and obstruction, leading to kidney failure. Definitive diagnosis requires identification of the characteristic histopathologic findings of large histiocytes with an eosinophilic granular cytoplasm admixed with intracytoplasmic or extracellular spherical Michaelis-Gutmann bodies, which are pathognomonic for the disease. Treatment is by prolonged antimicrobial therapy (8 to 12 weeks), with surgical intervention when necessary to relieve obstruction. Both TMP/SMX and fluoroquinolones have been effective. Anticholinergics and ascorbic acid are also sometimes given because they may increase cellular cyclic-GMP, restoring the defect in phagocytic function.

BIBLIOGRAPHY

Bent S, Nallamothu BK, Simel DL, et al: Does this woman have an acute uncomplicated urinary tract infection? *JAMA* 287:2701, 2002.

Cardenas DD, Hooton TM: Urinary tract infection in persons with spinal cord injury, *Arch Phys Med Rehab* 76:272, 1995.

Collins TR, Devries CR: Recurrent urinary tract infections in children: a logical approach to diagnosis, treatment, and long-term management, *Compr Ther* 23:44, 1997.

Fihn SD: Acute uncomplicated urinary tract infection in women, *N Engl J Med* 349:259, 2003.

Gould CV, Umscheid CA, Agarwal RK, et al: Guideline for prevention of catheter-associated urinary tract infection 2009, *Infect Control Hosp Epidemiol* 31:319, 2010.

Gupta K, Hooton TM, Naber KG, et al: International clinical practice guidelines for acute uncomplicated cystitis and pyelonephritis in women: a 2010 update by the IDSA and ESCMID Guidelines Committee, *Clin Infect Dis* 52:561, 2011.

Hooton TM: The current management strategies for community-acquired urinary tract infection, *Infect Dis Clin North Am* 17:303, 2003.

Hooton TM, Bradley SF, Cardenas DD, et al: 2009 International clinical practice guideline for the diagnosis, prevention and treatment of catheter-associated urinary tract infection in adults, *Clin Infect Dis* 50:625, 2010.

Johnson JR: Microbial virulence determinants and the pathogenesis of urinary tract infection, *Infect Dis Clin North Am* 17:261, 2003.

Johnssen TE: The role of imaging in urinary tract infections, *World J Urol* 22:392, 2004.

Lipsky BA, Byren I, Hooey CT: Treatment of bacterial prostatitis, *Clin Infect Dis* 50:1641, 2010.

Loffroy R, Guiu B, Watfa J, et al: Xanthogranulomatous pyelonephritis in adults: clinical and radiologic findings in diffuse and focal forms, *Clin Radiol* 2007.

Montini G, Tullus K, Hewitt I: Febrile urinary tract infections in children, *N Engl J Med* 365:239, 2011.

Nicolle LE: Uncomplicated urinary tract infection in adults including uncomplicated pyelonephritis, *Uro Clin North Am* 35:1, 2008.

Nicolle LE: Urinary tract infections in the elderly, *Clin Ger Med* 25:423, 2009.

Nicolle LE, Bradley S, Colgan R, et al: IDSA guidelines for the diagnosis and treatment of asymptomatic bacteriuria in adults, *Clin Infect Dis* 40:643, 2005.

Schaeffer AJ: Chronic prostatitis and the chronic pelvic pain syndrome, *N Engl J Med* 355:1690, 2006.

Scholes D, Hooton TM, Roberts PL, et al: Risk factors associated with acute pyelonephritis in healthy women, *Ann Intern Med* 142:26, 2005.

Sobel JD, Kauffman CA, McKinsey D, et al: Candiduria: a randomized, double-blind study of treatment with fluconazole or placebo. The National Institute of Allergy and Infectious Diseases Mycoses Study Group, *Clin Infect Dis* 30:19, 2000.

Stapleton A: Novel approaches to prevention of urinary tract infections, *Infect Dis Clin North Am* 17:457, 2003.

THE KIDNEY IN SPECIAL CIRCUMSTANCES

49 The Kidney in Infants and Children

Lawrence A. Copelovitch | Colin T. White | Susan L. Furth

KIDNEY DEVELOPMENT AND MATURATION

The development of the kidney begins in utero at approximately 5 to 6 weeks gestation and continues until nephron formation is complete at approximately 36 weeks gestation. Fetal urine production commences before the end of the first trimester, and by the third trimester becomes the primary component of the amniotic fluid, which is essential for normal pulmonary development. Although the full-term newborn has the same number of nephrons as an adult, the glomeruli and tubules of the infant kidney are immature. The neonatal tubule has diminished ability to concentrate or dilute the urine in response to different environmental or dietary conditions. Furthermore, the ability of the neonatal proximal tubule to reabsorb filtered HCO_3^- is less than that of adults. As a result, the average serum HCO_3^- concentration in preterm infants (16 to 20 mEq/L) is lower than in term infants (19 to 21 mEq/L), and it is lower than in older children and adults (24 to 28 mEq/L). Newborns often have higher serum potassium concentrations (6.5 to 7.0 mEq/L) than older children as a result of a decreased glomerular filtration rate (GFR) and a relative insensitivity of the neonatal tubule to aldosterone.

The GFR of the newborn kidney is only around 20 mL/min/1.73 m^2 in the first few days after birth, rising to approximately 40 mL/min/1.73 m^2 near the end of the first week after birth, and gradually reaching adult levels of 100 to 130 mL/min/1.73 m^2 by 2 years of age. The changes in GFR that occur after birth are the result of increased cardiac output and mean arterial blood pressure, a decrease in renal vascular resistance, and an increased surface area available for glomerular filtration. Concomitantly, blood flow is redistributed from the cortical-juxtamedullary glomeruli, which are larger but fewer in number than the more numerous glomeruli in the cortex.

In term neonates, the low GFR results in a serum creatinine (sCr) that remains similar to the mother's for the first 24 to 48 hours of life, and gradually settles to around 0.4 mg/dl at the fifth to seventh day of life. In preterm infants born at 28 to 30 weeks gestation, the GFR is only approximately 12 to 13 mL/min/1.73 m^2 within the first few days after birth, and the sCr may take longer to normalize. The full-term newborn kidney measures 4 to 5 cm in length and continues to grow until reaching 10 to 12 cm by adolescence. Although the glomeruli do grow in size, most of this renal parenchymal expansion results from tubular growth and maturation and from increased volume of the tubulointerstitial compartment.

ACUTE KIDNEY INJURY

Acute kidney injury (AKI) is defined as a sudden decrease in kidney function that compromises the normal regulation of fluid, electrolyte, and acid-base homeostasis. In practical terms, AKI is characterized by a reduction in the GFR, which results in an abrupt increase in the concentrations of sCr and blood urea nitrogen (BUN). In 2002, the Acute Dialysis Quality Initiative Group introduced the RIFLE criteria so as to stage AKI. RIFLE (acronym for *R*isk for kidney dysfunction, *I*njury to the kidney, *F*ailure of kidney function, *L*oss of kidney function, and *E*nd-stage renal disease) aimed to standardize the definition of AKI by stratifying patients based on changes in the sCr levels from baseline and/or abrupt decreases in urine output. The RIFLE criteria were found to be independent predictors of length of hospital stay, cost, morbidity, and mortality in adults. Subsequently, a modified pediatric RIFLE, or pRIFLE, was developed to stage AKI in children (Table 49.1).

As highlighted by the RIFLE criteria, the urine volume in AKI is variable: patients may be anuric, oliguric, and in some cases polyuric. AKI develops throughout a period of hours to days, whereas chronic kidney disease (CKD) develops over months to years. Short stature, renal osteodystrophy, delayed puberty, normocytic anemia, and hyperparathyroidism all suggest long-standing and advanced CKD rather than AKI. However, at a single point in an acute clinical presentation, it may be difficult to differentiate AKI from CKD without imaging studies, extensive laboratory testing for the aforementioned complications, and possibly a kidney biopsy. Furthermore, at the time of presentation, a patient with CKD may have superimposed AKI, referred to as acute on chronic kidney failure.

The likelihood of recovery from and appropriate treatment for AKI depends in part on the presence or absence of urine output, the quantity of urine output, the duration of anuria, and the underlying cause and severity of kidney injury. Quantifying the urine output is essential, as this predicts the clinical course and may aid in identifying the underlying insult. Oliguria is defined as urine output less than 1 mL/kg/h in infants and young children, and less than 0.5 mL/kg/h in older children. Patients with nonoliguric AKI have lower complication rates and higher survival rates than those with anuric or oliguric AKI. Causes of nonoliguric AKI include acute interstitial nephritis (AIN) or nephrotoxic renal insults, including aminoglycoside nephrotoxicity. In contrast, AKI in children with renal hypoperfusion injury, acute glomerulonephritis, or

Table 49.1   Pediatric-modified RIFLE (pRIFLE) Criteria

	eGFR	Urine Output
Risk	Decreased by 25%	Less than 0.5 mL/kg/hr for 8 hr
Injury	Decreased by 50%	Less than 0.5 mL/kg/hr for 16 hr
Failure	Decreased by 75% or less than 35 mL/min/1.73 m²	Less than 0.3 mL/kg/hr for 24 hr or anuric for 12 hr
Loss	Persistent failure greater than 4 wk	
End-stage	ESRD (greater than 3 mo)	

Adapted from Akcan-Arikan A, Zappitelli M, Loftis LL et al: Modified RIFLE criteria in critically ill children with acute kidney injury, Kidney Int 71:1028-1035, 2007 [10].
eGFR, Estimated glomerular filtration rate; *ESRD,* end-stage renal disease; *pRIFLE,* pediatric *R*isk for kidney dysfunction, *I*njury to the kidney, *F*ailure of kidney function, *L*oss of kidney function, and *E*nd-stage renal disease.

hemolytic uremic syndrome (HUS) is usually associated with oligoanuria. In infants, oliguric AKI normally occurs as a result of either renovascular accidents (renal artery or vein thrombosis) or ischemic acute tubular necrosis (ATN) from shock. The underlying cause of AKI may be classified as prerenal, intrinsic, or postrenal. It is important to note that many cases of AKI are multifactorial, especially in hospitalized children.

Prerenal AKI results from renal hypoperfusion caused by intravascular volume contraction, decreased effective circulating blood volume, or altered intrarenal hemodynamics. Intravascular volume contraction can be seen with volume depletion, acute blood loss, or extravascular accumulation of fluid (so-called third spacing of fluid). This is most often encountered in patients with the systemic inflammatory response syndrome (SIRS) or with hypoalbuminemia. Decreased effective blood circulation occurs when the true blood volume is normal or increased, but renal perfusion is decreased. This complicates left-sided heart failure, cardiac tamponade, or hepatorenal syndrome. Intrarenal afferent arteriolar vasoconstriction develops in hepatorenal syndrome, calcineurin toxicity, and nonsteroidal antiinflammatory drug (NSAID) use; intrarenal efferent arteriolar vasodilation occurs with the use of angiotensin-converting enzyme (ACE) inhibitors. In prerenal AKI, kidney function may be initially normal, but severe and/or prolonged renal hypoperfusion leads to tubular injury and intrinsic AKI.

Intrinsic renal injury or pathology may occur at the level of the renal vasculature, tubules, interstitium, or glomeruli. The basic mechanisms of such renal injuries include hypoperfusion and ischemic cell damage, toxin-mediated cell injury, and inflammation.

Vascular injury may occur in large vessels (e.g., renal artery or vein thrombosis) or in the microvasculature (e.g., HUS or thrombotic thrombocytopenic purpura, TTP). Direct tubular injury, also known as ATN, is the end result of either ischemic or toxin-mediated damage to the tubules. Ischemia-induced ATN is the result of renal hypoperfusion. If the

insult is prolonged and severe, prerenal AKI may progress to intrinsic AKI, which is no longer immediately reversible with restoration of renal perfusion. Toxin-mediated intrinsic AKI may be secondary to a large number of medications, including aminoglycosides, amphotericin, acyclovir, cisplatin, iodinated radiocontrast agents, and endogenous or exogenous toxins. Exogenous toxin-mediated AKI occurs from direct tubular damage (e.g., mercury) or from crystal formation (e.g., ethylene glycol and methanol poisoning). Endogenous toxins that can cause AKI are myoglobin, hemoglobin, and uric acid.

Inflammatory injury in the form of AIN most often occurs in the setting of medication exposures. Medications commonly associated with interstitial nephritis include extended-spectrum penicillins, NSAIDs, sulfonamides, and rifampin. AIN is also associated with infections, systemic diseases, tumor infiltrates, or genetic conditions. Acute glomerulonephritis is more common in school-age children, but is rare before 2 years of age. Postinfectious glomerulonephritis is the most common cause of acute glomerulonephritis and AKI in childhood; however, many other conditions produce a glomerulonephritic injury as well, including anti-glomerular basement membrane (anti-GBM) antibody disease, anti-neutrophil cytoplasmic antibody (ANCA) disease, lupus nephritis, IgA nephropathy, Henoch-Schönlein purpura (HSP) nephritis, and membranoproliferative glomerulonephritis (MPGN).

Despite the fact that congenital obstructive uropathies are among the most frequent causes of CKD in children, AKI itself is rarely the result of postrenal obstruction, except when this occurs in a solitary kidney either from aplasia, nephrectomy, or transplantation. More commonly in children with two functioning kidneys, postrenal AKI occurs in the setting of complete urethral or bladder neck obstruction, or in the unusual circumstance of bilateral ureteric obstruction. A variety of conditions can cause such unilateral or bilateral obstruction and subsequently lead to AKI, including calculi, ureteral blood clots, retroperitoneal fibrosis, neurogenic bladder, bladder or pelvic tumors, and urethral strictures or clot.

The major complications of AKI are related to either metabolic abnormalities or to fluid overload. The metabolic complications of AKI are hyperkalemia, metabolic acidosis, hypocalcemia, hyperphosphatemia, hyponatremia, and rarely uremia. Patients with oliguric or anuric AKI commonly present with hypervolemia and fluid overload. Hypertension is usually caused by salt and water overload, but may also be the result of changes in vascular tone or activation of the renin–angiotensin system due to parenchymal injury. If the fluid overload worsens, the child may develop pulmonary edema and/or congestive heart failure. Establishing fluid balance is perhaps the most challenging and critical step in managing AKI. Prerenal AKI is the most common situation in which intrinsic renal damage can be prevented. Any hypovolemic patient who presents with oligoanuric AKI has a potential prerenal component. The first step in managing this patient is fluid resuscitation with rapid infusion of isotonic saline. If the urine output does not increase after the patient is assessed to be euvolemic, intrinsic renal damage must be assumed. At this stage, in the absence of increased urine output, fluid restriction becomes essential to avoid hypertension, pulmonary edema, and congestive heart failure. Patients who present with nonoliguric

AKI may actually be polyuric and require greater than normal volumes of fluid to avoid intravascular volume depletion. Maintaining a euvolemic state, correcting electrolyte and acid-base disturbances, avoiding nephrotoxic agents, appropriately dosing medication for a reduced GFR, and providing adequate nutritional support are the essential principles for managing AKI. If volume or electrolyte management is unresponsive to medical therapy, or signs of uremia develop, dialysis should be initiated.

CHRONIC KIDNEY DISEASE

Chronic kidney disease is kidney damage of ≥3 months duration defined by either known pathology or markers of kidney injury, including abnormalities in blood, urine, or imaging tests. Importantly, the GFR may be normal early in CKD (Table 49.2) when diagnosis is important to retard progression and to prevent comorbid problems. The causes of CKD in infants, children, and adolescents are markedly different from those in adult patients. Diabetes and hypertension, which are the leading causes of CKD in adults, are associated with less than 0.1% of all end-stage renal disease (ESRD) in children. Approximately 60% of childhood CKD can be attributed to congenital anomalies of the kidney and urinary tract (CAKUT), including renal dysplasia, aplasia, hypoplasia, and/or obstructive uropathy. Other common causes include focal segmental glomerulosclerosis (FSGS) (5% to 10%), chronic glomerulonephritis (lupus nephritis, IgA nephropathy, HSP, or MPGN; 5% to 10%), ciliopathies (autosomal recessive polycystic kidney disease, nephronophthisis; 3% to 5%), and HUS (3% to 5%). Renovascular accidents, Alport syndrome, congenital nephrotic syndrome, primary hyperoxaluria, and cystinosis all remain rare but important causes of CKD in childhood.

In 2009, Schwartz et al derived a new equation for estimating GFR in children with CKD. The original Schwartz formula was developed in the mid-1970s, and designed to estimate GFR in children based on sCr, height, and an empiric constant. The new chronic kidney disease in children (CKiD) equation incorporates height, gender, sCr, cystatin C, and BUN to predict GFR with improved precision and accuracy in children with known CKD and measured GFR less than 75 mL/min/1.73 m^2:

$$eGFR = 39.1[\text{height in cm/sCr}]^{0.516}[1.8/\text{cystatin C}]^{0.294}$$
$$\times [30/\text{BUN}]^{0.169}[1.099]^{\text{Male}}[\text{height in cm}/1.4]^{0.188}$$

Furthermore, an updated constant of 0.413 for all children older than 1 year with known CKD was derived as a simplified and clinically useful CKiD bedside equation:

$$eGFR = 0.413[\text{height in cm}]/sCr$$

Accurate estimates of GFR can be extremely useful in appropriately staging CKD (see Table 49.2) to better identify and screen for the expected complications (Fig. 49.1).

Several aspects of the clinical history may indicate early CKD in infants and children, including abnormal antenatal ultrasound, oligohydramnios, polyhydramnios, polydipsia, polyuria, nocturia, and salt craving. However, many children are often asymptomatic or have vague, nonspecific complaints, including fatigue, headaches, or gastrointestinal symptoms. Failure to thrive, short stature, delayed puberty, pallor, and difficulty concentrating usually occur in the more advanced stages of CKD. Hypertension, left ventricular hypertrophy, and dyslipidemia are common findings in CKD, and these may occur at earlier stages in children with an underlying glomerular disorder (FSGS, glomerulonephritis, or HUS) as compared to those children with CAKUT. The primary metabolic abnormalities seen in advanced CKD include hyperkalemia, hyperphosphatemia, hypocalcemia, and metabolic acidosis. Renal osteodystrophy usually begins in CKD stage II to III as a result of reduced urinary phosphate excretion, elevated serum phosphorous levels and parathyroid hormone (PTH), hypocalcemia, and reduced circulating levels of activated vitamin D (1,25-dihydroxyvitamin D). Anemia typically develops in CKD stage III when the GFR drops below 40 to 60 mL/min/1.73 m^2 as a result of reduced renal production of erythropoietin.

The aims of treatment for CKD are fivefold: (1) treat the underlying condition whenever possible, (2) prevent the progression of the disease, (3) treat the complications of CKD, (4) provide the optimal conditions for normal growth and development, and (5) avoid further nephrotoxic insults. Hypertension and proteinuria are two risk factors independently associated with a more rapid progression of CKD. Consequently, treatment with ACE inhibitors or angiotensin receptor blockers (ARB) is indicated in many children with early to moderate CKD. The ESCAPE trial showed that over 5 years, children with CKD-associated hypertension treated with ACE inhibitors and intensified blood pressure control (target blood pressure below the 50th percentile for age, gender, and height) had delayed GFR loss as compared to children treated with ACE inhibitors with blood pressures targets in the conventional range (below the 90th percentile). In addition, ACE inhibitors reduced protein excretion by approximately 50% in all forms of nephropathy within the first 6 months in children with CKD. For patients with more advanced CKD, alternate antihypertensive agents might be required to avoid the risk of hyperkalemia.

The anemia of CKD is treated with recombinant human erythropoietin and iron supplementation. Renal osteodystrophy is primarily treated by restricting dietary phosphate intake, providing enteric phosphate binders, and administering calcitriol, a form of activated vitamin D (synthetic

Table 49.2 Stage of Chronic Kidney Disease

Stage	Description	GFR (mL/min/1.73 m^2)
1	Normal GFR	≥90
2	Mild CKD	60 to 89
3	Moderate CKD	30 to 59
4	Severe CKD	15 to 29
5	End-stage kidney failure	Less than 15 (or dialysis)

Adapted from Kidney Disease Outcomes Quality Initiative (K/DOQI): K/DOQI clinical practice guidelines for chronic kidney disease: evaluation, classification, and stratification. Executive summaries of 2000 updates. http://www.kidney.org/professionals/KDOQI/guidelines_ckd/toc.htm. CKD, Chronic kidney disease; GFR, glomerular filtration rate.

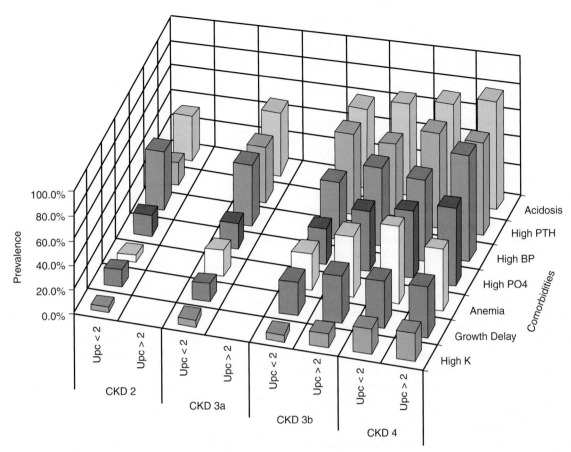

Figure 49.1   CKD comorbidities by stage and urine protein-to-creatinine ratio. CKD3 was divided into 3a (GFR 30 to 44 mL/min/1.73 m^2) and 3b (GFR 45 to 59 mL/min/1.73 m^2) for a more detailed analysis. *BP,* Blood pressure; *CKD,* chronic kidney disease; *GFR,* glomerular filtration rate; *K,* potassium; *PTH,* parathyroid hormone; *Upc,* urine protein-to-creatinine ratio. (Adapted from Furth SL, Abraham AG, Jerry-Fluker J et al: Metabolic abnormalities, cardiovascular risk factors and GFR decline in children with chronic kidney disease, *Clin J Am Soc Nephrol* 6:2132-2140, 2011.)

1,25-dihydroxyvitamin D). These interventions suppress parathyroid hormone secretion. Recombinant growth hormone therapy may be indicated for short stature after the provider ensures the child is receiving adequate calories and the secondary hyperparathyroidism and acidosis of CKD are adequately treated. Lifestyle choices that can hasten progression of CKD, including smoking, excessive body mass index, and frequent NSAID use, should all be avoided. Although protein restriction is commonly recommended in adults with CKD, children should target at least their required daily allowance of protein calories for appropriate growth.

HYPERTENSION

Hypertension in children older than 1 year is defined as systolic and/or diastolic blood pressure that is above the 95th percentile for age, gender, and height as defined by the *Fourth Report on the Diagnosis, Evaluation, and Treatment of High Blood Pressure in Children.* In children younger than 12 years, prehypertension is defined as systolic and/or diastolic blood pressure that is between the 90th and 95th percentile for age, gender, and height. In children aged 12 years and older, prehypertension is defined as blood pressure above 120/80 mm Hg, but below the 95th percentile for age, gender,

and height. Hypertension can be further staged according to severity. Stage 1 hypertension is defined as an average blood pressure level from the 95th percentile to 5 mm Hg above the 99th percentile. Stage 2 hypertension is defined as an average blood pressure that exceeds 5 mm Hg above the 99th percentile.

Ambulatory blood pressure monitoring (ABPM) has recently been introduced into the field of hypertension in children, and it has become a useful diagnostic tool. ABPM can help delineate some of the discrepancies observed between conventional blood pressure measurements in the office setting from measurements taken in a more natural environment. Patients with elevated blood pressures in the clinic but a normal ABPM study are currently designated as having isolated office hypertension, or white-coat hypertension. Those with normal conventional readings in clinic and an abnormal ABPM study are said to have masked hypertension.

Hypertension may also be classified by etiology. Essential hypertension, which is rarely seen in infants and younger children, is defined as hypertension without an otherwise identifiable cause. Secondary hypertension is an elevated blood pressure in the context of an identifiable underlying cause, such as intrinsic kidney disease, renovascular abnormalities, aortic coarctation, endocrinopathies, malignancies, central nervous system disease, medications, or a monogenetic form of hypertension. In general, the likelihood of identifying a secondary cause of hypertension is directly related to the degree of hypertension (stage 2), and is inversely related to the age of the child.

Renal parenchymal disorders, including glomerulonephritis, renal fibrosis, FSGS, renal dysplasia, and polycystic kidney disease, account for the vast majority of secondary causes of hypertension in children. Fibromuscular dysplasia and aortic coarctation are also relatively common causes, particularly in younger children. In neonates and premature infants, umbilical artery catheter-associated thromboembolism affecting the renal arteries is the most common cause of hypertension. Essential hypertension is usually characterized by prehypertension or stage 1 hypertension in adolescents, and is associated with obesity, a family history of hypertension, a sedentary lifestyle, and African-American race.

The evaluation of any child with hypertension largely depends on the likelihood of finding a secondary cause, and the extent of the evaluation should be individualized. Most younger children with hypertension, adolescents with stage 2 hypertension, and adolescents with stage 1 hypertension without obvious risk factors for essential hypertension will undergo an initial evaluation with a basic metabolic panel, urinalysis, and a kidney ultrasound. A cardiac echocardiogram may also be recommended to assess left ventricular mass as a sign of end-organ damage and to exclude the possibility of a coarctation. Management may be solely directed at lifestyle changes such as weight loss and dietary changes in the obese, sedentary, adolescent patient with mild hypertension; whereas children with secondary forms of hypertension almost always require pharmacotherapy. Several classes of antihypertensive agents are available for use in children, including ACE inhibitors, ARB, calcium channel blockers, and diuretics. Treatment is generally started as monotherapy at a low dose. The dose is then gradually increased, and additional medications added to avoid rapid reductions in blood pressure or other side effects. Monitoring of kidney function and electrolytes is often mandated by the choice of particular class of agents, for example, ACE inhibitors/ARB and/or diuretic, respectively. The long-term prognosis of pediatric hypertension primarily depends on the underlying etiology. Overall, there is an increased risk for future cardiovascular morbidity and mortality that may be modifiable with early recognition and treatment.

KEY BIBLIOGRAPHY

Akcan-Arikan A, Zappitelli M, Loftis LL, et al: Modified RIFLE criteria in critically ill children with acute kidney injury, *Kidney Int* 71:1028-1035, 2007.

Arora P, Kher V, Rai PK, et al: Prognosis of acute renal failure in children: a multivariate analysis, *Pediatr Nephrol* 11:153-155, 1997.

Copelovitch L, Meyers KEC, Kaplan BS: Acute renal failure. In Domico SF, Canning DA, Khoury A, editors: *The Kilalis-King-Belman textbook of clinical pediatric urology*, ed. 5, London, 2006, Informa Health Care, pp 7357-7366.

Copelovitch L, Warady BA, Furth SL: Insights from the Chronic Kidney Disease in Children (CKiD) Study, *Clin J Am Soc Nephrol* 6:2047-2053, 2011.

Falkner B: Hypertension in children and adolescents: epidemiology and natural history, *Pediatr Nephrol* 25:1219-1224, 2010.

Furth SL, Abraham AG, Jerry-Fluker J, et al: Metabolic abnormalities, cardiovascular risk factors and GFR decline in children with chronic kidney disease, *Clin J Am Soc Nephrol* 6:2132-2140, 2011.

Guignard JP: Measurement of glomerular filtration rate in neonates. In Polin RA, Fox WW, Abman SH, editors: *Fetal and neonatal physiology*, ed 3, Philadelphia, 2003, WB Saunders, pp 1205-1210.

Hoste EA, Kellum JA: RIFLE criteria provide robust assessment of kidney dysfunction and correlate with hospital mortality, *Crit Care Med* 34:2016-2017, 2006.

Kidney Disease Outcomes Quality Initiative (K/DOQI): K/DOQI clinical practice guidelines for chronic kidney disease: evaluation, classification, and stratification. Executive summaries of 2000 updates. http://www.kidney.org/professionals/KDOQI/guidelines_ckd/toc.htm.

Lurbe E, Alvarez J, Redon J: Diagnosis and treatment of hypertension in children, *Curr Hypertens Rep* 12:480-486, 2010.

Saland JM, Pierce CB, Mintsnefes MM, et al: Dyslipidemia in children with chronic kidney disease, *Kidney Int* 78:1154-1163, 2010.

Schwartz GJ, Haycock GB, Edelmann CM, et al: A simple estimate of glomerular filtration rate in children derived from body length and plasma creatinine, *Pediatrics* 58:259-263, 1976.

Schwartz GJ, Munoz A, Schneider MF, et al: New equations to estimate GFR in children with CKD, *J Am Soc Nephrol* 20:629-637, 2009.

Smith FG, Nakamura KT, Segar JL, et al: Renal function in utero. In Polin RA, Fox WW, Abman SH, editors: *Fetal and neonatal physiology*, ed 3, Philadelphia, 2003, WB Saunders, pp 1258-1260.

Thadhani R, Pascual M, Bonventre JV: Acute renal failure, *N Engl J Med* 334:1448-1460, 1996.

The ESCAPE Trial Group: Strict blood-pressure control and progression of renal failure in children, *N Engl J Med* 361:1639-1650, 2009.

The Fourth Report on the Diagnosis, Evaluation, and Treatment of High Blood Pressure in Children and Adolescents, National High Blood Pressure in Children and Adolescents: National High Blood Pressure Education Program Working Group on High Blood Pressure in Children and Adolescents, *Pediatrics* 114:555-576, 2004.

Woolf AS: Embryology. In Avner ED, Harmon WE, Niaudet P, editors: *Pediatric nephrology*, ed 5, Baltimore, 2004, Williams and Wilkins, pp 3-24.

Wuhl E, Mehls O, Schaefer F, et al: Antihypertensive and antiproteinuric efficacy of ramipril in children with chronic renal failure, *Kidney Int* 66:768-776, 2004.

Full bibliography can be found on www.expertconsult.com.

The Kidney in Pregnancy

50

Kavitha Vellanki | Susan Hou

Pregnancy produces dramatic changes in systemic hemodynamics, leading to an increase in total circulating blood volume and cardiac output and a decrease in systemic vascular resistance (SVR), resulting in a high output state with mildly reduced blood pressure (BP). The kidney experiences a marked increase in glomerular filtration rate (GFR) and renal plasma flow (RPF), which is critical for a favorable outcome in pregnancy. Understanding the adaptive changes that occur during pregnancy is crucial for differentiating and managing normal and compromised pregnancies.

ANATOMIC CHANGES DURING NORMAL PREGNANCY

During pregnancy, the kidney increases by 1 to 1.5 cm in length and by up to 30% in volume, reflecting increases in vascular and interstitial space without accelerated growth, a process akin to compensatory hypertrophy. Significant dilation and decreased peristaltic activity in the collecting system are noted as early as the third month of pregnancy, with more pronounced changes on the right side. Although the etiology is debated, hormonal changes in the initial period and compression of the ureters by the gravid uterus in the late gestational period are among the proposed causative mechanisms. Stasis of at least 200 mL of urine occurs in the collecting system. The increased susceptibility of pregnant women with asymptomatic bacteruria to acute pyelonephritis is attributed to urinary stasis. Magnetic resonance imaging can help in distinguishing physiologic hydronephrosis from obstruction in pregnancy; ultrasound is less reliable in such a setting. Structural changes generally resolve by 12 weeks postpartum, and persistent hydronephrosis beyond 12 to 16 weeks needs further workup (Box 50.1).

PHYSIOLOGIC CHANGES DURING NORMAL PREGNANCY

SYSTEMIC HEMODYNAMIC CHANGES

Pregnancy leads to vasodilation, and cardiac output increases by 40% to 50% above normal by 24 weeks of gestation. Plasma volume expands by 40% to 50%, whereas red blood cell mass increases by only 18% to 30%, resulting in a drop in hematocrit and leading to physiologic anemia of pregnancy. Despite the increase in blood volume and cardiac output, systemic BP decreases substantially and this decrease occurs despite an increase in many of the hormones that are generally associated with higher BP (a fourfold increase in

angiotensin, an eightfold increase in plasma renin, and a 10- to 20-fold increase in aldosterone). The pressor effects of these hormones are limited by profound reduction in SVR caused by the production of vasodilatory substances, such as prostacyclin, nitric oxide (NO), and relaxin. The lowest BP is seen between 16 to 20 weeks gestation, with a gradual increase towards term.

RENAL HEMODYNAMIC CHANGES

Glomerular filtration rate and RPF increase by approximately 50% with RPF being slightly higher than GFR. Hyperfiltration in pregnancy has been variously attributed to increased RPF, decreased oncotic pressure, and increased glomerular capillary Kf. Increase in GFR is noted as early as 4 weeks gestation, reaches peak level during the first half of pregnancy, and remains constant until term (Fig. 50.1). Despite a major increase in GFR, no long-term effects on glomerular function or structure are noted; this is true even in repetitive pregnancies with normal kidney function because of parallel reductions in both afferent and efferent arteriolar resistance with no change in intraglomerular pressure.

In women who previously had unilateral nephrectomy or kidney transplant, increases in GFR and RPF are often noted, because single kidneys can still adapt further as in normal pregnancy, although the changes are smaller and slower than in healthy women with two functioning kidneys.

METABOLIC CHANGES

Increased GFR leads to decreases in blood urea nitrogen (BUN) and serum creatinine levels. A BUN greater than 13 mg/dL or serum creatinine of 0.7 to 0.8 mg/dL is of concern in normal pregnancy and should be further investigated. Urinary protein excretion may increase but generally remains below 300 mg/24 hours. Total body water increases by 6 to 8 L, of which 4 to 6 L are extracellular. There is also a gradual cumulative retention of 900 mEq of sodium, the mechanisms of which remain unclear. A reset osmostat leads to a lower plasma osmolality (10 mOsm/L below normal) with a proportionate decrease in serum sodium by 4 to 5 mEq/L. Mild alkalemia from respiratory alkalosis and a compensatory decrease in serum bicarbonate to 18 to 22 mEq/L occur. Uric acid levels drop to 2.5 to 4 mg/dL from the combined effects of increased filtration and decreased tubular reabsorption. Serum levels and renal reabsorption of uric acid are significantly higher in pregnancies complicated by preeclampsia and intrauterine growth retardation (IUGR). Excretion of glucose increases soon

Box 50.1   Normal Adaptive Changes During Pregnancy

Structural Changes in the Kidney

Increase in kidney size by 1 to 1.5 cm
Dilation of the collecting system, more prominent on the right

Hormonal Changes

10- to 20-fold increase in aldosterone
8-fold increase in renin
4-fold increase in angiotensin

Systemic Hemodynamic Changes

Increased cardiac output by 40% to 50% of normal
Increased plasma volume by 40% to 50% of normal
Drop in SBP by ≈ 9 mm and DBP by 17 mm Hg (prominent in
    second trimester)
Resistance to pressor effect of angiotensin
Increased production of prostacyclin and nitric oxide

Renal Hemodynamic Changes

Increase in GFR and RPF by 50% above normal
Decrease in glomerular capillary oncotic pressure

Metabolic Changes

Decrease in BUN (to <13 mg/dL) and serum creatinine (to 0.4
    to 0.5 mg/dL)
Increase in total body water by 6 to 8 liters
Net retention of 900 mEq of sodium
Decrease in plasma osmolality by 10 mOsm/L
Decrease in serum sodium by 4 to 5 mEq/L
Mild respiratory alkalosis with compensatory metabolic acidosis
    (bicarb of 18 to 22 mEq/L)
Decrease in serum uric acid levels (to 2.5 to 4 mg/dL)
Glucosuria irrespective of blood glucose levels

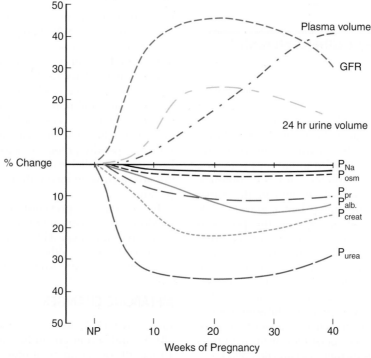

Figure 50.1   Physiologic changes induced in pregnancy. Increments and decrements in various parameters are shown in percentage terms with reference to the nonpregnant baseline. *GFR,* Glomerular filtration rate; *NP,* nonpregnant; P_{alb}, plasma albumin; P_{creat}, plasma creatinine; P_{Na}, plasma sodium; P_{osm}, plasma osmolality; P_{pr}, plasma proteins; P_{urea}, plasma urea. (From Davison JM: The kidney in pregnancy: a review, *J Royal Soc Med* 76:485-500, 1983.)

after conception and varies markedly even within a 24-hour period. Often, it does not correlate with blood glucose concentration or state of pregnancy. Normal glucose excretion returns within a week of delivery.

ASSESSMENT OF KIDNEY FUNCTION DURING PREGNANCY

Serum creatinine–based formulas are not accurate in calculating estimated GFR in pregnancy; accordingly, the guidance for application of MDRD formula excludes pregnant

women. Even in pregnant chronic kidney disease (CKD) patients, the MDRD equation underestimates "true" GFR as measured by inulin clearance by about 25 mL/min. Creatinine clearance (ClCr) measured in a 24-hour urine collection remains the most practical test to estimate GFR during pregnancy, although ClCr is expected to overestimate GFR by 10% to 20%, even in normal conditions. Estimating proteinuria during pregnancy by use of the urine-protein-to-creatinine ratio (UPCR) has been controversial, and 24-hour urine protein measurement remains the gold standard.

Table 50.1 Antihypertensive Medications in Pregnancy

Medication	Daily Dose	Side Effects/ Comments	Safety Label
Methyldopa	500 to 3000 mg in divided doses	First-line agent	Category B
Labetalol	200 to 1200 mg in divided doses	Widely used; efficacy and safety similar to methyldopa	Category B
Other beta blockers	Variable	IUGR and fetal bradycardia	Category C/D
Calcium channel blockers	Variable	Relatively safe	Category C
Diuretics	Variable	May cause diminished volume expansion	Category B/C
Clonidine	0.1 to 0.8 mg in divided doses	Limited data	Category C
Hydralazine	30 to 200 mg in divided doses	Widely used; not effective as a single agent	Category C
Minoxidil	2.5 to 10 mg in divided doses	Limited data	Category C
Spironolactone	Variable	Feminization of male fetus in animal studies; limited human data	Category C
Alpha blockers	Variable	Limited data	Category B/C
ACE inhibitors	Contraindicated	Renal dysplasia	Category D
ARBs	Contraindicated	Neonatal anuric renal failure	Category D

Category B: Animal studies show no fetal risk, but human data lacking.
Category C: Animal studies show fetal risk, but human data lacking.
Category D: Positive evidence of human fetal risk.
ACE, Angiotensin converting enzyme; *ARB,* angiotensin receptor blocker; *IUGR,* intrauterine growth retardation.

HYPERTENSIVE DISORDERS OF PREGNANCY

Hypertension in pregnancy is defined as BP ≥140/90 mm Hg, measured on at least two separate occasions. Hypertensive disorders occur in 6% to 8% of pregnancies and are the second leading cause of maternal mortality in the United States. To differentiate hypertensive disorders that predate pregnancy from a potentially more ominous disease peculiar to pregnancy, hypertensive disorders in pregnancy have been classified into four categories:

1. Chronic hypertension
2. Preeclampsia-eclampsia
3. Preeclampsia superimposed on chronic hypertension
4. Gestational hypertension

CHRONIC HYPERTENSION

Chronic hypertension is defined as hypertension that is present before pregnancy or that is diagnosed before 20 weeks of gestation or that is first diagnosed during pregnancy but does not resolve postpartum. Two thirds of women with pre-existing hypertension have a drop in BP between 13 and 20 weeks of gestation, and the diagnosis may not be apparent if they are first seen during this period. Women who do not have such a drop in BP are at risk for severe hypertension in third trimester and poor pregnancy outcomes. Chronic hypertension is associated with increased risk for IUGR, placental abruption, fetal mortality, and preeclampsia.

Data on specific BP targets in pregnancy are sparse, although hospitalization and early delivery rates are lower with antihypertensive medications. Since many safe antihypertensive medications are available, it is reasonable to treat mild hypertension in pregnancy, especially in women with kidney disease or other end organ damage. Because BP fluctuates during pregnancy, pregnant hypertensive women require close follow-up and should be taught to monitor their BP at home.

ANTIHYPERTENSIVE MEDICATIONS DURING PREGNANCY

Almost all antihypertensive medications cross the placenta (Table 50.1). Safety data are obtained from animal studies, retrospective review of human data, and long-term clinical experience.

Alpha-Methyldopa

Methyldopa has been used in pregnant women since 1960. It minimally affects uteroplacental blood flow and fetal hemodynamics and the major reported side effect is somnolence.

Calcium Channel Blockers

Once reserved for refractory hypertension, calcium channel blockers are now widely used as first-line antihypertensive agents in pregnancy. Nifedipine is most widely used and, like methyldopa, has minimal effect on uteroplacental blood flow. Profound hypotension has been reported with concurrent magnesium and nifedipine administration.

Beta-Adrenergic Blockers and Labetalol

Labetalol is the most widely used adrenergic blocker since it causes little adrenergic blockade in the newborn. Atenolol has been shown to decrease placental blood flow and affect fetal growth, whereas propranolol has been associated with neonatal bradycardia, hypoglycemia, and respiratory depression.

Hydralazine

Hydralazine is widely used but is ineffective as a single oral agent. Side effects have rarely been reported.

Angiotensin-Converting Enzyme (ACE) Inhibitors and Angiotensin Receptor Blockers (ARBs)

Second- and third-trimester exposure to ACE inhibitors is associated with oligohydramnios, renal dysplasia, and pulmonary hypoplasia. Similar problems are noted with ARBs. Even first-trimester exposure of ACE inhibitors is associated with increased congenital malformations. ACE inhibitors and ARBs should be avoided both during pregnancy and in women trying to conceive.

Diuretics

Some clinicians are averse to the use of diuretics in pregnancy because they aggravate the decreased intravascular volume seen with preeclampsia. In a metaanalysis involving more than 7000 normotensive pregnant women receiving diuretics, no increase in adverse fetal effects was noted. In settings where hypertension is related to volume expansion unrelated to pregnancy, diuretics frequently are needed for BP control and can be used with appropriate caution.

ACUTE TREATMENT OF SEVERE HYPERTENSION IN PREGNANCY

Hydralazine

Intravenous hydralazine in doses of 5 to 10 mg every 20 to 30 minutes is the drug of choice for hypertensive crisis in pregnancy.

Labetalol

Intravenous labetalol is the second most commonly used agent and is given either as a 20-mg loading dose followed by 20 to 30 mg every 30 minutes or as a 1- to 2-mg/min drip. The newborn should be monitored for bradycardia and hypotension.

Nifedipine

Short-acting nifedipine is still being used in a few centers to treat severe hypertension in pregnancy. It can be used when BP cannot be adequately controlled by hydralazine or labetalol.

SECONDARY HYPERTENSION

Secondary hypertension is a less common cause of hypertension in pregnancy than essential hypertension and preeclampsia. However, undiagnosed pheochromocytoma is associated with a maternal mortality rate as high as 50%. The diagnosis can be made by 24-hour urine measurements of epinephrine, norepinephrine, and their metabolites; values are unaltered in normal pregnancy or preeclampsia. Cocaine use can mimic pheochromocytoma and can be easily detected on toxic screen. Diagnosis of primary hyperaldosteronism is difficult because of alterations in renin and aldosterone secretions during pregnancy. Renovascular hypertension from fibromuscular dysplasia can lead to severe hypertension in pregnancy, and successful control of hypertension with angioplasty has been reported.

PREECLAMPSIA-ECLAMPSIA

Preeclampsia is a multisystem disease unique to human pregnancy and is the most frequently encountered glomerular complication in pregnancy. It is seen in approximately 5% of pregnancies in the United States, can occur even in molar pregnancies, and usually remits with removal of the placenta. Preeclampsia is characterized by new onset of hypertension (BP of ≥140/90 mm Hg) and proteinuria after 20 weeks of gestation, and is commonly associated with edema and hyperuricemia. Eclampsia is defined as the occurrence of seizures in a woman with preeclampsia in which the seizures cannot be attributed to other causes. Notably, preeclampsia is associated with increased lifetime risk for hypertension, ischemic heart disease, stroke, and venous thromboembolism.

RISK FACTORS

Preeclampsia is more common in first pregnancies and multigravidas with a new partner, suggesting that prior exposure to paternal antigens may have a protective role. This is further supported by higher rates of preeclampsia with shorter cohabitation periods prior to pregnancy, barrier method of contraceptive use, and pregnancies induced by artificial insemination with donated sperm. Other risk factors include multiple gestations, molar pregnancies, extremes of maternal age, family history or prior preeclampsia, and underlying maternal medical conditions such as hypertension, diabetes, CKD, obesity, and thrombophilias.

PATHOGENESIS

Placental abnormalities are universally noted in preeclampsia (Fig. 50.2). During pregnancy, trophoblasts migrate into uterine spiral arteries, transforming the thick muscular arteries into high-capacity vessels that permit greater blood flow to the uteroplacental unit. In preeclampsia, this process is incomplete and spiral arteries remain high-resistance vessels, leading to inadequate placental oxygen delivery, causing placental ischemia and release of factors that induce maternal vascular endothelial dysfunction. Whether placental ischemia alone is sufficient to cause preeclampsia is debatable because IUGR, also characterized by placental insufficiency, frequently occurs without preeclampsia.

Pregnancy is accompanied by increased production of vasodilator substances such as prostacyclin and NO. Despite the increased production of vasoconstrictors such as thromboxane and angiotensin, thromboxane increases less than prostacyclin, and there is resistance to the pressor effects of angiotensin. This balance is disrupted in preeclampsia. The ratio of thromboxane and prostacyclin is reversed, NO production is decreased, and sensitivity to the pressor effects of angiotensin returns before the onset of clinical symptoms.

Over the years, there has been intense effort to identify circulating factors that can explain the pathogenesis and ultimately lead to treatment of preeclampsia. Accumulating evidence points toward the role of placental antiangiogenic factors such as soluble fms-like tyrosine kinase-1 (sFlt1) and soluble endoglin (sEng) in pathogenesis of preeclampsia. sFlt1 is a soluble vascular endothelial growth factor (VEGF) receptor that binds to proangiogenic factors such as VEGF and placental growth factor (PlGF), neutralizing their effects. sEng is a soluble tumor growth factor (TGF) beta co-receptor that inhibits angiogenesis and induces vascular permeability and hypertension. Both sFlt1 and sEng have been shown to increase before onset of preeclampsia, with levels increasing precipitously just before the onset of clinical symptoms and generally normalizing several days after delivery, coinciding with improvement in proteinuria and hypertension. It is believed that preeclampsia occurs as a result of a decrease in growth factors such as VEGF and PlGF, along with overproduction of antiangiogenic factors such as sFlt1 and sEng. Although no screening test is yet proven accurate enough to predict preeclampsia, the use of a combination of the previously mentioned factors appears

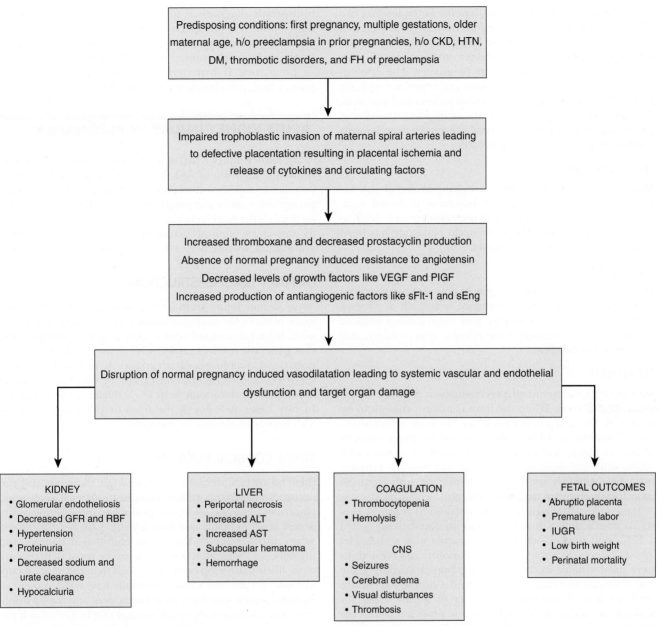

Figure 50.2   Pathogenesis of preeclampsia. *ALT,* Alanine aminotransferase; *AST,* aspartate aminotransferase; *CKD,* chronic kidney disease; *CNS,* central nervous system; *DM,* diabetes mellitus; *FH,* family history; *GFR,* glomerular filtration rate; *HTN,* hypertension; *IUGR,* intrauterine growth retardation; *PIGF,* placental growth factor; *RPF,* renal plasma flow; *sEng,* soluble endoglin; *sFlt-1,* soluble fms-like tyrosine kinase-1; *VEGF,* vascular endothelial growth factor.

promising. The most important clinical implications of these markers would be in diagnosing preeclampsia before the onset of overt symptoms, distinguishing preeclampsia from other causes of hypertension in patients with preexisting kidney disease, and developing therapeutic interventions that target their actions.

CLINICAL FEATURES

Preeclampsia is the most common cause of new-onset hypertension and proteinuria after 20 weeks of gestation. Edema is generally present, but 80% of pregnant women have edema, so this is not a diagnostic criterion. Preeclampsia is classified as severe in the presence of one of the following clinical features: alteration in mental status or stroke, BP >160/110 mm Hg, proteinuria >5 g/24 hours, oliguria, pulmonary edema, severe IUGR, or development of HELLP syndrome. HELLP syndrome is characterized by microangiopathic hemolytic anemia, elevated liver enzymes, and low platelets. It occurs in 10% to 20% of patients with preeclampsia. Other manifestations include pulmonary edema, cerebral edema, ascites, pleural effusion, retinal detachment, disseminated intravascular coagulation (DIC), and adult respiratory distress syndrome.

KIDNEY MANIFESTATIONS

The pathologic kidney lesion seen in preeclampsia is glomerular endotheliosis. The glomeruli are enlarged and swollen primarily as a result of hypertrophy of the intracapillary cells, which encroach on the capillary lumina, giving the appearance of bloodless glomeruli. Both GFR and RBF are decreased, the former more than the latter, leading to a 25% reduction in filtration fraction. Because GFR increases in pregnancy, serum creatinine levels in preeclampsia may still appear relatively normal. Proteinuria is generally non-selective and can appear late in pregnancy. The etiology of proteinuria is uncertain because podocytes are typically intact. There is impaired excretion of sodium and uric acid, the latter producing hyperuricemia, an important marker of preeclampsia. In contrast to normal pregnancy, preeclampsia is often associated with hypocalciuria.

FETAL OUTCOMES

Most babies of mothers with preeclampsia are at risk for preterm delivery, expedited to minimize maternal complications. Chronic placental hypoperfusion may lead to oligohydramnios and IUGR. Abruptio placentae has been reported with severe preeclampsia.

DIAGNOSIS

Diagnosis of preeclampsia, largely based on the characteristic clinical findings described earlier, is difficult in patients with underlying kidney disease and hypertension because these patients commonly have edema, hypertension, and proteinuria at baseline.

TREATMENT

Definitive management of preeclampsia is delivery of the placenta and fetus. When the fetus is mature enough to be delivered, the decision is easy. When the fetus is immature, careful monitoring of both the fetus and mother, treatment of hypertension, and prevention of maternal seizures with magnesium are critical. Continuous magnesium infusion must be cautiously used in kidney disease, with frequent monitoring of serum magnesium levels.

Data on low-dose aspirin for the prevention of preeclampsia are conflicting, although a recent metaanalysis suggested a 17% reduction of risk for preeclampsia with antiplatelet agents, largely consisting of low-dose aspirin; risk reductions were most notable in the high-risk group. Accordingly, the UK National Institute of Health and Clinical Excellence 2010 guidelines recommend 75 mg of aspirin daily for women at moderate to high risk for preeclampsia from 12 weeks of gestation until delivery. Data on the role of calcium in preventing preeclampsia are not convincing.

PREECLAMPSIA SUPERIMPOSED ON CHRONIC HYPERTENSION

Women with chronic hypertension who develop new-onset proteinuria after 20 weeks of gestation are diagnosed with superimposed preeclampsia. If such patients have proteinuria at baseline, diagnosis is difficult because proteinuria increases during pregnancy. These patients are considered preeclamptic if severe hypertension develops (≥160/110 mm Hg) in the latter half of pregnancy. Fetal outcomes are worse in hypertensive women with superimposed preeclampsia than in normotensive women developing preeclampsia.

GESTATIONAL HYPERTENSION

De novo BP elevation after mid-pregnancy and without proteinuria is classified as gestational hypertension. This nonspecific diagnosis is generally used only during pregnancy until a more specific diagnosis can be assigned. If preeclampsia has not developed and BP returns to normal by 12 weeks postpartum, it is called transient hypertension of pregnancy. If hypertension persists beyond 12 weeks postpartum, it is classified as chronic hypertension.

ACUTE KIDNEY INJURY IN PREGNANCY

Acute kidney injury (AKI) is a rare but serious complication. Although any form of AKI that affects adults in the general population can also affect pregnant women, a few causes are particularly common in pregnant women (Box 50.2). Prerenal azotemia is the most common cause of rise in serum creatinine in pregnancy, often occurring in the setting of hyperemesis gravidarum, uterine hemorrhage, or pyelonephritis.

URINARY TRACT OBSTRUCTION

Acute kidney injury from obstruction in pregnancy is seen more often in the setting of solitary kidney and polyhydramnios. Bilateral ureteral obstruction is a rare complication that generally resolves rapidly with delivery. AKI from functional hydronephrosis of pregnancy is rare but has been reported, and normalization of kidney function in lateral recumbent position may help in establishing the diagnosis. In rare cases, delivery of the fetus or percutaneous drain with nephrostomy may be required.

RENAL CORTICAL NECROSIS

Bilateral cortical necrosis is a pathologic diagnosis and can occur with pregnancy-related complications such as abruptio placentae, placenta previa, and prolonged intrauterine death. Severe renal ischemia and primary DIC have been proposed as the inciting agents leading to endothelial damage and thrombosis. Pregnant women with severe renal ischemia are more likely to develop cortical necrosis than the general population, and affected women generally have sudden onset of oliguria/anuria with flank pain, hematuria, and hypotension. Computed tomography or ultrasound can help establish the diagnosis by demonstrating hypoechoic or hypodense areas in the renal cortex. Many patients require dialysis with partial renal recovery seen in only to 20% to 40% of the cases.

Box 50.2   Causes of Acute Kidney Injury in Pregnancy

Volume depletion
    Hyperemesis gravidarum
    Postpartum bleeding
    Placental abruption
Sepsis
    Septic abortion
    Acute pyelonephritis
Severe preeclampsia
Bilateral cortical necrosis
Thrombotic microangiopathies (TTP-HUS)
Acute fatty liver of pregnancy
Urinary tract obstruction from gravid uterus

THROMBOTIC MICROANGIOPATHIES

Thrombotic thrombocytopenic purpura (TTP), hemolytic uremic syndrome (HUS), and severe preeclampsia with HELLP syndrome are important causes of AKI in late pregnancy.

TTP-HUS is characterized by unexplained thrombocytopenia and microangiopathic hemolytic anemia with kidney failure frequently present. Traditionally, TTP is considered when neurologic abnormalities are dominant, and HUS when there is profound kidney failure, especially in the postpartum period. TTP has been associated with deficiency of von Willebrand factor cleaving protease (ADAMTS 13) in nonpregnant states, but this association is not established in pregnancy. Mutations in genes encoding complement regulation have been associated with pregnancy-related HUS. Regardless, both TTP and HUS in pregnancy are treated with plasma exchange, and the dramatic decline in maternal mortality has been credited to its widespread use. Recurrence of TTP-HUS has been described both in subsequent pregnancies and in response to other inciting factors such as infections and drugs such as cyclosporine.

Distinguishing TTP-HUS from other microangiopathic syndromes, including severe preeclampsia accompanied by HELLP syndrome, can be difficult (Table 50.2). Thrombocytopenia, microangiopathic hemolytic anemia, AKI, proteinuria, and hypertension occur in both TTP-HUS and HELLP, although elevated liver enzymes are more common in HELLP syndrome, whereas elevated lactate dehydrogenase, prothrombin time, and partial thromboplastin time are more common in TTP-HUS.

ACUTE FATTY LIVER OF PREGNANCY

Acute fatty liver of pregnancy (AFLP) is a rare disorder that is unique to human pregnancy and characterized by microvesicular fatty infiltration of the hepatocytes with modest elevation of serum transaminases, increased bilirubin levels, and thrombocytopenia with or without DIC. AKI and hyperuricemia are common. Kidney biopsy findings in AFLP include acute tubular necrosis, fatty vacuolization of tubular cells, and occlusion of capillary lumens by fibrin-like material. Clinically, AKI may resemble hepatorenal syndrome with low fractional excretion of sodium and benign sediment, but the pathophysiology is likely distinct because elevated serum creatinine often precedes liver abnormalities. It typically presents in the third trimester with prodromal phase of nonspecific complaints such as nausea, vomiting, malaise, and epigastric pain. Jaundice appears a few days later, and patients can present with fulminant hepatic failure and encephalopathy. Definitive management is prompt delivery of the fetus. Both kidney and liver failure generally resolve postpartum with few patients requiring liver transplant.

PROTEINURIA

Proteinuria may be first detected during pregnancy, reflecting either preexisting or new-onset kidney disease. The most common cause of nephrotic range proteinuria in pregnancy is preeclampsia. Usually, a definitive diagnosis can wait until after pregnancy because nephrotic range proteinuria per se does not alter the natural course of pregnancy or fetal survival, as long as it is not associated with significant kidney failure or hypertension. The major exceptions are patients with either serologic evidence of lupus nephritis or profound hypoalbuminemia. In these cases, it is useful to know whether the underlying kidney disease can be effectively treated with corticosteroids during pregnancy. Low-dose diuretics are safe in pregnancy, but the safety of high-dose diuretics has not been established.

ACUTE PYELONEPHRITIS

Gestational pyelonephritis is a serious condition associated with IUGR, premature labor, septicemia, and, in severe cases, maternal death. AKI occurs in up to 25% of cases. Although the prevalence of asymptomatic bacteriuria is similar in both pregnant and nonpregnant women, 30% to 40% of pregnant women with untreated asymptomatic bacteriuria develop symptomatic urinary tract infection, including pyelonephritis. This risk is reduced by 70% to 80% if bacteriuria is eradicated. If a screening urine culture done at the first prenatal visit is negative, development of asymptomatic bacteriuria later in pregnancy is less likely in the absence of preexisting kidney disease. Cephalosporins and penicillins

---

Table 50.2   Features of Microangiopathic Syndromes Associated With Pregnancy

Features	HELLP	TTP	HUS	AFLP
Clinical onset	Third trimester	Any time	Postpartum	Third trimester
Unique to pregnancy	Yes	No	No	Yes
Underlying pathophysiology	Defective placentation	ADAMTS 13 deficiency	Mutations in genes regulating complement function	Defective mitochondrial beta-oxidation of fatty acids
Hypertension	Yes	Occasional	Yes	Frequently
Kidney failure	Yes	Yes	Yes	Yes
Thrombocytopenia	Present	Present	Present	Present
Liver function tests	Elevated	Normal	Normal	Elevated
Coagulation studies	Normal to high	High	Normal	Normal
Antithrombin III	Low	Normal	Normal	Low
Management	Delivery	Plasma exchange	Plasma exchange	Delivery

AFLP, Acute fatty liver of pregnancy; *HUS,* hemolytic uremic syndrome; *TTP,* thrombotic thrombocytopenic purpura.

are generally safe and effective. Treatment should be intravenous until the patient is afebrile and then continued for 14 days. Relapses of pyelonephritis can occur; accordingly, suppressive therapy with nitrofurantoin or a cephalosporin is recommended in women with normal and abnormal kidney function, respectively.

PREGNANCY IN CHRONIC KIDNEY DISEASE

Pregnancy in women with CKD may be complicated by hypertension/preeclampsia, worsening proteinuria, and premature delivery. The most serious concern for women with CKD who conceive is the potential for rapid loss of kidney function. The loss occurs irrespective of the cause of the underlying disease, with the risk increasing dramatically once a critical degree of baseline insufficiency is present. Failure to compensate increased GFR in the setting of the increased intraglomerular pressure is the most likely cause of such a rapid decline and cannot be predictably reversed once it occurs, even by terminating the pregnancy. Women who start dialysis for rapidly progressive kidney disease during pregnancy usually require continued dialysis postpartum. Despite the maternal risk for progressive kidney failure, the likelihood of the pregnancy resulting in a surviving infant is good. The most common adverse fetal outcomes noted are prematurity (40%-70%) and IUGR (20%-60%).

In many women, the initial diagnosis of CKD may occur during pregnancy; however, kidney biopsy typically is deferred until after pregnancy because of fear of increased risk for bleeding. When indicated, a kidney biopsy can be safely done with percutaneous ultrasound guidance in the usual prone position early in pregnancy or in lateral decubitus position later in pregnancy.

POLYCYSTIC KIDNEY DISEASE

Advanced kidney disease in women with polycystic kidney disease (PKD) generally develops after childbearing age. However, pregnant women with PKD experience an increased incidence of asymptomatic bacteriuria, more severe urinary tract infections, and an increase in the size and number of hepatic cysts due to estrogen stimulation. Women with intracranial aneurysms may be at increased risk for subarachnoid hemorrhage during labor.

GITELMAN AND BARTTER SYNDROMES

Increased requirement of potassium and magnesium supplementation in pregnant patients with underlying Gitelman syndrome and Bartter syndrome has been reported. Fetal survival is generally good, but these patients need frequent monitoring of their electrolytes.

LUPUS NEPHRITIS

Lupus nephritis is among the most variable and dangerous kidney diseases affecting pregnant women. Pregnancy-related immunologic and hormonal changes are associated with flares in approximately half of lupus nephritis patients, particularly in those with diffuse proliferative lesions. An increase in proteinuria or a decline in GFR, as well as the entire spectrum of life-threatening nonkidney manifestations such as cerebritis, pericarditis, and mesenteric vasculitis, can occur. Preeclampsia is a frequent complication (higher incidence in lupus nephritis compared with lupus patients with no kidney involvement) and often difficult to distinguish from a lupus nephritis flare. Fetal outcomes are generally good, with approximately 75% of pregnancies resulting in surviving infants when therapeutic abortions are excluded. Autoantibodies can cross the placenta, causing transient manifestations of lupus in the newborn. One of the classic manifestations in the neonate is congenital heart block associated with maternal anti-SSA antibody. Plasmapheresis has been attempted to clear anti-SSA antibodies without consistent success.

Although antiphospholipid antibody syndrome (APS) was initially considered wholly a part of the SLE syndrome, it has become increasingly evident that it can occur as a primary disease. APS is associated with a high risk for repeated abortions before 20 weeks gestation and unexpected intrauterine deaths in the second and third trimesters. Maternal complications include venous and/or arterial thrombosis, thrombocytopenia, pregnancy-induced hypertension, and preeclampsia. Management of APS consists of low-dose aspirin and heparin use.

New-onset lupus is an indication for biopsy during pregnancy since proliferative lupus nephritis requires prompt treatment, and first-line treatments are teratogenic (Table 50.3). Cyclosporine, azathioprine, and prednisone are considered safer in pregnancy than other agents, with cyclosporine probably being the most effective. For women with preexisting lupus nephritis, pregnancy is safest if the disease is in remission for 6 months on less than 10 mg daily prednisone, serum creatinine is less than 1.5 mg/dL, and BP is well controlled.

PREGNANCY IN DIALYSIS PATIENTS

Conception is rare in dialysis patients and is associated with poor fetal outcomes. Emerging data suggest that intensive dialysis results in better outcomes and may be a viable option for women whose reproductive years might otherwise be lost to CKD.

Menstrual irregularities generally begin as GFR falls below 15 mL/min, with amenorrhea typical at GFR below 5 mL/min. Early menopause is common, and, even in those patients who menstruate, cycles are often anovulatory. Numerous endocrine abnormalities have been suggested to play a role, including absent luteinizing hormone surge, shortened luteal phase, decreased progesterone and estradiol levels, and higher prolactin levels. Furthermore, lack of libido from medications, anemia, depression, and fatigue is common. Fertility rates are uncertain, ranging from 0.3% to 1% per year, with recent data suggesting improved conception rates. Conception rates appear significantly lower in women treated with peritoneal dialysis. Possibly, hypertonic solutions in the intraperitoneal space or compression of the fallopian tubes may interfere with transport of the ovum to the fallopian tube.

Pregnancy outcomes have significantly improved since the report of the first successful pregnancy in a dialysis patient

Table 50.3 Immunosuppressive Medications in Pregnancy*

Medication	Safety Label	Comments	Dosing Adjustments
Cyclosporine/tacrolimus	Category C	Increased incidence of maternal diabetes, hypertension, and preeclampsia	Higher doses required due to increased metabolism
Sirolimus	Category X	Contraindicated	Stopped 6 weeks before conception
Mycophenolic acid	Category X	Contraindicated	Stopped 12 weeks before conception
Azathioprine	Category D	Widely used despite being category D; low birth weights and leukopenia reported in newborns	No dosing adjustments required
Cyclophosphamide	Category D	Increased risk for congenital anomalies and childhood cancer	Used with caution
Rituximab	Category C	Limited human data; crosses placenta; B cell lymphocytopenia reported	Limited data

Category C: Animal studies show fetal risk, but human data lacking.
Category D: Positive evidence of human fetal risk.
Category X: Positive evidence of human fetal risk, and risks clearly outweigh potential benefits.
*Breastfeeding not recommended with any of the medications in this table.

Box 50.3 Management of Pregnant Hemodialysis Patients

Dialysis Dose

At least 20 hours of dialysis/week; goal BUN of <40 mg/dL

Dialysate Composition

Bicarbonate: 25 mEq/L
Calcium: 2.5 to 3.0 mmol/L with weekly Ca and Phos measurement
Sodium: 130 to 135 mEq/L based on serum Na

Diet/Vitamin Supplementation

Double dose of MVI
Folic acid 5 mg/daily
Unrestricted diet
Protein intake: 1.5 to 1.8 g/kg/day

Dry Weight

Assess weekly
Increases by 0.5 kg/week in second and third trimesters

Anemia

Increase in ESA and iron requirements
Target hemoglobin of 10 g/dL

Hypertension

Target postdialysis BP of 140/90 mm Hg

Diagnosis of Preeclampsia

Difficult to diagnose; must rely on worsening BP control
Aspirin 75 mg daily for prophylaxis of preeclampsia

Metabolic Bone Disease

Vitamin D analogs to maintain PTH levels, as in general dialysis patients
Oral phosphorus binders generally not required

---

in 1971. In 1998, only 50% of pregnancies in women conceiving after starting dialysis resulted in surviving infants. By 2002, there were enough data to suggest that 75% of infants would survive when dialysis was increased to 20 or more hours per week; however, premature labor remained a major issue. In 2008, one case series noted five of six pregnancies delivering after 36 weeks with nocturnal dialysis for an average 48 hours per week.

MANAGEMENT OF PREGNANT DIALYSIS PATIENTS

Because amenorrhea is common during dialysis, diagnosing pregnancy can be difficult. Beta HCG levels are elevated in the dialysis population and cannot be used to estimate gestational age or to diagnose molar pregnancy; accordingly, a pregnancy diagnosis should be confirmed with ultrasound. Medications should be carefully reviewed and teratogenic medications promptly discontinued. Hemodialysis should be intensified to more than 20 hours per week, targeting

predialysis BUN of 40 mg/dL (Box 50.3). Given such intense dialysis, unrestricted diet is allowed with daily protein intake increased to 1.1 g/kg/day because 10 to 15 g of amino acids can be lost in the dialysate. Dialysate calcium often needs to be increased to ensure adequate influx because of the increased requirements for fetal skeletal development, but this should be adjusted to PTH and ionized calcium levels. Anemia in pregnant dialysis patients usually worsens because of the loss of iron and red blood cells that occurs with frequent dialysis; thus increases in the requirements of erythropoietin and iron are expected. Twice the dose of multivitamins and folic acid of 5 mg are prescribed to satisfy the increased requirements for water-soluble vitamins (particularly folate) during pregnancy and to account for the increased losses with dialysis. Because weight should increase by 0.5 kg/week in the third trimester, weight gain should be expected. Determination of dry weight can be difficult and should be made by clinical examination and assessment of fetal growth. Pregnancy should be managed by a multi-disciplinary team that includes high-risk obstetricians and nephrologists.

PREGNANCY IN KIDNEY TRANSPLANT

Sexual dysfunction and infertility often reverse posttransplantation. Optimal contraception should be initiated during the peritransplant period. Since intrauterine devices need an intact immune system to function efficiently and high failure rates are associated with barrier methods, oral contraceptive pills may be the best choice, presuming that BP is adequately controlled. Alternatively, two barrier methods can be used in combination.

The optimal timing of pregnancy depends on the individual circumstances of the transplant recipient. Because women with CKD experience premature menopause, both chronologic age and risk for early menopause should be considered when planning for pregnancy posttransplant. The consensus opinion of the American Transplant Society is that pregnancy can be planned when the patient reaches 1 year posttransplantation, as long as the following criteria are met: adequate kidney function, stable immunosuppressive medication dosing in place, no rejection episodes in the past year, no recent infections that could jeopardize fetal survival, and no teratogenic medications being taken.

The major concerns are the effect of pregnancy on maternal allograft function and potential side effects of medications on fetal growth. Preeclampsia, premature delivery, low birth weight, and neonatal deaths are common in transplant recipients. Case-control studies have shown no increase in graft loss and do not indicate that pregnancy per se increases rejection risk; however, detection of rejection can be difficult because of pregnancy-related changes in renal physiology. When it doubt, kidney biopsy can be safely performed. Management of hypertension is important since many of these patients have chronic hypertension. Treatment recommendations are generally more aggressive than in the general pregnant population; targeting normotension is the goal.

All immunosuppressive medications cross the maternal-fetal circulation, and no choice exists other than to expose the fetus to the least offensive medications. Much remains to be learned about the pharmacokinetics and pharmacodynamics of immunosuppressive medications during pregnancy, and as expected, most of the available information is from retrospective review and clinical experience (see Box 50.3). Maintenance immunosuppression in pregnant transplant patients generally includes cyclosporine or tacrolimus, azathioprine, and prednisone. Mycophenolate should be avoided in transplant patients planning to become pregnant,

with azathioprine frequently used in its place. Antibodies used to treat rejection, such as thymoglobulin and alemtuzumab, cross the placenta. There is insufficient experience with these agents in pregnancy. Their use would seem preferable to losing the kidney, but this should be reserved for cases in which high-dose steroids are ineffective and a reasonable chance exists that the kidney can be salvaged.

BIBLIOGRAPHY

Abalos E, Duley L, Steyn DW, et al: Antihypertensive drug therapy for mild to moderate hypertension during pregnancy, *Cochrane Database Syst Rev* 2007.

Barua M, Hladunewich M, Keunen J, et al: Successful pregnancies on nocturnal home hemodialysis, *Clin J Am Soc Nephrol* 3:392-396, 2008.

Baumann MU, Nick A, Bersinger, et al: Serum markers for predicting preeclampsia, *Mol Aspects Med* 28:227-244, 2007.

Bobrie G, Liote F, Houillier P, et al: Pregnancy in lupus nephritis and related disorders, *Am J Kidney Dis.* 9:339, 1987.

Cornelis T, Odutayo A, Keunen J, et al: The kidney in normal pregnancy and preeclampsia, *Semin Nephrol* 31:4-14, 2011.

Davison JM: Changes in renal function in early pregnancy in women with one kidney. *Yale J Biol Med* 51:347-349, 1978.

Davison JM: The kidney in pregnancy: a review, *J Royal Soc Med* 76:485-500, 1983.

Duley L, Henderson-Smart DJ, Meher S, et al: Anti-platelet agents for preventing preeclampsia and its complications, *Cochrane Database Syst Rev* 2004.

Fakhouri F, Roumenina L, Provot F, et al: Pregnancy-associated hemolytic syndrome revisited in the era of complement gene mutations, *J Am Soc Nephrol* 21:859-867, 2010.

Hladunewich M, Hercz AE, Keunen J, et al: Pregnancy in end stage renal disease, *Semin Dialysis* 24:634-639, 2011.

Hou SH, Grossman SD, Madias NE: Pregnancy in women with renal disease and moderate renal insufficiency, *Am J Med* 78:185-194, 1985.

Imbasciati E, Gregorini G, Cabiddu G, et al: Pregnancy in CKD stages 3 to 5: fetal and maternal outcomes, *Am J Kidney Dis* 49:753-762, 2007.

Lindheimer MD, Davison JM, Katz AI: The kidney and hypertension in pregnancy: twenty existing years, *Semin Nephrol* 21:173-189, 2001.

Maynard SE, Karumanchi SA: Angiogenic factors and preeclampsia, *Semin Nephrol* 31:33-46, 2011.

McKay DB, Josephson MA: Pregnancy after kidney transplantation, *Clin J Am Soc Nephrol* 3:S117-S125, 2008.

National Collaborating Centre for Women's and Children Health: *Hypertension in pregnancy: the management of hypertensive disorders during pregnancy* London, 2010, Royal College of Obstetricians and Gynaecologists. Availablehttp://guidance.nice.org.uk/CG107/guidance.

Okundaye IB, Abrinko P, Hou S: A registry for pregnancy in dialysis patients, *Am J Kidney Dis* 31:766-773, 1998.

Report of the national high blood pressure education program working group on high blood pressure in pregnancy, *Am J Obstet Gynecol* 183:S1-S22, 2000; July.

Sibai BM, Grossman RA, Grossman SG: Effects of diuretics on plasma volume in pregnancies with long term hypertension, *Am J Obstet Gynecol* 150:831-835, 1984.

Singh Ajay K: Lupus nephritis and the anti-phospholipid antibody syndrome in pregnancy, *Kidney Int* 58:2240-2254, 2000.

Smith MC, Moran P, Ward MK, et al: Assessment of glomerular filtration rate during pregnancy using the MDRD formula, *BJOG* 115:109-112, 2008.

Kidney Disease in the Elderly

Ann M. O'Hare | C. Barrett Bowling | Manjula Kurella Tamura

51

AGE AND THE PREVALENCE OF CHRONIC KIDNEY DISEASE

The prevalence of chronic kidney disease (CKD) increases markedly with age. Among adults in the general population, prevalence increases from less than 5% for those under the age of 40, to 47% among those aged 70 and older—or one in every two people (Fig. 51.1). Although the high prevalence of CKD in older adults may in part reflect a high prevalence of comorbidities associated with CKD at older ages (e.g., diabetes and hypertension), a strong age-associated increase in the prevalence of CKD is present across a wide range of populations. The dramatic increase in prevalence of CKD at older ages largely reflects the relationship between the estimated glomerular filtration rate (eGFR) cut point of 60 mL/min/1.73 m^2 selected for defining disease and the distribution of eGFR within the population. Estimates of GFR in the general population follow a normal distribution with a median value around 80 to 90 mL/min/1.73 m^2. The midpoint of this distribution decreases with age, and, in the oldest age groups, the median eGFR moves close to 60 mL/min/1.73 m^2. In women without comorbidity participating in a community-based cohort study in the Netherlands, the median eGFR ranged from 90 mL/min/1.73 m^2 for those aged 18 to 24 years to 60 mL/min/1.73 m^2 for those aged 85 and older. Less than 5% of women aged 85+ without comorbidity had an eGFR close to 90 mL/min/1.73 m^2, the median value for the youngest age group. Among members of this cohort of similar ages, median levels of eGFR were lower for women compared with men and for people with versus those without other comorbidities, but these differences were far less dramatic than differences across age groups. In summary, median eGFR decreases with age, but there is a wide distribution of eGFR values among people of the same age.

The amount of urinary protein excretion also increases with age. However, both the distribution of albumin-to-creatinine ratio (ACR) and its relationship to the threshold value of 30 mg/g selected for defining CKD are quite different than for eGFR. Almost half of adults in the general population have an ACR below the level of detection, whereas values of 30 mg/g or higher occur in a small minority. Because the percentage of patients who meet ACR criteria for CKD varies less as a function of age than the percentage who meet eGFR criteria for CKD, the majority of older adults with CKD have a low eGFR without significant albuminuria, whereas the majority of younger adults with CKD have albuminuria but a normal eGFR (Fig. 51.2).

Prevalence estimates for CKD in older adults vary widely depending on the methods used to estimate GFR (Chapter 3).

The Cockroft-Gault and Modification of Diet in Renal Disease (MDRD) equations were not developed in populations that included a representative sample of older adults, and they have the disadvantage of relying on serum creatinine, which is a marker of both muscle mass and GFR. Small improvements in accuracy of GFR estimation can substantially impact the prevalence of CKD, because a disproportionately large number of patients with a low eGFR have levels that are only slightly under 60 mL/min/1.73 m^2. During the past several years, the Chronic Kidney Disease Epidemiology Collaboration (CKD-EPI) equation has supplanted the MDRD equation in clinical practice. Overall, use of this equation results in lower prevalence estimates of CKD in the general population compared with the MDRD equation, although this does not seem to be the case for older populations.

PROGRESSION TO END-STAGE RENAL DISEASE

Patients with CKD are at risk for progressive loss of kidney function and for ultimately developing end-stage renal disease (ESRD), traditionally defined as initiation of chronic dialysis or receipt of a kidney transplant. The burden of ESRD is particularly high in older adults: in the United States the mean age of new dialysis patients is 65 years, and the crude incidence of ESRD is highest among adults aged 75 and older. The high incidence of ESRD at older ages parallels the high prevalence of CKD in the elderly. However, among patients with similar levels of eGFR, those who are older are actually less likely to initiate kidney replacement therapy. This phenomenon likely reflects a number of different factors, including a greater competing risk of death, lower uptake of kidney replacement therapy, differences in the accuracy of eGFR estimates, and perhaps slower loss of kidney function among older compared with younger adults.

HIGH COMPETING RISK OF DEATH AT OLDER AGES

The incidence of ESRD increases exponentially as eGFR decreases. Mortality rates also increase with falling eGFR, but this increase is more linear and far less dramatic. Because the majority of patients with CKD have only moderate reductions in eGFR to the 45 to 59 mL/min/1.73 m^2 range, a time when the risk of death generally predominates over the risk of ESRD, most patients with CKD will die before they reach ESRD. At lower levels of eGFR, risk of ESRD eventually exceeds the risk of death for most patient

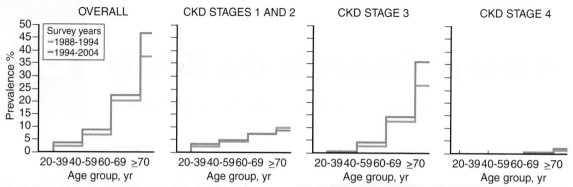

Figure 51.1   Stages of chronic kidney disease in the United States, 1988-1994 and 1994-2004. *CKD,* Chronic kidney disease. (Data from Coresh J, Selvin E, Stevens LA, et al: Prevalence of chronic kidney disease in the United States, *JAMA* 298:2038-2047, 2007.)

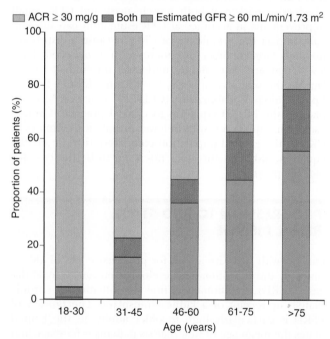

Figure 51.2   Proportions of patients with chronic kidney disease identified by albumin-to-creatinine ratio, estimated glomerular filtration rate, or both in the U.S. population. *ACR,* Albumin-to-creatinine ratio; *GFR,* glomerular filtration rate. (From James, MT, Hemmelgarn BR, Tonelli M et al: Early recognition and prevention of chronic kidney disease, *Lancet* 375:1296-1309, 2010 [adapted from McCullough PA, Li S, Jurkovitz CT et al: CKD and cardiovascular disease in screened high-risk volunteer and general populations: the Kidney Early Evaluation Program (KEEP) and National Health and Nutrition Examination Survey (NHANES) 1999-2004, *Am J Kidney Dis* 51(suppl 2): S38–S45, 2008].)

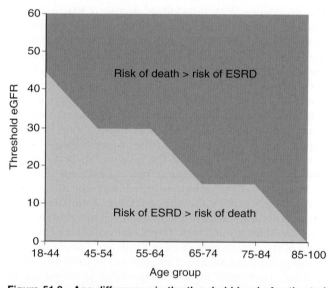

Figure 51.3   Age differences in the threshold level of estimated glomerular filtration rate at which risk of end-stage renal disease exceeds risk of death among a U.S. cohort of veterans. *eGFR,* Estimated glomerular filtration rate; *ESRD,* end-stage renal disease. (From O'Hare AM, Choi AI, Bertenthal D et al: Age affects outcomes in chronic kidney disease, *J Am Soc Nephrol* 18:2758-2765, 2007.)

groups; however, the threshold level of eGFR at which this transition occurs varies depending on age. For example, among a cohort of U.S. Veterans, the threshold level of eGFR at which the incidence of ESRD exceeded that of death was as high as 30 to 44 mL/min/1.73 m^2 for some younger age groups, but as low as 15 mL/min/1.73 m^2 for some older age groups (Fig. 51.3). Similar patterns are present when ESRD is defined more broadly to include patients who develop a sustained eGFR less than 15 mL/min/1.73 m^2 but do not receive kidney replacement therapy. The relationships among eGFR, ESRD, and the competing risk of

death are probably also modified by other factors such as level of proteinuria, sex, race, and other comorbidity. Thus it is likely that the threshold level of eGFR at which the risk of ESRD exceeds the risk of death among patients of the same age will vary across different populations.

AGE DIFFERENCES IN LOSS OF KIDNEY FUNCTION

The relationship between age and rate of loss of eGFR is less straightforward than the relationship between age and treated ESRD described earlier, and may vary depending on the method used to estimate progression, the method for ascertaining repeated measures of kidney function (e.g., systematic collection at regular intervals vs. as part of clinical care), and the population studied. Some studies, mostly in patients with early stages of CKD, have reported more rapid loss of kidney function among older compared with younger patients, whereas other studies, mostly among patients with lower levels of eGFR, have reported slower loss of kidney function at older ages. A recent study from Alberta, Canada,

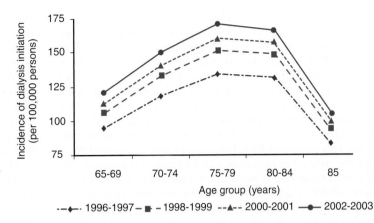

Figure 51.4 Incidence of treated end-stage renal disease by age group over time. (From Kurella M et al: Octogenarians and nonagenarians starting dialysis in the United States, *Ann Intern Med* 146:177-183, 2007.)

showed a similar incidence of kidney failure, defined as initiation of dialysis or a sustained eGFR less than 15 mL/min/1.73 m², for older and younger adults.

AGE DIFFERENCES IN END-STAGE RENAL DISEASE TREATMENT DECISIONS

Because most ESRD registries include only patients treated with kidney replacement therapy, little is known about those patients with advanced CKD who either prefer not to undergo dialysis or who are not offered dialysis. A growing number of single-center studies outside the United States have described relatively high rates of conservative management among older adults with advanced kidney disease. Joly et al reported that, among 146 consecutive patients aged 80 years or older who were referred to the renal unit at the Necker Hospital in Paris between 1989 and 2000 with an estimated creatinine clearance less than 10 mL/min, conservative nondialytic management was recommended in 37 (25%). Similarly, among 321 patients referred to a renal unit in Britain, palliative nondialytic care was recommended in 20%. Members of the nondialysis group were older, had lower functional status, and were more likely to have diabetes compared with the group in whom dialysis was recommended. An Australian study reported that older patients were more likely to receive information on conservative care and also were more likely to choose not to receive dialysis.

Because many elderly patients with advanced kidney disease are not referred to nephrologists, single-center studies in referred populations likely underestimate the number and percentage of elderly patients with advanced kidney disease who either prefer not to receive or are not offered dialysis. Using laboratory and administrative data from Alberta, Canada, Hemmelgarn et al found that, although the incidence of ESRD treated with dialysis was lower in older compared with younger patients with similar levels of eGFR, the incidence of a sustained eGFR less than 15 mL/min/1.73 m² not treated with dialysis was higher in older adults. These results suggest that there may be age differences in treatment practices for advanced kidney disease. However, this study could not provide information about whether or not older adults with a low eGFR were less likely to be treated with dialysis.

Little is currently known about treatment practices for advanced kidney disease in the United States. However, several lines of indirect evidence support the possibility that a substantial number of elderly U.S. patients with advanced CKD do not receive dialysis. First, across hospital referral regions in the United States, there are large differences in the incidence of treated ESRD among older adults that are not accounted for by differences in age, race, and sex. Hospital referral regions with the highest levels of healthcare spending in general have the highest incidence of treated ESRD. Furthermore, regional differences in the incidence of treated ESRD are most pronounced in the very elderly. Second, despite an increasing prevalence of CKD at older ages, the incidence of ESRD per million of population among U.S. adults peaks in the 75- to 79-year-old age group and decreases thereafter (Fig. 51.4). Similar trends across age groups appear to exist for treatment of acute kidney injury (AKI) among hospitalized patients. Hsu et al described age differences in the management of AKI among members of a large health maintenance organization in northern California from 1996 to 2003. Although the incidence of AKI not treated with dialysis increased linearly with age, the incidence of AKI treated with dialysis peaked among those aged 70 to 79 and declined at older ages. Collectively, these findings suggest that there may be age differences in treatment practices for advanced kidney disease in the United States.

CLINICAL SIGNIFICANCE OF MODERATE REDUCTIONS IN ESTIMATED GLOMERULAR FILTRATION RATE IN THE ELDERLY

Adults older than 70 years account for approximately one half of all U.S. adults with CKD; however, more than half of these older adults with CKD have only moderate reductions in eGFR into the 45 to 59 mL/min/1.73 m² range. In other words, older adults with moderate reductions in eGFR contribute significantly to the high overall prevalence of CKD in the U.S. population. For many of these older patients, an eGFR in this range falls close to the median value for their peers. Because eGFR is thought to decline as part of "normal" aging, some have questioned the clinical significance of such moderate reductions in eGFR in older adults.

Because death is far more common than progression to ESRD among patients with moderate reductions in eGFR, the debate about the clinical significance of eGFR in older adults has largely centered on mortality risk. Epidemiologic studies of CKD generally report the relative risk of death associated with a given level of kidney function compared with a referent category with "normal" kidney function. On a population level, the same increase in relative risk of death will be associated with a greater number of deaths in patients with higher background mortality rates (e.g., older patients). However, among individual patients, the same increase in the relative risk of death will translate into a smaller difference in life expectancy among those with more limited life expectancy. For example, a 10% increase in mortality risk translates into 1-year reduction in survival for a patient with a life expectancy of 10 years as compared with 1-month reduction in survival for a patient with a life expectancy of 10 months. This distinction becomes clinically relevant when considering mortality risk among older patients with very moderate reductions in eGFR in whom the relative risk of death is only modestly increased compared with the referent of patients with normal kidney function. Such modest increases in relative mortality risk may not translate into a meaningful difference in life expectancy in populations with very high baseline mortality rates.

Consistent with this possibility, some studies have demonstrated that the time to death (or relative hazard of death) associated with a given level of eGFR is attenuated at older ages. O'Hare and colleagues found that, in a large national cohort of veterans, at each level of eGFR the relative hazard of death was attenuated with increasing age. Members of this cohort age 65 and older with an eGFR in the range of 50 to 59 mL/min/1.73 m^2 (comprising nearly half of the cohort designated as CKD) did not have an increased relative risk of death compared with their age peers with an eGFR ≥60 mL/min/1.73 m^2. On the other hand, younger members of this cohort with moderate reductions in eGFR did have a higher risk of death compared with the referent group. Attenuation of the relative hazard of death associated with a given level of eGFR has been reported in several other cohorts, although in some of these cohorts there was some increase in risk for those with moderate reductions in eGFR relative to patients with higher levels of kidney function; this relationship was

dependent on the population studied, the level of eGFR and the referent category used, the equation used to estimate GFR, and whether analyses included information on level of proteinuria.

Given the very large numbers of older adults with modest reductions in eGFR and uncertainty about the clinical implications of such modest reductions, there is growing interest in efforts to distinguish high-risk from low-risk members of this group. Several studies have now suggested that information on other disease markers, such as level of proteinuria, eGFR trajectory, and cystatin C, are useful in identifying a higher risk subgroup within the large population of older adults with moderate reductions in eGFR.

COMORBIDITY AND GERIATRIC SYNDROMES AMONG OLDER ADULTS WITH CHRONIC KIDNEY DISEASE

Several earlier studies have considered whether CKD is associated with metabolic abnormalities among older adults. Two large studies showed that, similar to younger adults, lower eGFR was associated with a higher prevalence of anemia, hyperkalemia, acidosis, hyperphosphatemia, and hyperparathyroidism among older adults. Patients with CKD are also at higher risk for geriatric syndromes such as cognitive impairment, functional limitation, and falls. These syndromes are conceptualized as heterogeneous conditions that aggregate in older adults and result from a shared risk factor or factors. Geriatric syndromes contribute to frailty, a phenotype characterized as rendering the patient vulnerable to situational challenges, which in turn leads to disability, dependence, and death (Table 51.1). The burden of geriatric syndromes and frailty among older adults with CKD is quite high. For example, in several studies more than 20% of adults with stage 4 CKD had evidence of cognitive impairment and frailty, whereas, among dialysis patients over the age of 65, more than 30% have cognitive impairment, and more than

---

Table 51.1 Relevance and Significance of Select Geriatric Syndromes in Older Adults With Chronic Kidney Disease

Geriatric Syndromes	Relevance and Significance in Older Adults With CKD
Cognitive impairment	The prevalence and incidence of cognitive impairment increases at lower levels of eGFR and is common in older adults receiving chronic dialysis. In both the general population and in ESRD patients, cognitive impairment is associated with increased mortality.
Depressive symptoms	Depression is more common in patients with CKD and is associated with worsening kidney function and progression to ESRD. Among patients with ESRD, depression is associated with increased risk of mortality.
Falls	CKD complications such as neuropathy, muscle weakness, and anemia are associated with falls. CKD patients have a higher risk of fractures.
Polypharmacy	CKD patients take an average of eight medications and have decreased renal clearance of many drugs. Among older adults, polypharmacy is associated with increased mortality. Drug dosing is based on creatinine clearance, which may be a poor marker for kidney function in older adults with decreased muscle mass.
Poor physical performance	CKD is associated with poor physical performance. In the general population, poor physical performance predicts mortality and functional decline.
Frailty	Frailty is more prevalent in older adults with CKD than among those without CKD. Among dialysis patients, frailty is common even among younger patients and is associated with an increased risk of mortality.

CKD, Chronic kidney disease; *eGFR*, estimated glomerular filtration rate; *ESRD*, end-stage renal disease.

75% are frail. In contrast to the general population, geriatric syndromes and frailty are relatively common even among younger patients with CKD. These observations have led some investigators to describe CKD as a process of accelerated aging.

OUTCOMES AMONG OLDER ADULTS WITH ADVANCED CHRONIC KIDNEY DISEASE

Treatment options for advanced CKD are similar for older and younger adults. However, advanced age and the associated high burden of comorbidity and disability have important implications for determining the relative benefits and burdens of available treatment options. For some older adults, quality of life may be as important as length of life in making ESRD treatment choices.

DIALYSIS VERSUS CONSERVATIVE THERAPY

Median survival after dialysis initiation for adults ages 75 to 79, 80 to 84, 85 to 89, and ≥90 years is 1.7 years, 1.3 years, 0.9 years, and 0.6 years, respectively; however, considerable heterogeneity in survival exists among patients of similar ages, highlighting the limitations of using age alone to predict outcomes. For example, among adults ages 75 to 79 starting dialysis, 25% have a life expectancy of more than 3 years, whereas 25% have a life expectancy of less than 6 months. In addition to advanced age, a number of negative prognostic factors have been identified in epidemiological studies, including frailty or reduced functional status, low body weight or serum albumin concentration, number and severity of comorbidities, and late referral or unplanned dialysis initiation. Additionally, among patients who die within 6 months of starting dialysis, most die less than 3 months after starting. Validated prognostic models incorporating several of these factors have recently been developed and may help refine estimates of life expectancy.

Given these estimates and the slow rate of progression of CKD among many older adults, many are starting to question whether dialysis should be expected to extend life or improve quality of life for older adults with high levels of comorbidity and/or disability. Unfortunately, relatively little information is available about outcomes of conservative management among older adults with advanced CKD. Previous studies should be interpreted cautiously in light of the selection biases present (i.e., healthier patients are more likely to receive dialysis, and sicker patients are more likely to receive conservative management). Most, but not all, studies show that overall survival for patients selected for dialysis exceeds survival of patients selected for conservative management. However, the magnitude of this effect varies across studies. Among a French cohort of octogenarians, patients who initiated dialysis survived on average 20 months longer than those who received conservative therapy. In another study of septuagenarians reaching ESRD in the United Kingdom, those for whom dialysis was recommended survived 24 months longer than those for whom conservative therapy was recommended. However, those who chose dialysis also spent more days in the hospital and were more likely to die in the hospital. Notably, several studies suggest that there is a subgroup of older adults who do not experience a survival benefit from dialysis.

Older adults continue to experience a high burden of comorbidity and symptoms after starting dialysis. For example, older adults with ESRD are hospitalized approximately two times per year, or an average of 25 days per year. Functional decline is common and is especially prominent around the time of dialysis initiation or hospitalization. In one study of U.S. nursing home residents, there was a marked decline in functional status at the time of dialysis initiation. As a result, fewer than 13% of nursing home patients starting dialysis survived for 1 year and maintained their predialysis functional abilities. Similar patterns have been noted among ambulatory older adults starting chronic dialysis and among prevalent ESRD patients after hospitalization. Depression, cognitive impairment, and other geriatric syndromes are more common among older versus younger patients with ESRD. Adverse physical symptoms may also be prominent and interfere with daily functioning or quality of life.

Just as decisions to start dialysis vary nationally and internationally, so too do rates of dialysis withdrawal. Annually, 8% of U.S. dialysis patients withdraw from dialysis, a figure that rises to 13% among those over the age of 75. Comorbidity and recent hospitalizations are linked to dialysis withdrawal. Hospice use is low among patients with ESRD compared to other life-limiting conditions such as advanced dementia, heart failure, and cancer. In addition, fewer than half of all patients who withdraw from dialysis use hospice services before death. Low utilization may reflect restrictions on hospice for patients concurrently receiving dialysis as well as poor knowledge of hospice benefits.

Despite substantial morbidity, available data suggest quality of life is acceptable for many older adults receiving chronic dialysis. In the North Thames Study, older adults with ESRD had lower physical quality of life but mental quality of life that was similar to the age-matched general population. Similar results have been noted in the Dialysis Outcomes and Practice Patterns Study (DOPPS). In the HEMO trial, older adults with ESRD had similar changes in quality of life over 3 years to their younger counterparts. It should be noted that these studies included only prevalent dialysis patients, so it is possible that quality of life was overestimated because of the exclusion of sicker patients who withdrew from dialysis or died of other causes soon after initiating dialysis.

How should clinicians reconcile this information? One suggestion has been to rethink the process of obtaining informed consent for dialysis. This is especially true among patients with substantial comorbidity, disability, or cognitive impairment. Important elements of obtaining informed consent include discussions of anticipated prognosis and clearly delineating treatment alternatives. Although quality of life on dialysis is necessarily subjective, estimates of survival, functional status, and expected lifestyle changes can inform the decision-making process for many patients. A second suggestion has been to increase integration of palliative care services into routine dialysis care. Such an approach may help patients address the symptoms of ESRD and dialysis therapy, and prepare for end-of-life decisions.

TRANSPLANTATION

At the other end of the spectrum of ESRD treatment options, the demand for kidney transplantation continues to increase among older adults. Throughout the last 2 decades, the number of patients over the age of 60 on the U.S. kidney transplant waiting list has increased twentyfold, such that adults over the age of 60 now comprise approximately 30% of all wait-listed patients and 25% of all kidney transplant recipients. In these individuals, transplantation extends life by 1 to 4 years on average compared to remaining on dialysis. More recent studies suggest these benefits extend to selected patients over the age of 75. One study showed that kidney transplantation was cost effective for patients greater than age 65, but that the attractiveness of transplantation declined as waiting time increased. Short-term allograft survival is slightly lower among older adults, but is generally excellent.

The expanded criteria donor (ECD) list shortens waiting times at the cost of a higher risk of allograft loss. For older patients and those in regions with long waiting times, the benefits of an ECD kidney appear to outweigh the risks. As a result, this option is common among older transplant recipients. As the demand for transplantation among older adults rises, the selection of candidates and allocation of limited organs has become increasingly challenging. Perhaps as a result, the criteria for accepting an older patient to the transplant wait list vary greatly from center to center. Allocation of organs by more closely matching donor and recipient age has been implemented in Europe and is being considered in the United States.

MANAGEMENT OF OLDER ADULTS WITH CHRONIC KIDNEY DISEASE

The last decade has seen the evolution of a disease-based approach to CKD along with the development of clinical practice guidelines that both define CKD and provide an evidence-based approach to patient care. Clinical practice guidelines for CKD present a standardized approach to management, prioritizing interventions to reduce mortality and cardiovascular events and to prevent and slow disease progression at earlier stages of disease. At later stages of CKD, a greater focus is placed on management of disease complications and preparation for ESRD. The goal of clinical practice guidelines is to provide a simplified model to guide management rather than to address the many complex questions that may arise in individual patients. Contemporary guidelines for the management of patients with CKD do not distinguish between patients of different ages; however, at older ages, there is often tension between what might be recommended in clinical practice guidelines and what might be most beneficial for an individual patient.

HIGH BURDEN OF COMPLEX COMORBIDITY MAY COMPLICATE THE MANAGEMENT OF OLDER ADULTS WITH CHRONIC KIDNEY DISEASE

At older ages, patients often have more than one disease process. This is particularly true for older adults with CKD. The presence of multiple comorbid conditions may generate competing health priorities and conflicting treatment recommendations. Clinical practice guidelines rarely acknowledge the possibility that patients may have more than one condition, and most do not provide guidance on how to manage the multiple competing health priorities

that often arise in older adults with complex comorbidity. Boyd et al provided a hypothetical case to illustrate how disease-based guidelines may be harmful in older adults with complex comorbidity (Fig. 51.5). In an older patient with a fairly standard set of comorbidities, these authors modeled the onerous pharmacologic and nonpharmacologic treatment regimen with multiple potential drug interactions and competing treatment priorities that would result if all relevant practice guidelines were followed.

DIFFERENCES IN OUTCOMES AMONG OLDER AND YOUNGER PATIENTS WITH CHRONIC KIDNEY DISEASE MAY IMPACT TREATMENT EFFECTS

Guidelines for patients with CKD assume a uniform relationship between level of kidney function and clinical outcomes among patients of all ages; however, the relative and absolute frequency of different clinical outcomes varies among older and younger patients with the same levels of eGFR. Such differences in outcomes are likely to impact the benefit of many recommended interventions for individual patients. For example, although interventions intended to lower cardiovascular risk have the potential to prevent the greatest number of events among high-risk groups (e.g., older patients with CKD), in patients with more limited life expectancy such interventions will provide less substantial overall gains in life expectancy or event-free survival. Similarly, interventions to slow progression to ESRD may prevent the greatest number of cases of ESRD in older adults, due to the higher crude incidence of ESRD at older ages; however, the benefit of interventions to prevent nondeath outcomes such as ESRD may be more limited in patients with a shorter life expectancy who are less likely to survive long enough to experience the relevant outcome. Similar principles apply to several treatment decisions undertaken to prepare optimally for ESRD. A patient who is unlikely to survive to the point of initiating chronic dialysis is unlikely to benefit from interventions to prepare for ESRD (e.g., vascular access placement). Thus, clinical practice guidelines and the evidence on which these are based must be interpreted within the context of each patient's life expectancy, baseline risk for the outcome of interest, and their goals and preferences.

LIMITED EVIDENCE TO SUPPORT RECOMMENDED INTERVENTIONS IN OLDER ADULTS WITH CHRONIC KIDNEY DISEASE

Evidence for interventions recommended in clinical practice guidelines are often based on the results of clinical trials that did not enroll a representative sample of older adults. Thus the benefits and harms of many recommended interventions are unknown in older adults. It can be difficult to extrapolate available evidence from younger trial populations to real-world populations of older adults if there are systematic differences between these populations. Similar to the general population, evidence supporting the efficacy for many recommended interventions is often lacking in older adults with CKD. For example, most trials of angiotensin converting enzyme (ACE) inhibitors and angiotensin receptor blockers (ARB) cited in support of contemporary practice guidelines for the use of these agents in CKD did not enroll any adults older than 70.

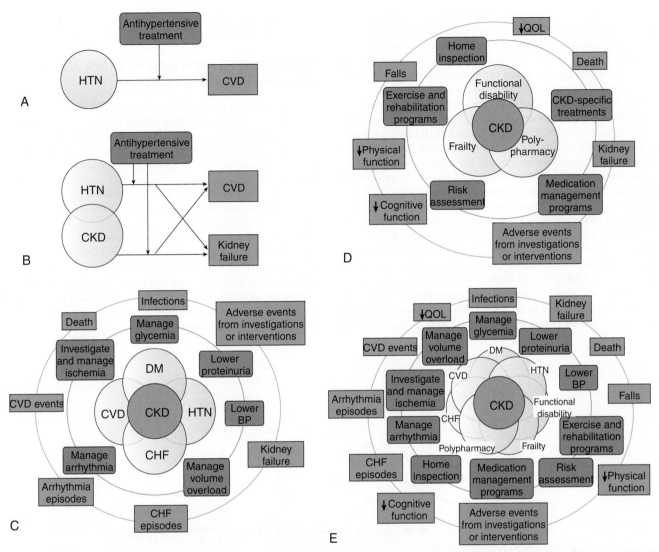

Figure 51.5   Disease models increase in complexity with increasing numbers of disease conditions, treatments, and outcomes considered, such as in patients with chronic kidney disease (CKD) or of older age. Circles indicate diseases, rectangles outcomes, and rounded rectangles treatments. Disease models show treatment of **(A)** hypertension (HTN) without CKD; **(B)** HTN in patients with CKD; **(C)** CKD and a cluster of additional common comorbid conditions; **(D)** CKD along with a cluster of geriatric syndromes; and **(E)** CKD in older patients, incorporating clusters of common comorbid conditions as well as geriatric syndromes (the overlap of **C** and **D**). *BP,* Blood pressure; *CHF,* congestive heart failure; *CKD,* chronic kidney disease; *CVD,* cardiovascular disease; *DM,* diabetes mellitus; *QOL,* quality of life. (From Uhlig K, Boyd C: Guidelines for the older adult with CKD, *Am J Kidney Dis* 58:162-165, 2011.)

Additionally, the relevance of these trials to older adults with CKD is especially uncertain, because most researchers selected for patients with proteinuria whereas the majority of older adults with CKD have a low eGFR without substantial proteinuria. A subgroup analysis among older participants in the Reduction in Endpoints in NIDDM with the Angiotensin-II Antagonist Losartan (RENAAL) study (which enrolled adults with diabetes and proteinuria) suggests that renin-angiotensin system blockade slows progression to ESRD in older adults with diabetes and proteinuria; however, the results of another trial, the Antihypertensive and Lipid Lowering Therapy to Prevent Heart Attack Trial (ALLHAT), may be of much greater relevance to the majority of older adults with CKD. ALLHAT differed from most other trials examining the effect of ACE inhibitors and ARB on progression of kidney disease, as approximately half of

the participants in this trial with CKD were 70 years of age or older, and participants were not selected for proteinuria (in fact, the trial did not even ascertain level of proteinuria). Among ALLHAT participants with CKD, lisinopril was no more effective than either chlorthalidone or amlodopine in slowing progression to ESRD. Thus, in evaluating the relative benefits and harms of different interventions recommended for older adults with CKD, clinicians should consider the strength of available evidence and its relevance to individual older patients.

HETEROGENEITY IN HEALTH STATUS, LIFE EXPECTANCY, AND PREFERENCES

The large degree of heterogeneity in health status, life expectancy, and preferences among older adults may be difficult to accommodate within the disease-based framework embodied in clinical practice guidelines. The disease-based approach assumes a direct causal relationship between clinical signs and symptoms and underlying disease pathophysiology. Thus, treatment plans often target pathophysiologic mechanisms relevant to the disease process with the goal of improving disease-related outcomes. Outcomes prioritized by a disease-based approach to CKD include survival, cardiovascular events, and progression to ESRD; however, these outcomes might not always be meaningful to individual patients. For patients with limited life expectancy, interventions intended to lengthen life might not be as important as those that allow them to maintain independence, maintain or improve quality of life, or optimize pain control—outcomes that may not always be tied to a specific underlying disease process. When faced with competing health priorities, patients may be willing to make tradeoffs to achieve those outcomes that matter most to them. Because those outcomes prioritized by clinical practice guidelines for CKD may not align with those outcomes that matter most to an individual older patient with CKD, eliciting individual patient goals and priorities is a crucial step in determining

the relevance and potential benefits of guideline-recommended treatment strategies for individual patients.

INDIVIDUALIZED APPROACH TO OLDER ADULTS WITH CHRONIC KIDNEY DISEASE

The individualized approach avoids some of the inherent tensions that arise when applying a strict disease-based approach to complex older patients (Fig. 51.6). The individualized approach prioritizes outcomes that matter to the patient and that can be modified by available interventions. Whereas the disease-oriented approach assumes that signs and symptoms can be explained by one or more underlying disease processes and are best addressed by interventions targeting those processes, the individualized approach embraces the notion that signs and symptoms might not be directly explained by an underlying disease process and might reflect a variety of different intrinsic and extrinsic processes. Under the individualized approach, signs and symptoms are often considered legitimate targets for intervention, in many instances requiring complex multifaceted interventions that do not target a specific underlying disease process.

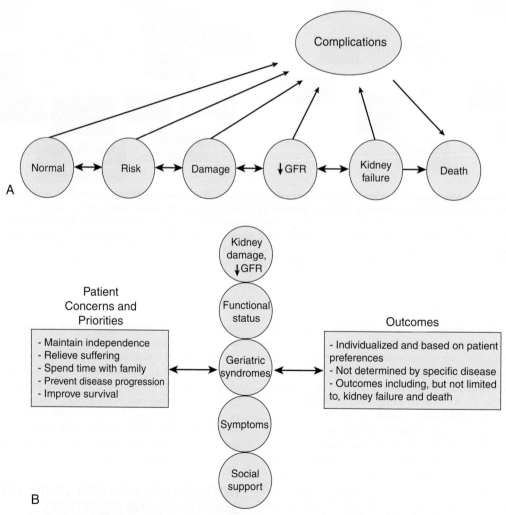

Figure 51.6 Conceptualization of (A) disease-based and (B) individualized approaches to chronic kidney disease. *GFR,* Glomerular filtration rate. (From Bowling CB, O'Hare AM: Managing older adults with CKD: individualized versus disease-based approaches, *Am J Kidney Dis* 59:293-302, 2012.)

OPTIMIZING INDIVIDUALIZED TREATMENT DECISIONS IN OLDER ADULTS WITH CHRONIC KIDNEY DISEASE

Many older adults with CKD will benefit from some interventions recommended under a disease-oriented approach. Information on prognosis and the comparative effectiveness of different therapies is often very helpful in structuring individualized treatment plans and helping patients to evaluate the benefits and harms of interventions recommended under a disease-based approach. Walter and Covinsky developed a framework to support individualized decisions about cancer screening in older adults. This framework uses information on life expectancy and baseline risk of dying from a screen-detectable cancer to generate quantitative estimates of each patient's likelihood of developing the outcome of interest during their remaining lifetime, thus determining how much they will benefit from interventions to prevent this outcome. Because patients may weigh the same information on risks and benefits differently, patient preferences are critical in determining how quantitative information on life expectancy, baseline risk of disease outcomes, and the efficacy of clinical interventions will ultimately inform treatment decisions.

A similar approach could be used to evaluate the benefit of recommended treatments in older adults with CKD. In applying this approach, it is important to recognize that, although the presence and severity of CKD carries prognostic significance in older adults, many other factors can impact prognosis, leading to substantial heterogeneity in life expectancy despite similar levels of kidney function. In addition, whereas life expectancy and disease-related outcomes such as slowing progression of kidney disease are often important, other outcomes such as independence and quality of life may matter more to patients. By accounting for differences in prognosis, baseline risk, and patient goals and preferences, the individualized approach is expected to yield diverse treatment plans in older adults with very similar levels of kidney function.

ACKNOWLEDGMENTS

Support was provided through a Beeson Career Development Award from the National Institute on Aging to Manjula Kurella Tamura and the Birmingham/Atlanta GRECC Special Fellowship in Advanced Geriatrics and John A. Hartford Foundation/Southeast Center of Excellence in Geriatric Medicine to C. Barrett Bowling.

KEY BIBLIOGRAPHY

Bowling CB, O'Hare AM: Managing older adults with CKD: individualized versus disease-based approaches, *Am J Kidney Dis* 59:293-302, 2012.

Boyd CM, Darer J, Boult C, et al: Clinical practice guidelines and quality of care for older patients with multiple comorbid diseases: implications for pay for performance, *JAMA* 294:716-724, 2005.

Coresh J, Selvin E, Stevens LA, et al: Prevalence of chronic kidney disease in the United States, *JAMA* 298:2038-2047, 2007.

Hemmelgarn BR, James MT, Manns BJ, et al: Rates of treated and untreated kidney failure in older vs younger adults, *JAMA* 307:2507-2515, 2012.

Jassal SV, Chiu E, Hladunewich M: Loss of independence in patients starting dialysis at 80 years of age or older, *N Engl J Med* 361:1612-1613, 2009.

Johansen KL, Chertow GM, Jin C, et al: Significance of frailty among dialysis patients, *J Am Soc Nephrol* 18:2960-2967, 2007.

Kurella M, Chertow GM, Fried LF, et al: Chronic kidney disease and cognitive impairment in the elderly: the health, aging, and body composition study, *J Am Soc Nephrol* 16:2127-2133, 2005.

Kurella M, Covinsky KE, Collins AJ, et al: Octogenarians and nonagenarians starting dialysis in the United States, *Ann Intern Med* 146:177-183, 2007.

Kurella Tamura M, Covinsky KE, Chertow GM, et al: Functional status of elderly adults before and after initiation of dialysis, *N Engl J Med* 361:1539-1547, 2009.

Kurella Tamura M, Tan JC, O'Hare AM: Optimizing renal replacement therapy in older adults: a framework for making individualized decisions, *Kidney Int* 82:261-269, 2012.

Murray AM, Arko C, Chen SC, et al: Use of hospice in the United States dialysis population, *Clin J Am Soc Nephrol* 1:1248-1255, 2006.

Murtagh FE, Marsh JE, Donohoe P, et al: Dialysis or not? a comparative survival study of patients over 75 years with chronic kidney disease stage 5, *Nephrol Dial Transplant* 22:1955-1962, 2007.

O'Hare AM, Bertenthal D, Covinsky KE, et al: Mortality risk stratification in chronic kidney disease: one size for all ages? *J Am Soc Nephrol* 17:846-853, 2006.

O'Hare AM, Choi AI, Bertenthal D, et al: Age affects outcomes in chronic kidney disease, *J Am Soc Nephrol* 18:2758-2765, 2007.

O'Hare AM, Kaufman JS, Covinsky KE, et al: Current guidelines for using angiotensin-converting enzyme inhibitors and angiotensin II-receptor antagonists in chronic kidney disease: is the evidence base relevant to older adults? *Ann Intern Med* 150:717-724, 2009.

O'Hare AM, Rodriguez RA, Hailpern SM, et al: Regional variation in health care intensity and treatment practices for end-stage renal disease in older adults, *JAMA* 304:180-186, 2010.

Rao PS, Merion RM, Ashby VB, et al: Renal transplantation in elderly patients older than 70 years of age: results from the Scientific Registry of Transplant Recipients, *Transplantation* 83:1069-1074, 2007.

Uhlig K, Boyd C: Guidelines for the older adult with CKD, *Am J Kidney Dis* 58:162-165, 2011.

Walter LC, Covinsky KE: Cancer screening in elderly patients: a framework for individualized decision making, *JAMA* 285:2750-2756, 2001.

Wetzels JF, Kiemeney LA, Swinkels DW, et al: Age- and gender-specific reference values of estimated GFR in Caucasians: the Nijmegen Biomedical Study, *Kidney Int* 72:632-637, 2007.

Full bibliography can be found on www.expertconsult.com.

CHRONIC KIDNEY DISEASE AND ITS THERAPY

52 Pathophysiology of Chronic Kidney Disease

William L. Whittier | Edmund J. Lewis

HOW IS CHRONIC KIDNEY DISEASE DEFINED?

Chronic kidney disease (CKD) is currently defined by abnormal measurements of the actual or estimated glomerular filtration rate (GFR) for a minimum of 3 months (Box 52.1). The GFR is the rate of plasma flow filtered across the glomerular basement membrane (GBM). In practice, GFR commonly is estimated using serum creatinine, with a rise in serum creatinine most often signifying a reduction in GFR. Because the serum creatinine is a product of metabolism and muscle breakdown, its level can vary, not just due to changes in GFR, but also in conditions of body mass differences (i.e., malnutrition) or excessive muscle breakdown (i.e., rhabdomyolysis). Creatinine-based GFR estimating equations attempt to correct for these nonkidney factors. The rationale behind GFR estimation using serum creatinine, as well other methods, to estimate and measure kidney function are detailed in Chapter 3, with the caveat that there is no perfect marker of GFR.

The definition of CKD also includes situations in which the GFR is normal, but pathology in the kidney is still present, such as radiographically imaged cysts in polycystic kidney disease or early glomerular disease manifested clinically by isolated proteinuria. These definitions and the staging of CKD are discussed in more detail in Chapter 53.

In the United States, it has been estimated that approximately 15% of the adult population has CKD, based on the definitions just mentioned. It is clear that the great majority of these patients do not reach end-stage renal disease (ESRD) in their lifetimes. Many of these patients have relatively stable kidney function and are more likely to die *with* rather than *of* CKD. However, for patients who initiate dialysis to treat chronic kidney failure, there is, on average, 75% mortality by 5 years. This mortality risk varies based on several comorbidities: a young patient without diabetes mellitus (DM) will have less risk than an older patient with DM and heart failure. Cardiovascular disease is the main cause of death in patients with CKD, with manifestations including coronary, cerebral, and peripheral vascular disease, arrhythmias, heart failure, and sudden death (Chapter 56).

The most common causes of CKD and ESRD (Table 52.1) are diabetic nephropathy (Fig. 52.1) and hypertensive nephrosclerosis. Primary glomerular diseases (i.e., IgA nephropathy, membranous glomerulonephritis), secondary glomerular diseases (i.e., lupus nephritis, amyloidosis), tubulointerstitial, vascular, cystic, and hereditary kidney diseases are all much less common. Each of these has specific pathophysiologic mechanisms for kidney damage, and therefore the treatments developed for these diseases are different, aimed at controlling or reversing the primary disease process.

The idea, then, that CKD could be generalized into one disease process is an oversimplification, because the primary processes causing kidney damage are protean. However, the pathophysiology of progression of many of these disorders involves similar pathways and, more important, generic treatments aimed at slowing this progression have been applied across a wide variety of kidney diseases effectively and safely. Over the last 20 years, specific treatments have been developed and proven to delay progression to ESRD, and other therapies continue to be studied. Therefore recognizing CKD as an entity, as early as possible, becomes important to help implement therapy, which may delay or reverse this progression and attempt to reduce the associated high risk for mortality.

PATHOPHYSIOLOGIC MECHANISMS OF CHRONIC KIDNEY DISEASE

The pathophysiology of CKD is complex and in large part dependent on the primary cause. After a primary acute or chronic insult occurs, such as in diabetic nephropathy or lupus nephritis, many common pathways are activated to perpetuate glomerular and tubulointerstitial injury (Fig. 52.2). These harmful adaptations, occurring as a result of an initial injury, can be broadly categorized into those that are hemodynamically mediated or those that are nonhemodynamic.

HEMODYNAMIC INJURY

Much of the work in hemodynamic-mediated injury stems from the animal model of 5/6 nephrectomy. Following unilateral nephrectomy and 2/3 removal of the contralateral kidney in rats, hypertension, proteinuria, and progressive decline in GFR ensue. Pathologic examination of the remaining tissue exhibits hyperfiltration injury, as evidenced by glomerular hypertrophy and focal segmental glomerular sclerosis (FSGS). The process occurs at a linear rate in proportion to the greater reduction in kidney mass. Micropuncture techniques reveal an increase in renal plasma flow and hyperfiltration of the remaining nephrons. Systemic hypertension and glomerular hypertension, from activation of the renin-angiotensin-aldosterone system (RAAS), cause progressive glomerular damage and proteinuria. As a result of these changes, afferent arteriolar tone decreases less than efferent tone. This net efferent vasoconstriction

Box 52.1   Important Characteristics of Chronic Kidney Disease

1. Chronic kidney disease (CKD) is currently defined by a reduction in glomerular filtration rate over a period of time or evidence of kidney damage.
2. The most common causes of CKD are diabetes mellitus and hypertension, and less frequent causes are primary glomerular, tubulointerstitial, and cystic diseases.
3. The pathophysiology of chronic kidney damage is related to the underlying disease, but it is accelerated by glomerular hypertension, systemic hypertension, inflammation, and fibrosis.
4. Risk factors for progression are hypertension, proteinuria, and recurrent acute kidney injury.
5. Treatment for CKD is disease specific, but several generalized methods can be applied to almost all kidney diseases. The goal is slowing or reversing progression, with therapies aimed at correcting the pathophysiologic patterns. These involve blocking the renin-angiotensin-aldosterone system (RAAS) with medications, controlling blood pressure, and reducing proteinuria when present. This goal is attempted while also targeting cardiovascular risk reduction. Novel methods, which require further study, involve attacking the inflammatory and fibrotic effects of the pathophysiology.

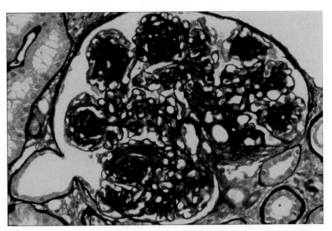

Figure 52.1 Glomerulus from a patient with overt diabetic nephropathy, termed "The Face of the Enemy" by Dr. Edmund J. Lewis. There is marked expansion with nodular glomerular sclerosis, consistent with Kimmelstiel-Wilson nodules. Note the hypertrophied glomerulus, prominent mesangium, and aneurysmal features of the capillary walls, giving the appearance of a daisy flower (methenamine silver stain; magnification × 230).

Table 52.1   Frequency of Primary Disease Causing End-Stage Renal Disease

Disease	Percentage (%)
Diabetes mellitus type 1	3.9
Diabetes mellitus type 2	41.0
Hypertension	27.2
Primary glomerulonephritis	8.2
Tubulointerstitial	3.6
Hereditary or cystic	3.1
Secondary glomerulonephritis or vasculitis	2.1
Neoplasm or plasma cell dyscrasias	2.1
Miscellaneous	4.6
Unknown	5.2

increases intraglomerular and filtration pressure further, perpetuating hyperfiltration injury. Animal models of other kidney diseases, such as that of diabetic nephropathy in the rat, reveal similar pathophysiologic changes of glomerular hypertension, hypertrophy, and hyperfiltration.

These maladaptive hemodynamic effects are mediated by the RAAS (Figs. 52.2 and 52.3). With nephron loss, adaptation leads to release of renin from the juxtaglomerular apparatus due to decreased perfusion pressure and low solute delivery to the macula densa. Renin converts angiotensinogen to angiotensin I, which, under the influence of angiotensin converting enzyme (ACE), is converted to angiotensin II (AII). AII, in addition to increasing aldosterone production from the adrenal gland, is the main perpetrator of glomerular hemodynamic maladaptation. Through an increase in sympathetic activity, AII is a potent vasoconstrictor, especially predominant in the postglomerular arterioles. It also exhibits a role in salt and water retention, both directly through proximal tubular sodium reabsorption and indirectly

through aldosterone dependent distal sodium reabsorption. Finally, it stimulates the posterior pituitary to release antidiuretic hormone (ADH).

The net effect of all of these mechanisms is an integral component of autoregulation, helping to maintain GFR when perfusion is decreased. However, in the setting of nephron loss through a primary kidney insult or CKD, the effect of continuous AII overactivity is perpetual maladaptation by creating systemic and, notably, glomerular hypertension. This glomerular hypertension increases the filtration fraction, increases the radius of the pores in the GBM through an increase in hydrostatic pressure, and eventually results in clinical proteinuria and glomerular destruction.

The best example of a human model of decreased nephron mass or number would be in the setting of a solitary kidney, or unilateral renal agenesis. Ashley and Mostofi originally reported 232 patients with unilateral renal agenesis in the 1960s, and, although the pathology was not described, 16% of the patients died from kidney failure. Later, in the 1980s, autopsy series and case series confirmed the association of unilateral renal agenesis with hypertension, proteinuria, progressive kidney disease, glomerulomegaly, and FSGS (Fig. 52.4). Besides renal agenesis, another human example is the condition known as oligomeganephronia. This is a form of congenital renal hypoplasia in which the number of nephrons is reduced. The glomeruli hypertrophy to compensate for the reduced nephron number. The sequelae of this include hypertension, proteinuria, and FSGS related to hyperfiltration as well as progressive kidney failure. Other clinical human examples of disease that support this mechanism of kidney injury include obesity-related glomerulomegaly and nephropathy, dysplastic solitary kidney, or partial nephrectomy in the setting of a solitary kidney.

Since animal models and human congenital diseases of reduced nephron mass lead to hemodynamic maladaptation and morphologic evidence of FSGS, it is natural to speculate that a transplant donor would be at risk for this same pathophysiology. Fortunately, the development of

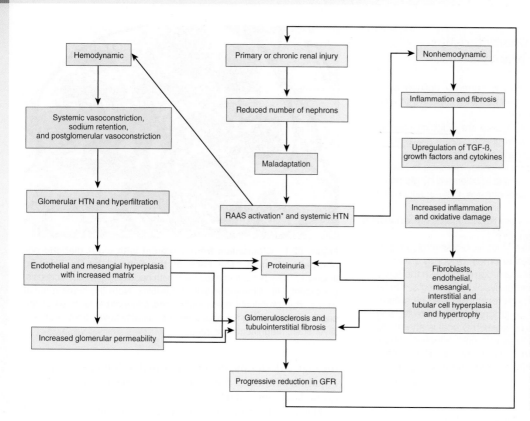

Figure 52.2 Schematic diagram of the pathogenesis of progressive chronic kidney disease. After a primary or chronic injury occurs, activation of the RAAS leads to hemodynamic and nonhemodynamic injury. *GFR,* Glomerular filtration rate; *RAAS,* renin-angiotensin-aldosterone system; *TGFβ,* transforming growth factor-β. *See Figure 52.3 for details of the RAAS activation.

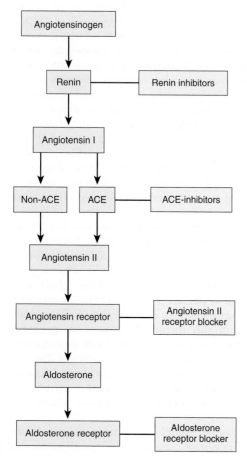

Figure 52.3 Schematic representation of renin-angiotensin-aldosterone activation and targeted therapies that interrupt the pathway. *ACE,* Angiotensin converting enzyme.

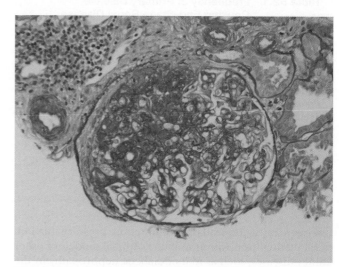

Figure 52.4 Hypertrophied glomerulus with sclerotic segment encompassing almost 50% of the glomerular surface area from a patient with unilateral dysplastic kidney, hypertension, and proteinuria. The uninvolved segment of the glomerulus has patent capillaries and normal architecture. The glomerular diameter was measured to be 270 μm (periodic acid-Schiff stain; magnification × 230). Normal glomerular diameter is 144 ± 11 μm.

hypertension or kidney damage in the remaining kidney in transplant donors is infrequent. This may reflect extensive screening of potential donors, resulting in a sufficiently healthy population with minimal vascular disease, such that the donor can readily compensate for a 50% reduction in kidney mass. Similar results are seen in experimental models, where adult rats with unilateral nephrectomy rarely develop hypertension or kidney disease; however,

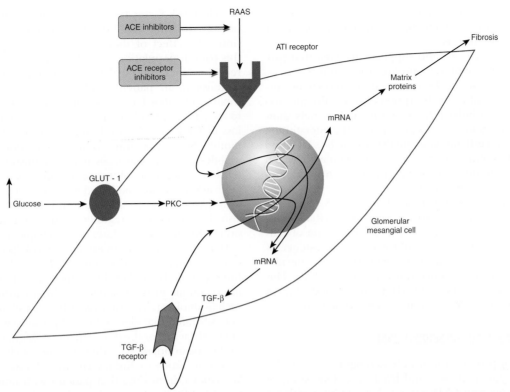

Figure 52.5   Schematic representation of a glomerular mesangial cell in chronic kidney disease due to diabetic nephropathy. Activation of RAAS upregulates TGF-β, which leads to matrix accumulation, inflammation, and fibrosis. Hyperglycemia also perpetuates this fibrosis via increased activity of PKC (protein kinase C). Through interruption of this cascade, ACE inhibitors and angiotensin receptor blockers are effective treatments, delaying progression of chronic kidney disease in diabetic nephropathy. *AT-I,* Angiotensin I; *GLUT-1,* glucose transporter; *mRNA,* messenger ribonucleic acid; *RAAS,* renin-angiotensin-aldosterone system; *TGF-β,* transforming growth factor-β.

when a solitary kidney is removed in immature rats, the glomerular lesion FSGS manifests in the remaining kidney. Therefore hemodynamic injury may be present or apparent only when the kidney is undergoing normal growth. Another explanation of this benign clinical course in patients donating a kidney is that the development of clinical pathology is directly linked to the length of time and degree of reduction of nephron mass. Indeed, there are studies demonstrating an increased risk for hypertension, proteinuria, and progressive kidney disease in patients who have more than a 50% reduction in kidney mass, such as those with bilateral partial nephrectomy for carcinoma, and a greater likelihood of progressive kidney disease with a longer duration of nephron mass reduction.

NONHEMODYNAMIC INJURY

Besides the hemodynamic effects of systemic vasoconstriction, sodium retention, and postglomerular vasoconstriction, activation of the RAAS leads to several nonhemodynamic maladaptive pathways (see Fig. 52.2), which can lead to inflammation and fibrosis. AII has been demonstrated in high concentrations in virtually every compartment of the kidney in CKD, including the mesangial cells, endothelial cells, podocytes, the urinary space (Bowman capsule), and the tubulointerstitium.

Activation of the RAAS eventually results in fibrosis and a progressive decline in GFR. This fibrosis manifests with upregulation of several growth factors and their receptors,

such as connective tissue growth factor (CTGF), epidermal growth factor (EGF), insulin-like growth factor-1 (IGF-1), platelet-derived growth factor (PDGF), vascular endothelial growth factor (VEGF), transforming growth factor-β (TGF-β), and monocyte chemotactic protein-1 (MCP-1). The activation of these factors by AII and aldosterone leads to cellular proliferation and hypertrophy of glomerular endothelial and epithelial cells, mesangial cells, tubulointerstitial cells, and fibroblasts. AII and TGF-β also upregulate other factors that lead to the overproduction of extracellular matrix, such as type 1 procollagen, plasminogen activator inhibitor 1, and fibronectin. In addition, excess adhesion molecules, such as integrins or vascular cellular adhesion molecule 1, allow the increased extracellular matrix and hypercellularity to accumulate and persist. This leads to cell proliferation, extracellular matrix accumulation, adhesion of these cells, and functional changes with eventual fibrosis (Fig. 52.5).

Inflammation is also a key component in the progression of kidney disease (see Fig. 52.2). This may seem obvious in diseases in which inflammation is the primary insult, such as postinfectious glomerulonephritis or severe lupus nephritis, because it is apparent by light microscopy of kidney biopsy specimens. However, inflammation is an important factor in the progression of almost all types of kidney diseases and is mediated in part by the RAAS. AII recruits T cells and macrophages by stimulating endothelin-1 (ET-1) and increases production of nuclear factor κ-light-chain-enhancer of activated B cells (Nf-κB); these molecules release cytokines, creating more inflammation. Increased expression of TGF-β also creates cellular recruitment. Finally, free radical oxygen species lead to additional injury, which enables further inflammation and fibrosis.

Experimental evidence also supports the idea that proteinuria itself contributes to progressive nephrosclerosis. Through hyperfiltration, the increased glomerular permeability to albumin allows reabsorption of more albuminuria by the proximal tubular cells. Experimental models show that when this protein becomes prevalent in the interstitium, macrophages and inflammatory mediators, such as ET-1 and MCP-1 as well as other chemokines, are upregulated, which eventually leads to inflammation and subsequent tubulointerstitial and glomerular fibrosis.

Through primary stimulation of the RAAS, predominantly through TGF-β, a cascade of events occurs that begins with inflammation, is perpetuated by accumulation of cells and matrix, is exacerbated by adhesion and persistence of these cells and matrix, and ends with injury, glomerulosclerosis, and tubulointerstitial fibrosis (see Fig. 52.2). This creates a progressive course of CKD, proteinuria, decline in GFR, and a vicious cycle of continuous RAAS activation.

RISK FACTORS FOR PROGRESSION

Risk factors for progression include demographic variables such as older age, male sex, and black race. One study of younger patients with CKD estimated the lifetime risk for ESRD for a 20-year-old person to be 7.8% for black women, 7.3% for black men, 1.8% for white women, and 2.5% for white men. Although the possible reasons for these factors are complex, they are not modifiable. Conversely, hypertension, proteinuria, and recurrent acute kidney injury (AKI) are all potentially modifiable factors that deserve attention (Box 52.2).

Via increased activity of the RAAS, hypertension is a dominant force continuing the cycle of progressive CKD. In patients who have diabetic nephropathy from type 2 DM, the most common cause of CKD, elevated blood pressure

is a clear risk factor for a precipitous decline in GFR and, notably, treating this hypertension reduces this progression. The effect of therapy is even more pronounced in this patient population when treatment is with angiotensin receptor blockade (Fig. 52.6). Early in the 1980s, Mogensen established, in patients with diabetic nephropathy, that treating elevated blood pressure (mean 162/103 mm Hg) to an achieved level of 144/95 mm Hg reduced the rate of loss of GFR from 1.23 mL/min/month to 0.49 mL/min/month. Since that time, other observational studies and well-designed clinical trials have demonstrated that hypertension is clearly a risk factor for progressive ESRD in diabetic nephropathy, and blood pressure reduction, especially with RAAS blockade, attenuates this risk (see Fig. 52.6 and also the section on Treatment and Prevention of Progression of Kidney Disease, later in this chapter).

Hypertension is also an established risk factor for progression of nondiabetic kidney disease. The Multiple Risk Factor Intervention Trial (MRFIT), which used multiple medical interventions to treat patients of high cardiovascular risk, such as smoking, hypertension, obesity, and hyperlipidemia, demonstrated that elevated blood pressure was an independent risk factor for the development of kidney failure. Other studies of nondiabetic kidney disease, such as the African American Study of Kidney Disease (AASK), reveal a similar pattern, indicating that patients with nondiabetic CKD benefited from a lower achieved blood pressure, especially if proteinuria was present. Similarly, observational studies suggest slower progression in patients with other causes of CKD, such as polycystic kidney disease, when blood pressure is controlled.

Proteinuria, similar to hypertension, is a well-established risk factor for progression of CKD. In patients with overt diabetic nephropathy, the degree of baseline proteinuria is directly correlated with a more progressive decline in GFR (Fig. 52.7). This is also true in nondiabetic kidney diseases, such as IgA nephropathy or severe lupus nephritis. In the Modification of Diet in Renal Disease (MDRD) study, a population that was predominantly nondiabetic, those with proteinuria had the highest risk for progressive kidney disease. The Ramipril Efficacy in Nephropathy (REIN) study similarly noted that, in nondiabetic CKD, the baseline level of proteinuria was the strongest predictor of kidney failure, independent of the baseline GFR. Even in patients with earlier stages of CKD, with an estimated GFR of >60 mL/min/1.73 m², those that demonstrate albuminuria by ≥2+ on dipstick or >300 mg albumin/g of creatinine are over three times more likely to double the serum creatinine over time compared with those with levels consistent with microalbuminuria (30-300 mg albumin/g creatinine). This trend is also true when comparing patients who have microalbuminuria with those who have urine albumin levels less than 30 mg/g.

Despite these robust data, controversy exists as to whether proteinuria is truly a pathogenic risk factor or just a marker of kidney disease severity. If proteinuria were a simple manifestation of advanced disease, such as a cough in the setting of pneumonia, then treating the symptom would have minimal to no effect on improving the disease outcome. However, targeting and reducing proteinuria is highly effective at improving kidney outcomes, both in diabetic (see Fig. 52.7) and nondiabetic kidney diseases (see Treatment and Prevention of Progression of Kidney Disease, later).

Box 52.2   Risk Factors for the Development or Progression of Kidney Disease

Proteinuria
Hypertension
Episodes of acute kidney injury
Underlying cause of kidney disease (e.g., diabetic nephropathy)
Obesity
Hyperlipidemia
Smoking
High-protein diet
Metabolic acidosis
Hyperphosphatemia
Hyperuricemia
African-American or Native American race
Male gender
Older age
Family history of DM, CKD, or ESRD
Low birth weight

CKD, Chronic kidney disease; *DM,* diabetes mellitus; *ESRD,* end-stage renal disease.

The idea that recurrent or episodic AKI leads to progressive chronic kidney dysfunction is a sound one based on the pathophysiology of the disease (see Fig. 52.2). Multiple studies have now shown that, in patients with preexisting CKD, AKI is a risk factor for the development of chronic kidney failure. The degree of preexisting CKD, severity of AKI, advanced age, presence of DM, and low serum albumin amplify this risk. In a retrospective study by Ishani and colleagues, the hazard ratio of developing ESRD for older adult patients (>67 years) who had CKD without AKI was 8.4, whereas for those patients who had CKD and AKI, the hazard ratio for progressing to ESRD was 41.2.

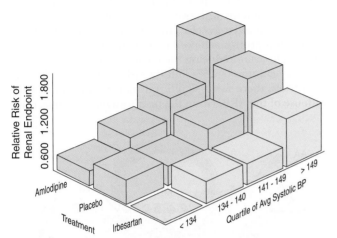

Figure 52.6 Simultaneous impact to quartile of achieved systolic blood pressure and treatment modality on the relative risk for reaching a renal endpoint (doubling of baseline serum creatinine or ESRD, defined as serum creatinine ≥6.0 mg/dL or renal replacement therapy). *Avg,* Average. (Reproduced with permission from Pohl MA, Blumenthal S, Cordonnier DJ et al: Independent and additive impact of blood pressure control and angiotensin II receptor blockade on renal outcomes in the irbesartan diabetic nephropathy trial: clinical implications and limitations, *J Am Soc Nephrol* 16:3031, 2005.)

Knowledge that AKI affects CKD is important so that future therapies can be evaluated and developed in an attempt to retard this progression. It is also relevant at present, as minimizing episodes of iatrogenic AKI in CKD patients can often be achieved. It is sensible to avoid, if possible, situations that may cause AKI, such as iatrogenic hypotension or nephrotoxic injury from polypharmacy, iodinated contrast exposure, atheroemboli, and nonsteroidal antiinflammatory agents in vulnerable patients.

Many other factors have been associated with a progressive decline in GFR (see Box 52.2). The primary kidney disease impacts the rate of progression, as glomerular diseases and polycystic kidney diseases tend to progress faster than most tubulointerstitial diseases. Although evidence establishing hyperlipidemia, tobacco dependence, or obesity as risk factors is not as robust as that pointing to hypertension or proteinuria, these associations do exist, and targeting these risk factors when present is prudent.

TREATMENT AND PREVENTION OF CHRONIC KIDNEY DISEASE PROGRESSION

Based on the underlying pathophysiology, therapies have been developed and studied in an attempt to safely slow or reverse the vicious cycle of RAAS activation, glomerular hypertension, systemic hypertension, proteinuria, inflammation, and progressive fibrosis (Table 52.2). In addition, therapies have targeted other clinically modifiable risk factors, all with the goal of safely reducing or reversing the progression of CKD.

ANTAGONISM OF THE RENIN-ANGIOTENSIN-ALDOSTERONE SYSTEM

Based on the animal models of 5/6 nephrectomy and diabetic glomerulosclerosis, it is plausible that interruption of the RAAS cascade (see Fig. 52.3) could lead to renoprotection. In animal models, AII selectively causes hemodynamic

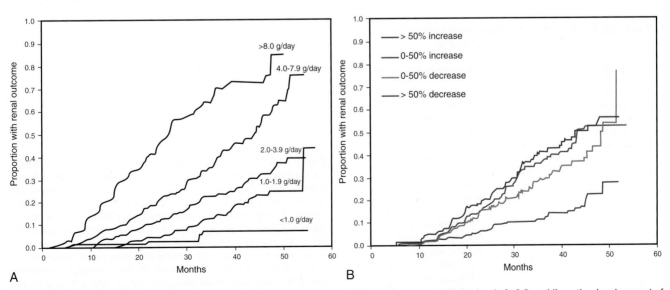

Figure 52.7   A, Kaplan-Meier analysis of doubling of a baseline serum creatinine level, serum creatinine level of ≥6.0 mg/dL, or the development of ESRD by baseline proteinuria values. **B,** Kaplan-Meier analysis of doubling of a baseline serum creatinine level, serum creatinine level of ≥6.0 mg/dL, or the development of ESRD by level of proteinuria change in the first 12 months. (Reproduced from Atkins RC, Briganti EM, Lewis JB et al: Proteinuria reduction and progression to renal failure in patients with type 2 diabetes mellitus and overt nephropathy, *Am J Kidney Dis* 45:283, 285, 2005.)

mediated injury through efferent arteriolar vasoconstriction, whereas the use of angiotensin-converting enzyme (ACE) inhibitors and angiotensin receptor blockers (ARBs) effectively dilates the efferent arteriole, leading to glomerular relaxation and subsequent reduction in glomerular hypertrophy and injury (Fig. 52.8). RAAS blockade also mediates improvements in systemic hypertension, which further reduces glomerular hypertension. In addition to the hemodynamic reduction in glomerular damage, blockade of the RAAS in animals has been shown to impair the inflammatory and fibrosing effects of the various cytokines, including TGF-β. The net effect of RAAS antagonism is therefore renoprotective on multiple levels: hemodynamic, antifibrotic, and antiproteinuric.

Lewis and colleagues tested the hypothesis that this could lead to renoprotection in humans in 1993. In a randomized controlled clinical trial, 409 patients with overt type 1 diabetic nephropathy received either the ACE inhibitor captopril or placebo with achievement of equivalent systemic blood pressures between the two groups. The results of this study were a dramatic 43% reduction in the doubling of the serum creatinine, as well as a significant reduction in the time to death, dialysis, or transplantation with captopril compared with placebo. Thus for the first time in human patients, ACE inhibitors established renoprotection and remission in advanced diabetic nephropathy.

RAAS blockade has also been evaluated in type 2 diabetic nephropathy. In the Irbesartan for Microalbuminuria in Type 2 Diabetes (IRMA-2) trial, of patients with type 2 DM, preserved GFR, and microalbuminuria, irbesartan was more effective at reducing the progression to overt proteinuria from microalbuminuria than placebo at identical blood pressure levels. Two large randomized studies subsequently validated the use of angiotensin receptor blockers in overt type 2 diabetic nephropathy. In the Irbesartan Diabetic Nephropathy Trial (IDNT), 1715 hypertensive patients with overt diabetic nephropathy (median baseline serum creatinine 1.67 mg/dL; median baseline urine protein excretion

2.9 g/24 hours) were randomized to receive one of three different treatment regimens: irbesartan 300 mg daily, the calcium channel blocker amlodipine 10 mg daily, or placebo. The achieved blood pressure was not different among the three groups. With irbesartan, the risk for reaching the composite endpoint of doubling of the serum creatinine, ESRD, or death was 20% lower than compared with placebo and 23% lower compared with amlodipine. In addition to use of the ARB, lower systolic blood pressure was also associated with a decreased relative risk in doubling the serum creatinine or ESRD (see Fig. 52.6). Analogous results were demonstrated with the ARB losartan in the Reduction in Endpoints in NIDDM with the Angiotensin-II Antagonist Losartan (RENAAL) trial. In this randomized controlled trial, 1513 patients with overt type 2 diabetic nephropathy were randomized to receive either losartan or placebo. Once again, both groups achieved equivalent blood pressure levels, with losartan reducing the incidence of doubling of the serum creatinine by 25% and the risk for ESRD by 28%. In both trials, there was a significant reduction in proteinuria with use of the ARB. Given the nearly identical results, these

Table 52.2　Therapies for Slowing Progression of Chronic Kidney Disease

Proven Benefit	Preliminary Evidence
Angiotensin converting enzyme inhibitors	Aldosterone receptor antagonists
Angiotensin receptor antagonists	Renin inhibitors
Blood pressure control	Dietary measures, exercise
Blood pressure goal between 120 and 140 mm Hg systolic and 80 and 90 mm Hg diastolic	Weight loss in obesity
	Smoking cessation
Proteinuria reduction	Glycemic control in diabetes mellitus
	Reduction of hyperuricemia, hyperlipidemia, hyperphosphatemia
	Acid-base balance
	Novel therapies
	Endothelin-1 antagonists
	Pirfenidone
	Vitamin D
	Inhibitors of advanced glycation end products

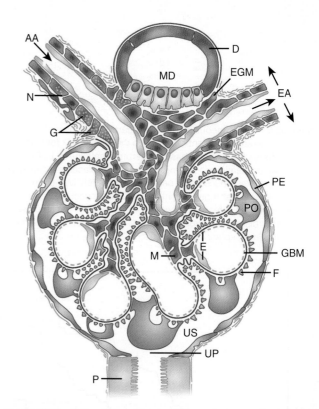

Figure 52.8　Schematic representation of glomerular hemodynamic changes with blockade of the renin-angiotensin-aldosterone system. Angiotensin converting enzyme (ACE) inhibitors and angiotensin receptor blockers (ARBs) blunt the intrarenal arteriolar effects of angiotensin II, which leads to net dilation of the efferent arteriole (EA) (*black arrows*) and reduction in glomerular hypertension. This reduction in glomerular capillary pressure reduces glomerular hyperpermeability, leading to a reduced urinary protein excretion and renoprotection. *AA,* Afferent arteriole; *D,* distal tubule; *E,* endothelial cell; *EGM,* extraglomerular mesangial cell; *F,* foot process; *G,* juxtaglomerular granular cell; *GBM,* glomerular basement membrane; *M,* mesangial cell; *MD,* macula densa; *N,* sympathetic nerve endings; *P,* proximal tubule; *PE,* parietal epithelial cell; *PO,* epithelial podocyte; *UP,* urinary pole; *US,* urinary space.

trials provide remarkable attestation for the use of ARBs for renoprotection in overt diabetic nephropathy.

In addition to systemic and glomerular hypertension, proteinuria is also reduced in patients with diabetic nephropathy treated with RAAS blockade. In both IDNT and RENAAL, baseline proteinuria was directly related to developing the endpoint of doubling of the serum creatinine or ESRD. More important, those patients that had a decrease in proteinuria experienced improved kidney outcomes (see Fig. 52.7), emphasizing that proteinuria may be an independent risk factor to the development of progressive kidney disease, and reducing proteinuria is an appropriate surrogate target for an overall benefit in kidney outcomes.

Similar results are seen in nondiabetic kidney disease, where a metaanalysis by Jafar and colleagues demonstrated that RAAS inhibition slows progression, particularly in individuals with proteinuria exceeding 1000 mg/day. To confirm this finding, investigators for the REIN trial randomized 352 proteinuric patients with hypertension but without diabetic nephropathy to receive either the ACE inhibitor ramipril or conventional antihypertensive therapy, achieving identical blood pressure control in both groups. Notably, patients randomized to receive ramipril had a 50% lower risk for progression to ESRD during the 3 years of follow-up. Similar to prior findings, patients who had greater degrees of proteinuria and received ramipril had less marked decline in GFR compared with patients receiving conventional antihypertensive therapy.

In summary, clinical trial data reveal that inhibition of the RAAS with ACE inhibitors or ARBs provides the strongest renoprotection available to date, especially in patients with diabetic nephropathy or proteinuric CKD not due to DM, and these agents should be first-line therapy in these clinical settings. Critically, advanced CKD does not preclude their use.

The question that naturally follows is whether additive or dual blockade would provide synergistic renoprotection. At the present time, most of the trials performed with dual blockade with use of either ACE inhibitors, angiotensin receptor blockers, renin inhibitors, or aldosterone antagonists have broadly demonstrated reduction in proteinuria. However, whether there will be a long-term benefit of dual therapy on "hard" outcomes, such as a decrease in the rate of decline of GFR or a decrease in the incidence of kidney failure, remains unknown. Currently, dual blockade of the RAAS cannot be recommended, and it may incur harm (see Proteinuria Reduction, later), particularly in individuals without substantial proteinuria. In addition, care must be taken to monitor and treat the potential development of hyperkalemia when using any agent to block the RAAS. Given the fact that many of these patients have a decreased GFR and an inability to excrete potassium, maximally blocking the RAAS at multiple sites may contribute to hyperkalemia; accordingly it is prudent to check the serum potassium 7 to 14 days after initiating therapy with these agents.

BLOOD PRESSURE CONTROL

Blockade of the RAAS exerts its beneficial effect by reducing glomerular hypertension while simultaneously reducing systemic blood pressure. This clearly makes them first-line agents in most patients with hypertension and CKD. Observational studies and randomized controlled trials have shown that lowering blood pressure in patients with hypertension and CKD slows the rate of disease progression. The ideal goal blood pressure in patients with CKD, however, remains controversial. Present guidelines suggest the target of <130/80 mm Hg for patients with CKD or DM, a lower goal than that which is recommended for the general population (<140/90 mm Hg). This is based on several studies revealing that "intensive" blood pressure control has substantial benefits in CKD for the treatment of nephropathy and/or cardiovascular disease. Notably, blood pressure control often requires at least two to four antihypertensive medications, including an agent to block the RAAS and usually a diuretic.

How far should blood pressure be lowered, and is there a detrimental effect in lowering blood pressure too much in patients with CKD? This concern was raised in 1988, when the concept of the "J-curve" was introduced. The J-curve implies that lowering blood pressure reduces cardiovascular disease and death to a point, below which a plateau is achieved where lower blood pressure no longer confers a benefit and actually may result in increased risk for adverse events. A post hoc analysis of the IDNT trial described the J-curve in diabetic nephropathy: worse outcomes were seen in patients with overt diabetic nephropathy at both high and very low systolic blood pressures. The lowest risk for kidney outcomes was seen at achieved systolic blood pressures between 120 and 130 mm Hg, and the risk for death was increased below an achieved systolic blood pressure of 120 mm Hg. In 2010, investigators for the Action to Control Cardiovascular Risks in Diabetes (ACCORD) trial reported the results of a trial consisting of 4733 patients with type 2 DM, relatively preserved kidney function (serum creatinine ≤1.5 mg/dL), and either increased cardiovascular disease risk or a history of cardiovascular disease. These patients were randomized to an intensive systolic blood pressure goal of <120 mm Hg compared with a systolic blood pressure goal of <140 mmHg. The achieved blood pressure in the intensive group was 119/64 mm Hg; in the standard control group, it was 134/71 mm Hg. Over an average follow-up of nearly 5 years, there was no difference in cardiovascular disease or stroke between the two groups; however, the intensive therapy arm demonstrated more hypotension, higher serum creatinine, and lower estimated GFR, as well as a tenfold higher rate of hyperkalemia, suggesting that the beneficial effects of hypertension treatment reach a plateau somewhere between a systolic blood pressure of 120 and 140 mm Hg. Additional evidence for a plateau exists in patients without diabetic nephropathy from the follow-up data of the AASK trial, where there was no difference in outcomes, including doubling of serum creatinine, ESRD, or death in patients with the lower achieved blood pressure, unless proteinuria (defined as a urine protein/creatinine ratio of >0.22 g of protein per g of creatinine) was present at baseline.

Accordingly, lowering blood pressure to <120/80 mm Hg in patients with CKD or diabetic nephropathy with pharmacologic therapy is not warranted. Consistent blood pressures above 140/90 mm Hg should be treated, and the first-line agent in people with diabetes or with proteinuria should be an ACE inhibitor or ARB. The exact blood pressure goal in patients with CKD remains controversial, but the present guideline of <130/80 mm Hg for patients with diabetic nephropathy and/or proteinuria is reasonable.

LIFESTYLE MODIFICATION

Based on the pathophysiology for acute and chronic kidney disease, glomerular hyperfiltration due to altered hemodynamics plays a role. Theoretically, decreasing elevated intraglomerular pressure by any means may have a benefit. Dietary protein restriction is a proposed method, and in the animal model of 5/6 nephrectomy, dietary protein restriction demonstrated reduced kidney injury by decreasing afferent arteriolar vasodilation, glomerular hypertension, and oncotic pressure. Unfortunately, contrary to RAAS blockade, human studies on dietary protein restriction have not shown substantial benefits.

The current recommended diet for people with diabetes, consisting of low sodium, low fat, and moderately low protein with high fiber, has been shown to decrease blood pressure in patients with hypertension and type 2 DM in the absence of CKD or proteinuria. Based on available evidence, a prudent diet for a patient with CKD is to limit protein intake to approximately 0.8-1.0 g/kg of body weight per day and to limit dietary sodium to <2.4 g a day. This is discussed in further detail in Chapter 54. Additionally, as discussed in Chapter 25, control of blood glucose levels in patients who have DM is important to reduce microvascular and cardiovascular complications, although few data support intensive glycemic control for reducing the rate of GFR decline in patients with diabetic nephropathy.

Obesity and obesity-related glomerulopathy are increasing in prevalence. Obesity is a risk factor for developing CKD, and in patients who already have documented CKD, obesity is a risk factor for progression. Preexisting albuminuria is exacerbated by weight gain and decreases with weight loss. This finding fits well into the model of hyperfiltration and glomerular hypertension with subsequent proteinuria; however, more evidence is needed to determine the relationship of obesity with a progressive decline in GFR.

Hyperlipidemia, similar to obesity, may be a modifiable risk factor to slow progressive CKD. Hyperlipidemia may contribute to CKD progression through proinflammatory and profibrotic mechanisms, considering the fact that low-density lipoproteins (LDL) have these properties. Animal models reveal that rats fed high-cholesterol diets exhibit a greater degree of glomerulosclerosis and interstitial disease compared with those fed a low-cholesterol diet. In the same animal models, 3-hydroxy-3-methyl-glutaryl-CoA reductase inhibitors (statins) have been shown to limit inflammatory cytokines and adhesion molecules and slow the progression of kidney disease. Observational studies in humans also support this hypothesis; however, unlike blockade of the RAAS, human clinical trials investigating the use of statin therapy to decrease the progression of CKD have been discouraging. In the Study of Heart and Renal Protection (SHARP) trial, 6247 patients with moderate to severe CKD were randomized to receive a statin and ezetimibe or placebo, and although there was a cardiovascular benefit, no difference was seen in the development of kidney failure in the active therapy arm.

PROTEINURIA REDUCTION

In patients with or without a reduced GFR, proteinuria is an independent risk factor for progressive kidney injury.

Prospective randomized controlled trials in humans with advanced overt diabetic nephropathy have shown that higher levels of proteinuria at baseline are a powerful predictor of eventual decline in GFR (see Fig. 52.7). This is also true in patients who excrete lower levels of albumin in the urine (consistent with microalbuminuria). Furthermore, the ability to successfully reduce levels of proteinuria with the use of ACE inhibitors or ARBs is predictive of a more benign course in patients with diabetic nephropathy (see Fig. 52.7), as well as other proteinuric kidney diseases, including hypertensive nephrosclerosis, IgA nephropathy, membranous glomerulonephritis, and severe lupus nephritis.

Therefore reducing proteinuria to the lowest possible amount would seem beneficial. However, in one study, in which patients with vascular disease or high-risk DM were randomized to receive either the ARB telmisartan or the ACE inhibitor ramipril, or both, combination therapy reduced albuminuria to a greater degree than therapy alone, but it was associated with a greater decline in estimated GFR. In another study of overt diabetic nephropathy, the renin inhibitor aliskiren was found to lower proteinuria to a greater degree when used in combination with losartan compared with losartan alone; however, a follow-up study of dual therapy with aliskiren and valsartan was halted early because of increased risk for stroke, kidney complications, hyperkalemia, and hypotension in the dual therapy group. Therefore, although lowering proteinuria is beneficial, blocking the RAAS system at multiple different sites (see Fig. 52.3) to do so may not achieve added benefit. Before recommending this therapy, positive long-term kidney outcomes in dual therapy studies need to be demonstrated.

Notably, the level of protein excretion may be helpful in defining optimal blood pressure goals. Nondiabetic patients in the MDRD trial, the AASK trial, and the REIN trial with higher levels of proteinuria had a greater benefit from a lower blood pressure goal. In the REIN study, the beneficial effect in the intensive blood pressure arm was more pronounced with use of ACE inhibitors.

NOVEL METHODS

Novel therapies attempting to reduce the progression of chronic kidney disease exist; these target the inflammatory and/or fibrotic effects that occur in the pathophysiology of CKD progression. Pirfenidone is a novel agent that targets the fibrosing pathway of CKD and has beneficial effects in animal models of CKD and diabetic nephropathy. However, positive, large, long-term human clinical trials showing a reduction in the progression of CKD have not yet been completed. Endothelin antagonists are another promising area for the future as ET-1 contributes to kidney damage via both vasoconstrictive properties as well promotion of interstitial fibrosis. Animal models have demonstrated a benefit of endothelin antagonists with a reduction in proteinuria and improvement in creatinine clearance. At present, positive safety and efficacy data from clinical trials evaluating these agents is lacking.

Another novel medication, pyridoxamine, exerts its effect through antioxidant properties and impairment in advanced glycation end products (AGEs). Pyridoxamine has been evaluated in a multicenter randomized controlled trial of patients with overt diabetic nephropathy. In that trial, the drug failed to reduce GFR loss at 1 year, but there was a stabilization noted in the group of patients with the most preserved baseline kidney function. Sulodexide, a glycosaminoglycan, was rigorously tested in clinical trials of patients with diabetic nephropathy and failed to show a benefit.

Treatment of hyperuricemia, hyperphosphatemia, and vitamin D deficiency and maintaining appropriate acid-base balance with sodium bicarbonate therapy have been shown in observational studies and/or small clinical trials to be associated with a reduction in albuminuria and/or the progression of CKD. These therapies may hold promise for the future, but validated long-term controlled trials are currently lacking.

CARDIOVASCULAR RISK REDUCTION

The leading cause of death in patients with CKD is cardiovascular disease. Hypertension, sodium and volume retention, anemia, hyperphosphatemia, high prevalence of DM and vascular disease, and electrolyte disturbances including hyperkalemia are all reported risk factors that may contribute to this effect. Based on this, it may be prudent to reduce this risk with lifestyle modifications, smoking cessation, use of aspirin, and pharmacologic therapy for hypertension, dyslipidemia, albuminuria, and hyperglycemia (when present), because there appears to be synergy between cardiovascular disease development and the progression and development and progression of CKD.

CONCLUSIONS

The pathophysiology of CKD is largely dependent on the primary insult, but common pathways exist across almost all subsets of kidney disorders. This includes hemodynamic-mediated hyperfiltration and eventual nephron loss, as well as inflammatory and cellular mediated fibrosis. Much of the pathophysiology arises from maladaptation to autoregulation with hyperactivation of the RAAS. Theoretically, blocking these pathways will interrupt this progression; in fact, the most robust clinical evidence for slowing or reversing the progression is with disruption of the RAAS system. Controlling blood pressure, lowering proteinuria, avoiding AKI, and attempting cardiovascular risk reduction are important goals for the physicians treating patients with CKD. Exciting novel therapies are eagerly anticipated, but these must be tested through rigorous clinical study for safety, tolerability, and efficacy.

BIBLIOGRAPHY

Agodoa LY, Appel L, Bakris GL, et al: Effect of ramipril vs amlodipine on renal outcomes in hypertensive nephrosclerosis: a randomized controlled trial, *JAMA* 285:2719-2728, 2001.

Ashley DJ, Mostofi FK: Renal agenesis and dysgenesis, *J Urol* 83:211-230, 1960.

Atkins RC, Briganti EM, Lewis JB, et al: Proteinuria reduction and progression to renal failure in patients with type 2 diabetes mellitus and overt nephropathy, *Am J Kidney Dis* 45:281-287, 2005.

Baigent C, Landray MJ, Reith C, et al: The effects of lowering LDL cholesterol with simvastatin plus ezetimibe in patients with chronic kidney disease (Study of Heart and Renal Protection): a randomised placebo-controlled trial, *Lancet* 377:2181-2192, 2011.

Brenner BM, Cooper ME, de ZD, et al: Effects of losartan on renal and cardiovascular outcomes in patients with type 2 diabetes and nephropathy, *N Engl J Med* 345:861-869, 2001.

Brenner BM, Meyer TW, Hostetter TH: Dietary protein intake and the progressive nature of kidney disease: the role of hemodynamically mediated glomerular injury in the pathogenesis of progressive glomerular sclerosis in aging, renal ablation, and intrinsic renal disease, *N Engl J Med* 307:652-659, 1982.

Cushman WC, Evans GW, Byington RP, et al: Effects of intensive blood-pressure control in type 2 diabetes mellitus, *N Engl J Med* 362:1575-1585, 2010.

GISEN Group: (Gruppo Italiano di Studi Epidemiologici in Nefrologia). Randomised placebo-controlled trial of effect of ramipril on decline in glomerular filtration rate and risk of terminal renal failure in proteinuric, non-diabetic nephropathy, *Lancet* 349:1857-1863, 1997.

Hemmelgarn BR, Manns BJ, Lloyd A, et al: Relation between kidney function, proteinuria, and adverse outcomes, *JAMA* 303:423-429, 2010.

Ishani A, Xue JL, Himmelfarb J, et al: Acute kidney injury increases risk of ESRD among elderly, *J Am Soc Nephrol* 20:223-228, 2009.

Jafar TH, Stark PC, Schmid CH, et al: Progression of chronic kidney disease: the role of blood pressure control, proteinuria, and angiotensin-converting enzyme inhibition: a patient-level meta-analysis, *Ann Intern Med* 139:244-252, 2003.

Klag MJ, Whelton PK, Randall BL, et al: Blood pressure and end-stage renal disease in men, *N Engl J Med* 334:13-18, 1996.

Klahr S, Levey AS, Beck GJ, et al: The effects of dietary protein restriction and blood-pressure control on the progression of chronic renal disease. Modification of Diet in Renal Disease Study Group, *N Engl J Med* 330:877-884, 1994.

Lewis EJ, Hunsicker LG, Bain RP, Rohde RD: The effect of angiotensin-converting-enzyme inhibition on diabetic nephropathy. The Collaborative Study Group, *N Engl J Med* 329:1456-1462, 1993.

Lewis EJ, Hunsicker LG, Clarke WR, et al: Renoprotective effect of the angiotensin-receptor antagonist irbesartan in patients with nephropathy due to type 2 diabetes, *N Engl J Med* 345:851-860, 2001.

Mann JF, Schmieder RE, McQueen M, et al: Renal outcomes with telmisartan, ramipril, or both, in people at high vascular risk (the ONTARGET study): a multicentre, randomised, double-blind, controlled trial, *Lancet* 372:547-553, 2008.

Mogensen CE: The effect of blood pressure intervention on renal function in insulin-dependent diabetes, *Diabete Metab* 15:343-351, 1989.

Parving HH, Brenner BM, McMurray JJ, et al: Cardiorenal end points in a trial of aliskiren for type 2 diabetes, *N Engl J Med* 367:2204-2213, 2012.

Parving HH, Lehnert H, Brochner-Mortensen J, Gomis R, Andersen S, Arner P: The effect of irbesartan on the development of diabetic nephropathy in patients with type 2 diabetes, *N Engl J Med* 345:870-878, 2001.

Pohl MA, Blumenthal S, Cordonnier DJ, et al: Independent and additive impact of blood pressure control and angiotensin II receptor blockade on renal outcomes in the irbesartan diabetic nephropathy trial: clinical implications and limitations, *J Am Soc Nephrol* 16:3027-3037, 2005.

Tonelli M, Muntner P, Lloyd A, et al: Using proteinuria and estimated glomerular filtration rate to classify risk in patients with chronic kidney disease: a cohort study, *Ann Intern Med* 154:12-21, 2011.

53 Staging and Management of Chronic Kidney Disease

Lesley A. Inker | Andrew S. Levey

Chronic kidney disease (CKD) is a growing worldwide public health problem, characterized by increasing prevalence, high cost, and poor outcomes. The poor outcomes of CKD are not restricted to progression of kidney disease leading to chronic kidney failure, but also include increased risk for acute kidney injury (AKI), cardiovascular disease (CVD), and mortality, as well as a wide variety of other complications.

In 2002, the Kidney Disease Outcomes Quality Initiative (KDOQI) of the National Kidney Foundation (NKF) sponsored guidelines for the definition, classification, evaluation, and risk stratification of CKD. The purpose of these guidelines was to create uniform terminology to improve communications among all involved in the care and management of CKD, including patients, physicians, researchers, and policymakers. The guidelines were adopted with minor modification by Kidney Disease: Improving Global Outcomes (KDIGO) in 2005. In response to controversy and accumulation of new data, KDIGO sponsored a Controversies Conference in 2009, which recommended maintaining the definition of CKD but modifying the classification, ultimately leading to new guidelines in 2012. The goals of this chapter are to describe the conceptual model for the progression of CKD, the revised KDIGO guidelines for the definition and stages of CKD, and the associated prevalence and clinical action plan, with emphasis on the role of nephrologists in the care of these patients.

DEFINITION AND STAGING OF CHRONIC KIDNEY DISEASE

COURSE OF CHRONIC KIDNEY DISEASE

Figure 53.1 shows a conceptual model for the course of CKD, and Table 53.1 outlines the outcomes. This model describes the natural history of CKD, beginning with antecedent conditions associated with increased risk for developing kidney disease, followed by the stages of CKD (kidney damage, decreased glomerular filtration rate [GFR], and kidney failure), and associated complications.

Risk factors for development of CKD include exposure to factors that cause kidney disease, such as hypertension, diabetes, autoimmune diseases, and kidney stones, and characteristics that increase susceptibility to kidney disease, such as older age, minority racial and ethnic status, and reduced nephron mass. The mechanisms underlying increased susceptibility have not been completely described or proven. For example, minority race or ethnicity may imply an underlying genetic tendency, or it may be a marker for lack of access to health care. Susceptibility factors may explain why a family history of kidney disease, regardless of the cause, places an individual at increased risk for development of kidney disease.

The horizontal arrows in Figure 53.1 indicate transitions among kidney outcomes. The arrows pointing from left to right emphasize the progressive nature of CKD. However, the rate of progression is variable, and not all CKD progresses; thus, not all patients with CKD develop kidney failure. Interventions in earlier stages may slow or prevent the progression to later stages. Early stages of kidney disease may be reversible, and individuals with kidney failure can revert to earlier stages through kidney transplantation, shown as dashed arrowheads pointing from right to left. Studies suggest that CKD is a risk factor for development of AKI, and that episodes of AKI may increase the risk for progression of CKD. The earlier stages and the risk factors for progression to higher stages can be identified, permitting improvement in outcome by prevention, earlier detection, and initiation of therapies that can slow progression and prevent the development of kidney failure.

The diagonal arrows emphasize complications of CKD other than kidney outcomes. Metabolic and endocrine complications of decreased GFR, including anemia, bone and mineral disorders, malnutrition, and neuropathy, have long been recognized as consequences of kidney failure, but these abnormalities may appear with lesser reduction in GFR. Similarly, nephrotic syndrome occurs in patients with marked albuminuria, but hyperlipidemia and hypercoagulability may be observed with lesser increases in albuminuria. It is well accepted that both decreased GFR and albuminuria are associated with an independent risk of CVD and all-cause mortality. More recently, recognized complications are threats to patient safety from systemic toxicity from drugs and procedures, as well as an increased risk of infections and impaired cognitive and physical function. Strategies for prevention, early detection, and treatment of CKD complications may prolong survival and improve quality of life even if there is no effect on kidney disease progression.

DEFINITION OF CHRONIC KIDNEY DISEASE

Chronic kidney disease is defined as either kidney damage or GFR of less than 60 mL/min/1.73 m² of body surface area lasting for longer than 3 months (90 days). CKD can be diagnosed without knowledge of its cause (Table 53.2).

Kidney damage can be within the parenchyma, large blood vessels, or collecting systems, and it is usually inferred from markers rather than direct examination of kidney tissue. As discussed later, the markers of kidney damage often provide

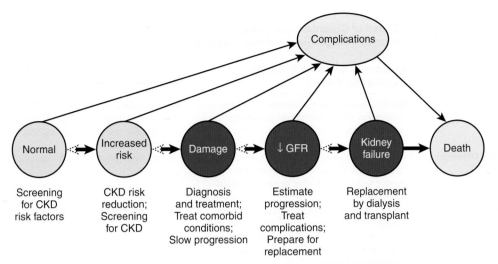

Figure 53.1   Conceptual model for chronic kidney disease. The continuum of development, progression, and complications of chronic kidney disease (CKD) and strategies to improve outcomes. *Dark green circles,* Stages of CKD; *light green circles,* potential antecedents of CKD; *lavender circles,* consequences of CKD; *thick arrows between circles,* development, progression, and remission of CKD. *Complications* refers to all complications of CKD, including complications of decreased glomerular filtration rate and cardiovascular disease. Complications may also arise from adverse effects of interventions to prevent or treat the disease. *Horizontal arrows pointing from left to right* emphasize the progressive nature of CKD. *Dashed arrowheads pointing from right to left* signify that remission is less frequent than progression. (Reproduced with modifications from the National Kidney Foundation: K/DOQI clinical practice guidelines for chronic kidney disease: evaluation, classification, and stratification. *Am J Kidney Dis* 39[2 Suppl 1]:S1-266; 2002, and Levey AS, Stevens LA, Coresh J: Conceptual model of CKD: applications and implications, *Am J Kidney Dis* 53:S4-S16, 2009.)

Table 53.1   Outcomes of Chronic Kidney Disease and Relationship to Kidney Disease Characteristics

	Kidney Disease Characteristics		
Outcomes of CKD	**GFR**	**Albuminuria**	**Cause**
Kidney Outcomes			
CKD progression (GFR decline and worsening albuminuria)	+	+++	+++
AKI	+++	+	+
Chronic kidney failure	+++	+	+++
Complications (Current and Future)			
CVD and mortality	+++	+++	++
Systemic drug toxicity	+++	+	+
Metabolic/endocrine (anemia, bone and mineral disorders, malnutrition, and neuropathy)	+++	+	+
Infections, cognitive impairment, frailty	++	++	++

AKI, Acute kidney injury; *CKD,* chronic kidney disease; *CVD,* cardiovascular disease; *GFR,* glomerular filtration rate.
Number of + indicates the strength of the risk relationship between the kidney disease characteristic and the outcome.

Table 53.2   Definition of Chronic Kidney Disease

Criteria for CKD*	
Markers of Kidney Damage	• Albuminuria greater than 30 mg/day • Urine sediment abnormalities • Electrolyte and other abnormalities caused by tubular disorders • Pathologic abnormalities • Imaging abnormalities • History of kidney transplantation
Decreased GFR	• GFR less than 60 mL/min/1.73 m²

CKD, Chronic kidney disease; *GFR,* glomerular filtration rate.
*Either of the listed items for more than 3 mo.

abnormalities in urine sediment (e.g., tubular cells or casts), abnormal findings on imaging studies (e.g., hydronephrosis, asymmetry in kidney size, polycystic kidney disease, small echogenic kidneys), and abnormalities in blood and urine chemistry measurements (those related to altered tubular function, such as renal tubular acidosis). A history of kidney transplantation is also defined as a marker of kidney damage, and patients with a functioning transplant are considered to have CKD, irrespective of the presence of other markers of kidney damage or the level of GFR.

Decreased GFR, specifically GFR less than 60 mL/min/1.73 m², lasting more than 3 months is defined as CKD, irrespective of age. The level of GFR is usually accepted as the best overall index of kidney function in health and disease. GFR less than 60 mL/min/1.73 m² represents the loss of half or more of the adult level of normal kidney function, and it is associated with an increased prevalence of systemic complications. The normal level of GFR varies according to age, gender, and body size.

a clue to the likely site of damage within the kidney and, in association with other clinical findings, the cause of kidney disease. Because most kidney diseases in North America are caused by diabetes or hypertension, persistent albuminuria is the principal marker. Other markers of damage include

Table 53.3 Classification of Cause of Chronic Kidney Disease Based on Presence or Absence of Systemic Disease and Location of Pathologic-Anatomic Findings

	Examples of Systemic Diseases Affecting the Kidney	Examples of Primary Kidney Diseases
Glomerular Diseases	Diabetes, autoimmune diseases, systemic infections, drugs, neoplasia (including amyloidosis)	Diffuse, focal, or crescentric proliferative glomerulonephritis; focal and segmental glomerulosclerosis; idiopathic membranous nephropathy; minimal change disease
Tubulointerstitial Diseases	Systemic infections, autoimmune diseases, sarcoidosis, drugs, urate, environmental toxins (lead, aristolochic acid), neoplasia (myeloma)	Urinary tract infections, stones, obstruction
Vascular Diseases	Decreased perfusion (heart failure, liver disease, renal artery disease), atherosclerosis, hypertension, ischemia, cholesterol emboli, vasculitis, thrombotic microangiopathy, systemic sclerosis	ANCA-associated vasculitis; fibromuscular dysplasia
Cystic and Congenital Diseases	Polycystic kidney disease, Alport syndrome, Fabry disease, oxalosis	Renal dysplasia, medullary cystic disease
Diseases Affecting the Transplanted Kidney	Recurrence of native kidney disease (diabetes, oxalosis, Fabry disease)	Chronic rejection; calcineurin inhibitor toxicity; BK virus nephropathy; recurrence of native kidney disease (glomerular disease)

ANCA, Antineutrophil cytoplasm antibody.

NOTE: Genetic diseases are not considered separately, because some diseases in each category are now recognized as having genetic determinants.

Normal GFR is approximately 120 to 130 mL/min/1.73 m² in a young adult, and declines with age by approximately 1 mL/min/1.73 m² per year after the third decade. More than 25% of individuals aged 70 years and older have GFR of less than 60 mL/min/1.73 m²; whether this results from normal aging or the high prevalence of systemic vascular diseases that cause kidney disease remains controversial. Whatever its cause, GFR less than 60 mL/min/1.73 m² in the elderly is an independent predictor of adverse outcomes such as death and CVD. As in younger patients, adjustment of drug doses is required in elderly patients with this level of GFR.

Kidney failure is defined either as a GFR less than 15 mL/min/1.73 m² or a need to start kidney replacement therapy (dialysis or transplantation). A number of terms refer to severe decrease in kidney function, which is not synonymous with kidney failure. *Uremia* is defined as elevated concentrations within the blood of urea, creatinine, and other nitrogenous end products of amino acid and protein metabolism that are normally excreted in the urine. The *uremic syndrome,* the terminal clinical manifestation of kidney failure, is the group of symptoms, physical signs, and abnormal findings on diagnostic studies that result from the failure of the kidneys to maintain adequate function. *End-stage renal disease* (ESRD) generally refers to kidney failure treated by dialysis or transplantation, regardless of the level of kidney function, and is used administratively in the United States and elsewhere. The availability of dialysis and transplantation for treatment of kidney failure varies around the world. ESRD might not include patients with kidney failure who are not treated with dialysis or transplantation.

STAGES OF CHRONIC KIDNEY DISEASE

The NKF-KDOQI classification system for stages of CKD was based on the severity of the disease defined only by the level of GFR. The KDIGO classification is based on the cause of the disease and level of albuminuria as well as the level of GFR. The more detailed classification adopted by KDIGO relates more closely to prognosis. The cause of disease is generally classified according to the presence of absence of systemic diseases (secondary or primary) and the presumed location of the pathologic-anatomic lesions (glomerular, tubulointerstitial, vascular, cystic, or disease in the kidney transplant) (Table 53.3). Categories for GFR and albuminuria levels are shown in Tables 53.4 and 53.5. Figure 53.2A shows the two-dimensional grid developed for the 2009 KDIGO Controversies Conference relating the risk of kidney outcomes and mortality to level of GFR and albuminuria. The green, yellow, orange, and red shaded categories represent patients at low, moderate, high, and very high risk of kidney outcomes and mortality, respectively.

PREVALENCE

Figure 53.2B shows the prevalence estimates derived from a single measurement of serum creatinine to estimate GFR and albumin-to-creatinine ratio (ACR) during National Health and Nutrition Examination Surveys (NHANES) from 1988 to 2006. The prevalence of ACR greater than 30 mg/g or GFR less than 60 mL/min/1.73 m² (gray shaded area) is approximately 13.8% of the U.S. adult population. The proportion of participants in the groups at moderate, high, and very high risk (as categorized in Fig. 53.2A) is about 73%, 18%, and 9%, respectively, representing a prevalence in the general population of about 10%, 2%, and 1%, respectively. This prevalence is more than 50 times greater than the prevalence of treated ESRD of approximately 0.2% reported by the United States Renal Data System during this interval. Because kidney disease usually begins late in life

Table 53.4   Categories of Chronic Kidney Disease by the Level of Glomerular Filtration Rate and Corresponding Clinical Action Plan

Category	GFR Levels (mL/min/1.73 m²)	Terms	Clinical Action Plan
G1*	Greater than 90	Normal or high	Diagnose and treat the cause Treat comorbid conditions Evaluate for CKD risk factors Start measures to slow CKD progression Start measures to reduce CVD risk
G2*	60 to 89	Mildly decreased[†]	Estimate progression
G3a	45 to 59	Mildly to moderately decreased	Adjust medication dosages as indicated
G3b	30 to 44	Moderately to severely decreased	Evaluate and treat complications
G4	15 to 29	Severely decreased	Prepare for kidney replacement therapy (transplantation and/or dialysis) if appropriate
G5	Less than 15	Kidney failure (add D if treated by dialysis)	Start kidney replacement therapy (if uremia present)

CKD, Chronic kidney disease; *CVD*, cardiovascular disease; *GFR*, Glomerular filtration rate.
*GFR stages G1 or G2 without markers of kidney damage do not fulfil the criteria for CKD.
[†]Relative to young adult level
NOTE: GFR in mL/min/1.73 m² may be converted to mL/s/1.73 m² by multiplying by 0.01667.

Table 53.5   Categories of Chronic Kidney Disease by the Level of Albuminuria and Corresponding Clinical Action Plan

Category	AER (mg/day)	Approximately Equivalent ACR (mg/mmol)	(mg/g)	Terms	Clinical Action Plan
A1	Less than 30	Less than 3	Less than 30	Normal to mildly increased	Diagnose and treat the cause Treat comorbid conditions Evaluate for CKD risk factors Start measures to slow CKD progression Start measures to reduce CVD risk
A2	30 to 299	3 to 30	30 to 299	Moderately increased*	Treatment with renin-angiotensin system blockers and lower blood pressure goal if hypertensive
A3	Greater than 300	≥30	Greater than 300	Severely increased	Treat nephrotic syndrome (if present)

ACR, Albumin-to-creatinine ratio; *AER*, albumin excretion rate; *CKD*, chronic kidney disease; *CVD*, cardiovascular disease.
*Relative to young adult level.

and progresses slowly, most people in the earlier stages of CKD die before reaching kidney failure. In these patients, the burden of CKD is reflected in the complications of earlier stages, including increased mortality and morbidity, reduced quality of life, and high cost.

DIAGNOSIS, EVALUATION, AND MANAGEMENT

Chronic kidney disease care is directed by the cause, as well as by the level of GFR and albuminuria (see Tables 53.3, 53.4, and 53.5). Four key points must be emphasized. First, the action plan for each GFR and albuminuria stage includes recommended care for the cause of disease, as well as addressing factors associated with progression to more advanced stages. Second, the action plan is cumulative, in that recommended care at each stage of disease includes care for earlier stages.

Third, care for patients with CKD requires multiple interventions, and the coordinated, multidisciplinary effort of primary-care physicians, allied healthcare workers, and other specialists in addition to nephrologists. Fourth, the management of each stage of disease must take into consideration kidney outcomes and complications. The stage-specific clinical action plan is a guide, but not a replacement, for the physician's assessment of the needs of each specific patient. Figure 53.3 provides a 5-step overview of the diagnosis and evaluation of CKD. More details regarding evaluation and management are discussed in other chapters.

DIAGNOSIS

As part of routine checkups, all patients should be evaluated to determine whether they are at increased risk for developing CKD. Those deemed at high risk should at minimum

A

GFR stages, description and range (mL/min per 1.73 m²)			Albuminuria stages, description and range (mg/g)				
			A1 Optimal and high-normal		A2 High	A3 Very high and nephrotic	
			<10	10–29	30–299	300–1999	≥2000
G1	High and optimal	>105					
		90–104					
G2	Mild	75–89					
		60–74					
G3a	Mild-moderate	45–59					
G3b	Moderate-severe	30–44					
G4	Severe	15–29					
G5	Kidney failure	<15					

B

GFR stages, description and range (mL/min/ 1.73 m²)			Albuminuria stages, description and range (mg/g)				
			A1		A2	A3	
			Optimal	High-normal	High	Very high	All
			<10	10–29	30–299	>300	
G1	Optimal	>105	23.6%	5.7%	1.9%	0.1%	31.4%
		90–104	20.0%	4.7%	1.7%	0.3%	26.7%
G2	Mild	75–89	17.3%	4.1%	1.6%	0.2%	23.0%
		60–74	8.2%	2.7%	1.3%	0.1%	12.2%
G3a	Mild-moderate	45–59	2.5%	1.1%	0.8%	0.2%	4.7%
G3b	Moderate-severe	30–44	0.6%	0.4%	0.4%	0.2%	1.5%
G4	Severe	15–29	0.1%	0.1%	0.1%	0.1%	0.4%
G5	Kidney failure	<15	0.0%	0.0%	0.0%	0.1%	0.1%
All			72.2%	18.8%	7.8%	1.3%	100.0%

Figure 53.2 A, Composite ranking for relative risks by glomerular filtration rate and albuminuria (Kidney Disease: Improving Global Outcomes, 2009). Colors reflect the ranking of relative risk by glomerular filtration rate (GFR) and albuminuria. *Green,* No chronic kidney disease (CKD); *yellow,* moderate risk; *orange,* high risk; *red,* very high risk. The ranks were assigned for five outcomes (all-cause mortality, cardiovascular disease mortality, end-stage renal disease, acute kidney injury, and CKD progression) from a metaanalysis of general population cohorts, and they were averaged across all five outcomes for the 28 GFR and albuminuria categories (GFR greater than 15 mL/min/1.73 m² and albuminuria less than 2000 mg/g). The categories with mean rank numbers 1 to 8 are green, mean rank numbers 9 to 14 are yellow, mean rank numbers 15 to 21 are orange, and mean rank numbers 22 to 28 are red. Color for twelve additional cells with diagonal hash marks is extrapolated based on results of the metaanalysis of CKD cohorts. The highest level of albuminuria is termed *nephrotic* to correspond with nephrotic-range albuminuria, and it is expressed here as greater than 2000 mg/g. Albuminuria is expressed as albumin-to-creatinine ratio (ACR). Column and row labels are combined to be consistent with the number of estimated GFR (eGFR) and albuminuria stages agreed on at the conference. (Reproduced from Levey AS et al: The definition, classification and prognosis of chronic kidney disease: a KDIGO Controversies Conference report, *Kidney Int* 80:17-28, 2011.) **B, Prevalence of chronic kidney disease in the United States by glomerular filtration rate and albuminuria.** *Grey shading* represents chronic kidney disease (CKD) defined by glomerular filtration rate (GFR) or albuminuria (13.8%). Cells show the proportion of adult population in the United States. Data from the National Health and Nutrition Examination Survey (NHANES) 1988-06 (N = 18 026). GFR is estimated with the CKD-EPI (epidemiology) equation and standardized serum creatinine. Albuminuria is established by one measurement of albumin-to-creatinine ratio (ACR); thus proportions for GFR greater than 60 mL/min per 1.73 m² exceed those reported based on persistence of albuminuria. Values in cells might not total to values in margins because of rounding. Category of very high albuminuria includes nephrotic range. (Reproduced from Levey AS, Coresh J: Chronic kidney disease, *Lancet* 379:165-180, 2012.)

				Albuminuria stages, description and range (mg/g)				
				A1		A2	A3	
				Optimal and high-normal		High	Very high and nephrotic	
				<10	10–29	30–299	300–1999	≥2000
GFR stages, description and range (mL/min/ 1.73 m²)	G1	High and optimal	>105					
			90–104					
	G2	Mild	75–89					
			60–74					
	G3a	Mild-moderate	45–59					
	G3b	Moderate-severe	30–44					
	G4	Severe	15–29					
	G5	Kidney failure	<15					

C

Figure 53.2, cont'd   C, Management of chronic kidney disease by glomerular filtration rate and albuminuria stages. Management for all patients includes identifying the clinical diagnosis, slowing the progression of chronic kidney disease (CKD), and reducing the risk for cardiovascular disease. Therapies focusing on complications of decreased glomerular filtration rate (GFR) are shown as horizontal lines; therapies focused on complications of albuminuria are shown as vertical lines (see Tables 53.4 and 53.5). Width of lines corresponds to intensity of management.

have a measurement of serum creatinine concentration to estimate GFR and an assessment of albuminuria. The recommended method for assessing albuminuria is measurement of the ACR in an untimed ("spot") urine sample. Current guidelines suggest testing in patients with hypertension, diabetes, CVD, cancer, human immunodeficiency virus (HIV) infection, and before imaging procedures with iodine-based or gadolinium-based contrast. Clinical practice also includes measurement of serum creatinine with GFR estimation as part of the basic metabolic panel for patients with acute illness or before planned invasive procedures. At present, there are few data regarding the optimal frequency of testing for CKD in high-risk individuals, although annual testing is recommended in patients with hypertension, diabetes, and HIV. Until evidence is available, it is reasonable to suggest that others at increased risk be tested at least every 3 years.

EVALUATION

The goals of evaluation are to identify the duration and cause of kidney disease, to assess severity based on the levels of GFR and albuminuria, and to determine the risk for progression of kidney disease and of complications. In patients in whom CKD has been diagnosed, evaluation starts with a thorough history and physical examination to detect any signs and symptoms that may be clues to the etiology of kidney disease and, in particular, any reversible or treatable causes (e.g., uncontrolled hypertension, use of nonsteroidal antiinflammatory drugs). Medications should be reviewed to identify those that can cause kidney

toxicity and others that must be adjusted based on GFR. The physical examination should include particular attention to details such as blood pressure, fundoscopy, and vascular examination. Laboratory tests should be performed to detect other markers of damage or functional disturbances (e.g., urine specific gravity, urine pH, urine sediment examination, serum electrolytes). Imaging studies should be performed if indicated based on clinical clues. Ultrasonography can be performed to detect anatomic abnormalities and to exclude obstruction of the urinary tract. Further testing may be indicated if there is concern about anatomic abnormalities. It has been recommended that individuals with GFR less than 60 mL/min/1.73 m² should have measurements of hemoglobin as well as serum calcium, phosphate, albumin, and parathyroid hormone, but these measures are often not abnormal until GFR is less than 45 mL/min/1.73 m². Laboratory evaluation should also include a search for traditional CVD risk factors, such as a lipid profile, and possibly tests for nontraditional risk factors such as insulin resistance and inflammation. Additional studies may be necessary to evaluate symptoms of CVD more fully or to detect asymptomatic CVD in patients with multiple risk factors.

As discussed earlier, many elderly individuals meet the criteria for a diagnosis of CKD because of estimated GFR less than 60 mL/min/1.73 m². In the absence of risk factors for CKD, albuminuria, or other markers of kidney damage, patients with isolated decreased GFR may be at low risk for progression to kidney failure, but are at increased risk for CKD complications and for CVD. In such patients, clinicians may elect to defer some parts of the evaluation for

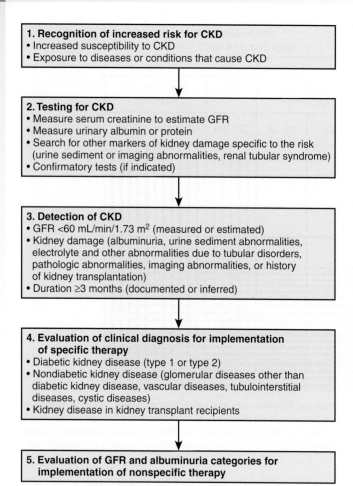

Figure 53.3   Detection and evaluation of chronic kidney disease. *CKD,* Chronic kidney disease; *GFR,* glomerular filtration rate.

CKD; however, a search for reversible causes of decreased GFR, adjustment of medication dosages for decreased GFR, appropriate attention to CVD risk-factor management, and subsequent monitoring of estimated GFR are appropriate measures.

EVALUATION OF DURATION

Kidney diseases and disorders may be acute or chronic depending on their duration. The distinction between acute and chronic is arbitrary, but is useful in clinical practice. KDIGO defines chronicity as duration longer than 3 months (90 days), and the term *acute kidney diseases and disorders* (AKD) could be used to describe kidney disease with duration less than 3 months, including AKI. The duration of kidney disease may be documented or inferred based on the clinical context. For example, a patient with decreased kidney function or kidney damage in the midst of an acute illness, without previous documentation of kidney disease, may be inferred to have AKD. A patient with similar findings in the absence of an acute illness may be inferred to have CKD. In both cases, repeat ascertainment of kidney function and kidney damage is recommended for accurate diagnosis. The timing of the evaluation depends on clinical judgment, with earlier evaluation for patients suspected of having AKD and later evaluation for patients suspected of having CKD.

EVALUATION OF CAUSE

Identification of the cause of kidney disease enables treatments directed at the etiology, such as infection, drug toxicity, autoimmune disease, or obstruction of the urinary tract. In addition, the cause of kidney disease has implications for the rate of progression and the risk of complications. In clinical practice, CKD is most often detected as decreased estimated GFR during evaluation and management of other medical conditions. Thus, cause of disease is generally established by recognition of the clinical setting and the presence or absence of markers of kidney damage. A simplified classification emphasizes diseases in native kidneys (diabetic or nondiabetic in origin) and diseases in transplanted kidneys. Diabetic nephropathy is the largest single cause of kidney failure in the United States, accounting for approximately one third of new cases. Its earliest manifestation is albuminuria with normal or elevated GFR. Nondiabetic kidney disease includes glomerular, vascular, tubulointerstitial, and cystic kidney disorders. Clinical judgment should determine whether additional methods are necessary to characterize kidney disease, including imaging studies, other urine or serum markers, or biopsy of the kidney. For many patients with CKD (especially older patients with hypertension or diabetes and no evidence of the other disorders mentioned earlier), the cause will be unknown and presumed to be a result of vascular disease. In these cases, management will be based primarily on levels of GFR and albuminuria.

EVALUATION OF GLOMERULAR FILTRATION RATE

Current guidelines focus on estimated GFR rather than serum creatinine alone for a variety of reasons. Serum creatinine is affected by factors other than GFR. Consequently, there is a wide range of "normal" serum creatinine, and in many patients GFR must decline by approximately 50% before serum creatinine rises above this threshold. This is particularly important in the elderly, in whom the serum creatinine does not reflect the age-related decline in GFR because of a concomitant decline in muscle mass and creatinine production. For these reasons, it is difficult to use the serum creatinine alone to estimate the level of GFR, especially to detect earlier stages of CKD. GFR estimating equations are discussed in Chapter 3.

EVALUATION OF ALBUMINURIA

The KDIGO guidelines focus on albuminuria rather than proteinuria for several reasons. Albumin is the principal component of urinary protein in most kidney diseases; recent recommendations for measurement of urine proteins emphasize quantification of albuminuria rather than total protein; and, as noted before, recent epidemiologic data demonstrate a strong graded relationship of the quantity of urine albumin with both kidney and CVD risk. The ratio of concentrations of albumin-to-creatinine in a spot urine specimen has now replaced 24-hour excretion rates as the preferred method for initial evaluation of albuminuria. Use of such a ratio corrects for variations in urinary protein concentration because of urinary concentration, and is far more convenient than timed urine collections. A "positive" result for a spot urine ACR is greater than 30 mg/g, although this does not take into account variation in creatinine excretion by age, gender, and race. If a more accurate assessment is required, confirmation may be sought by measurement of albumin excretion

Table 53.6 Albuminuria and Proteinuria Measures

Measure	Categories		
	Normal to Mildly Increased	Moderately Increased	Severely Increased
AER (mg/24 hr)	Less than 30	30 to 300	Greater than 300
PER (mg/24 hr)	Less than 150	150 to 500	Greater than 500
ACR			
(mg/mmol)	Less than 3	3 to 30	Greater than 30
(mg/g)	Less than 30	30 to 300	Greater than 300
PCR			
(mg/mmol)	Less than 15	15 to 50	Greater than 50
(mg/g)	Less than 150	150 to 500	Greater than 500
Protein reagent strip	Negative to trace	Negative to positive	Positive or greater

ACR, Albumin-to-creatinine ratio; *AER,* albumin excretion rate; *PCR,* protein-to-creatinine ratio; *PER,* protein excretion rate.

Urine ACR may be divided into more than three categories. The normal urinary ACR in young adults is less than 10 mg/g; ACR 10 to 29 mg/g is high normal. Urine ACR greater than 2000 mg/g is accompanied by signs and symptoms of nephrotic syndrome (low serum albumin, edema, and high serum cholesterol).

Relationships between excretion rates and concentration ratios with urine creatinine are inexact. Excretion of urinary creatinine indicates muscle mass and varies with age, gender, race, diet, and nutritional status, and generally exceeds 1.0 g/day in healthy adults; therefore, the numeric value for urinary ACR (mg/g) is usually less than the rate of urinary albumin excretion (mg/day). Rates of 30 to 300 mg/day and greater than 300 mg/day correspond to microalbuminuria and macroalbuminuria, respectively.

Relationships between urinary albumin and total protein are inexact. Normal urine contains small amounts of albumin, low-molecular-weight serum proteins, and proteins that are from renal tubules and the lower urinary tract. In most kidney diseases, albumin is the main urine protein, comprising about 60% to 90% of total urinary protein when total protein is very high. Values corresponding to normal, high-normal, high, very high, and nephrotic-range total protein are approximately less than 50, 50 to 150, 150 to 500, greater than 500, and greater than 3500 mg/g, respectively.

Threshold values for standard international (mg/mol) and conventional units (mg/g) are not exact. Conversion factor for ACR: 1.0 mg/g = 0.113 mg/mmol.

rate in a timed urine collection. Table 53.6 provides a rough guide to measures of urine albumin and total protein in spot and timed urine collections that correspond to the KDIGO albuminuria stages. Further discussion of albuminuria and proteinuria is provided in Chapter 5.

MANAGEMENT

The essential features of management according to GFR and albuminuria stages are shown in Tables 53.4 and 53.5, and Figures 53.1 and 53.2C: treating specific causes of kidney disease; treating other reversible conditions causing kidney damage or decreased GFR; slowing progression of kidney disease by use of ACE inhibitors and ARBs and a lower blood-pressure goal in patients with higher levels of albuminuria; assuring medication safety by avoiding drugs that are toxic to the kidney and adjusting doses of drugs that are excreted by the kidney in patients with decreased GFR; treating metabolic and endocrine complications of decreased GFR; treating the nephrotic syndrome; treating CVD and its risk factors; and preparing for kidney replacement therapy in patients with severely decreased GFR.

Patient education is central to the management strategy. CKD is often asymptomatic, and patients may not understand the importance of multidrug regimens and laboratory testing without explicit education. Complete management requires behavioral change by the patient, which may include lifestyle alterations, self-monitoring of blood pressure, and adherence to medication regimens and medical follow-up. Patient education is also important with respect to avoiding medications that are toxic to the kidneys. Patients must be aware that any drug or herbal remedy may

be directly nephrotoxic or may require a dosage adjustment for the level of kidney function.

HEALTHCARE STRUCTURE FOR TREATMENT OF CHRONIC KIDNEY DISEASE

NEPHROLOGY REFERRAL

Chronic kidney disease can be a life-threatening condition. Nephrologists have multiple roles in the diagnosis and care of patients at all stages of CKD, including determining the cause of CKD, recommending specific therapy, suggesting treatments to slow progression in patients who have not responded to conventional therapies, identifying and treating kidney disease–related complications, and preparing for dialysis.

Recommendations for referral to a kidney disease specialist are not universal, as specific practice patterns are dependent on healthcare systems and available resources in a geographic region. The strongest evidence regarding the importance of referral to a nephrologist is for management of GFR stages 4 and 5 (GFR less than 30 mL/min/1.73 m^2). Late referral to a nephrologist (i.e., less than 3 months before the start of dialysis therapy) has been associated with higher mortality after the initiation of dialysis. It is therefore recommended by many organizations, regardless of the healthcare system or geographic region, that all patients with GFR stage 4 be referred to a nephrologist. During GFR stage 4, it is important to prepare the patient for the possible onset of kidney failure (GFR stage 5). Preparation involves estimating the risk of progression to kidney failure,

Table 53.7   Recommendations for Referral to Specialists for Consultation and Comanagement of Chronic Kidney Disease

GFR less than 30 mL/min/1.73 m²	Kidney disease specialist
ACR greater than 300 mg/g	Kidney disease specialist
Hematuria not from urologic conditions	Kidney disease specialist
Inability to identify a presumed cause of CKD	Kidney disease specialist
Increased risk for progression of kidney disease	Kidney disease specialist
GFR decline greater than 30% within 4 mo without explanation	Kidney disease specialist
Difficult to manage complications of CKD such as anemia requiring erythropoietin stimulating therapy, or abnormalities of bone and mineral metabolism requiring phosphorus binders or vitamin D preparations	Kidney disease specialist
Hyperkalemia (serum potassium concentration greater than 5.5 mEq/L)	Kidney disease specialist
Resistant hypertension (BP greater than 130/80 mm Hg despite adherence to a three-drug antihypertensive regimen that includes a diuretic)	Kidney disease or hypertension specialist
Difficult-to-manage drug complications	Kidney disease or hypertension specialist
Acute presentations of CVD	CVD specialist
Complex or severe chronic CVD conditions	CVD specialist
Age less than 18 yr	Pediatric kidney disease specialist

Adapted from National Kidney Foundation: KDOQI clinical practice guidelines for hypertension and antihypertensive agents in chronic kidney disease. Reproduced from Am J Kidney Dis, 43: *S1-S268, 2004.*
ACR, Albumin-to-creatinine ratio; *BP,* blood pressure; *CKD,* chronic kidney disease; *CVD,* cardiovascular disease; *GFR,* glomerular filtration rate.

holding discussions regarding kidney replacement therapy (dialysis and transplantation), and instituting conservative therapy for those who are not willing or are unable to undergo kidney replacement therapy. In patients who elect replacement therapy, timely creation of vascular access for hemodialysis, home dialysis training, and donor evaluation for preemptive transplantation should occur during GFR stage 4. For patients with CKD in GFR stages 1 to 3 (GFR greater than 30 mL/min/1.73 m²), only a subset is likely to require referral to a specialist. Table 53.7 lists clinical criteria for referral to specialists.

BIBLIOGRAPHY

Bayliss EA, Bhardwaja B, Ross C, et al: Multidisciplinary team care may slow the rate of decline in renal function, *Clin J Am Soc Nephrol* 6:704-710, 2011. Epub January 27, 2011.

Coresh J, Selvin E, Stevens LA, et al: Prevalence of chronic kidney disease in the U.S. during 1988-1994 and 1999-2004, *JAMA* 298:2038-2047, 2007.

Eckardt KU, Berns JS, Rocco MV, et al: Definition and classification of CKD: the debate should be about patient prognosis—a position statement from KDOQI and KDIGO, *Am J Kidney Dis* 53:915-920, 2009.

Gupta SK, Eustace JA, Winston JA, et al: Guidelines for the management of chronic kidney disease in HIV-infected patients: recommendations of the HIV Medicine Association of the Infectious Diseases Society of America, *Clin Infect Dis* 40:1559-1585, 2005.

Inker LA, Coresh J, Levey AS, et al: Estimated GFR, albuminuria, and complications of chronic kidney disease, *J Am Soc Nephrol* 22:2322-2331, 2011.

Ishani A, Xue JL, Himmelfarb J, et al: Acute kidney injury increases risk of ESRD among elderly, *J Am Soc Nephrol* 20:223-228, 2009.

James MT, Hemmelgarn BR, Tonelli M: Early recognition and prevention of chronic kidney disease, *Lancet* 375:1296-1309, 2010.

Johnson D: *The CARI Guidelines: Early Chronic Kidney Disease 2011, When to Refer for Specialist Renal Care.* Available. http://www.cari.org.au/DNT%20workshop%202011/6%20Specialist%20Renal%20Care_Early%20CKD_DNT.pdf Accessed December 8, 2011.

Levey AS, Coresh J: Chronic kidney disease, *Lancet* 379:165-180, 201210.1016/S0140-6736(11)60178-5. Epub August 12, 2012.

Levey AS, Coresh J, Balk E, et al: National Kidney Foundation practice guidelines for chronic kidney disease: evaluation, classification, and stratification, *Ann Intern Med* 139:137-147, 2003.

Levey AS, de Jong PE, Coresh J, et al: The definition, classification and prognosis of chronic kidney disease: a KDIGO Controversies Conference report, *Kidney Int* 80:17-28, 2011. Epub December 8, 2010; doi:10.1038/ki.2010.483.

Levey AS, Eckardt K, Tsukamoto Y, et al: Definition and classification of chronic kidney disease: a position statement from Kidney Disease: Improving Global Outcomes (KDIGO), *Kidney Int* 67:2089-2100, 2005.

Levey AS, Stevens LA, Coresh J: Conceptual model of CKD: applications and implications, *Am J Kidney Dis* 53:S4-S16, 2009.

Levey AS, Stevens LA, Schmid CH, et al: for the CKD-EPI (Chronic Kidney Disease Epidemiology Collaboration)A new equation to estimate glomerular filtration rate, *Ann Intern Med* 150:604-612, 2009.

Levin A, Hemmelgarn B, Culleton B, et al: Guidelines for the management of chronic kidney disease, *CMAJ* 179:1154-1162, 2008.

National Kidney Foundation: K/DOQI clinical practice guidelines for chronic kidney disease: evaluation, classification, and stratification, *Am J Kidney Dis* 39(2 Suppl 1):S1-S266, 2002.

National Kidney Foundation: K/DOQI clinical practice guidelines on hypertension and antihypertensive agents in chronic kidney disease, *Am J Kidney Dis* 43:S1-290, 2004.

Sarnak M, Levey A, Schoolwerth A, et al: Kidney disease as a risk factor for development of cardiovascular disease: a statement from the American Heart Association Councils on Kidney in Cardiovascular Disease, High Blood Pressure Research, Clinical Cardiology, and Epidemiology and Prevention, *Circulation* 42:1050-1065, 2003.

Uhlig K, Levey AS: Developing guidelines for chronic kidney disease: we should include all of the outcomes, *Ann Intern Med* 156:599-601, 2012.

Vassalotti JA, Stevens LA, Levey AS: Testing for chronic kidney disease: a position statement from the National Kidney Foundation, *Am J Kidney Dis* 50:169-180, 2007.

Nutrition and Kidney Disease

54

D. Jordi Goldstein-Fuchs | Amy Frances LaPierre

Nutrition assessment, monitoring, and intervention are critical components in caring for patients with chronic kidney disease (CKD). Reflecting altered metabolism, CKD stages 1 through 5 have distinct nutritional requirements warranting specific evaluation and treatment. In addition, individual patients have unique nutritional issues as a result of their metabolism, underlying kidney disease, CKD stage, genetics, and environment. This chapter reviews the nutritional issues associated with CKD and interventions currently recommended for optimizing nutrition and overall health, with a focus on individualized care.

PROTEIN AND CALORIES

Malnutrition, defined in this chapter as hypoalbuminemia and/or a body mass index of less than 18 kg/m^2, is common in people with CKD. The prevalence of mild to moderate malnutrition (serum albumin, 3.5 to 3.7 g/dL) ranges between 18% and 59% for dialysis patients. Approximately 8% to 37% of patients are severely malnourished (serum albumin, <2.5 g/dL). Factors contributing to malnutrition include anorexia, metabolic acidosis, protein and amino acid losses into dialysate, and comorbid illnesses. Ultimately, malnutrition and wasting may lead to loss of vigor, poor rehabilitation, poor quality of life, and death.

Protein requirements for adults receiving hemodialysis are affected by several factors related to the dialysis process itself, such as the type of dialyzer membrane (biocompatible or incompatible) and dialyzer reuse. Reported mean amino acid losses per hemodialysis session are 7.2 g when a traditional cellulose membrane is used, 6.1 g with a low-flux polymethylmethacrylate membrane, and 8.0 g with a high-flux polysulfone membrane. Patients receiving continuous ambulatory peritoneal dialysis (CAPD) lose approximately 5 to 12 g of total protein per day in addition to 2 to 4 g of free amino acids. Additional factors in determining protein requirements include alterations in amino acid metabolism and gut absorption. For example, loss of amino acids during hemodialysis is believed to alter the intracellular amino acid pools and affect protein metabolism. Metabolic acidosis, common in dialysis patients, also may induce muscle catabolism. These factors contribute to the higher protein requirement of dialysis patients; accordingly, the recommended dietary protein intake for dialysis patients is 1.2 to 1.3 g per kilogram of body weight per day.

The optimal dietary protein intake for patients with CKD stages 1 through 4 is controversial. The 2000 National Kidney Foundation Kidney Disease Outcomes Quality Initiative (NKF-KDOQI) Clinical Practice Guidelines for Nutrition in Chronic Renal Failure suggest that patients whose glomerular filtration rate (GFR) is between 25 and 55 mL/min/1.73 m^2 should eat at least 0.8 g of protein per kilogram body weight per day. Patients with a GFR less than 25 mL/min/1.73 m^2 and not receiving dialysis should target 0.6 g/kg/day. For patients with CKD stage 4 to 5 unable to tolerate this level of protein restriction, protein intake can be increased to 0.75 g/kg/day.

Although data on the optimal quantity of dietary protein for CKD patients are not defined, high protein intake is associated with glomerular hyperfiltration. This hyperfiltration may increase the rate of GFR loss. With general population trends suggesting that increasing protein intake to 25% to 30% of total calories facilitates weight management, it is possible that many individuals with CKD could be protein loading. Accordingly, when optimizing individual diet plans, nutrition education and assessment of diet intake are complicated. Important aspects of CKD care need to be integrated into the medical management plan.

Fifty percent of protein ingested by CKD patients should be of high biologic value (i.e., containing a high proportion of essential amino acids). The biologic value of a protein expresses the percentage of absorbed nitrogen that is retained by the body for growth and maintenance. If an adequate amount of high-biologic-value protein is not consumed, negative nitrogen balance may result in an increase in blood urea nitrogen (BUN) secondary to tissue catabolism. Intake of dietary protein above these recommendations can result in excess urea nitrogen generation and glomerular hyperfiltration.

A similar situation results when calorie intake is inadequate. Once protein requirements are met, carbohydrates and fats are needed to provide the remainder of the calorie requirement. Inadequate dietary intake of carbohydrates and fats leads to protein catabolism for energy and accumulation of nitrogenous wastes in the bloodstream. Calorie requirements of stable patients with CKD stages 1 through 4 who are consuming 0.8 g/kg/day of protein are thought to be comparable to those of normal healthy persons. Nitrogen balance becomes more positive as energy intake is increased. This is a beneficial effect, because adequate calorie intake allows protein to be used for protein catabolism rather than for energy. Therefore CKD patients on lower-protein diets are advised to consume more calories, up to 30 to 35 kcal/kg/day. Because many patients with advanced CKD may have inadequate protein intake, they can become malnourished by the time dialysis is started. Factors contributing to the incidence of malnutrition before initiation of kidney replacement therapy include hospitalizations and severity of comorbid complications. The daily caloric intake

Table 54.1   Daily Nutrient Recommendations for Patients With Chronic Kidney Disease Stages 1 Through 5

Nutrient	Stages 1-4	Hemodialysis	Peritoneal Dialysis
Protein	GFR >30 mL/min/1.73 m^2: ≥0.8 g/kg/day GFR 15-29 mL/min/1.73 m^2: 0.6-0.75 g/kg/day Nephrotic syndrome: 0.8-1.0 g/kg/day	≥1.2 g/kg/day with at least 50% HBV	≥1.2-1.3 g/kg/day with at least 50% HBV
Energy (if patient is <90% or >115% of median standard weight, use aBWef)	35-40 kcal/kg, depending on nutritional status and stress factors	≥60 year: 30-35 kcal/kg <60 year: 35 kcal/kg	≥60 year: 30-35 kcal/kg including dialysate calories <60 year: 35 kcal/kg including dialysate calories
Phosphorus	10-20 mg/g of protein or 600-800 mg/day	900 mg/day or <17 mg/kg/day	900 mg/day or <17 mg/kg/day
Sodium	Varies with cause of CKD; usually "no added salt" (i.e., 2-4 g/day)	2000-3000 mg/day (88-130 mmol/day)	Individualized based on physical examination; in CAPD and APD, 3000-4000 mg/day (130-175 mmol/day)
Potassium	Usually not restricted until GFR is <10 mL/min/1.73 m^2	40 mg/kg or approximately 2000-3000 mg/day (50-80 mmol/day)	Generally unrestricted with CAPD and APD: approximately 3000-4000 mg/day (80-105 mmol/day) unless serum level is increased or decreased
Fluid	As indicated by clinical status	500-1000 mL/day plus daily urine output	In CAPD and APD, approximately 2000-3000 mL/day based on clinical status; unrestricted if weight and blood pressure are controlled and residual kidney function is 2-3 L/day
Calcium	800 mg/day or as needed to maintain goal serum levels	Same as for CKD stages 1-4	Same as for CKD stages 1-4
Vitamins and minerals	RDA for vitamin B complex and C; individualize zinc, iron, calcium, and vitamin D	Vitamin C, 60-100 mg; vitamin B$_6$, 5-10 mg; folic acid, 0.8-1 mg; DRI for others; individualize zinc, calcium, iron, and vitamin D	Same as for hemodialysis

aBWef, Adjusted edema-free body weight; *APD,* automated peritoneal dialysis; *CAPD,* continuous ambulatory peritoneal dialysis; *CKD,* chronic kidney disease; *DRI,* dietary reference intake; *GFR,* glomerular filtration rate; *HBV,* high biologic value; *NAS,* no added salt; *RDA,* recommended dietary allowance.

recommended for CKD stage 5 is 35 kcal/kg of ideal body weight for individuals younger than 60 years of age and 30 to 35 kcal/kg for those 60 years or older. Exceptions are obese (>120% of ideal body weight) and malnourished persons, with the latter group requiring more calories for repletion. Table 54.1 summarizes nutrient recommendations for stable adult patients with CKD stages 1 through 5.

Critically, both overweight status and obesity are significant risk factors for CKD, defined by both albuminuria and/or reduced glomerular filtration rate. Accordingly, lifestyle modifications with a focus on diet and exercise likely have a major role in CKD prevention and treatment (Fig. 54.1).

ALTERED NUTRIENT REQUIREMENTS

SODIUM AND WATER

Healthy kidneys maintain sodium balance by adjusting sodium excretion in response to dietary intake. Until late stages of CKD, an adaptive mechanism permits continued sodium excretion and maintenance of balance. The remaining nephrons excrete a higher percentage of filtered sodium, with the effect being decreased fractional reabsorption of

sodium by the renal tubules and increased fractional excretion. Although the decision to implement dietary sodium restriction depends on the individual patient's fluid status, urinary sodium excretion, and the presence or absence of hypertension, because of the beneficial effects of a lower sodium intake on overall cardiovascular health, dietary sodium restriction is more commonly initiated during earlier stages of disease than has been in the past. The current recommendation for advanced CKD is to ideally lower intake to 1500 mg per day.

During kidney replacement therapy, urine output continues to decline, with most patients eventually becoming anuric. Accordingly, fluid intake must be controlled and individually prescribed. Balance of both sodium and water is maintained by matching dietary intake to the removal by dialysis plus any losses incurred via residual kidney function. Concurrent medications, particularly diuretics, also may play a role on overall sodium and fluid balance.

POTASSIUM

As GFR declines, the ability of the tubules to secrete potassium decreases. Nephron adaptation occurs to maintain potassium balance by increasing the amount secreted by the

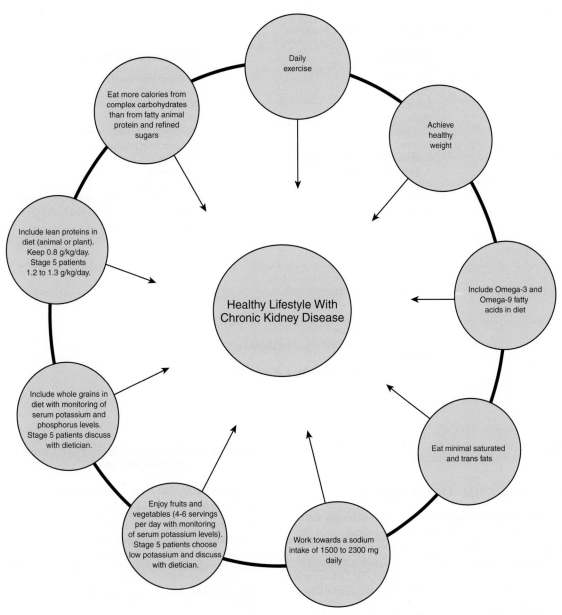

Figure 54.1   Healthy nutrition and lifestyle concepts for patients with chronic kidney disease stages 1 through 5.

remaining tubules, with systemic compensation reflected in increased stool and sweat potassium content. As much as 20% to 50% of ingested potassium can appear in the stool when the GFR is less than 5 mL/min/1.73m². These two adaptations are sufficient to maintain potassium balance with normal potassium intake (100 mEq/day, or 3.9 g/day) if the GFR is greater than 10 mL/min/1.73 m² and the urine output is at least 1000 mL/day. At lower GFR levels, potassium restriction is necessary to maintain serum levels in the normal range of 3.5 to 5.0 mEq/L. Medications will also influence overall potassium balance: ACE inhibitors, angiotensin receptor blockers, and aldosterone receptor blockers routinely prescribed for hypertensive patients with kidney disease or cardiovascular disease can potentiate hyperkalemia as kidney disease progresses, even affecting potassium levels in dialysis patients.

Dietary potassium restriction for hemodialysis patients is required to avoid hyperkalemia. Potassium accumulates in the body between dialysis treatments unless the patient has adequate gastrointestinal or urinary losses. Hyperkalemia results from eating potassium-dense foods or potassium supplements, or it can be secondary to catabolism, hemolysis, or acidemia. Table 54.2 identifies a variety of high-potassium foods. When counseling patients about intake of potassium or other dietary components, it is important to use educational materials that have been modified to incorporate culturally specific foods.

The recommended potassium intake for hemodialysis patients is 51 to 77 mEq/day (2 to 3 g/day). Patients performing peritoneal dialysis therapy can tolerate a more liberal dietary intake of potassium (77 to 102 mEq/day, or 3 to 4 g/day) or, in some cases, an unrestricted intake. Potassium requirements in CKD stages 1 through 4 are based on the individual's disease, metabolism, serum potassium levels, and medications. Patients with type 4 renal tubular acidosis and those receiving drugs that interfere with the

Table 54.2   Foods Containing High Levels of Potassium

Fruits	Vegetables	Beverages and Other Foods
Apricots	Artichokes	Bran and bran products
Avocado	Beans, dried	Chocolate
Banana	Broccoli	Coconut
Cantaloupe	Brussels sprouts	Granola
Casaba melon	Escarole	Low-sodium baking powder or soda
Dried fruits (dates, figs, raisins, prunes)	Endive	Milk and milk products (ice cream, yogurt—2 cups)
Honeydew	Greens (Swiss chard, collard, beet, dandelion, mustard)	Molasses
Mango	Kale	Nuts/seeds
Nectarine	Kohlrabi	Peanut butter
Orange	Lentils	Salt substitute or "lite" salt (containing potassium)
Papaya	Legumes	Potassium chloride—DO NOT USE
Rhubarb	Lima beans	Snuff/chewing tobacco
Juice of fruits listed	Mushrooms	
Tangelo	Parsnips	
Watermelon	Potatoes (french fries, chips, baked, mashed, boiled, sweet potatoes, yams)	
	Pumpkin	
	Rutabaga	
	Spinach, Swiss chard	
	Salt-free vegetable juice (ALL vegetable juices)	
	Tomatoes	
	Winter squash (acorn, butternut, Hubbard)	

renin-angiotensin-aldosterone system may need more rigorous potassium restriction to avoid hyperkalemia.

PHOSPHORUS, CALCIUM, AND VITAMIN D

The kidney filters approximately 7 g of phosphorus daily, of which 80% to 90% is reabsorbed by the tubules and the remainder excreted in the urine. In early stages of CKD, hyperphosphatemia is prevented by an adaptive decrease in tubular phosphate resorption. Not until the GFR falls to less than 20 mL/min does hyperphosphatemia usually become clinically evident.

As CKD progresses, the damaged kidneys are unable to respond to parathyroid hormone (PTH) or phosphatonins to increase phosphorus excretion. Serum phosphorus levels rise, and dietary restriction becomes necessary. Dietary phosphorus restriction to 800 to 1000 mg/day, or 17 mg/kg of body weight per day, is commonly recommended. Tables 54.3 and 54.4 provide examples of foods that are high in phosphorus content.

Although dietary phosphate is present in highest concentration in animal proteins and dairy products, phosphorus additives also add significantly to dietary phosphate burden. Phosphorus additives aid in water-holding capacity, increase pH to slow discoloration of meats, reduce cooking losses, retard oxidative rancidity, aid microbial protection, and enhance textural properties. Manufacturers are not required to list the phosphorus content on food labels, and the phosphorus load of additives does not show up on nutrient databases used to analyze the macro- and micronutrients of foods, unlike naturally occurring phosphorus. However, the International Food Additives Council provides a "Phosphates Use in Foods" table

Table 54.3   Foods Containing High Levels of Phosphorus

Legumes, Nuts and Seeds, Whole Grains	Meat and Other Foods	Dairy and Beverages
Beans (navy, kidney, lima, pinto)	Chocolate	Beer
Soybeans	Dried fruit	Colas: Coke, Pepsi, Dr. Pepper
Black-eyed peas	Molasses	Eggnog
Lentils	Beef liver, calf liver	Hot chocolate
Peanut butter	Liver sausage	Milk
Nuts	Liverwurst	Casseroles
Coconuts	Beef, bottom round	Cheese
Pumpkin seeds	Pork, fresh	Cream soups
Sunflower seeds	Veal, cubes, rib roast	Custard
Bran, bran flakes, bran muffins		Ice cream
Brown rice		Pudding
Wheat germ		Yogurt
Raisin bran, 100% bran		
100% whole grain		

(http://www.foodadditives.org/phosphates/phosphates_used_in_food.html), identifying the specific ingredient providing additional phosphorus.

Because of the ubiquitous nature of dietary phosphate, dietary restriction alone typically is not sufficient to maintain normal serum levels. Phosphate-binding medications (e.g., calcium salts, sevelamer, lanthanum carbonate), which bind to dietary phosphorus and prevent its absorption in

Table 54.4   Hidden Sources of Phosphorus and Alternatives*

Hidden Sources of Phosphorus	Suggested Alternatives
Disodium phosphate	Use fresh meat products.
Monosodium phosphate	Use natural (not processed)
Sodium hexametaphosphate	cheeses, in very small amounts.
	Prepare pancakes, waffles,
Potassium tripolyphosphate	biscuits, and breads from raw ingredients, not ready-made
Trisodium triphosphate	mixes with unknown contents.
Sodium tripolyphosphate	Limit the obvious sources of
Tetrasodium pyrophosphate	phosphorus, such as dairy foods, colas, beans, nuts,
Phosphoric acid	and chocolate.

*It is important for both patients and clinicians to be familiar with the hidden sources of phosphorus in food products that are not typically identified on the nutrient food label. This table lists some forms of phosphorus that are included in the ingredient lists of many foods, as well as some suggestions for limiting the intake of foods that contain them.

the gastrointestinal tract, are frequently required. For a discussion of vitamin D and secondary hyperparathyroidism, see Chapter 55.

WATER AND FAT-SOLUBLE VITAMINS

Adult dialysis patients usually have low blood levels of water-soluble vitamins unless they take a vitamin supplement. Causes include losses into the dialysate, restrictive diets, anorexia and reduced food intake, and alterations in metabolism. Accordingly, supplementation is indicated. Specifically, higher daily doses of pyridoxine (B_6, 10 mg), folate (0.8-1 mg), and ascorbic acid (60 mg) are recommended for dialysis patients. The same amounts are recommended for patients in earlier stages of CKD, except that 5 mg of vitamin B_6 is recommended. The increased vitamin B_6 requirement for dialysis patients is evidenced by low plasma and red blood cell pyridoxine levels and low plasma levels of the vitamin's coenzyme, pyridoxine phosphate.

Identification and treatment of nutritional vitamin D [25(OH)D] deficiency is suggested by many providers. The incidence of vitamin D deficiency in CKD patients has been reported to be as high as 59%. Serum levels of 25(OH)D can be checked and patients supplemented when levels are found to be below 32 ng/mL. Supplementation dose is dependent on the whether insufficiency or deficiency exists. Serum levels should be monitored every 6 months, or more frequently in supplemented patients, to ensure both repletion as well as avoidance of toxicity.

Vitamin A and retinol-binding protein are normally cleared by the kidneys, and therefore may accumulate as kidney function deteriorates. Vitamin A supplementation should be avoided to prevent vitamin A toxicity. Vitamin K replacement is not indicated unless intestinal flora are suppressed by antibiotic therapy. Vitamin E supplementation has not been shown to be beneficial. Special vitamin

supplements for dialysis patients that meet these requirements are available over the counter or by prescription.

MINERALS AND TRACE ELEMENTS

The dietary requirements for trace elements are not known, and with the exception of iron, supplementation is not usually recommended. Adequacy of diet, medications, and the nutritional and medical status of patients with any stage of CKD determine the need for supplementation of minerals.

Hypermagnesemia may be present because magnesium is primarily excreted by the kidneys under normal circumstances. As the "renal diet" tends to contain less magnesium than a typical American diet, active restriction of dietary magnesium is usually not necessary to maintain normal serum levels. Hypermagnesemia has been induced by ingestion of magnesium-containing antacids, enemas, and laxatives. Hypomagnesemia can also occur, particularly in patients treated with immunosuppressants following transplantation, or who have had inadequate intake from anorexia or increased gastrointestinal losses.

The requirement for iron is affected by intake, dialysis-induced blood losses, frequency of laboratory testing, impaired intestinal iron absorption, and occult gastrointestinal bleeding. All of these factors are likely to cause iron deficiency anemia. Monitoring iron status and the treatment of iron deficiency is discussed in detail in Chapter 57. For patients with CKD stages 1 through 4 who may require oral iron therapy, ferrous gluconate, ferrous fumarate, or ferrous sulfate may be recommended. Ferrous gluconate contains 12% elemental iron, ferrous fumarate 33%, and ferrous sulfate 20%. Ferrous gluconate is often better tolerated. Maximal absorption occurs if the iron supplements are taken on an empty stomach, but individuals who experience gastric upset may take them with food. Tea, coffee, milk, cereals, dietary fiber, eggs, and antacids should not be taken with iron, because they impair absorption. Intestinal iron absorption is enhanced if iron is taken with vitamin C (200 mg vitamin C or more per 30 mg of elemental iron).

Low plasma zinc levels observed in dialysis patients may be the result of dietary restriction of protein, impaired zinc absorption, redistribution of the body pool of zinc, or a decrease in zinc binding to plasma protein. Uremic symptoms of hypogeusia, sexual impotence, and anorexia have been reported to improve after subjects were given zinc supplementation in clinical trials, but routine zinc replacement is not usually prescribed. The effects of aluminum retention are a concern for dialysis patients. Accumulation of aluminum in cerebral gray matter may be responsible for the dialysis encephalopathy syndrome. Aluminum also may accumulate in bone, possibly contributing to bone disease. These problems have largely disappeared since the routine use of aluminum-containing phosphate binders was abandoned. Nonetheless, chronic use of medications containing aluminum should be avoided in patients with advanced CKD or end-stage renal disease.

CARNITINE

L-Carnitine (1-3-hydroxy-4-*N*-trimethylaminobutyrate) is an amino acid whose main function is to transfer long-chain fatty acids from the cytoplasm through the inner membrane of the mitochondria for oxidation. Carnitine deficiency can result in inefficient energy production and impaired oxidation of long-chain fatty acids. The high prevalence of cardiomyopathy, skeletal myopathy, dyslipidemia, and erythropoietin resistance that characterizes the dialysis population has prompted evaluation of carnitine deficiency. Routine L-carnitine therapy is not currently recommended because of the lack of consistent data demonstrating improvement in clinical outcomes. Carnitine supplementation may be indicated for patients who present with muscle weakness and fatigue associated with low plasma carnitine levels for which no other cause can be identified.

NUTRITION ASSESSMENT AND MANAGEMENT OF CHRONIC KIDNEY DISEASE

Current nutrition assessment and management in adult dialysis patients relies on analysis of biochemical parameters as reflected by blood indices, including BUN, creatinine, total protein, albumin, potassium, phosphorus, calcium, sodium, cholesterol, triglycerides, glucose, and alkaline phosphatase, many of which are measured monthly. Other important elements of the nutrition assessment include anthropometric measurements, physical and clinical evaluations, and food intake information. These data, in the context of a patient's previous values and trends, are incorporated with the patient's estimated dry weight (i.e., the weight at which the patient is free of detectable peripheral edema and has normal blood pressure without postural hypotension), interdialytic fluid weight gains, and blood pressure measurements to evaluate nutrition and fluid status.

BLOOD UREA NITROGEN

Dietary protein intake and the predialysis BUN concentration are highly correlated when patients are clinically stable; accordingly, BUN can be used to indirectly monitor the patient's protein intake. Optimal BUN values for adult dialysis patients are in the range of 60 to 80 mg/dL, whereas values above 100 mg/dL suggest excessive dietary protein intake, inadequate dialysis, catabolism, or gastrointestinal bleeding. Values below 60 mg/dL suggest inadequate protein intake, anabolism, residual kidney function, or intense dialysis. Because the BUN is dependent on factors in addition to dietary protein intake, laboratory and clinical parameters should be considered in conjunction with BUN for nutrition management.

Decreases in serum albumin concentration and dry weight are important indicators of nutritional status, but there may be a lag of a few months between a compromised protein intake and these changes. The determination of protein intake can provide an earlier clue. One of the methods of assessing protein intake is the normalized protein catabolic rate (nPCR). In CKD stages 1 through 4, the nPCR is calculated by multiplying the BUN by the rate of urea nitrogen generation in milligrams per minute (equivalent to total body water) and adding urinary urea nitrogen. For CKD stage 5, nPCR is derived from predialysis and postdialysis BUN levels, since urinary urea nitrogen values are

not typically available. This calculation assumes that the urea generation rate can be used to estimate nPCR because urea is the primary product of protein catabolism. It also assumes that nPCR equals dietary protein intake when the patient is in nitrogen balance. The desired range of nPCR for chronic dialysis patients—hence the necessary dietary protein intake—is 1.2 to 1.3 g/kg of dry body weight. If a patient is catabolic (as evidenced by weight loss, decreased serum albumin, or onset of medical illness), the nPCR is greater than dietary protein intake, whereas an anabolic patient's nPCR is less than protein intake.

Protein balance can be calculated from the difference between dietary protein intake and nPCR. This method is best used to monitor nitrogen balance of noncatabolic patients because catabolized protein can be both exogenous (i.e., derived from the diet) and endogenous. The nPCR should be incorporated into the nutrition assessment procedure for all stages of CKD. For CKD stages 1 through 4, nitrogen balance should be determined if a patient presents with a deleterious change in nutritional status or appetite (e.g., hypoalbuminemia, weight loss). In hemodialysis, nPCR should be determined as part of the monthly Kt/V calculation.

SERUM PROTEINS

Levels of serum total protein, transferrin, albumin, and prealbumin are all commonly used for nutrition assessment of visceral protein stores. In patients with CKD of any stage, the reliability of these parameters for nutritional status is questionable because of the metabolic and fluid derangements associated with the uremic state. All serum protein levels are affected by hydration status. Of these three serum proteins, albumin is most often used to assess visceral stores, likely reflecting the wide availability of the albumin assay and the association between albumin and clinical outcomes (although this association may be mediated by non-nutritional factors). A twofold increase in the relative risk for death has been reported for hemodialysis patients with serum albumin levels between 3.5 to 4.0 g/dL, compared with those with levels of 4.0 to 4.5 g/dL, whereas patients with serum albumin concentration of 2.5 g/dL may be at 20-fold higher risk for death. Serum albumin has a long half-life (18 to 20 days) and is often a late marker of malnutrition. However, low serum albumin levels are often accompanied by abnormal levels of other indices that reflect malnutrition (e.g., anthropometrics, total lymphocyte count, ferritin), and usually indicate a state of poor nutrition These other markers are influenced by factors such as fluid balance, iron status, and anemia so that no one marker can be relied upon to assess nutritional status, and a panel of indices reflecting the various compartments is required to complete a nutrition assessment. In addition, non-nutritional factors, including inflammation, affect serum albumin metabolism in patients with CKD. In states of inflammation, hepatic synthesis of C-reactive protein and other positive acute-phase reactant proteins is prioritized over albumin synthesis. Hence, albumin is a negative acute-phase reactive protein, and serum levels fall as a result of reduced hepatic albumin synthesis.

Serum prealbumin has a shorter half-life (2 days) than albumin and, for this reason, has been considered to be a more sensitive nutritional measure. Although it may be falsely elevated in CKD because of decreased renal catabolism, prealbumin levels lower than 30 mg/dL in dialysis patients are associated with increased mortality. In addition, because prealbumin has been directly correlated with changes in nutritional status, it can be useful for longitudinal monitoring of a patient with stable kidney function.

Insulin-like growth factor-1 (IGF-1), a serum protein with mitogenic properties and insulin-like activities, may be a sensitive biochemical indicator of nitrogen balance. A serum IGF-1 concentration below 200 ng/mL likely indicates poor nutritional status. Moreover, current research suggests that treatment with recombinant human IGF-1 may induce an anabolic response in malnourished dialysis patients. Additional research is needed before definitive recommendations can be offered in regard to IGF-1 supplementation.

SODIUM, POTASSIUM, PHOSPHORUS, AND CALCIUM

Serum chemistries are typically monitored monthly in chronic hemodialysis patients. The nonserum parameters, such as interdialytic weight gain and pre- and postdialysis blood pressure, are recorded at each dialysis treatment. Causes of fluctuations in these values must be determined and discussed with the patient in relation to potential nutritional interventions. Disorders of calcium and phosphorus are discussed in detail in Chapter 11, and the approach to mineral and bone disorder, including binder, vitamin D analogue, and calcimimetic use, is discussed in Chapter 55.

LIPIDS

Although they are difficult to achieve, normal cholesterol and triglyceride values are the goal for nondialysis CKD patients. Whereas total fat intake as a percentage of calories is important, the fatty acid composition of dietary fat also plays a role in prevention of cardiovascular disease (CVD). Saturated and trans fatty acids are known to modify serum lipoprotein patterns toward those associated with higher CVD risk (i.e., elevated total cholesterol, low-density lipoproteins, and triglycerides, plus reduced high-density lipoproteins). The exact percentage of calories that should be obtained from carbohydrates and fats varies according to nutritional status, level of kidney function, and presence of comorbid conditions (e.g., diabetes) in an individual patient. In general, however, the recommendation for CKD patients is to keep fat calories to less than 30% of total calories. This is similar to the recommendation for the general population.

However, it is not just quantity of fat that is important to the diet intake, but quality of fat as well. Both omega-3 (n-3) and omega-9 (n-9) fatty acids have been demonstrated to be beneficial in regards to improving lipid profiles and ameliorating proinflammatory mechanisms of injury associated with chronic diseases, including CVD. This latter mechanism pertains particularly to the n-3 polyunsaturated fatty acids (PUFAs), which exert antithrombotic, antiproliferative, and antiaggregatory platelet effects. The major n-3 PUFAs are eicosapentaenoic acid (EPA), docosapentaenoic acid (DPA), and docosahexaenoic acid (DHA).

Large randomized interventional trials have reported reductions in sudden cardiac death with n-3 supplementation

Table 54.5 Potassium and Phosphorus Content in Dietary Sources of n-3 PUFA

Food Source	Omega 3 (mg per 3- to 4-ounce serving)	Phosphorus (mg)	Potassium (mg)
Seafood			
Canned tuna	170-240 mg	130	202
Cod	150-240 mg	293	246
Scallops	180-340 mg	362	267
Clams	250 mg	168	39
Shrimp	290 mg	207	96
Crab	270-400 mg	155	301
Pollock	450 mg	188	303
Flounder or sole	480 mg	214	136
Lake trout	600 mg	230	409
Salmon	1100 mg	170	416
Albacore tuna	1600 mg	283	448
Herring	1700 mg	201	278
Sardines	1800 mg	417	338
Mackerel	2200 mg	184	267
Oils			
Olive	100 mg	*	*
Soybean	900 mg	*	*
Canola	1300 mg	*	*
Walnut	1400 mg	*	*
Cod liver oil	2800 mg	*	*
Flaxseed	6900 mg	*	*
Other Sources			
Tofu	300 mg in 4 ounces	76	165
Soybeans	500 mg in ½ cup	248	794
Flaxseeds	1800 mg in 1 ounce	647	820
Walnuts	2600 mg in 1 ounce	98	125

*Negligible.

in the general population. Some studies show improvement in hypertension in CKD patients ingesting diets enriched in n-3 PUFAs; early findings suggest that they improve patency of hemodialysis vascular access. The KDOQI Clinical Practice Guidelines for Cardiovascular Disease in Dialysis Patient recommends further research to identify n-3 PUFA supplementation guidelines, but given the promising preliminary evidence of its benefits, it is a therapeutic option that is easily integrated into a patient's diet. The doses described below can be considered safe in CKD patients:

- For patients without documented coronary heart disease (CHD), eat a variety of fatty fish at least twice weekly.
- For patients with documented CHD, consume about 1 gram of EPA+DHA daily, preferably from fatty fish. Fish oil in capsule form can also be considered.

It is important to be aware of the potassium and phosphorus content of the dietary sources of n-3 PUFA. Table 54.5

identifies foods high in omega-3 fatty acids, and includes the potassium and phosphorus content of these foods.

For those individuals who do not tolerate dietary fish or oral omega-3 fatty acid supplements, a reasonable opinion-based recommendation included in the KDOQI Clinical Guidelines for Diabetes and CKD is to distribute the percentage of fat calories as follows: 10% omega-3 fatty acids, 10% omega-9 fatty acids, 5% omega-6 fatty acids, and 5% saturated fatty acids. This would translate into a diet that used fats predominantly derived from canola and olive oils, with minimal use of butter, lard, and other vegetable oils.

GLUCOSE

Abnormal carbohydrate metabolism is frequently observed in CKD patients, especially those with infection, peripheral insulin resistance, and late-stage CKD. This contrasts with lower insulin or sulfonylurea dosages required in late-stage CKD, reflecting decreased insulin clearance by the kidneys. Therefore close monitoring of blood glucose, insulin requirements, and diet is necessary in all stages of CKD. Glycemic control is further discussed in Chapter 25.

Patients undergoing peritoneal dialysis may develop glucose intolerance and gain weight due to glucose absorbed from the dialysate. Calculation of energy requirements for peritoneal dialysis patients must take into consideration the amount of glucose absorbed during the procedure (see Chapter 59). To estimate the amount of calories obtained from the dialysis procedure, the total grams of dextrose used over 24 hours is multiplied by 3.4 kcal/g (or 3.7 kcal/g for anhydrous dextrose). This result is then multiplied by the estimated absorption rate of 70%. For example, if a patient uses one 2-liter bag of 1.5% dextrose, one 2-liter bag of 4.25% dextrose, and one 2-liter bag of 2.5% dextrose in 24 hours, the total grams of dextrose used is 30 + 85 + 50 = 165 g. The amount of calories absorbed from the dialysate is then calculated as follows: 165 g × 3.4 kcal/g × 70% = 393 kcal absorbed.

ANTHROPOMETRY

Anthropometry includes measurements of body weight (estimated dry weight for dialysis patients), height, triceps skinfold, abdominal circumference, calf circumference, midarm muscle circumference, elbow breadth, and subscapular skinfold. These values provide information about the distribution of body fat and skeletal muscle mass, and over time, identify nutritional deficiencies or excesses in calorie and protein reserves compared with standardized percentiles. One of the problems with using anthropometric measurements to assess the nutrition status in CKD is that reference values are derived from healthy individuals. This is a potential pitfall given the known alterations in body composition associated with uremia and the presence of edema. Anthropometry is usually performed on the nondominant arm, but in hemodialysis patients the dominant arm is used if the contralateral arm has a vascular access in place. To minimize the interference of edema, measurements should be made during the last hour of dialysis. For routine care, anthropometric measurements are recommended every 3 to 6 months.

Neck circumference, reflecting upper body subcutaneous fat, is another anthropometric measurement that is receiving increasing attention because of its association with cardiovascular risk. The utility of this measurement in CKD populations is currently being evaluated. Other methods of assessing body composition include dual-energy x-ray absorptiometry (DEXA) and bioelectrical impedance. These techniques are accurate, but at present their use is limited to research purposes because of equipment availability, radiation dose, patient acceptance, and cost.

PHYSICAL AND CLINICAL EVALUATION

Wasting syndrome, a protein-calorie malnutrition state that is prevalent in the dialysis population, is sometimes seen in earlier CKD stages as well. It is characterized by decreased relative body weight (patient's body weight divided by "normal weight" for the same age range, height, gender, and skeletal frame size), skinfold thickness (adipose store), arm muscle mass, and total body nitrogen, as well as signs of macronutrient and micronutrient deficiencies (e.g., hair loss; dry, flaky skin).

Another method used to assess protein-energy status is subjective global assessment (SGA). SGA requires evaluation of subjective and objective patient information, including the medical history and physical examination. Based on this evaluation, patients are classified into various nutritional status categories ranging from well-nourished to severely malnourished. This technique was originally devised for nutrition assessment of general surgery patients, but it has been validated for use in peritoneal dialysis patients as well. KDOQI recommended the SGA as part of routine nutrition monitoring.

PATIENT-REPORTED FOOD INTAKE

Obtaining patient-reported food intake is an important component of the nutritional care of patients with CKD. In addition to providing the opportunity to quantify food intake, food records reveal sources of problems related to food intake and tolerance, food habits, patterns, and allergies. The interactive nature of reported food intake provides the dietitian with an opportunity to establish rapport with each patient. All of this information can be used to formulate an individual meal plan to help patients meet their nutritional needs. Reported food intake can be obtained in the form of a 24-hour recall, a multiple-day food record, diet history (retrospective general review of usual intake), or food frequency (how often foods from each food group are eaten and which specific foods within each group are included in the diet). The optimal method remains unknown because these have not been widely studied in the CKD patient population. Recently, a Food Frequency Questionnaire was found useful in evaluating the dietary intake of a cohort of hemodialysis patients.

Regardless of the reporting method, data should include current nutrient intake, factors that affect intake (e.g., difficulty chewing or swallowing, other physical impediments to adequate intake, nausea, vomiting, diarrhea, allergies), current medications, food preferences, cultural influences, meal patterns, meals eaten away from home, and portion sizes. Fluid intake, including solid foods with high water content, should be reported in the same detail. Whenever possible, diet information should be collected directly from the patient. Otherwise, family members or caregivers may be interviewed.

INTRADIALYTIC NUTRITION SUPPORT

In addition to nutritionally supporting patients with acute illnesses, intravenous or intraperitoneal nutrition is sometimes used as an intervention for malnutrition in patients receiving maintenance dialysis. For hemodialysis patients, intravenous amino acids, carbohydrates, and fats are infused directly into the venous drip chamber of the hemodialysis circuit during treatment. This therapy is referred to as intradialytic parenteral nutrition (IDPN). The formulations utilized are lower in dextrose concentration and do not include fatty acids. In peritoneal dialysis, a bag of dextrose dialysate is fortified with an amino acid solution and can be given as a final fill for CCPD patients and drained after a 4- to 6-hour dwell. It can also be administered as a 4- to 6-hour dwell for CAPD patients (see Chapter 59). This approach is termed intraperitoneal nutrition (IPN).

The benefit of both IDPN and IPN therapy as an intervention for malnutrition and hypoalbuminemia is uncertain, and insurance coverage for IDPN and IPN is sporadic. Currently, Medicare Part D and broader commercial insurance plans will pay for IDPN/IPN therapy in accordance with the following criteria:

Protein Malnutrition
- Patient given intensive dietary counseling, emphasizing need for increased protein and/or calorie intake, for a minimum of 1 month with no evidence of clinical improvement (i.e., rise in serum albumin and/or weight)
- Initiation of oral supplementation attempted with no improvement in albumin levels and/or weight gain after 1 to 2 months
- Average serum albumin <3.5 g/dL for 3 months
- Progressive decline in serum albumin to <3.5g/dL over 3 months
- nPCR <0.8 or documentation of inadequate protein intake

Calorie Malnutrition
- Current weight <90% of IBW/DBW
- BMI <18
- Weight loss >5% over 3 months

Whether or not IDPN and IPN therapies confer nutritional and overall benefit to dialysis patients requires randomized clinical trials. The same is true in regard to the role of oral nutrition supplementation during hemodialysis treatments.

DIET AND NUTRITION FOR CHRONIC KIDNEY DISEASE

The 2010 Guidelines for Americans include recommendations that target risk reduction for cardiovascular disease. Can these be applied to the CKD population? The guidelines include recommendations to decrease overweight and obesity and to include fruits, vegetables, whole grains, low-fat dairy, lean protein foods, and vegetable oils while limiting saturated fatty acids, trans-fatty acids, cholesterol, excess sugars, sodium, and refined grains. With an emphasis on reducing cardiovascular risk, it is prudent to apply these healthy lifestyle guidelines (which also incorporate achieving a healthy weight and participating in physical exercise) to CKD patients. Monitoring for hyperkalemia and hyperphosphatemia should be included, with diet modified if needed. For CKD stages 1 through 4, medications can also be adjusted to help accomplish nutrition goals while potentially reducing risk for kidney disease progression. Figure 54.1 demonstrates nutrition concepts that can be applied to patients with CKD in an individualized manner by the nephrology dietitian. The keys to successful nutrition management are education, individualized application, and monitoring.

BIBLIOGRAPHY

American Heart Association: *Fish 101*. Available at http://www.heart.org/HEARTORG/GettingHealthy/NutritionCenter/Fish-101_UCM_305986_Article.jsp. Accessed February 19, 2012.

Beddhu S, Cheung AK, Larive B, et al: Hemodialysis (HEMO) Study Group: inflammation and inverse associations of body mass index and serum creatinine with mortality in hemodialysis patients, *J Ren Nutr* 17:372-380, 2007.

Bossola M, Tazza L, Giungi S, et al: Artificial nutritional support in chronic hemodialysis patients: a narrative review, *J Ren Nutr* 20:213-223, 2010.

Cuppari L, Garcia-Lopes MG: Hypovitaminosis D in chronic kidney disease patients: prevalence and treatment, *J Ren Nutr* 19:38-43, 2009.

Flock MR, Kris-Etherton PM: Dietary guidelines for Americans 2010: implications for cardiovascular disease, *Curr Atheroscler Rep* 13:499–507.

Friedman A: Omega-3 fatty acid supplementation in advanced kidney disease, *Sem Dialysis* 20:396-400, 2010.

Hingorjo MR, Qureshi MA, Mehdi A: Neck circumference as a useful marker of obesity: a comparison with body mass index and waist circumference, *J Pak Med Assoc* 62:36-40, 2012. Jan.

Ikizler A: Effects of hemodialysis on protein metabolism, *J Ren Nutr* 15:39-43, 2005.

Moe SM, Zidehsarai MP, Chambers MA, et al: Vegetarian compared with meat dietary protein source and phosphorus homeostasis in chronic kidney disease, *Clin J Am Soc Nephrol* 6:257-264, 2011.

National Kidney Foundation: NKF-K/DOQI clinical practice guidelines for nutrition in chronic renal failure, *Am J Kidney Dis* 35(Suppl 2):S1-S140, 2000.

National Kidney Foundation: NKF-K/DOQI clinical practice guidelines for chronic kidney disease: evaluation, classification, and stratification, *Am J Kidney Dis* 39(Suppl 1):S1-S266, 2002.

National Kidney Foundation Kidney Disease Outcomes Quality Initiative: Clinical practice guidelines for cardiovascular disease in dialysis patients. State of the science: novel and controversial topics in cardiovascular diseases, *Am J Kidney Dis* 45(Suppl 3):S90-S97, 2005.

National Kidney Foundation Kidney Disease Outcomes Quality Initiative: Clinical practice guide and clinical practice recommendations for diabetes and chronic kidney disease, *Am J Kidney Dis* 49(Suppl 2):S12-S154, 2007.

Navaneethan SD, Kirwan JP, Arrigain S, et al: Overweight, obesity and intentional weight loss in chronic kidney disease: NHANES, *Int J Obes (Lond)* 36:1585-1590, 1999-2006.

Nigwekar SU, Bhan I, Thadhani R: Ergocalciferol and cholecalciferol in CKD, *Am J Kidney Dis* 60:139-156, 2012.

Pentec Health: *Clinical criteria for IDPN and IPN*. Available, http://www.pentechealth.com/product_rns_criteria.html. Accessed February 19, 2012.

Presi SR, Massaro JM, Hoffmann U, et al: Neck circumference as a novel measure of cardiometaoblic risk: the Framingham Heart Study, *J Clin Endocrinol Metab* 95:3701-3710, 2010.

Sigrist M, Levin A, Tejani AMJ: Systematic review of evidence for the use of intradialytic parenteral nutrition in malnourished hemodialysis patients, *J Ren Nutr* 20:1-7, 2010.

Tanner RM, Brown TM, Muntner P: Epidemiology of obesity, the metabolic syndrome, and chronic kidney disease, *Curr Hypertens Rep* 14:152-159, 2012.

Tareen N, Partins D, Zadshir A, et al: The impact of routine vitamin supplementation on serum levels of 25 (OH) D3 among the general adult population and patients with chronic kidney disease, *Ethn Dis* 15(4 Suppl 5):102-106, 2005.

55 Bone Disorders in Chronic Kidney Disease

L. Darryl Quarles

Chronic kidney disease (CKD) alters the regulation of calcium, phosphate, and vitamin D homeostasis, leading to secondary hyperparathyroidism, elevations in serum fibroblast growth factor 23 (FGF23), metabolic bone disease, soft-tissue calcifications, and other metabolic derangements that have a significant impact on morbidity and mortality. Although metabolic bone disease, reductions in circulating $1,25(OH)_2$ vitamin D, hyperphosphatemia, hypocalcemia, and abnormalities of parathyroid function are historically the main clinical manifestations of disordered mineral metabolism in CKD, elevated FGF23, extraskeletal and vascular calcifications, and the impact of nontraditional risk factors on cardiovascular disease and mortality are increasingly recognized as important aspects of CKD. Earlier interventions and stringent management guidelines to control serum parathyroid hormone (PTH), calcium, and phosphorus concentrations have been proposed for patients with CKD by the National Kidney Foundation (NKF) Kidney Disease Outcomes Quality Initiative (K/DOQI), but there is lack of consensus regarding the best approach to treat abnormalities in mineral metabolism effectively and safely, and to prevent the complications associated with these abnormalities. In addition to active vitamin D analogues, calcimimetic drugs that target the calcium sensing receptor in the parathyroid gland are available to suppress PTH. There is similar lack of consensus on other issues, such as the clinical significance of low circulating 25(OH)D levels in people with CKD (which represents vitamin D deficiency in those without CKD); the dose and route of active vitamin D analogue required to treat secondary hyperparathyroidism; and the relative role of calcium and noncalcium phosphate binders to control serum phosphate. The importance of vitamin D pathways in regulating innate immunity and cardiovascular function, in addition to its more traditional role in regulating mineral metabolism, are also being recognized as exacerbating hyperphosphatemia and increasing FGF23. Treatment with vitamin D has also proven ineffective in attenuating the severity of left ventricular hypertrophy (LVH) in CKD. Finally, emerging knowledge about the endocrine functions of bone (and specifically the role of the phosphaturic and vitamin D regulating hormone FGF23 in LVH, cardiovascular mortality, and glomerular filtration rate [GFR] loss) has led to a reexamination of the pathogenesis and treatment of disordered mineral metabolism in CKD.

PATHOGENESIS OF ABNORMAL MINERAL METABOLISM AND SECONDARY HYPERPARATHYROIDISM IN CHRONIC KIDNEY DISEASE

An increase in circulating PTH concentrations is the hallmark of secondary hyperparathyroidism. The major metabolic abnormalities leading to the increase in PTH are diminished production of $1,25-(OH)_2D_3$ (calcitriol, the activated form of vitamin D), decreased serum calcium, and increased serum phosphorus. In normal subjects, PTH is responsible for maintaining the serum calcium concentration within a narrow range through direct actions on the distal tubule of the kidney to increase calcium resorption and on bone to increase calcium and phosphate efflux (Fig. 55.1). In addition, some PTH effects are mediated by its effect on the production of calcitriol by the kidney via stimulation of Cyp27b1, the enzyme that converts inactive 25 hydroxyvitamin D to active $1,25(OH)_2D$. The net effects of PTH's bone and kidney actions are to create the positive calcium balance that is necessary to maintain calcium homeostasis. To prevent a concomitant positive phosphate balance resulting from the skeletal effects of PTH and the gastrointestinal actions of calcitriol, PTH acts secondarily to increase renal phosphorus excretion, mostly by decreasing activity of the sodium phosphate cotransporter in the proximal renal tubule.

Parathyroid disease in CKD is a progressive disorder characterized by both increased PTH secretion and growth in the number of the PTH-secreting chief cells (hyperplasia). Elevations in serum PTH levels first become evident when the GFR falls to less than 60 mL/min/1.73 m². This occurs before hyperphosphatemia, reduction in calcitriol levels, or hypocalcemia is detectable by routine laboratory measurements. This delay in detectable serum chemistry abnormalities is presumably caused by the actions of increased PTH to restore homeostasis. PTH levels increase progressively as kidney function declines, such that all untreated subjects reaching stage 5 CKD (GFR less than 15 mL/min/1.73 m² or dialysis) would be expected to have elevated PTH levels.

The initial event leading to secondary increments in PTH has traditionally been assigned to primary reductions in $1,25(OH)_2D$ levels caused by decreased production by the diseased kidney. More recent data implicate an initial role of elevated FGF23 in the genesis of secondary hyperparathyroidism in CKD. In this scenario, increments in FGF23 reduce $1,25(OH)_2D$ production by suppressing Cyp27b1 activity in the proximal tubule, and possibly enhance $1,25(OH)2D$ catabolism through increased Cyp24 activity. Cross-sectional studies in humans and serial studies of animal models with CKD suggest that increments in serum FGF23 precede elevations of PTH, and correlate with reductions in circulating $1,25(OH)_2D$ concentrations. However, the respective roles of FGF23 and PTH remain controversial, because FGF23 has been shown to suppress (not stimulate) PTH in certain experimental settings, and PTH appears to stimulate FGF23

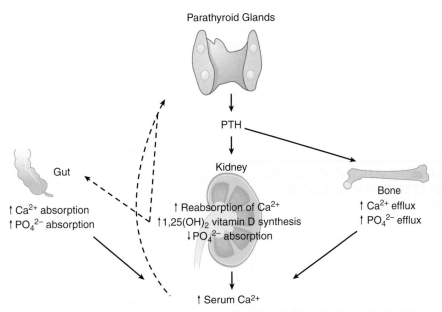

Figure 55.1   Regulation of systemic calcium homeostasis. Parathyroid hormone (PTH) is a calcemic hormone that targets the kidney to promote renal calcium conservation and the bone to increase efflux of calcium and phosphorus. PTH-mediated production of 1,25(OH)$_2$D$_3$ (activated vitamin D) by the kidney increases gastrointestinal calcium and phosphate absorption. The phosphaturic actions of PTH on the kidney cause it to excrete the excess phosphate that accompanies calcium absorption by the intestines and calcium efflux from bone. Changes in calcium, 1,25(OH)$_2$D$_3$, and phosphate levels exert feedback on the parathyroid glands *(dotted line)*. In chronic kidney disease (CKD) elevations of serum fibroblast growth factor 23 (FGF23) is an early event leading to suppression of 1,25(OH)$_2$D production and possibly increased catabolism. FGF23-mediated suppression of 1,25(OH)$_2$D may be the initiating event leading to secondary hyperparathyroidism. In advanced CKD, elevations of PTH appear to stimulate FGF23 further. Elevated levels of serum phosphate and FGF23 are associated with increased mortality in CKD.

expression in CKD as evidenced by the effect of parathyroidectomy to lower circulating FGF23 levels.

FGF23, a key regulator of phosphate and vitamin D homeostasis, is perhaps the initial adaptive response to CKD and may also play a role in cardiovascular complications as well as progression of kidney disease. Gene transcription of FGF23 in mouse models is regulated both by systemic factors, such as hyperphosphatemia and elevated 1,25-(OH)$_2$D$_3$ levels, and by local bone-derived factors. FGF23 knockout mice are hyperphosphatemic and display soft tissue and vascular calcifications, growth retardation, and bone mineralization abnormalities. FGF23 is expressed mainly in osteocytes in bone and, to a much lesser extent, in the bone marrow, the ventrolateral thalamic nucleus, the thymus, and lymph nodes. FGF23 promotes phosphate excretion by inhibition of sodium-dependent phosphate resorption. It also inhibits 1α-hydroxylase activity in the proximal tubule, leading to a decrease in calcitriol synthesis. FGF23 may also act in the heart through "off-target effects" to activate FGF receptors (FGFR) in the absence of its co-receptor a-Klotho, or on the kidney through "on-target" effects on FGFR:Klotho complexes to regulate genes, such as the suppression of ACE2. In addition, FGF23 has been implicated in the pathogenesis of kidney fibrosis. In any case, FGF23 levels are increased early in CKD and correlate with the degree of hyperphosphatemia. Moreover, treatment with vitamin D analogues elevates FGF23 levels. Further studies are needed to determine how to interpret the significance of FGF23 levels in CKD.

Unless adequately treated, secondary hyperparathyroidism progresses inexorably, with the frequency of parathyroidectomy proportional to the number of years on dialysis. The

difficulty in treating hyperparathyroidism is partly because of the massive hyperplasia and possibly adenomatous transformation of the parathyroid gland that occurs as a result of the chronic stimulation of PTH production in CKD. Enlarged, hyperplastic parathyroid glands retain some responsiveness to calcium-mediated PTH suppression in secondary hyperparathyroidism. As this responsiveness is lost because of reductions in extracellular calcium-sensing receptor (CaSR) and vitamin D receptor (VDR) expression as well as autonomous adenomatous transformation of the parathyroid gland, hypercalcemia develops in some patients. This is referred to as *tertiary* hyperparathyroidism.

Three molecular targets have been identified that regulate parathyroid gland function, including the G protein–coupled CaSR, the VDR, and the FGF23 receptor, which is constituted by the FGFR:Klotho complex. The molecular identity of the putative extracellular phosphate sensor remains undefined. Calcium acting through the CaSR is the major regulator of PTH transcription, secretion, and parathyroid gland hyperplasia. Calcitriol, which acts on the VDR in the parathyroid gland to suppress PTH transcription, but not PTH secretion, has overlapping functions with the CaSR. It appears, however, that the physiologic role of the VDR in regulating parathyroid gland function may be subordinate to that of calcium. In this regard, secondary hyperparathyroidism and bone abnormalities in VDR-deficient mice can be corrected by normalizing the serum calcium concentration. Extracellular phosphate also has direct effects on parathyroid production, apparently through the regulation of PTH messenger RNA (mRNA) levels, possibly by increasing posttranscriptional PTH mRNA message stability. Hyperphosphatemia may indirectly affect PTH production by lowering ionized calcium through chelation and suppressing 1α-hydroxylase and, hence, calcitriol production by the kidney. Finally, FGF23 has recently been shown to target the parathyroid gland via FGFR:Klotho complexes and to suppress PTH secretion. The actions of FGF23 on the parathyroid gland remain to be further elucidated, because most states of FGF23 excess are associated with elevations of PTH, and stimulation of FGFR pathways would be expected to lead to cell hyperplasia.

HISTOLOGIC CLASSIFICATIONS OF BONE DISEASE ASSOCIATED WITH CHRONIC KIDNEY DISEASE

Bone is a dynamic tissue that undergoes repetitive cycles of removal and replacement. Osteoclasts, under the influence of paracrine and systemic factors, resorb bone, whereas osteoblasts fill in the resorptive cavities with new extracellular matrix that undergoes mineralization. This process is also regulated by physiochemical properties as well as proteins that either inhibit or promote the mineralization process. A subset of osteoblasts become embedded in the bone matrix to form an interconnected network of cells (osteocytes) that also respond to systemic and local stimuli to secrete factors regulating the bone remodeling process. During growth, new trabecular bone is added to the long bones beneath the growth plate, and factors that affect bone remodeling can also impact growth-plate morphology, leading to rickets. In adults, bone disease can manifest as too little (osteopenia) or too much (osteosclerosis) bone, high or low states of bone turnover, and impaired mineralization.

PTH through PTH receptors, $1,25(OH)_2D$ through vitamin D receptors, and calcium and phosphate through effects on mineralization of bone extracellular matrix can all impact bone health. Osteoblast-mediated bone formation entails generation of a collagen matrix that undergoes mineralization controlled by a complex interplay between factors promoting and inhibiting mineralization. Bone formation is coupled to osteoclast-mediated bone resorption through osteoblastic paracrine pathways involving the secretion of a receptor activator of nuclear factor-κB ligand (RANKL), which stimulates osteoclast formation, function, and survival. Osteoblasts also secrete osteoprotegerin (OPG), which bind to RANKL to inhibit bone resorption. Denosumab, a monoclonal antibody that binds to RANKL and mimics the effects of OPG, is used to treat osteoporosis. Osteocytes also regulate bone formation through the production and secretion of sclerostin (SOST), which inhibits Wnt signaling pathways and promotes bone formation.

The circulating level of PTH is the primary determinant of bone turnover in CKD and is a major determinant of the type of bone disease present. PTH receptors are present in both osteoblasts and osteocytes. PTH suppresses SOST expression and stimulates cAMP as well as other pathways leading to increased osteoblast-mediated bone formation. Long-term exposure to high circulating concentrations of PTH leads to increased bone resorption. In contrast, more short-term, intermittent exposure to PTH can result in increased bone formation in excess of bone resorption. Intermittent PTH administration is the basis for use of teriparatide to treat osteoporosis. In addition, $1,25(OH)_2D$, at

least in experimental settings, promotes mineralization and stimulates bone resorption. The specific types of histologic changes also depend on the age of the patient, the duration and cause of kidney failure, the type of dialysis therapy used, the presence of acidosis, vitamin D status, accumulation of metals such as aluminum, and other conditions affecting mineralization of the extracellular matrix.

Bone disease associated with CKD (Fig. 55.2) has traditionally been classified histologically according to the degrees of abnormal bone turnover and impaired mineralization of the extracellular matrix. These histologic changes in bone have been best studied in dialysis patients. The current categories are as follows:

1. Secondary hyperparathyroidism (high-turnover bone disease or osteitis fibrosa).
2. Mixed uremic bone disease (a mixture of high-turnover bone disease and osteomalacia).
3. Osteomalacia (defective mineralization).
4. Adynamic bone disease (decreased rates of bone formation without a mineralization defect).

High-turnover bone disease caused by excess PTH is characterized by greater number and size of osteoclasts and an increase in the number of resorption lacunae with scalloped trabeculae, as well as abnormally high numbers of osteoblasts. There is an increased amount of osteoid (unmineralized bone), which may have a woven appearance that reflects a disordered collagen arrangement under conditions of rapid matrix deposition. The excess in osteoid surfaces that accompanies increased bone turnover has been described as mixed uremic bone disease, but it may reflect a normal response to increased turnover rather than superimposed defective mineralization. Peritrabecular fibrosis (and even marrow fibrosis), reflecting PTH stimulation of osteoblastic precursors, is observed in severe disease.

Osteomalacia is characterized by prolongation of the mineralization lag time as well as by increased thickness, surface area, and volume of osteoid. Osteomalacia was formerly linked to aluminum toxicity from both contamination of water in dialysates and use of aluminum-based phosphate binders. Other causes of osteomalacia that may be present in CKD patients include 25-hydroxyvitamin D deficiency (secondary to poor dietary vitamin D and calcium intake, and lack of exposure to sunlight because of poor mobility and extended hospitalizations), metabolic acidosis (which inhibits both osteoblasts and osteoclasts), and hypophosphatemia (e.g., in Fanconi syndrome).

Adynamic bone disease is a low-turnover bone state that has received increased attention. Bone mineralization is best assessed using tetracycline-labeled bone biopsies. Tetracycline is deposited in newly mineralized bone. Two doses of tetracycline spaced by a known time interval can be administered before bone biopsy. Subsequent measurement of the width of the mineralized bone deposited between the luminescent tetracycline bands on biopsy reflects the rate of bone mineralization. In bone biopsy series, as many as 40% of hemodialysis patients and 50% of peritoneal dialysis patients have adynamic bone disease. In this disorder, the amount of osteoid thickness is normal or reduced, and there is no mineralization defect. The main findings are decreased numbers of osteoclasts and osteoblasts and very low rates of bone formation as measured by tetracycline labeling. High

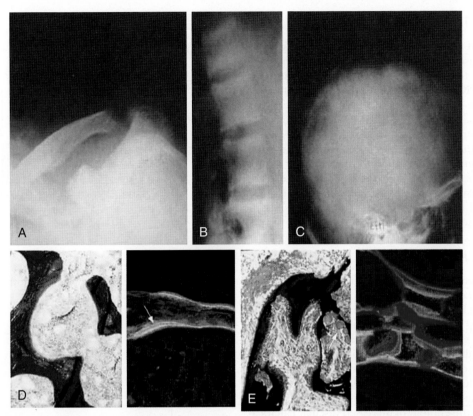

Figure 55.2   Radiographic and histologic features of bone disease associated with chronic kidney disease (CKD). A, Radiographic findings of severe erosion of the distal clavicle resulting from secondary hyperparathyroidism. **B,** Example of "rugger-jersey spine" resulting from sclerosis of the end plates associated with hyperparathyroidism. **C,** "Pepper-pot skull" with areas of erosion and patchy osteosclerosis associated with hyperparathyroidism. **D,** Histologic appearance of normal bone. On the left, a section stained with Goldner Masson trichrome stain shows mineralized lamellar bone (*blue*) and adjacent nonmineralized osteoid surfaces (*red-brown*). On the right, a Villanueva-stained section viewed under fluorescent light shows tetracycline labeling of freshly formed bone. Double staining (*arrow*) indicates amount of new bone laid down during the interval between the two periods of tetracycline administration. **E,** Histologic appearance of osteitis fibrosa in a patient with stage 5 CKD and elevated parathyroid hormone levels. On the left, Goldner Masson trichrome stain shows increased numbers of multinucleated osteoclasts at resorptive surfaces (*black arrow*) and extensive bone-marrow fibrosis (*light blue staining of marrow*). On the right, tetracyline labeling shows marked increases in the osteoid (*orange-red staining*) and in sites of new bone formation as measured by the yellow-green bands below the osteoid surfaces. (**A-C** from Martin KJ, Gonzalez EA, Slatopolsky E: Renal osteodystrophy. In Brenner BM, editor: *Brenner and Rector's the kidney*, ed 7, Philadelphia, 2004, Saunders, p 2280, with permission.)

serum calcium levels sometimes seen in adynamic bone disease may in part be secondary to high oral calcium loads and suppression of PTH when calcium-based phosphate binders are used. There may also be a decreased ability of bone to buffer calcium loads. The main risk factors for adynamic bone disease are peritoneal dialysis, older age, corticosteroid use, and diabetes. It is thought that adynamic bone disease represents a state of relative hypoparathyroidism in CKD.

Based on limited bone histologic data, approximately 40% of blacks and 20% of whites have high turnover disease, with the remainder having normal or low bone turnover in spite of elevated circulating PTH levels. However, this longstanding classification of CKD-associated bone disease has been questioned. One concern is that mixed uremic bone disease may not represent a distinct entity, because increased turnover is most often accompanied by variable degrees of reversible mineralization deficit. Another problem is the uncertainty about the existence of adynamic bone disease, which in reality represents a low rate of bone formation that overlaps the normal range and is probably caused by subnormal PTH secretion accompanying an excess of calcium and/or vitamin D treatment. Thus, adynamic bone disease

may not be a naturally occurring separate disease, but a consequence of overtreatment of hyperparathyroidism with calcium and calcitriol. Recently, the Kidney Disease: Improving Global Outcomes (KDIGO) initiative recommended a simpler classification, called Turnover, Mineralization, and Volume (TMV). Especially if specific therapies that target each of these characteristics are developed, this classification could prove useful; however, treatments are at present directed toward maintaining serum PTH levels in a range that: (1) prevents osteitis fibrosa and increased cortical porosity on one end of the spectrum, and (2) avoids low-turnover osteopenia (adynamic bone) at the other end.

CLINICAL MANIFESTATIONS OF BONE DISEASES ASSOCIATED WITH CHRONIC KIDNEY DISEASE

Most patients with CKD and mildly elevated circulating levels of PTH are asymptomatic. When clinical features of bone disease are present, they can be classified into musculoskeletal and extraskeletal manifestations.

MUSCULOSKELETAL MANIFESTATIONS

Fractures, tendon rupture, and bone pain resulting from metabolic bone disease, muscle pain and weakness, and periarticular pain are the major musculoskeletal manifestations associated with CKD. The most clinically significant effect of metabolic bone disease in CKD is hip fracture, which has a high incidence among stage 5 CKD patients and is associated with an increased risk for death. There is a roughly 4.4-fold increase in hip fracture risk in dialysis patients compared to the general population. Both high and low serum values of PTH are associated with increased fracture risks. The utility of measurements of bone mineral density (BMD) as an indicator of fracture risk has not been established in CKD as in the general population.

EXTRASKELETAL MANIFESTATIONS

The most important advance in the understanding of the clinical significance of disordered bone and mineral metabolism in CKD has been the recognition that it is a systemic disorder affecting soft tissues, particularly blood vessels, heart valves, and skin. Cardiovascular disease accounts for approximately half of all deaths of dialysis patients (see Chapter 56). Coronary and peripheral vascular calcifications occur frequently in stage 5 CKD, and increase as a function of the number of years on dialysis. Gaining a better understanding of the etiology of increased vascular calcification and how it may influence clinical cardiovascular events is of critical importance.

Several patterns of vascular calcification have been described. The first occurs as focal calcification associated with lipid-laden foam cells that are seen in atherosclerotic plaques. These calcifications may increase both the fragility and the risk for rupture of plaques. Some have questioned the role of calcification in the pathogenesis of the atherosclerotic vascular lesions, raising the possibility that it is an epiphenomenon. The second pattern of vascular calcification is diffuse; it is not associated with atherosclerotic plaques and occurs in the media of vessels. This pattern is seen with aging, diabetes, and progressive kidney failure. This so-called Mönckeberg's sclerosis was thought to be of little clinical significance for many years, but its effects of increasing blood vessel stiffness and reducing vascular compliance, which result in a widened pulse pressure, increased cardiac afterload, and LVH, are potential mechanisms that could contribute to cardiovascular morbidity (Fig. 55.3). Coronary calcium load as detected by electron-beam computed tomography (EBCT) has not been shown to correlate in dialysis patients with the degree of coronary vessel stenosis, suggesting that medial calcification is a disease entity separate from atherosclerosis in these patients.

The exact mechanisms of vascular medial calcification probably reflect the combined effects of decreased mineralization inhibitors, such as matrix Gla protein (a calcification inhibitor known to be expressed by smooth muscle cells and macrophages in the artery wall) and increased mineralization inducers. It is now clear that vascular calcification is an active, cell-mediated process. Accumulating evidence suggests that vascular smooth muscle cells undergo a phenotypic transition to an osteoblast-like cell that is important in driving the calcification process. Elevated serum phosphorus causes upregulation

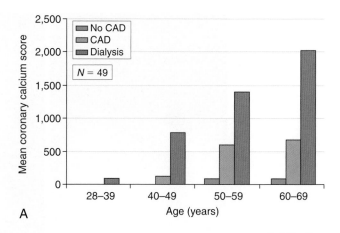

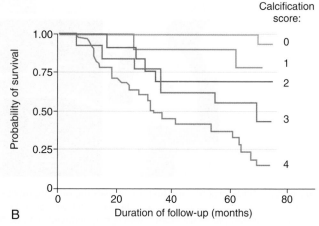

Figure 55.3   Increased risk of death and cardiovascular calcification in dialysis patients. A, Calcium score was determined by electron-beam computed tomography (EBCT). The mean coronary artery calcium score was significantly higher in hemodialysis patients than in nondialysis patients with documented cardiovascular disease. **B,** Risk of death in hemodialysis patients increases as a function of a calcification score measured ultrasonographically. (*P* is less than 0.0001 for comparisons among all curves). *CAD,* Calcium artery disease. (**A** from Braun J, Oldendorf M, Moshage W, et al: Electron beam computed tomography in the evaluation of cardiac calcifications in chronic dialysis patients. *Am J Kidney Dis* 27:394-401, 1996, with permission from the National Kidney Foundation. **B** from Blacher J, Guerin AP, Pannier B, et al: Arterial calcification, arterial stiffness, and cardiovascular risk in end-stage renal disease. *Hypertension* 38:938, 2001, with permission.)

of a type III sodium-dependent phosphate cotransporter Pit-1 (POU1F1) in smooth muscle cells. The resulting increased intracellular phosphorus upregulates core binding factor alpha 1 (Cbfa1/RUNX2), a transcription factor believed to be critical in mediating this phenotypic switch to osteoblast-like cells. Concomitantly, bone matrix proteins, such as osteopontin and osteocalcin, are found only in calcified vessels. Clinically, an increased calcium-phosphorus product (obtained by multiplying a patient's serum calcium concentration, preferably corrected for albumin, by the serum phosphorus level, both expressed in milligrams per deciliter) is associated with an increased risk of vascular and visceral calcification.

An emerging area of study concerns how uremia may affect the vascular calcification process, independent of its effects on serum phosphorus. For example, the glycoprotein fetuin-A, which is downregulated during the acute phase response, is an important inhibitor of calcification. Patients on hemodialysis have lower serum fetuin-A levels than do controls. Higher cardiovascular mortality was associated in univariate analysis with lower fetuin-A levels in hemodialysis patients, but this association did not persist after correction for accompanying risk factors by multivariate analysis.

The contribution of vitamin D to vascular calcification is controversial and debated. Some studies suggest that calcitriol can modulate vascular smooth muscle growth and influence vascular calcification by upregulation of the VDR and increased calcium uptake into smooth muscle cells. Vitamin D treatment enhances the extent of arterial calcification in animals that are also given warfarin to inhibit γ-carboxylation of the matrix Gla protein. On the other hand, in several large retrospective clinical studies, hemodialysis patients treated with active vitamin D analogues had lower mortality rates than patients not treated with active vitamin D compounds. These observational studies were potentially confounded by other variables, and randomized trials evaluating the role of vitamin D in survival in ESRD are needed to confirm this hypothesis—especially because all vitamin D analogues are associated with dose-dependent increases in serum calcium and serum phosphate, factors associated with vascular calcifications and increased mortality.

Calciphylaxis, or calcemic uremic arteriolopathy, is another form of vascular calcification that is observed primarily, although not exclusively, in stage 5 CKD. The prevalence is not well established, but it has been reported to occur in 1% to 4% of dialysis patients. Calciphylaxis manifests with extensive calcifications of the skin, muscles, and subcutaneous tissues. Most often, skin lesions occur on the breast, abdomen, and thighs. Unusual presentations, such as necrosis of the tongue and of the penis, as well as visceral involvement of the lungs, pancreas, and intestines, have been described. Examination may not only show a violaceous rash, skin nodules, skin firmness, and eschars, but also livedo reticularis and painful hyperesthesia of the skin. Nonhealing ulcerations of the skin and gangrene resistant to medical therapy often lead to amputation, uncontrollable sepsis, and death. Histologically, there is extensive medial calcification of small arteries, arterioles, capillaries, and venules, as well as intimal proliferation, endovascular fibrosis, and sometimes thrombosis. Whether the molecular pathogenesis of calciphylaxis is similar to that of Mönckeberg's sclerosis is not clear. Cases reported to be associated with very high PTH levels improved after parathyroidectomy. However, there are other cases in which the PTH levels were only mildly elevated. Interestingly, in the EVOLVE study, the use of cinacalcet in addition to standard therapy for secondary hyperparathyroidism reduced the incidence of calciphylaxis. Other risk factors for calciphylaxis are obesity, advancing age, female gender, diabetes mellitus, warfarin use, recent trauma, hypotension, and calcium ingestion. Anecdotal reports suggest that sodium thiosulfate, bisphosphonate therapy, daily hemodialysis, hyperbaric oxygen treatment, and normalization of serum phosphate levels may improve outcomes.

RELATIONSHIP BETWEEN DISORDERED MINERAL METABOLISM AND MORTALITY IN CHRONIC KIDNEY DISEASE

Cardiovascular and all-cause mortality are high in CKD. In addition to traditional cardiovascular risk factors associated with underlying diseases leading to CKD and inflammation associated with CKD, abnormalities of bone and mineral metabolism are linked to increased mortality. In particular, hyperphosphatemia and elevated FGF23 concentrations show the strongest association with increased mortality.

All associative studies to date have shown that elevation of serum phosphorus is an independent risk factor for increased mortality in patients undergoing chronic maintenance hemodialysis as well as CKD patients not yet on dialysis. Because increases in serum phosphorus greater than 3.5 mg/dl are independently associated with an incremental risk for mortality in CKD, current recommendations emphasize keeping serum phosphate in the normal range. Some studies suggest that better control of serum phosphate, as well as use of noncalcium compared to calcium-based phosphate binders to control hyperphosphatemia, may be associated with improved outcomes. In addition, PTH in the 400 to 600 pg/mL range, hypercalcemia, and elevated alkaline phosphatase are associated with increased mortality in maintenance hemodialysis patients. However, the EVOLVE study, which compared the use of cinacalcet with standard therapy with active vitamin D analogues and phosphate binders, only showed a 7% nonsignificant survival benefit.

Most important, elevated serum FGF23 is associated with increased LVH and mortality in CKD and ESRD. The increased mortality risk is independent of concomitant hyperphosphatemia in ESRD. Since high-dose active vitamin D analogues increase serum phosphate and FGF23 concentrations, associative studies indicating that treatment with active vitamin D analogues impart a survival advantage need to be reexamined. Indeed, the recently completed PRIMO study failed to show an effect of paracalcitol on left ventricular mass.

MUSCULOSKELETAL ABNORMALITIES NOT RELATED TO DISORDERED CALCIUM AND PHOSPHATE HOMEOSTASIS: AMYLOIDOSIS

Patients who have been on dialysis for many years are at risk for developing osteoarticular amyloid depositions that consist of β_2-microglobulin (β_2M). This protein, which is found in the cell membrane and serves to stabilize the major histocompatibility complex (MHC) class I antigen on cell surfaces, is normally released into the plasma with cell turnover and cleared by the kidney. Severe forms of β_2M-deposition disease manifest as a destructive spondyloarthropathy, often in the cervical and lumbar spine, and can lead to spinal instability and vertebral compression. Magnetic resonance imaging (low-signal intensity on both T1- and T2-weighted images) is important in distinguishing this entity from other destructive spinal processes. Carpal tunnel syndrome and arthritis are more frequent manifestations of β_2M amyloid deposition. β_2M deposits are found in periarticular areas, joints, and tendon sheaths. Bone cysts, especially in regions next to large joints where tendons insert (e.g., hip, proximal humerus, proximal tibia), can be seen on radiography. There is no effective treatment except for kidney transplantation to prevent ongoing bony damage from amyloidosis. High-flux hemodialysis or hemofiltration with increased clearance of β_2M compared to conventional dialysis may be beneficial (see Chapter 58).

DIAGNOSIS OF BONE DISEASES ASSOCIATED WITH CHRONIC KIDNEY DISEASE

BIOCHEMICAL PARAMETERS

Abnormal parathyroid gland function is assessed by measurement of random circulating PTH levels. Full-length PTH has a half-life of 2 to 4 minutes. PTH is cleaved into an inactive C-terminal fragment, an active N-terminal fragment, and inactive midregion fragments in the peripheral tissues. These PTH fragments are normally excreted by the kidney and have a prolonged half-life in kidney failure. A two-site immunoreactive assay is currently used to measure circulating PTH concentrations. This "intact PTH" assay uses two antibodies: one detects an epitope near the N-terminal end, and the other detects the C-terminal end. The assay actually detects the full-length bioactive PTH (1-84) (i.e., amino acid residues 1 through 84) and PTH fragments such as PTH (7-84). The PTH fragment PTH (7-84) may lack biologic activity or may potentially have distinct biologic actions. It may have hypocalcemic effects in vivo, and it has been shown to inhibit osteoclastic bone resorption in vitro. Newer, second-generation immunoreactive PTH assays ("whole PTH" or "bio-intact PTH") have been developed that recognize amino acid residues 1 through 4 of the N-terminal region of PTH and specifically detect full-length PTH (1-84). PTH levels using the whole PTH assay are approximately 50% to 60% lower than those measured with the intact PTH assay. The best way to use this more specific assay has not been determined. The normal range of the intact PTH assay is 10 to 65 pg/mL in patients with normal kidney function. However, because of end-organ resistance to PTH seen in the later stages of CKD, possibly mediated by a decrease in PTH receptors on osteoblasts, the recommended target PTH levels are greater than the upper limit of the normal range in dialysis patients. The previously recommended target ranges for serum intact PTH are 35 to 70 pg/mL, 70 to 110 pg/mL, and 150 to 300 pg/mL for CKD stages 3, 4, and 5, respectively, reflecting the progressive resistance to PTH as CKD progresses (Table 55.1). Because of the lack of standardization of PTH assays, more recent KDIGO recommendations suggest following trends in PTH when values are less than 600 pg/mL, and initiating treatment when values are trending upward. The long-term impact of this more conservative management strategy remains to be determined. This approach may minimize oversuppression of PTH and low-turnover bone disease, but it includes the risk of undersuppression of parathyroid gland hyperplasia leading to progression of secondary to tertiary hyperparathyroidism.

PTH levels are a direct measure of parathyroid gland function and an indirect measure of bone remodeling. PTH levels greater than 300 pg/mL correlate with the bony changes of secondary hyperparathyroidism and/or osteitis fibrosis. However, these observations are primarily derived from older studies in which patient demographics differed from those of today's dialysis population and before the widespread use of active vitamin D analogues. Patients with adynamic bone disease usually have intact PTH levels lower than 150 pg/mL, but these values also occur in subjects with normal bone.

PTH is only a crude, indirect measure of bone turnover, because factors other than PTH can affect bone. The utility of PTH levels as an indicator of bone turnover can be increased by assessment of bone-specific alkaline phosphatase levels, which correlate with the degree of osteoblastic

---

Table 55.1   Kidney Disease Outcomes Quality Initiative, Kidney Disease: Improving Global Outcomes (KDIGO), and Japanese Society of Dialysis Therapy (JSDT) Clinical Practice Guidelines for Bone Metabolism and Disease in Chronic Kidney Disease

CKD Stage	GFR Range (mL/min/1.73 m^2)	Phosphorus (mg/dl)	Calcium (Corrected, mg/dl)	Ca × P (mg^2/dl^2)	Intact PTH (pg/mL)
	Recommended Target Serum Values				
	K/DOQI				
3	30 to 59	2.7 to 4.6	8.4 to 10.2	—	35 to 70
4	15 to 29	2.7 to 4.6	8.4 to 10.2	—	70 to 110
5	Less than 15, dialysis	3.5 to 5.5	8.4 to 9.5	Less than 55	150 to 300
	KDIGO				
5	Less than 15, dialysis	Normal range	Normal range	Not recommended	150 to 600 (2 to 9 × normal)
	JSDT				
5	Less than 15, dialysis	3.5 to 6	8.4 to 10	Not recommended	60 to 180

Modified from National Kidney Foundation: Kidney Disease Outcomes Quality Initiative. Clinical practice guidelines for bone metabolism and disease in chronic kidney disease. Am J Kidney Dis 43:S1-S201, 2004.
CKD, Chronic kidney disease; *Ca × P,* calcium-phosphorus product; *GFR,* glomerular filtration rate; *JSDT,* Japanese Society of Dialysis Therapy; *KDIGO,* Kidney Disease: Improving Global Outcomes; *K/DOQI,* Kidney Disease Outcomes Quality Initiative; *PTH,* parathyroid hormone.

activity. Other biochemical markers of bone turnover are being developed that may provide a more accurate assessment of osteoblast and osteoclast activity in bone. For example, serum tartrate-resistant acid phosphatase 5b levels correlate well with histologic indices of osteoclasts and may serve as a specific marker for osteoclastic activity in CKD patients with bone disease. Efforts to correlate the different subtypes of bone disease with various markers of bone remodeling in both dialysis and predialysis patients are areas of ongoing research.

BONE BIOPSY

Although rarely done today, the gold standard for assessing and diagnosing the various types of bone disease in patients with CKD is an iliac crest bone biopsy with double tetracycline labeling. Bone histomorphometric analysis of the biopsy specimen includes assessment of bone and fibrosis volumes, amount of osteoid and mineralization, and number of osteoblasts and osteoclasts seen on bony surfaces. Bone biopsies should be considered in the setting of atraumatic fracture with no other clear underlying cause, suspected aluminum toxicity to confirm the presence of osteomalacia before chelation therapy or parathyroidectomy in patients with severe musculoskeletal symptoms and/or hypercalcemia with intermediate (100 to 500 pg/mL) intact PTH levels, and to confirm the diagnosis of adynamic bone disease.

IMAGING

In general, radiographic studies are not indicated in the diagnosis of the bone disorders associated with CKD, although certain radiographic changes can be seen (see Fig. 55.2A through C). Increased osteoblast function, especially in the setting of severe elevations of PTH, can lead to increased trabecular bone volume and accounts for the sclerotic changes that manifest as a "rugger-jersey spine" on radiography. Osteoclast-mediated bone resorption of secondary hyperparathyroidism results in cortical thinning and the classic radiographic evidence of subperiosteal, intracortical, and endosteal bone resorption. Subperiosteal erosions are best seen at the distal ends of the phalanges and clavicles and at the sacroiliac joints. Radiographically, expansile lytic lesions (brown tumors) can be seen in severe osteitis fibrosis. Pseudofractures, which appear as wide, radiolucent bands perpendicular to the bone long axis, can be seen in osteomalacia.

There is no accurate correlation between BMD as measured by dual-energy X-ray absorptiometry (DEXA) and the type of CKD-associated bone disease present. Osteoporosis is defined as a BMD that is at least 2.5 standard deviations lower than the mean BMD of a young adult of the same gender. Although patients with CKD typically have lower BMDs than the general population, the interpretations of DEXA scans are further complicated in secondary hyperparathyroidism because of focal areas of osteosclerosis, the presence of extraskeletal calcifications, and the variable presence of osteomalacia. However, analysis of BMD at distal sites, such as the ultradistal radius, or hip may be useful in assessing fracture risk in CKD. BMD may also be considered in patients who have undergone kidney transplantation, or who have known risk factors or previous fractures and are candidates for osteoporosis therapy.

TREATMENT OF DISORDERED BONE AND MINERAL METABOLISM IN CHRONIC KIDNEY DISEASE

The treatment of disordered mineral metabolism in CKD is directed toward normalizing serum calcium, phosphate, PTH, and metabolic acidosis while minimizing the risks associated with the therapies. In the United States, the types of treatment chosen are influenced by the economic constraints of the healthcare system, which limits the frequency of hemodialysis in most patients to three treatments per week. Clinical practice guidelines for bone metabolism and disease in CKD stages 3, 4, and 5 have been developed by several organizations and are outlined in Table 55.1.

These recommendations are influenced by data linking an elevated serum phosphorus concentration or calcium-phosphorus product to increased mortality, and by the growing concern that excessive calcium exposure may increase the risk of cardiovascular calcification. Achieving these targets with current treatment regimens is difficult. For example, in a survey of 288 facilities that included 749 dialysis patients treated with vitamin D therapy, only 29% had average intact PTH levels within the defined target range. When serum calcium, phosphorus, and calcium-phosphorus products were included, the number of stage 5 CKD patients currently achieving K/DOQI guidelines for all these parameters was even lower. Nonetheless, these guidelines are a first step toward standardizing the approach to this difficult disorder.

The various tools for treating hyperphosphatemia and secondary hyperparathyroidism include dietary phosphorus restriction, calcium-based and non–calcium-based phosphate binders, calcitriol or other active vitamin D analogues, calcimimetics, daily or nocturnal hemodialysis, and parathyroidectomy.

CONTROLLING SERUM PHOSPHORUS

Dietary phosphorus restriction (800 to 1000 mg/day) is difficult to attain but should be initiated for all subjects with stage 5 CKD. Dairy products, nuts, beer, and chocolate all have a high content of phosphorus (see Chapter 54). For patients who are undergoing thrice-weekly dialysis and are receiving adequate nutrition, dietary phosphate restriction will be inadequate to correct the positive phosphate balance, especially in the presence of concurrent active vitamin D therapy, which increases phosphorus absorption from the gut. More frequent and prolonged hemodialysis (see Chapter 58) has been associated with lower serum phosphorus levels, but with thrice-weekly hemodialysis, phosphate binders are almost invariably required.

The choice of phosphate binder (i.e., calcium-containing vs. nonaluminum, non–calcium-containing) depends on many considerations, including the binder's efficacy, side effects, and cost. For many years, calcium-based phosphate binders were the mainstay of therapy to control serum phosphate levels. Commonly used calcium-based phosphate binders include calcium carbonate and calcium acetate. Calcium carbonate contains 500 mg of elemental calcium in a 1250-mg tablet, whereas calcium acetate contains 169 mg of elemental calcium in one 667-mg tablet. Calcium citrate should not be used as a phosphate binder, because citrate increases aluminum absorption from the gut. Calcium-based phosphate binders should be taken with meals to maximize binding of ingested phosphorus in the gut. When they are taken in the fasting state, more calcium is absorbed systemically and less phosphorus is bound. The concomitant use of active vitamin D sterols increases calcium absorption and the risk of hypercalcemia. Whereas the risk of calcium loading in relation to mortality remains to be established, the K/DOQI recommendations in stage 5 CKD are to limit the total dose of calcium-based phosphate binders to 1500 mg elemental calcium per day and the total intake of elemental calcium to 2000 mg/day. Calcium acetate has greater phosphorus-binding capacity than calcium carbonate, potentially allowing the use of lower doses of calcium binder. However, various small trials have not shown significant differences in the prevalence of hypercalcemia between these two compounds.

Vascular calcifications have been documented by EBCT in the coronary arteries of dialysis patients before 30 years of age. This, taken with growing concern about the possible clinical consequences of vascular calcifications, has led to the greater use of noncalcium binders. Sevelamer is a noncalcium phosphate binder containing cross-linked polyallylamine hydrochloride. It acts as an ion exchange polymer to bind phosphorus in the gut, but is less effective than calcium on a weight basis. However, in human trials, sevelamer, when titrated to meet serum phosphorus goals, appeared equal in efficacy to the calcium-containing binders. Sevelamer has also been shown to decrease serum cholesterol and low-density lipoproteins, and increase high-density lipoproteins in stage 5 CKD patients. Sevelamer has been associated with fewer arterial calcifications than calcium-based phosphate binders in dialysis patients. Whether this effect is due to less calcium loading, the lipid-lowering effect, or mild acidosis induced by sevelamer has not been established. Sevelamer hydrochloride-induced acidosis has been attributed to the replacement of bicarbonate for chloride on the polymer and also to sevelamer's binding of short-chain fatty acids in the large intestines. The net effect of acidosis on vascular calcification in vivo is not fully understood. Sevelamer carbonate may address this issue. Sevelamer is more costly than calcium binders and may be associated with gastrointestinal side effects at higher doses that can limit its use in some individuals. Nevertheless, regimens using vitamin D analogues to raise calcium and suppress PTH, along with sevelamer to lower phosphorus, are effective in controlling both the skeletal and extraskeletal complications of stage 5 CKD.

The effect of sevelamer on cardiovascular mortality remains a critical question. Recent prospective trials comparing the effect of sevelamer versus calcium-containing phosphate binders on mortality produced equivocal results. One small, randomized trial with 127 incident hemodialysis patients monitored for a mean of 44 months demonstrated a significant overall survival advantage for sevelamer, although specific cardiovascular mortality was not assessed. The larger, open-labeled Dialysis Clinical Outcomes Revisited (DCOR) trial, which randomly assigned 2103 patients to either sevelamer or calcium-containing binders with a mean follow-up of 20.3 months, failed to show a difference in cardiovascular mortality between the two groups.

In subgroup analysis of the DCOR results, patients older than 65 years who were treated with sevelamer had a lower all-cause mortality, but not lower cardiovascular mortality. In addition, patients who remained in the study for longer than 2 years on treatment with sevelamer had a decrease in all-cause mortality. The short duration of follow-up, the high drop-out rate, and the fact that the study was not powered statistically to detect differences in specific causes of death are limitations of this study. Further investigations are needed to determine whether sevelamer in fact decreases cardiovascular events and cardiovascular mortality.

Although they are the most effective binders, aluminum-containing phosphate binders are not often used because of the potential for systemic aluminum absorption and subsequent neurologic, hematologic, and bone toxicity. Absorption of aluminum is increased by the concomitant use of sodium citrate for metabolic acidosis. Because of the potential for long-term toxicity, aluminum-containing antacids should be used only for a short period (less than 4 weeks) and only for severe hyperphosphatemia that is refractory to other treatments.

Another non–calcium-based phosphate binder is lanthanum carbonate. Lanthanum, like aluminum, is a trivalent cation with an ability to chelate dietary phosphate, but it has low systemic absorption. In a phase III trial over a 1-year period, lanthanum carbonate controlled serum phosphorus levels to an extent comparable to high-dose calcium carbonate. Mild gastrointestinal symptoms were the most common side effect in the lanthanum group. Lanthanum, unlike sevelamer, is an effective binder even in the acidic environment of the gut and does not bind bile acids. Adherence may be better than with calcium-based binders or sevelamer as a result of a lower pill burden. Because there is accumulation of small amounts of lanthanum in bone, it is important to continue to assess its side effects in long-term studies. Polynuclear iron compounds that form insoluble complexes with phosphate are under early investigation.

ACTIVATING THE CALCIUM-SENSING AND VITAMIN D RECEPTORS TO SUPPRESS PARATHYROID HORMONE HYPERFUNCTION

VITAMIN D ANALOGUES

Treatment with $1,25\text{-}(OH_2)D_3$ (calcitriol) or an active vitamin D analogue (paricalcitol, doxercalciferol, alfacalcidol, or 22-oxacalcitrol) is also a means of controlling secondary hyperparathyroidism. By binding to the VDR on parathyroid tissues, the vitamin D analogue suppresses PTH production. There is not uniform agreement about the route, dose, and type of active vitamin D analogue that should be given. Some of the available vitamin D analogues cause less hypercalcemia than calcitriol, possibly because of decreased intestinal effect on calcium absorption. The "second-generation" analogue paricalcitol has generated interest as studies suggest that it leads to less elevation of serum calcium and phosphorus as well as a greater PTH suppression than calcitriol. When paricalcitol was compared to calcitriol in a large observational study of hemodialysis patients, its use was associated with significantly lower mortality. Although this study initially raised questions about the extent to which efforts to control secondary hyperparathyroidism with vitamin D analogues might cause harm, subsequent retrospective studies suggested improved survival in dialysis patients treated with active vitamin D analogues compared to patients who did not receive vitamin D at all. However, a recent analysis of a large international dialysis database supported the possibility that the effect of vitamin D may represent a patient selection bias. Prospective clinical trials are needed to determine whether vitamin D therapy offers a survival advantage in dialysis patients.

The current recommendations are to administer active vitamin D sterols to all patients undergoing hemodialysis or peritoneal dialysis who have serum intact PTH values greater than 300 pg/mL, provided that their serum phosphorus is less than 5.5 mg/dl and their total serum calcium, corrected for serum albumin, is less than 9.5 mg/dl. Equipotent intravenous doses of calcitriol, paricalcitol, and doxercalciferol for PTH suppression are 0.5, 2.5, and 5.0 mcg, respectively, for PTH suppression. Whereas intermittent intravenous administration of active vitamin D analogues is common in the United States, in other countries daily oral therapy is more common. It remains to be established which approach is more effective in lowering serum PTH and reducing toxicity. Typical doses of calcitriol are 0.5 to 4.0 mcg intravenously after each hemodialysis session. Calcitriol can also be administered intraperitoneally. Typical oral doses are 0.25 to 1.0 mcg/day. No data support the use of higher doses of vitamin D, which are associated with elevations of calcium and phosphorus.

Stage 5 CKD patients whose PTH levels drop to less than 150 pg/mL during treatment for secondary hyperparathyroidism require a reduction in their active vitamin D analogue or phosphate binders. In patients with suspected osteomalacia, the risk for aluminum toxicity should be assessed. In patients with presumed adynamic bone disease, vitamin D analogues or phosphate binders can be decreased enough to allow the intact PTH level to drift up to levels within the target range. Individuals who develop hypercalcemia while taking vitamin D analogues can be switched to a lower calcium dialysate bath, and their vitamin D dose can be decreased or stopped.

Treatment with 25-(OH)D$_3$ is recommended in the K/DOQI guidelines for stage 5 CKD patients who have levels of 25-(OH)D$_3$ lower than 30 ng/mL. However, the utility of this treatment is not well established, because these patients would not be expected to convert this intermediate to calcitriol. Also, recent studies have suggested that it is difficult to normalize serum 25-(OH)D$_3$ levels in patients with ESRD with typical replacement doses of ergocalciferol. Nevertheless, the cost and risk of adverse side effects of nutritional vitamin D supplementation are small, and the potential effects of 25(OH)D on innate immunity and other cellular functions may warrant hormonal replacement therapy in patients with low circulating 25(OH)D levels.

CALCIMIMETICS

Calcimimetics offer a novel approach for treating secondary hyperparathyroidism without using active vitamin D analogues or raising serum calcium levels. Calcimimetics are CaSR agonists that act on the parathyroid gland by allosterically increasing the sensitivity of the receptor to calcium. Cinacalcet, the first available drug of this group, was approved by the U.S. Food and Drug Administration (FDA)

in 2004 to treat secondary hyperparathyroidism in patients with stage 5 CKD. Treatment with cinacalcet causes significant decreases in PTH without elevating serum calcium or phosphorus concentrations (Fig. 55.4). In fact, there is usually a reduction in serum calcium and a tendency toward reduced serum phosphorus with calcimimetics. In one study, the use of cinacalcet resulted in approximately 41% of patients attaining the PTH and calcium-phosphorus product goals recommended by the K/DOQI guidelines, compared with fewer than 10% achieving these targets in the group treated with phosphate binders and vitamin D analogues alone. Additional studies are needed to evaluate the effect of cinacalcet in altering the natural history of parathyroid gland hyperplasia. Prospective trials examining the impact of lowering the calcium-phosphorus product with calcimimetics in combination with active vitamin analogues, however, did not reduce vascular calcifications. Preliminary results from the EVOLVE (Evaluation of Cinacalcet Therapy to Lower Cardiovascular Events) study also failed to show a benefit of cinacalcet in reducing mortality in subjects with ESRD. These studies reflect the difficulty in demonstrating survival benefits from interventions directed at correcting the abnormalities of mineral metabolism in CKD.

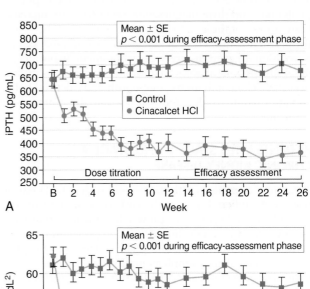

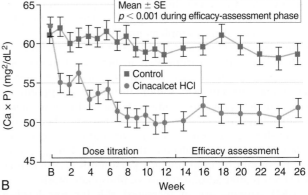

Figure 55.4 Suppression of serum parathyroid hormone (PTH) levels (A) by cinacalcet without elevation of the serum calcium-phosphorus product (Ca × P) (B) in hemodialysis patients with secondary hyperparathyroidism not adequately controlled by treatment with phosphate binders and vitamin D analogues. *iPTH,* Intact parathyroid hormone; *SE,* standard error. (From Block GA, Martin KJ, de Francisco AL, et al: Cinacalcet for secondary hyperparathyroidism in patients receiving hemodialysis. *N Engl J Med* 350:1516-1525, 2004, with permission.)

PARATHYROIDECTOMY

As a remaining option for patients with uncontrolled hyperparathyroidism, parathyroidectomy should be considered for persistently elevated intact PTH levels (greater than 800 pg/mL) associated with hypercalcemia and/or hyperphosphatemia despite medical management, and for calciphylaxis or severe bone pain and fractures in the presence of elevated intact PTH levels. Either a subtotal parathyroidectomy or a total parathyroidectomy with forearm gland implantation can be performed. Some surgeons favor the latter procedure to avoid the need for repeated invasive neck surgery if hyperparathyroidism recurs. Glands can be removed from the forearm if necessary. Both subtotal and total parathyroidectomy with implantation are effective methods, and there are no studies comparing these approaches. Nonetheless, there is a 15% to 30% recurrence rate of hyperparathyroidism after complete or partial parathyroidectomy. Percutaneous ethanol injection into the gland as an ablation procedure for hyperparathyroidism refractory to medical management is performed in some centers in lieu of surgical parathyroidectomy. "Hungry bone" syndrome is a frequent complication of parathyroidectomy, especially when markedly elevated PTH values are acutely reduced. This syndrome is characterized by hypocalcemia, hypophosphatemia, and hypomagnesemia secondary to increased bone uptake of these three ions after removal of the resorptive influence of PTH. For unclear reasons, hyperkalemia is occasionally seen. If severe or symptomatic hypocalcemia develops, treatment with a continuous calcium infusion is necessary. Concomitant treatment with oral calcitriol before and after parathyroidectomy may mitigate the hungry bone syndrome.

PATIENTS WITH STAGE 3 AND STAGE 4 CHRONIC KIDNEY DISEASE

Treatment of patients with stage 3 and stage 4 CKD has not been well studied; however, the early development of parathyroid gland hyperplasia caused by chronic stimulation suggests that treatment should focus on prevention of parathyroid gland hyperplasia. Phosphate restriction, phosphate binders, and calcium supplementation are the mainstays of treatment in stages 3 and 4 CKD. Metabolic acidosis causes an efflux of calcium from bone as bone buffers hydrogen ions with carbonate release. Chronic metabolic acidosis should be corrected with sodium bicarbonate supplementation. The need for and timing of therapy with active vitamin D analogues in stages 3 and 4 CKD have not been firmly established. Treatment with active vitamin D analogues, ideally with agents less calcemic than calcitriol (e.g., paricalcitol), should be used only for persistently elevated intact PTH levels after administration of phosphate binders.

CKD patients are at increased risk for low levels of 25-hydroxyvitamin D for several potential reasons, including lack of sunlight if chronically ill or bedridden, poor oral intake of foods containing vitamin D, lower skin production of vitamin D_3 in elderly patients secondary to lower skin content of 7-dehydrocholesterol, and the presence of nephrotic syndrome causing loss of 25-hydroxyvitamin D and vitamin D–binding protein in the urine. Although the level of 25-hydroxyvitamin D in CKD that is diagnostic of hypovitaminosis D has not been firmly established, levels less than 30 ng/mL are associated with rising PTH levels. Stage 3 and 4 CKD patients with vitamin D levels lower than 30 ng/mL should be supplemented with ergocalciferol (vitamin D_2) or cholecalciferol (vitamin D_3). In patients without CKD, correction of vitamin D deficiency increases BMD and decreases the incidence of fractures. Cinacalcet has not been well studied in patients with CKD stages 3 and 4, and is not approved by the FDA for these patients.

BISPHOSPHONATES

The use of bisphosphonates in patients with ESRD is poorly studied, and these agents are not widely prescribed in this setting because of concern that their use may exacerbate adynamic bone disease. In CKD, bisphosphonates may exacerbate kidney failure. In kidney transplant recipients, bisphosphonate may protect against immunosuppression-induced bone loss and prevent fracture. Limited data suggest that the bisphosphonates alendronate and risedronate are safe and effective for reducing fracture incidence in osteoporotic patients with CKD.

KIDNEY TRANSPLANTATION

The bony changes of secondary hyperparathyroidism improve after transplantation; however, in patients with severe hyperparathyroidism before transplantation, elevated serum levels of PTH can persist for as long as 10 years. The incidence of parathyroidectomy remains high after kidney transplantation, probably reflecting the irreversible hyperplasia of parathyroid tissue that occurs during the course of CKD. It is not uncommon for patients to develop hypophosphatemia after kidney transplantation. This reduction in serum phosphorus may be mediated by persistent hyperparathyroidism and by other variables unrelated to PTH, such as increased levels of FGF23 that also reduce renal tubular reabsorption of phosphate. Typically, phosphate supplementation is reserved for severe hypophosphatemia (less than 1.5 mg/dl). More aggressive use of phosphate supplementation may exacerbate secondary hyperparathyroidism. Transplantation also prevents, but does not reverse, bone damage from amyloidosis caused by β_2M deposition. Symptoms of amyloidosis frequently abate after transplantation, perhaps because of concomitant steroid therapy.

Although successful kidney transplantation corrects many of the conditions that lead to disordered mineral metabolism associated with kidney failure, the prednisone used to prevent rejection results in increased bone fragility, osteoporosis, and increased fracture rates. Other risk factors for fractures in this population include the presence of pretransplantation fracture, diabetes mellitus, and older age. In fact, the risk of fractures is greater in kidney transplant recipients than in patients on dialysis. There is an early rapid decrease in BMD during the first year after transplantation, as measured by DEXA scan, and then a slower, ongoing BMD loss similar to that observed in otherwise similar people without kidney failure. DEXA scans have been recommended in kidney transplant patients at the time of the transplantation and then yearly, at least for the first several years after transplant. In contrast to the general population, however, there is no clear evidence that low BMD by DEXA correlates with increased fracture risk in kidney transplant recipients. Calcium and vitamin D supplementation may be effective in counteracting the effects of glucocorticoids to reduce gastrointestinal calcium absorption. Studies have shown that calcium supplementation used with active vitamin D compounds preserves BMD at least early in the posttransplant period, but data showing that such treatment reduces fracture incidence are lacking. Intravenous bisphosphonate administered at the time of transplantation and periodically within the first year thereafter appears to decrease the rate of bone loss as measured by BMD. However, given the concern for bisphosphonate-induced adynamic bone disease in this population and the lack of data on reduced facture incidence with this approach, there are currently no consensus recommendations on the use of bisphosphonates in kidney recipients. Decisions should be individualized, and caution should be maintained.

Avascular necrosis is another complication of kidney transplantation. It most typically occurs in the femoral heads or other weight-bearing joints, and is characterized by the collapse of surface bone and cartilage. The pathogenesis of this disorder is not clear, but it is probably related to prednisone therapy. Magnetic resonance imaging is the most sensitive technique to evaluate patients with hip pain after transplantation for the presence of avascular necrosis. Surgical therapies include core decompression and hip replacement.

An often severe bilateral pain in the feet, ankles, or knees that begins within 3 months after transplantation characterizes posttransplantation distal limb syndrome. It is associated with elevated alkaline phosphatase levels and evidence of bone marrow edema and/or hemorrhage and is determined by magnetic resonance imaging of the affected areas. The condition, which is thought to result from intraosseous hypertension and has been associated with calcineurin inhibitors, is usually self-limited, resolving spontaneously within 6 months. Some patients have pain relief after the calcineurin inhibitor dose is lowered or a calcium channel blocker is added.

BIBLIOGRAPHY

Block GA: Association of serum phosphorus and calcium × phosphate product with mortality risk in chronic hemodialysis patients: a national study, *Am J Kidney Dis* 31:607-617, 1998.

Block GA, Klassen PS, Lazarus JM, et al: Mineral metabolism, mortality, and morbidity in maintenance hemodialysis, *J Am Soc Nephrol* 15:2208-2218, 2004.

Block GA, Martin KJ, de Francisco AL, et al: Cinacalcet for secondary hyperparathyroidism in patients receiving hemodialysis, *N Engl J Med* 350:1516-1525, 2004.

Block GA, Raggi P, Bellasi A, et al: Mortality effect of coronary calcification and phosphate binder choice in incident hemodialysis patients, *Kidney Int* 71:438-441, 2007.

Bricker NS, Fine LG: Uremia: formulations and expectations. The trade-off hypothesis: current status, *Kidney Int* 8:S5-S8, 1978.

Brown EM, Gamba G, Riccardi D, et al: Cloning and characterization of an extracellular Ca^{2+}-sensing receptor from bovine parathyroid, *Nature* 366:575-580, 1993.

Chertow GM, Burke SK, Raggi P, et al: Sevelamer attenuates the progression of coronary and aortic calcification in hemodialysis patients, *Kidney Int* 62:245-252, 2002.

D'Haese PC, Spasovski GB: A multicenter study on the effects of lanthanum carbonate (Fosrenol) and calcium carbonate on renal bone disease in dialysis patients, *Kidney Int* 85:S73-S78, 2003.

Drueke TB: β_2-Microglobulin and amyloidosis, *Nephrol Dial Transplant* 15:17-24, 2000.

Faul C, Amaral AP, Oskouei B, et al: FGF23 induces left ventricular hypertrophy, *J Clin Invest* 121:4393-4408, 2011.

Gutierrez OM, Mannstadt M, Isakova T, et al: Fibroblastic growth factor 23 and mortality among patients undergoing hemodialysis, *N Engl J Med* 359:584-592, 2008.

Malluche HH, Mawad HW, Monier-Faugere MC: Renal osteodystrophy in the first decade of the new millennium: analysis of 630 bone biopsies in black and white patients, *J Bone Miner Res* 26:1368-1376, 2011.

Suki WN, Zabaneh R, Cangiano JL, et al: Effects of sevelamer and calcium-based phosphate binders on mortality in hemodialysis patients, *Kidney Int* 72:1130-1137, 2007.

Teng M, Wolf M, Lowrie E, et al: Survival of patients undergoing hemodialysis with paricalcitol or calcitriol therapy, *N Engl J Med* 349:446-456, 2003.

Teng M, Wolf M, Ofsthun MN, et al: Activated injectable vitamin D and hemodialysis survival: a historical cohort study, *J Am Soc Nephrol* 16:1115-1125, 2005.

Thadhani R, Appelbaum E, Pritchett Y, et al: Vitamin D therapy and cardiac structure and function in patients with chronic kidney disease: the PRIMO randomized controlled trial, *JAMA* 307:674-684, 2012.

The EVOLVE Trial Investigators: Effect of cinacalcet on cardiovascular disease in patients undergoing dialysis, *N Engl J Med* 367:2482-2494, 2012.

Quarles LD, Lobaugh B, Murphy G: Intact parathyroid hormone overestimates the presence and severity of parathyroid-mediated osseous abnormalities in uremia, *J Clin Endocrinol Metab* 75:145-150, 1992.

Raggi P, Chertow GM, Torres PU, et al: The Advance study: a randomized study to evaluate the effects of cinacalcet plus low-dose vitamin D on vascular calcifications in patients on hemodialysis, *Nephrol Dial Transplant* 26:1327-1339, 2011.

Sprague SM, Llach F, Amdahl M, et al: Paricalcitol versus calcitriol in the treatment of secondary hyperparathyroidism, *Kidney Int* 63:1483-1490, 2003.

Stehman-Breen CO, Sherrard DJ, Alem AM, et al: Risk factors fractures for hip fracture among patients with end-stage renal disease, *Kidney Int* 58:2200-2205, 2000.

Sugarman JR, Frederick PR, Frankenfield DL, et al: Developing clinical performance measures based on the Dialysis Outcomes Quality Initiative Clinical Practice Guidelines: process, outcomes and implications, *Am J Kidney Dis* 42:806-812, 2003.

Weisinger JR, Carlini RG, Rojas E, et al: Bone disease after renal transplantation, *Clin J Am Soc Nephrol* 6:1300-1313, 2006.

56 Cardiac Function and Cardiovascular Disease in Chronic Kidney Disease

Daniel E. Weiner | Mark J. Sarnak

Cardiovascular disease is the leading cause of mortality across the spectrum of chronic kidney disease (CKD), with increased risk seen in individuals with microalbuminuria as well as in those with reduced glomerular filtration rate (GFR). Cardiovascular disease takes multiple forms in individuals with CKD, with atherosclerotic and arteriosclerotic vessels, heart failure, and structural changes including left ventricular hypertrophy (LVH) and valvular diseases common in all CKD stages. The risk of cardiovascular disease outcomes increases as kidney function declines, with the risk of cardiovascular disease death in dialysis patients 10 to 20 times that of the general population. This chapter focuses largely on individuals with reduced GFR, acknowledging that albuminuria both indicates CKD and is a very strong predictor of cardiovascular disease risk at all levels of kidney function, most notably in individuals with CKD stages 1 through 3a where metabolic sequelae of reduced GFR have not yet substantially manifest.

EPIDEMIOLOGY OF CARDIOVASCULAR DISEASE IN CHRONIC KIDNEY DISEASE

STAGES 3 TO 4 CHRONIC KIDNEY DISEASE

Manifesting with cardiac ischemia, heart failure, and arrhythmia, cardiovascular disease is overwhelmingly the leading cause of morbidity and mortality in individuals with CKD. Among individuals with reduced GFR, there is a progressive increase in the age-standardized incidence of cardiovascular disease events as kidney function declines, such that, compared to an age-standardized baseline rate of 21 cardiovascular events per 1000 person-years in individuals with estimated glomerular filtration rate (eGFR) greater than 60 mL/min/1.73 m^2, rates increase to 37, 113, 218, and 366 events per 1000 person-years among people with estimated GFR of 45 to 59 (CKD stage 3a), 30 to 44 (CKD stage 3b), 15 to 29 (CKD stage 4), and less than 15 mL/min/1.73 m^2 (CKD stage 5), respectively. Even in analyses that adjust for demographic and socioeconomic risk factors as well as cardiovascular risk factors such as diabetes, hypertension, and dyslipidemia, the risk of a cardiovascular event is dramatically increased at lower GFR (Fig. 56.1). This risk relationship is independent of a person having pre-existing cardiovascular disease (Fig. 56.2).

Prevalence of cardiovascular disease in people with CKD is similarly high. For example, in population screening programs administered by the National Kidney Foundation, 12% to 20% of individuals with eGFR between 30 and 59 mL/min/1.73 m^2 (stage 3 CKD) state that they have had a previous "heart attack or stroke" versus 5% to 10% for those with eGFR of 60 mL/min/1.73 m^2 or greater. In analyses adjusted for similar risk factors as those mentioned earlier, both reduced eGFR and microalbuminuria (indicating CKD stages 1 to 2) were independently associated with prevalent cardiovascular disease. Likewise, in pooled community cohorts, cardiovascular disease was prevalent in 31.3% of individuals with eGFR between 15 and 60 mL/min/1.73 m^2 (stage 3 to 4 CKD) versus 14.4% with eGFR ≥60 mL/min/1.73 m^2. Cardiovascular disease may be subclinical in CKD populations; in Chronic Renal Insufficiency Cohort (CRIC) participants undergoing cardiac computed tomography, there was a graded increased risk of coronary calcification with both lower eGFR and higher levels of albuminuria, even in individuals with no known history of cardiovascular disease. Similarly, in the elderly, the frequency of advanced atherosclerotic lesions increased as eGFR decreased (33.6% for eGFR ≥60 mL/min/1.73 m^2, 41.7% for CKD stage 3a, 52.3% for CKD stage 3b, and 52.8% for CKD stage 4).

LVH is also highly prevalent in CKD stages 3 and 4, likely reflecting pressure and volume overload. In one cross-sectional study of 175 patients with CKD, LVH was present in 27% of patients with creatinine clearance above 50 mL/min, 31% of patients with creatinine clearance between 25 and 49 mL/min, and 45% of patients with creatinine clearance below 25 mL/min. LVH was even more common in the African-American Study of Kidney Disease and Hypertension (AASK) cohort, where 69% of the population had LVH based on echocardiographic criteria. These findings contrast with a prevalence of LVH of less than 20% in older adults in the general population.

Both incident and prevalent heart failure are common in people with CKD. In the Atherosclerosis Risk in Communities study, individuals with eGFR less than 60 mL/min/1.73 m^2 at baseline were at twice the risk of incident heart failure hospitalization and death compared to those with eGFR of ≥90 mL/min/1.73 m^2, regardless of the presence of baseline coronary disease. Similarly, heart failure is highly prevalent in CKD. Among adult members of a large group-model health maintenance organization in the northwestern United States, 6.0% of individuals with predominantly early stage 3 CKD had a diagnostic code for heart failure versus 1.8% in an age- and sex-matched population.

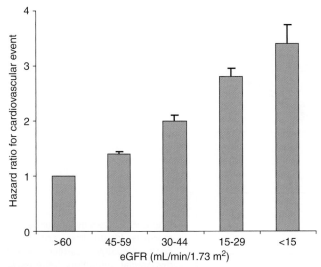

Figure 56.1 Hazard ratios for cardiovascular events according to the baseline estimated glomerular filtration rate. Adjusted for baseline age, sex, income, education, coronary disease, chronic heart failure, stroke or transient ischemic attack, peripheral artery disease, diabetes, hypertension, dyslipidemia, cancer, hypoalbuminemia, dementia, liver disease, proteinuria, previous hospitalizations, and subsequent dialysis requirement. *eGFR,* Estimated glomerular filtration rate. (Plotted using data in Go AS et al: Chronic kidney disease and the risks of death, cardiovascular events, and hospitalization, *N Engl J Med* 351:1296-1305, 2004.)

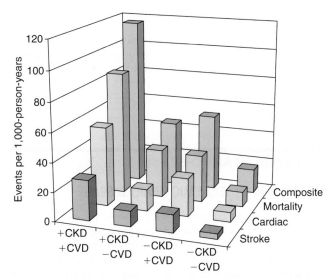

Figure 56.2 Unadjusted event rates for individuals with and without baseline chronic kidney disease (estimated glomerular filtration rate of 15 to 59 mL/min/1.73 m²) and cardiovascular disease. Cardiac events include myocardial infarction and fatal coronary disease. Stroke includes both fatal and nonfatal stroke events. Mortality includes all causes of death, and the composite outcome includes any cardiac, stroke, or mortality event. *CKD,* Chronic kidney disease; *CVD,* cardiovascular disease. (Reprinted with permission from Weiner DE et al: Cardiovascular outcomes and all-cause mortality: exploring the interaction between CKD and cardiovascular disease, *Am J Kidney Dis* 48:392-401, 2006.)

Other structural heart diseases seen commonly in CKD include aortic valve, mitral valve, and mitral annular calcification. Mitral valve or annular calcification was present in 20% of individuals with reduced kidney function (roughly stage 3 to 4 CKD) in the Framingham Offspring Study,

and there was an independent statistically significant 60% increased odds of prevalent mitral annular calcification compared to those with eGFR ≥60 mL/min/1.73 m². The Framingham Heart Study and other studies also have shown an increased prevalence of aortic valve calcification in individuals with CKD; however, this association is attenuated after adjustment for other risk factors.

STAGE 5 CHRONIC KIDNEY DISEASE/DIALYSIS

In dialysis patients, incident cardiovascular disease is common, with similar cardiovascular mortality rates in a 20-year-old dialysis patient and an 80-year-old individual from the general population (Fig. 56.3). This likely reflects a high prevalence of cardiovascular disease (22.5% of individuals initiating dialysis in the United States in 2006 had known coronary disease) as well as a high case-fatality rate compared to the general population. Even in the absence of clinically apparent coronary disease, subclinical coronary disease may be common. In a study of 30 incident asymptomatic dialysis patients with no known coronary disease history, cardiac catheterization showed significant coronary disease in 16 patients (10 of whom had diabetes mellitus), including 5 with luminal narrowing greater than 90%. Of note, only 2 of these 5 patients had dipyridamole thallium scintigraphy results suggestive of ischemia. This small but provocative report should be reproduced in a larger, more generalizable population.

The incidence and prevalence of LVH and heart failure are also extremely high in dialysis patients. More than 30% of participants in the Frequent Hemodialysis Network studies, a group that overall was healthier than the general dialysis population, had LVH at study entry (defined using cardiac magnetic resonance imaging). Based on United States Renal Data System (USRDS) administrative data, approximately 25% of hemodialysis and 18% of peritoneal dialysis patients will be diagnosed with heart failure annually, whereas approximately 55% of prevalent hemodialysis patients are identified as having a history of heart failure.

Hemodialysis patients also have a high prevalence of valvular calcification; in one study, 45% of subjects had calcification of the mitral valve and 34% of subjects had calcification of the aortic valve, compared with expected prevalence of 3% to 5% in the general population. Overall, studies have demonstrated rates of mitral annular calcification ranging from 30% to 50% in hemodialysis patients.

TYPES OF CARDIOVASCULAR DISEASE

Cardiovascular disease in individuals with CKD has a variety of manifestations, chiefly comprising atherosclerosis, arteriosclerosis, and cardiomyopathy/valvular disease (Table 56.1). In most cases, clinically apparent cardiovascular disease reflects the interplay among these manifestations. Atherosclerosis is defined as an occlusive disease of the vasculature that occurs because of the deposition of lipid-laden plaques, and arteriosclerosis is defined as nonocclusive remodeling of the vasculature accompanied by a loss of arterial elasticity. Both of these conditions may manifest with ischemic heart disease and heart failure. Certain risk factors, including dyslipidemia, primarily predispose an individual to development

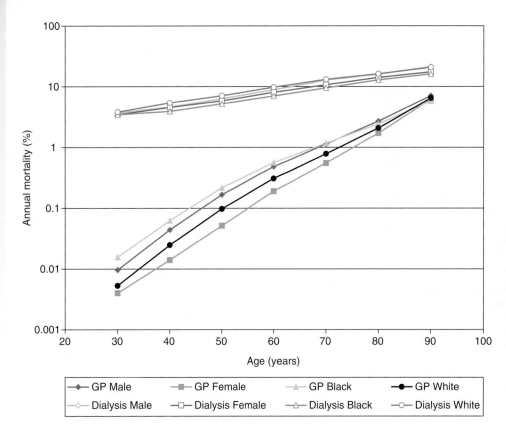

Figure 56.3 **Cardiovascular disease mortality (death from arrhythmia, cardiomyopathy, cardiac arrest, myocardial infarction, atherosclerotic heart disease, and pulmonary edema) in the general population compared with patients with chronic kidney failure treated by dialysis.** *GP,* General population. (Reprinted with permission from Foley RN, Parfrey PS, Sarnak MJ: Clinical epidemiology of cardiovascular disease in chronic renal disease, *Am J Kidney Dis* 32:S112-S119, 1998.)

and progression of atherosclerosis, whereas others, including elevated calcium-phosphorus product, may predispose to arteriosclerosis. Volume overload and anemia may primarily predispose an individual to cardiac remodeling and LVH, whereas hypertension, which is common at all stages of CKD, is associated with all of these disease manifestations. Over time, the interplay among these manifestations may yield both segmental perfusion defects due to disease affecting larger coronary arteries as well as insufficient subendocardial perfusion secondary to cardiac hypertrophy (causing increased demand) and capillary dropout. The end result is myocyte death.

RISK FACTORS FOR CARDIOVASCULAR DISEASE

Much of the increased burden of cardiovascular disease in CKD is a result of increased prevalence of both traditional and nontraditional cardiovascular disease risk factors. Traditional risk factors were identified in the Framingham Heart Study as conferring increased risk of cardiovascular disease in the general population. Nontraditional risk factors are factors that were not defined in the initial reports of the Framingham Heart Study that increase in prevalence as kidney function declines and that are hypothesized to be cardiovascular disease risk factors in patients with CKD (Table 56.2). All CKD stages, even stages 1 and 2 where microalbuminuria is present but GFR is preserved, have been independently associated with cardiovascular disease in epidemiologic studies. Although CKD may directly cause cardiovascular disease through mechanisms that include fluid retention, anemia, and abnormal mineral metabolism,

it is also probable that CKD represents a risk state in which factors associated with the development of CKD, including diabetes, hypertension and possibly dyslipidemia, account for the enhanced cardiac risk. In the latter hypothesis, the presence of CKD is a marker of the severity and duration of these other risk factors.

ISCHEMIC HEART DISEASE

PREDICTION OF ISCHEMIC HEART DISEASE

The Framingham coronary heart disease prediction equations use traditional risk factors including age, sex, diabetes, blood pressure, and lipid levels to estimate cardiac risk in the general U.S. population. However, use of these well-accepted prediction equations to assign cardiac risk to patients with CKD may be problematic, as risk factors that are at least in part dependent on intact nutrition (e.g., serum cholesterol) and cardiac health (e.g., systolic and diastolic blood pressure) appear to have different relationships with adverse outcomes. Accordingly, although many of the traditional risk factors that predict coronary heart disease in the general population are important risk factors in the late-stage CKD population, the relative importance of each risk factor may be different. In particular, diabetes in individuals with CKD is a more powerful marker of cardiac risk than it is in the general population, perhaps reflecting the fact that diabetes severe enough to cause kidney damage is also capable of causing systemic vascular disease.

In dialysis patients, the Framingham equations fail altogether, although older individuals and those with diabetes do have higher cardiovascular event rates. In hemodialysis

Table 56.1   Types of Cardiac Disease in Chronic Kidney Disease

CVD Type	Pathologic or Structural Manifestation	Risk Factors	Indicators/Diagnostic Test	Clinical Sequelae
Arterial Disease	Atherosclerosis: Luminal narrowing of arteries because of plaques	Dyslipidemia Diabetes mellitus Hypertension Other traditional and nontraditional risk factors	Inducible ischemia on nuclear imaging Cardiac catheterization	Myocardial infarction Angina Sudden cardiac death Heart failure
	Arteriosclerosis: Diffuse dilatation and wall hypertrophy of larger arteries with loss of arterial elasticity	Hypertension Volume overload Hyperparathyroidism Hyperphosphatemia Other factors predisposing to medial calcification	Vascular calcification Increased pulse pressure Aortic pulse wave velocity Cardiac computed tomography Other arterial imaging	Myocardial infarction Angina Sudden cardiac death Heart failure LVH
Cardiomyopathy	LV Hypertrophy: Adaptive hypertrophy to compensate for increased cardiac demand	Pressure overload Increased afterload because of hypertension, valvular disease, and arteriosclerosis Volume overload Volume retention because of progressive kidney disease ± anemia	Echocardiography Cardiovascular magnetic resonance imaging	Myocardial infarction Angina Sudden cardiac death Heart failure
	Decreased LV contractility	Ischemic heart disease Hypertension LVH Other traditional and nontraditional risk factors	Echocardiography	Cardiorenal syndrome* Sudden cardiac death Heart failure Myocardial infarction Angina
	Impaired LV relaxation	Hypertension Anemia and volume overload Abnormal mineral metabolism Other arteriosclerosis risk factors Other traditional and non-traditional risk factors	Echocardiography	Heart failure Myocardial infarction Angina Sudden cardiac death
Structural Disease	Pericardial effusion	Delayed or insufficient dialysis	Echocardiography	Heart failure Hypotension
	Aortic and mitral valve disease	CKD stages 3 through 5 Abnormal calcium/phosphate/PTH metabolism Aging Dialysis vintage	Echocardiography	Aortic stenosis Endocarditis Heart failure
	Mitral annular calcification	CKD Stages 3 through 5 Abnormal calcium/phosphate/PTH metabolism	Echocardiography Uniform echodense rigid band located near the base of the posterior mitral leaflet	Arrhythmia Embolism Endocarditis Heart failure
	Endocarditis	Valvular disease Chronic venous catheters	Echocardiography	Arrhythmia Heart failure Embolism
Arrhythmia	Atrial fibrillation	Ischemic heart disease Cardiomyopathy	Electrocardiography	Hypotension Embolism
	Ventricular arrhythmia	Ischemic heart disease Cardiomyopathy Electrolyte abnormalities	Electrocardiography Electrophysiology study	Sudden cardiac death

CKD, Chronic kidney disease; *CVD,* cardiovascular disease; *LV,* left ventricle; *LVH,* left ventricular hypertrophy; *PTH,* parathyroid hormone.
*Cardiorenal syndrome is reviewed in Chapter 29.

Table 56.2	Traditional and Nontraditional Cardiac Risk Factors in Chronic Kidney Disease

Traditional Risk Factors	Nontraditional Factors
Older age	Albuminuria
Male	Lipoprotein (a) and apo (a) isoforms
Hypertension	Lipoprotein remnants
Higher LDL cholesterol	Anemia
Lower HDL cholesterol	Abnormal mineral metabolism
Diabetes	Extracellular fluid volume overload
Smoking	Electrolyte imbalance
Physical inactivity	Oxidative stress
Menopause	Inflammation
Family history of cardiovascular disease	Malnutrition
Left ventricular hypertrophy	Thrombogenic factors
	Sleep disturbances
	Altered nitric oxide/endothelin balance
	Sympathetic overactivity

Revised from Sarnak MJ et al: Kidney disease as a risk factor for development of cardiovascular disease: a statement from the American Heart Association Councils on Kidney in Cardiovascular Disease, High Blood Pressure Research, Clinical Cardiology, and Epidemiology and Prevention, Circulation 108:2154-2169, 2003.
HDL, High-density lipoprotein; *LDL,* low-density lipoprotein.

patients, there is little increase in mortality risk at even the highest systolic blood pressures, whereas lower systolic blood pressures (less than 120 mm Hg) are associated with the highest risk of mortality. These altered relationships do not speak to pathophysiology, but rather likely reflect current health status and cardiac and nutritional reserve.

DIAGNOSIS OF ISCHEMIC HEART DISEASE

No single diagnostic test has proven optimal for identifying ischemic heart disease in patients with CKD, and each has pitfalls specific to CKD that may affect sensitivity and specificity. Currently, a functional assessment of perfusion that includes cardiac imaging is likely the best initial option to identify cardiac ischemia. These options include exercise or pharmacologic nuclear stress tests as well as exercise or pharmacologic stress echocardiography. Importantly, the ability to perform exercise stress testing is often limited by comorbid conditions in the CKD population. Overall, dobutamine stress echocardiography, assuming adequate institutional expertise and based on limited data, may have higher specificity and at least equivalent or higher sensitivity than pharmacologic nuclear stress tests for detecting angiographically apparent coronary lesions, while additionally providing information on valvular and other structural disease. Critically, there is no absolute contraindication to cardiac catheterization in patients with CKD, including those already on dialysis, although preservation of existing kidney function is an important consideration in all stages of kidney disease, including those receiving hemodialysis and especially those treated with peritoneal

dialysis. With careful management and conservative use of iodinated contrast (see Chapter 37), many individuals with stage 3 and stage 4 CKD can avoid significant contrast nephropathy.

PREVENTION AND TREATMENT OF ISCHEMIC HEART DISEASE

STAGES 3 TO 4 CHRONIC KIDNEY DISEASE

In the earlier stages of CKD, there is a moderate body of data, predominantly derived from subgroup analyses of larger clinical trials, demonstrating benefits with many interventions that are favorable in the general population. Therefore, currently accepted treatment strategies for primary prevention of cardiac disease in individuals with CKD stages 3 to 4 mirror those seen in the general population, while exercising caution to minimize therapies with increased risk in patients with CKD.

In individuals with CKD stages 3 to 4, dyslipidemia (Table 56.3), hypertension, and diabetes likely should be treated to current general population guidelines, as therapies directed to these conditions appear not only to reduce the risk of cardiac disease but also reduce the risk of progression to kidney failure. Blood pressure management is discussed in detail in Chapter 66, and diabetes and diabetic nephropathy in Chapter 25. Individualized care is important given the challenges associated with therapies. For example, there is an increased risk of hyperkalemia with blockade of the renin-angiotensin-aldosterone system that needs to be balanced against the benefits of this therapy in the individual patient. Other concerns include an increased risk of rhabdomyolysis seen with dual statin and fibrate therapy, and this combination should be avoided in advanced CKD.

Most interventions for acute management as well as both primary and secondary prevention of coronary disease remain inadequately studied in advanced CKD, but, based on general population experience, many may be useful. Best studied are lipid lowering therapies, with the Study of Heart and Renal Protection (SHARP) demonstrating a significant benefit for primary prevention of cardiovascular disease events in individuals with CKD stage 3b to 4 (see Table 56.3). The benefits of other common interventions are less certain. For example, low-dose aspirin use in individuals with known cardiovascular disease or a high-burden of cardiac risk factors is likely beneficial; however, data on more aggressive antiplatelet therapy with agents including glycoprotein IIb/IIIa inhibitors or clopidogrel following myocardial infarction or in the setting of acute coronary syndromes suggest that there may be a substantial risk of bleeding in individuals with advanced CKD, resulting in an overall equivocal benefit.

The better choice between medical management versus invasive management of coronary disease in advanced CKD remains uncertain. Given existing data, an individualized approach may be optimal for CKD stage 3b and 4 patients with multivessel coronary artery disease, with options including intensive medical therapy as a first-line treatment. Percutaneous interventions and coronary artery bypass grafting may be deferred to a later time or used as part of a more aggressive first-line approach based on an individual patient's symptom burden, longer term prognosis, and lifestyle values.

Table 56.3   Randomized Controlled Studies of Lipid Lowering Therapies Specifically in Chronic Kidney Disease

Study	Intervention	Population	Median Follow-Up	Primary Outcome	Risk of Primary Outcome	Risk of All-Cause Mortality
4D	Atorvastatin 20 mg daily (vs. placebo)	1255 participants Age 18 to 80 yr Type 2 diabetes Hemodialysis for less than 2 yr LDL 80 to 190 mg/dl	4.0 yr	Composite of death from cardiac causes,* fatal stroke, nonfatal MI, or nonfatal stroke	HR = 0.92 (0.77 to 1.10)	RR = 0.93 (0.79 to 1.08)
AURORA	Rosuvastatin 10 mg daily (vs. placebo)	2776 participants Age 50 to 80 yr Hemofiltration or hemodialysis for more than 3 mo	3.8 yr	Composite of death from cardiovascular causes, nonfatal MI, or nonfatal stroke	HR = 0.96 (0.84 to 1.11)	HR = 0.96 (0.86 to 1.07)
ALERT	Fluvastatin 40 mg daily with dose increase permitted (vs. placebo)	2102 participants Age 30 to 75 yr More than 6 mo from transplant Stable kidney graft function No recent MI Total cholesterol 155 to 348 mg/dl	5.4 yr	Major adverse cardiac event, defined as cardiac death, nonfatal MI, or coronary revascularization procedure	RR = 0.83 (0.64 to 1.06)	RR = 1.02 (0.81 to 1.30)
SHARP	Simvastatin 20 mg daily + ezetimibe 10 mg daily (vs. placebo)	9270 participants Age 40+ yr No previous MI or coronary revascularization Creatinine more than 1.7 mg/dl (men) or more than 1.5 mg/dl (women)	4.9 yr	Composite of coronary death,† nonfatal MI, ischemic stroke, or any revascularization procedure	RR = 0.83 (0.74 to 0.94)	RR = 1.02 (0.94 to 1.11)
	Subgroups within SHARP‡	Nondialysis (n = 6247)	Not reported	As above	RR = 0.78 (0.67 to 0.91)	Not reported
		Hemodialysis (n = 2527)			RR = 0.95 (0.78 to 1.15)	
		Peritoneal Dialysis (n = 496)			RR = 0.70 (0.46 to 1.08)	

4D, German Diabetes Dialysis Study; *ALERT,* assessment of Lescol in renal transplantation; *AURORA,* a study to evaluate the use of Rosuvastatin in subjects in regular hemodialysis: an assessment of survival and cardiovascular events; *HR,* hazard ratio; *LDL,* low-density lipoprotein; *MI,* myocardial infarction. *RR,* risk ratio; *SHARP,* Study of Heart and Renal Protection.

Data in parentheses represent 95% confidence intervals. HR and RR report the relationship between treatment vs. placebo, with values below 1 favoring treatment and above 1 favoring placebo.

*In 4D, death from cardiac causes comprised fatal myocardial infarction (death within 28 days after a myocardial infarction), sudden death, death due to congestive heart failure, death due to coronary heart disease during or within 28 days after an intervention, and all other deaths ascribed to coronary heart disease. Patients who died unexpectedly and had hyperkalemia before the start of the three most recent sessions of hemodialysis were considered to have had sudden death from cardiac causes.

†In SHARP, the original primary outcome included cardiac death, defined as death due to hypertensive heart disease, coronary heart disease, or other heart disease; the analytic plan was modified before data analysis to focus on death due to coronary heart disease rather than cardiac death.

‡In SHARP, there was no statistically significant difference in the risk of the primary outcome between dialysis and nondialysis patients ($p = 0.25$) or between hemodialysis and peritoneal dialysis patients ($p = 0.21$).

STAGE 5 CHRONIC KIDNEY DISEASE/DIALYSIS

To date, clinical trial data demonstrating a significant survival benefit with accepted cardiovascular disease therapies in the dialysis population are lacking, although data from the United States and from Australia do suggest that the rates of cardiovascular disease death in dialysis patients have decreased during the past several years for reasons that remain uncertain. The overall failure to find specific interventions that significantly reduce the cardiovascular disease burden in individuals treated with maintenance dialysis most likely reflects the fact that there are numerous competing causes of death in these patients, and addressing single risk factors may be insufficient to reduce mortality.

Lipid management has been best studied, with two large, adequately powered clinical trials both showing no benefit associated with statins in hemodialysis patients. A third trial enrolled both late-stage CKD and dialysis patients and demonstrated an overall benefit (see Table 56.3); peritoneal dialysis patients remain inadequately studied. Based on these results, we do not recommend routinely initiating statin therapy in hemodialysis patients. In patients with known coronary disease, individual decision making based on life expectancy would be suggested.

Current practice for other cardiovascular risk modifying therapy is chiefly based on observational data and extrapolations from the non-CKD population. In individuals receiving dialysis, interventions directed at blood pressure and diet are challenging given the difficulty of maintaining blood pressure in a narrow range as well as the catabolic nature of the dialysis milieu. Additionally, some risk factors associated with adverse events in the general population appear to be protective in the dialysis population. For example, higher blood pressure and obesity both are associated with better survival in dialysis patients, probably because they reflect greater cardiac and nutritional reserves, respectively. Other challenges with risk-factor management include difficulty with ascertainment. For example, blood pressure measurements are often unreliable because of the presence of dialysis access and arterial calcification, home and ambulatory blood pressure measurements are infrequently used for clinical care, and glycated hemoglobin measurements may not accurately reflect diabetes control.

Despite a lack of definitive supporting evidence, the following targets are reasonable based predominantly on clinical practice guidelines extracting data from the nondialysis population: (1) predialysis blood pressure goal of less than 140/90 mm Hg, optimally accomplished by achieving appropriate dry weight and then with pharmacologic therapy, provided there is no substantial orthostatic hypotension or symptomatic intradialytic hypotension; (2) serum LDL cholesterol goal of less than 100 mg/dl in individuals with known atherogenic disease and reasonable life expectancy; and (3) modest glycemic control based on frequent glucose assessments, assuming that hypoglycemia can be avoided. In some patients, tighter control of cardiovascular disease risk factors may be advisable and cost effective, although tools to identify dialysis patients who are most likely to benefit from these interventions remain insufficient. Finally, smoking cessation efforts are essential in all stages of CKD. As with earlier stages of CKD, ischemic heart disease can be treated successfully with invasive therapies in dialysis patients; however, the risk of complications is higher in patients with CKD. Accordingly, the optimal strategy remains unknown, and a policy of shared decision making is suggested.

LEFT VENTRICULAR HYPERTROPHY AND HEART FAILURE

DIAGNOSIS OF LEFT VENTRICULAR HYPERTROPHY AND HEART FAILURE

Diagnosis of LVH is readily accomplished with echocardiography, an inexpensive, noninvasive, and widely available test. Cardiac function should be assessed in the euvolemic state, as both significant volume depletion and overload may reduce left ventricular inotropy. Accordingly, in dialysis patients, two-dimensional echocardiography is likely to be most informative if performed on the interdialytic day. Although three-dimensional echocardiography may be useful to assess left ventricle (LV) structure as it avoids the use of geometric assumptions of LV shape that are required to estimate LV mass and volume, the increasing availability of cardiac magnetic resonance imaging likely makes this modality the most accurate assessment of LV structure. Screening echocardiography is currently recommended for

incident dialysis patients; however, there is no evidence that this improves clinical outcomes.

Heart failure and the cardiorenal syndrome are extensively discussed in Chapter 29. Heart failure is a clinical syndrome characterized by specific symptoms, including dyspnea and fatigue, and signs, including edema and rales. Although this constellation of signs and symptoms may be consistent with heart failure, these symptoms also occur in many individuals with CKD and may simply reflect volume overload. Regardless of the specific cause, individuals with persistent or recurrent volume overload have poor clinical outcomes overall. Importantly in hemodialysis patients, where preload is rapidly changing and fluid overload is managed with ultrafiltration, hypotension may be the only manifestation of heart failure.

TREATMENT OF LEFT VENTRICULAR HYPERTROPHY AND HEART FAILURE

Potentially modifiable risk factors for LVH include anemia, hypertension, extracellular volume overload, abnormal mineral metabolism including hyperphosphatemia and secondary hyperparathyroidism, and, on rare occasions, arteriovenous fistulae that are causing high-output heart failure. Definitive clinical trials evaluating the effect on mortality of modification of these risk factors for development and regression of LVH are not currently available, leading to reliance on surrogate outcomes. Whereas angiotensin converting enzyme (ACE) inhibitor and angiotensin receptor blocker (ARB) therapy may result in a favorable surrogate outcome, namely left ventricular mass reduction, randomized trials in CKD targeting normalization of hemoglobin levels with recombinant human erythropoietin had no effect on the similar surrogate outcome of LVH or left ventricular mass. Critically, no trials in CKD stages 3 to 4 have demonstrated a reduction in cardiac outcomes or mortality with these interventions when they are used for the purpose of treating or preventing LVH. In hemodialysis patients enrolled in the Frequent Hemodialysis Network study, those who received more frequent hemodialysis experienced a significant improvement in LV mass, suggesting a critical role for consistent volume control.

Heart failure therapy differs by CKD stage, as diuretics are a mainstay of therapy in predialysis patients, whereas fluid overload in dialysis patients is treated with ultrafiltration. Chronic therapy for heart failure in CKD stages 3 through 5 has not been adequately studied; therefore, recommendations are either extrapolated from the general population or are based on small trials. Notably, ACE inhibitors and ARBs likely have both cardiac and kidney benefits independent of their blood-pressure lowering effects in CKD stages 1 to early stage 4, with limited data suggesting some improvement in LV geometry as well as cardiovascular outcomes associated with these medications. Potential further benefits associated with aldosterone blockade (e.g., spironolactone) are currently being studied, with a potential limitation of hyperkalemia, especially when used in conjunction with ACE inhibitors or ARBs. Beta-blocking agents, another mainstay of heart-failure therapy in the general population, are also beneficial in patients with CKD, with evidence supporting carvedilol use to reduce mortality risk in dialysis patients with left ventricular dysfunction. Cardiac glycosides (e.g., digoxin) are frequently used in heart failure in the general population where they decrease morbidity but not mortality. Although there are no specific studies of cardiac glycosides in CKD, they should be used judiciously if at all in these patients, with careful attention to dosage, drug levels, and potassium balance.

ARRHYTHMIA AND SUDDEN CARDIAC DEATH

Arrhythmias are extremely common in individuals with CKD, likely reflecting the high prevalence of structural heart disease, ischemic heart disease, and electrolyte abnormalities. Atrial fibrillation is the most common arrhythmia, with prevalence estimates for paroxysmal and permanent atrial fibrillation as high as 30% in individuals with advanced CKD, including dialysis patients. Ventricular arrhythmias are probably also exceedingly common, although true rates cannot be determined. Prevalent dialysis patients have cardiovascular disease mortality rates of more than 80 deaths per 1000 person years, with cardiac arrest and arrhythmia accounting for more than 60% of events.

There are few data on prevention and treatment of arrhythmia and sudden cardiac death in the CKD or dialysis population, with most current treatment recommendations for individuals not treated with dialysis mirroring those seen in the general population. Although an increasing number of late-stage CKD and dialysis patients are receiving implantable cardioverter-defibrillators (ICDs) to prevent sudden cardiac death, there are no trial data that have shown a survival benefit or demonstrated cost effectiveness. Critically, ICD and other cardiac device wires typically traverse the left subclavian vein and may predispose to central stenosis, adversely affecting hemodialysis vascular access options. Given the high incidence of sudden cardiac death, one sensible preventative strategy for ambulatory settings where CKD patients are treated, including clinics and dialysis facilities, is to ensure the presence of an automated external defibrillator (AED) and that clinic personnel are trained in its use.

STROKE

Cerebrovascular disease is also common in individuals with CKD (see Fig. 56.2), with a higher incidence of both ischemic and hemorrhagic events than seen in the general population. Critically, even in the absence of clinically evident strokes, both silent lesions and substantial brain white matter disease may be present. Not surprisingly, the presence of cardiovascular disease is associated with cerebrovascular manifestations in individuals with CKD, including worse cognitive function.

Although not specifically studied, stroke prevention and treatment strategies for patients with earlier stages of CKD likely should follow general population guidelines, including management of traditional risk factors and the use of antithrombotic agents as indicated. For example, among individuals with CKD stage 3 participating in the Stroke Prevention in Atrial Fibrillation 3 trials, warfarin use based on general population recommendations was associated with a considerable reduction in the incidence of embolic stroke without a substantial increase in adverse events. In contrast, clinical trial data are absent in dialysis patients, where the risk of bleeding complications and falls are substantially higher. In cohort data from dialysis populations, there appears to be an increased risk of death in patients treated with warfarin for primary stroke prevention in the setting of atrial fibrillation. Given the frequency with which atrial fibrillation occurs in individuals with kidney failure as well as the indication biases involved in the decision to treat dialysis patients with warfarin in these cohorts, warfarin for stroke prophylaxis in the dialysis population is another area that urgently requires an adequately powered clinical trial to inform management decisions.

BIBLIOGRAPHY

Baigent C, Landray MJ, Reith C, et al: The effects of lowering LDL cholesterol with simvastatin plus ezetimibe in patients with chronic kidney disease (Study of Heart and Renal Protection): a randomised placebo-controlled trial, *Lancet* 377:2181-2192, 2011.

Chronic Kidney Disease Prognosis Consortium: Association of estimated glomerular filtration rate and albuminuria with all-cause and cardiovascular mortality in general population cohorts: a collaborative meta-analysis, *Lancet* 375:2073-2181, 2010.

Cice G, Ferrara L, D'Andrea A, et al: Carvedilol increases two-year survival in dialysis patients with dilated cardiomyopathy: a prospective, placebo-controlled trial, *J Am Coll Cardiol* 41:1438-1444, 2003.

Collins AJ, Foley RN, Chavers B, et al: United States Renal Data System 2011 Annual Data Report: Atlas of chronic kidney disease & end-stage renal disease in the United States, *Am J Kidney Dis* 59(1 Suppl 1):A7, e1-420, 2012.

deFilippi CWS, Rosanio S, Tiblier E, et al: Cardiac troponin T and C-reactive protein for predicting prognosis, coronary atherosclerosis, and cardiomyopathy in patients undergoing long-term hemodialysis, *JAMA* 290:353-359, 2003.

Fox CS, Larson MG, Vasan RS, et al: Cross-sectional association of kidney function with valvular and annular calcification: the Framingham heart study, *J Am Soc Nephrol* 17:521-527, 2006.

Fox CS, Muntner P, Chen AY, et al: Use of evidence-based therapies in short-term outcomes of ST-segment elevation myocardial infarction and non-ST-segment elevation myocardial infarction in patients with chronic kidney disease: a report from the National Cardiovascular Data Acute Coronary Treatment and Intervention Outcomes Network registry, *Circulation* 121:357-365, 2010.

Go AS, Chertow GM, Fan D, et al: Chronic kidney disease and the risks of death, cardiovascular events, and hospitalization, *N Engl J Med* 351:1296-1305, 2004.

Hart RG, Pearce LA, Asinger RW, et al: Warfarin in atrial fibrillation patients with moderate chronic kidney disease, *Clin J Am Soc Nephrol* 6:2599-2604, 2011.

Ohtake T, Kobayashi S, Moriya H, et al: High prevalence of occult coronary artery stenosis in patients with chronic kidney disease at the initiation of renal replacement therapy: an angiographic examination, *J Am Soc Nephrol* 16:1141-1148, 2005.

Palmer SC, Di Micco L, Razavian M, et al: Effects of antiplatelet therapy on mortality and cardiovascular and bleeding outcomes in persons with chronic kidney disease: a systematic review and meta-analysis, *Ann Intern Med* 156:445-459, 2012.

Raggi P, Boulay A, Chasan-Taber S, et al: Cardiac calcification in adult hemodialysis patients: a link between end-stage renal disease and cardiovascular disease? *J Am Coll Cardiol* 39:695-701, 2002.

Roberts MA, Polkinghorne KR, McDonald SP, et al: Secular trends in cardiovascular mortality rates of patients receiving dialysis compared with the general population, *Am J Kidney Dis* 58:64-72, 2011.

Sarnak MJ: Cardiovascular complications in chronic kidney disease, *Am J Kidney Dis* 41(Suppl 5):11-17, 2003.

Sarnak MJ, Levey AS, Schoolwerth AC, et al: Kidney disease as a risk factor for development of cardiovascular disease: a statement from the American Heart Association Councils on Kidney in Cardiovascular Disease, High Blood Pressure Research, Clinical Cardiology, and Epidemiology and Prevention, *Circulation* 108:2154-2169, 2003.

Umana E, Ahmed W, Alpert MA: Valvular and perivalvular abnormalities in end-stage renal disease, *Am J Med Sci* 325:237-242, 2003.

Wang LW, Fahim MA, Hayen A, et al: Cardiac testing for coronary artery disease in potential kidney transplant recipients: a systematic review of test accuracy studies, *Am J Kidney Dis* 57:476-487, 2011.

Weiner DE, Tabatabai S, Tighiouart H, et al: Cardiovascular outcomes and all-cause mortality: exploring the interaction between CKD and cardiovascular disease, *Am J Kidney Dis* 48:392-401, 2006.

Weiner DE, Tighiouart H, Elsayed EF, et al: The Framingham predictive instrument in chronic kidney disease, *J Am Coll Cardiol* 50:217-224, 2007.

Wright RS, Reeder GS, Herzog CA, et al: Acute myocardial infarction and renal dysfunction: a high-risk combination, *Ann Intern Med* 137:563-570, 2002.

Anemia and Other Hematologic Complications of Chronic Kidney Disease

Jay B. Wish

ANEMIA

EPIDEMIOLOGY AND PATHOGENESIS

Anemia is defined by the World Health Organization as a hemoglobin (Hb) concentration of less than 13.0 g/L in adult men and nonmenstruating women, and less than 12.0 g/dl in menstruating women. The incidence of anemia in patients with chronic kidney disease (CKD) increases as the glomerular filtration rate (GFR) declines. Population studies such as the National Health and Nutrition Examination Survey (NHANES) by the National Institutes of Health and the Prevalence of Anemia in Early Renal Insufficiency (PAERI) study suggest that the incidence of anemia is less than 10% in CKD stages 1 and 2, 20% to 40% in CKD stage 3, 50% to 60% in CKD stage 4, and more than 70% in CKD stage 5.

The pathogenesis of anemia in patients with CKD is multi-factorial (Box 57.1), but the contribution of erythropoietin (EPO) deficiency becomes greater as GFR declines. Hypoxia inducible factor (HIF), which is produced in the kidneys and other tissues, is a substance whose spontaneous degradation is retarded in the presence of decreased oxygen delivery because of anemia or hypoxemia. The sustained presence of HIF leads to signal transduction and the synthesis of EPO. In normal patients, plasma EPO levels increase dramatically in response to anemia. Because of their loss of functioning mass, the kidneys in patients with CKD fail to increase EPO production in response to anemia or other conditions that decrease oxygen delivery.

The kidneys produce about 90% of circulating EPO, and loss of EPO production in the setting of CKD is the primary cause of anemia in these patients. EPO binds to receptors on erythroid progenitor cells in the bone marrow, specifically the burst-forming units (BFU-E) and colony-forming units (CFU-E). The absence of EPO causes these cells to undergo programmed death or apoptosis, which is mediated by Fas ligand. In the presence of EPO, these erythroid progenitors differentiate into reticulocytes and red blood cells (RBCs).

Figure 57.1 demonstrates the complex interactions among EPO; proinflammatory cytokines such as interleukin 1 (IL-1), tumor necrosis factor-α (TNF-α), IL-6, and interferon-γ (IFN-γ); hepcidin; and iron in the production of RBCs. Hepcidin is a peptide produced by the liver that interferes with RBC production by decreasing iron availability for incorporation into erythroblasts. Hepcidin gene expression is upregulated by IL-6 and iron overload, and downregulated by TNF-α and iron deficiency. At the cell surface of macrophages and jejunal cells (and probably other cells), hepcidin binds to ferroportin, the membrane-embedded iron exporter, resulting in internalization and degradation of the complex. This inhibits iron transport across the cell membrane, trapping it in macrophages, and preventing it from being absorbed from the intestine. Hepcidin activity is probably the basis for most of the "anemia of chronic disease" syndromes, and it contributes to the anemia in patients with CKD when inflammation and infection are present. However, in anemic CKD patients without inflammation or infection, EPO deficiency plays a much greater role than hepcidin.

The evidence for inhibition of RBC production by uremic toxins in patients with CKD is poor, as most of these patients have an appropriate erythropoietic response to exogenously administered EPO if they are iron replete and free of inflammation or infection. It has been demonstrated that RBC survival is decreased from 120 days in normal individuals to 60 to 90 days in patients with CKD. This may be a result of RBC trauma from microvascular disease as well as decreased resistance to oxidative stress. The reduction of EPO in patients with CKD also contributes to neocytolysis, a physiologic process that leads to hemolysis of the youngest RBCs in the circulation.

CLINICAL MANIFESTATIONS

The major clinical manifestations of anemia in patients with or without CKD are fatigue (both with exercise and at rest), decreased cognitive function, loss of libido, and decreased sense of well-being. These symptoms tend to occur when the Hb is less than 10 g/dl, and they are more severe at lower Hb levels. More insidious are the cardiac complications of anemia, which may occur when the patient is otherwise asymptomatic and contribute to the adverse cardiovascular morbidity and mortality outcomes observed among patients with CKD. In patients with underlying coronary artery disease, anemia may lead to an exacerbation of angina because of decreased myocardial oxygen delivery. Decreased peripheral oxygen delivery because of anemia leads to peripheral vasodilation, increased sympathetic nervous system activity, increased heart rate and stroke volume, and, ultimately, left ventricular hypertrophy (LVH). LVH strongly correlates with adverse outcomes (hospitalization and mortality) in patients with CKD. A decrease in Hb of 0.5 g/dl below normal correlates with a 32% increase in LVH risk, whereas a 5 mm Hg increase in systolic blood pressure correlates with only an 11% increase in LVH risk. Most anemic CKD patients treated with erythropoiesis-stimulating agents (ESAs) report a decrease in subjective symptoms and improved quality of life (QoL), but evidence supporting regression of LVH, fewer clinical cardiac events, or decreased mortality with ESA treatment is not compelling (see later discussion).

LABORATORY EVALUATION

Because the prevalence of anemia even among patients with stages 1 and 2 CKD is as high as 10%, the consequences of anemia are severe, and treatment is available, the 2006 National Kidney Foundation (NKF) Kidney Disease Outcomes Quality Initiative (K/DOQI) clinical practice guidelines recommended annual screening for all patients with CKD (regardless of stage) for anemia. If anemia is present (defined as Hb less than 13.5 g/dl in adult men and Hb less than 12.0 g/dl in adult women), then further evaluation should be undertaken to determine the cause of the anemia. This evaluation should include a complete blood count including RBC indices, reticulocyte count, serum ferritin concentration, and transferrin saturation (TSAT) or reticulocyte Hb content (CHr). The anemia of EPO deficiency is normocytic (normal mean corpuscular volume, MCV) and normochromic (normal mean corpuscular Hb concentration, MCHC). A low MCV (microcytosis) is suggestive of iron deficiency, but may be seen in hemoglobinopathies such as thalassemia. A high MCV (macrocytosis) is suggestive of vitamin B_{12} or folate deficiency. If the MCV is elevated, vitamin B_{12} and folate levels should be assessed.

The serum ferritin level correlates with iron bound to tissue ferritin in the reticuloendothelial system. Serum ferritin does not carry or bind to iron, and its function is unknown. Serum ferritin is also an acute phase reactant, and it increases in the setting of acute or chronic inflammation independent of tissue iron stores. The TSAT is a measure of circulating iron available for delivery to the erythroid marrow, and is calculated by dividing the serum iron concentration by the total iron binding capacity (TIBC). The TIBC correlates with the serum level of transferrin, which is the major iron-carrying protein in the blood. A TSAT of less than 16% in an anemic patient with CKD is consistent with absolute or functional iron deficiency, both of which are characterized by decreased delivery of iron to the erythroid marrow. Absolute iron deficiency occurs in the setting of decreased total body iron stores and is accompanied by a serum ferritin level of less than 25 ng/mL in men and less than 12 ng/mL in women. Functional iron deficiency is seen in patients with a low TSAT and a normal or elevated serum ferritin. It may be a result of the pharmacologic stimulation of RBC production by ESAs, which causes iron demand by the erythroid marrow to outstrip the ability of the reticuloendothelial system to release iron to circulating transferrin. Functional iron deficiency may also result from the action of hepcidin in the setting of inflammation or infection. The hallmark of functional iron deficiency anemia is that it responds to the administration of intravenous iron supplements, with an

---

Box 57.1   Factors That Cause or Contribute to Anemia in Patients With Chronic Kidney Disease

Insufficient production of endogenous EPO
Iron deficiency
Acute and chronic inflammatory conditions
Severe hyperparathyroidism
Aluminum toxicity
Folate deficiency
Decreased survival of RBCs

EPO, Erythropoietin; *RBCs,* red blood cells.

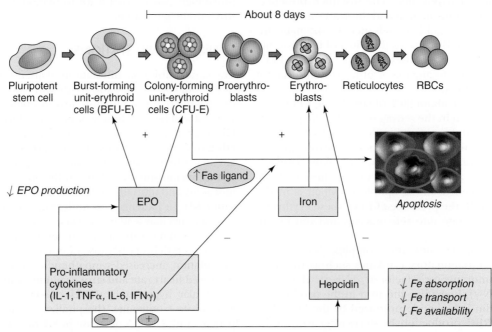

Figure 57.1   Erythropoiesis in chronic kidney disease. *EPO,* Erythropoietin; *Fe,* iron; *IFN,* interferon; *IL,* interleukin; *RBCs,* red blood cells; *TNF,* tumor necrosis factor. (Courtesy Iain Macdougall, MD.)

increase in Hb level and/or a decrease in ESA requirements despite the normal or elevated serum ferritin concentration. If the anemic patient with a low TSAT and a normal or high serum ferritin level does not respond to intravenous iron, the presumptive diagnosis is reticuloendothelial blockade, meaning that hepcidin has completely prevented the release of iron from macrophages to circulating transferrin. It should be noted that although the diagnosis of iron depletion is based on a serum ferritin concentration of less than 25 ng/mL, and that of iron deficient erythropoiesis is based on a TSAT of less than 16%, anemic CKD patients with considerably higher serum ferritin and TSAT levels often respond to iron supplements (see Iron Therapy, later).

The reticulocyte count is a useful and inexpensive test to distinguish anemia caused by underproduction of RBCs from that caused by RBC loss or destruction. In the setting of EPO deficiency, RBC production is decreased and most anemic patients would be expected to have a decreased absolute reticulocyte count (less than 40,000 to 50,000 cells per mL of whole blood). An elevated reticulocyte count is inconsistent with EPO deficiency, and an evaluation for hemolysis and blood loss should be undertaken.

Although it would seem that demonstration of a decreased blood EPO level would secure the diagnosis of EPO deficiency, routine testing for EPO levels in anemic patients with CKD is not recommended. The reason is that patients who respond to exogenous ESAs may have a normal or even an elevated EPO concentration, which may nevertheless be inappropriately low for the severity of their anemia. Furthermore, the test is expensive. Therefore, it is recommended that EPO deficiency be a diagnosis of exclusion (i.e., negative evaluation for other treatable causes of anemia) in the anemic CKD patient. However, a cause other than EPO deficiency should also be considered if the severity of the anemia is disproportionate to the degree of reduction in kidney function, or if leukopenia and/or thrombocytopenia are present.

ERYTHROPOIESIS-STIMULATING AGENTS

After other treatable causes of anemia have been excluded, and a diagnosis of EPO deficiency is inferred, the treatment of choice for many anemic patients with CKD is an ESA. Recombinant human erythropoietin (rHuEPO, or epoetin) has been available since 1989, and has revolutionized the treatment of anemia in patients with CKD who previously depended on blood transfusions and androgens. Although absorption of epoetin administered subcutaneously is incomplete with degradation of some of the protein before it reaches the circulation, the slower absorption and sustained serum epoetin levels make this route of administration 20% to 30% more efficient than a comparable intravenously administered dose. Nonetheless, the vast majority of patients undergoing hemodialysis in the United States receive their epoetin by the intravenous route because of the convenience of administration into the extracorporeal blood circuit. One possible additional motivation for intravenous administration is the association between cases of pure red cell aplasia (PRCA) in Europe and subcutaneous administration of the Eprex formulation of epoetin alfa (discussed later).

Patients with CKD who are not yet on dialysis and patients undergoing peritoneal dialysis usually receive epoetin subcutaneously. The package insert for epoetin recommends thrice-weekly dosing, because the clinical trials that were submitted for approval by the U.S. Food and Drug Administration (FDA) involved hemodialysis patients who received the drug with each treatment. For CKD patients not on dialysis and peritoneal dialysis patients, thrice-weekly dosing is not practical. It is more painful because of the subcutaneous route, and not necessary since clinical trials in these patients have shown epoetin administered every 1 to 2 weeks equally effective. Epoetin is effective in maintaining target Hb levels in 76% of CKD patients not on dialysis when administered as infrequently as every 4 weeks. Darbepoetin alfa is a bioengineered epoetin molecule with two additional N-linked carbohydrate side chains. It has a longer half-life and duration of action than epoetin. As with epoetin, studies have demonstrated that darbepoetin is effective in maintaining target Hb levels when administered as infrequently as every 4 weeks in selected patients. There appears to be no difference in subcutaneous versus intravenous administration in terms of efficacy. The side effect profile of darbepoetin is virtually identical to that of epoetin; both agents are associated with the development or exacerbation of hypertension in 20% to 30% of patients. The mechanism for the hypertension is multifactorial and related to increased RBC mass, attenuation of the peripheral vasodilation associated with anemia, and, perhaps, a direct inhibitory effect on vascular endothelial vasodilatory mediators such as nitric oxide and prostaglandins. The existence or exacerbation of hypertension is not a contraindication to ESA therapy; rather, the hypertension should be treated with more aggressive pharmacologic therapy, increased ultrafiltration on dialysis, and/or a decrease in the ESA dose to slow the rate of Hb rise and to allow for physiologic vasomotor adaptation. There is no evidence that the rate of vascular access thrombosis is increased in hemodialysis patients when ESA treatment is employed to maintain Hb levels within the currently recommended target range. All other side effects reported with ESA therapy are no greater than with placebo.

Peginesatide is a pegylated polypeptide with high affinity to the EPO receptor and no homology to native human EPO. It is effective for increasing Hb when administered once monthly. In phase 3 clinical trials in dialysis patients, peginesatide demonstrated similar efficacy and safety to epoetin. Peginesatide was approved by the FDA in March 2012 for treatment of anemia in patients with end-stage renal disease (ESRD) on dialysis, but voluntarily recalled by the manufacturer in February 2013 after post-marketing reports of fatal anaphylactic reactions (three deaths among 25,000 patients treated). The cause of these reactions remains unclear as of this writing, but it is considered unlikely that peginesatide will return to the market.

PURE RED CELL APLASIA

Pure red cell aplasia is a form of aplastic anemia that is caused by the production of antierythropoietin antibodies induced by administration of exogenous ESAs. The diagnosis of PRCA should be suspected in a patient with a sudden weekly drop in Hb of approximately 1 g/dl, or a weekly transfusion requirement and low reticulocyte count (less than 20,000 cells/μL) despite a high dose of ESA for several months. In contrast to classic aplastic anemia, the white blood cell and platelet counts are preserved in PRCA. A definitive diagnosis of PRCA is made by the demonstration of antierythropoietin antibodies in the blood, or a bone marrow examination showing normal cellularity and less than 4% erythroblasts. Treatment includes discontinuation of the ESA and immunosuppressive therapy (e.g., cyclophosphamide); most patients respond after several months and do not relapse after the immunosuppressive therapy is discontinued. A cluster of PRCA cases in Europe was traced almost exclusively to subcutaneous administration of a form of epoetin alfa stabilized with Tween 80. This additive was never used in the United States where PRCA has always been rare. With removal of this preparation from the European market, the incidence of PRCA fell dramatically. Because it has no homology to native or recombinant EPO, peginesatide has been shown to be effective in the treatment of PRCA, but it has not been approved by the FDA for that indication.

TARGET HEMOGLOBIN LEVEL

The target Hb level for anemic patients with CKD treated with ESAs has been controversial, because observational studies have disagreed with the results of interventional trials. Based on studies of epoetin efficacy in the early 1990s that compared outcomes in untreated patients with hematocrit (Hct) values in the mid-20s with those in treated patients with Hct values in the mid-30s, the first version of the NKF-K/DOQI anemia guidelines (1997) had an opinion-based recommendation that the target Hct for epoetin-treated patients should be 33% to 36%. However, a number of observational studies from the United States Renal Data System (USRDS) and large dialysis chain databases suggested that the benefits of higher Hct or Hb levels extend to levels greater than 39% and 13 g/dl, respectively, with QoL increasing directly across the spectrum of Hct/Hb levels. In 1998, results from the Normal Hematocrit Study, which randomized 1223 hemodialysis patients with underlying cardiac disease receiving epoetin to a target Hct of 30% versus a target Hct of 42%, became available. The study was terminated early because of the low likelihood that the patients randomized to the higher Hct would show better outcomes. The patients in the higher Hct group had a relative risk of 1.3 (confidence interval, 0.9 to 1.9) for the primary endpoints of death or myocardial infarction. Furthermore, patients in the higher Hct group had a significantly greater incidence of vascular access thrombosis. Based on this study, the 2001 version of the NKF-K/DOQI anemia guidelines recommended a target Hb of 11 to 12 g/dl in ESA-treated anemic patients with CKD.

The Cardiovascular Risk Reduction by Early Anemia Treatment with Epoetin Beta (CREATE) study randomly assigned 603 patients with GFRs between 15 and 35 mL/min/1.73 m^2 and a baseline Hb of 11 to 12.5 g/dl to one of two groups. Group 1 patients were immediately treated with epoetin beta to a target Hb of 13 to 15 g/dl. Group 2 patients were treated only when their Hb fell to less than 10.5 g/dl with a target Hb of 10.5 to 11.5 g/dl. There was no difference between the two groups in the primary endpoint (time to first cardiovascular event). Although there was no difference in the rate of decline in GFR between the two groups, more patients in group 1 required dialysis. Patients

in group 1 also had better general health and improved physical function, based on standard survey instruments. There was no difference between the two groups in combined adverse events.

The Correction of Hemoglobin and Outcomes in Renal Insufficiency (CHOIR) study was a much larger study in which 1432 patients with stage 4 CKD were randomized to a target Hb of 11.3 g/dl versus 13.5 g/dl. The average follow-up period was 16 months, and the study was terminated early because of safety concerns in the higher Hb group. The primary endpoint was a composite of death, myocardial infarction, hospitalization for congestive heart failure (without renal replacement therapy), and stroke. The patients in the higher Hb group had a significantly higher incidence of the composite endpoint, congestive heart failure, death, and hospitalization (cardiovascular and all-cause). There was no difference between the groups in rates of stroke, myocardial infarction, renal replacement therapy, or QoL.

Based of the results of the CHOIR and CREATE studies, the FDA changed the package insert for epoetin and darbepoetin to add a boxed warning regarding the risks for death and serious cardiovascular events when ESAs are administered to achieve target Hb levels of 13.5 to 14.5 g/dl versus 10.0 to 11.3 g/dl. It was also stated that the physician should "individualize dosing to achieve and maintain Hb levels within the range of 10 to 12 g/dl" in patients with CKD. The FDA recommendations not withstanding, in 2007 the NKF-K/DOQI anemia workgroup published an updated recommendation that the Hb target for ESA-treated CKD patients should be 11.0 to 12.0 g/dl, and a guideline (moderately strong evidence) that the Hb target should not exceed 13 g/dl.

The Trial to Reduce Cardiovascular Events with Aranesp Therapy (TREAT) study was published in 2009. TREAT examined the use of darbepoetin in anemic patients with type 2 diabetes and nondialysis CKD. Unlike the CHOIR and CREATE studies, the TREAT study had a placebo arm. Important outcomes that were considered included death, cardiovascular events, progression of kidney disease, and QoL. Group 1 was treated with darbepoetin to a Hb target of 13 g/dl, and group 2 was not administered any ESA unless the Hb level decreased to less than 9 g/dl. Other than a higher incidence of stroke in the high Hb group, cardiovascular events and deaths were similar in both arms. Fatigue scores were lower among patients in the high Hb arm, but the other QoL scores were similar in both groups. Unsurprisingly, there were more blood transfusions in the placebo group. A finding of some concern was that patients with a history of cancer were more likely to die of cancer if randomized to the higher Hb target. The findings of the CHOIR, CREATE, and TREAT studies are summarized in Table 57.1.

In 2011, the FDA substantially changed the product information for epoetin and darbepoetin, eliminating the target Hb range of 10 to 12 g/dl and adding a new boxed warning regarding the risk of death, myocardial infarction, stroke, venous thromboembolism, thrombosis of vascular access, and tumor progression and recurrence. Other elements of the 2011 FDA guidelines are summarized in Box 57.2. The elimination of a target Hb range for ESA therapy, which had generally driven the development and use of standardized ESA dose titration protocols, and the substitution of

Table 57.1   Large Randomized Studies of Erythropoiesis-Stimulating Agents in Anemic Chronic Kidney Disease Patients

	NHS	CHOIR	CREATE	TREAT
Year Published	1998	2006	2006	2009
Location	United States	United States	Europe	International
ESA	Epoetin alfa	Epoetin alfa	Epoetin beta	Darbepoetin alfa
CKD Stage and Comorbidity	Dialysis with cardiac disease	Nondialysis	Nondialysis	Nondialysis with type 2 diabetes
Number of Patients	1223	1432	603	4038
High Hb Target (g/dl)	14 (Hct 42)	13.5	13 to 15	13
Low Hb target (g/dl)	10 (Hct 30)	11.3	10.5 to 11.5	9
CV Endpoints	RR 1.3 (CI 0.9 to 1.9)	Higher in high Hb group	No difference	No difference except higher stroke in high Hb group
Progression of CKD	Not applicable	No difference	More in high Hb group	No difference
Cancer Deaths	Not noted	Not noted	Not noted	Higher in high Hb group among patients with previous cancer
QoL	Better in high Hb group	No difference	Better in high Hb group	No difference except less fatigue in high Hb group

CHOIR, Correction of Hemoglobin and Outcomes in Renal Insufficiency; *CI,* confidence interval; *CKD,* chronic kidney disease; *CREATE,* Cardiovascular Risk Reduction by Early Anemia Treatment with Epoetin; *CV,* cardiovascular; *ESA,* erythropoiesis-stimulating agent; *Hb,* hemoglobin; *NHS,* Normal Hematocrit Study; *QoL,* quality of life; *RR,* risk ratio; *TREAT,* Trial to Reduce Cardiovascular Events with Aranesp Therapy.

Box 57.2   U.S. Food and Drug Administration Guidelines on Use of Erythropoiesis-Stimulating Agents in Patients With Chronic Kidney Disease

In controlled trials, patients experienced greater risks for death, serious adverse cardiovascular reactions, and stroke when administered ESAs to target a Hb level of greater than 11 g/dl .

No trial has identified a Hb target level, ESA dose, or dosing strategy that does not increase these risks.

Use the lowest ESA dose sufficient to reduce the need for RBC transfusions.

Physicians and patients should weigh the possible benefits of decreasing transfusions against the increased risks of death and other serious cardiovascular adverse events.

Do not increase the dose more frequently than once every 4 wk. Decreases in dose can occur more frequently. Avoid frequent dose adjustments.

If the Hb rises rapidly (e.g., more than 1 g/dl in any 2-wk period), reduce the dose of ESA by 25% or more as needed to reduce rapid responses.

For patients who do not respond adequately (Hb increase less than 1 g/dl after 4 wk of therapy), increase the dose by 25%.

For patients who do not respond adequately over a 12-wk escalation period, increasing the ESA dose further is unlikely to improve response and may increase risks.

Use the lowest dose that will maintain a Hb level sufficient to reduce the need for RBC transfusions. Evaluate other causes of anemia. Discontinue ESA if responsiveness does not improve.

For Patients Not on Dialysis:

Consider initiating ESA treatment only when the Hb level is less than 10 g/dl, AND

The rate of Hb decline indicates the likelihood of requiring RBC transfusion, AND

Reducing the risk of allosensitization and/or other RBC transfusion related risks is a goal.

If the Hb level exceeds 10 g/dl, reduce or interrupt the dose of ESA.

For Patients on Dialysis:

Initiate ESA treatment when the Hb level is less than 10 g/dl.

If the Hb level approaches or exceeds 11 g/dl, reduce or interrupt the dose of ESA.

The intravenous route is recommended for patients on hemodialysis.

ESA, Erythropoiesis-stimulating agent; *Hb,* hemoglobin; *RBC,* red blood cell.

---

a recommendation for "individualization" of ESA therapy with the goal of transfusion avoidance has led to considerable confusion and controversy within the nephrology community. Especially challenging is the FDA recommendation that ESA therapy in CKD patients not on dialysis not be initiated until the Hb is less than 10 g/dl, and that the dose be reduced or interrupted if Hb rises to greater than 10 g/dl.

Given the stated goal of minimizing transfusions, perhaps the FDA should have simply recommended Hb target ranges of 9 to 10 g/dl and 9 to 11 g/dl in the nondialysis and dialysis CKD populations, respectively, since anemia management protocols are probably here to stay. Nonetheless, the concept of individualization in therapy is appropriate to properly balance the risk and benefit. Transfusion avoidance is a higher priority to avoid allosensitization in patients who are candidates for kidney transplantation. The QoL benefits of ESA therapy and higher Hb levels vary with patients' comorbidities, psychologic structures, functional levels, and expectations. Ideally, the goals of ESA therapy should incorporate the effect of treatment on patients' perception of their QoL using instruments that focus attention on the specific domains that are affected by anemia. The improvement in each of these domains, including fatigue, energy level, sense of vitality, and physical functioning, should be assessed on an individual basis to determine the Hb target range for each patient.

In 2012, the Kidney Disease: Improving Global Outcomes (KDIGO) Clinical Practice Guideline for Anemia in CKD was published. The KDIGO recommendations regarding target Hb level for patients receiving ESA therapy are summarized in Box 57.3. It should be noted that the KDIGO guideline acknowledges a QoL benefit from ESA therapy, which the FDA does not. The international 2012 KDIGO anemia guideline replaces the 2006-2007 K/DOQI anemia guideline as the most current evidence basis for treatment of anemia in patients with CKD in the United States.

NEW AGENTS

Following the expiration of patents on epoetin in 2014, it is anticipated that a number of new ESAs will enter the U.S. market. These include Mircera (methoxy polyethylene glycol-epoetin beta), which has already been approved by the FDA for use in both nondialysis and dialysis CKD

> ### Box 57.3   Key KDIGO Recommendations Regarding Target Hemoglobin Level in Patients Receiving Erythropoiesis-Stimulating Agent Therapy
>
> For adult CKD nondialysis patients with Hb less than 10 g/dl, it is suggested that the decision to initiate ESA therapy is individualized based on the rate of fall of Hb, previous response to iron therapy, risk of needing transfusion, risks related to ESA therapy, and presence of symptoms attributable to anemia.
>
> For adult CKD patients on dialysis, it is suggested that ESA therapy is used to avoid having the Hb concentration fall below 9 g/dl by starting ESA therapy when the Hb is 9 to 10 g/dl. Individualization of therapy is reasonable as some patients may have improvements in QoL at higher Hb concentration, and ESA therapy may be started above 10 g/dl.
>
> In general, it is suggested that ESAs are not used to maintain Hb concentration above 11.5 g/dl in adult patients with CKD.
>
> Individualization of therapy will be necessary as some patients experience improvements in QoL at Hb concentrations above 11.5 g/dl and will be prepared to accept the risks.
>
> In all adult patients it is recommended that ESAs not be used intentionally to increase the Hb above 13 g/dl.
>
> ---
>
> *CKD,* Chronic kidney disease; *ESA,* erythropoiesis-stimulating agent; *KDIGO,* Kidney Disease: Improving Global Outcomes; *QoL,* quality of life.

---

patients, and has been extensively used in other parts of the world for a number of years. As with peginesatide, the pegylation of the molecule retards its metabolism and allows for once-monthly dosing. Biosimilar ESAs, which are lower-cost "generic" versions of biopharmaceutical parent compounds, are undergoing clinical trials in the United States and are already extensively used in other parts of the world. A novel approach to anemia treatment under development includes agents that potentiate HIF activity by inhibiting the prolyl hydroxylase (PH) enzyme that normally degrades HIF. This stimulates the production of endogenous EPO, even in patients with ESRD, suggesting that significant EPO production can be induced in nonrenal tissues. These agents also downregulate hepcidin production, which may make them more effective than conventional ESAs for treating patients with underlying inflammation. Moreover, the HIF-PH inhibitors can be taken orally, which makes them potentially attractive to CKD patients not on dialysis, and those on home dialysis who would otherwise have their ESA administered subcutaneously.

IRON THERAPY

Iron deficiency frequently coexists with EPO deficiency as a cause of anemia in patients with CKD who are not undergoing hemodialysis, and it almost universally develops in patients on hemodialysis because of blood losses in the extracorporeal circuit, frequent blood testing, oozing from vascular access sites after the dialysis needles are withdrawn, and vascular access procedures. CKD patients not on hemodialysis may develop iron deficiency because of inadequate oral iron intake resulting from dietary protein restriction or loss of a taste for red meat. Even if iron deficiency is not present at the time of initial anemia evaluation, it often develops after the initiation of ESA therapy, because the stimulation of new RBC production exhausts existing iron stores. Therefore, it is important to regularly monitor iron status with serum ferritin and TSAT levels monthly during initiation of ESA therapy and every 3 months after a stable Hb level has been achieved. As mentioned earlier, the target serum ferritin and TSAT levels for patients receiving ESAs are higher than those used to diagnose iron deficiency in the general population because of the phenomenon of functional iron deficiency induced by ESA-stimulated bone marrow RBC production. The target serum ferritin level recommended by the 2006 NKF-K/DOQI anemia guidelines is ≥200 ng/mL for hemodialysis patients and ≥100 ng/mL for nonhemodialysis patients receiving ESAs. The target TSAT level is ≥20% in patients receiving ESAs with or without hemodialysis.

Supplemental iron can be administered orally or intravenously. Oral iron may be sufficient to achieve target iron parameters in nonhemodialysis CKD patients, because they do not have the ongoing blood losses of patients undergoing hemodialysis. However, even in nonhemodialysis CKD patients, oral iron may be ineffective because of adherence issues, side effects, and the magnitude of iron deficit. Commonly prescribed oral ferrous iron salts (sulfate, fumarate, gluconate) must be oxidized by stomach acid to the ferric form before they can be absorbed by the small intestine. This step may be impaired if stomach acid is buffered by food or an antacid, or if the patient is taking a histamine-2 blocker or proton pump inhibitor. Therefore, oral iron salts should be administered 1 hour before or 2 hours after a meal. The minimal effective oral iron dose to repair iron deficiency is 200 mg of elemental iron daily, but each 325-mg tablet of ferrous sulfate contains only 65 mg of elemental iron, requiring an iron-deficient patient to take at least three tablets daily in divided doses. The bioavailability of oral iron salts is only 1% to 2% of the administered dose in patients with elevated serum ferritin, so even an adherent patient may be unable to repair an iron deficit with an oral agent. Finally, oral iron salts are associated with gastrointestinal side effects such as epigastric pain and constipation that may further limit compliance.

For nonhemodialysis patients with iron deficiency unresponsive to oral iron and for all hemodialysis patients receiving ESAs whose iron parameters are at or below target levels, intravenous iron therapy is recommended. Four forms of intravenous iron are available in the United States: iron dextran, iron sucrose, iron gluconate, and ferumoxytol. Iron dextran is the least expensive, but it has been associated with fatal anaphylactic reactions leading to a "black box" warning by the FDA and the need for a test dose of 25 mg at the time of the first administration. The absence of a reaction to the test dose makes it less likely, but it does not guarantee that the patient will not have an anaphylactic reaction to a therapeutic dose of iron dextran. An advantage of iron dextran is that it can be administered in dosages as high as 1000 mg in a single session. This may be a consideration for nonhemodialysis patients with limited access to a healthcare facility to receive intravenous iron, and it preserves veins for future hemodialysis vascular access, because fewer infusions are required. Iron sucrose and iron gluconate have never been associated with a fatal anaphylactic reaction and do not require a test dose. However, they can be administered to a maximum of only 250 to 300 mg per session, so a nonhemodialysis patient with severe iron deficiency will require several infusions to replete iron stores. Iron sucrose and iron gluconate are preferred in hemodialysis patients whose regular visits and access to the circulation through the extracorporeal circuit make smaller and more frequent dosing appropriate. Iron sucrose and iron gluconate have been associated with nonfatal anaphylactic reactions, hypotension, and nausea/vomiting. For iron dextran, sucrose, and gluconate, slower infusion rates and smaller doses in a single session are associated with a lower incidence of side effects.

There are two intravenous iron preparations, ferumoxytol and ferric carboxymaltose, that can be given in rapid infusion doses of 500 to 1000 mg. Ferumoxytol is approved by the FDA for administration of 510 mg in less than 1 minute. A second dose can be administered 3 to 8 days later in a patient with TSAT less than 20%. Ferric carboxymaltose can be given in a single dose as high as 1000 mg, but this is not yet approved by the FDA although it has been in use in other parts of the world. These agents have potential appeal to nonhemodialysis CKD patients with iron deficiency because they would allow decreased frequency and duration of clinic visits to receive intravenous iron therapy, and they would preserve veins for future hemodialysis vascular access. The safety profiles of ferumoxytol and ferric carboxymaltose appear to be similar to those of iron sucrose and gluconate, with serious adverse events occurring in 0.4% to 0.6% of treatments. Characteristics of available intravenous iron preparations are summarized in Table 57.2.

The Dialysis Patients' Response to IV Iron with Elevated Ferritin (DRIVE) study examined the efficacy of intravenous iron administration in hemodialysis patients who had Hb less than 11 g/dl on adequate ESA therapy, TSAT less than 25%, and serum ferritin of 500 to 1200 ng/mL. The study showed that administration of eight 125-mg doses of iron gluconate resulted in more efficient erythropoiesis, a more rapid rise in Hb levels, a decrease in ESA requirements, and adverse events similar to those in a control group that received no intravenous iron. These findings suggest that there is a spectrum of responsiveness to intravenous iron that extends to patients with serum ferritin levels as high as 1200 ng/mL.

Concerns have been raised about the potential toxicity of intravenous iron supplements, including cellular and vascular damage from oxidative stress and impaired white blood cell function based on in vitro studies. There has been

Table 57.2   Intravenous Iron Preparations Available in the United States

Generic Name	Brand Name	Labeled Dosing for Iron Deficiency	IV Administration Time	Test Dose Required?
Iron dextran	Dexferrum INFeD	1000 mg in 10 divided doses or total dose as a single IV infusion	Infusion rate should not exceed 500 mL/hours	Yes
Iron sucrose	Venofer	1000 mg in 10 divided doses (hemodialysis)	5 minutes undiluted; 15 minutes if diluted in saline	No
		1000 mg in 5 divided doses (nondialysis)	Undiluted over 5 minutes or infused over 30 to 60 minutes	
		1000 mg in 2 doses of 300 mg and 1 dose of 400 mg (peritoneal dialysis)	300 mg infused over 1.5 hours 400 mg infused over 2.5 hours	
Iron gluconate	Ferrlecit Nulecit	1000 mg in 8 divided doses (hemodialysis only)	60 minutes diluted in saline	No
Ferumoxytol	Feraheme	510 mg × 2 doses	Undiluted over 17 seconds, 5 to 8 days apart	No

IV, Intravenous.

evidence of increased urinary excretion of markers of tubular injury, but not increased albuminuria, in CKD patients receiving intravenous iron sucrose. However, observational studies have not demonstrated increased hospitalizations or mortality in hemodialysis patients receiving an average of less than 400 mg of intravenous iron per month, and intravenous iron therapy was not identified as a risk factor for bacteremia in hemodialysis patients in a multivariate analysis. Serial liver biopsies in patients with hemochromatosis showed no significant organ injury when the serum ferritin level was less than 2000 ng/mL. The 2006 K/DOQI anemia guidelines suggested that decisions regarding intravenous iron therapy in patients with serum ferritin levels greater than 500 ng/mL should weigh ESA responsiveness, Hb concentration, TSAT level, and the patient's clinical status.

RESISTANCE TO ERYTHROPOIESIS-STIMULATING AGENTS AND ADJUVANT THERAPY

ESA resistance has been defined as failure to achieve Hb greater than 11 g/dl despite an epoetin dose of greater than 500 units/kg/wk or the equivalent of another ESA. The causes of ESA resistance are the same as the causes of anemia in CKD (see Box 57.1), with the obvious exception of EPO deficiency and with the addition of PRCA. After iron deficiency, the most common cause of ESA resistance in patients with CKD is inflammation/infection. This is often associated with high levels of acute phase reactants such as serum ferritin, C-reactive protein, and erythrocyte sedimentation rate, but the source of the inflammation/infection may not be readily apparent. It has been demonstrated that hemodialysis patients who use catheters for vascular access have lower mean Hb levels and higher mean ESA doses, which probably reflects the inflammatory state induced by the presence of the catheter and its biofilm, even in the absence of positive cultures for pathogens.

Although the intention-to-treat analyses of the CHOIR and TREAT studies conclude that higher target Hb levels are associated with increased cardiovascular events, secondary analyses of these studies implicate the higher ESA doses received by the patients in the higher Hb arms. The conclusion is that ESA doses should not be uptitrated indefinitely in patients who fail to achieve target Hb levels, because the risk of ESA therapy far exceeds the benefit in such patients. For patients who have not responded adequately over a 12-week escalation period, the FDA recommends that increasing the dose further is unlikely to improve response and may increase risks. For CKD patients not on dialysis, an epoetin dose ceiling of 300 units/kg/wk (or the equivalent of another ESA) should be considered, whereas the dose ceiling for dialysis patients should be 450 units/kg/week (or equivalent dose of another ESA).

There is insufficient evidence to support the use of adjuvants to ESA therapy, such as L-carnitine and vitamin C, in the management of anemia in patients with CKD. Although androgens were widely used to increase Hb levels in dialysis patients in the pre-ESA era, their use is not recommended because of insufficient evidence to support their efficacy in patients receiving adequate doses of ESAs and because of the potential for long-term toxicity.

Despite the use of adequate doses of ESA and iron therapy, transfusions with RBCs are sometimes required in the setting of ESA resistance or acute blood loss. Transfusions are considered a last resort because of the potential development of sensitization affecting future transplantation candidacy and the small risk of blood-borne infections. There is no single Hb concentration that necessitates transfusion, and the decision of whether and when to transfuse should be made based on the patient's individual situation, including comorbid illnesses, symptoms, acuity of Hb decrease, and potential for future transplantation as well as the Hb level.

OTHER HEMATOLOGIC MANIFESTATIONS OF KIDNEY DISEASE

ABNORMALITIES OF HEMOSTASIS

Patients with advanced stages of CKD typically have normal results on coagulation studies and normal platelet counts, but they exhibit an increased bleeding tendency because of defects in platelet function. This is manifested by a prolonged bleeding time, abnormal studies of platelet aggregation and adhesiveness, and decreased release of platelet factor 3. There may also be an abnormal interaction between platelets and vascular endothelium, mediated by decreased activity of von Willebrand factor (vWF) as well as increased release of endothelial nitric oxide and prostacyclin in uremia. The clinical manifestations of these abnormalities include an increased tendency and increased duration of bleeding after trauma and in the setting of serosal inflammation. This often manifests as epistaxis, bleeding with tooth brushing, and easy bruisability, but it can result in life-threatening gastrointestinal hemorrhage or hemorrhagic pericarditis. The bleeding diathesis is only partially corrected by dialysis, and larger molecules that accumulate in the setting of kidney failure, such has parathyroid hormone, have also been implicated. The anemia may also contribute to the bleeding diathesis of uremia, as higher RBC counts push platelets closer to the vessel wall, making them more effective. Treatment of anemia with RBC transfusion and/or ESAs to Hb greater than 10 g/dl improves the bleeding diathesis. Platelet function improves after the initiation of ESA therapy but before the Hb rises, suggesting that ESAs may improve platelet function directly.

The treatment of choice for bleeding episodes in uremic patients is to provide adequate dialysis with minimal or no anticoagulation, and to initiate ESA therapy. If bleeding continues or if the patient is at risk for bleeding from an invasive procedure, then treatment with desmopressin (DDAVP) should be considered. DDAVP is a synthetic form of antidiuretic hormone that has minimal vasopressor activity and is used in the treatment of diabetes insipidus. The mechanism of its action in the setting of uremic bleeding is thought to be related to the release of vWF from endothelial cells and platelets. The dose of DDAVP is 0.3 mcg/kg intravenously or 3 mcg/kg intranasally, and it can be repeated 1 to 2 times before tachyphylaxis develops. The onset of action is immediate, and the duration of action is 4 to 8 hours. More than half of patients treated with DDAVP respond with an improvement in bleeding time, and the reason for the lack of response in other patients is unknown. Because of the tachyphylaxis, it is recommended that DDAVP be administered only once, immediately before an invasive procedure (and not the day before). DDAVP tachyphylaxis appears to abate after 48 hours, and twice-weekly therapy has been shown effective in some patients with chronic bleeding.

Conjugated estrogens (Premarin) act to reduce bleeding for up to 14 days, but the onset of action takes 6 hours. The dose is 0.6 mg/kg daily for 5 consecutive days, and this regimen has been effective in controlling gastrointestinal bleeding associated with ateriovenous malformations in uremic patients. The mechanism of action may be related to inhibition of vascular nitric oxide production.

Like DDAVP, cryoprecipitate provides vWF, but it is less convenient to use and carries the risk of blood-borne infections. The onset of action of cryoprecipitate is 1 hour, and its effect peaks at 12 hours. The dose is 10 units and can be repeated as necessary. The response to cryoprecipitate is highly variable, and it should be reserved for life-threatening hemorrhage.

The platelet hemostatic defect in uremia does not appear to protect against vascular access thrombosis, which is a common problem in hemodialysis patients. The use of antiplatelet agents such as aspirin and clopidogrel to preserve vascular access may be associated with an unacceptably high rate of bleeding and is not recommended. Use of these agents for conventional indications, such as coronary artery and cerebrovascular disease, is not contraindicated in patients with CKD, although the benefit must be weighed against risk. Similarly, heparin and warfarin are frequently needed for conventional indications in patients with CKD, but the use of these agents superimposes a risk of bleeding on the underlying abnormalities of platelet function. It is estimated that the incidence of venous thrombotic and thromboembolic disease (exclusive of vascular access thrombosis) in patients with CKD is twice that of the general population. This is attributed to the complications of nephrotic syndrome with increased plasma fibrinogen and decreased plasma antithrombin III levels, the presence of systemic lupus with circulating "anticoagulants" such as antiphospholipid antibodies, elevated levels of homocysteine, venous injury from previous catheter placement, and the continued presence of intravascular "foreign bodies" such as dialysis catheters and arteriovenous grafts. Increased experience with enoxaparin in patients with CKD has simplified anticoagulation in certain settings, because monitoring of the partial thromboplastin time is not required. The dose of enoxaparin for CKD patients with GFR less than 30 mL/min/1.73 m^2 is 1 mg/kg subcutaneous daily for deep venous thrombosis (DVT) and acute coronary syndromes, or 30 mg daily subcutaneous for DVT prophylaxis.

ABNORMALITIES OF LEUKOCYTES

Except for a transient decrease in circulating granulocytes during the first 15 to 30 minutes of hemodialysis with older, unmodified cellulosic membranes, the white blood cell count of patients with uremia tends to be normal. The decrease in circulating granulocytes during unmodified cellulosic membrane hemodialysis is caused by alternative complement pathway activation, which leads to microleukoagglutination and margination of granulocytes in the pulmonary circulation. This may be responsible for the transient hypoxia that is sometimes observed during hemodialysis, and it is completely reversed by the end of the dialysis treatment. The function of granulocytes, including chemotaxis, adherence, phagocytosis, and production of reactive oxygen species, is altered in uremia; these changes may also be exacerbated by exposure to unmodified cellulosic membranes. Impaired granulocyte function is associated with increased susceptibility to infection with encapsulated bacteria, such as *Staphylococcus*, contributing to the high incidence of these infections in dialysis patients.

Monocyte and lymphocyte function are also impaired in uremia, leading to a decrease in cellular-type immunity. This may manifest as an increased susceptibility to viral infections such as influenza, decreased response to vaccinations, and anergy to immunologic skin testing. The latter phenomenon makes it important to place control skin tests (e.g., mumps, streptokinase/streptodornase) when evaluating the response to tuberculosis skin tests. The activity of autoimmune diseases such as systemic lupus erythematosus may be attenuated after uremia supervenes. An impairment of cytokine release decreases the febrile response to pathogens in uremic patients, so that infections may go unnoticed and may become more serious before diagnosis. The clinical implication is that symptoms suggestive of infection must trigger an aggressive diagnostic and therapeutic response in this vulnerable population.

BIBLIOGRAPHY

Besarab A, Bolton WK, Browne JK, et al: The effects of normal as compared with low hematocrit values in patients with cardiac disease who are receiving hemodialysis and erythropoietin, *N Engl J Med* 339:584-590, 1998.

Besarab A, Coyne D: Iron supplementation to treat anemia in patients with chronic kidney disease, *Nat Rev Nephrol* 6:699-710, 2010.

Besarab A, Goodkin DA, Nissenson AR: The normal hematocrit study—follow-up, *N Engl J Med* 358:433-444, 2008.

Coyne D: From anemia trials to clinical practice: understanding the risks and benefits when setting goals of therapy, *Semin Dialysis* 21:212-216, 2008.

Coyne DW, Kapoian T, Suki W, et al: DRIVE Study Group: ferric gluconate is highly efficacious in anemic hemodialysis patients with high serum ferritin and low transferrin saturation: results of the Dialysis Patients' Response to IV Iron with Elevated Ferritin (DRIVE) Study, *J Am Soc Nephrol* 18:975-984, 2007.

Drueke TB, Locatelli F, Clyne N, et al: Normalization of hemoglobin level in patients with chronic kidney disease and anemia, *N Engl J Med* 355:2071-2984, 2006.

Fishbane S, Nissenson AR: Anemia management in chronic kidney disease, *Kidney Int* 78(Suppl 117):S3-S9, 2010.

Horl WH: Clinical aspects of iron use in the anemia of kidney disease, *J Am Soc Nephrol* 18:382-393, 2007.

Kidney Disease: Improving Global Outcomes (KDIGO) Anemia Work Group: KIDGO Clinical Practice Guideline for Anemia in CKD, *Kidney Int*, 2012.

Kliger A, Fishbane S, Finkelstein FO: Erythropoietic stimulating agents and quality of a patient's life: individualizing anemia treatment, *Clin J Am Soc Nephrol* 7:354-357, 2012.

Lewis EF, Pfeffer MA, Feng A, et al: Darbeopetinalfa impact on health status in diabetes patient with kidney disease: a randomized trial, *Clin J Am Soc Nephrol* 6:845-855, 2011.

Macdougal IC, Ashenden M: Current and upcoming erythropoiesis-stimulating agents, iron products and other novel anemia medications, *Adv Chronic Kidney Dis* 16:117-130, 2009.

Macdougall IC, Rossert J, Casadevall N, et al: A peptide-based erythropoietin-receptor agonist for pure red-cell aplasia, *N Engl J Med* 361:1848-1855, 2009.

Manns BJ, Tonelli M: The new FDA labeling for ESA—implications for patients and providers, *Clin J Am Soc Nephrol* 7:348-353, 2012.

National Kidney Foundation: K/DOQI clinical practice guidelines and clinical practice recommendations for anemia in chronic kidney disease, *Am J Kidney Dis* 47(Suppl 3):S1-S145, 2006.

National Kidney Foundation: K/DOQI clinical practice guidelines and clinical practice recommendations for anemia in chronic kidney disease: 2007 update of hemoglobin target, *Am J Kidney Dis* 50:471-530, 2007.

Pfeffer M, Burdmann E, Chen C, et al: A trial of darbepoetinalfa in type 2 diabetes and chronic kidney disease, *N Engl J Med* 361:2019-2032, 2009.

Singh AK, Szczech L, Tang KL, et al: Correction of anemia with epoetinalfa in chronic kidney disease, *N Engl J Med* 355:2085-2098, 2006.

Szczech LA, Burnhart HXS, Inrig JK, et al: Secondary analysis of the CHOIR trial: epoetin-alfa dose and achieved hemoglobin outcomes, *Kidney Int* 74:791-798, 2008.

Wish JB: Assessing iron status: beyond serum ferritin and transferrin saturation, *Clin J Am Soc Nephrol* 1(Suppl 1):54-58, 2006.

KIDNEY REPLACEMENT THERAPIES: DIALYSIS AND TRANSPLANTATION

58 Hemodialysis

Raymond M. Hakim

Hemodialysis is an extracorporeal therapy that is prescribed to reduce the signs and symptoms of uremia and to replace partially a number of the key functions of the kidneys when kidney function is no longer sufficient to maintain the patient's well-being or life. Although hemodialysis is one of several therapies (peritoneal dialysis, hemodiafiltration, transplantation) that can be used for the treatment of acute or chronic end-stage renal disease (ESRD), this chapter focuses primarily on hemodialysis.

PRINCIPLE FUNCTIONS OF HEMODIALYSIS

Hemodialysis used in the treatment of ESRD is effective in (a) reducing the concentration of uremic toxins, particularly small and medium-sized molecules, primarily by diffusion; (b) reducing excess fluid volume by convection; and (c) correcting some of the metabolic abnormalities, such as acidosis and hyperkalemia, by use of dialysate solutions with variable solute concentrations. The two major components of the hemodialysis procedure that will be discussed are the dialyzer and the dialysate.

DIALYZER

STRUCTURE

The most commonly used device for the performance of hemodialysis is the hollow fiber dialyzer, comprised of several thousand bundles of hollow fibers. These hollow fibers are made of thin, semipermeable membranes and are encased in a plastic tubing device that allows blood to be pumped from the patient into the inside of these hollow fibers while an aqueous solution, the dialysate, is pumped outside these hollow fibers, typically in the opposite direction of the blood flow, to maximize the diffusion gradients across the membranes.

There are generally two types of dialysis membranes (Fig. 58.1); the first are called "low-flux" membranes and are made up of fibers with small pore sizes, which allow the diffusion of small solutes such as urea and water, but do not allow the passage of larger molecules such as β2-microglobulin. "High-flux" membranes have larger pore sizes and allow the passage of larger molecules such as β2-microglobulin, and because of these larger pore sizes, the rate of water transfer (ultrafiltration coefficient) is much higher than that for low-flux membranes.

The manufacturing process of these membranes is such that, regardless of whether it is a low-flux or a high-flux membrane, the pore sizes are not uniform, and there is a distribution of pore sizes that allows the diffusion or removal of differently sized molecules at different rates (Fig. 58.2). It is important to note that the distribution of pore sizes for high-flux membranes is such that it does not allow for the passage of albumin.

PRINCIPAL FUNCTIONS OF THE DIALYZER

Diffusion

Diffusion describes the movement of solutes from a milieu with high concentrations across a semipermeable membrane into a milieu where it is in lower concentration. The rate and amount of solute that diffuses across the membrane in either direction depends on the difference in concentration between the blood and dialysate compartments, the molecular size of the solute, the characteristics of the membrane including its surface area, thickness, and porosity, and the conditions of flow (e.g., turbulent or smooth). These membrane characteristics are generally labeled "mass transfer characteristic" or "coefficient of diffusion," and are specific for the membrane used and the solute under consideration.

Using urea as the prototype solute, hemodialysis allows the movement of urea from the blood compartment, where it is in high concentration, to the dialysate compartment across the hollow fiber membranes. Thus, as blood is pumped and traverses through the dialyzer inside hollow fibers, urea concentration of the blood is reduced; concurrently, the urea concentration of the dialysate increases as it traverses outside the hollow fibers in the opposite direction. If the blood and dialysate were to flow in the same direction, then the urea concentration gradient between the blood and dialysate compartments would be considerably reduced at the exit site of the dialyzer, whereas a countercurrent flow ensures maximum difference in concentration and therefore higher flux of solute from the blood compartment; accordingly, most dialysis procedures use countercurrent flow of blood and dialysate.

The principles of diffusion apply not only to urea and other solutes that have a higher concentration in the blood than dialysate, but also to the diffusion of substances that have a higher concentration in the dialysate than blood. An example of the latter is the diffusion of bicarbonate from the dialysate into the blood compartment. A useful way to express the diffusion of a substance across the dialysis membrane is termed "clearance," analogous to the clearance of solutes in the native kidney.

$$K = \frac{Q_B(C_A - C_v)}{C_A}$$

The clearance of solute from the blood compartment (K, in mL/min) is expressed as the difference in the amount

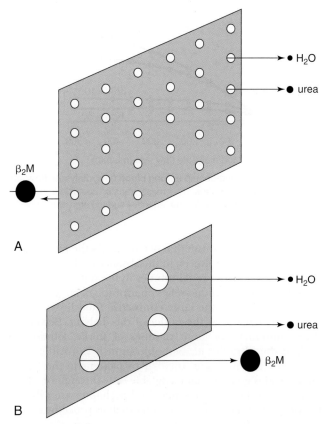

A

B

Figure 58.1 Schematic diagrams of low-flux and high-flux membranes. A, Low-flux membranes have small pores that are highly permeable to small solutes such as water and urea (60 Da) but restrict the transport of middle molecules such as β2-microglobulin (β2M). Because of their small pores, they also tend to have low ultrafiltration coefficients, although the ultrafiltration coefficient can be increased by increasing the surface area of the membrane. A low-flux membrane can be either high efficiency or low efficiency for urea transport, depending on its surface area and, to a lesser extent, its thickness. **B,** High-flux membranes have large pores that facilitate the transport of middle molecules such as β2M in addition to small molecules. Their ultrafiltration coefficients are high. A high-flux membrane can be either high efficiency or low efficiency, depending on its surface area and, to a lesser extent, its thickness. (Reproduced with permission from Cheung A: Hemodialysis and hemofiltration. In Greenberg A, editor: *Primer on kidney diseases,* ed 3, Philadelphia, 2001, National Kidney Foundation/Saunders, ch 47.)

of a solute at the inlet ($Q_B \times C_A$, where Q_B is the blood flow rate in mL/min and C_A is the concentration in mg/mL at the inlet or "arterial" side of the dialyzer) and the amount of solute at the outlet ($Q_B \times C_V$, where C_v is the concentration at the outlet or "venous" side of the dialyzer), divided by the concentration at the inlet (C_A).

Convection

The simple equation for solute clearance does not take into account convective clearance of solutes. Convection refers to the mass transport of solutes along with the fluid it is dissolved in (plasma water) and is driven by the higher hydrostatic pressures in the blood compartment generated by the blood pump. The amount of solute removed by convection is not dependent on the concentration of the solute, but rather on the difference in hydrostatic pressure between the blood and dialysate compartment and the characteristic of the membrane, termed the "sieving coefficient."

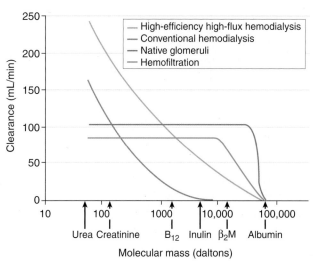

Figure 58.2 Solute clearance profile of various membranes. The curves are constructed based partially on data and partially on theoretical projection. The actual values may vary depending on the surface area of the membrane and operating conditions (e.g., blood flow rate). The curve for native glomeruli represents the summation of all the glomeruli in two normal kidneys. "Glomeruli" instead of "kidneys" are used because tubular reabsorption substantially lowers the kidney clearance of certain solutes, such as urea and glucose. Clearance of solutes by diffusion (via either conventional or high-efficiency/high-flux dialysis) deteriorates rapidly with increase in molecular mass of the solute. In contrast, clearance by convection (hemofiltration or glomeruli) remains constant over a wide range of molecular mass. *B12,* Vitamin B12; *β2M,* β2-microglobulin. (Reproduced with permission from Cheung A: Hemodialysis and hemofiltration. In Greenberg A, editor: *Primer on kidney diseases,* ed 4, Philadelphia, 2005, National Kidney Foundation/Saunders, ch 90.)

The relative contribution of convective transport to overall clearance depends on the pore size of the membrane as well as the size and charge of the solute. In general, the relative contribution of convective transport to the overall clearance for small molecules, such as urea, is minor, but it is more substantial for larger molecules (e.g., $β_2$ microglobulin) because of the low diffusive clearance of these large molecules.

Therefore, a more complete representation of solute clearance incorporating both diffusion and convection is:

$$K = \frac{Q_{Bi} \times C_A - Q_{Bo} \times C_V}{C_A} \approx \frac{Q_{Bo}\,(C_A - C_V)}{C_A} + Q_{uf}$$

where Q_{uf} is the difference between Q_{Bi} (inlet blood flow) and Q_{Bo} (outlet blood flow) and is termed ultrafiltration rate (UFR) in mL/min.

Because any solute removed from the blood compartment appears in the dialysate, another expression of solute clearance (K) that includes both convective and diffusive removal is based on the measurement of the concentration of that solute at the outlet of the dialysate; this is true for all solutes that are not already present in dialysate. This can be represented as

$$K = \frac{Q_{DO} \times C_{DO}}{C_A}$$

where Q_{DO} is the dialysate flow rate at the outlet (mL/min), C_{DO} is the concentration of the solute in the dialysate (mg/mL) at the outlet, and C_A is the concentration (mg/mL) in the blood at the inlet. Because this represents the net loss of the

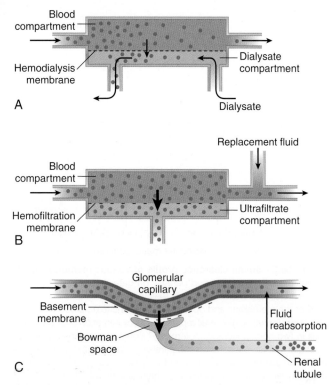

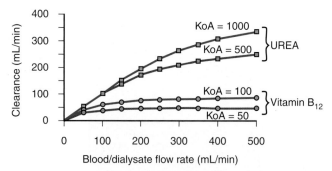

Figure 58.4   The relationship among blood flow, dialysate flow, and membrane characteristics. The mass transfer coefficient is usually represented as KoA where A is the effective surface area of the specific dialyzer.

Figure 58.3   Schematic representation of solute and fluid transport across the semipermeable artificial membranes and glomerular basement membrane. A, Hemodialyzer. The plasma concentration of solutes (*solid circles*) in the blood inlet is high. Because of diffusive loss across the semipermeable hemodialysis membrane (*dotted line*), the plasma concentration in the blood outlet is much lower. The thin arrow across the dialysis membrane represents a small amount of fluid loss (which is not necessary for solute removal). A high dialysate flow rate is used to maintain the concentration gradient across the dialysis membrane for solute removal. **B,** Hemofilter. Plasma concentrations of solutes in the blood compartment remain unchanged as blood travels the length of the fiber and are similar to their concentrations in the ultrafiltrate. The hemofiltration membrane (*broken line*) has relatively large pores, which allow the necessary removal of a large volume of fluid (*heavy arrow*). Replacement fluid is infused into the blood outlet to lower the plasma concentration of solutes and compensate for the fluid loss. **C,** Glomerulus. Analogous to hemofiltration, plasma concentration of solutes remains unchanged throughout the length of the glomerular capillary and is similar to that in Bowman space. Fluid removal across the glomerular basement membrane (*broken curve*) is large (*heavy arrow*). Reabsorption of fluid from the renal tubules lowers the plasma concentration of the solutes. (Reproduced with permission from Cheung A: Hemodialysis and hemofiltration. In Greenberg A, editor: *Primer on kidney diseases,* ed 4, Philadelphia, 2005, National Kidney Foundation, Saunders, ch 90.)

solute (both diffusive and convective) and does not depend on the extent of partitioning of the solute between plasma water and red blood cells or on calculation of the sieving coefficient of the membrane, it is the more easily used and accurate measurement of solute clearance.

Hemofiltration

A technique that allows for the removal of solutes as well as plasma water primarily or solely by convection (i.e., without diffusion) is called *hemofiltration*. In this technique, there is no dialysate flow, and the ultrafiltrate has the same composition as plasma water. Conceptually, this technique mirrors

the clearance mechanism that occurs across the native glomerulus (Fig. 58.3). However, in the absence of fluid reabsorption mediated by the renal tubules in the native kidney, the hemofiltration technique relies on infusion of large amounts of fluids to replace the large convective fluid losses, generally middialyzer or at the outlet of the dialyzer. Because of the requirement of large volumes of sterile solutions to replace the ultrafiltrate, hemofiltration is not widely used for the treatment of chronic dialysis patients in the United States, and is commercially available only through one manufacturer in the United States. In this chapter, we will limit the detailed discussion to the hemodialysis procedure.

Net Clearance

Although the previous equations predict that the clearance of a substance will increase as blood flow (Q_B) and/or dialysate flow (Q_D) increase, in reality the clearance of solutes increases linearly with increases in blood and/or dialysate flow only up to a point before leveling off (Fig. 58.4). This plateau is reached at different clearance values depending on the size of the solute and the specific membrane characteristics (porosity, thickness, surface charge, the chemical composition of the membrane, and so forth). The summative membrane characteristics are called the mass transfer coefficient (Ko). The mass transfer coefficient is specific for the membrane used and the solute being considered; for dialyzers, this is usually represented as KoA, where A is the effective surface area of the specific dialyzer. Manufacturers generally provide the KoA of the different solutes for the specific dialyzer, and the clearance of specific solutes at different blood and dialysate can be calculated from such values. However, it is important to keep in mind that these KoA values are determined by manufacturers in aqueous solutions, and will result in a higher calculated value for these solute clearances than is observed clinically.

Another important caveat in the relationship between higher clearance and higher blood flow rate is the fact that, in the clinical setting, blood flow rate measured by the blood pump may not accurately represent the actual blood flow rate flowing through the hollow fibers of the dialyzer. For example, in cases where the size of the needle used in the inlet bloodline (arterial fistula needle) is too small or the hemodialysis vascular access is malfunctioning because of an inlet stenosis, it is possible that the volume of blood that is delivered by each rotation of the blood pump may be less than predicted, and therefore the blood flow rate noted

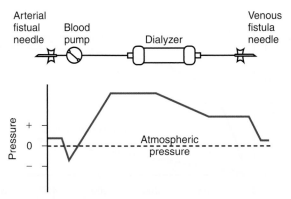

Figure 58.5   The dialysis circuit, with positive and negative pressures at different points in the circuit.

on the dialysis machine (which is calculated from the rotation of the blood pump) may overestimate both the blood flow rate and the resulting solute clearance calculation.

A practical implication of these observations is that, although the clearance of most solutes theoretically increases with higher blood and dialysate flow rates, in practice the maximum prescribed blood flow rate should not exceed a rate at which the negative pre-pump pressure (Fig. 58.5) is greater than –250 mm Hg, not only because this reduces effective clearance (and may also indicate access malfunction) but also because there is higher likelihood of red blood cell lysis, presumably from the sudden change between the negative pressures in the blood tubing before the blood pump and the rapid rise in hydrostatic pressures after the pump.

Finally, although these limitations to blood flow rate do not apply to dialysate flow, there are also practical limits to increasing the dialysate flow rate; not only is the expense of preparing water for dialysate preparation increased, but, because of the limitation of the mass transfer coefficient for specific solutes and specific dialysis membranes, the optimal combination of dialysate flow is approximately 1.5 to 2.0 times the true blood flow rate inside the hollow fibers. Thus, if the maximum blood flow rate (above which the negative arterial pressure prepump exceeds –250 mm Hg) is 350 mL/min, then the optimal dialysate flow is around 600 to 700 mL/min.

Assessing the Dialysis Dose

If clearance is defined as the amount of solute removed by the dialysate at any one time, then the total amount of solute removed during a dialysis procedure can be calculated from Kt, where K, the clearance in mL/min, is multiplied by the time (t) of the procedure in minutes; this assumes that the clearance (K) remains constant throughout the time of the procedure. The other variable that determines the net impact of solute removal from the patient by hemodialysis is the volume of distribution of the solute. Thus, the dose of dialysis is usually defined as Kt/V, where V is the volume of distribution of that particular solute. Urea has been the index molecule used to define the dose of dialysis, because it is easily measured, it is small and therefore diffuses readily across a dialysis membrane, and, importantly, its volume of distribution (total body water) can be calculated from the weight of the patient. Thus, the dose of dialysis traditionally

is defined in terms of urea, rather than other solutes, and the K in the earlier equation typically refers to urea clearance.

A simpler but conventional measure of dialysis dose is urea reduction rate (URR). The URR is also based on urea but avoids the need to define or measure clearance or determine the volume of distribution. The URR usually is expressed as percent reduction, defined as

$$\% \, URR = \frac{(C_{pre} - C_{post})}{C_{pre}} \times 100$$

where C_{post} is the urea concentration at the completion of dialysis, and C_{pre} is the urea concentration before the start of dialysis. This is traditionally expressed as a percentage. Because both calculations of dialysis dose are dependent on changes in urea concentration, there is a nonlinear relationship between Kt/V and URR, which is best represented by the equation:

$$Kt/V = 0.04 \times URR \, (\%) - 1.2$$

Solute Clearance Other Than Urea

Although solute clearance by diffusion is dependent on the size of the solute molecule, other considerations, such as the electrical charge of the molecule and its effective size, also impact the net transfer of uremic solutes across the membrane. One example is the clearance of phosphate. Phosphate (PO_4) is a uremic toxin that accumulates as kidney failure progresses. Although phosphate has a low molecular weight and, based on its molecular size, would be expected to be easily cleared by high-flux dialysis membranes, in reality phosphate is cleared rather poorly during dialysis because of its high negative charge and the large number of water molecules that circulate with the phosphate moiety; additionally, because of the large intracellular reservoirs of phosphate and slow transfer from the intracellular to the plasma compartment, net phosphate clearance by dialysis is poor. This results in a time-dependent slow clearance during conventional dialysis, with moderate clearance and declining removal during the first 2 hours of standard hemodialysis, and negligible removal afterward. However, as discussed later, the removal of phosphates is higher during longer dialysis treatments, such as occurs with nocturnal dialysis (approximately 8 hours), because the longer dialysis time allows the time-dependent transfer of phosphate from intracellular to the plasma compartment; accordingly, patients treated with nocturnal dialysis often require fewer or no phosphate binders.

Extracellular Volume Control (Ultrafiltration)

Another important function of hemodialysis is the removal of excess fluid that accumulates in the absence of effective kidney function. The major driving force that determines the rate of ultrafiltration or convective flow is the difference in hydrostatic pressure between the blood compartment and the dialysate compartments across the dialysis membrane; this is called the transmembrane pressure (TMP). Modern dialysis equipment adjusts these hydrostatic pressure gradients by varying the negative ("suction") pressure in the dialysate compartment rather than increasing the pressure in the blood compartment; this avoids the potential for increased lysis of red blood cells. Although the traditional "low-flux" dialysis membrane exhibited a linear relationship between the TMP and the amount of fluid removed, the commonly used high-flux membranes have much larger pore sizes, allowing more rapid UFRs and more rapid transfer of plasma water from the blood compartment to the dialysate. However, as this rapid transfer of plasma water occurs at the inlet of the dialyzer, the concentration of protein (oncotic pressure) rapidly rises in the blood compartment; because these proteins are also negatively charged, there is a corresponding development of a "concentration polarization," whereby there is a rapid increase in negatively charged plasma protein concentration at the membrane surface (inside the blood compartment). This has the effect of disproportionately increasing the oncotic pressure at the interface between the blood compartment and the surface of the membrane. The high oncotic pressure at the surface of these high-flux membranes inhibits further ultrafiltration to the extent that, toward the blood outlet of high-flux dialysis membranes, "reverse filtration" may occur, with dialysate solutions moving across the membrane into the blood compartment. This reverse filtration phenomenon is more likely to occur in membranes with large pore sizes (high-flux membranes) that allow more rapid ultrafiltration than in low-flux membranes, and it also results in a nonlinear relationship between the rate of ultrafiltration and TMP in dialysis using a high-flux membrane as shown in Figure 58.6.

Because of this nonlinear relationship, the UFR is currently determined by accurately measuring the dialysate inflow and outflow rates in a closed-loop circuit rather than manually adjusting the TMP. An accurate fluid pump is used to remove fluid at the desired UFR; as fluid is removed from this closed-loop circuit, a negative pressure is generated in the dialysate loop that allows the ultrafiltration of exactly the same amount of fluid from the blood compartment. In this way, the rate of ultrafiltration is no longer dependent on the high-flux ultrafiltration characteristics of the membrane, but rather is dependent on the UFR set by the operator (Fig. 58.7).

DIALYSATE

In addition to removal of uremic solutes by diffusion and correction of extracellular volume by ultrafiltration, a third function of hemodialysis is to correct a number of metabolic abnormalities that result from the absence of kidney function. Although there are numerous abnormalities in the concentration of various metabolites that result from kidney failure, acid-base (bicarbonate) balance and potassium concentration are examples of the use of various dialysate solutions to correct such abnormalities.

BICARBONATE

In the absence of kidney function, the acidic moieties that are typically the product of metabolism accumulate in the blood and, after exhausting other available buffers, are neutralized by ambient serum bicarbonate molecules, resulting in metabolic acidosis with serum bicarbonate levels typically ranging from 15 to 17 mEq/L in patients with chronic kidney disease (CKD) stage 5 before initiation of dialysis.

One of the functions of dialysis is to compensate for this metabolic acidosis by replenishing blood bicarbonate. Most often, this is accomplished using formulations of dialysate solutions with bicarbonate concentrations, generally between 30 and 32 mEq/L. This "higher than normal"

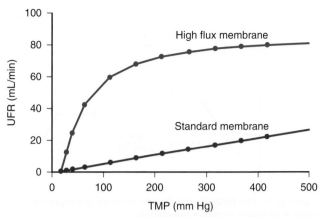

Figure 58.6 The relationship between ultrafiltration rate (UFR) and transmembrane pressure (TMP) for different types of dialysis membranes.

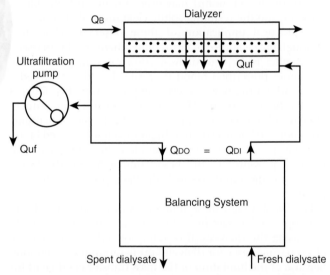

Figure 58.7 Schematic diagram of the "closed-loop" ultrafiltration control used with high-flux membranes.

bicarbonate concentration is needed not only to provide a concentration gradient from the dialysate to the blood compartment, but also to allow the patient to have an intradialysis bicarbonate "reserve." Thus the patient on dialysis cycles during every dialysis from a state of mild metabolic acidosis with respiratory compensation at the beginning of dialysis to a state of mild metabolic alkalosis (and compensatory hypoventilation) at the end of dialysis.

Sodium bicarbonate is used as the source of bicarbonate in the dialysate. However, this product cannot simply be added as a component of dialysate, because the presence of other electrolytes needed in the dialysate (specifically calcium and magnesium) would result in their precipitation as carbonates, thereby reducing the concentration of all three components. Current dialysate delivery technology requires the preparation of two separate dialysate streams, one called "acid concentrate," which combines all the ingredients of dialysate except sodium bicarbonate, and a second stream that contains sodium bicarbonate and sodium chloride. These two concentrates are then separately diluted with treated water and combined together just before reaching the dialysate inlet, resulting in a modestly alkalotic (pH = 7.8) dialysate solution.

One important detail in the choice of dialysate bicarbonate levels is the presence of acetate in the formulation of the "acid concentrate" mentioned earlier. Depending on the manufacturer and whether the concentrate is liquid or powder, most "acid concentrates" contain 4 to 8 mEq/L of acetate (acetic acid) to maintain an acidic milieu and to prevent precipitation of calcium and magnesium salts. It is important that the prescription for the dialysate bicarbonate take into consideration the concentration of the acetate, because the acetate is rapidly metabolized (Krebs cycle) to bicarbonate on a 1:1 ratio. Thus, when the dialysate prescription is for a "bicarbonate level of 35 mEq/L," the effective total buffer in the dialysate may be as high as 42 mEq/L, depending on the amount of acetate; this may result in marked postdialysis alkalemia. There are ongoing studies about the optimal concentration of total buffer, but most observation data suggest that a total buffer of around 35 to 37 mEq/L is optimal; ideally, such a concentration should be adjusted for each patient, depending on their dietary intake, protein catabolic rate, and the resulting predialysis and postdialysis bicarbonate level.

POTASSIUM

Similar therapeutic considerations apply to the prescription of dialysate potassium (K) levels. In the absence of kidney function, potassium (and other electrolytes such as magnesium) accumulates in the blood; accordingly, an important function of dialysis is to reduce the potassium concentration between dialysis episodes to a level that prevents significant predialysis hyperkalemia while avoiding significant hypokalemia after dialysis.

Because potassium removal depends on the difference in potassium concentration between the blood and the dialysate, in concept the simplest way in which potassium removal can be maximized is to use a dialysate potassium concentration of 0 mEq/L. Critically, "0K" dialysate should be avoided, as its use results in an early and very rapid decline in serum potassium concentrations, exceeding the rate at which serum potassium can be replenished from intracellular stores, and potentially predisposing to cardiac arrhythmias or cardiac arrest. In the opinion of the author, the optimal dialysate potassium for almost all patients is 2 or 3 mEq/L, and, for patients with a high predialysis potassium level, the best (safest) option is still to use a dialysate potassium of 2 or 3 mEq/L while extending the dialysis duration to remove more potassium but at a slower rate, which reduces the risk of arrhythmias.

PREPARING PATIENTS FOR MAINTENANCE HEMODIALYSIS

PATIENT EDUCATION AND CHOICE OF THERAPY

It is important to emphasize that the selection of hemodialysis therapy should be a joint decision by the patient and the physician that follows a full discussion about other available kidney replacement therapy options (peritoneal dialysis, home hemodialysis, cadaveric or living-related transplantation) as well as the option of no invasive therapeutic intervention. Such a discussion provides the nephrology team with an opportunity to advise the patient about the medical aspects and the advantages and disadvantages of each modality, accounting for individual patient factors, including patient age, underlying kidney diagnosis and other medical conditions, and family and social conditions. Although the final decision should always take into account the patient's preferences, in the opinion of the author, the nephrologist has the responsibility not only to discuss fully the therapeutic options available but also to offer advice and recommendations about the available choices.

If the patient is competent to make decisions, and the patient and physician are in agreement, there is little that should stand in the way of carrying out their choice, be it for or against the initiation of dialysis. Anecdotally, it should be noted that, particularly among older patients who present with very advanced kidney disease, many refuse to consider dialysis treatment while in the office, but they seldom refuse it when confronting acute pulmonary edema or pericarditis; thus, the relationship between the CKD patient and the nephrology team ideally should be longstanding to allow full discussion of the therapeutic options, the necessary time for the psychological acceptance of the therapy before dialysis is urgently needed, and sufficient time for the creation of a functional native arteriovenous (AV) fistula for repetitive blood access.

30-20-10 Program for Dialysis Preparation

In the United States, more than 40% of patients who initiate dialysis do so without previous active follow-up by nephrologists, even though most patients have had some interaction with the healthcare system before kidney failure. Even for patients who are followed by nephrologists, there may be reluctance by the patient and even by the nephrologist to discuss fully the therapeutic options for treating kidney failure. Unless such discussion occurs, the patient will typically end up on hemodialysis—ill-prepared, resentful, and depressed.

A number of publications have highlighted the advantages of using the 30-20-10 "rule of thumb" for an orderly process of patient referral to a nephrologist and initiation of kidney replacement therapy. According to this guideline, at a glomerular filtration rate (GFR) of 30 mL/min, patients should be referred for active follow-up with a nephrologist, preferably jointly with the referring physician. The 30-20-10 "rule of thumb" further suggests that when the patient's GFR is around 20 mL/min, an AV fistula should be placed in patients who have not already elected an alternative kidney replacement modality while therapeutic options continue to be actively discussed with the patient (and family). Finally, at a GFR of around 10 mL/min, an informed choice of kidney replacement modality (including conservative therapy) should be in place for initiation when medically indicated.

Although opinions differ on this topic, this author's recommendation is that an AV fistula be placed at a GFR of 20 mL/min even in patients who elect peritoneal dialysis (PD) as an initial therapy (because of the relatively high rate of PD technique failure) and in those who desire cadaveric transplantation, because the wait-time for such transplantation can be several years.

Psychological Factors in Dialysis Initiations

Patients who are informed about the probable need to initiate dialysis often undergo the same reactions as those patients being informed about any life-threatening illness; most undergo the stages of grief that have been described by Kubler-Ross—denial, anger, bargaining, depression, and finally acceptance of this lifelong chronic hardship.

It is essential to allay the anxiety and fear common in patients nearing kidney failure. Whenever possible, family members should be included in the decision-making process, and all members of the nephrology team, including the nephrologist, nurses, social workers, transplant coordinators, and dieticians, should participate in this process. If possible, patients and interested family members should visit the dialysis unit well before requiring dialysis, as this simple exercise may help alleviate many of their fears and misconceptions. Because most patients also anticipate much pain during dialysis, it should be stressed that almost no pain is involved. The need for compliance with diet, fluid intake, medications, and dialysis schedules should be stressed, and the patient should be empowered to participate in his or her own care, helping to ensure compliance and improve satisfaction. For patients presenting with an acute need to start dialysis, one option to consider is to frame dialysis initiation specifically as a trial, stressing that the decision to initiate is temporary and should not be binding.

Choice of Treatment Modalities

Several factors influence modality choice. Patient age is most apparent. For example, infants and children have high morbidity on long-term hemodialysis or peritoneal dialysis; accordingly, kidney transplantation offers the greatest likelihood of successful growth and development. On the other hand, morbidity and mortality for elderly patients may be higher with transplant than with dialysis, particularly in the absence of a living donor. The cause of kidney failure is an element that needs to be integrated into the selection of treatment options; for example, patients with brittle diabetes or previous abdominal surgery may benefit from thrice weekly in-center hemodialysis, whereas those with cirrhosis or severe cardiomyopathy may be treated more successfully with peritoneal dialysis or daily hemodialysis regimens. When multiple dialysis modalities are equally possible from a medical point of view, practical issues such as the presence of a supportive family environment, work habits, and economic factors (e.g., availability of transportation, housing issues, and distance from dialysis centers) often favor one modality over another.

VASCULAR ACCESS

Preparation and Timing of Vascular Access

Whichever option the patient chooses (except in cases of well-matched living-related transplantation that can be preplanned), it is recommended for all patients approaching the need for dialysis initiation that an AV fistula be created at a GFR of around 20 mL/min. Even if the patient's initial choice is peritoneal dialysis, a "backup" AV fistula in these patients can be valuable for long-term care, as many peritoneal dialysis patients will lose their PD catheters temporarily at least once because of infection or mechanical failure, and multiple PD catheter losses frequently occur in individual PD patients. Each PD catheter loss may require a hemodialysis treatment for several weeks, in part accounting for the high dropout rate of patients on PD therapies (25% to 30%

on an annual basis). However, if a synthetic graft is all that is possible because of poor native vasculature, backup access is not recommended, because the risk-to-benefit ratio of synthetic grafts is unacceptably high in this situation.

Native AV fistulas have a significantly lower incidence of infection, and their half-life, if they are well developed before their use, is much longer than that of synthetic grafts. In some medical centers, access-related problems account for 30% to 40% of all nephrology admissions, representing a medical, emotional, and economic burden to the patient; thus the presence of either rapidly progressing or already advanced kidney disease should prompt AV fistula creation well before the expected date of initiation of dialysis. Central vein catheters, even if placed for a short time, are associated with a high risk of infection and adversely impact the longevity of any subsequent AV fistula or graft.

The following recommendations are useful guidelines:

1. A vascular access surgeon should evaluate patients with progressive kidney function decline at the earliest opportunity to determine the best sites for vascular access (this should occur no later than at a GFR of around 20 mL/min, according to the 30-20-10 rule of thumb). Early placement of AV fistulas not only allows for the development of the fistula (which generally takes 6 to 8 weeks on average), but also allows for needed interventions, including placement of a second fistula if the initial fistula does not mature. Studies show that in approximately 50% of cases of AV fistula creation, a second procedure is required before the fistula is usable for hemodialysis because of the associated central venous stenosis, particularly in patients who previously had central venous catheters.
2. Although access should be planned first in the nondominant arm, sites should be preserved in the other arm as well. The use of the nondominant arm is preferred, particularly for self-dialysis, as it makes self-cannulation more likely. Radial arteries and cephalic veins should be preserved except in life-threatening situations. In particular, use of radial arteries for nonessential "arterial lines" as well as the use of peripherally inserted central catheters (PICC lines) should be discouraged. Whenever possible, phlebotomy should be limited to veins over the dorsum of the hand and the ulnar side of the forearm. If absolutely necessary, median antecubital veins may be punctured with small butterfly needles. Intravenous lines should spare the cephalic vein. If long-term outpatient infusions are required, consider using tunneled internal jugular catheters rather than PICC lines.
3. In hospitalized patients, sites that are being preserved should be marked with a black felt-tipped pen as a reminder to all. A notice on the wall above the patient's bed is also helpful.
4. Patients should be educated to preserve their own vasculature.

TYPES OF ARTERIOVENOUS FISTULAS

Radiocephalic Arteriovenous Fistulas

A standard vascular access now preferred by most access surgeons is a distal cephalic vein to radial artery end-to-side anastomosis near the wrist. Again, the preservation of both cephalic veins from the time of kidney disease diagnosis

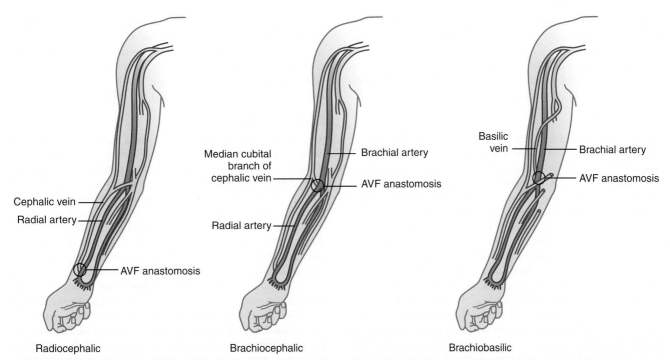

Figure 58.8 **Anatomy of the upper-extremity vasculature.** Vessels named are instrumental for the creation of hemodialysis fistula and grafts for vascular access. *AVF,* Arteriovenous fistula. (Adapted with permission from Allon M, Robbin ML: Increasing arteriovenous fistulas in hemodialysis patients: problems and solutions, *Kidney Int* 62:1109-1124, 2002.)

is critical, because the radiocephalic fistula is the optimal first option, thus preserving upper-arm veins for later use (Fig. 58.8).

Brachiocephalic and Brachiobasilic Fistulas

The next best approach is a more proximal fistula also employing the patient's own vasculature, as described in Figure 58.8. Upper-arm fistulas tend to have higher flow and therefore are more vulnerable to aneurysmal dilation; additionally, patients may have more difficulty self-cannulating upper-arm access. Nevertheless, in patients without adequate forearm cephalic veins, brachiocephalic or brachiobasilic AV fistulas should still be placed approximately 6 months in advance of the time when dialysis is anticipated. A final, less common option is a proximal radial artery fistula.

Access in Problem Patients

In patients who cannot receive either a forearm or an upper-arm fistula using their own vasculature, a synthetic graft may be placed in the forearm. Either a distal radial artery to basilic vein (straight) graft or a loop from the brachial artery to the basilic vein should be considered. Synthetic grafts are more prone to infection and clotting than fistulas using endogenous vessels. Therefore, synthetic grafts should not be placed in anticipation of future dialysis need until generally 3 to 4 weeks before initiation of dialysis, with the recognition that optimal timing can be a challenge.

Catheters

Because kidney disease is often "silent," it is inevitable that some patients will present with clear indications for initiation of dialysis but without a permanent access. In such cases, if hemodialysis is elected, dialysis initiation requires the placement of a catheter, preferably in the internal jugular vein. Because of the much higher propensity for infections, catheter malfunction and inadequate blood flow through these catheters, and the risk of developing vein stenosis along the path of the catheter, it is critical that a permanent access plan be developed and implemented as soon as it is determined that the patient has chronic (and not acute) kidney failure. Ideally, the placement of permanent access, preferably an AV fistula, should take place during the initial hospital admission and before the patient is discharged to the dialysis unit.

Another option is to place a PD catheter and to continue to dialyze such patients in an outpatient setting while educating the patient and their family members about the technique of PD dialysis as well as other therapeutic options. Finally, if the age and medical condition of the patient permit, living-related transplantation should be pursued.

INITIATION OF HEMODIALYSIS

Assuming that hemodialysis is the modality of choice, what is the optimal dialysis prescription? This section briefly discusses different dialysis techniques, including short daily hemodialysis and nocturnal hemodialysis, with a focus on conventional, thrice weekly, in-center dialysis, as this remains the most common hemodialysis strategy. The dialysis dose, the time needed to optimize kidney replacement therapy, and strategies for accomplishing this are reviewed. To place common hemodialysis strategies into context, current in-center hemodialysis regimens average less than 3.5 hours per procedure and tend to provide less than 10 mL/min of creatinine clearance for the patient on an intermittent basis. Considering that this level is below the level at which hemodialysis is initiated, it is clear that the delivery of dialysis is inadequate and likely allows for shortened survival. It is therefore not surprising that the annual mortality rate of patients on such therapy is more than 20%, and that the 5-year survival of ESRD patients is less than many forms of cancer. Several factors should be considered in the prescription of dialysis to optimize outcomes.

DIALYSIS TIME

It is possible to estimate the minimum dialysis time that a patient may need to achieve a specific target Kt/V or URR, taking into consideration the patient's residual kidney function (RKF). For the hypothetical 70-kg person, the first step is to calculate the volume of urea distribution, which is total body water. For men, this is assumed to be 60% of body weight (42 L), whereas in women it is assumed to be 55% of body weight (38.5 L). The next step is to determine the clearance of the dialyzer at specific "blood" and dialysate flow rates. An in vitro evaluation of urea clearance is usually included in the package insert of the dialyzer, accounting for the surface area of the dialyzer, the solution flow rate, and other dialyzer factors. However, since this is an in vitro assessment based on an aqueous solution, it is reasonable to assume that the in vivo urea clearance is approximately 80% of the reported in vitro clearance. Accordingly, assuming the in vitro urea clearance at a "blood flow" of 300 mL/min and dialysate flow of 500 mL/min is 250 mL/min, then the presumed in vivo urea clearance is $250 \times 0.8 = 200$ mL/min, at a blood flow of 300 mL/min.

If the goal of therapy is to achieve a minimum Kt/V of 1.2, as recommended by Kidney Disease Outcomes Quality Initiative (KDOQI) guidelines, then the minimum time needed for this patient to achieve a Kt/V of 1.2 is:

$$t = \frac{1.2 \times 42\,\text{L}}{0.2\,\text{L/min}} = 252 \text{ min or 4 h and 12 min}$$

Although larger surface-area dialyzer and higher blood flow rates are means of reducing dialysis duration, based on these data as well as emerging evidence regarding the risks of exceeding an UFR of 10 mL/kg/h, it is strongly recommended that, after the first several sessions, the maintenance dialysis time should be prescribed at no less than 4 hours thrice weekly.

Recently, retrospective analyses of large data sets from the United States and other countries have highlighted the impressive survival benefit of patients dialyzed for 4 or more hours. Possible explanations include theoretical benefits of an increase in the dose of dialysis as well as a decrease in the rate of ultrafiltration to below 10 mL/kg/h, which has been found to be associated with better cardiovascular stability. A final important reason for starting patients at 4 hours is psychological; after a patient is initiated on dialysis for less than 4 hours, there is a strong reluctance on the part of many patients to increase the dialysis duration, regardless of the reason.

For stable CKD patients with progressive kidney failure who may have their initial hemodialysis in the outpatient setting, it would be reasonable to consider starting such patients for 2 hours in the first session, 3 hours in the second session, and 4 hours in the third session to avoid possible disequilibrium; however, the goal of at least a 4-hour treatment should be achieved as quickly as possible.

Finally, for patients initiating dialysis with a catheter and without a developing AV fistula or graft, it is recommended that the dialysis time be extended by 30 minutes (to 4.5 hours), with clear communication that dialysis time may be reduced to 4 hours only if and when a permanent access is used routinely for dialysis, and the catheter is removed.

RESIDUAL KIDNEY FUNCTION

Almost all patients initiating dialysis have some RKF and urine output. Although residual function provides additional (and continuous) clearance of solutes and water, the initiation of hemodialysis leads to a relatively rapid loss of RKF, possibly reflecting dialysis-associated hypotension and ischemic kidney injury, progression of the underlying kidney disease, or the inflammatory burden associated with the dialysis procedure itself. Studies have shown that in most patients, RKF is reduced close to zero within approximately 3 months following dialysis initiation. Therefore, although it is common to initiate dialysis at shorter times when taking into account the endogenous clearance of solutes from the RKF, we recommend against such a process, since the loss of RKF is fairly rapid, the measurement of RKF (requiring intradialytic urine collection at around 48 hours) is burdensome, and, most important, there is strong resistance among patients who initiate dialysis with a shorter duration to extend their treatment when RKF is lost. Accordingly, it is the author's suggestion that RKF should not be considered when the prescription for dialysis is considered.

TARGET OR "DRY" WEIGHT AND RATE OF ULTRAFILTRATION

A critical item for patients initiating dialysis is the establishment of a target weight, which is the weight that the patient needs to achieve at the end of dialysis and at which the patient is close to euvolemia—the so-called "dry weight." Although patients who present with dependent peripheral edema or pulmonary edema have excess fluid volume that can be easily targeted, often it is difficult to determine the target dry weight on clinical examination.

For the rare patient who is not on antihypertensive medications, the achievement of near normal blood pressure may be one of the signs of achieving target weight; however, most CKD patients receive multiple blood-pressure medications, complicating the use of blood-pressure readings as an index of euvolemia. Blood-pressure medications also complicate the achievement of the target weight, because these medications may predispose patients to hypotension during fluid removal. Accordingly, achievement of target weight based on clinical assessment is often a process of trial and error that subjects patients to frequent episodes of hypotension.

Recently, two devices have become available to help in determining target weight. The first (Bioimpedance) can be used on the patient during dialysis by applying electrodes to the skin and measuring the electrical impedance of tissue as fluid is removed during dialysis via ultrafiltration. As of this writing, the use of bioimpedance devices to determine target or "dry weight" has not received FDA clearance in the United States. The second device, called the "crit-line," provides a continuous measure of online hematocrit. The principle of this device is that ultrafiltration can be temporarily halted toward the end of dialysis, followed by assessment of the rate of fluid transfer into the vascular space, which is indicated by a decline in hematocrit from hemodilution. Substantial declines in hematocrit indicate the need to lower the postdialysis target weight.

The attempt to determine target weight should not distract from another important consideration, namely the determination and prescription of UFRs—the rate at which fluid is removed from the total body water. Recent literature suggests that rates of ultrafiltration that exceed 10 mL/kg/h (approximately 700 mL/h for the 70 kg person) are often associated with cardiovascular instability, hypotension, and cramps. Therefore, if the target weight of the patient after dialysis is more than 3 kg (3 L) lower than the patient's predialysis weight, additional dialysis sessions or increasing dialysis time (to allow the achievement of target weight without exceeding the range of 10 mL/kg/h UFR) should be strongly considered.

DOSE OF DELIVERED DIALYSIS

As discussed earlier, the dose of delivered dialysis is traditionally determined by changes in urea concentration before and after dialysis. Although urea is no longer considered the principal "uremic toxin," urea concentration in the blood and subsequent urea clearance with dialytic therapy correlate reasonably well with the changes observed clinically. Furthermore, urea is easily measured in the blood and dialysate, is evenly distributed in total body water, and rapidly diffuses from intracellular to extracellular and vascular spaces. Therefore, it is reasonable to assume that changes in urea concentration during dialysis reflect the dose of dialysis.

Using urea as the accepted marker of the dose of dialysis, the DOQI guidelines established by the National Kidney Foundation in consensus with the Renal Physician Association and National Institutes of Health recommend that achievement of a urea Kt/V index of at least 1.2 represents the minimum accepted dose of thrice weekly hemodialysis. On the basis of limited long-term studies and no clinical trial data, the best patient outcomes appear associated with Kt/V values of 1.2 to 1.4, to be achieved in no less than 4 hours (as discussed previously) and at UFRs that do not exceed 10 mL/kg/h. The determination of URR or Kt/V depends critically on the accurate determination of urea pre- and postdialysis, and the accurate determination of dialysis time. It is therefore important to be aware of the potential errors that could be introduced in determining each of these measures.

Potential Errors in Predialysis Urea Measurement

Blood for predialysis urea is generally collected after insertion of the access needle in the patient's vascular access, or it is drawn directly from the catheter. If the blood sample is drawn from a catheter or a recently flushed bloodline, there is a strong likelihood that the blood sample will be diluted with residual saline solution, unless approximately 5 mL of blood is drawn and set aside, and then the blood sample for urea measurement is drawn. Therefore, the technique and methodology of blood sample drawing should be evaluated to ensure that there is no dilution of the predialysis blood urea sample.

Potential Errors in Postdialysis Urea Measurement

The postdialysis urea blood sample must be drawn from the "arterial" (intake) needle and must be drawn either at least 2 minutes after dialysis is terminated (preferred) or toward the end of dialysis after the dialysate flow is stopped and the blood pump has been slowed to 50 mL/min for at least 5 minutes to avoid recirculation. *Recirculation* of blood at the end of dialysis not only refers to the possibility of mixing the blood from the inlet (arterial) and outlet (venous) blood that occurs commonly when the needle tips are close to each other (less than 1 inch apart), particularly when blood flow is high, but also refers to a phenomenon called *cardiopulmonary recirculation*. Cardiopulmonary recirculation occurs throughout a dialysis session and can be illustrated by the following observation: when tested, the urea concentration of the blood entering the dialyzer is often different from the urea concentration of the blood in distant peripheral tissues, because the dialyzed blood (which has low urea) concentration dilutes the blood entering the right atrium from the tissues, and it takes several minutes for this blood in the right atrium to be "pumped" or distributed to the peripheral tissues. This cardiopulmonary recirculation is more pronounced in patients dialyzed with high urea clearance dialysis (large dialyzer surface area or rapid blood flow) and in patients with low cardiac output. In many patients, the solute (urea) concentration at the arterial (inlet) bloodline rises by approximately 10% over a 3-minute period after dialysis is discontinued, and blood samples drawn immediately after termination of dialysis will have artificially lower urea concentration, resulting in overestimation of urea reduction and Kt/V compared to blood samples drawn after the urea concentration is uniformly distributed throughout the patient. It is therefore important to emphasize the need for prescribing exactly how the postdialysis urea sample needs to be drawn, specifically that one should either wait for 2 minutes after dialysis has ended (preferred) or reduce the blood flow to 50 mL/min for 5 minutes, with the dialysate turned off, before the postdialysis blood is sampled.

Potential Errors in Treatment Time

Although treatment time is generally considered to be the difference between the dialysis start time and termination time, actual treatment time may be significantly lower than "clock time," reflecting factors such as time taken to reach maximum blood flow, alarm interruptions, and other interruptions, such as time for patients to use bathrooms. Modern dialysis machines report either actual dialysis time or blood volumes processed, the latter based on the rotation of the blood pump (with its attendant caveat mentioned earlier).

ANTICOAGULATION PRESCRIPTIONS

The contact of the blood with "foreign" surfaces such as the dialyzer membrane triggers the coagulation cascade. In the absence of anticoagulants, this results in blood clotting inside the dialyzer hollow fibers leading initially to loss of dialyzer surface area, and eventually to loss of appreciable volumes of patient blood in the clotted dialyzer. Because the coagulation cascade is triggered as soon as blood is in contact with foreign surfaces, anticoagulation must be effective before such blood–membrane contact. The most commonly used anticoagulant is unfractionated heparin; initial dosing is most often weight based (approximately 50 units/kg), administered as a bolus immediately following needles insertion and establishment of access patency. Because it is important to allow the heparin to reach systemic circulation, an interval of approximately 3 minutes following the administration of heparin should elapse before the blood is allowed to reach the extracorporeal circuit via the blood pump. If blood reaches the dialyzer membrane before full anticoagulation, it is likely that local clotting inside the fibers will occur, reducing the available dialyzer membrane surface area and therefore the clearance of uremic toxins.

Because of the steady decline in heparin concentration and level of anticoagulation during dialysis (via both heparin metabolism and adsorption on the extracorporeal surface), it is recommended that a continuous infusion of low doses of heparin be administered throughout most of the treatment at a rate of approximately 1000 units/h. For patients with permanent accesses (AV fistula or graft), it is also recommended that this continuous heparin be discontinued approximately 30 minutes before the end of dialysis to facilitate timely hemostasis of the vascular access after the withdrawal of the needles at the termination of dialysis. For patients dialyzed with a catheter, continuous heparin may be prescribed until the end of the treatment to reduce the risk of clotting of the catheter tips, because "hemostasis" of the catheter at the termination of dialysis is not required.

Although these recommendations are not based on extensive studies, they are clinically effective in most patients. In patients who may be using warfarin anticoagulation for other reasons, the dose of heparin should be reduced although not eliminated, as heparin and warfarin have different mechanisms of action on the coagulation cascade. In a small fraction of patients, heparin results in significant thrombocytopenia and alternative methods of anticoagulation need to be considered.

FREQUENCY OF DIALYSIS

Thrice weekly dialysis, with each session lasting a few hours, was established somewhat arbitrarily as the standard for maintenance hemodialysis in the 1970s, primarily for practical reasons including patient and staff convenience. Because of technological advances in the delivery of dialysis, the dialysis procedure has become much safer, with greater availability of equipment suitable for home use; accordingly, regimens with different frequencies and different times of day are being explored. Nevertheless, thrice weekly, daytime in-center hemodialysis remains by far the most common regimen.

Nocturnal Dialysis

Because of the need to have several episodes of patient turnover during the day (to accommodate the number of patients who need to be dialyzed), nephrologists who wanted to prescribe dialysis times of 6 to 8 hours initiated nocturnal dialysis, wherein patients begin their dialysis treatment in the evening, spending 6 to 8 hours receiving dialysis (generally while sleeping). This can be performed either in-center or at home. Such prolonged dialysis allows for an increase in the total dose of dialysis (Kt/V often approximately 2.5 for nocturnal dialysis) with much slower rates of ultrafiltration and diffusive clearance. Data are accumulating that demonstrate that nocturnal dialysis is associated with better blood pressure control with a reduced requirement for antihypertensive medications, less intradialytic hypotension, and reduced hospitalization and mortality. Because the total solute clearance also increases, nocturnal dialysis is also associated with better phosphorus control with a reduced requirement for phosphorus binders.

There is a slow but steady increase in the number of dialysis facilities that provide nocturnal dialysis, because these facilities can accommodate more patients (both during the day and night), with minimal or moderate marginal cost; however, patient acceptance, nurse recruitment, and the need for physician visits at night are some of the barriers for this therapy. Nocturnal dialysis can also be performed at home, but the fear of catastrophic events, such as severe hypotension and needle dislodgement while the patient is asleep, has limited this strategy. Of note, devices that are activated by red blood cells and awaken the patient if there is a blood leak recently have become available; these may improve the safety of nocturnal dialysis procedure, both in-center and at home.

Short Daily Hemodialysis and Hemofiltration

An alternative to nocturnal dialysis that still increases the weekly number of dialysis hours is short daily hemodialysis, which is most often performed 5 or 6 times weekly for approximately 3 hours per session. This modality may result in improved blood pressure control and reduced left ventricular hypertrophy, along with a significant reduction in mortality.

One modification of this short daily hemodialysis regimen, called hemodiafiltration, was recently introduced, whereby hemofiltration replaces the usual process of having blood and dialysate flow countercurrent across a dialysis membrane as described earlier. This therapy is now available commercially, can be used at home, and requires the provision of the hemofilter as well as sterile replacement fluid. The advantage of daily hemofiltration is that it does not require dialysate preparation, and, possibly because this technique allows the removal of higher molecular weight uremic solutes, hemofiltration may improve patient outcomes. Potential disadvantages include the requirement for daily treatments and the need for home delivery of large volumes of fluid on a regular basis. Another noted disadvantage of daily dialysis therapies is that the frequent cannulation of the AV fistula may lead to an increase in the frequency of procedures for access repair.

Whether through nocturnal or daily hemodialysis, both of which are associated with improved survival and improvements in other intermediate outcomes (see Chapter 60), it is clear that more attention needs to be paid to dialysis duration if patient outcomes are to improve. Recent data clearly demonstrate that the adequacy of hemodialysis should not be solely based on URR or Kt/V (which can be accomplished in shorter times, using large surface-area dialyzers), but also should take into account the cumulative weekly dialysis time, as well as the rate of ultrafiltration, with short daily dialysis better approximating the continuous daily clearance of the native kidneys.

BIBLIOGRAPHY

Chertow GM, Levin NW, Kliger AS, et al: In-center hemodialysis six times per week versus three times per week, N Engl J Med 363: 2287-2300, 2010.

Culleton BF, Walsh M, Klarenbach SW, et al: Effect of frequent nocturnal hemodialysis vs conventional hemodialysis on left ventricular mass and quality of life: a randomized controlled trial, JAMA 298:1291-1299, 2007.

Eknoyan G, Beck GJ, Cheung AK, et al: Hemodialysis (HEMO) Study Group: effect of dialysis dose and membrane flux in maintenance hemodialysis, *N Engl J Med* 347:2010-2019, 2002.

El Ters M, Schears GJ, Taler SJ, et al: Association between prior peripherally inserted central catheters and lack of functioning arteriovenous fistulas: a case-control study in hemodialysis patients, *Am J Kidney Dis* 60:601-608, 2012.

Finkelstein FO, Story K, Firenek C, et al: Perceived knowledge among patients cared for by a nephrologist about chronic kidney disease and end-stage renal disease therapies, *Kidney Int* 58:235-242, 2011.

Foley RN, Gilbertson DT, Murray T, et al: Long interdialytic interval and mortality among patients receiving hemodialysis, *N Engl J Med* 365:1099-1107, 2011.

Goldstein MB, Jindal KK, Levin A, et al: The adequacy of hemodialysis: assessment and achievement. In Jacobson HR, Striker GE, Klahr S, editors: *The principles and practice of nephrology*, St. Louis, 1995, Mosby. ch 97.

Grootman MP, Van den Dorpal MA, Bots ML, et al: Effect of online hemodiafiltration on all cause mortality and cardiovascular outcomes, *J Am Soc Nephrol* 23:1087-1096, 2012.

Lacson E, Lazarus JM, Himmelfarb J, et al: Balancing fistula first with catheters last, *Am J Kidney Dis* 50:379-395, 2007.

Lacson E Jr, Brunelli SM: Hemodialysis treatment time: a fresh perspective, *Clin J Am Soc Nephrol* 6:2523-2530, 2011.

Lacson E Jr, Wang W, DeVries C, et al: Effects of a nationwide predialysis educational program on modality choice, vascular access, and patient outcomes, *Am J Kidney Dis* 58:235-242, 2011.

Lacson E Jr, Wang W, Zebrowski, et al: Outcomes associated with intradialytic oral nutritional supplements in patients undergoing maintenance hemodialysis: a quality improvement report, *Am J Kidney Dis* 60:591-600, 2012.

McIntyre CW, Rosensky SJ: Starting dialysis is dangerous, *Kidney Int* 82:382-387, 2012.

Mehrotra R, Agarwal R: End stage renal disease and dialysis: nephrology re-assessment. NephSAP, volume 11, November 2012. Available at http://www.asn-online.org/education/nephsap/active.aspx. (Accessed May 24, 2013.)

Owen WF, Lew NL, Liu Y, et al: The urea reduction ratio and serum albumin concentration as predictors of mortality in patients undergoing hemodialysis, *N Engl J Med* 329:1001-1006, 1993.

Rosensky SJ, Eggers P, Jackson K, et al: Early start of hemodialysis may be harmful, *Arch Intern Med* 171:396-403, 2011.

Shen JI, Winklelmayer WC: Use and safety of unfractionated heparin for anticoagulation during maintenance hemodialysis, *Am J Kidney Dis* 60:463-486, 2012.

Solid CA, Carlin C: Timing of arteriovenous fistula placement and medical costs during dialysis initiation, *Am J Nephrol* 35:498-508, 2012.

Spiegel DM: Avoiding harm and achieving optimal dialysis outcomes—the dialysate component, *Adv Chronic Kidney Dis* 19:166-170, 2012.

Suri RS, Nesrallah GE, Mainra R, et al: Daily hemodialysis: a systematic review, *Clin J Am Soc Nephrol* 1:33-42, 2006.

59 Peritoneal Dialysis

Anand Vardhan | Alastair J. Hutchison

Peritoneal dialysis (PD), hemodialysis, and kidney transplantation are the cornerstones of kidney replacement therapy. These modalities are not mutually exclusive, and during a lifetime of therapy, patients may transfer from one modality to another, often returning to the original form in due course. In the 1950s and 1960s, peritoneal dialysis was used predominantly to manage acute kidney injury, and patients with end-stage renal disease (ESRD) were treated almost exclusively by hemodialysis and occasionally by intermittent peritoneal dialysis (IPD). The introduction in 1976 of continuous ambulatory peritoneal dialysis (CAPD) transformed this paradigm. There was a dramatic rise in the use of peritoneal dialysis internationally during the 1980s and 1990s, especially in the developing world. This has not been the case in the United States, where usage declined by approximately 6.5% each year between 1996 and 2000, and by 2.4% each year between 2000 and 2004. In 2004, the incident rate for new peritoneal dialysis patients in the United States was 21.6 per million population. It has remained relatively steady since then and was 21.9 per million population in 2009.

Although many comparisons have been made between hemodialysis and peritoneal dialysis, the focus has shifted more recently to where a therapy is delivered (i.e., home-based or hospital-based). The advantages of home-based therapies for some patients are becoming apparent. Home-based therapies are popular in Canada, Netherlands, Iceland, Finland, Denmark, Australia, New Zealand, Mexico, and Hong Kong, where more than 20% of dialysis patients are treated with home therapies. PD accounts for almost 80% of patients on dialysis in Hong Kong and about 65% of patients in Mexico. Contrary to prior concepts of self-care requiring a fully capable patient, PD has expanded in some countries to become the therapy of choice for older adults and those with multiple comorbidities. The introduction of assisted PD has made home treatment more widely available, with patients receiving varying degrees of assistance by a trained health professional in their home.

Acute-start PD is used in many parts of the world, especially for patients with single-organ acute kidney injury requiring dialysis, as well as for "late presenters" with end-stage kidney disease (ESKD).

PRINCIPLES OF PERITONEAL DIALYSIS

THE PERITONEAL MEMBRANE

With peritoneal dialysis, the peritoneal membrane is used as the dialyzing surface. The visceral peritoneal membrane tightly covers the intestine and mesentery, whereas the parietal peritoneum lines the remaining surfaces of the abdominal cavity. The peritoneal membrane consists of a single layer of mesothelial cells overlying an interstitium in which the blood and lymphatic vessels lie. The mesothelial cells are covered by microvilli that markedly increase the nominal surface area ($2\ m^2$) of the peritoneum, but the effective peritoneal surface area available for dialysis is estimated to be about one third of this.

SOLUTE MOVEMENT

Peritoneal dialysis primarily represents solute and fluid exchange across the peritoneal membrane between the peritoneal capillary blood and the dialysis solution that is instilled into the peritoneal cavity. There is also a small amount of fluid and solute resorption via the lymphatics. Solute movement occurs as a result of both diffusion and convective transport, whereas fluid shifts relate largely to osmosis created by the addition of osmotic agents to the dialysis solutions. During peritoneal dialysis, solutes such as urea, creatinine, and potassium move from the peritoneal capillaries across the peritoneal membrane to the peritoneal cavity, whereas other solutes, such as lactate and bicarbonate, usually move in the opposite direction. Solute movement is mainly by diffusion and is therefore based on the concentration gradient of the solute between dialysate and blood. Solutes also move across the peritoneal membrane by convection, which is defined as the movement of solutes as a result of fluid flux.

FLUID MOVEMENT

Standard peritoneal dialysis fluid contains varying concentrations of glucose, in the form of dextrose, as the osmotic agent. Therefore the dialysate is hyperosmolar in relation to serum, causing fluid efflux (ultrafiltration) to occur. The volume of ultrafiltration depends on the concentration of glucose solution used for each exchange, the length of time the fluid dwells in the peritoneal cavity, and the individual patient's peritoneal membrane characteristics (discussed later). With increasing dwell time, transperitoneal glucose absorption diminishes the dialysate glucose concentration and the osmotic gradient. In most patients, ultrafiltration is consequently decreased with long dwell times, such as with the overnight dwell on CAPD or the long daytime dwell on automated peritoneal dialysis (APD).

The crucial physiologic components of the peritoneal dialysis system are peritoneal blood flow and the peritoneal membrane. Components that can be manipulated to maximize solute and fluid removal are dialysate volume, dwell time, and number of exchanges per day. Various techniques and regimens have emerged in the field of peritoneal dialysis as a consequence of increased understanding of peritoneal membrane transport characteristics or permeability in relation to the amount of solute and fluid to be removed.

MEASURING SOLUTE AND FLUID TRANSPORT TO DETERMINE PERITONEAL MEMBRANE CHARACTERISTICS

Peritoneal dialysis effectively removes substances with low molecular weights, such as creatinine, urea, and potassium that are not in the infused dialysis fluid. With increasing dwell time, solutes move across the peritoneal membrane toward concentration equilibrium, and the ratio of dialysate to serum solute levels approaches 1.0. Because the peritoneal membrane has a net negative charge, negatively charged solutes, such as phosphate, move across it more slowly than positively charged solutes of similar size, such as potassium. Macromolecules such as albumin cross the peritoneum by mechanisms that are not completely understood—most likely via lymphatics and through large pores in the capillary membranes. During a dwell, the osmotic gradient created by the dialysate within the abdominal cavity declines as the glucose is absorbed. In time, this can result in fluid reabsorption into the systemic circulation because of the added effects of intraperitoneal hydrostatic pressure and intravascular oncotic pressure. Continuous lymphatic absorption also diminishes net fluid removal.

The rate of movement of small solutes between dialysate and blood differs from one patient to another. Peritoneal function characteristics are monitored by the peritoneal equilibration test (PET) (Fig. 59.1). In this standardized test, 2 L of dialysate containing 2.5 g/dL glucose is infused, and the ratio of dialysate to plasma creatinine (D/PCr ratio) at the end of a 4-hour dwell is calculated. With this test, each patient's peritoneal membrane can be categorized as having high (D/PCr >0.81), high-average (0.65 to 0.81), low-average (0.50 to 0.65), or low (<0.5) peritoneal transport capability. Use of 2 L of dialysate containing 4.25 g/dL glucose for a 4-hour dwell permits assessment of ultrafiltration failure; an effluent volume of less than 2400 mL is diagnostic.

Removal of fluid and solutes is highly dependent on the type of transporter status as described by the PET (Fig. 59.2). Patients with a high D/PCr ratio (high transporters) have rapid clearance of small molecules, but poor ultrafiltration because of rapid glucose absorption and dissipation of the osmotic gradient between dialysate and blood. These patients require short-dwell peritoneal dialysis regimens to achieve adequate fluid removal. In addition, because the volume of fluid removed also contributes to the solute clearance of equilibrated dialysate via convection, high transporters also have reduced solute clearance over long dwells because of low drain volumes. Patients with a low D/PCr ratio (low transporters) have low clearance rates for solutes and usually require more dialysis exchanges, increased volume per exchange, or both to avoid uremic symptoms once residual kidney function is lost. Ultrafiltration in this category of patient is relatively better. Most patients have high-average to low-average peritoneal transport characteristics and do well on either CAPD or APD.

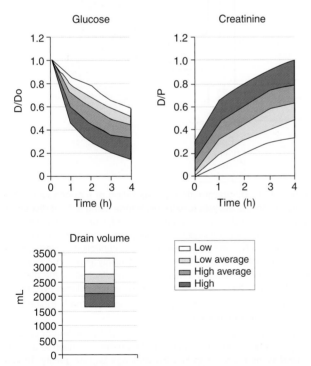

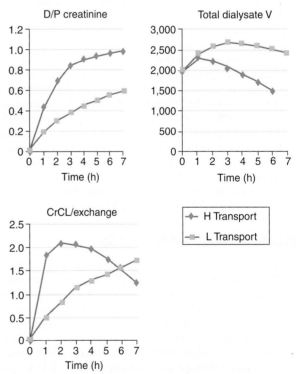

Figure 59.1 The peritoneal equilibration test (PET) measures the peritoneal transport characteristics of glucose from the peritoneal fluid to plasma and of creatinine from plasma to the peritoneal fluid. The instilled peritoneal fluid volume for the PET is 2 L. D/D_0 represents the ratio of dialysate glucose concentration (D) at a given time point to the dialysate glucose concentration at time 0 (D_0). D/P represents the ratio of dialysate (D) to plasma (P) concentrations. The rate of transport of these molecules depends on the permeability of the membrane: the higher the permeability (high transporter), the more rapid the transport of glucose, with dissipation of the osmotic gradient and therefore less drain volume.

Figure 59.2 The profiles of intraperitoneal dialysate volume (V) and solute transport (CrCl/exchange), in relation to dwell time in hours, vary in high transporters (H) and low transporters (L). These profiles are used in prescription setting of dwell times and fluid volumes. For long-dwell continuous ambulatory peritoneal dialysis (CAPD), high transporters show both low fluid removal and low CrCl, compared with low transporters. *CrCl,* Creatinine clearance; *D/P creatinine,* dialysate-to-plasma creatinine ratio.

TECHNIQUES OF PERITONEAL DIALYSIS

CONTINUOUS AMBULATORY PERITONEAL DIALYSIS

CAPD is perhaps the most uncomplicated method of carrying out dialysis. It involves the manual instillation of up to 3 L of dialysis fluid in the peritoneal cavity through an indwelling abdominal catheter four to five times a day. This typically means three or four short dwells during the day and a long dwell overnight. In adults, the total volume of fluid exchanged in a day typically ranges from 8 to 10 L. Thus dialysis occurs continuously throughout the entire 24-hour period and patients are free to engage in daily activities between exchanges. The prescription specifies the type of dialysis fluid, volume to be used, dwell time, and number of exchanges. It may be varied according to patient size, peritoneal permeability, and residual kidney function.

Peritoneal dialysis fluid is instilled by gravity into the peritoneal cavity and drained after a dwell period of several hours, depending on the number of exchanges planned in the 24-hour period. The basic CAPD system, which has remained largely unchanged for almost 3 decades, consists of a plastic bag containing 0.5 to 3.0 L of dialysis fluid, a transfer set (tubing between the catheter and the plastic bag), and a permanent, indwelling Silastic catheter, which is implanted so that the tip of the intraperitoneal portion lies in the pelvis. Because the connection between the bag and the transfer set is interrupted three to five times a day to facilitate fluid exchange (approximately 1500 exchanges per year), the procedure must be carried out using a strict, aseptic, nontouch technique that the patient or helper performs at home. The most common connection device used today is based on a Y-disconnect system. It consists of a filled bag and an empty bag of the same size with a Y-shaped junction that can be connected to the PD catheter. Once the connection has been made, this device allows drainage of the effluent from the abdomen through the connection into the empty bag, before fresh dialysate is instilled. This ensures "flushing out" of any accidental touch contamination in the tubing before infusion of new fluid into the peritoneal cavity (Fig. 59.3). This system reduces the incidence of infection and also relieves the patient from carrying the empty bag and transfer set, thus improving the psychological aspects and quality of life of CAPD patients.

AUTOMATED PERITONEAL DIALYSIS

Automated peritoneal dialysis is a broad term that refers to all forms of peritoneal dialysis that utilize a mechanical device (called a cycler) for instillation and drainage of dialysis fluid. In its simplest, earliest form (known as intermittent peritoneal dialysis [IPD]), it was delivered in hospitals intermittently for prolonged periods of up to 24 hours, exchanging 20 to 60 L of dialysis fluid for either acute kidney injury or maintenance therapy in end-stage disease. IPD is quite uncommon now because most cycler-assisted exchanges are carried out overnight by patients at home during sleep to allow freedom of movement during the day. More elaborate APD regimens (illustrated in Table 59.1) include:

- Continuous cycling peritoneal dialysis (CCPD), which provides three to four exchanges during the night and one during the day (a reversal of the CAPD regimen)

- Nocturnal intermittent peritoneal dialysis (NIPD), which provides rapid exchanges during the night, with no fluid in situ during the day (NIPD with "dry day")
- Nocturnal peritoneal dialysis plus one or two exchanges during the day to allow for increased small-solute and fluid clearance (NIPD with "wet day")
- Tidal peritoneal dialysis (TPD), in which only a portion of fluid in the abdomen is drained at the end of a cycle before it is filled again. The proportion of fluid removed can be set on the cycler and is usually between 50% and 85%. The less the proportion of fluid removed, the more rapid the cycling requirement and the greater the total volume of dialysate used. The concept behind tidal PD is to allow continuous fluid-membrane contact to improve dialysis efficiency. In practice, however, tidal settings are often used to relieve abdominal pain at the end of the drain cycle and to prevent catheter malfunction rather than improve dialysis efficacy.

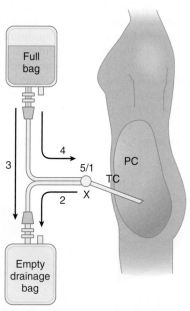

Figure 59.3   Diagrammatic representation of a continuous ambulatory peritoneal dialysis (CAPD) exchange using a Y-set disconnect system. The Y-set consists of tubing with a full bag of dialysate at one end and an empty drainage bag at the other, placed on the floor. Fluid flow is by gravity, and the direction of flow is controlled by clamps on the tubing. Between exchanges, the peritoneal cavity (PC) contains dialysate and only a short, capped extension tubing attached to the peritoneal Tenckhoff catheter (TC). The exchange procedure includes five steps:

1. To begin the exchange, the patient connects the Y tubing to the short extension tubing at X.
2. Keeping the clamp on the full bag closed, the patient or caregiver opens the clamp on the peritoneal catheter extension to allow the fluid in the PC to drain into the drainage bag by gravity. Time required: 10-15 minutes.
3. The patient then closes the clamp on the peritoneal catheter extension tubing and opens the clamp on the full bag, allowing fresh fluid to "flush" the tubing of air and any contamination into the drainage bag. Time required: a few seconds (count of 5).
4. Next, the patient closes the clamp on the drainage bag and opens the clamp on the peritoneal catheter extension tubing, allowing fresh dialysis fluid into the PC via the TC. Time required: 10 minutes.
5. The final step is to close the clamp on the peritoneal catheter extension tubing, disconnect the Y tubing, and cap the short extension tubing.

Table 59.1 Regimens Used in Peritoneal Dialysis

Type of Dialysis*	Number of Daytime Exchanges	Number of Nighttime Exchanges	Volume of Exchanges (L)
CAPD	2-3	1-2[†]	1.0-3.0
CCPD	1	3-5	1.0-3.0
NIPD	0	3-5	2.0-3.0
NIPD with "wet day"	1-2	3-5	2.0-3.0
TPD	0	4-20	1.0-2.0
IPD	5-10	5-10	1.0-2.0

CAPD, Continuous ambulatory peritoneal dialysis; *CCPD*, continuous cycling peritoneal dialysis; *IPD*, intermittent peritoneal dialysis; *NIPD*, nocturnal intermittent peritoneal dialysis; *TPD*, tidal peritoneal dialysis.

*All regimens except CAPD use a cycler machine and are therefore variants of automated peritoneal dialysis.

[†]If an additional exchange is needed during CAPD to achieve adequate dialysis, a mechanical exchange device can be used to perform the exchange during the night while the patient is asleep.

Table 59.2 Composition and Physical Properties of Peritoneal Dialysis Fluids (Including Osmotic Agents Used)

Agent/Physical Property	Amount/Value
Sodium	132-133 mEq/L
Chloride	95-101 mEq/L
Calcium	2.5-3.5 mEq/L
Magnesium	0.5 mEq/L
Buffer[§]	
Lactate	36.5-40 mEq/L
Bicarbonate	0-34 mEq/L
Osmotic agent[‡]	
Glucose	1.5, 2.5, or 4.25 g/dL*
Amino acids	1.1 g/dL[†]
Icodextrin	7.5 g/dL
pH	5.2-7.4
Osmolarity	282-485 mOsmol/L

*Glucose-based solutions with low levels of glucose degradation products (GDPs) and physiologic pH are available and are being used increasingly.

[†]Amino acid solutions are used infrequently in practice. Electrolyte values reflect the ionic concentration.

[‡]Current osmotic agents include glucose, icodextrin, and amino acids; these are not typically present together.

[§]Either bicarbonate or lactate serves as the buffer, typically in a total concentration not exceeding 40 mEq/L

APD regimens usually entail an increased number of short-dwell exchanges to enhance solute and fluid removal. The cycler delivers a set number of exchanges over 8 to 10 hours, with the last fill constituting the long day dwell. This day dwell may be necessary to provide additional dialysis to achieve solute and fluid removal targets. The most obvious advantage of APD is that it eliminates the need for intensive manual involvement since most of the dialysis occurs at night during sleep. In essence, APD entails only two procedures daily: an initial connection of the catheter to the machine and a disconnection at the end of dialysis. APD is increasingly being used in the United States and Europe in lieu of CAPD, with a trend to increased use in developing countries as well. This trend may be related to the convenience of performing the dialysis connections and to the new cycler models that are smaller, lighter, and less expensive. In the past, APD tended to be offered only to patients who had been identified by PET as "high transporters" and therefore required shorter dwell times. However, lifestyle issues and freedom from daytime exchanges are now major factors in modality selection for both patient and physician.

PERITONEAL DIALYSIS SOLUTIONS

GLUCOSE-BASED PERITONEAL DIALYSIS SOLUTIONS

Standard peritoneal dialysis solutions (Table 59.2) contain varying concentrations of glucose as the osmotic agent, electrolytes, and buffers such as sodium, magnesium, calcium, chloride, and lactate. Lactate was initially used as the buffer in preference to the more physiologic bicarbonate for technical reasons, because the low pH of lactate prevented caramelization of the glucose while autoclaving for sterilization during the manufacturing process. The biocompatibility of these solutions has been intensively studied, and there is now no doubt that their unphysiologically low pH, high osmolarity, and content of glucose degradation products

(GDPs) generated during manufacturing and autoclaving are harmful to peritoneal cells in vitro. These effects are implicated in peritoneal neovascularization, collagen production, and peritoneal thickening, all of which may contribute to loss of peritoneal function. More physiologic solutions use bicarbonate as the buffer and are dispensed in twin bags that contain the glucose and bicarbonate solutions in separate compartments. At the point of use, the two solutions are mixed by breaking a protective seal to produce a dialysate with a neutral pH and low GDP content. Alternative osmotic agents such as icodextrin and a mixture of amino acids have also been developed and are in routine use worldwide. These are discussed in greater detail later in this chapter, and, due to the sentiment that their more physiologic constitution may result in better preservation, are increasingly utilized, with cost the major limiting factor.

ICODEXTRIN DIALYSIS SOLUTION

Although glucose remains the most common osmotic agent in use because of its relatively low immediate toxicity, low cost, and ease of manufacture, two alternative osmotic agents, icodextrin and amino acid-based solutions, have interesting and attractive properties. Icodextrin is a starch-derived glucose polymer that produces ultrafiltration by exerting colloid oncotic pressure when administered intraperitoneally. A 7.5% solution is almost isosmolar to serum but produces sustained ultrafiltration over a period of up to 12 hours, with minimal absorption of icodextrin. The volume of ultrafiltrate is comparable to that produced by a hyperosmolar 4.25% glucose dialysate without the accompanying calorie load or glucose exposure to the peritoneal membrane. It improves fluid balance because it can be left for the long overnight dwell in CAPD and for the long daytime dwell in APD. It serves to achieve sustained ultrafiltration irrespective of transporter status or situations of peritoneal inflammation (e.g., peritonitis). The current license limits the amount of icodextrin used to one exchange per day, ranging usually from 1 L to 2.5 L depending on patient size and need for ultrafiltration. Notably, small amounts of complex carbohydrate are absorbed into the circulation via the lymphatic system, and on regular daily use they reach a steady-state plasma level in 7 to 10 days. These complex carbohydrates are hydrolyzed in part to maltose by circulating amylase, and maltose levels of around 1.4 mg/mL are observed with no significant impact on plasma osmolality. The long-term adverse effects of this are not known but are not thought to be harmful. Of critical importance, the maltose in the circulation interferes with blood glucose measurement in patients with diabetes using home blood glucose monitoring equipment. Blood glucose measurement therefore must be done with a glucose-specific method to prevent maltose interference. In case of any doubts, the manufacturer(s) of the monitor and test strips should be contacted to seek clarification, because falsely high readings can result in insulin overdose and are linked to accidental deaths in peritoneal dialysis patients. Most antibiotics are compatible with icodextrin and can be administered dissolved in this solution during the long dwell.

AMINO ACID–BASED DIALYSIS SOLUTIONS

Amino acid–based solutions intend to provide nutritional supplementation during peritoneal dialysis dwells. The commercially available solution is a mixture of 15 amino acids in a concentration of 1.1%. The solution also contains standard concentrations of sodium, calcium, magnesium, chloride, and lactate. The amino acids act as the osmotic agent and are absorbed across the peritoneal membrane during the dwell to a variable extent. The evidence to support improvement in nutrition, as well as overall outcomes, is not compelling, but this dialysate can be used in malnourished patients both for nutritional supplementation and reduction of glucose exposure. Used in combination with icodextrin, it has the potential to preserve peritoneal membrane integrity while reducing excessive glucose absorption. A 2 L bag contains approximately 25% of the daily protein requirement of a 70 kg adult. Successful utilization of the amino acids is dependent on an adequate calorie load, and amino acid dialysate (Nutrineal) should be instilled after the patient has had a meal. In CAPD regimens, Nutrineal is usually administered after the midday meal, and in APD regimes it can be the first exchange on the cycler. One exchange per day of 2 to 2.5 L is recommended, and a maximum of two exchanges may be used. Amino acid–based dialysate should be avoided in severe uremia, disorders of amino acid metabolism, severe liver disease, acidosis, hypokalemia, and hypersensitivity.

PERITONEAL CATHETERS

The access for peritoneal dialysis is a catheter inserted into the abdominal cavity using local anesthetic with sedation. General anesthesia is usually reserved for patients with previous abdominal surgery and complicated insertions, but practices vary by center. The catheter can be inserted surgically under direct vision through a minilaparotomy, percutaneously using the Seldinger technique, or with peritoneoscopic or laparoscopic guidance. There are numerous catheter designs, such as the Swan neck catheter (said to undergo less catheter tip migration and have fewer exit-site infections) and curled catheters. None offers a significant proven advantage over the original double-cuffed Silastic Tenckhoff catheter, and this original and simple design remains the most commonly used catheter. The intraabdominal portion of the catheter has multiple perforations through which dialysate flows. Most catheters are double cuffed. With the deep cuff placed in a paramedian position in the rectus muscle, the extraperitoneal portion of the catheter is tunneled through the subcutaneous tissue to exit the skin, pointing laterally and caudally. The superficial cuff is located inside the subcutaneous tunnel, 2 to 3 cm from the exit site. Peritoneal dialysis can be initiated immediately after catheter placement if it is urgently required, provided that exchange volumes are small and the patient is kept recumbent. In practice, dialysis typically has been deferred for approximately 4 weeks after insertion to allow the surgical wound and exit site to heal properly. The surgical wound is secured in an occlusive dressing postoperatively and left untouched usually for 10 days, at which point patient training for exit-site care commences and plans for training to perform CAPD or APD are made. Some providers will use hemodialysis as a temporary measure if necessary until peritoneal dialysis is initiated, whereas a minority will initiate urgent start peritoneal dialysis, using low volumes in the supine position.

MANAGEMENT OF PERITONEAL DIALYSIS

PERITONEAL DIALYSIS PRESCRIPTION

In determining the appropriate prescription for an individual patient, one needs to account for the fixed components at the time, including residual kidney function, peritoneal membrane permeability, and the size of the patient, as well as the variable components of dialysate volume, dwell times, concentration of glucose, and number of exchanges. A prescription entails modifications of the variable components to arrive at a regimen that provides for adequate solute and fluid removal to meet clinical needs while maintaining reasonable quality of life. Setting a peritoneal dialysis prescription is outlined in Figure 59.4. Dialysis adequacy regarding solute removal, fluid status, nutritional status, and clinical well-being are monitored regularly (see later discussion), and the prescription is modified accordingly.

The overall clearance capacity of the peritoneum for small solutes is limited by the volume of dialysate that can be provided daily. Many CAPD patients are prescribed four exchanges of 2 L of dialysate per day. Four 2 L CAPD exchanges per day with 2 L daily net ultrafiltration represents a drain volume of 70 L/week, which is inadequate in the absence of significant residual kidney function for most patients, especially those who weigh more than 80 kg. Initially, most patients have residual kidney function that contributes to the total solute clearance. As kidney function is gradually lost, patients require either larger exchange volumes (2.5 or 3.0 L) and/or additional exchanges to avoid

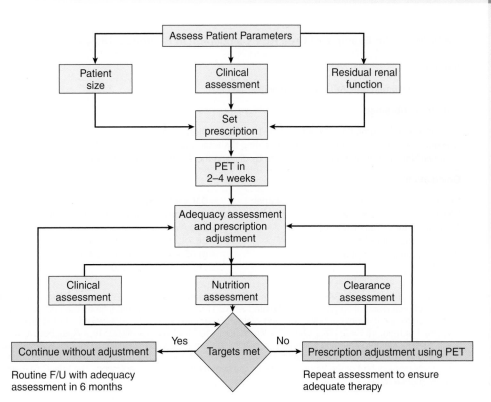

Figure 59.4 Algorithm for prescription setting. After the initial peritoneal equilibration test (PET) at 2 to 4 weeks, the prescription is altered according to the membrane permeability results. For high transporters, short-dwell automated peritoneal dialysis (APD) is appropriate; for high-average and low-average transporters, continuous ambulatory peritoneal dialysis (CAPD) would suffice. *F/U,* Follow-up.

uremic symptoms and reach the target values of urea Kt/V and creatinine clearance. In a CAPD regimen, the fifth exchange may be provided by use of an automated device that functions at night. However, this technique is in decline because it effectively introduces a mini-APD machine, and most patients and physicians would opt to switch completely at this point from CAPD to APD. Larger patients should be started on exchange volumes of 2.5 to 3.0 L. APD can achieve higher clearance of small solutes, but it may necessitate one or two day dwells ("wet day") in addition to three or four nocturnal exchange volumes of 2.5 to 3.0 L each.

PERITONEAL DIALYSIS ADEQUACY

Adequacy of peritoneal dialysis is determined by clinical assessment, solute clearance measurements, nutritional status, and fluid removal. The well-dialyzed patient has a good appetite, no nausea, and minimal fatigue. In contrast, the uremic patient is anorectic with dysgeusia, nausea, and complaints of fatigue. In addition to these clinical parameters, two biochemical measures are used to assess adequacy of solute removal:

1. An index of peritoneal urea removal, expressed as Kt/V, is urea clearance (K) multiplied by time (t) and related to total body water volume, which is assumed to be the urea distribution volume (V). Kt is obtained by multiplying the ratio of effluent dialysate to plasma urea nitrogen concentration (D/P$_{urea}$) by the 24-hour effluent drain volume. Kidney urea clearance is added to this value to yield the total daily body clearance. The daily value is multiplied by 7 to provide a weekly value. V can be estimated as 60% of weight in males, or 55% of weight in females. A typical calculation is given in Table 59.3.

2. Creatinine clearance (CrCl) is provided by both peritoneal clearance and residual kidney function. Peritoneal CrCl is again obtained from a 24-hour collection of dialysate, but to this is added an estimate of the glomerular filtration rate (GFR) achieved by the residual kidney function. By tradition, residual kidney clearance is determined by averaging CrCl and urea nitrogen clearance as an estimate of the GFR. This is performed to correct for tubular secretion of creatinine, which substantially overestimates GFR at low levels of kidney function. An adjustment for body surface area is also usually applied.

Although the validity of these measurements and calculations continues to cause some controversy, they have become the accepted methods of estimating dialysis adequacy, and various national and international organizations have set minimum targets for both CrCl and urea clearance based on them. However, it is sometimes difficult for patients to achieve one or both targets, and doubt remains about the precise level at which the targets should be set. The National Kidney Foundation Kidney Disease Outcomes Quality Initiative (KDOQI) Practice Guidelines for Peritoneal Dialysis were published in 1997 and updated in 2006. Largely as a result of one large, well-conducted, and randomized prospective study (ADEMEX), which showed no survival advantage with the higher dialysis dose, the target minimum Kt/V for urea was reduced from 2.0 to 1.7 and the target total weekly CrCl from 60 L to 50 L in the 2006 KDOQI guideline. Several guidelines have since emerged including the United Kingdom Renal Association Guidelines, the European Renal Best Practice, and the International Society for Peritoneal Dialysis Guidelines, all with similar recommendations. It is thought that failure to achieve this target is likely to lead to uremic symptoms, decreased protein intake, and an increase in mortality, but conclusive evidence is lacking because investigators

Table 59.3   An Example of Urea Kt/V Calculation in Peritoneal Dialysis

Patient
70-kg adult woman on CAPD (four exchanges/day)

Data to be obtained

24-hr dialysate volume [(4 × 2 L infusion) + 1 L net ultrafiltrate = 9 L]
D/P ratio for urea (0.9), determined by collecting the total drained dialysate for 24 hr
Residual kidney urea clearance, determined by dividing the 24-hr urine urea nitrogen by the BUN (20 L/wk, which corresponds to 2 mL/min)

Calculation

Peritoneal urea clearance/day (D/P × volume)	$= 0.9 \times 9 \text{ L} = 8.1 \text{ L}$
Weekly peritoneal urea clearance	$= 8.1 \text{ L/day} \times 7 \text{ days/wk} = 56.7 \text{ L/wk}$
Residual kidney urea clearance	$= 20 \text{ L/wk}$
Total urea clearance (Kt)	$= 56.7 \text{ L/wk} + 20 \text{ L/wk} = 76.7 \text{ L/wk}$
Volume of urea distribution (V)*	$= (0.55 \times \text{Weight in kg}) = 38.5 \text{ L}$
Weekly Kt/V	$= 76.7 \text{ L} \div 38.5 \text{ L} = 2.0$

BUN, Blood urea nitrogen; *CAPD,* continuous ambulatory peritoneal dialysis; *D/P ratio,* dialysate-to-plasma creatinine ratio.
*Volume of urea distribution (V) can be estimated as 0.60 (men) or 0.55 (women) times the body weight in kilograms. However, it is more accurate to use the formula of Watson and Watson, which takes into account weight (in kilograms), height (in centimeters), sex, and age (in years). For men, V(L) = 2.477 + (0.3362 × Weight) + (0.1074 × Height) − (0.09516 × Age). For women, V(L) = −2.097 + (0.2466 × Weight) + (0.1069 × Height). The data collection for creatinine clearance (CrCl) is similar to that for Kt/V. However, the urinary component of CrCl is usually corrected for creatinine secretion by averaging it with the urinary urea clearance. The peritoneal CrCl is simply calculated by dividing the creatinine content of the 24-hr dialysate by the serum creatinine concentration. The total CrCl (peritoneal + kidney) is normalized to 1.73 m² body surface area.

are naturally reluctant to test the point at which reducing the dialysis "dose" produces clinical symptoms. Although current targets may indicate the minimum solute clearance targets required to achieve an acceptable long-term clinical outcome, some patients need more dialysis to prevent uremic symptoms. In addition, it must always be remembered that the term *dialysis adequacy* is restricted to the description of solute removal adequacy only and does not encompass the other aspects of care. Control of hypertension, maintenance of fluid balance, maximal cardiovascular risk reduction, and management of comorbidities can hugely influence outcome in any dialysis patient, but, even here, conclusive, randomized, prospective studies are lacking. Despite these issues, anuric patients can usually be adequately managed on peritoneal dialysis by appropriate prescription adjustments, including the use of APD regimens and icodextrin.

It is now well recognized that residual kidney function is extremely important in providing adequate solute and fluid clearance. Most studies show that residual kidney function correlates with improved morbidity and mortality, and its preservation forms an important part of the management for a peritoneal dialysis patient. To preserve residual kidney function, nephrotoxic drugs such as aminoglycosides and nonsteroidal antiinflammatory agents should be avoided whenever possible, and episodes of hypotension from any cause should be corrected as rapidly as possible. Residual kidney function is better preserved in patients receiving peritoneal dialysis than in those receiving hemodialysis, so peritoneal dialysis may be the better initial therapy option for end-stage kidney failure.

FLUID REMOVAL WITH PERITONEAL DIALYSIS

Although peritoneal dialysis patients benefit from continuous daily fluid removal, it is generally accepted that most patients continue to have mild fluid overload to some extent. This reflects the fact that the "dry weight" is difficult to achieve with precision. Whether this state of continuous mild overload is more or less harmful than the thrice-weekly rapid variation in fluid status experienced by a hemodialysis patient is unknown, but the problem tends to become more troublesome in the long term when residual kidney function is lost and peritoneal dialysis ultrafiltration capacity is reduced. It appears that fluid removal has a more significant impact on outcome than solute clearance. Net ultrafiltration of at least 750 mL/day is associated with better survival in anuric patients, although the exact reason is unclear. Greater emphasis is now placed on optimizing fluid status, and algorithms are available that help the physician manage fluid overload in CAPD patients (Fig. 59.5). The use of icodextrin for the longest dwell achieves better fluid balance and results in improvement in left ventricular indices.

NUTRITION IN THE PERITONEAL DIALYSIS PATIENT

On the basis of anthropometric studies, as many as 40% of peritoneal dialysis patients are believed to be protein malnourished . This condition is in part due to losses of amino acids and approximately 8 to 12 grams of protein each day in the dialysate; additionally, peritonitis markedly increases dialysate protein losses. Patient appetite may be suppressed by absorbed dialysate glucose, uremia, and a sense of abdominal fullness, resulting in lower dietary intake. Both the Kt/V and the weekly CrCl correlate, albeit weakly, with dietary protein intake, suggesting that a certain minimum dose of dialysis is required for adequate protein intake. The serum albumin level is inversely related to both mortality and hospitalization in peritoneal dialysis patients, although it must be remembered that serum albumin is greatly influenced by inflammation and is a poor marker of nutritional status when used alone. High protein intake of at least

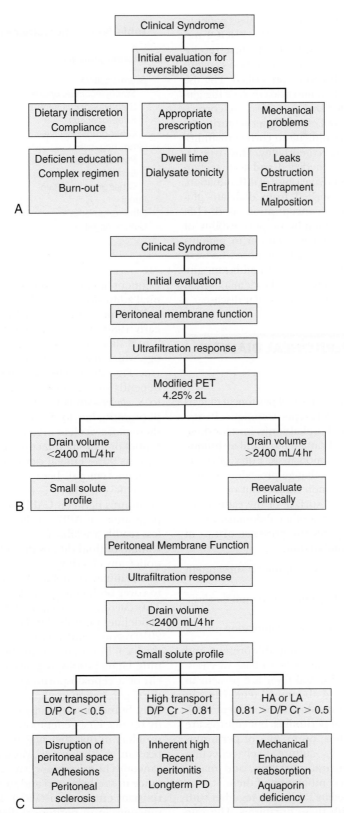

Figure 59.5 Evaluation of the clinical syndrome of fluid overload. **A,** This initially entails the evaluation and search for reversible causes. **B,** After reversible causes are excluded, it is appropriate to evaluate peritoneal membrane function using the modified peritoneal equilibration test (PET) with 2 L of 4.25% glucose. **C,** Algorithm for further evaluation and treatment based on the small solute profile. For high-transport patients, the therapy is outlined. For low-transport patients peritoneal dialysis may not be possible and peritoneal sclerosis should be excluded, especially encapsulating peritoneal sclerosis. *D/P Cr,* Ratio of dialysate to plasma creatinine; *HA,* high-average transport; *LA,* low-average transport; *PD,* peritoneal dialysis.

1.2 g/kg/day is recommended for peritoneal dialysis patients, but many ingest only 0.8 to 1.0 g/kg/day. The KDOQI recommendations are that such patients should first receive dietary counseling and education; if protein intake remains inadequate, oral supplements should be prescribed. The use of amino acid dialysate (in which amino acids replace the glucose) has been tried on a limited basis as a means of correcting protein malnutrition, but proof of its long-term nutritional benefit is lacking. It is especially difficult to correct malnutrition related to inflammation and comorbidity. This "type II" malnutrition may well be cytokine mediated, and its correction necessitates eliminating the underlying cause of inflammation.

The number of calories absorbed from dialysate glucose depends on the dextrose concentration used (1.5, 2.5, or 4.25 g/dL) and on the membrane permeability of the patient. Excessive weight gain is common in patients undergoing peritoneal dialysis, especially in those who were already overweight at the start of dialysis. In addition, glucose absorption frequently results in dyslipidemia, which may contribute to atherosclerotic cardiovascular disease.

COMPLICATIONS OF PERITONEAL DIALYSIS

PERITONITIS

Peritonitis remains a major complication of peritoneal dialysis despite advances in equipment and aseptic technique. Peritonitis accounts for 15% to 35% of hospital admissions for these patients and is the major cause of catheter loss and technique failure resulting in transfer to hemodialysis. Entry of bacteria into the catheter during an exchange procedure (touch contamination) is the most common source, but organisms can also track along the external surface of the catheter or migrate into the peritoneum from another abdominal viscus.

Diagnosis of peritonitis requires the presence of two of the following criteria in any combination:

- Organisms identified on Gram staining or subsequent culture
- Cloudy fluid (white cell count >100/mm³; >50% neutrophils)
- Symptoms and signs of peritoneal inflammation

Cloudy dialysate effluent is almost invariably present, and abdominal pain is present in about 80% to 95% of cases. Gastrointestinal symptoms, chills, and fever are present in as many as 25% of the cases, and abdominal tenderness in 75%. Bacteremia is rare. Gram staining of the effluent is seldom helpful, except with fungal peritonitis, but cultures are usually positive. In many centers, up to 20% of peritonitis episodes result in a "no growth" culture, likely reflecting suboptimal sample collection, transportation, and inadequate culture techniques, or a combination of these.

Causes of peritonitis are listed in Table 59.4, together with the frequency of infection with these organisms. The rate of peritonitis with *Staphylococcus epidermidis* has decreased since the introduction of the Y-set and the flush-before-fill technique, and *Staphylococcus aureus* and enteric organisms now account for a larger proportion of peritonitis episodes than in the past. Because patients infected with these organisms are more symptomatic than those with *S. epidermidis* peritonitis, peritonitis has become a less

Table 59.4   Microorganisms Causing Peritonitis

Microorganisms	Frequency (%)
Gram-positive	
Staphylococcus epidermidis	30-40
Staphylococcus aureus	15-20
Streptococcus	10-15
Other gram-positive	2-5
Gram-negative	
Pseudomonas	5-10
Enterobacter	5-20
Other gram-negative	5-7
Fungi	2-10
Other organisms	2-5
Culture negative	10-30

frequent but more severe complication, often requiring hospital admission.

Peritonitis rates, originally very high in the late 1970s and early 1980s, have decreased to less than one episode every 2 to 3 dialysis years, owing to improvements in connectology, which have decreased the risk for touch contamination (see Fig. 59.3). The catheter removal rate for peritonitis depends on the infecting microorganism. Peritonitis due to *S. epidermidis* is less likely to result in catheter loss than peritonitis due to *S. aureus* or *Pseudomonas aeruginosa*. If these more virulent organisms are associated with a catheter tunnel or exit-site infection, the catheter loss rate can be as high as 90%. Fungal peritonitis almost invariably requires catheter removal, because a medical cure can only rarely be achieved. There is no apparent difference in rates of peritonitis between CAPD and APD. However, detection of peritonitis on APD can be delayed because the effluent is less readily available for inspection after each drain, and the volume of fluid dilutes the cells so that the patient may not notice any clouding.

The initial treatment of peritonitis is empiric and designed to cover both gram-positive cocci and gram-negative bacilli. The current International Society for Peritoneal Dialysis Guidelines published in Peritoneal Dialysis International in 2010 recommend a center-specific empiric therapy based on the local history of sensitivities of organisms causing peritonitis. Gram-positive organisms may be covered by vancomycin or a cephalosporin, and gram-negative organisms by a third generation cephalosporin or aminoglycoside empirically. Subsequent therapy should be tailored to the sensitivity results. First-generation cephalosporins pose a potential problem in that they may not adequately cover methicillin-resistant staphylococci, whereas widespread empiric use of vancomycin raises concerns about the promotion of resistance in staphylococci and the development of vancomycin-resistant enterococci (VRE). However, the long half-life of vancomycin in peritoneal dialysis patients makes it simple to administer, and it is widely used. Aminoglycoside levels should be monitored to avoid accelerated loss of residual kidney function and vestibulo-ototoxicity; however, because these antibiotics also have a relatively long-half life in peritoneal dialysis patients, the traditional advice regarding peak and trough levels is invalid, and these values probably tell the physician nothing about intraperitoneal levels.

Table 59.5   Antibiotics and Dosing Schedules for Intraperitoneal Use (Unless Otherwise Stated)

Antibiotic	Initial Dose (mg/L)*	Subsequent Doses	
		Each Exchange (mg/L)	Once Daily (mg)
Ampicillin	125	125	No data
Aztreonam	1000	250	1000
Cefazolin	500	125	500
Ceftazidime	500	125	1000
Fluconazole	200 mg PO	—	200 PO
Aminoglycosides†	20	4	20
Metronidazole	500 mg PO/IV	—	500 PO/IV tid
Vancomycin	15-30 mg/kg	25	15-30 mg/kg q5-7d

*Once-daily antibiotic dosing with the long dwell is preferred to the addition of antibiotic to each exchange and has been shown to be efficacious for cefazolin, cephalothin, and ceftazidime. Patients receiving automated peritoneal dialysis (APD) may be changed to a continuous ambulatory peritoneal dialysis (CAPD) schedule; if they remain on an APD schedule, antibiotics are added to each exchange.

†This group includes gentamicin, tobramycin, and netilmicin (same doses for all). Penicillins and aminoglycosides are incompatible and should not be administered in the same bag.

Table 59.5 provides a list of antibiotics used in IPD and their dosing schedules. Antibiotics are usually administered intraperitoneally once a day in the long-dwell exchange (overnight in CAPD and during the daytime long dwell in APD). They can also be given continuously in every exchange. The dosage may need adjustment if residual kidney function is significant. Duration of therapy depends on the organisms and the severity of the peritonitis; it is usually 14 days for *S. epidermidis* infections and 3 weeks for most other infections.

It should be possible (in up to 80% of cases) to achieve complete cure without having to resort to catheter removal. Persistent symptoms beyond 96 hours can occur in 10% to 30% of episodes, and cure is only possible by removal of the catheter. Cure may be obtained if antibiotics alone are continued beyond 96 hours without catheter removal, but this poses a high risk for damage to the peritoneum, and neither the short-term bacterial outcome nor the long-term peritoneal membrane effect is good. Therefore if there is no clear evidence of improvement (i.e., reduction in abdominal pain, falling dialysis fluid cell count, visual clearing of the peritoneal dialysis effluent) after 96 hours of treatment with appropriate antibiotic therapy, the catheter should be removed as soon as possible. In a study in which antibiotics were continued for 10 days for "resistant" peritonitis without clearing of the fluid and without catheter removal, one third of the patients died; another one third lost ultrafiltration, necessitating discontinuation of peritoneal dialysis; and only one third were able to continue with peritoneal dialysis. Relapsing peritonitis, defined as an episode that occurs within 4 weeks of completion of therapy of a prior episode with the same organism, occurs in about 10% to

15% of episodes. The term *recurrent peritonitis* is used when a second episode occurs within 4 weeks of completion of therapy but with a different organism. Catheter removal in these cases ultimately occurs in as many as 15% of these cases, and death has been reported in 1% to 3%.

Peritonitis results in a marked increase in acute peritoneal protein losses and a transient decrease in ultrafiltration due to the increased permeability to the dialysate dextrose. Although peritoneal membrane changes are usually transient in the setting of acute peritonitis, peritoneal fibrosis (often referred to as sclerosis) may be involved in severe episodes or as a cumulative effect of multiple episodes of peritonitis (see later discussion).

PERITONEAL CATHETER EXIT SITE AND TUNNEL INFECTION

Peritoneal catheter infections can involve the exit site (erythema or purulent drainage), the tunnel (edema, erythema, or tenderness over the subcutaneous pathway), or both simultaneously. *S. aureus* is the most common cause of exit site and tunnel infections; *Pseudomonas* is the next most frequent organism. *S. aureus* exit site infections are difficult to treat and frequently progress to tunnel infections and peritonitis, in which case catheter removal is required for eradication. *S. aureus* nasal carriage is associated with an increased risk of *S. aureus* catheter infection. Treatment of nasal carriers with intranasal mupirocin twice daily for 5 days each month, mupirocin applied daily to the exit site regardless of carrier status, or oral rifampin 600 mg/day for 5 days every 12 weeks has been shown to be effective in reducing *S. aureus* catheter infections. The application of mupirocin at the exit site as part of routine exit site care has resulted in a dramatic reduction of exit site infections and peritonitis related to *S. aureus*. Bacteriologic monitoring of the peritoneal dialysis population for *S. aureus* carriage is unnecessary when this approach is adopted, but concern exists that it may in the future encourage growth of resistant organisms. *P. aeruginosa* catheter exit site infections are very difficult to resolve, frequently relapse, and often necessitate catheter replacement.

CATHETER MALFUNCTION, HERNIAS, AND FLUID LEAKS

The most important noninfectious complications during peritoneal dialysis are abdominal wall–related hernias, leakages of dialysis fluid, and inflow and outflow malfunction. Before peritoneal dialysis treatment is started, all significant abdominal wall–related hernias should be corrected. With the presence of 2 to 3 L of dialysate in the abdominal cavity, intraabdominal pressure is increased, and preexisting hernias will worsen during peritoneal dialysis treatment. The most frequently occurring hernias after commencement of peritoneal dialysis are incisional, umbilical, and inguinal hernias. Significant hernias should be repaired surgically, and IPD may be continued postoperatively using low dwell volumes in a supine position.

Leakage of peritoneal fluid is related to catheter implantation technique, trauma, or patient-related anatomic abnormalities. It can occur early (<30 days) or late (>30 days) after implantation, and it may have various clinical manifestations depending on whether the leak is external or subcutaneous. Early leakage is usually external, appearing as fluid through the wound or the exit site. Late leakage may develop at the site of any incision and entry into the peritoneal cavity. The exact site of the leakage can be determined by computed tomography after infusion of 2 L of dialysis fluid containing radiocontrast material. Scrotal or labial edema can be a sign of an early or late fluid leak, usually through a patent processus vaginalis. Therapy usually entails a period off peritoneal dialysis during which the patient is maintained on hemodialysis or on limited, low-volume peritoneal dialysis in the supine position as necessary. For recurrent leaks, surgical repair is essential. Leakage of fluid into the subcutaneous tissue is sometimes occult and difficult to diagnose. It may manifest as diminished drainage, which might be mistaken for ultrafiltration failure. Computed tomography and abdominal scintigraphy may identify the leak.

Outflow-inflow obstruction is the most frequently observed early event, occurring within 2 weeks after implantation of the catheter, although it may also be seen later, coincident with other problems such as peritonitis. One-way outflow obstruction is the most frequent problem and is characterized by poor flow and failure to drain the peritoneal cavity. Common causes include both intraluminal factors (blood clot, fibrin) and extraluminal factors (constipation, occlusion of catheter holes by adjacent organs or omental wrapping, catheter tip dislocation out of the true pelvis, incorrect catheter placement at implantation). An abdominal radiograph is useful in localizing the peritoneal dialysis catheter tip for malposition and evaluating stool burden. Depending on the cause, appropriate therapy may entail laxatives to clear the bowels, heparinized saline flushes and urokinase instillation into the catheter to relieve blockages, manipulation under fluoroscopy guidance (using a stiff wire or stylet with a "whiplash" technique), and laparoscopic revision or open replacement of the catheter in cases of catheter displacement.

PERITONEAL MEMBRANE CHANGES: ENCAPSULATING PERITONEAL SCLEROSIS AND ULTRAFILTRATION FAILURE

The peritoneum exposed to peritoneal dialysis reacts to the new environment. There is thickening of the peritoneal interstitium and basement membrane reduplication, both in the mesothelium and in the capillaries. These changes occur in response to the nonphysiologic composition of standard dialysis solutions and also from the direct actions of glucose and GDPs, which form advanced glycation end products (AGEs), and related changes in the peritoneal membrane. Changes in peritoneal microvessels and neovascularization occur, analogous to those seen in diabetic retinopathy, with deposition of type IV collagen. Other conditions that are important in the pathogenesis of peritoneal thickening are recurrent acute peritonitis, chronic inflammatory reactions mediated by uremic or low-level bacterial activation of peritoneal macrophages, and intraperitoneal production of proinflammatory and profibrotic cytokines such as vascular endothelial growth factor, interleukin 6, and transforming growth factor-β.

Data from an international biopsy registry showed that thickening of the membrane usually occurs after a period

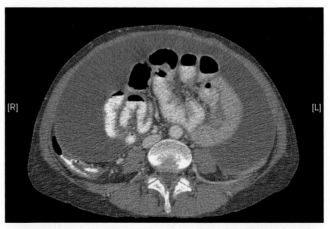

Figure 59.6　Portal phase abdominal CT following intravenous and oral contrast. The patient is an adult female who was previously on peritoneal dialysis for more than 5 years and was converted to haemodialysis recently for PD technique failure and presented with ascites, features of intermittent intestinal obstruction, and loss of appetite and weight. The scan shows large-volume ascites with peritoneal thickening and enhancement. The bowel loops are tethered to the root of the mesentery suggestive of a diagnosis of encapsulating peritoneal sclerosis.

of 4 to 5 years of peritoneal dialysis and is associated with increasing severity of vasculopathy, although there is considerable interpatient variability with some patients showing only relatively minor changes even after more than 5 years on dialysis. For patients who have been undergoing peritoneal dialysis for more than 5 years, it is prudent to be vigilant for signs of a sudden increase in peritoneal permeability, particularly in association with raised inflammatory markers or vague gastrointestinal symptoms. These signs may indicate development of the rare condition known as encapsulating peritoneal sclerosis (EPS), which is characterized by dense fibrosis and thickening of the peritoneum with bowel adhesions and encapsulation (Fig. 59.6).

The pathogenesis of EPS is complex, and no single etiologic factor has been identified; factors such as multiple episodes of peritonitis, use of high-glucose dialysis solutions, and genetic predisposition have been proposed, with little substantiating evidence. Although EPS is rare, its incidence rises significantly after 5 years of peritoneal dialysis therapy. EPS is a serious, life-threatening condition with variable reported mortality that probably depends on severity at the time of diagnosis. One series reported a 60% death rate within 4 months after presentation with intestinal obstruction. Progressive loss of ultrafiltration and sudden development of high-transporter status may be early warning signs in some patients. However the designation "EPS" should be reserved for the point at which encapsulation has clearly occurred. Clinically, the features are those of ileus or frank intestinal obstruction. Diarrhea is also observed when partial obstruction spontaneously resolves. Gut motility is compromised as a result of binding of the intestinal loops to the parietal peritoneum and abdominal wall by an aggressive fibrotic process. Treatment consists of resting the bowel with total parenteral nutrition and surgical enterolysis for obstructive symptoms, which is best undertaken at specialized centers. Surgical enterolysis can take from 4 to 8 hours to achieve a successful result without causing perforation, but may result in rapid recovery of gastrointestinal function. Some advocate cessation of peritoneal dialysis and conversion to hemodialysis, but others suspect that such a change may exacerbate the fibrotic process. There are anecdotal reports of use of antifibrotic agents such as tamoxifen or immunosuppressive agents, with limited success.

Net ultrafiltration failure is the most important transport abnormality in patients undergoing long-term peritoneal dialysis. On the basis of clinical symptoms, its prevalence has been reported to increase from 3% after 1 year on CAPD to about 30% after 6 years. Ultrafiltration failure is defined as net ultrafiltration of less than 400 mL after a 4-hour dwell using 2 L of 4.25% glucose-containing dialysate. This condition is associated with a large peritoneal vascular surface area and impaired aquaporin channel–mediated water transport. It is best managed with frequent, short dwells and elimination of long dwells, such as with nocturnal APD, combined with daytime icodextrin. Because icodextrin is such a large molecule, its reabsorption is relatively unaffected by membrane permeability. It exerts colloid oncotic pressure and is able to maintain gradual but sustained ultrafiltration for 12 hours or longer. Improvement of peritoneal function can be brought about by minimizing glucose exposure (i.e., using glucose-free dialysate), providing peritoneal rest (being "dry" during the day on APD), using solutions that are low in GDPs, and using icodextrin, which has been shown to extend peritoneal dialysis therapy time in patients with loss of ultrafiltration. Mortality in this group is higher than for other patients on peritoneal dialysis, probably because of poor fluid control, which adds to the overall cardiovascular risk. Ultrafiltration failure also leads to increased protein loss in the dialysate, which compromises nutrition.

DIABETIC PATIENTS ON PERITONEAL DIALYSIS

Diabetic glomerulosclerosis is the most common cause of kidney failure among peritoneal dialysis patients. Most diabetic patients require insulin while they are on peritoneal dialysis, even if they did not require it before the initiation of dialysis. This is partly the result of glucose absorption from the dialysate and associated weight gain. Insulin can be given to peritoneal dialysis patients via the intraperitoneal route, the subcutaneous route, or a combination of both. If given intraperitoneally, the total daily dose of insulin required must be increased because insulin adsorbs onto the polyvinylchloride bags. Patients undergoing APD usually require long-acting subcutaneous insulin (with or without intraperitoneal regular insulin) for adequate glucose control. Injection of insulin into dialysis fluid bags confers a theoretical risk for bacterial contamination and subsequent peritonitis, although no evidence of this consequence has been reported. Nevertheless, it is a rarely used route of insulin administration for diabetic patients at present.

OUTCOMES OF PERITONEAL DIALYSIS

Survival of patients treated with peritoneal dialysis is similar to those treated with hemodialysis, with peritoneal dialysis possibly slightly better during the first 2 years of dialysis therapy. Several observational studies from Canada and Europe

have suggested a survival advantage in commencing dialysis therapy with peritoneal dialysis and then changing to hemodialysis when the therapy fails, rather than starting on hemodialysis first. Beginning with peritoneal dialysis maximizes the advantages that it confers during the first few years of dialysis in terms of preserving residual kidney function and better fluid control. If patient preference and medical conditions allow, peritoneal dialysis may well be the most appropriate initial dialysis therapy when a patient requires renal replacement therapy.

Patient and technique survival with peritoneal dialysis continue to improve. According to the latest United States Renal Data System (USRDS) Report in 2011, the 6- and 12-month survival probabilities remain unchanged since 1996 in the hemodialysis population at 0.84 and 0.74, respectively. The survival probabilities over the same periods for peritoneal dialysis have improved from 0.89 to 0.93 at 6 months and from 0.79 to 0.85 at 1 year. In contrast, 5-year survival has improved for both modalities: from 0.29 to 0.34 for hemodialysis and from 0.29 to 0.40 for peritoneal dialysis. Risk factors for death among patients undergoing peritoneal dialysis include increasing age, presence of cardiovascular disease or diabetes mellitus, decreased serum albumin level, poor nutritional status as determined by anthropometric measurements, and inadequate dialysis. The leading causes of death are cardiovascular disease and infections.

Patients transfer from peritoneal dialysis to hemodialysis for many reasons, including peritonitis or exit site infection, catheter malfunction, inability to perform the dialysis procedure, and inadequate clearance or ultrafiltration (particularly with loss of residual kidney function) (see Fig. 59.5). In many cases, the patient who loses a catheter because of peritonitis or a catheter infection elects to switch to hemodialysis permanently. The increasing use of the Y-set and flush-before-fill systems is associated with improved technique survival on CAPD, primarily due to lower peritonitis rates. It is hoped that long-term outcomes will improve with greater emphasis on maintenance of residual kidney function, greater use of more physiologic peritoneal dialysis solutions, and the use of peritoneal dialysis in an integrated renal replacement treatment program as an equally important modality to hemodialysis and perhaps as the first-line dialytic treatment for most patients with ESRD.

Transplantation is the goal for many patients undergoing dialysis. The allograft and patient survival rates of transplanted peritoneal dialysis patients are similar to those of transplanted hemodialysis patients, but there is reduced delayed graft function in the peritoneal dialysis group. Delayed graft function, in combination with graft rejection, is a strong predictor of graft survival. If the transplant does not initially function, peritoneal dialysis may be continued provided that the peritoneal cavity was not breached during surgery. The peritoneal dialysis catheter is usually left in place for several weeks until the graft is functioning well.

USE OF PERITONEAL DIALYSIS IN AN INTEGRATED RENAL REPLACEMENT THERAPY PROGRAM

The use of peritoneal dialysis worldwide varies from 2% or 3% to more than 80% of the dialysis population in different countries. Such discrepancies cannot be explained by medical variables alone. Major reasons include such nonmedical factors as economic considerations and physician biases and prejudices, which have a strong impact on the therapy options suggested to patients. A decline in the use of peritoneal dialysis has been seen in many Western countries, partly related to lack of patient choice because there are fewer nephrologists and centers specializing in the delivery of peritoneal dialysis. However, interest in home-based therapies is on the rise as evidence of its superiority over in-center hemodialysis accumulates. The concept of "PD first" is gaining consensus, and peritoneal dialysis is widely recommended as the preferred modality to commence kidney replacement therapy because it preserves residual kidney function, preserves vascular access, and results in outcomes that are as good or better than hemodialysis in the initial years while the patient awaits a kidney transplant. In a lifetime, a patient is likely to utilize each of the three modalities, possibly more than once. For instance, a patient may begin with PD, move to hemodialysis, and then have a transplant, perhaps returning to peritoneal dialysis after graft failure.

PERITONEAL DIALYSIS FOR ACUTE KIDNEY INJURY

Intermittent peritoneal dialysis can be successfully used to manage acute kidney injury. In the past, acute PD was performed using a rigid peritoneal catheter, which was inserted percutaneously using a stylet, without a subcutaneous tunnel. PD exchanges would be commenced immediately to provide renal replacement and ultrafiltration; however, an increased risk for fluid leakage and peritonitis led to its disuse. In critical illness, bedside insertion of a Tenckhoff catheter using the Seldinger technique under local anesthesia is equally straightforward and carries a much smaller risk for infection. Rapid exchanges are performed to maximize clearance of small solutes—up to one exchange per hour, ideally using an APD machine. More frequent exchanges are unlikely to improve solute clearance, and they introduce a large "down time," when the peritoneum is mostly empty in between dwells. The patient may be kept on APD for 48 hours or even longer, or IPD may be performed daily for 10 to 12 hours. Although these procedures are extremely effective for volume control and are better tolerated in hemodynamically unstable patients than is hemodialysis, clearance of small solutes may be inadequate in catabolic patients or patients undergoing total parenteral nutrition who are receiving large protein loads. In addition, in the intensive care unit setting, the risk for peritonitis remains, although it should be remembered that central venous hemodialysis catheters also carry significant risks for bacteremia and other complications. Nevertheless, peritoneal dialysis has been largely replaced by hemodialysis and continuous venovenous hemofiltration or hemodiafiltration for the management of acute kidney injury. In the recent past, several publications, most of them from Europe, have described positive outcomes in single-organ system failure treated with acute peritoneal dialysis.

ASSISTED PERITONEAL DIALYSIS

Although patients have been receiving assistance one way or another for as long as peritoneal dialysis has been in existence, so-called assisted peritoneal dialysis (aPD) is increasingly recognized as a distinct dialysis modality. Assistance may be provided by trained members of the family, paid nurses, or health care professionals, depending on the setup of the health care system. Often, staff members at intermediate care facilities, assisted-living centers, and nursing homes are trained to carry out aPD for their residents. The advantages of aPD over in-center hemodialysis for older adults include independence from the hospital and slower removal of solute and fluid, reducing the likelihood of cardiovascular instability. In addition, older adult patients on aPD are less likely to suffer from malnutrition. Other patient groups who may be suitable for aPD include those with physical disabilities (e.g., rheumatoid arthritis), patients requiring terminal care (with disseminated malignancy or severe intractable heart failure), those with learning disabilities, and or those who are slow to learn simply because of language barriers.

Assistance can also be provided for CAPD, although this requires three or four visits daily. This model has been prevalent in France since the late 1970s. Assisted automated peritoneal dialysis (aAPD) is gaining in popularity as more older patients are being accepted for dialysis. Various degrees of assistance can be provided; one model includes a daily visit from the health care worker to the patient's home. During the visit, the health care worker will strip down and set up the cycler (each morning); review and dress the PD catheter exit site if required; check blood pressure, weight, and blood glucose if the patient has diabetes; document patient progress and communicate any variance to the dialysis unit; and maintain adequate stocks of dialysis fluids. This level of assistance greatly simplifies the role of dialysis patients, who simply connect their catheter to the machine before going to bed at night and disconnect it in the morning.

KEY BIBLIOGRAPHY

Abu-Alfa AK, Burkart J, Piraino B, et al: Approach to fluid management in peritoneal dialysis: a practical algorithm, *Kidney Int Suppl* S8-16, 2002.

Brown EA, Davies SJ, Rutherford P, et al: Survival of functionally anuric patients on automated peritoneal dialysis: the European APD Outcome Study, *J Am Soc Nephrol* 14:2948-2957, 2003.

Brown EA, Johansson L, Farrington K, et al: Broadening Options for Long-term Dialysis in the Elderly (BOLDE): differences in quality of life on peritoneal dialysis compared to haemodialysis for older patients, *Nephrol Dial Transplant* 25:3755-3763, 2010.

Davies SJ, Woodrow G, Donovan K, et al: Icodextrin improves the fluid status of peritoneal dialysis patients: results of a double-blind randomized controlled trial, *J Am Soc Nephrol* 14:2338-2344, 2003.

de Freitas D, Jordaan A, Williams R, et al: Nutritional management of patients undergoing surgery following diagnosis with encapsulating peritoneal sclerosis, *Perit Dial Int* 28(3):271-276, 2008 May-Jun.

Garcia-Lopez E, Lindholm B, Davies S: An update on peritoneal dialysis solutions, *Nat Rev Nephrol* 2012.

Gokal R: Peritoneal dialysis in the 21st century: an analysis of current problems and future developments, *J Am Soc Nephrol* 13(Suppl 1): S104-S116, 2002.

Li PK, Szeto CC, Piraino B, et al: Peritoneal dialysis-related infections recommendations: 2010 update, *Perit Dial Int* 30:393-423, 2010.

Lo WK, Ho YW, Li CS, et al: Effect of Kt/V on survival and clinical outcome in CAPD patients in a randomized prospective study, *Kidney Int* 64:649-656, 2003.

Mujais S, Nolph K, Gokal R, et al: Evaluation and management of ultrafiltration problems in peritoneal dialysis. International Society for Peritoneal Dialysis Ad Hoc Committee on Ultrafiltration Management in Peritoneal Dialysis, *Perit Dial Int* 20(Suppl 4):S5-21, 2000.

Mupirocin Study Group: Nasal mupirocin prevents Staphylococcus aureus exit-site infection during peritoneal dialysis. Mupirocin Study Group, *J Am Soc Nephrol* 7:2403-2408, 1996.

National Kidney Foundation: K/DOQI Guidelines on Peritoneal Dialysis Adequacy, *NATIONAL KIDNEY FOUNDATION*, 2007. 23-2-2012.

Paniagua R, Amato D, Vonesh E, et al: Effects of increased peritoneal clearances on mortality rates in peritoneal dialysis: ADEMEX, a prospective, randomized, controlled trial, *J Am Soc Nephrol* 13:1307-1320, 2002.

Qi H, Xu C, Yan H, et al: Comparison of icodextrin and glucose solutions for long dwell exchange in peritoneal dialysis: a meta-analysis of randomized controlled trials, *Perit Dial Int* 31:179-188, 2011.

Summers AM, Abrahams AC, Alscher MD, et al: A collaborative approach to understanding EPS: the European perspective, *Perit Dial Int* 31(3):245-248, 2011 May-Jun.

Uttley L, Vardhan A, Mahajan S, et al: Decrease in infections with the introduction of mupirocin cream at the peritoneal dialysis catheter exit site, *J Nephrol* 17:242-245, 2004.

Williams JD, Craig KJ, Topley N, et al: Morphologic changes in the peritoneal membrane of patients with renal disease, *J Am Soc Nephrol* 13:470-479, 2002.

Woodrow, G and Davies, S. UK Renal Association Peritoneal Dialysis Guidelines 2009-2012. UK Renal Association Website. 30-7-2010. 27-1-2012.

Full bibliography can be found on www.expertconsult.com.

60 Outcomes of Kidney Replacement Therapies

Rajnish Mehrotra | Kamyar Kalantar-Zadeh

Patients with chronic kidney disease (CKD) stage 5, also known as end-stage renal disease (ESRD), often require either kidney transplantation or maintenance dialysis to sustain life. In general, the paucity of living and deceased donors and the medical ineligibility of many ESRD patients for transplantation substantially limit the number of patients who can receive a kidney transplant. In contrast, many countries around the world have made a social compact to make maintenance dialysis therapy available to every ESRD patient. Thus, maintenance dialysis is the dominant method of treatment for ESRD.

It is estimated that there are almost 2 million ESRD patients treated with maintenance dialysis worldwide. Furthermore, an imminent increase of the global dialysis patient census is expected given the exponential growth of dialysis patient populations in such emerging economies as China. It is believed that currently more than 80% of dialysis patients worldwide are treated with in-center hemodialysis (HD), generally delivered thrice weekly; most of the rest are treated with home peritoneal dialysis (PD). In the last 5 to 10 years, variations in the conventional method of delivery of different therapies, but particularly HD, are increasingly being used, creating a veritable menu of kidney replacement therapies from which patients can choose (Box 60.1). Notwithstanding the myriad options, the median life expectancy of ESRD patients starting dialysis therapy still remains short, ranging from 3 to 5 years, prompting increased interest in determining if the method of delivery of kidney replacement therapy affects the survival of ESRD patients. This chapter reviews the contemporary studies comparing the survival of patients treated with different kidney replacement modalities.

MAINTENANCE DIALYSIS OR KIDNEY TRANSPLANTATION

For many patients, a functioning kidney transplant is less intrusive in their daily lives than maintenance dialysis and, hence, offers a substantial lifestyle advantage. However, these advantages are partially counterbalanced by the short-term surgical risks and longer-term medical risks from lifelong immunosuppression. Studies suggest that, despite these short- and longer-term risks, ESRD patients who receive a kidney transplant have a longer life expectancy when compared to individuals with equivalent health status who remain on the waiting list for a deceased donor organ. The survival advantage with a successful transplant extends even to transplants where the kidney is harvested from "extended criteria" deceased donors

and in individuals whose age or coexisting medical conditions would have precluded them from being considered as donors previously. Furthermore, the earlier in the course of ESRD that a patient receives a kidney transplant, the longer the allograft functions. These observational reports are limited given systematic differences in individuals who receive a kidney transplant versus those who remain on the waiting list or those who receive an organ transplant earlier in the course of the disease that cannot be fully accounted for in statistical models. Although it is important to recognize these limitations, it is equally important to acknowledge that a clinical trial comparing kidney transplantation with maintenance dialysis in general or the various different dialysis modalities separately is unlikely to be undertaken. Accordingly, the substantial lifestyle advantages along with the possibility of increased longevity make a compelling case for ensuring that every eligible ESRD patient can undergo a kidney transplant as early as feasible given the constraints imposed by the availability of living donors and waiting time for a deceased donor transplant.

HEMODIALYSIS OR PERITONEAL DIALYSIS

Both HD and PD require significant but different adaptations to patients' lifestyles. First, HD requires high-flow access to the bloodstream. Second, except for some recent trends, virtually all the patients treated with HD are treated in a dialysis facility, and, throughout the developed world, HD is most commonly provided thrice weekly for 3 to 4 hours per session. Because of transportation needs and time to achieve vascular access hemostasis after treatment, in-center HD requires a total commitment of at least 4 to 5 hours thrice weekly. Variations from this general approach are increasingly being used and include differences in length and/or frequency of each treatment session (e.g., short daily HD of 2.5 to 4.0 hours, long thrice weekly HD sessions of 5 to 7 hours each) as well as site where dialysis is performed (home vs. in-center including conventional vs. nocturnal).

PD, in contrast, is almost exclusively performed at home. Although patients traditionally perform four exchanges every day with continuous ambulatory peritoneal dialysis (CAPD), it is increasingly being performed with the use of a cycler at night, referred to as automated peritoneal dialysis (APD). APD usually requires patients to be connected to the machine for 8 to 10 hours with or without a daytime manual exchange. Thus, the flexibility of dialyzing at home with PD is counterbalanced by the need to perform dialysis daily.

<table>
<tr><td>

Box 60.1   Various Forms of Kidney Replacement Therapies Used in End-Stage Kidney Disease

In-Center Hemodialysis (HD)

Thrice Weekly

Standard duration (3 to 4+ hours)
Diurnal, long-duration
Nocturnal, long-duration

Frequent

Hemodiadiltration (HDF)

Online HDF

Home HD

Diurnal, thrice weekly with conventional machines
Frequent with conventional or low-flow machines
Frequent, long-duration nocturnal

Peritoneal Dialysis (PD)

Continuous ambulatory PD
Automated PD

Kidney Transplantation

Living related or unrelated donor
Deceased donor

</td></tr>
</table>

The necessary lifestyle adjustments for either dialysis modality are extremely important when considering studies that have compared the outcomes of HD and PD patients. It is widely accepted that randomized, controlled clinical trials are the gold standard when comparing the outcomes of patients treated with two different therapies; however, the disparate effects of each treatment on patients' lifestyles have stymied efforts to undertake randomized, controlled comparisons of HD and PD thus far. For example, the clinical trial comparing these two modalities in the Netherlands was abandoned for futility, because more than 90% of eligible patients, when the two treatment modalities were explained, had a preference for one modality over the other, and they refused to be randomized (Table 60.1). In this clinical trial, patients randomized to HD had a slightly better health-related quality of life, but these findings have substantially limited external validity. There is currently another effort to conduct a randomized, controlled comparison of HD and PD in China (Clinicaltrials.gov identifier: NCT01413074), which aims to randomize 1370 patients; all-cause mortality is the primary outcome measure, enrollment began in June 2011, and follow-up is expected to be completed by August 2016. Until then, one has to depend on observational studies to compare the survival of HD and PD patients.

In the decades since the advent of widespread use of PD for treatment of kidney failure, numerous single- and multicenter observational studies have compared outcomes of patients treated with PD to those treated with HD. Despite differences among individual studies, analyses of survival data from national registries of patients who started treatment during the 1990s show a few common themes; specifically, patients who started treatment with PD had a lower death risk for the first 1 to 2 years but a higher long-term risk. The apparent "early survival advantage" with PD was greater and of longer duration for younger and healthier patients, particularly among nondiabetics with no additional comorbidity. In contrast, there was little if any apparent "early survival advantage" with PD among older and sicker patients, and there appeared to be a higher long-term death risk.

Additionally, since the mid-1990s, there has been a differential change in outcome of patients treated with the two dialysis therapies such that improvements in survival of patients treated with PD have outpaced those seen for patients treated with HD (Fig. 60.1). This differential improvement in outcomes appears worldwide, with data emerging from the United States, France, Australia, New Zealand, Canada, and Taiwan. The reasons for these differential changes over time are unclear, but they highlight the importance of considering an "era effect," or secular trend, in addition to the complexities in comparing the HD and PD outcomes mentioned earlier. The results of observational studies that have compared the outcomes of HD and PD patients who started treatment after 2000 are summarized in Table 60.2. These contemporary studies, even though nonrandomized, have more diligently attempted to account for potential bias when comparing two therapies as different as HD and PD, with some applying advanced statistical tools such as propensity scores and/or marginal structural models. Notwithstanding the sophistication of statistical models used, the risk for residual confounding persists. Stated differently, it remains uncertain whether differences in outcomes of patients treated with the two therapies are a result of the dialysis modality or simply reflect the differences in outcomes of patients treated with HD and PD. With this caveat, these studies suggest that the "early survival advantage" with PD described in studies of earlier cohorts may be attributable to the high risk of death for patients who start HD with central venous catheters and disproportionate representation of late-referred patients in the HD cohort. In other words, the "early survival advantage" with PD may not be a direct benefit of the dialysis modality but rather a result of differences in patients who choose PD rather than HD. More importantly, these studies demonstrate that the 4-, 5-, and 10-year survival of patients treated with HD and PD in different parts of the world with different PD utilization rates are similar (Fig. 60.2). Additionally, there are studies that demonstrate equivalent outcomes with HD and PD in subgroups of patients, such as those infected with hepatitis C, those with atheroembolic disease, or those returning to dialysis after a failed kidney transplant. Two studies seem to be the exception to the theme of equivalency of outcomes with HD and PD. One study, with data from the European registry, showed a robust survival advantage for patients who started treatment with PD, whereas a study from France showed a higher death risk among ESRD patients with congestive heart failure treated with PD.

It is important to mention that the studies discussed earlier primarily compare thrice-weekly in-center HD with PD. There are no data that have compared the survival of patients treated with PD to those with alternative HD regimens, including home or frequent HD.

Table 60.1   Summary of Randomized, Controlled Trials Undertaken to Compare Various Kidney Replacement Therapies

First Author (Publication Yr)	Control Group	Intervention Group	Sample Size	Primary Outcome Measures	Key Results
Thrice-Weekly In-Center HD vs. PD					
Korevaar (*Kidney Int* 2003)	Thrice-weekly HD	PD	38	Quality-adjusted life yr score	95% of eligible subjects refused to be randomized, limiting external validity; in first 2 yr, HD associated with slightly better quality-adjusted life yr score
Thrice-Weekly In-Center HD vs. Frequent In-Center HD					
Chertow (*N Engl J Med* 2010)	2.9 treatments/wk, mean duration 213 min	5.2 treatments/wk, mean duration 154 min	245	Death or 12-mo change in left ventricular mass; death or 12-mo change in physical health score	Frequent HD associated with significant benefits with respect to both coprimary outcomes and improved control of blood pressure and serum phosphorus but higher incidence of vascular access procedures
Thrice-Weekly HD vs. Frequent Nocturnal Home HD					
Culleton (*JAMA* 2007)	3 treatments/wk, in-center	5 to 6 treatments/wk, at least 6 hr per treatment	51	6-mo change in left ventricular mass	Nocturnal HD associated with significant improvement in primary outcome, as well as kidney-specific domains of quality of life, blood pressure, and mineral metabolism
Rocco (*Kidney Int* 2011)	2.9 treatments/wk, mean duration 256 min, home	5.1 treatments/wk, mean duration 379 min	87	Death or 12-mo change in left ventricular mass; death or 12-mo change in physical health score	No significant effect of nocturnal home hemodialysis or either of the two coprimary outcomes, but associated with improved control of hypertension and hyperphosphatemia; trend toward increased vascular access events
Thrice-Weekly Low-Flux HD vs. Postdilution Online HDF					
Grooteman (*J Am Soc Nephrol* 2012)	Low-flux in-center HD	Postdilution online HDF with 6 L/hr convective clearances with high-flux dialyzers	714	All-cause mortality	No significant difference in all-cause mortality or cardiovascular events; post hoc analyses showed that patients with higher convective clearances had lower all-cause mortality
Continuous Ambulatory vs. Automated PD					
De Fijter (*Ann Intern Med* 1994)	Continuous ambulatory PD	Automated PD	82	Patient and technique survival, time to first peritonitis, and hospital admission and catheter removal rates	Significantly fewer hospitalizations, and peritonitis rate with automated PD; no difference in patient or technique survival or time to first peritonitis
Bro (*Perit Dial Int* 1999)	Continuous ambulatory PD	Automated PD	34	Health-related quality of life	No difference in quality of life; too few events to assess the effect on clinical outcomes; automated PD patients reported more time for work, family, and social activities

HD, Hemodialysis; *HDF,* hemodiafiltration; *PD,* peritoneal dialysis.

ALTERNATIVE HEMODIALYSIS REGIMENS

The length of each session and the frequency of treatment used in conventional HD regimens were primarily based on feasibility and convenience, and thrice-weekly treatment regimens necessarily entail one 3-day interval between HD treatments. Several observational studies have indicated that the death risk of patients is highest during this long interdialytic interval. Similarly, several studies have demonstrated an inverse association between length of each HD session and patient survival. This has led to an increasing use of HD with a frequency higher than thrice weekly and/or treatment duration longer than 3 to 4 hours per session (see Box 60.1). Three recent randomized, controlled clinical trials have tested two of these

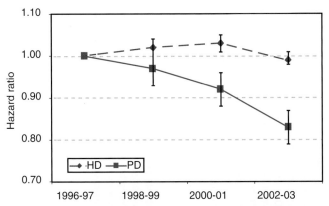

Figure 60.1   Change in 1-year risk of death or transfer to another dialysis modality for all incident hemodialysis and peritoneal dialysis patients in the United States. Data are expressed as hazards ratio with 95% confidence interval for three time periods, 1998 to 1999, 2000 to 2001, and 2002 to 2003, with incident patients in 1996 to 1998 as reference. *HD,* Hemodialysis; *PD,* peritoneal dialysis. (Reproduced with permission from Khawar O et al: Is the declining use of long-term peritoneal dialysis justified by outcome data? *Clin J Am Soc Nephrol* 2:1317-1328, 2007.)

alternative regimens (see Table 60.1). Patients treated with both short-daily in-center and nocturnal home HD achieved significant reductions in blood pressure, antihypertensive medications, serum phosphorus levels, and use of phosphate binders. Furthermore, patients randomized to short-daily in-center HD showed significant improvements in each of the two coprimary composite outcomes—death or change in left ventricular mass, and death or change in physical health composite on a quality of life measure. In contrast, the results of the two clinical trials of nocturnal home HD have been inconsistent. Although the smaller clinical trial from Canada showed a salutary effect of the treatment on left ventricular mass, there was no significant improvement in either of the two coprimary composite outcomes in the trial undertaken by the Frequent Hemodialysis Network (death or change in left ventricular mass; death or change in physical health composite). More importantly, the latter study illustrated yet again the challenges in randomizing patients to two therapies, with the investigators achieving only one third of their enrollment goal. These data support the notion that intensive HD regimens are superior in improving a variety of intermediate outcomes, but whether they will lower death risk remains to be determined in larger studies.

At least six recent observational studies have evaluated the survival of patients treated with alternative HD regimens of varying combinations of increased length of each session and/or frequency (Table 60.3). Three of these studies demonstrate a lower death risk with nocturnal HD, whether performed thrice weekly in-center or at home, when compared to patients treated with thrice-weekly, conventional duration, in-center HD. Furthermore, outcomes for patients treated with nocturnal home HD appear to be equivalent to those seen for deceased donor transplant recipients. A small but consistent survival advantage has also been reported for patients treated with short-daily home HD using the low-flow NxStage system. There are

no studies that have compared the outcomes of patients treated with these alternative HD regimens to those treated with PD. These data are quite encouraging, but, as discussed earlier, caution needs to be exercised when interpreting observational studies comparing treatments with disparate effects on patients' lifestyle. Furthermore, the overall health and functional status of patients starting treatment with these alternative HD regimens is considerably better than even those treated with PD, and these differences cannot readily be accounted for by matching or other statistical adjustments. Thus, there is substantial uncertainty as to whether the survival benefit seen in observational studies is attributable to the dialysis modality or reflects other characteristics of patients treated with these alternative HD regimens.

In summary, although additional observational studies and comparative effectiveness analyses are expected, it is highly unlikely that a randomized trial testing the efficacy of any of these alternative HD regimens, adequately powered for mortality, will be undertaken in the near future. Thus, providers should be aware of the proven benefits of these alternative HD regimens on important intermediate measures, and should ensure that patients are offered the wide range of HD treatment options.

ONLINE HEMODIAFILTRATION

Hemodiafiltration (HDF) combines both hemofiltration (HF) and HD in a single procedure. Whereas in the United States HDF is mostly performed in intensive care units, many other countries have adapted this modality for outpatient therapy, mostly known as "online" HDF. Online HDF, where replacement fluid is prepared from ultrapure dialysate, can be performed safely thanks to recent technologic advances; however, in some countries, including the United States, government restrictions prohibit the use of online HDF. HDF was initially performed in adults in 1977, and later used in children in the early 1980s. The use of HDF allows significantly higher convective clearances to be combined with the diffusive dialysis clearances, resulting in a better tolerated treatment session. However, in a recent randomized, controlled trial, there was no difference in outcomes of patients treated with HDF or conventional HD regimens.

VARIATIONS IN PERITONEAL DIALYSIS REGIMENS

As indicated earlier, PD can be performed either as CAPD or APD. In addition to the different lifestyle implications, APD is more expensive than CAPD. In most of the developed world, APD has become the dominant PD modality, driven largely by lifestyle considerations. On the other hand, PD patients in the developing world, including the emerging economies, are almost exclusively treated with CAPD primarily for economic reasons. There are potential medical differences between the two PD modalities that have been considered, with several studies suggesting that APD is associated with a more rapid decline in residual kidney function. Moreover, there is concern that frequent nighttime exchanges with APD may lead to inadequate

Table 60.2 Observational Studies Comparing Mortality in Incident Hemodialysis and Peritoneal Dialysis Patients since 2000

First Author (Publication Yr)	Cohort Period, Country	Sample Size	Statistical Approach	Follow-up Duration	Key Results
Liem (*Kidney Int* 2007)	1987 to 2002, Netherlands	16,643 (HD 10,841; PD 5802)	Cox proportional hazards model	Up to 16 yr	In younger diabetic and nondiabetic patients, lower risk for PD patients for the first 15 mo; no difference thereafter. In older nondiabetics, lower risk for PD patients in the first 6 mo, but higher risk after the first 15 mo. In older diabetics, no difference in early death but higher risk for PD patients after the first 15 mo.
Huang (*Perit Dial Int* 2008)	1995 to 2002, Taiwan	48,629 (HD 45,820; PD 2809)	Cox proportional hazards model	Up to 6 yr	Overall similar 5-yr (HD, 54%; PD, 56%) and 10-yr survival (HD, 34%; PD, 35%); subgroup analysis showed higher risk for death among all diabetics and older nondiabetics (greater than 55 yr)
Sanabria (*Kidney Int Suppl* 2008)	2001 to 2003, Colombia	923 (HD 437; PD 486)	Cox proportional hazards model	Up to Dec 2005	No difference in overall adjusted mortality rates between HD and PD; lower death risk for young, nondiabetic patients treated with PD but similar outcomes in all other groups
McDonald (*J Am Soc Nephrol* 2009)	1991 to 2005, Australia and New Zealand	25,287 (HD 14,733; PD 10,554)	Cox proportional hazards model, including analyses in propensity-score quartiles	Up to 31 Dec 2005	Overall 11% lower risk for death for PD patients in the first yr, but 33% higher risk after the first 12 mo; early survival advantage with PD seen only in young patients without comorbidities. In the most recent cohort (2004), no difference in long-term mortality of HD and PD patients
Weinhandl (*J Am Soc Nephrol* 2010)	2003, USA	6337 pairs (HD 6337; PD 6337)	Propensity-score matched cohort	Up to 4 yr	Overall mortality risk was 8% lower for PD patients. Similar adjusted 4-yr survival (HD, 48%; PD, 47%)
Mehrotra (*Arch Intern Med* 2011)	1996 to 2004, USA	684,426 (HD 620,020; PD 64,406)	Marginal structural model	Up to 5 yr	In 2002 to 2004, no significant difference in the 5-yr adjusted survival of HD and PD patients (35% and 33%, respectively). Lower risk for death for younger, nondiabetic PD patients; higher death risk for older diabetics—particularly those with additional comorbidity—treated with PD
Perl (*J Am Soc Nephrol* 2011)	2001 to 2008, Canada	38,512 (HD, 31,100; PD, 7412)	Proportional and nonproportional piecewise exponential survival model	Up to 5 yr	First yr mortality of HD patients who started dialysis with a fistula or graft was similar to those with PD but significantly higher for those HD patients who started with central venous catheters; during entire follow-up period, HD patients with fistula/graft had lower and those with central venous catheters higher death risk than PD patients
Quinn (*J Am Soc Nephrol* 2011)	1998 to 2006, Ontario, Canada	6573 (HD, 4538; PD, 2035)	Cox proportional hazards model	Up to 31 Dec 2005	No significant difference in early or late mortality of HD and PD patients who started dialysis electively as outpatients and had at least 4 mo of predialysis nephrology care
Tranyor (*Nephrol Dial Transplant* 2011)	1982 to 2006, Scotland	3197 (HD, 2107; PD, 1090)	Cox proportional hazards model	Through 31 Dec 2006	No significant difference in survival of nondiabetic transplant-listed patients treated with either HD of PD
Van de Luijtgaarden (*Nephrol Dial Transplant* 2011)	1998 to 2006, ERA-EDTA Registry	15,828 (HD, 12,731; PD, 3097)	Cox proportional hazards model	Up to 3 yr	18% lower 3-yr death risk in patients starting treatment with PD; survival benefit greater in those with no underlying comorbidity and no difference in death risk in those with comorbidity
Yeates (*Nephrol Dial Transplant* 2012)	1991 to 2004, Canada	46,839 (HD, 32,531; PD, 14,308)	Cox proportional hazards model	Up to 31 Dec 2007	For the 2001 to 2004 cohort, PD patients had a lower death risk than HD patients for the first 2 yr, but there was no difference in death risk thereafter

ERA-EDTA, European Renal Association, European Dialysis and Transplant Association; *HD*, hemodialysis; *PD*, peritoneal dialysis.

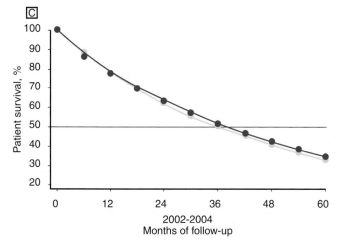

Figure 60.2   Five-year survival of patients treated with hemodialysis and peritoneal dialysis from 2002 to 2004. (Reproduced with permission from Mehrotra R et al: Similar outcomes with hemodialysis and peritoneal dialysis in patients with end-stage renal disease, *Arch Intern Med* 171:110-118, 2011.)

volume removal compared to that achieved with CAPD. However, evidence for these potential adverse effects of APD is, at best, inconsistent. Nevertheless, it is important to determine if the medical outcomes with CAPD and APD are equivalent.

Two randomized, controlled trials that have compared CAPD and APD were unable to demonstrate any significant differences in any medical outcomes (see Table 60.1). However, the sample sizes were small, and, thus, these studies were inadequately powered to determine relevant differences in outcomes by modality. In recent years, at least seven large observational studies have examined the relative outcomes with CAPD and APD (Table 60.4). The preponderance of evidence suggests that there is no overall difference in either all-cause mortality or technique survival in patients treated with CAPD and APD (Fig. 60.3), although APD may offer a survival advantage in the high/fast transporter subgroup of patients.

Thus, because the available data seem to support no significant differences in the medical outcomes of patients treated with CAPD and APD, it follows that lifestyle and economic considerations will continue to drive the differential use of the two PD modalities in different parts of the world.

Table 60.3   Observational Studies of Alternative Hemodialysis Regimens

First Author (Publication Yr)	Treatment Group	Comparator Group	Key Results
Nocturnal In-Center HD			
Lacson (*Clin J Am Soc Nephrol* 2010)	655 patients, 3 HD sessions/wk, mean duration 470 min	15,334 patients, 3 HD sessions/wk, mean duration 222 min	No significant difference in adjusted death risk but lower hospitalizations in patients treated with nocturnal in-center HD
Lacson (*J Am Soc Nephrol* 2012)	746 patients, 3 HD sessions/wk, mean duration 471 min	2062 propensity-score matched conventional HD patients	Nocturnal in-center HD associated with 25% lower death risk
Frequent, Diurnal Home HD			
Johansen (*Kidney Int* 2009)	43 patients, median 5 HD sessions/wk, 2.8 h/session, majority with Aksys machine	Propensity-score matched in-center HD patients from the United States Renal Data System	No difference in death risk or composite outcome of death, acute myocardial infarction, or stroke, with frequent, diurnal home HD
Weinhandl (*J Am Soc Nephrol* 2012)	1873 patients treated with Nxstage One HD system	9365 propensity-score matched in-center HD patients from the United States Renal Data System	Home HD with NxStage One system associated with 13% lower risk for all-cause mortality and 8% lower risk of cardiovascular mortality
Nocturnal or Long-Duration Home HD			
Johansen (*Kidney Int* 2009)	94 patients, median 6 sessions/wk, 8 hr/session	Propensity-score matched in-center HD patients from the United States Renal Data System	Significantly lower death risk with nocturnal home HD; no difference in hospitalizations
Pauly (*Nephrol Dial Transplant* 2009)	177 patients, 3 to 7 sessions/wk, 6 to 8 hr/session	533 matched deceased donor and 533 matched living donor kidney transplant recipients	Survival of nocturnal home HD patients similar to that of deceased donor transplant recipients but inferior to that of living donor transplant recipients
Nesrallah (*J Am Soc Nephrol* 2012)	338 patients, 4.8 sessions/wk, mean duration 441 min	1388 matched patients from Dialysis Outcomes and Practice Patterns study participants, 3.0 sessions/wk, mean duration 236 min	45% lower death risk in patients treated with intensive home HD

HD, Hemodialysis.

Table 60.4 Observational Studies of Continuous Ambulatory Peritoneal Dialysis and Automated Peritoneal Dialysis

First Author (Publication Yr)	Cohort Period, Country	Data Source	Sample Size (CAPD vs. APD)	Follow-up Duration	Outcomes Comparison between CAPD and APD	
					Patient Survival	**Technique Survival**
Mujais (*Kidney Int Suppl* 2006)	2000 to 2003, USA	Baxter Healthcare Corporation On-Call system	Total 40,869	Through Jun 2005	No difference	Better in APD group
Badve (*Kidney Int* 2008)	1999 to 2004, Australia and New Zealand	ANZDATA Registry	2393 vs. 1735	Though Mar 2004	No difference	No difference
Sanchez (*Kidney Int Suppl* 2008)	2003 to 2005, Mexico	Single center	139 vs. 98	Through Dec 2005	Better in APD group	Better in APD group
Mehrotra (*Kidney Int* 2009)	1996 to 2004, USA	USRDS	42,942 vs. 23,439	Through Sep 2006	No difference	No difference
Michels (*Clin J Am Soc Nephrol* 2009)	1997 to 2006, Netherlands	NECOSAD	562 vs. 87	Through Aug 2007	No difference	No difference
Johnson (*Nephrol Dial Transplant* 2010)	1999 to 2004, Australia and New Zealand	ANZDATA Registry	High transporters (142 vs. 486) Low transporters (n = 196)		Lower death risk with APD for high transporters and higher risk for low transporters	No difference
Cnossen (*Perit Dial Int* 2011)	2001 to 2008, USA	Renal Research Institute	179 vs. 441		No difference	No difference

ANZDATA, Australia and New Zealand Dialysis and Transplant; *APD,* automated peritoneal dialysis; *CAPD,* continuous ambulatory peritoneal dialysis; *NECOSAD,* Netherlands Cooperative Study on the Adequacy of Dialysis; *USRDS,* United States Renal Disease System.

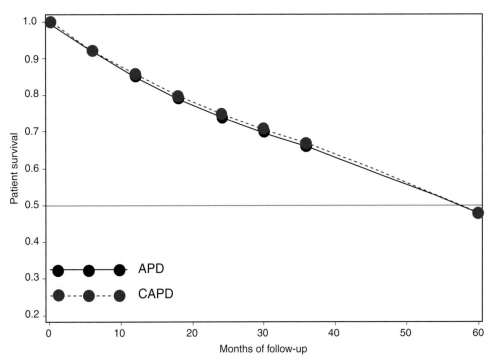

Figure 60.3 Comparison of survival of patients treated with continuous ambulatory and automated peritoneal dialysis in the United States from 1996 to 2004. *APD,* Automated peritoneal dialysis; *CAPD,* continuous ambulatory peritoneal dialysis. (Reproduced with permission from Mehrotra R et al: The outcomes of continuous ambulatory and automated peritoneal dialysis are similar, *Kidney Int* 76:97-107, 2009.)

DIALYSIS MODALITY IN CHILDREN

Most children with ESRD who need dialysis before receiving a kidney transplant are treated with PD, although a significant proportion is treated with in-center and home HD therapies. Despite interest and feasibility of online HDF in children, the majority of pediatric dialysis units across the world still perform HD using highly permeable membranes, allowing back filtration in the filter and therefore a degree of convective flow (i.e., internal HDF). Notwithstanding the general assumption that transplant is the best option for children, there are currently no convincing data as to which of the dialysis modalities offer a better outcome in children who are awaiting a kidney transplant.

IMPLICATIONS FOR DIALYSIS MODALITY SELECTION

Understanding the differences in outcomes with the various kidney replacement therapies will help providers advise individual patients as they weigh their choices for the treatment of kidney failure. A diagnosis of ESRD and the need for dialysis is stress provoking and sometimes devastating, with approximately 10% of patients having a constellation of symptoms consistent with posttraumatic stress disorder. Structured interviews and focus groups of ESRD patients indicate that, when considering dialysis modalities, many are confronting their mortality and worrying about being a burden on others; patients and their families seek knowledge about treatment options, are concerned about actual or perceived lack of choice, and weigh alternatives to determine what effect the treatment will have on their lifestyles. It is against this background of emotional turmoil that practitioners should juxtapose the paucity of adequately powered randomized, controlled trials to determine the effect of any given dialysis therapy on hard outcomes and the uncertainty of attribution from observational studies. It appears reasonable to conclude that, for most ESRD patients, there are no compelling medical reasons to choose one dialysis therapy over another. Instead, the primary goal of the healthcare provider should be to provide iterative education about different treatment options and to allow the patient to choose the kidney replacement therapy that best allows him or her to lead a fulfilling and productive life.

BIBLIOGRAPHY

Chertow GM, Levin NW, Beck GJ, et al: In-center hemodialysis six times per week versus three times per week, *N Engl J Med* 363:2287-2300, 2010.

Culleton BF, Walsh M, Klarenbach SW, et al: Effect of frequent nocturnal hemodialysis vs conventional hemodialysis on left ventricular mass and quality of life: a randomized controlled trial, *JAMA* 298:1291-1299, 2007.

Fenton SS, Schaubel DE, Desmeules M, et al: Hemodialysis versus peritoneal dialysis: a comparison of adjusted mortality rates, *Am J Kidney Dis* 30:334-342, 1997.

Foley RN, Gilbertson DT, Murray T, et al: Long interdialytic interval and mortality among patients receiving hemodialysis, *N Engl J Med* 365:1099-1107, 2011.

Grooteman MP, van den Dorpel MA, Bots ML, et al: Effect of Online Hemodiafiltration on All-Cause Mortality and Cardiovascular Outcomes, *J Am Soc Nephrol* 23:1087-1096, 2012.

Johansen KL, Zhang R, Huang Y, et al: Survival and hospitalization among patients using nocturnal and short daily compared to conventional hemodialysis: a USRDS study, *Kidney Int* 76:984-990, 2009.

Khawar O, Kalantar-Zadeh K, Lo WK, et al: Is the declining use of long-term peritoneal dialysis justified by outcome data? *Clin J Am Soc Nephrol* 2:1317-1328, 2007.

Korevaar JC, Feith GW, Dekker FW, et al: Effect of starting hemodialysis compared with peritoneal dialysis in patients new on dialysis treatment: a randomized controlled trial, *Kidney Int* 64:2222-2228, 2003.

Lacson E Jr, Xu J, Suri R, et al: Survival with three-times weekly in-center nocturnal versus conventional hemodialysis, *J Am Soc Nephrol* 23:687-695, 2012.

McDonald SP, Marshall MR, Johnson DW, et al: Relationship between dialysis modality and mortality, *J Am Soc Nephrol* 20:155-163, 2009.

Mehrotra R, Chiu YW, Kalantar-Zadeh K, et al: Similar outcomes with hemodialysis and peritoneal dialysis in patients with end-stage renal disease, *Arch Intern Med* 171:110-118, 2011.

Mehrotra R, Chiu YW, Kalantar-Zadeh K, et al: The outcomes of continuous ambulatory and automated peritoneal dialysis are similar, *Kidney Int* 76:97-107, 2009.

Mehrotra R, Kermah D, Fried L, et al: Chronic peritoneal dialysis in the United States: declining utilization despite improving outcomes, *J Am Soc Nephrol* 18:2781-2788, 2007.

Morton RL, Tong A, Howard K, et al: The views of patients and carers in treatment decision making for chronic kidney disease: systematic review and thematic synthesis of qualitative studies, *BMJ* 340:c112, 2010.

Nesrallah GE, Lindsay RM, Cuerden MS, et al: Intensive hemodialysis associates with improved survival compared with conventional hemodialysis, *J Am Soc Nephrol* 23:696-705, 2012.

Rocco MV, Lockridge RS Jr, Beck GJ, et al: The effects of frequent nocturnal home hemodialysis: the Frequent Hemodialysis Network Nocturnal Trial,, *Kidney Int* 80:1080-1091, 2011.

Vonesh EF, Snyder JJ, Foley RN, et al: The differential impact of risk factors on mortality in hemodialysis and peritoneal dialysis, *Kidney Int* 66:2389-2401, 2004.

Weinhandl ED, Foley RN, Gilbertson DT, et al: Propensity-matched mortality comparison of incident hemodialysis and peritoneal dialysis patients, *J Am Soc Nephrol* 21:499-506, 2010.

Weinhandl ED, Liu J, Gilbertson DT, et al: Survival in daily home hemodialysis and matched thrice-weekly in-center hemodialysis patients, *J Am Soc Nephrol* 23:895-904, 2012.

Wolfe RA, Ashby VB, Milford EL, et al: Comparison of mortality in all patients on dialysis, patients on dialysis awaiting transplantation, and recipients of a first cadaveric transplant, *N Engl J Med* 341:1725-1730, 1999.

Selection of Prospective Kidney Transplant Recipients and Donors

Greg Knoll | Todd Fairhead

Kidney transplantation is the treatment of choice for most patients with end-stage renal disease (ESRD) because it prolongs survival, improves quality of life, and is less costly than the alternative therapy of dialysis. However, only a small percentage of ESRD patients actually receive a transplant; many patients are not suitable candidates, and for those patients who are eligible, there are simply not enough organs available. As the primary contact for patients with advanced chronic kidney disease (CKD), as well as for those already on dialysis, nephrologists are in a unique position to counsel and guide patients through the transplantation process. A thorough understanding of who is suitable for transplantation and the required evaluation will facilitate this process.

WHO SHOULD BE CONSIDERED FOR KIDNEY TRANSPLANTATION?

There are very few absolute contraindications for kidney transplantation. All patients should be evaluated by their nephrologist for transplant suitability, and potentially referred to a transplant center for further evaluation. Eligibility should not be based on age, gender, race, or socioeconomic status. Given that donor kidneys are a rare and limited resource, a patient must be expected to survive beyond current waiting times for transplantation. Careful evaluation of physiologic age, medical comorbidities, and functional status will help determine whether a patient may be eligible for transplantation. Box 61.1 lists the contraindications for transplantation.

TIMING OF REFERRAL

Both mortality and graft outcomes are improved with early transplantation. Patients who receive a preemptive kidney transplant have a superior outcome as compared with patients who undergo dialysis treatments before receiving a transplant. Similarly, length of exposure to dialysis affects transplant outcomes and mortality. Improved outcomes are inversely related to duration on dialysis. Thus, to allow adequate time to complete the required medical tests before transplantation and to facilitate potential preemptive transplantation, patients with CKD should be referred to a kidney transplant center early in their disease course. Many potential transplant recipients are medically complex. Determining suitability for transplantation may require multiple specialist visits and medical tests. This process may take 6 to 12 months to complete and should be factored into the overall referral time. For patients with potential living donors, appropriate time should be allocated for donor workup as well.

In the United States, the United Network for Organ Sharing (UNOS) allows listing for transplantation when a patient's estimated glomerular filtration rate (eGFR) falls below 20 mL/min, whereas organizations in other countries have established stage 5 CKD (eGFR below 15 mL/min) as the upper limit for listing. Thus patients should be referred for transplantation evaluation when they have stage 4 CKD (eGFR below 30 mL/min) that is progressing. In many programs, transplantation assessment is initiated with referral to a multidisciplinary kidney replacement therapy planning clinic. In these clinics, transplant eligibility is considered, and teaching is provided alongside planning for dialysis initiation. It is important to recognize that certain barriers to transplant referral have been identified. Access to transplantation may be decreased for patients of certain ethnicities, those with lower socioeconomic status and/or education level, or those living a greater distance from a transplant referral center.

MEDICAL EVALUATION FOR TRANSPLANTATION

A complete medical, surgical, and psychosocial history is required upon consideration for transplantation. A thorough physical examination may identify abnormalities that affect transplant suitability, such as poor dentition or diminished arterial pulses. Table 61.1 lists the minimum investigations required before transplantation. Additional testing based on medical comorbidities may be necessary. Each coexisting illness should be evaluated for its potential effect on transplant outcome. In addition, total disease burden and functional capacity must be factored into a final decision. Both the American Society of Transplantation (2001) and the Canadian Society of Transplantation (2005) have published clinical practice guidelines for the eligibility of kidney transplant recipients. Because little evidence is available to guide the evaluation process, most recommendations are based on expert opinion.

GENERAL CONSIDERATIONS

Advanced age is not a contraindication to transplantation. At present, patients over 65 years of age are the fastest-growing group of wait-listed potential recipients. Death-censored graft outcomes are similar or better in these older adult recipients. With advanced age, special attention should be paid to pretransplant medical comorbidities, functional status, and quality of life. The cost of maintaining a proposed recipient on the waiting list is not insignificant. A patient's capacity to survive beyond current waiting list times to transplantation and beyond must be considered. The technical aspects of the transplant surgery limit transplantation in extremely young children. However, this should not delay transplant workup, and preemptive transplantation should be considered when possible.

OBESITY

Patients with extreme obesity are susceptible to an increased risk for transplant-related complications, including delayed graft function, wound complications, and infections, as well as an increased risk for new-onset diabetes after transplantation. Additionally, long-term graft failure rates and mortality are higher among obese recipients when compared with otherwise comparable recipients. As such, many transplant programs avoid transplanting patients with extreme obesity. Individual programs limit transplantation to individuals under a certain body mass index (BMI), usually 40 kg/m². In patients with a BMI between 30 and 39 kg/m², weight-loss counseling should be provided. Bariatric surgery may be considered in individuals with a BMI greater than 40 kg/m².

KIDNEY DISEASE

Many kidney diseases recur after transplantation. Recent analyses suggest that allograft failure secondary to recurrent disease is now the third-most common reason for graft failure, only behind rejection and death with a functioning graft. In an analysis of the Australia and New Zealand Dialysis and Transplant Registry (ANZDATA), allograft loss due to recurrent disease occurred in 8.4% of patients with biopsy-proven glomerulonephritis who received a kidney transplant. Similarly, when the Mayo Clinic retrospectively analyzed specific causes of kidney allograft loss, recurrent disease was diagnosed in 14.3% of all lost allografts. An additional 6.5% of graft loss was due to glomerular pathology that could not be classified as recurrent because of incomplete clinical information. Despite this, the risk for recurrence rarely precludes transplantation, and allograft failure from recurrence is rare in first 5 years posttransplant. In the ANZDATA analysis, the overall 10-year incidence of allograft loss was similar among transplant recipients with glomerulonephritis versus those with other causes of kidney failure, and no risks were identified that would preclude transplantation. It is important to counsel prospective transplant recipients about the risk for recurrent disease. Table 61.2 shows the incidence of recurrence of different forms of kidney disease.

IgA nephropathy may recur in up to 60% of allograft biopsies; however, clinically significant recurrence (with elevated creatinine or proteinuria) develops in only 30% of kidney transplants. Furthermore, clinical recurrence tends

Box 61.1 Contraindications to Kidney Transplantation

Chronic illness with life expectancy less than 1 year
Active malignancy with short life expectancy
Active infection
Poorly controlled psychosis
Medical nonadherence or active substance abuse

Table 61.1 Proposed Workup for Potential Kidney Transplant Candidates

Test	Comments
Physical examination	Attention to dentition, arterial pulses
Tissue typing	ABO blood type, HLA identification, PRA
Viral serology	CMV, EBV, VZV, HSV, HCV, HBV, HIV, HTLV, VDRL
Cardiac testing	ECG
	Echocardiogram
	Risk stratification if high risk
Imaging	Chest radiograph
	Abdominal ultrasound or imaging equivalent
	Arterial vascular imaging if high risk (Doppler ultrasound, CT scan, angiogram)
Female-specific	Breast exam and mammogram
	Pap smear
Male-specific	Prostate exam
Consultations	Transplant surgeon
	Cardiologist (if high-risk)
	Social worker

CMV, Cytomegalovirus; *EBV,* Epstein-Barr virus; *ECG,* electrocardiogram; *HBV,* hepatitis B virus; *HCV,* hepatitis C virus; *HIV,* human immunodeficiency virus; *HLA,* human leukocyte antigen; *HSV,* herpes simplex virus; *HTLV,* human T-lymphotropic virus; *VDRL,* venereal disease research laboratory (test); *VZV,* varicella zoster virus.

Table 61.2 Risk for Recurrence and Graft Loss After Transplantation

Type of Glomerulonephritis	Risk for Clinically Relevant Recurrence (% of patients)	Risk for Graft Failure 5-10 Years Posttransplant (% of patients)
IgA nephropathy	15%-50%	10%
FSGS	30%	20%
Membranous nephropathy	40%	15%
MPGN type I	30%-50%	15%
MPGN type II	80%	30%
ANCA glomerulonephritis	10%-15%	5%
SLE	5%	3%
Anti-GBM	<5%	Rare
Fibrillary/immunotactoid glomerulopathy	>50%	Unknown

ANCA, Anti-neutrophil cytoplasmic antigen; *FSGS,* focal segmental glomerulosclerosis; *GBM,* glomerular basement membrane; *MPGN,* membranoproliferative glomerulonephritis; *SLE,* systemic lupus erythematosus.

to be late, and graft loss due to IgA nephropathy occurs in only 10% of patients. Focal segmental glomerulosclerosis (FSGS) can recur in up to 30% of transplant recipients and is more common in those with primary FSGS. In patients with a previously failed allograft due to recurrent FSGS, risk for recurrence rises to as high as 50% to 80%. In many cases, recurrence appears to be secondary to a circulating permeability factor that affects podocyte foot process and glomerular slit diaphragm integrity. Plasma exchange may reduce proteinuria and prolong the life of the allograft. Recently, the circulating permeability factor was proposed to be soluble urokinase-type plasminogen activator receptor (suPAR), giving hope for more definitive treatments for recurrent FSGS in the future. Membranous nephropathy can recur in up to 40% of cases posttransplant. Unlike in the nontransplanted kidney, spontaneous remission is rare and graft failure can occur in as many as 50% of cases by 10 years. Rituximab may limit proteinuria and allograft damage after recurrence.

Membranoproliferative glomerulonephritis (MPGN) has a high rate of recurrence posttransplantation, with type I recurring in 30% to 50% of patients and type II recurring in over 80% of patients. The presence of serum monoclonal proteins and low complement levels at the time of transplantation are risks for MPGN recurrence. Recurrence of MPGN is usually early in the transplant course and associated with proteinuria. The risk for graft loss from MPGN type I is approximately 15% at 10 years, whereas it is as high as 90% after 5 years in MPGN type II. Recurrence of rapidly progressive glomerulonephritis is rare if disease is quiescent at the time of transplantation. In patients with anti-glomerular basement membrane (anti-GBM) disease, the absence of circulating anti-GBM antibodies should be confirmed before considering transplantation. Although the presence of anti-neutrophil cytoplasmic antibodies (ANCA) does not preclude transplantation, patients should achieve a clinical remission period in which they are not taking immunosuppressive medications before transplantation. Similarly, a positive serostatus in patients with systemic lupus erythematosus (SLE) does not preclude transplantation; however, active disease should be quiescent. Recurrence of lupus nephritis is rare (<20%), possibly because of protection from immunosuppressive transplant medications. Glomerular diseases with organizing deposits such as amyloidosis, fibrillary, and immunotactoid glomerulonephritis can all recur with rates greater than 50%. With both primary and secondary forms of amyloidosis, transplantation is often limited by severe cardiac disease; early death from cardiovascular disease or infection is quite high. Total burden of amyloidosis needs to be considered before transplantation.

Genetic forms of kidney disease may affect the transplanted allograft. Rarely, patients with Alport disease can develop antibodies against type IV collagen leading to a condition similar to Goodpasture disease. Patients with primary oxalosis are highly susceptible to rapid oxalate deposition in the transplanted kidney without treatment. These patients are best managed with concurrent liver transplantation and supplementation with orthophosphate and pyridoxine. Patients with kidney failure secondary to sickle cell nephropathy can be safely transplanted with good results, providing their overall health allows transplantation.

INFECTION

Presence of an active infection—bacterial, fungal, or viral—is a contraindication for transplantation. All potential recipients should be screened for chronic infections during the transplant evaluation and assessed for acute infection at the time of transplantation. Clinical and occult dialysis access-related infections in indwelling peritoneal dialysis catheters and tunneled hemodialysis catheters need to be fully treated before transplantation.

Efforts to protect immunosuppressed recipients should occur before transplantation. Transplant candidates should be immunized against seasonal influenza, hepatitis B virus (HBV), and pneumococcal pneumonia. Additionally, vaccination against human papilloma virus and primary (chickenpox) and secondary (shingles) *Varicella zoster* infection should be considered in high-risk recipients. Although efficacy of immunization is notably poor in the ESRD population, risk for infection posttransplant is high.

Cytomegalovirus (CMV) can be transmitted via kidney transplant, and commonly leads to disease if untreated. Measuring a potential recipient's CMV serostatus is important before transplantation, but a negative serostatus does not preclude receipt of a kidney transplant from a CMV-positive donor. Additionally, potential recipients and donors should be screened for Epstein-Barr virus (EBV) and herpes simplex virus (HSV) before transplant. Those recipients with an EBV-mismatched kidney transplant should undergo EBV virus screening for posttransplant lymphoproliferative disorder (PTLD), whereas HSV-mismatched patients may be offered acyclovir for prophylaxis.

Tuberculosis (TB) infection is common in immunosuppressed kidney transplant patients, and may approach 15% in TB endemic areas. Risk factors for developing TB after transplant include a positive tuberculin skin test reaction before transplant, prior residence in a TB-endemic area, a chest radiograph suggestive of prior TB, and older age. Before transplantation, all potential recipients should undergo tuberculin skin testing and a chest radiograph. High-risk patients should undergo prophylactic TB treatment for 6 to 12 months in the absence of documented prior treatment. It is probably safe to proceed with transplantation after beginning prophylactic TB treatment, but evidence is lacking.

Although once considered an absolute contraindication, kidney transplantation in HIV-positive recipients has become possible in the current era of highly active antiretroviral therapy (HAART). Patient and allograft survival in this population is acceptable and no worse than other high-risk groups (e.g., older recipients), although incidence of acute rejection is increased. Patients with HIV should be referred to a transplant center with experience managing this infection. In general, HIV RNA should be undetectable and CD4 count should be greater than 200 mm^3 before consideration for transplant.

In the modern era of immunosuppression, allograft loss due to BK (polyoma) virus has emerged as an important threat to graft survival. Polyoma virus infection is ubiquitous in the general population, with overimmunosuppression thought to be responsible for clinically evident disease. Limited evidence suggests that retransplantation in patients who have suffered a previous allograft failure from BK virus may be successful; thus BK virus should not preclude retransplantation.

MALIGNANCY

Immunosuppression likely promotes tumor growth and increases the risk for cancer recurrence. As allograft survival lengthens, death from malignancy continues to increase. Thus active malignancy is an absolute contraindication to transplantation, with the exception of superficial squamous cell and basal cell skin cancers. In patients with a history of malignancy, a waiting period between successful treatment of cancer and transplantation is recommended. The length of this waiting period depends on the type of malignancy and the risk for recurrence. In general, a waiting period of 2 years is recommended for most types of cancer. In high-risk malignancies such as breast cancer, colon cancer, melanoma, and invasive and/or symptomatic renal cell cancer, a waiting period of 5 years is recommended. Small, incidentally discovered renal cell cancers and cervical cancer in situ do not require any waiting period. Multiple myeloma is a contraindication for transplantation unless considered concurrently with an allogeneic bone marrow transplant.

Although life expectancy is shortened in dialysis-dependent prospective kidney transplant recipients, most programs perform pretransplant malignancy screening. Screening should be based on clinical practice guidelines for the general population as part of a periodic health examination. All patients should receive a chest radiograph, abdominal ultrasound, and age-appropriate colon cancer screening as part of their workup. Women should undergo breast examination, pelvic exam, and Pap smear as dictated by their age. Men should receive a prostate examination if symptomatic. Additionally, patients who have received cyclophosphamide in the past should be considered for urine cytology and cystoscopy to rule out bladder malignancy.

CARDIOVASCULAR DISEASE

Cardiovascular disease is the leading cause of death in patients on dialysis and in kidney transplant recipients, with diabetics at particular risk. Therefore all potential transplant recipients should be carefully evaluated for the presence of heart disease before listing. At a minimum, patients should be assessed for signs and symptoms of cardiovascular disease and undergo an ECG and echocardiogram. Patients with progressive angina symptoms or a myocardial infarction within 6 months should not be offered transplantation. In patients with severe and irreversible coronary artery disease, projected life expectancy must be balanced against the risks of transplant surgery. It is worth noting that left ventricular dysfunction due to uremic cardiomyopathy is not a contraindication to transplantation and frequently improves after surgery. In patients at high risk for underlying coronary disease (including men over age 40, women over age 50, patients with diabetes, patients with multiple traditional cardiovascular risk factors), noninvasive testing may be performed to identify underlying disease. Patients with positive noninvasive stress test results may be referred for angiography and potential revascularization before transplantation.

At present, cardiac risk stratification of potential kidney transplant candidates is guided by little supporting evidence.

Although data demonstrate that noninvasive testing can accurately diagnose coronary artery disease in patients with diabetes and in CKD patients without diabetes, subsequent management varies widely from center to center. Current guidelines from the American College of Cardiology (ACC)/American Heart Association (AHA) recommend revascularization only in symptomatic patients with high-risk cardiac lesions. In two clinical trials that examined preoperative revascularization versus medical management in moderate to high-risk individuals, perioperative event rates and mortality did not differ. It should be noted that patients with advanced CKD have not been studied in this context, nor has the question of life expectancy after organ transplant in individuals with a significant burden of coronary artery disease been directly addressed. With prolonged waiting times, cardiovascular disease in high-risk individuals may progress. Many programs perform periodic noninvasive rescreening in wait-listed patients; however, the value of this practice is unknown, and newly detected disease is only variably acted upon.

Modifiable risk factors for cardiovascular disease should be managed appropriately in prospective kidney transplant recipients. Blood pressure should be treated to a target of at least 140/90 mm Hg and smoking cessation should be encouraged. The utility of treating dyslipidemia in dialysis patients has recently come into question; however, control of LDL cholesterol should be considered in high-risk individuals.

CEREBROVASCULAR DISEASE

After transplantation, recipients are at an increased risk for cerebrovascular disease when compared with pretransplant patients or the general population. Patients with symptomatic transient ischemic attacks or a recent stroke should be symptom free for 6 months before transplantation. Consideration of carotid endarterectomy should be given to those individuals with known carotid stenosis. Screening of asymptomatic patients is unclear. Again, modifiable risk factors, including smoking and blood pressure, should be addressed before transplant.

LIVER DISEASE

Because progressive liver disease causes significant morbidity and mortality in transplant patients, all prospective recipients should be screened. In patients with liver disease not caused by viral hepatitis, liver function testing and a liver biopsy should be considered to assess severity of disease. The patient's immunosuppressed state in the posttransplantation period permits viral replication that can accelerate chronic viral hepatitis. Therefore all patients should be screened for HBV and hepatitis C virus (HCV) infection. In patients with significant liver disease and/or cirrhosis, consideration of combined liver-kidney transplant may be an option.

Patients with positive hepatitis B surface antigen (HBsAg) should undergo testing for hepatitis B viral load by PCR, hepatitis B early antigen (HBeAg), and hepatitis D virus (HDV). Patients with evidence of active viral replication (HBeAg-positive, or hepatitis B viral load–positive) should forgo transplantation until HBV is effectively treated. Those with both HBV and HDV should not be considered for transplantation because of the risk for severe liver disease.

In patients with chronic active hepatitis and elevated liver enzymes, liver biopsy should be performed, and posttransplant antiviral therapy (e.g., lamivudine) should be considered. Transplant outcomes are generally worse in patients who are HBsAg-positive as compared with those who are not. The decision whether to transplant can be difficult, and specialist assistance may be required.

HCV infection can lead to accelerated liver disease after transplantation. All prospective transplant recipients who have serologic evidence of HCV exposure should undergo HCV load testing by PCR and liver biopsy. Although patients with HCV have worse outcomes after transplant when compared with those without infection, outcomes are improved over remaining on dialysis. Treatment of HCV after transplantation is limited by the high risk for immunologic rejection with interferon-alpha. Efforts should be made to eradicate HCV with antiviral therapy before transplantation. Patients with HCV may be able to accept a kidney from an HCV-positive donor; however, this remains controversial.

PULMONARY DISEASE

Patients with pulmonary disease are at increased risk for perioperative respiratory complications. Thus patients with severe, irreversible lung disease, including severe chronic obstructive pulmonary disease (COPD), cor pulmonale, and those needing supplemental oxygen, should not be offered kidney transplantation. Current smokers and patients with known lung disease should undergo pulmonary function testing for risk stratification before transplantation. Smokers who undergo transplantation are at risk for increased perioperative events and have poor long-term outcomes as compared with nonsmokers. All smokers should be offered smoking cessation aids and counseling as necessary to encourage smoking cessation.

THROMBOTIC RISK

Patients with a history of venous or arterial thromboembolic disease may be at risk for perioperative graft loss due to thrombosis. Screening for genetic risks of thrombosis should be considered in those individuals with a positive medical history, and a plan for perioperative anticoagulation should be constructed. Patients with a history of SLE should be screened for antiphospholipid antibodies. Inherited disorders of complement may lead to atypical hemolytic uremic syndrome (HUS), with recurrent disease occurring in up to 25% to 50% of allografts. Screening for genetic abnormalities may allow for an individualized perioperative plan including plasma exchange and/or calcineurin inhibitor avoidance, which may lessen recurrence risk.

UROLOGIC EVALUATION

Patients with a history of lower urinary tract abnormalities, bladder dysfunction, or recurrent urinary tract infections require urologic investigation and voiding cystourethrogram. In addition, high-risk patients, such as those with diabetes, should be screened with a postvoid residual. Efforts should be made to preserve the native bladder, and self-intermittent catheterization is preferable to urinary diversion with ureteroiliostomy. Patients with significant exposure to cyclophosphamide should be screened with cystoscopy

to rule out malignancy. Pretransplant nephrectomy should be considered in patients with severe reflux or recurrent nephrolithiasis with recurrent infection, difficult-to-control hypertension, severe nephrotic syndrome, and symptomatic polycystic kidneys.

PSYCHOLOGICAL EVALUATION

All prospective transplant recipients should undergo screening to identify cognitive or psychological impairments that may alter their ability to provide informed consent or their ability to follow medical protocols after transplantation. Medication nonadherence remains a major cause of graft loss. However, identification of individuals at risk is difficult and not often apparent during the transplant workup. In general, one should be cautious in restricting access to transplantation in those at risk for nonadherence. Patients with addiction or a history of chemical dependency should be offered counseling and rehabilitation. Many programs require a period of abstinence before a patient is put on the waiting list. Those individuals with major psychiatric illness should receive appropriate psychiatric care with the recognition of potential medication interactions and side effects.

IMMUNOLOGIC CONSIDERATIONS BEFORE TRANSPLANTATION

Tissue compatibility between donor and recipient is determined by matching ABO blood type, human leukocyte antigen (HLA), and/or major histocompatibility complex (MHC). Blood and HLA tissue typing is performed on all suitable transplant candidates at the time of wait-listing. For the most part, the donor kidney must be ABO compatible with the recipient. Although HLA matching is desired, it is rarely achieved because of the tremendous allelic polymorphisms present in the MHC genes. In kidney transplantation, HLA A, B, and DR are thought to be most important in histocompatibility. Both early rejection and long-term allograft survival are affected by HLA matching, with a zero antigen mismatched kidney having a decreased risk for rejection and better long-term survival as compared with a six antigen mismatched kidney.

A major barrier to transplantation is the development of antibodies against HLA epitopes, called sensitization. Anti-HLA antibodies are formed during exposure to foreign HLA through blood transfusions, pregnancy, and prior transplantation. The presence of anti-HLA antibodies against a donor HLA-type precludes transplantation because of the extreme risk for hyperacute rejection and graft failure. Thus all candidates on the waiting list are screened for the presence of anti-HLA antibodies at least every 3 months.

Screening for anti-HLA antibodies is performed through serologic testing (by mixing donor lymphocytes with recipient serum) or, now more routinely, through solid phase assays such as flow cytometry or the Luminex platform. An estimate of a recipient's anti-HLA antibody burden can be estimated by mixing recipient serum with a panel of lymphocytes representing random donors from the general population. The percentage of lymphocytes that react to recipient antibodies is called panel-reactive antibody (PRA), and provides an estimate of the likelihood of finding a suitable donor within the population. A high PRA means it will be more difficult to find a compatible donor. In addition, a high PRA is associated with worse graft survival, even if the final cross-match against the donor is negative. Using solid-phase assays, most transplant centers are now able to determine the specificity of a recipient's anti-HLA antibodies. A list of unacceptable HLA antigens can then be compiled for a recipient. Comparing this profile to the donor's HLA type to assess tissue histocompatibility is termed a virtual cross-match. Solid-phase assays to detect anti-HLA antibodies are much more sensitive than serologic detection, and can often identify low-titer antibodies that were previously undetectable. Even with a negative cross-match, presence of low titer antibodies against donor HLA is associated with antibody-mediated rejection and higher rates of graft loss.

At the time of transplantation, a final cross-match is completed to ensure tissue compatibility. Recipient serum is mixed with donor tissue. A positive cross-match indicates the presence of donor-specific anti-HLA antibodies (DSA) and predicts hyperacute rejection. Because not all positive cross-match results are due to antibodies that cause hyperacute rejection, further laboratory tests may be necessary before transplantation. In patients with a high PRA, the cross-match is often performed using historical sera with the highest PRA value. Recipients with a current negative cross-match but a historical positive cross-match may undergo transplantation, but they are at a higher risk for antibody-mediated rejection.

Patients with a high PRA are disadvantaged and often have prolonged waiting times because of the limited number of compatible donors. Strategies to lower a patient's PRA to increase the probability of finding a suitable donor are constantly evolving. Noninvasive strategies, such as enrollment in a living donor–paired exchange program, have increased access for mismatched living donor pairs (see later). Strategies to decrease or eliminate anti-HLA or anti-ABO antibodies may include targeting of either the antibodies or the B cell/plasma cell clones that produce the antibodies. Use of plasmapheresis and high-dose intravenous immunoglobulin (IVIG) has been used successfully to greatly reduce or eliminate anti-HLA antibodies. Rituximab and bortezomib (and, rarely, splenectomy) have been used to target B cells and plasma cells. Although these strategies have allowed successful transplantation with ABO-incompatible or positive cross-match donors, the risk for antibody-mediated rejection and graft loss remains increased.

DECEASED DONOR ORGANS

Because of the shortage of deceased donor organs, novel sources of kidneys for transplantation continue to be explored. Expanded criteria donor (ECD) kidneys include those from donors over the age of 60 or from donors between 50 and 59 years old with two of the following: cerebrovascular accident as the cause of death, hypertension, or terminal serum creatinine greater than 1.5 mg/dL. ECD kidneys have a 1.7-fold higher probability of graft failure 2 years after transplantation as compared with standard criteria donor (SCD) kidneys; however, early access to transplantation may benefit potential transplant recipients. In patients over the age of 65 or patients over the age of 40 with diabetes and prolonged deceased donor transplant wait times, receipt of an

ECD kidney confers a survival advantage over waiting for an SCD kidney. Younger, healthier kidney transplant candidates may be better served by waiting for an SCD kidney. UNOS permits all wait-listed candidates to declare whether they are willing to accept an ECD kidney. Patients willing to receive an ECD kidney are also eligible to receive SCD kidneys.

In North America, the majority of organs are collected from deceased donors meeting the criteria for brain death. More recently, organs have been collected from donors not meeting the criteria for brain death, but whose death is determined by cardiac criteria (donation after cardiac death, or DCD). Organ procurement in DCD donors can be controlled or uncontrolled. In controlled DCD donation, consent for donation is obtained before death, and life support is withdrawn in a controlled fashion in the operating room. An uncontrolled donor dies before consent for organ donation and attempts are made to preserve the organs until consent can be obtained. DCD donor kidneys suffer a higher rate of delayed graft function; however, long-term outcomes appear to be similar to those achieved with SCD kidneys.

ALLOCATION OF DECEASED DONOR ORGANS IN THE UNITED STATES

UNOS and the Organ Procurement and Transplant Network (OPTN) allocate donated kidneys in the United States. Patients who are medically ready for transplantation may be placed on the UNOS waiting list for a deceased donor kidney. Kidneys are allocated by policies designed to balance equity and efficacy. Only a brief overview of this process will be provided; policies can be viewed in more detail online (http://optn.transplant.hrsa.gov/policiesAndBylaws/policies.asp).

Deceased donor kidneys are allocated by ABO blood type—thus ABO-O donor kidneys are available only to O recipients. This allocation is followed for A, B, and AB kidneys also. There is mandatory national sharing of zero-antigen mismatched kidneys with pediatric recipients or adults with a PRA greater than 20% because of the proven enhanced allograft survival benefit. Otherwise, donor kidneys are first offered locally, then regionally, and then nationally. All potential recipients on the UNOS waiting list are allocated points, which determine their priority for transplantation. Patients with more points receive higher priority. Points are awarded for length of waiting time, quality of DR antigen match, degree of sensitization and PRA, medical urgency, and pediatric recipient status. Details of the point system for kidney allocation can be reviewed at the OPTN website (see earlier).

Current allocation policies are not without criticism. At present, the allocation policy does not take into account factors associated with allograft and recipient survival, resulting in less efficient organ utilization. Patients with a low probability of long-term survival have equal access to younger SCD kidneys, or "ideal" donors. New organ allocation policies that attempt to maximize lifetime benefit are now being discussed. A donor profile index, time on dialysis, and an estimation of recipient survival after transplantation are all being considered for incorporation into a new allocation algorithm. These considerations could result in kidneys being matched to the recipient based on expected survival of the kidney and the recipient. With the new proposals, concern remains that certain groups may be disproportionately disadvantaged.

LIVING KIDNEY DONATION

Although the number of deceased donors has increased significantly since 1990 (Fig. 61.1), this has not kept pace with the increased number of patients being added to the kidney transplant waiting list. As such, wait times have increased dramatically, to the point where it is difficult to accurately calculate median wait times in certain regions. Looking at it another way, only 30% of candidates will have received a kidney transplant within 3 years of being placed on the wait list. The lack of access to deceased donor organs, as well as the superior outcomes with live donors, has resulted in the increased usage of living kidney donors for transplantation. In the 15 years from 1990 to 2005, the number of living kidney donors used in the United States increased dramatically (see Fig. 61.1). Since 2005 this growth has slowed somewhat, but there were still more than 6500 living kidney donors used for transplantation in 2010 alone.

Living kidney donation offers several potential advantages over deceased donor transplantation. First, the procedure is elective and scheduled, thus ensuring that both donor and recipient are in optimal medical condition. The planned nature of the operation also facilitates the use of preemptive transplantation (i.e., kidney transplantation without prior dialysis), which has been associated with both improved patient and allograft survival. Second, the incidence of delayed graft function (need for dialysis in the first week posttransplantation) is much lower for recipients of living donor kidneys. In 2009, only 3.4% of living donor kidney recipients had delayed graft function, compared with 24% of deceased donor transplant patients. Finally, patient and allograft survival rates are superior for living donor kidneys compared with deceased donors. In the most recently available data, patients who received a living donor kidney transplant in 2008 had a 1-year allograft survival of 96% compared with 92% for deceased donor recipients. For patients who received a living donor kidney transplant in 2004, the 5-year patient survival was 93% compared with only 85% for deceased donor recipients. Similarly, for those who received a living donor transplant in 2004, the 5-year allograft survival was 83% compared with only 70% for recipients of deceased donor kidney transplant.

LIVING DONOR EVALUATION PROCESS

Living donation is a unique medical situation in which the patient (donor) undergoes an operation with risk yet receives no direct medical benefit from the procedure. Many donors do, however, report benefits such as an improved sense of well-being from seeing a friend or relative thrive after transplantation. Given the exceptional circumstances surrounding living donation, it is crucial that informed consent be obtained in an open and thoughtful manner. Consent should be obtained for both the evaluation process and the surgical procedure itself. The potential donor needs to understand that the evaluation process requires a series of tests—and that the results of some of these tests may be abnormal. Certain test results may prompt disclosure to another agency (e.g., HIV-positive test results reported to public health) or may impact future insurability (e.g., significant proteinuria). Other points that should be fully discussed as part of the informed consent process are outlined in Box 61.2.

After informed consent, the evaluation consists of a psychosocial and medical assessment. The psychosocial assessment must be conducted by an appropriate professional

Box 61.2 Key Points of Informed Consent Process for Living Kidney Donors

Living kidney donors should understand the following items as part of the informed consent process:

- Consent may be withdrawn at any time.
- The evaluation process and operation both involve risk.
- Abnormalities discovered during the evaluation might impact future insurability or may require reporting to another agency (e.g., positive HIV test).
- There is a small but real risk for death with live donor nephrectomy (3.1 per 10,000 donors).
- All donors will lose kidney function postoperatively, but the actual amount is difficult to predict.
- Living donors have developed ESRD, but the risk appears no greater than for the general population.

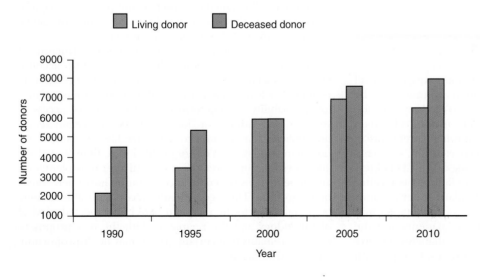

Figure 61.1 **Living and deceased organ donors in the United States.** (Data accessed on February 13, 2012, from www.optn.transplant.hrsa.gov).

with experience in living kidney donation. This person will vary from site to site, but is most often a social worker, clinical psychologist, or psychiatrist. Important components of the psychosocial assessment are outlined in Box 61.3. Significant concerns with any of these factors may preclude donation or require further assessment by other health care professionals (e.g., psychiatrist).

The medical assessment should be conducted by a surgeon or physician (ideally both) with expertise in living kidney donation. The goal of the medical evaluation is to determine (a) the overall health of the potential donor and whether he or she is fit for surgery; (b) the current kidney health of the potential donor and his or her risk for kidney disease or medical complications in the future; (c) the presence of any conditions that may result in disease transmission (e.g., infection) to the recipient; and (d) the immunologic compatibility of the potential donor with the intended recipient. The tests required to address these components of the medical evaluation are listed in Box 61.4.

Before proceeding with specific testing, a medical history and physical examination is required for all living donors. The history should focus on conditions related to overall health and fitness for surgery, such as the presence of cardiovascular disease, liver disease, pulmonary disease, or hematologic conditions (bleeding disorders or thrombosis). Significant abnormalities in any of these areas may preclude donation or require more specialized testing and/or referral to another consultant.

AGE OF THE LIVING KIDNEY DONOR

Age is an important consideration when assessing living kidney donors. Most programs will not allow living donors younger than 18 years of age, and 15% of transplant centers require donors to be at least 21 years old. On the opposite end of the age spectrum, wide variation exists in practice. The most common upper age limit for living donors is 65 years old, and this cutoff was reported at 21% of American transplant centers in a 2007 survey. Notably, 59% of programs reported that no upper age limit was in effect at their center. Despite these survey results, between 1992 and 2011, there were only 1200 living kidney donors 65 years of age or older in the United States, with approximately 100 per year in the past few years.

The age of the living donor is important for three main reasons. First, advanced age may lead to inferior graft outcomes in the recipient. This question has been addressed in a few recent analyses, and fortunately, the results are encouraging. A large analysis using the United States Renal Data System (USRDS) registry showed that transplant patients who received a kidney from a living donor older than 55 years of age had a risk for graft loss similar to those who received a kidney from a living donor 55 years of age or younger (adjusted relative risk 1.00; 95% confidence interval [CI] 0.47 to 2.13). It is important to note that graft survival from these older living donors was actually superior to younger standard criteria *deceased* donors. A subsequent analysis showed that recipients of live kidneys from donors above the age of 70 had similar graft survival to those who received standard criteria allografts from 50- to 59-year-old deceased donors (hazard ratio 1.19; 95% CI 0.87 to 1.63).

A second reason for the importance of the age of living donors is related to comorbidity. Advanced age is often

---

Box 61.3 Key Points to Be Addressed in the Psychosocial Assessment of Living Kidney Donors

Capacity suitable for informed consent

No evidence of coercion to donate

Social support network adequate to assist with recovery from surgery

Financial stablity to take time off from work and cover expenses

High-risk behavior (e.g., IV drug use) that might increase risk for disease transmission to the recipient

Current or previous psychiatric disorders that might influence decision making or response to adverse outcomes

---

Box 61.4 Medical Assessment of Living Kidney Donors

1. General donor health and immediate surgical risk
   - Complete blood count, prothrombin time or international normalized ratio (INR), partial thromboplastin time
   - HCG for women of childbearing potential
   - Electrolytes, transaminases, bilirubin, calcium, phosphorus, albumin
   - Chest radiograph and electrocardiogram
2. Current kidney health and future disease risk
   - Serum creatinine
   - Fasting blood glucose, total cholesterol, HDL-cholesterol, LDL-cholesterol, triglycerides
   - Urinalysis, urine culture
   - Proteinuria measurement: albumin-creatinine ratio (ACR), protein-creatinine ratio (PCR), or 24-hour urine collection for total protein and/or albumin
   - Kidney function measurement: 24-hour urine collection for creatinine clearance or measured GFR using an exogenous marker (inulin; radioactive or cold iothalamate, iohexol, DTPA, or EDTA)
   - CT or MR angiogram
3. Potential disease transmission to recipient
   - Cytomegalovirus (CMV), herpes simplex virus (HSV), and Epstein Barr virus (EBV) antibody
   - Human immunodeficiency virus (HIV)
   - Human T lymphotropic virus (HTLV)
   - HBV surface antigen, core antibody, and surface antibody
   - HCV virus antibody
   - Rapid plasma reagin test for syphilis
   - Papanicolaou test for women
   - Mammogram for women over 40 years
   - Prostate-specific antigen for men over 50 years (40 years if African-American or positive family history)
   - Colon cancer screen for donors over 50 years (fecal occult blood testing or visualization with colonoscopy, virtual colonoscopy, or flexible sigmoidoscopy)
4. Immunologic compatibility with recipient
   - ABO blood type
   - Human leukocyte antigen (HLA) typing

associated with increased comorbidity, which may lead to more perioperative complications at the time of the donor nephrectomy. Other than a longer hospital stay (median difference, 1 day), living donors older than 60 years of age do not have a significant difference in minor complications (e.g., UTI), major complications (e.g., re-operation), or even death following nephrectomy. In an analysis of 80,347 live donors, the 90-day mortality rate was 3.1 per 10,000 donors, and this rate was not significantly different for donors above or below 60 years of age. In addition, the long-term survival to 12 years was actually greater for donors older than 60 years compared with an age-matched cohort of nondonors who did not have contraindications to live donation.

Finally, age is important when considering live donors because it influences the amount of time that the donor is at risk to develop ESRD or other complications that might negatively affect someone with a solitary kidney. For example, a 22-year-old overweight African-American man with predia-betes has a significant risk for developing overt diabetes and ESRD given the many potential years of life ahead of him. Although being overweight and having prediabetes are not absolute contraindications to donation on their own, this young man may not be an appropriate donor because of his future risk for disease. In contrast, a 63-year-old white female with well-controlled hypertension on one medication might be a suitable donor given that her lifetime risk for kidney failure is much lower than that for a younger patient without risk factors.

KIDNEY FUNCTION

Ninety percent of programs in the United States use a 24-hour urine collection for creatinine clearance as the measure of kidney function, with the remainder using a direct measure of GFR, such as a radioisotopic clearance. Estimating equations based on the serum creatinine (e.g., CKD-EPI or MDRD study equations) should *not* be used in potential living donors because they systematically underestimate true GFR in healthy populations. The threshold for declining donors based on GFR or creatinine clearance is somewhat controversial with varied practice. Approximately two thirds of American centers exclude donors with a creatinine clearance less than 80 mL/min/1.73 m², whereas 25% require the value to be within two standard deviations of the mean creatinine clearance for the donor's age. See Table 61.3 for creatinine clearance values in the normal population.

From the perspective of the transplant recipient, it is crucial to ensure that kidney mass and function are adequate to prevent premature graft loss. This can usually be achieved when the donor's creatinine clearance is above 80 mL/min/1.73 m², which explains why this cutoff is commonly used. Lower values can provide adequate kidney mass and may be appropriate for certain recipients (e.g., older adults). However, from the perspective of the living donor, the appropriate clearance threshold might be somewhat different. It is well known that GFR declines with age, and thus a creatinine clearance of 80 mL/min/1.73 m² in a 20-year-old is very different from a clearance of 80 mL/min/1.73 m² in a 65-year-old donor. For 20-year-olds, this cutoff is well below two standard deviations of the mean for their age, and nephrectomy (with a further loss of GFR) may put them at increased risk for ESRD given their long potential lifetime. For 65-year-old donors, a clearance of 80 mL/min/1.73 m²

is within the normal range for their age, and the risk for ESRD is much less given that they have fewer years of life remaining. For these reasons, it is preferred to individualize donor acceptance using age-based creatinine clearance or GFR values, with consideration also given to the intended recipient, rather than using rigid cutoffs.

BLOOD PRESSURE

Sitting blood pressure should be measured at least two times in any potential living donor. Ambulatory blood pressure monitoring should be considered if isolated office hypertension is suspected. Hypertension was previously considered a contraindication to donation, but practice is now quite varied. Only 47% of programs exclude donors with normal blood pressure on one antihypertensive medication; 36% continue to exclude only those with persistently borderline blood pressure values. The increased acceptance of hypertensive donors is based on favorable data from select, mostly white, patients with well-controlled hypertension who have undergone living donation. Limited outcome data are available from hypertensive donors in other populations who may be at higher risk (e.g., African-Americans). The Amsterdam forum on the care of the live kidney donor suggests that patients with easily controlled blood pressure who meet other criteria (i.e., age >50 years, GFR >80 mL/min, no proteinuria) may be acceptable as live kidney donors. Until further data are available, the use of living donors with hypertension should be restricted to white donors.

PROTEINURIA

The 24-hour urine collection is still used by most programs (75%) to assess for proteinuria, but spot urine protein or albumin (PCR or ACR) measurements are becoming more commonly used. Mildly abnormal values should be repeated, especially if patients were acutely ill with fever or were exercising before testing. Younger donors (<30 years) may have orthostatic proteinuria, and this condition can be ruled out if protein excretion is normal (<50 mg per 8 hours) during the supine period and elevated when in the upright position. The threshold for excluding donors based on proteinuria is not consistent among centers. Whereas 36% of programs exclude donors

Table 61.3	Measured Creatinine Clearance According to Age			
Age (yr)	Mean Creatinine Clearance (mL/min/1.73 m²)	SD	Mean – SD	Mean – 2 SD
17-24	140	12	128	116
25-34	140	21	119	98
35-44	133	20	113	93
45-54	127	17	110	93
55-64	120	16	104	88
65-74	110	16	94	78
75-84	97	16	81	65

Used with permission of the American Society of Nephrology; previously published in Kher A, Mandelbrot DA: The living kidney donor evaluation: focus on renal issues Clin J Am Soc Nephrol 7:366-371, 2012.

with greater than 150 mg/day of total protein, 44% require proteinuria to be greater than 300 mg/day before exclusion. The Amsterdam guideline recommends a higher threshold of 300 mg/day before excluding donors. Albuminuria more closely reflects glomerular disease and is a better predictor of cardiovascular events. Given the strong link with proteinuria and kidney disease, it seems prudent to exclude any donor with abnormal albuminuria (>30 mg/day) or total proteinuria greater than 300 mg/day. A lower threshold may be needed in cases of familial kidney disease, borderline blood pressure, or other abnormalities such a microscopic hematuria.

HEMATURIA

Isolated microscopic hematuria should be confirmed with repeat urinalysis including microscopy to verify the presence of red blood cells as the cause of dipstick hematuria. Urine culture should be performed to rule out infection, and menstrual contamination should always be considered in premenopausal women. Imaging will rule out a structural kidney cause, but most donors must undergo cystoscopy to rule out local bladder causes. Finally, glomerular hematuria from IgA nephropathy, hereditary nephritis, or thin basement membrane nephropathy must be considered in an otherwise healthy donor. These conditions can only be diagnosed by kidney biopsy, and this test should be considered if the donor understands the risks and is motivated to continue the evaluation. The most common practice (43% of programs) is to accept donors with hematuria only if urologic evaluation and kidney biopsy are both negative. However, 21% of programs would exclude patients with hematuria (>10 RBC/HPF) regardless of these investigations.

DIABETES

Given the risk for diabetic nephropathy, established diabetes is a contraindication to donation. All donors should have a fasting blood glucose performed to rule out undiagnosed diabetes, impaired fasting glucose, or prediabetes. Patients at increased risk for diabetes (e.g., history of gestational diabetes, first-degree relative with diabetes, BMI >30) should have an oral glucose tolerance test or glycated hemoglobin test. Potential donors with impaired fasting glucose need to be assessed on a case-by-case basis; young patients or those with other risk factors such as obesity, hypertension, or dyslipidemia should be excluded from donation.

OBESITY

Obesity (BMI >30) is associated with short-term surgical complications following nephrectomy, as well as an increased risk for future medical conditions such as diabetes, hypertension, and dyslipidemia. Fifty-two percent of programs exclude donors with a BMI greater than 35, whereas 20% exclude those with BMI above 40. A recent study found that obesity was associated with more hypertension and dyslipidemia after a mean follow-up of 11 years, but was not significantly different from an obese control group who did not donate. In addition, obese donors had a GFR that was similar to nonobese donors, and were not at increased risk for long-term deterioration in kidney function. Not all patients with an elevated BMI have central obesity, and potential donors should be examined for body habitus and muscle mass before excluding based on BMI alone. Another option is to have donors lose weight to a certain target before proceeding with surgery, with appropriate support and counseling to prevent immediate weight gain postnephrectomy.

NEPHROLITHIASIS

Kidney stones are a very common occurrence, with as many as 19% of men and 9% of women having a symptomatic kidney stone in their lifetime. The majority of these stones are composed of calcium oxalate. Improved imaging techniques have increased the ability to detect small, asymptomatic kidney stones as well. As such, nephrolithiasis is not an uncommon problem in potential living donors. The major concern for the living donor is recurrence postnephrectomy, which could result in obstruction of the single remaining kidney and lead to kidney failure. The majority of programs (53%) accept donors with a history of kidney stones as long as the metabolic workup is normal. Another consideration is age at onset and time since symptomatic episode. Younger patients are at an increased risk for recurrence, given their long projected lifespan. Patients whose stone episode was remote (>10 years) are at decreased risk for recurrence. Patients with a history of stone disease or stones on imaging should have a metabolic workup done, including serum calcium and bicarbonate to rule out metabolic acidosis. A 24-hour urine collection (preferably on two occasions) should be performed to assess calcium, oxalate, uric acid, and citrate excretion. Patients who should be excluded as donors include those with recurrent stones and those at high risk for recurrence. These include patients with metabolic abnormalities (e.g., hypercalciuria), chronic diarrhea/malabsorption, gout, cysteine, uric acid, or struvite stones.

Limited data are available to guide the selection of living kidney donors. Most studies to date have been single-center or small in sample size, have had a relatively short duration of follow-up, and notably, may have been biased by not including all donors in follow-up. As such, donor selection is often made using personal opinion or center-based protocols. Contraindications to living donation have recently been published and are presented in Table 61.4. It is important to assess potential donors individually and to use the information available as a guide. Younger donors have a much higher lifetime risk for developing complications such as diabetes or ESRD, and the evaluation should be conducted with this in mind. Similarly, older donors have a much lower lifetime risk for complications and may be appropriate for donation with certain conditions (e.g., hypertension). Further research concentrating on complete and long-term follow-up, especially involving those with medical abnormalities, is needed to enrich the data available to make evidence-based decisions in living kidney donation.

Table 61.4   Absolute and Relative Contraindications to Living Kidney Donation

Absolute Contraindications	Relative Contraindications
Age <18 yr	Age 18–21 yr
Mentally incapable of making informed decision	Creatinine clearance <2 SD below mean for age
Uncontrolled hypertension, or hypertension with end organ damage	Albuminuria or proteinuria
	Hypertension in non-Caucasian race
Diabetes	Hypertension in young donor
BMI >35 kg/m^2	Prediabetes in young donor
Untreated psychiatric conditions	BMI >30 kg/m^2
Nephrolithiasis with high likelihood of recurrence	Bleeding disorder
	History of thrombosis or embolism
Evidence of donor coercion	Nephrolithiasis
Active malignancy or incompletely treated malignancy	History of malignancy, especially if metastatic
Persistent infection	Significant cardiovascular disease

Used with permission of the American Society of Nephrology; previously published in Kher A, Mandelbrot DA: The living kidney donor evaluation: focus on renal issues Clin J Am Soc Nephrol 7:366-371, 2012.

BIBLIOGRAPHY

Briganti EM, Russ GR, McNeil JJ, et al: Risk of renal allograft loss from recurrent glomerulonephritis, *N Engl J Med* 11(347):103-109, 2002.

Delmonico FA: Report of the Amsterdam Forum on the Care of the Live Kidney Donor: Data and Medical Guidelines, *Transplantation* 79:S53-S66, 2005.

De Vriese AS, De Bacquer DA, Verbeke FH, et al: Comparison of the prognostic value of dipyridamole and dobutamine myocardial perfusion scintigraphy in hemodialysis patients, *Kidney Int* 76:428-436, 2009.

Dew MA, Jacobs CL, Jowsey SG, et al: Guidelines for the psychosocial evaluation of living unrelated kidney donors in the United States, *Am J Transplant* 7:1047-1054, 2007.

Fairhead T, Knoll G: Recurrent glomerular disease after kidney transplantation, *Curr Opin Nephrol Hypertens* 19:578-585, 2010.

Frassetto LA, Tan-Tam C, Stock PG: Renal transplantation in patients with HIV, *Nat Rev Nephrol* 5:582-589, 2009 Oct.

Gaston RS, Danovitch GM, Adams PL, et al: The report of a national conference on the wait list for kidney transplantation, *Am J Transplant* 3:775-785, 2003.

Gill J, Bunnapradist S, Danovitch GM, et al: Outcomes of kidney transplantation from older living donors to older recipients, *Am J Kidney Dis* 52:541-552, 2008.

Gill JS, Ma I, Landsberg D, et al: Cardiovascular events and investigation in patients who are awaiting cadaveric kidney transplantation, *J Am Soc Nephrol* 16:808-816, 2005.

Kasiske BL, Cangro CB, Hariharan S, et al: The evaluation of renal transplant candidates: clinical practice guidelines, *Am J Transplant* supp 2 Vol 1, 2001.

Kher A, Mandelbrot DA: The living kidney donor evaluation: focus on renal issues, *Clin J Am Soc Nephrol* 7:366-371, 2012.

Knoll G, Cockfield S, Blydt-Hansen T, et al: Canadian Society of Transplantation: consensus guidelines on eligibility for kidney transplantation, *CMAJ* 8(173):S1-S25, 2005.

Lefaucheur C, Suberbielle-Boissel C, Hill GS, et al: Clinical relevance of preformed HLA donor-specific antibodies in kidney transplantation, *Am J Transplant* 8:324-331, 2008.

Lentine KL, Schnitzler MA, Brennan DC, et al: Cardiac evaluation before kidney transplantation: a practice patterns analysis in Medicare-insured dialysis patients, *Clin J Am Soc Nephrol* 3:1115-1124, 2008.

Organ Procurement and Transplantation Network (OPTN) and Scientific Registry of Transplant Recipients (SRTR): *OPTN / SRTR 2010 Annual Data Report*, Rockville, Md, 2011, Department of Health and Human Services, Health Resources and Services Administration, Healthcare Systems Bureau, Division of Transplantation.

Segev DL, Muzaale AD, Caffo BS, et al: Perioperative mortality and long-term survival following live kidney donation, *JAMA* 303:959-966, 2010.

Rule AD, Larson TS, Bergstralh EJ, et al: Using serum creatinine to estimate glomerular filtration rate: accuracy in good health and in chronic kidney disease, *Ann Intern Med* 141:929-937, 2004.

Tavakol MM, Vincenti FG, Assadi H, et al: Long-term renal function and cardiovascular disease risk in obese kidney donors, *Clin J Am Soc Nephrol* 4:1230-1238, 2009.

U.S. Renal Data System, USDRS 2011 Annual Data Report: *Atlas of Chronic Kidney Disease and End-Stage Renal Disease in the United States*, Bethesda, Md, 2011, National Institutes of Health, National Institute of Diabetes and Digestive and Kidney Diseases.

Wang JH, Kasiske BL: Screening and management of pretransplant cardiovascular disease, *Curr Opin Nephrol Hypertens* 19:586-591, 2010 Nov.

Posttransplantation Monitoring and Outcomes

62

Jagbir S. Gill

The management of kidney transplant recipients is complex and spans a wide range of clinical scenarios. Posttransplant care begins in the immediate postsurgical period and continues through the various phases that make up the natural history of kidney transplantation. Whereas the early phases of care focus primarily on postsurgical management, monitoring of allograft function, and optimization of immunosuppression, later phases of care extend this focus to include ongoing assessment and management of factors that contribute to chronic allograft dysfunction, allograft loss, and death with a functioning graft. The nuances of posttransplant care have changed significantly over time as our understanding of the natural history of transplantation has evolved, the case-mix of transplant recipients has become more complex, and new technologies to monitor transplant recipients have emerged. In this chapter, we will review the major aspects of posttransplant care through this continuum in the current era of transplantation.

RECIPIENT AND DONOR CHARACTERISTICS

With changes in the demographics of the population with end-stage renal disease (ESRD) and improvements in technologies and immunosuppression, the benefits of kidney transplantation are now offered to patients who previously would not have been eligible. With these successes come increased challenges and complexities in posttransplant care, along with a greater need to individualize care for various subgroups of kidney transplant recipients. For instance, older adult patients are the fastest-growing segment of kidney transplant recipients, with patients 65 years of age and older accounting for more than 16% of all recipients in the United States in 2009. The complexities of pre- and posttransplant care are unique in older adult recipients because they are more likely to have a greater burden of comorbid disease and a higher risk for death with a functioning allograft. However, the risk for acute allograft rejection is lower in older transplant recipients as a result of immunosenescence, which may allow for decreased use of immunosuppression. Therefore posttransplant care must be tailored to risks and outcomes within individual populations. Also, with the increased success of desensitization strategies, both HLA- and ABO-incompatible transplantation are realities in our current era, but these cases require more intense follow-up given their higher risk for rejection and allograft loss. Other high-risk recipient groups include human immunodeficiency virus (HIV)-positive recipients, repeat transplant recipients, and multiorgan transplant recipients, each of which bring unique challenges to posttransplant care.

Similarly, the characteristics of deceased donors have changed over time, further complicating early posttransplant care. In the face of increasing demand for transplantation, organs from higher-risk deceased donors are routinely transplanted in selected recipients. Expanded criteria donors (ECDs) include donors 60 years of age or older and those aged 50 to 59 years with two or more high-risk characteristics, including long-standing hypertension, a terminal serum creatinine above 1.5mg/dL, or death due to a cerebral vascular accident. Recipients who receive ECD kidneys have an increased risk for delayed graft function (DGF) and a 70% increased risk for allograft loss from any cause, compared with recipients who receive kidneys from deceased donors aged 18 to 39 years with no comorbidities. Organs from ECDs are allocated only to recipient populations that continue to derive a significant survival benefit from transplantation, such as older adult and diabetic transplant candidates. In addition, kidneys are increasingly transplanted from donors after cardiac death (DCDs), as opposed to donors after brain death. In fact, DCDs now contribute nearly 12% of all organs in the United States. Not surprisingly, kidneys from DCDs are subject to a greater degree of ischemic injury at the time of donation, often resulting in DGF. However, long-term allograft and patient survival remain similar in recipients of kidneys from DCDs or from donors after brain death.

THE FIRST WEEK

Most kidney transplant recipients have a hospital duration ranging from 4 to 7 days following surgery. In the acute postoperative phase, care of the transplant recipient involves assessment for immediate graft function, management of potential surgical complications, and treatment of postoperative fluid and electrolyte shifts.

The details of kidney transplantation surgery vary depending on whether the donor kidney is from a living donor or a deceased donor, as well as the specific anatomy of a given recipient. In general, the surgery involves engraftment in the iliac fossa with vascular anastomoses between the donor renal artery to the recipient external iliac artery and the donor vein to the external iliac vein. Perioperative complications that may require surgical exploration and management include bleeding and thrombosis of the renal artery or vein.

Assessment of graft function involves quantifying urine output (keeping the baseline urine output of the recipient in mind) and following serum chemistries every 12 to 24 hours. Immediate graft function is denoted by a rapid drop in serum creatinine levels and urine output in excess of 100 mL/hour, and is expected in all living donor kidney transplant recipients and in most recipients of deceased donor kidneys. Immediate graft function is less likely in recipients of kidneys from ECDs and DCDs, and in cases with prolonged cold ischemic times (>24 hours).

DGF is typically denoted as the requirement for dialysis within the first week posttransplant and occurs in less than 5% of living donor transplant recipients, 22% of standard criteria deceased donor recipients, 32% of ECD recipients, and over 37% of DCD recipients. In addition to donor factors, the duration of cold ischemic time and warm ischemic time are important predictors of DGF. Dialysis is initiated based on volume status and metabolic parameters. Either hemodialysis or peritoneal dialysis may be performed depending on the patient's baseline dialysis modality. In the case of peritoneal dialysis, it is important to confirm that the peritoneum was not breached during the surgery before resumption of dialysis.

Although the cause of DGF is usually acute ischemic tubular injury, alternate causes (including vascular thrombosis and early acute rejection) need to be considered. Therefore a Doppler kidney ultrasound to assess for blood flow in the allograft is recommended within hours of a clinical change in allograft function. Elevated resistive indices may suggest either tubular injury or rejection; thus, the baseline risk for rejection and duration of DGF should be considered in assessing the cause of early graft dysfunction. If rejection is suspected or DGF persists beyond 1 week, an allograft biopsy should be performed.

Reduced exposure to calcineurin inhibitors (CNIs) in the setting of DGF is recommended to avoid further tubular injury associated with CNI nephrotoxicity, but this must be balanced with the risk for rejection. The use of induction immunosuppressive agents is recommended if CNIs are to be reduced or avoided in the setting of DGF. There are few data to support a uniform approach to immunosuppression in the setting of DGF, but some centers prefer to use T lymphocyte–depleting antibodies (thymoglobulin) for induction, along with immediate initiation of an antimetabolite (mycophenolate) and corticosteroids, with delayed introduction of CNI only once there is evidence of graft function. The majority of DGF cases recover within 1 to 3 months, but numerous studies have demonstrated inferior allograft survival in patients who have developed DGF.

Fluid and electrolyte management is a key component of early postoperative care. Hemodynamic extremes of hypotension and volume overload should be avoided in older adult patients and in those with compromised cardiac function. Electrolyte shifts, including hypercalcemia and hypophosphatemia associated with secondary hyperparathyroidism and hypomagnesemia associated with diuretic use, may be seen early posttransplantation and should be managed accordingly.

OUTPATIENT CARE

Following discharge from the hospital, transplant recipients are closely followed by the transplant center. The frequency of monitoring is greatest during the first 3 months, as the risk for rejection is highest during this period. Patients are followed twice weekly during the first month posttransplant and then weekly for the remainder of the first 3 months, with the frequency of visits gradually reduced to every 4 to 8 weeks by the end of the first year.

Routine posttransplant monitoring includes a follow-up history and physical examination along with measurement of serum chemistries, a complete blood count, liver enzymes, whole blood CNI levels, and urinalysis. Spot albumin-to-creatinine ratios are also periodically monitored. Preemptive viral screening and monitoring are indicated for the first 3 to 6 months at variable frequencies depending on the patient's risk for infection.

IMMUNOSUPPRESSION

Immunosuppression after transplant consists of induction therapy, followed by lifelong maintenance immunotherapy. Chapter 63 provides greater details on specific induction and maintenance agents, including their side effect profiles. Induction therapy is administered at the time of transplantation and includes intravenous methylprednisolone, along with either an anti-CD25 antibody (basiliximab) or a T lymphocyte–depleting antibody (the polyclonal antibody thymoglobulin). Alemtuzumab is a monoclonal antibody used in the management of chronic lymphocytic leukemia that results in potent lymphocyte depletion, and has been increasingly used as an induction agent in kidney transplantation.

Maintenance immunosuppression typically consists of triple immunosuppressive therapy with a CNI, an antimetabolite, and low-dose corticosteroids. Until the early 2000s, azathioprine was the preferred posttransplantation antimetabolite; however, mycophenolic acid (MPA) agents more selectively target lymphocytes, resulting in superior efficacy in preventing acute rejection and increased patient tolerability. Rapamycin has been studied as an alternative to CNIs or for use in combination with CNIs. Although concerns regarding wound healing and nephrotoxicity have minimized the use of rapamycin as a primary de novo immunosuppressant agent after transplantation, data suggesting a reduced risk for malignancies with the use of rapamycin have renewed interest in this agent, particularly for patients with recurrent skin cancers posttransplant. Belatacept is a recently approved intravenously administered costimulatory blocker that binds CD80 and CD86 on the surface of antigen presenting cells to inhibit T cell activation and promote anergy and apoptosis. The optimal indication for this agent remains unclear and will likely be refined in the coming years.

IMMUNOSUPPRESSIVE PROTOCOLS

The majority of transplant recipients are maintained on triple immunosuppressive therapy including CNI, MPA, and corticosteroids. Low rates of acute rejection and growing concern with the adverse effects of these agents, including chronic CNI nephrotoxicity, have led to strategies to minimize immunosuppressive exposure. Minimization of CNI and corticosteroid exposure has been most frequently studied, but ongoing debate continues, countering the merits of immunosuppression minimization with the increasingly recognized importance of chronic immune-mediated injury.

Posttransplant corticosteroid exposure has been reduced significantly, with prednisone doses rapidly tapered to 5 to 10 mg daily within the first 4 to 6 weeks after surgery. Late withdrawal of corticosteroids has been largely abandoned in the face of numerous studies demonstrating an increased risk for rejection when corticosteroids are withdrawn beyond 3 to 6 months posttransplant. Early corticosteroid withdrawal or avoidance strategies, however, have demonstrated largely favorable outcomes. A metaanalysis of 34 studies, including 5637 patients receiving steroid withdrawal or avoidance regimens, found that steroid avoidance reduced the risk for hyperlipidemia, hypertension, and new-onset diabetes after transplantation. Woodle and colleagues conducted a multicenter randomized controlled trial of early corticosteroid withdrawal (within 7 days) compared with low-dose maintenance corticosteroids in a CNI- and MPA-based regimen. The early steroid withdrawal group had an increased rate of biopsy-proven acute rejection and chronic allograft nephropathy, but no difference was found in the composite primary endpoint of death, graft loss, or severe acute rejection through 5 years. When examined separately, graft and patient survival were also not different. Although steroid exposure should be minimized whenever possible, corticosteroid avoidance or early withdrawal should be reserved for patients at low risk for rejection and only with careful and frequent posttransplant monitoring.

LONG-TERM DRUG DOSING AND MONITORING

Because of inter- and intrapatient variability in the bioavailability and absorption of CNI, routine whole blood drug level monitoring is essential. Trough levels of CNI correlate well with drug exposure and clinical events, particularly for tacrolimus. However, evidence exists that peak drug levels (2 hours after dose) of cyclosporine correlate better with drug exposure and clinical events, including acute rejection. As a result, certain centers have adopted peak level, or "C2" monitoring, for cyclosporine. Although specific therapeutic targets may vary depending on concomitant immunosuppression, levels are typically kept highest in the first month after transplant, with a gradual reduction over the next 6 months. In interpreting drug levels, it is important to remember that different labs may use different assays, resulting in different results.

Routine therapeutic drug level monitoring is not recommended for MPA, because trough levels do not correlate well with clinical efficacy and the repeat measurements required to appropriately calculate the area under the curve are labor intensive and not feasible for routine measurement. Target doses (2 g daily for mycophenolate mofetil and 1440 mg daily for mycophenolate sodium) are based on clinical trials demonstrating efficacy at these doses. Transient dose reduction or temporary discontinuation of MPA is recommended in cases of significant diarrheal symptoms or profound leukopenia. However, full doses should be resumed after resolution of symptoms, if tolerated, because prolonged dose reductions or discontinuations are associated with inferior allograft survival.

ADVERSE EFFECTS AND DRUG INTERACTIONS

Adverse effects of immunosuppressant medications should be assessed during each follow-up visit. Significant effects of corticosteroids include cataracts, bone loss and fractures, avascular necrosis, hypertension, weight gain, dyslipidemia, glucose intolerance, mood lability, and acne. MPAs may confer bone marrow toxicity (leukopenia, anemia), gastric reflux, diarrhea, and pancreatitis. CNIs may cause acute and chronic nephrotoxicity, although the impact of CNIs on chronic graft function is being increasingly questioned. Other significant effects of CNIs include hypomagnesemia, hyperkalemia, hyperuricemia, neurotoxicity (e.g., tremor), and rarely, thrombotic microangiopathy. Tacrolimus is more strongly associated with new-onset diabetes after transplantation than cyclosporine, whereas cyclosporine is more commonly associated with cosmetic changes, including gingival hyperplasia and hirsutism.

The narrow therapeutic and toxic window for CNIs in addition to the high potential for altered metabolism from interference of the cytochrome 450 (CYP450) mechanism mandate careful examination and recognition of potential drug interactions. Common CYP450 drug inhibitors (which will increase CNI levels) and inducers (which will lower CNI levels) are outlined in Table 62.1. New drugs should be introduced with care, and drug levels should be carefully monitored, when indicated. MPA is not metabolized via the

Table 62.1	Selected Common Drug Interactions With Calcineurin Inhibitors
Increases CNI Level (Inhibits Enzyme)*	**Decreases CNI Level (Stimulates Enzyme)***
Calcium channel blockers Diltiazem Verapamil	**Antibiotics** Rifabutin Rifampin
Antiarrhythmics Amiodarone	**Antiepileptics** Phenobarbital Phenytoin
HIV protease inhibitors Ritonavir Saquinavir Indinavir	Carbamazepine **Herbal substances** St. John's wort
Azole antifungal agents Ketoconazole Clotrimazole Itraconazole Voriconazole	
Antibiotics Erythromycin base Synercid (quinupristin and dalfopristin)	
Antidepressants Fluvoxamine	
Other agents Grapefruit juice	

HIV, Human immunodeficiency virus.
*Listed drugs interact with the calcineurin inhibitors (CNI) cyclosporine and tacrolimus because they are metabolized by the cytochrome P450 CYP3A4 isoenzyme.

CYP450 enzyme pathway, and there are fewer drug interactions compared with CNI; however, any drugs that may potentiate leukopenia should not be used in conjunction with these agents.

ALLOGRAFT DYSFUNCTION

The immune response to an allograft involves (1) recognition of foreign antigens, (2) activation of recipient lymphocytes, and (3) effector mechanisms leading to rejection of the allograft. The human major histocompatibility complex (MHC) is a cluster of genes on chromosome 6 that encodes human leukocyte antigens (HLA) in addition to other agents critical in controlling the immune response; MHC is the key factor in the initiation of the immune response to an allograft. The HLA antigens are the major barriers to transplantation, and allogeneic donor HLA antigens are the main targets of the immune system in rejection of the graft. However, the role of non-HLA antigens in inciting an immune response and subsequent rejection is increasingly being realized.

ACUTE ALLOGRAFT DYSFUNCTION

A 15% to 20% increase in serum creatinine from baseline suggests graft dysfunction and warrants a thorough evaluation, including an assessment of risk factors for acute kidney injury, an ultrasound of the allograft, and often an allograft biopsy. Nonimmune causes of allograft dysfunction should be ruled out, including CNI nephrotoxicity, acute interstitial nephritis, pyelonephritis, ischemic injury, recurrent native kidney disease, and BK nephropathy. Supratherapeutic CNI levels and the presence of isometric tubular vacuolization or arteriolar hyalinosis on biopsy (Fig. 62.1) strongly suggest acute CNI nephrotoxicity, although an allograft biopsy is not usually required for diagnosis since a reduction in CNI dose will quickly improve kidney function. Recurrent native kidney disease rates vary depending on the original cause of ESRD and require allograft biopsy for diagnosis. BK polyomavirus nephropathy may cause graft injury with a high risk for subsequent graft loss, but a histologic diagnosis is often difficult.

The Banff classification has standardized criteria for allograft pathology, including those for acute rejection (Box 62.1). The glomeruli, tubules, interstitium, and vessels should be examined for the presence of inflammation and lymphocyte infiltration. Interstitial inflammation with lymphocytes is scored from 0 (absent) to 3 (severe). Tubulitis is the definitive aspect of acute cellular rejection and is quantified from mild (t1) to severe (t3). Vessel wall infiltration, or arteritis, represents a greater severity of rejection (grade II) and ranges from mild/moderate (v1) to severe (v2). Although lymphocyte infiltration in the glomeruli may accompany acute rejection, it is not a criterion of rejection.

Treatment of acute cellular rejection includes intravenous pulse corticosteroids, intensification of maintenance immunosuppression, and polyclonal antilymphocyte antibodies (thymoglobulin) in more severe cases. Although recovery from acute rejection has improved dramatically over time, an episode of acute rejection (even if successfully treated) significantly increases the risk for early graft loss.

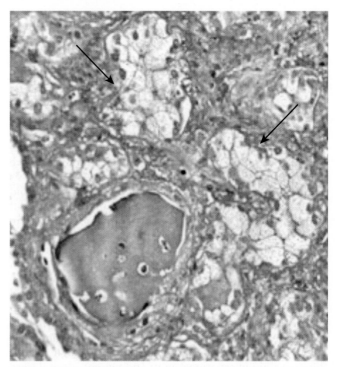

Figure 62.1 Pathology of acute CNI nephrotoxicity showing isometric tubular vacuolization *(arrows).*

Antibody-mediated rejection (AMR) involves the production of antidonor antibodies by plasma cells, either from memory or naive B cells or from those that existed before transplantation. These donor-specific antibodies (DSAs) interact with allograft vascular endothelium, resulting in complement activation, cell death, loss of vascular integrity, and subsequent ischemic injury. In addition to the presence of circulating DSA, the diagnosis of AMR requires the presence of immunopathologic staining for the complement component C4d in peritubular capillaries and histologic evidence of acute or chronic tissue injury. These histologic findings may include acute tubular injury, vasculitis, and peritubular capillary inflammation.

The importance of DSA appears to extend beyond the acute rejection episode; chronic exposure to low levels of DSA (even in the absence of a clinical episode of AMR) may lead to chronic AMR. As a result, the treatment of AMR primarily targets DSA and the subsequent complement activation that it ultimately induces. Plasmapheresis and high-dose intravenous immune globulin (IVIG) aim to lower DSA levels through removal or inactivation, respectively. Anti-CD20 agents (rituximab) aim to reduce antibody levels by depleting B lymphocytes and preventing the maturation of new DSA-producing plasma cells. The proteasome inhibitor bortezomib causes apoptosis of normal plasma cells and has had favorable results in the treatment of AMR in small single-center uncontrolled studies. Although its benefit is largely unproven, bortezomib may be considered in refractory cases of AMR.

CHRONIC ALLOGRAFT DYSFUNCTION

A gradual decline in kidney function manifested by a slowly rising creatinine, increasing levels of proteinuria,

---

Box 62.1 Banff 2007 Criteria for Allograft Pathology

1. **Normal**
2. **Antibody-mediated changes** (may coincide with categories 3, 4, and 5)

   C4d deposition without morphologic evidence of active rejection

   C4d+, presence of circulating antidonor antibody, no signs of acute or chronic TCMR or ACMR

   Acute antibody-mediated rejection

   C4d+, presence of circulating antidonor antibodies, morphologic evidence of acute tissue injury such as (type/grade):

   I. ATN-like minimal inflammation

   II. Capillary and glomerular inflammation (ptc/g>0) and/or thromboses

   III. Arterial -v3*

   Chronic active antibody-mediated rejection

   C4d+, presence of circulating antidonor antibodies, morphologic evidence of chronic tissue injury such as glomerular double contours and/or peritubular capillary basement membrane multilayering and/or interstitial fibrosis/tubular atrophy and/or fibrosis.
3. **Borderline changes**

   Suspicious for acute T-cell–mediated rejection. No intimal arteritis, but foci of tubulitis (t1, t2, or t3) with minor interstitial inflammation (i0 or i1) or interstitial infiltration (i2, i3) with mild (t1) tubulitis (t1, i1 or greater)
4. **T-cell–mediated rejection** (TCMR; may coincide with 2, 5, and 6)

   Acute T cell mediated rejection (type/grade)

   IA. Significant interstitial infiltration (i2; >25% of parenchyma affected) and foci of moderate tubulitis (t2; >4 mononuclear cells/tubular cross section or group of 10 tubular cells)

   IB. Significant interstitial infiltration (i2; >25% of parenchyma affected) and foci of severe tubulitis (t3; >10 mononuclear cells/tubular cross-section or group of 10 tubular cells)

   IIA. Mild-to-moderate intimal arteritis (v1)

   IIB. Severe intimal arteritis comprising >25% of the luminal area (v2)

   III. Transmural arteritis and/or arterial fibrinoid change and necrosis of medial smooth muscle

   Chronic active T-cell–mediated rejection

   Chronic allograft arteriopathy (arterial intimal fibrosis with mononuclear cell infiltration)
5. **Interstitial fibrosis and tubular atrophy,** no evidence of any specific etiology (grade)

   I. Mild interstitial fibrosis (ci1) and tubular atrophy (ct1); <25% of cortical area affected

   II. Moderate interstitial fibrosis (ci2) and tubular atrophy (ct2); 26%-50% of cortical area affected

   III. Severe interstitial fibrosis (ci3) and tubular atrophy (ct3); >50% of cortical area affected
6. **Other:** changes not considered to be due to rejection—acute and/or chronic (may coincide with categories 2, 3, 4, and 5)

ATN, Acute tubular necrosis; *C4d+,* activated complement component C4d; *cg,* glomerulopathy; *ci,* interstitial fibrosis; *ct,* tubular atrophy; *g,* glomerulitis; *i,* interstitial infiltration; *ptc,* peritubular capillaritis; *t,* tubulitis; *v,* vessel wall infiltration or arteritis.
*Degrees of lymphocyte infiltration are scored 0 (absent) to 3 (severe).

---

and worsening hypertension denotes chronic allograft dysfunction and typically precedes chronic allograft loss. Chronic allograft loss is defined as allograft failure that occurs after 1 year posttransplant. For years, the term *chronic allograft nephropathy* was cited as the most common cause of chronic allograft loss, without a clear understanding of its underlying etiology. In the 2005 Banff reclassification, this term was abandoned and replaced with the term *interstitial fibrosis and tubular atrophy (IF/TA)* to more accurately represent the histologic findings associated with chronic allograft loss, without ascribing any specific cause to the histologic changes. A number of histologic changes may be seen in chronic failing allografts, including vascular changes (endothelial inflammation and intimal thickening), glomerular changes (glomerular capillary wall thickening, often with a double contour appearance—termed transplant glomerulopathy), and interstitial fibrosis with tubular atrophy. Many of these histologic changes are associated with inferior allograft survival. For instance, transplant glomerulopathy carries one of the worse prognoses with 5-year graft survival rates of less than 50% from the time of diagnosis. The Banff classification grades the degree of IF/TA (I, II, III) according to the severity of interstitial fibrosis (mild, moderate, severe) and tubular atrophy (mild to severe), but these grades have not been precisely correlated with allograft outcomes.

It is clear from long-term protocol biopsy studies that the underlying causes of these histologic changes are multifactorial and include both immune-mediated and non-immune–mediated processes, such as chronic CNI nephrotoxicity, recurrent disease, and subclinical and overt chronic antibody-mediated rejection.

Chronic CNI nephrotoxicity was first described in the 1970s and is attributed to the renal vasoconstrictive effects of CNI and direct tubular toxicity. The histologic hallmarks of chronic CNI nephrotoxicity are largely nonspecific and include stripped interstitial fibrosis, glomerular sclerosis, and arteriolar hyalinosis (the only specific finding of CNI nephrotoxicity). CNI nephrotoxicity has been touted as a key contributor to chronic allograft dysfunction, but recent studies have suggested a more prominent role for immune-mediated injury in chronic allograft dysfunction, bringing into question the safety of CNI minimization posttransplantation. Therefore the relative importance of CNI nephrotoxicity and chronic rejection remains an active source of debate.

Chronic active antibody-mediated rejection is a subset of AMR and is characterized by the presence of circulating DSA and histologic evidence of chronic allograft injury, including transplant glomerulopathy, peritubular capillary basement membrane multilayering, and interstitial fibrosis and tubular atrophy. The mechanism and treatment of chronic antibody-mediated damage is not precisely defined, but it is recognized as a key therapeutic target in reducing the risk for chronic allograft loss.

ASSESSMENT OF ALLOGRAFT DYSFUNCTION

Current strategies to monitor allograft function are limited to serum creatinine, proteinuria, and surveillance allograft biopsies in some programs. Unfortunately, aside from the invasive procedure of an allograft biopsy, these are late markers of allograft dysfunction and are inadequate to detect early immune injury, subclinical rejection, and chronic allograft inflammation, all of which are increasingly recognized as important contributors of chronic allograft function.

Allograft biopsy remains the gold standard for early detection of allograft changes since histologic rejection can be seen before changes in serum creatinine. However, the impact of interventions that are guided solely by biopsy findings remains unclear, with a recent randomized study demonstrating no effect with treatment. Ultimately, the invasive nature of a biopsy and patient reluctance limit the widespread use of surveillance biopsies. Therefore novel noninvasive markers of immune-mediated injury and chronic inflammation are needed.

DSAs are routinely monitored *before* transplantation because they correlate with increased rates of subclinical and clinical AMR in the early posttransplant period. In the setting of AMR, DSA levels may also be a useful therapeutic target and can be monitored during these treatment regimens, although the precise therapeutic targets are unknown. De novo DSAs posttransplant have also been associated with higher transplant failure rates and may occur before proteinuria or changes in serum creatinine. Therefore some have advocated for routine monitoring of DSAs posttransplant. However, the cost-effectiveness of routine DSA monitoring, particularly in stable low-risk and intermediate-risk patients, remains unclear.

A number of unique biomarkers have been studied to detect acute rejection and early allograft injury, including urinary markers related to cytotoxic T lymphocytes (granzyme A/B, perforin, Fas ligand, serpin B9), regulatory T cells (FOXP3), CD4 T cells (chemokines, TIM-3), and markers of renal tubular injury (NGAL, A1M, cleaved B2M). Although a number of promising observations have been made, most of these markers still require further validation to document their clinical applicability and usefulness.

INFECTIOUS COMPLICATIONS

PROPHYLAXIS AND MONITORING

The risk for infection is related to the overall level of immunosuppression, recipient factors, donor factors, and community exposures. Strategies to minimize infection after transplant include pretransplant vaccination and a combination of universal posttransplant prophylaxis (e.g., perioperative antibiotic prophylaxis) and preemptive therapy (e.g., monitoring and treating for viremic states).

Universal prophylaxis is given to all patients for a defined time period, and includes the administration of perioperative antibiotics and low-dose trimethoprim-sulfamethoxazole

(TMP-SMZ) for 6 months to lifetime after transplant to prevent *Pneumocystis jirovecii* pneumonia (formerly known as PCP), *Toxoplasma gondii*, many *Nocardia* and *Listeria* species, and common urinary and respiratory pathogens. Patients intolerant to TMP-SMZ may receive either atovaquone or dapsone instead.

Preemptive therapy utilizes quantitative assays at predetermined intervals to detect early infection, with initiation of therapy when there is a positive assay. Preemptive therapy is often used in monitoring for cytomegalovirus (CMV), Epstein-Barr virus (EBV), BK polyomavirus, and viral hepatitis, depending on donor and recipient factors.

APPROACH TO POSTTRANSPLANT INFECTIONS

Clinical presentations of infectious disease may be variable and atypical in immunosuppressed patients. Therefore, workup for a suspected infection should be broad and may include blood and urine cultures, a chest radiograph, and bronchoscopic evaluation when investigating pulmonary infiltrates. In cases where the source of infection is unclear, the threshold for initiation of broad-spectrum antibiotics should be low. Consideration of donor-derived infections, latent viral infections, and new opportunistic infections, factoring in the timing posttransplant, is important in developing a differential diagnosis.

A detailed approach to and management of infectious complications posttransplant are outlined in Chapter 64 and will not be discussed in this chapter, with the exception of human BK polyomaviruses. The human polyomavirus BK (BKV) causes BK nephropathy in up 10% of kidney transplant recipients. BKV may be harbored within the recipient or in the uroepithelium of the donor, with reactivation and replication upon immunosuppression. Renal tubular epithelial invasion produces an inflammatory response similar to acute rejection, with resultant atrophy and fibrosis. A creeping increase of serum creatinine, along with BKV viruria and viremia, is often the only clinical sign of BK nephropathy. Therefore preemptive screening is essential. BKV PCR should be performed once every 3 months for the first 2 years posttransplant, and then annually until the fifth year. Viremic patients should have immunosuppressive doses reduced and undergo an allograft biopsy if there is evidence of kidney dysfunction. In patients with sustained viremia despite a reduction in immunosuppression, adjunctive therapy with cidofovir, leflunomide, IVIG, and fluoroquinolones may be considered, although these treatments remains largely unproven.

HEMATOLOGIC COMPLICATIONS

Common causes of hematologic complications after transplant are outlined in Table 62.2. Nearly half of kidney transplant recipients will be anemic within the first 6 months posttransplant, with 10% to 40% remaining anemic at 1 year, irrespective of graft function. Within days of kidney transplantation, erythropoietin levels increase as a result of the functioning allograft, with an early surge to supraphysiologic levels in the first 2 to 3 weeks. Despite this, anemia may persist because of a number of factors, including baseline anemia, surgical blood loss, iron deficiency, allograft dysfunction, and viral illness. In addition, a number of drugs introduced

Table 62.2 Hematologic Complications Post Kidney Transplantation

Hematologic Complication	Cause(s)
Anemia	Allograft dysfunction (early or late posttransplant)
	Iron deficiency
	Blood loss
	EPO resistance
	Immunosuppressive medications (mycophenolic acid agents, azathioprine, rapamycin)
	Other medications (trimethoprim-sulfamethoxazole, valganciclovir, ganciclovir, ACE inhibitors)
	Infections (parvovirus B19, CMV, BK polyomavirus, tuberculosis, varicella zoster virus)
	Comorbid conditions (e.g., cardiovascular disease, peripheral vascular disease)
	Hemolytic anemia (minor ABO incompatibility, rhesus D unmatching, autoimmune anemia)
Leukopenia	Immunosuppressive medications (mycophenolic acid agents, azathioprine, rapamycin, thymoglobulin, alemtuzumab)
	Other medications (valganciclovir, ganciclovir, trimethoprim-sulfamethoxazole)
	Infections (cytomegalovirus, tuberculosis, and overwhelming bacterial infections)
Thrombocytopenia	Immunosuppressive medications (thymoglobulin, alemtuzumab, azathioprine, rapamycin)
	Other medications (antibiotics, antiviral agents, heparin)
	Infection
	HUS/TTP (CNI use)
	Autoimmune thrombocytopenia

posttransplant may cause anemia, including antimetabolites (mycophenolic acid, azathioprine), antiviral agents, antibiotics (e.g., TMP-SMX), and ACE inhibitors. Although some agents, such as ACE inhibitors, may result in isolated anemia, most of these drugs typically impact other cell lines as well.

Workup of posttransplant anemia should include iron studies, a reticulocyte count, and an assessment of other cell lines. If the etiology remains unclear or involves more than one cell line, a hematologist should be consulted. Parvovirus B19 should also be considered with unexplained isolated anemia.

Leukopenia, with or without anemia, is most often associated with immunosuppressive or antiviral medications. Dose reductions or discontinuation usually improve medication-related cytopenias within a matter of days to weeks. If cytopenias persist, alternate etiologies should be explored. Anemia and thrombocytopenia, with or without allograft dysfunction, may indicate hemolytic uremic syndrome. This may be secondary to CNI or recurrent HUS-TTP, and generally portends a poor prognosis warranting therapy with plasmapheresis.

METABOLIC COMPLICATIONS

Many of the metabolic abnormalities that contribute to renal osteodystrophy in ESRD patients, such as phosphate retention, secondary hyperparathyroidism, decreased calcitriol synthesis, and β_2-microglobulin (β_2M) accumulation, are reversed with transplantation; however, a degree of hyperparathyroidism may persist. Persistent uncontrolled hyperparathyroidism-associated hypercalcemia increases the risk for posttransplant bone disease and contributes to vascular calcifications. In cases of severe symptomatic or persistent hypercalcemia, parathyroidectomy may be indicated. The use of calcimimetics posttransplant is not well established, with trials ongoing to examine their use in this setting. To date, cinacalcet therapy has been shown to effectively normalize serum calcium levels, but the impact on PTH and serum phosphorous levels has been variable.

Hypophosphatemia after transplantation is induced by phosphate wasting in the urine as a result of hyperparathyroidism and PTH-independent pathways, such as persistent elevations of FGF-23. Plasma phosphate levels below 1.0 mg/dL can cause muscle weakness and possibly osteomalacia, and should be reversed with supplementation. Osteopenia and osteonecrosis posttransplant are caused by multiple factors, including persistent uremia-induced abnormalities in calcium homeostasis and acquired defects in mineral metabolism induced by immunosuppressive medications. Measures to prevent and treat posttransplant bone disease include minimizing corticosteroid exposure, providing supplemental calcium, treating vitamin D deficiency, and encouraging weight-bearing exercise. Antiresorptive agents may be considered, but data on their benefits in kidney transplant recipients are lacking.

POSTTRANSPLANT MALIGNANCY

Incidence rates of malignancies at 1 and 3 years posttransplant compared with the general population are outlined in Table 62.3. Kidney transplant recipients have a higher incidence of most cancers posttransplant, but the risks are particularly high for certain viral-mediated malignancies, including EBV-related posttransplant lymphoproliferative disease (PTLD), skin and lip cancers, and HHV-8-associated Kaposi sarcoma. In addition, certain malignancies are more common in patients with kidney disease, such as kidney and urinary tract malignancies. Risk factors for cancer after transplant include advanced recipient age, white race, male sex, and prior history of cancer. Recipients with prior cancers must be disease-free for an established time before transplantation, and should be monitored more intensively after transplantation.

Successful treatment of malignancy relies on regular screening and early detection. Typically, malignancy-screening guidelines from the general population are applicable in the posttransplant setting and should be coordinated annually after transplant. Cancers of the skin are the most common malignancies in adult kidney transplant recipients and include squamous and basal cell carcinomas, malignant melanomas, and Merkel cell tumors. Kidney transplant recipients have a 250-fold and 10-fold increased incidence of squamous cell carcinoma and basal

Table 62.3 Age-Adjusted Cancer Rates* in Male and Female Transplant Recipients Compared With the U.S. Population

	Cancer Rates in Men			Cancer Rates in Women		
Type of Cancer	U.S. Population	1 Year Posttransplant	3 Years Posttransplant	U.S. Population	1 Year Posttransplant	3 Years Posttransplant
Skin Cancers						
Melanoma	19.0	60.4	131.3	12.1	99.9	63.5
Nonmelanoma skin	24.0	2017.1	2160.2	14.3	851.6	1320.5
Lymphomas						
Hodgkin's lymphoma	3.2	37.9	98.6	2.5	11.5	93.5
NHL	22	882	150.7	15.7	667.5	456.7
Gastrointestinal						
Colon	66.4	137.2	107.7	48.5	91.1	137.0
Esophagus	8.8	17.4	21.3	2.2	3.6	6.2
Hepatobiliary	9.4	33.5	39.2	5.4	83.2	24.3
Pancreas	12.3	19.8	12.4	9.6	25.1	44.1
Small intestine	2.0	3.8	4.1	1.4	25.1	0
Stomach	11.0	38.9	4.1	5.1	23.7	21.4
Genitourinary						
Bladder	38.3	148.9	60.9	10.0	69.0	36.3
Kidney	16.0	671.0	226.1	8.4	767.7	122.9
Prostate	162.0	477.4	265.8	–	–	–
Testes	5.5	21.3	20.4	–	–	–
Cervix	–	–	–	9.4	9.4	53.7
Ovary	–	–	–	16.2	29.5	42.4
Uterus	–	–	–	0.7	51.7	21.5
Vulvovaginal	–	–	–	3.0	14.6	26.5
Other						
Breast	1.5	6.8	6.0	134.1	343.4	144.3
Lung	89.1	149.4	202.8	53.4	141.8	194.1
CNS	7.9	15.1	36.3	1.7	8.9	21.0
Kaposi sarcoma	1.5	55.0	26.1	0.1	56.0	6.2

Modified from Table 3 in Kasiske BL, Snyder J, Gilbertson DT, et al: Cancer after kidney transplantation in the United States, Am J Transplant 4:905-913, 2004.
CNS, Central nervous system; *NHL,* non-Hodgkin's lymphoma.
*Rates per 100,000 for U.S. population. Rates per 100,000 person-years for transplant recipients. All rates standardized to the 2000 U.S. census population.

cell carcinoma, respectively, compared with the general population. Patients should be counseled to minimize sun exposure, use protective clothing and sunscreen regularly, and perform annual self-examinations for skin lesions. Suspicious lesions should be biopsied, and patients with recurrent lesions should be routinely followed by a dermatologist.

EBV-associated PTLD is characterized by lymphoproliferation, and includes clinical syndromes ranging from infectious mononucleosis to life-threatening malignancies. Of note, PTLD remains relatively uncommon in kidney transplant recipients (1%-2%), typically occurring in the context of primary EBV infection within the first year posttransplant. Additional risk factors for PTLD include young recipient age, CMV mismatch or disease, and the use of

T lymphocyte–depleting antibody. Universal prophylaxis for EBV is not recommended. However, antiviral prophylaxis (acyclovir or ganciclovir) may be considered for EBV-negative recipients with EBV-positive donors because it may result in a reduced rate of PTLD. Prophylaxis with IVIG has been shown to reduce the incidence of non-Hodgkin's lymphoma posttransplant in retrospective studies, but prospective randomized controlled trials in pediatric patients have been inconclusive. High viral loads often predate the clinical presentation of PTLD; therefore, frequent EBV viral load monitoring is recommended in high-risk populations. If viremia occurs in the absence of other clinical signs of PTLD, reduction of immunosuppression and initiation of antiviral therapy may be indicated. Most PTLD cases are non-Hodgkin's lymphomas of B cell origin and are CD20-positive. Mortality rates with PTLD are greater than 50%, with increased age, elevated lactate dehydrogenase levels, multiorgan involvement, and the presence of constitutional symptoms predicting a higher risk for death. The importance of clonality in PTLD is often debated, with monoclonal B cell lymphomas considered more malignant and resistant to treatment compared with polyclonal lymphomas. Treatment involves reduction of immunosuppression and typically includes administration of an anti-CD20 agent (rituximab), with or without additional cytotoxic therapies.

Immunosuppressive reduction should be considered in all patients with malignancy posttransplant, but it should be reviewed in each case to balance the risks for rejection and recurrent malignancy. The role of mTOR in malignancies has been the subject of increased study in the last decade. Indeed, rapamycin has been shown to suppress the growth and proliferation of certain tumors in various animal models. Small studies in humans have suggested that rapamycin may confer a reduced risk for malignancy compared with CNIs, particularly in skin and renal cancers. However, in an analysis of Medicare claims data for transplant recipients in the United States, de novo use of rapamycin was associated with an increased risk for PTLD. Although further studies are clearly needed to delineate the benefits of rapamycin in reducing the risk for posttransplant malignancy, many centers currently consider converting patients with recurrent malignancies to a rapamycin-based immunosuppressive regimen.

CARDIOVASCULAR RISK FACTORS

Cardiovascular death is the leading cause of allograft loss and accounts for nearly 60% of deaths posttransplant. Risk factors for coronary disease after transplantation include the traditional risk factors of increased age, diabetes mellitus, hypertension, cigarette smoking, and hyperlipidemia, as well as proteinuria, reduced kidney function, elevated lipoprotein(a) levels, elevated CRP and IL6 levels, and obesity, particularly in the context of the metabolic syndrome (Table 62.4).

METABOLIC SYNDROME

The constellation of central obesity, dyslipidemia, hypertension, and fasting hyperglycemia is called metabolic syndrome and is associated with an increased risk for diabetes mellitus, proteinuria, reduced kidney function, and cardiovascular disease in the general population. Numerous studies have reported a high prevalence of metabolic syndrome both before and after transplantation. In one U.S. study, the pretransplant prevalence of metabolic syndrome was 57.2% in nondiabetic recipients, and metabolic syndrome pretransplant was an independent risk factor for new-onset diabetes after transplantation (NODAT) in 31.4% of recipients. After transplantation, metabolic syndrome has been reported in up to 63% of recipients and is associated with worse kidney function and allograft survival. Among the various components of metabolic syndrome, systolic hypertension and hypertriglyceridemia have been reported to have the greatest negative impact on long-term allograft function.

Table 62.4 Cardiovascular Risk Factors Post Kidney Transplantation

Cardiovascular Risk Factor	Contributing Factors Posttransplant
Hypertension	Volume overload Calcineurin inhibitors Corticosteroids Allograft dysfunction Renal artery stenosis
Obesity	Liberalization of dietary restrictions Persistent physical inactivity Chronic corticosteroid use
Dyslipidemia	Corticosteroids may cause elevations in LDL and total cholesterol, but are associated most strongly with hypertriglyceridemia posttransplant Calcineurin inhibitors are associated with elevated total cholesterol and LDL levels and reductions in HDL levels independent of corticosteroid use Rapamycin is mostly associated with hypertriglyceridemia
Diabetes	Calcineurin inhibitors (especially tacrolimus) are associated with hyperglycemia and NODAT Corticosteroids are associated with hyperglycemia and NODAT Rapamycin is associated with hyperglycemia and NODAT Chronic hepatitis C infection is associated with pre- and posttransplant diabetes possibly due to HCV-induced islet cell dysfunction and liver dysfunction associated with insulin resistance
Reduced kidney function	Immune- and non-immune–mediated allograft injury with resultant chronic kidney disease
Elevated homocysteine	Homocysteine levels continue to rise post kidney transplantation and may be associated with cyclosporine use

NODAT, New-onset diabetes after transplantation.

OBESITY

Pretransplant obesity (BMI >30) increases the risk for surgical wound infections, allograft loss, and cardiovascular disease posttransplant. Weight gain is common posttransplant, particularly in women, African-Americans, low-income patients, and recipients with pretransplant obesity. All transplant recipients should receive counseling on the importance on diet and exercise. Pharmacologic agents and surgical options for weight loss may be considered in morbidly obesity patients both before and after transplantation.

HYPERTENSION

Hypertension is seen in 60% to 80% of all transplant recipients and is associated with worse allograft survival. In the early posttransplant period, volume management, allograft function, and changes to baseline antihypertensive therapy may contribute to hypertension. Immunosuppressive agents, including CNIs and corticosteroids, may further exacerbate hypertensive states. For instance, cyclosporine increases both systemic and renal vascular resistance and induces renal vasoconstriction via increased release of vasoconstrictors, such as endothelin.

The presence of atherosclerotic disease and complications during organ procurement and transplantation increase the risk for transplant renal artery stenosis (RAS). In addition, CMV infection and DGF have been found to be associated with RAS. Therefore in cases of refractory hypertension posttransplant, particularly when associated with unexplained allograft dysfunction, RAS should be considered. As in the nontransplant setting, ACE inhibitor–induced reversible decline in kidney function may be suggestive of RAS. Blood pressure targets are variable and depend on comorbid disease, including diabetic status and presence of proteinuria. The KDIGO guideline for care of the kidney transplant recipient suggests maintaining blood pressure at less than 130/80 mm Hg.

Calcium channel blockers, ACE inhibitors, and beta blockers may all be considered first-line antihypertensive agents posttransplant, with selection of a specific agent dependent on other patient-specific factors. A recent Cochrane Group metaanalysis of randomized trials found that only calcium channel blockers reduced graft loss and improved GFR compared with placebo, whereas ACE inhibitors more effectively reduced proteinuria. Notably, the renoprotective benefits of ACE inhibitors posttransplant have not been confirmed.

DYSLIPIDEMIA

The Assessment of Lescol in Renal Transplantation (ALERT) trial was a large multicenter study of stable transplant recipients who received either fluvastatin (Lescol) or placebo with the outcome of lowering LDL cholesterol and reducing the risk for cardiac events. After 5 years of follow-up, the fluvastatin group had lower total and LDL cholesterol and fewer cardiac deaths and nonfatal MIs, but there was no difference in major adverse cardiac events. It is important to note that despite concerns regarding increased risks for statin-induced rhabdomyolysis due to CNI coadministration, no increased risk for rhabdomyolysis was noted in the statin arm of the trial. Therefore, although the mortality benefit of statins posttransplant remains unproven, statins remain the drug of choice for the treatment of dyslipidemia in transplant recipients.

NEW-ONSET DIABETES AFTER TRANSPLANTATION

The incidence of NODAT has been variably reported, but recent studies note a prevalence of 16% at 1 year posttransplant. The development of NODAT confers a 46% increased risk for graft loss and an 87% increased risk for death posttransplant, with a tripling of the risk for cardiovascular death. The reason for an increased risk for graft loss remains unclear, but it may be due to a combination of diabetic nephropathy and the implications of reduced immunosuppression to avoid NODAT.

In addition to traditional risk factors for diabetes (older age, obesity, preexisting glucose intolerance, and a family history of diabetes mellitus), risk factors for NODAT

include the type and degree of immunosuppression, African-American race, level of HLA matching, chronic hepatitis C infection, and the cause of ESRD, with some reports suggesting a higher risk associated with polycystic kidney disease. Calcineurin inhibitors, particularly tacrolimus, may cause pancreatic beta cell dysfunction and contribute to insulin resistance. Cyclosporine is less diabetogenic than tacrolimus, and some centers have advocated the use of cyclosporine in patients at high risk for developing NODAT. Alternatively, reduced doses of CNI are recommended to minimize the risk for NODAT. However, no comparative studies have been conducted to demonstrate the benefit and safety of cyclosporine-based immunosuppression or low-dose CNI in patients at high risk for NODAT. Rapamycin is also diabetogenic, and has been shown to worsen glycemic control after conversion from a CNI.

Corticosteroids cause hyperglycemia through a number of mechanisms in a dose-dependent manner. Therefore, rapid reduction of prednisone to maintenance doses (5-10 mg/day) significantly improves hyperglycemia. However, the relative benefit of complete steroid withdrawal versus maintenance with low-dose prednisone has not been consistently demonstrated.

All transplant recipients should have fasting blood glucose levels checked weekly for the first month, and then at 3, 6, and 12 months thereafter. Impaired fasting blood glucose results should be further evaluated with an oral glucose tolerance test. HbA1C assessment should be used to direct therapy in patients with NODAT. Hyperglycemic patients should receive counseling on diet and lifestyle modification, and be initiated on therapy if hyperglycemia persists. All oral hypoglycemic agents have been found to be safe and effective posttransplant; however, the metabolism and adverse effects of each drug should be considered in relation to immunosuppressant medications and the level of allograft function.

BIBLIOGRAPHY

Engels EA, Pfeiffer RM, Fraumeni JF, et al: Spectrum of cancer risk among US solid organ transplant recipients, *JAMA* 306:1891-1901, 2011.

Fishman JA: Infection in solid-organ transplant recipients, *N Engl J Med* 357:2601-2614, 2007.

Gloor J, Cosio F, Lager DJ, et al: The spectrum of antibody-mediated renal allograft injury: implications for treatment, *Am J Transplant* 8:1367-1373, 2008.

Ho J, Wiebe C, Gibson IW, et al: Immune monitoring of kidney allografts, *Am J Kidney Dis* 60:629-640, 2012.

Holdaas H, Fellstrom B, Jardine AG, et al: Effect of fluvastatin on cardiac outcomes in renal transplant recipients: a multicentre, randomised, placebo-controlled trial, *Lancet* 361:2024-2031, 2003.

Hricik DE: Metabolic syndrome in kidney transplantation: management of risk factors, *Clin J Am Soc Nephrol* 6:1781-1785, 2011.

Humar A, Michaels M: AST ID Working Group on Infectious Disease Monitoring: American Society of Transplantation recommendations for screening, monitoring and reporting of infectious complications in immunosuppression trials in recipients of organ transplantation, *Am J Transplant* 6:262-274, 2006.

Humar A, Morris M, Blumberg E, et al: Nucleic acid testing (NAT) of organ donors: is the 'best' test the right test? A consensus conference report, *Am J Transplant* 10:889-899, 2010.

Kasiske B, Cosio FG, Beto J, et al: Clinical practice guidelines for managing dyslipidemias in kidney transplant patients: a report from the Managing Dyslipidemias in Chronic Kidney Disease Work Group of the National Kidney Foundation Kidney Disease Outcomes Quality Initiative, *Am J Transplant* 4(Suppl 7):13-53, 2004.

Kasiske BL, Snyder J, Gilbertson DT, et al: Cancer after kidney transplantation in the United States, *Am J Transplant* 4:905-913, 2004.

Kidney Disease: Improving Global Outcomes (KDIGO) Transplant Work Group. KDIGO clinical practice guideline for the care of kidney transplant recipients, *Am J Transplant* 9(Suppl 3):S1-S157, 2009.

Mannon RB: Immune monitoring and biomarkers to predict chronic allograft dysfunction, *Kidney Int Suppl* S59-S65, 2010.

Merion RM, Ashby VB, Wolfe RA, et al: Deceased-donor characteristics and the survival benefit of kidney transplantation, *JAMA* 294:2726-2733, 2005.

Nankivell BJ, Borrows RJ, Fung CL, et al: The natural history of chronic allograft nephropathy, *N Engl J Med* 349:2326-2333, 2003.

Nickerson P: Post-transplant monitoring of renal allografts: are we there yet? *Curr Opin Immunol* 21(5):563-568, 2009.

OPTN/SRTR 2010 Annual Data Report: Rockville, Md. Department of Health and Human Services, Health Resources and Services Administration, Healthcare Systems Bureau, Division of Transplantation, 2011.

Solez K, Colvin RB, Racusen LC, et al: Banff 2007 classification of renal allograft pathology: updates and future directions, *Am J Transplant* 8:753-760, 2008.

Stegall MD, Gloor JM: Deciphering antibody-mediated rejection: new insights into mechanisms and treatment, *Curr Opin Organ Transplant* 15:8-10, 2010.

Vincenti F, Larsen C, Durrbach A, et al: Costimulation blockade with belatacept in renal transplantation, *N Engl J Med* 353:770-781, 2005.

Woodle ES, First MR, Pirsch J, et al: A prospective, randomized, double-blind, placebo-controlled multicenter trial comparing early (7 day) corticosteroid cessation versus long-term, low-dose corticosteroid therapy, *Ann Surg* 248:564-577, 2008.

63 Immunosuppression in Transplantation

Sindhu Chandran | Flavio G. Vincenti

The central issue in organ transplantation remains the suppression of allograft rejection. Understanding the physiology of the immune response to a transplanted organ and developing targeted immunosuppressive drugs are keys for successful graft function.

PHYSIOLOGY OF IMMUNORECOGNITION

The immune system evolved to discriminate self from nonself, and this response against nonself consists of an array of receptor-mediated sensing and effector mechanisms broadly described as innate and adaptive. Innate immunity is primitive, does not require priming, and is of relatively low affinity but broadly reactive. Adaptive immunity is antigen-specific, depends on antigen exposure or priming, and can be of very high affinity. The major effectors of innate immunity are complement, granulocytes, monocytes/macrophages, natural killer (NK) cells, mast cells, and basophils. The major effectors of adaptive immunity are B and T lymphocytes.

A transplant between genetically distinct individuals of the same species is called an allogeneic graft, or an allograft. The immune response to an allograft requires three elements: recognition of foreign antigens, activation of antigen-specific lymphocytes, and the effector phase of graft rejection. The recognition of antigens as peptide fragments bound to major histocompatibility complex (MHC) molecules, known as human leukocyte antigens (HLA) in humans, is the central event in the initiation of an alloresponse. HLA molecules (Fig. 63.1) are highly polymorphic, follow Mendelian codominant inheritance, and constitute the principal antigenic barrier to transplantation. The degree of HLA matching between the donor and the recipient plays an important role in graft survival, and HLA matching has been incorporated into kidney allocation. In addition, non-HLA molecules, such as MHC class I–related chain A (MICA), are recognized as playing a significant role in rejection, particularly in recipients of well–MHC-matched kidneys.

There are two types of HLA molecules: class I and class II. Class I HLA molecules are expressed on all nucleated cells, whereas class II molecules are usually expressed only on antigen presenting cells (APCs), which include dendritic cells, B lymphocytes, and macrophages. Cytokines such as interferon-γ induce, upregulate, and broaden HLA expression, so that all cells in a graft can become potential targets of the immune response. Ischemia-reperfusion injury in the graft leads to the production of inflammatory cytokines and recruitment of macrophages, and acute rejection episodes are more common in grafts with prolonged ischemia times. Recipient T cells may respond directly to peptides/HLA complexes presented by donor APCs in the graft or to donor HLA peptides presented on the recipient's own APCs (Fig. 63.2). Acute rejection of an allograft is believed to be primarily dependent on direct allorecognition, whereas the indirect pathway may play a larger role in chronic rejection.

T cells are critically important in the rejection of allogeneic grafts. CD4 T cells (helper T cells) are thought to mediate the initial recognition of an allograft and to help amplify and coordinate the subsequent immune response, including providing help to CD8 (effector) T cells. T cell recognition of the alloantigen occurs via binding of the T cell receptor (TCR)/CD3 complex on the T cells surface to the peptide/MHC complex on APCs. This is referred to as *signal 1*, and leads to phosphorylation of TCR-associated proteins and downstream activation of several pathways, including calcineurin, protein kinase C, and mitogen-activated protein (MAP) kinase pathways.

The calcineurin pathway has been best characterized, and involves the activation of calcineurin (a phosphatase) by an increase in cytosolic calcium. Calcineurin dephosphorylates nuclear factor of activated T cells (NFAT), allowing NFAT to translocate from the cytoplasm to the nucleus. NFAT binds to regulatory sequences and increases gene transcription of several cytokines, including interleukin (IL)-2, a T cell growth factor, as well as IL-4, interferon-gamma (IFN-γ), and tumor necrosis factor-α (TNF-α).

Although the specificity of the immune response is determined by signal 1, a costimulatory signal, or *signal 2*, which occurs though accessory molecules, is essential for T cell activation. The most potent of these signals regulating T cell clonal expansion and differentiation is provided by the B7/CD28 family of molecules (Fig. 63.3). B7-1 (CD80) and B7-2 (CD86) are ligands on APCs that bind to CD28, expressed on most T cells. Engagement of CD28 increases the production of IL-2 and other cytokines, and results in T cell proliferation. CD80 and CD86 also regulate T cells by binding another antigen on T cells called cytotoxic T-lymphocyte antigen-4 (CTLA-4), which inhibits T cell proliferation. A costimulatory interaction between CD40 on APCs and CD40 ligand (CD154, CD40L) on T cells is also critical for activation of APCs and upregulation of B7 expression on T cells. One way to induce T cell anergy in vitro is to provide the T cell with an antigen specific signal through the TCR (signal 1) in the absence of CD28 engagement (signal 2). However, in most in vivo models of B7 blockade, anergy has been difficult to demonstrate, possibly due to the complexity of costimulation that involves multiple stimulatory and inhibitory signals.

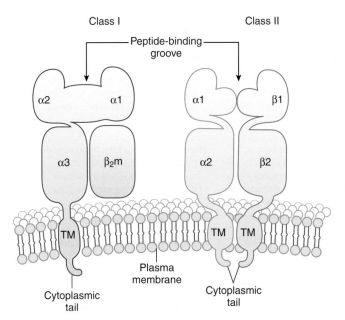

Figure 63.1 Structure of HLA class I and class II molecules. Beta$_2$-microglobulin (β_2m) is the light chain of the class I molecule. The α chain of the class I molecule has two peptide-binding domains (α1 and α2), an immunoglobulin-like domain (α3), the transmembrane region (TM), and the cytoplasmic tail. Each of the class II α and β chains has four domains: the peptide-binding domain (α1 or β1), the immunoglobulin-like domain (α2 or β2), the transmembrane region, and the cytoplasmic tail. (From Klein J, Sato A: The HLA System, *N Engl J Med* 343:702-709, 2000.)

Antigen-specific activation of T cells, particularly CD4 T cells, leads to the production of cytokines, recruitment of monocytes, and proliferation of CD8 T cells, NK cells, and B cells. CD8 T cells cause cell death in the graft through the release of soluble cytotoxic factors (granzymes and perforin) as well as upregulated Fas ligand on T cells which binds to Fas (CD95) on target cells and triggers apoptosis.

In addition to T cells, B cells and the humoral arm of the immune system play a major role in acute and chronic graft injury. Antibodies produced by the differentiation of B cells into plasma cells cause cell injury through complement fixation or antibody-dependent cellular cytotoxicity. Hyperacute rejection occurs when preformed recipient antibodies to donor HLA antigens or ABO blood group antigens result in complement activation, intravascular coagulation, and graft necrosis within 24 hours of transplantation. Although cross-matching and ABO blood typing have virtually eliminated hyperacute rejection, B cells and plasma cells continue to play an important role in subsequent

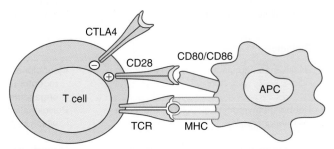

Figure 63.3 Signal 1 and signal 2. (From Vincenti F: Costimulation blockade in autoimmunity and transplantation, *J Allergy Clin Immunol* 121:299-306, 2008.)

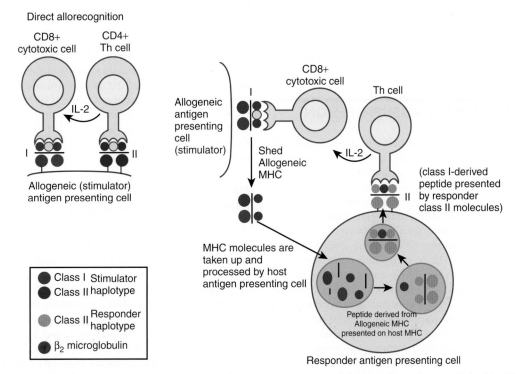

Figure 63.2 Diagrammatic representation of the direct and indirect pathways of allorecognition. (From Rogers NJ, Lechler RI: Allorecognition, *Am J Transplant* 1:97-102, 2001.)

Table 63.1 Commonly Used Induction and Maintenance Immunosuppressive Agents

Drug	Phase of Use	Mechanism of Action	Side Effects
Glucocorticoids: methylprednisolone (Solumedrol), prednisone (Deltasone)	Induction and maintenance	Binds cytosolic receptors and heat shock proteins, and blocks transcription of IL-1, IL-2, IL-3, IL-6, TNF-α, and IFN-γ	Hypertension, hyperglycemia, dyslipidemia, osteoporosis, impaired wound healing, cosmetic effects
Small Molecules			
Calcineurin inhibitors: cyclosporine (Sandimmune, Neoral, Gengraf), tacrolimus (Prograf)	Maintenance	Forms a complex with cyclophilin or FK-binding protein, which binds to calcineurin, preventing dephosphorylation of regulatory proteins and decreasing transcription of IL-2, IL-4, IFN-γ, and TNF-α; also increases TGF-β, which inhibits IL-2	Tremor, nephrotoxicity, hypertension, hyperglycemia, hyperuricemia, hyperlipidemia (CsA), hirsutism (CsA), gingival hyperplasia (CsA), hair loss (tacrolimus)
Azathioprine (Imuran, Azasan)	Maintenance	Purine analog that blocks DNA, RNA, and protein synthesis	Marrow suppression, pancreatitis
Mycophenolate mofetil (Cellcept), mycophenolic acid (Myfortic)	Maintenance	Inhibits IMPDH (inosine monophosphate dehydrogenase), preventing de novo guanosine nucleotide synthesis	Diarrhea, marrow suppression, teratogenic
mTOR inhibitors: sirolimus (Rapamune), everolimus (Zortress)	Maintenance	Forms a complex with FK-binding protein-12, which blocks p70 S6 kinase, causing G1 cell cycle arrest	Hyperlipidemia, hyperglycemia, thrombocytopenia, impaired wound healing, interstitial pneumonitis, teratogenic
Biologics			
Basiliximab (Simulect)	Induction	Monoclonal antibody to CD25 (IL-2 receptor α chain), which blocks IL-2 engagement	Rare infusion reactions
Rabbit antithymocyte globulin (Thymoglobulin)	Induction	Polyclonal antithymocyte antibody, which depletes T cells	Cytokine release syndrome, serum sickness, thrombocytopenia, prolonged lymphopenia
Alemtuzumab (Campath)	Induction	Monoclonal antibody to CD52, which depletes T cells, B cells, and NK cells	Cytokine release syndrome, prolonged lymphopenia
Belatacept (Nulojix)	Maintenance	CTLA-4-Ig fusion protein, which competes with CD28 for CD80/86 binding, inhibiting T cell costimulation	Rare infusion reactions

antibody-mediated rejection (AMR), and may be important mediators of chronic graft injury and late graft loss.

STRATEGIES FOR IMMUNOSUPPRESSION

The first attempts at immunosuppression used total-body irradiation. Subsequently, azathioprine was introduced in the early 1960s, and soon thereafter was routinely accompanied by prednisolone in an immunosuppressive regimen. The polyclonal antilymphocyte antibody preparations became available in the mid-1970s. The introduction in the early 1960s, of cyclosporine in the early 1980s dramatically improved 1-year graft survival rates from 50% to over 80%, and in 1985, OKT3, a monoclonal antibody to CD3, was introduced for the treatment of acute rejection. In the 1990s, tacrolimus and mycophenolate mofetil emerged as alternatives to cyclosporine and azathioprine, anti–IL-2 receptor antibodies were approved for induction, and sirolimus became available. In 2011, belatacept was approved as the first biologic agent for use in maintenance immunotherapy. Commonly used immunosuppressants and their mechanisms of action are listed in Table 63.1.

Transplant immunosuppression is guided by three key principles. First, multiple agents directed at different molecular targets within the alloimmune response are used simultaneously to maximize synergy and efficacy while minimizing toxicity. Second, greater immunosuppression (induction) is needed for early engraftment or to treat established rejection than for long-term graft maintenance. And third, continuous vigilance is essential to identify rejection, drug toxicity, and infection so that the immunosuppressive regimen can be modified appropriately.

MECHANISMS OF ACTION OF IMMUNOSUPPRESSIVE DRUGS

T cells have historically been the major target of immunosuppression. The three signal model of T-cell activation and subsequent cellular proliferation provides a useful guide to the sites of action of the major immunosuppressive agents (Fig. 63.4). Signal 1 is the antigen-specific signal provided by the interaction of the MHC/peptide complex on APCs with the T cell receptor/CD3 complex. Signal 2 is a non–antigen-specific costimulatory signal provided by the engagement of B7 on APCs with CD28 on the T cell. These two signals activate intracellular pathways leading to the production of IL-2 and other cytokines. Stimulation of the IL-2 receptor (CD25) leads to activation of mTOR, a protein kinase, and

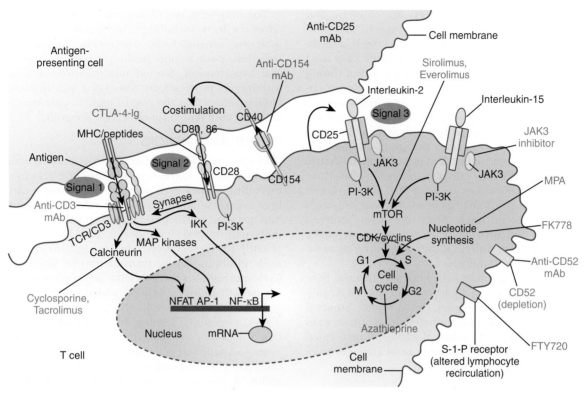

Figure 63.4   Individual immunosuppressive drugs and sites of action in the three-signal model. *MAP,* Mitogen-activated protein; *MPA,* mycophenolic acid; *NFAT,* nuclear factor of activated T cells. (From Halloran PF: Immunosuppressive drugs for kidney transplantation, *N Engl J Med* 351:2715-2729, 2004.)

provides signal 3, which triggers cell proliferation. Therapies targeting antibody-mediated injury are directed against B cells, plasma cells, and complement activation. In general, all drugs in current clinical use have been more effective at suppressing primary than memory immune responses.

INDUCTION THERAPY

High intravenous doses of corticosteroids are used as part of nearly all induction immunosuppression protocols. Induction therapy with biologic agents is used to delay the use of nephrotoxic calcineurin inhibitors and/or to intensify the initial immunosuppressive therapy in patients at high immunologic risk (i.e., broadly sensitized, African-American, or pediatric patients, or individuals receiving a repeat transplant). Biologic agents for induction therapy are currently used in over 80% of kidney transplant recipients, and are divided into two groups: depleting agents and immune modulators.

Depleting agents diminish the recipient's lymphocyte population at the time of transplantation, and induction with these agents has been shown to improve graft survival. Antithymocyte globulin (ATG), a polyclonal antilymphocyte preparation directed against T cells and approved for the reversal of acute rejection (usually rabbit-derived thymoglobulin), is used off-label as the most common induction agent in kidney transplantation. It is interesting to note that ATG also causes sustained and rapid expansion of regulatory T cells, which play an important part in maintaining immune homeostasis and limiting antigraft immunity. The standard dose of rabbit-derived thymoglobulin is 1.5 mg/kg

daily for 4 to 10 days. Alemtuzumab (Campath-1H) is a humanized anti-CD52 monoclonal antibody that targets lymphocytes, monocytes, macrophages, and NK cells, and causes prolonged B and T cell depletion. Alemtuzumab is also increasingly used off-label as induction therapy (in about 10% of kidney transplants), particularly as part of steroid-sparing protocols. It is usually given as a single dose of 30 mg intraoperatively when infusion-related events are often masked by general anesthesia. ATGAM, an equine antithymocyte globulin, is rarely used in the United States because of its poorer efficacy. OKT3, a murine monoclonal antibody to CD3, was associated with significant acute side effects (cytokine release syndrome) and was withdrawn from the market.

Depleting agents can elicit major side effects, including fever, chills, and hypotension. The polyclonal agents are xenogeneic proteins. Cell death and cytokine release peak with the first infusion and diminish substantially with subsequent doses. Premedication with corticosteroids, acetaminophen, and an antihistamine along with slow infusion (over 4-6 hours) through a large-diameter vessel minimize reactions. Other side effects include leukopenia, thrombocytopenia, serum sickness, glomerulonephritis, and rarely, anaphylaxis. In the long term, depleting agents have been associated with a higher incidence of infections and malignancy, particularly posttransplant lymphoproliferative disorders (PTLD).

Immune-modulating induction agents do not deplete T cells, with the possible exception of T regulatory cells, but rather block IL-2–mediated T cell activation. Daclizumab

(Zenapax) and basiliximab (Simulect) are chimeric and humanized monoclonal antibodies, respectively, that bind to the α chain of the IL-2 receptor, thus blocking IL-2 mediated responses. Daclizumab has a longer half-life ($T_{1/2}$) than basiliximab (20 days versus 7 days), and the typical dosing schedule results in longer saturation of the IL-2Rα on circulating T cells (120 days versus 30 to 45 days). However, saturation of the IL-2Rα may not prevent rejection, and was noted to be similar in patients with or without an acute rejection episode. Rejection in patients despite IL-2R blockade may occur through a mechanism that bypasses the IL-2 pathway as a result of cytokine-cytokine receptor redundancy (i.e., IL-7, IL-15). Both drugs are fairly well tolerated, and no cytokine release syndrome has been observed, although anaphylaxis may occur rarely. Since the manufacturer's withdrawal of daclizumab from the market in October 2008, basiliximab is the only anti-IL2R antibody currently available for use as induction therapy.

More aggressive approaches to induction therapy have been used in patients with high levels of anti-HLA antibodies, donor-specific antibodies, or previous humoral rejection. These include plasmapheresis and intravenous immune globulin (IVIG) to reduce the levels of preformed antibodies, and rituximab, a chimeric anti-CD20 monoclonal antibody, to selectively deplete B cells.

MAINTENANCE IMMUNOTHERAPY

The basic immunosuppressive protocols use multiple drugs simultaneously. Therapy typically involves a calcineurin inhibitor (CNI), glucocorticoids, and mycophenolate mofetil (MMF), each directed at a discrete site in T cell activation. Protocols employing rapid steroid withdrawal (within 1 week) are being used in over a third of kidney transplant recipients with good short-term results, although the effects on long-term graft function are unknown. Azathioprine has mostly fallen out of favor, but it is still used during pregnancy and sometimes as part of low-cost regimens. Sirolimus and everolimus have been used mostly in de novo or conversion regimens that spare/minimize CNI exposure. Maintenance biologic therapy with belatacept, in combination with a steroid and an antiproliferative agent, permits complete avoidance of calcineurin inhibition and has been associated with superior kidney function and improved metabolic parameters in recipients with low immunologic risk.

GLUCOCORTICOIDS

Glucocorticoids are used in high doses both as part of induction protocols and for the treatment of acute rejection episodes, and in low doses for maintenance immunosuppression. Steroids exert broad antiinflammatory effects on multiple components of cellular immunity, but have little effect on humoral immunity. They lyse (in some species) and redistribute lymphocytes, causing a rapid transient lymphopenia. To effect long-term responses, steroids bind to intracellular receptors and downregulate the transcription of numerous genes such as IL-1, IL-2, IL-3, IL-6, TNF-α, and IFN-γ, thereby inhibiting T cell activation. Neutrophils and monocytes display poor chemotaxis and decreased lysosomal enzyme release. Additionally, steroids curtail the activation of NF-κB, thus increasing the apoptosis of activated cells.

The long-term use of steroids is associated with several adverse effects, including growth retardation in children, avascular osteonecrosis, osteopenia, increased risk for infection, poor wound healing, cataracts, hyperglycemia, and hypertension. Steroid minimization (avoidance and withdrawal) protocols are associated with improved metabolic parameters at the cost of higher acute rejection rates and unknown long-term effects on the graft.

CALCINEURIN INHIBITORS

Cyclosporine A (CsA) ushered in the modern era of organ transplantation, increasing the rates of early engraftment, extending kidney graft survival, and making cardiac and liver transplantation possible. Cyclosporine and tacrolimus are structurally unrelated agents that bind to distinct molecular targets (cyclophilin and FK-binding protein [FKBP] 12, respectively), blocking calcineurin and selectively inhibiting signal transduction in activated T cells. Cyclosporine also increases the expression of transforming growth factor-β (TGF-β), which inhibits IL-2 and the generation of cytotoxic T cells.

CsA, a lipophilic and highly hydrophobic cyclic polypeptide of 11 amino acids, is produced by the fungus *Beauveria nivea*. CsA supplied in the original soft gelatin capsule (Sandimmune) is absorbed slowly, with 20% to 50% bioavailability. A modified microemulsion formulation (Neoral) with improved bioavailability has become the most widely used preparation. Generic preparations of both are available and are bioequivalent to the original formulation, but not to each other. The initial dose is usually 10 to 15 mg/kg/day, divided into two doses. Administration of CsA with food delays and decreases its absorption, and can lower the area under the drug concentration curve (AUC) by 13% and peak concentration by 33%. The elimination of cyclosporine from the blood is generally biphasic, with a terminal $T_{1/2}$ of 5 to 18 hours. It is metabolized extensively in the gut and the liver by CYP3A and P-glycoprotein. CsA and its metabolites are excreted principally through the bile into the feces, with 6% being excreted in urine. Dosage adjustments are required for hepatic dysfunction, but not for reduced glomerular filtration rate. Trough CsA levels (C0 level) are poorly reflective of the AUC and thus are not an accurate indication of CsA exposure in individual patients. Drug levels 2 hours after Neoral dose administration (C2 levels) have shown better correlation with the AUC, but are difficult to obtain in routine clinical practice.

The principal adverse reactions to CsA therapy are kidney dysfunction and hypertension. Tremor, hirsutism, hyperlipidemia, hyperuricemia, and gingival hyperplasia are also frequently encountered. Nephrotoxicity occurs in the majority of patients, and is the major reason for cessation or modification of therapy. It causes a dose-related, reversible renal vasoconstriction that particularly affects the afferent arteriole. CsA-enhanced TGF-β expression may be responsible for the development of interstitial fibrosis in the kidney, as well as its effect on the proliferation of tumor cells. Thrombotic microangiopathy (TMA) is an uncommon but distinct form of CNI-induced endothelial toxicity. It can be systemic or limited to the kidney, and it usually responds to withdrawal of the CNI.

Tacrolimus (FK506; Prograf) is a macrolide antibiotic produced by *Streptomyces tsukubaensis*. Because of perceived slightly greater efficacy and ease of blood level monitoring, tacrolimus has become the preferred CNI in most transplant centers. It is indicated for the prophylaxis of solid-organ allograft rejection, and is also used as rescue therapy in patients who develop rejection episodes despite maintaining therapeutic levels of CsA. Oral bioavailability is about 25%, and $T_{1/2}$ of tacrolimus is 8 to 12 hours. Like CsA, it is extensively metabolized in the gut and liver by CYP3A and the majority is excreted in the feces. The recommended initial oral dose is 0.2 mg/kg/day in two divided doses. Trough tacrolimus levels seem to correlate better with the drug AUC and with clinical events than they do for CsA. The first generic tacrolimus product gained FDA approval in August 2009. Dose requirements and trough levels are similar between brand and generic tacrolimus, but postconversion monitoring is prudent because patients may require dose titration. Care should also be taken when switching from one generic version to another. Similar to CsA, nephrotoxicity is a limiting factor with tacrolimus. Neurotoxicity (e.g., tremor, headache, paresthesias, seizures), hyperglycemia, hypomagnesemia, and gastrointestinal (GI) complaints tend to occur more commonly in patients on tacrolimus as compared with CsA, whereas elevations in uric acid and LDL cholesterol are less common. Diarrhea and alopecia are common in patients on both tacrolimus and mycophenolate. Unlike CsA, tacrolimus does not cause hirsutism or gingival hyperplasia.

Both CsA and tacrolimus are extensively metabolized by hepatic microsomal enzymes, especially CYP3A, as well as via P-glycoprotein, and interact with a wide variety of commonly used drugs. These interactions have been better characterized for CsA, but usually apply to both drugs. CYP3A inhibitors can decrease CsA metabolism and increase blood CsA concentrations (Table 63.2). These include calcium channel blockers (e.g., verapamil, diltiazem), antifungal agents (e.g., fluconazole, ketoconazole), antibiotics (e.g., erythromycin), human immunodeficiency virus protease inhibitors (e.g., ritonavir), and other drugs (e.g., amiodarone). Grapefruit

juice inhibits CYP3A and the P-glycoprotein multidrug efflux pump, and can increase the blood concentrations of both CNIs. In contrast, hepatic microsomal inducers such as some antibiotics (e.g., nafcillin, rifampin), anticonvulsants (e.g., phenobarbital, phenytoin), and St. John's wort can decrease CsA and tacrolimus blood levels. CsA and tacrolimus also affect the concentration of other drugs by competing for the hepatic microsomal system and plasma protein binding, and they decrease the clearance of drugs such as statins, digoxin, and methotrexate. Close monitoring of drug levels and attention to dosage is required when such combinations are used. CNI nephrotoxicity can also be exaggerated by the combination with amphotericin, aminoglycosides, and nonsteroidal antiinflammatory drugs.

Voclosporin (VCS, ISA 247) is a small molecule analog of cyclosporine with higher potency. A phase 2 study showed similar efficacy and comparable kidney function in patients receiving voclosporin as compared with tacrolimus, with a lower incidence of hyperglycemia. It remains unclear whether it will be further developed and marketed for use in transplantation.

ANTIPROLIFERATIVE AGENTS

Azathioprine (Imuran) is an imidazolyl derivative of 6-mercaptopurine, which inhibits de novo purine synthesis. Cell proliferation is thereby inhibited, impairing a variety of lymphocyte functions. Azathioprine was the first chemical immunosuppressive agent used in organ transplantation, but it has been mostly superseded by mycophenolate in current clinical practice. Oral bioavailability of azathioprine is about 50%, and it is metabolized by oxidation and methylation in the liver and/or erythrocytes. The major side effect is myelosuppression, which can be severe if it is used in combination with allopurinol. Allopurinol inhibits the enzyme xanthine oxidase, which converts azathioprine to inactive 6-thiouric acid. Other adverse effects of azathioprine include hepatotoxicity, alopecia, GI toxicity, pancreatitis, and increased risk for neoplasia.

Table 63.2   Notable Drug Interactions With Cyclosporine

Drug Class	Agents	Effect on Cyclosporine Level
Anticonvulsants	Barbiturates, phenytoin, carbamazepine, oxcarbazepine	↓
Antibiotics	Nafcillin, IV trimethoprim, imipenem, cephalosporins, terbinafine	↓
	Clarithromycin, erythromycin, telithromycin	↑
Antifungals	Terbinafine	↓
	Ketoconazole, fluconazole, itraconazole, voriconazole	↑
Antimycobacterials	Rifampin, rifabutin (to a lesser extent)	↓
	Pyrazinamide	↑
Antiretrovirals	Efavirenz, etravirine, nevirapine	↓
	Atazanavir, boceprevir, darunavir, delavirdine, fosamprenavir, indinavir, ritonavir, saquinavir, telaprevir	↑
Antiarrhythmics	Amiodarone, dronedarone, quinidine	↑
Calcium channel blockers	Diltiazem, nicardipine, verapamil	↑
Food and herbs	St. John's wort	↓
	Grapefruit juice	↑
Glucocorticoids	Methyprednisolone, prednisone	May ↓ or ↑ via CYP3A4 induction or competitive inhibition
Miscellaneous	Bosentan, octreotide, orlistat	↓
	Carvedilol, bromocriptine, metoclopramide, cimetidine	↑

Mycophenolate mofetil (MMF; Cellcept) is a prodrug that is rapidly hydrolyzed to the active drug mycophenolic acid (MPA), a selective, noncompetitive, reversible inhibitor of inosine monophosphate dehydrogenase (IMPDH). B and T cells lack nucleotide salvage pathways, are highly dependent on de novo purine synthesis for cell proliferation, and are therefore selectively inhibited by this drug. MMF is indicated for the prophylaxis of transplant rejection, and is typically used in combination with a CNI and glucocorticoids. In addition, it has benefits in the treatment of acute and chronic rejection, which arise from its ability to inhibit the recruitment and interaction of mononuclear cells and to prevent the development and progression of proliferative arteriolopathy, respectively. The typical starting dose is 1 g twice daily, although a higher dose (1.5 g twice daily) may be recommended for African-American recipients. The parent drug is cleared from the blood within a few minutes, and MPA in turn is conjugated to glucuronide (MPAG) before excretion in bile. Enterohepatic cycling of MPAG occurs, producing a second peak at 5 to 6 hours, after which MPAG is excreted in the urine. Although oral bioavailability is about 90% with a $T_{1/2}$ of 12 hours, plasma concentrations of MPA after a single dose in kidney transplant patients within the first month are about half of those found in healthy volunteers or long-term transplant recipients. A generic version of MMF was approved in 2009 and can be safely substituted for Cellcept. As with the use of tacrolimus and cyclosporine generics, it is important to ensure that patients consistently receive the same generic product, that patients and clinicians are aware when substitutions occur, and that enhanced vigilance is provided during the transition.

The principal toxicities of MMF are GI and hematologic. These include leukopenia, anemia, diarrhea, abdominal pain, and vomiting. An enteric-coated form of MPA (Myfortic) is also available, which anecdotally has superior GI tolerability, although this has not been convincingly demonstrated in controlled studies. There is also an increased incidence of certain infections with MMF, especially sepsis associated with CMV and an association with progressive multifocal leukoencephalopathy (PML) caused by JC virus. Because of the higher potency of CsA in interrupting enterohepatic circulation, the combination of MMF with tacrolimus leads to higher AUC for MPA and is more immunosuppressive than when it is used in combination with CsA. The use of MMF in pregnancy is associated with congenital malformations and increased risk for pregnancy loss. Women of childbearing potential must adhere to a Risk Evaluation and Mitigation Strategy (REMS) and use effective contraception while taking MMF.

Sirolimus (Rapamycin; Rapamune) is a macrocyclic lactone produced by *Streptomyces hygroscopicus*. It also forms a complex with FKBP-12, but unlike with tacrolimus, this complex binds to and inhibits the protein kinase mTOR leading to a cell-cycle arrest in G1 phase. Sirolimus is indicated for the prophylaxis of kidney transplant rejection, usually in combination with a reduced dose of a CNI and glucocorticoids. Particular attention has focused on its use in protocols employing early or late CNI withdrawal or minimization, although enthusiasm has dampened for early use because of higher rates of acute rejection, possibly due to expansion of CD8 memory T cells. However, sirolimus has also been associated with the expansion of CD4 regulatory T cells, and may therefore find utility as part of regimens to promote transplant tolerance. One unique advantage is its antitumor effect, which arises from its inhibition of angiogenesis and G1 to S cell cycle transition. mTOR inhibition has shown clinical benefit in both primary and metastatic Kaposi sarcoma and renal cell carcinoma, and it shows promise in the treatment of other solid and hematologic malignancies.

Sirolimus is absorbed rapidly after an oral dose, and bioavailability is about 15%. It is extensively metabolized in the liver by CYP3A4 and P-glycoprotein. The blood $T_{1/2}$ after multiple doses in stable kidney transplant patients is 62 hours. It is usually dosed once daily, with target trough blood levels of 5 to 15 ng/mL. Interactions of sirolimus are common with drugs that are metabolized or transported by CYP3A4 and P-glycoprotein (see Table 63.2). In healthy volunteers, concomitant administration of sirolimus and CsA (as Neoral) increased the AUC for sirolimus by 230% compared with sirolimus alone. It is therefore recommended that sirolimus be administered 4 hours after the morning CsA dose. Everolimus is closely related chemically and clinically to sirolimus, but has a shorter $T_{1/2}$ (23 hours) and therefore a shorter time to achieve steady-state drug concentrations. The toxicities and reported drug interactions appear to be the same.

The major adverse effects of sirolimus in the early post-transplant period arise from its antiproliferative actions, including impaired wound healing and wound dehiscence, prolonged delayed kidney graft function, and a higher incidence of lymphoceles. Hypercholesterolemia and hypertriglyceridemia, hyperglycemia, bone marrow suppression, oral ulcers, and GI side effects are well known. Rarely, it can cause localized limb edema, angioedema, and interstitial pneumonitis. Sirolimus given alone does not produce acute or chronic decreases in kidney function. However, it can cause direct tubular and podocyte toxicity resulting in hypokalemia, de novo proteinuria, and nephrotic syndrome. In combination with standard doses of CNI, there is a potentiation of nephrotoxicity that is not completely explained by their pharmacokinetic interaction. For this reason, it is recommended that the CNI dose be reduced when sirolimus is added. Sirolimus is embryotoxic, and its use is contraindicated in pregnancy. Women must use effective contraception while on sirolimus. Reversible oligospermia and reduced testosterone levels have also been described.

BIOLOGICS FOR MAINTENANCE IMMUNOSUPPRESSION

Abatacept (CTLA4-Ig) contains the binding region of CTLA4 and the constant region of human IgG_1, and it competitively inhibits CD28 (Fig. 63.5). However, CTLA4-Ig was less effective when used in nonhuman primate models of kidney transplantation. Belatacept (LEA29Y; Nulogix) is a second-generation CTLA4-Ig with two amino acid substitutions, which has higher affinity for CD80 (twofold) and CD86 (fourfold), yielding a 10-fold increase in potency. Preclinical studies showed that belatacept did not induce tolerance but did prolong graft survival. In clinical trials, belatacept was initially administered intravenously every 2 weeks, then every 4 or 8 weeks without CNIs. It showed comparable efficacy to CsA, and was associated with superior kidney function and metabolic parameters. Belatacept received FDA approval in 2011 for maintenance immunotherapy in kidney transplantation. In clinical trials, the more intense regimen was associated with more infections and PTLD, and therefore it is not approved for use in EBV-negative patients.

A second costimulatory pathway involves the interaction of CD40 on activated T cells with CD40 ligand (CD154) on APCs. Two humanized anti-CD154 monoclonal antibodies have been used in clinical trials in kidney transplantation and autoimmune diseases, but were associated with thromboembolic events. An alternative approach using monoclonal antibodies to CD40 is currently being tested in transplantation, autoimmune diseases, and lymphomas.

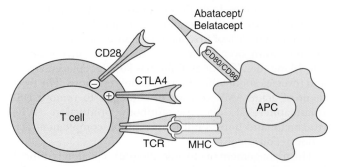

Figure 63.5 Abatacept and belatacept bind to CD80 and CD86 and block costimulation. (From Vincenti F: Costimulation blockade in autoimmunity and transplantation, *J Allergy Clin Immunol* 121:299-306, 2008.)

SMALL MOLECULES

Cytokine receptors are enticing targets for modulation by new small molecules. Janus kinases (JAK) are important cytoplasmic tyrosine kinases involved in cell signaling. Tofacitinib (CP-690550) inhibits JAK3, which is expressed on NK cells, activated T cells, B cells, and myeloid cells. In clinical trials, it was noninferior to tacrolimus in terms of rejection rates and graft survival. It also showed a lower rate of hyperglycemia but a trend toward more infections, including CMV and polyomavirus. Sotrastaurin (AEB071) inhibits multiple protein kinase C isoforms, leading to decreased T cell activation, but it showed poor efficacy in preventing rejection after CNI withdrawal in clinical trials.

TARGETING B CELLS AND HLA ANTIBODY

Most of the advances in transplantation can be attributed to drugs designed to inhibit T cell responses. As a result, T cell–mediated acute rejection has become much less of a problem, whereas B cell responses such as AMR and other effects of DSA have become more evident. Current strategies include B cell depletion, modulation of B cell activation and survival, plasma cell depletion, antibody removal, and inhibition of antibody effector function (Fig. 63.6).

Rituximab (Rituxan), a chimeric monoclonal antibody directed against CD20 on B cells, causes rapid sustained depletion of circulating and lymphoid B cells for over 6 months. Since CD20 is not found on pro-B cells or plasma cells, rituximab does not prevent regeneration of B cells

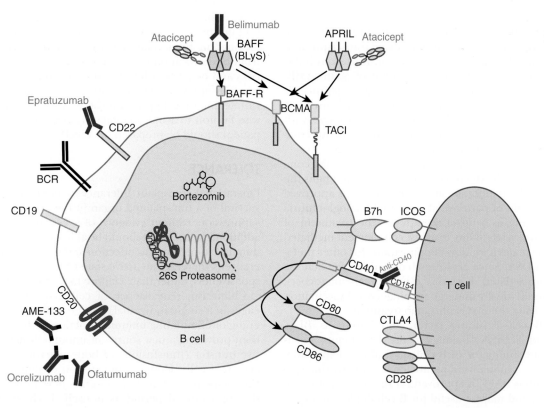

Figure 63.6 Novel strategies targeting humoral alloimmunity. (From Webber A, Hirose R, Vincenti F: Novel strategies in immunosuppression: issues in perspective, *Transplantation* 91:1057-1064, 2011.)

from precursors and does not directly affect immunoglobulin levels, although some studies have reported a reduction in DSA. It has been used pretransplant to reduce high levels of preformed anti-HLA or ABO antibodies, as well as posttransplant to treat acute AMR. It has not yet been rigorously tested in clinical trials. Infusion reactions can occur and are usually prevented by premedication. Rare cases of PML have been associated with its use. Newer fully human and humanized monoclonal anti-CD20 antibodies are currently being tested for the treatment of lymphomas. In early studies, these are less immunogenic, more efficacious, and can overcome rituximab resistance.

IVIG is a preparation of human polyclonal IgG (95%) derived from the pooled plasma of adults. The mechanism of action of high-dose IVIG in immune modulation is complex and involves multiple pathways. It provides antiidiotypic antibodies, reduces the expression and function of Fc receptors on leukocytes and endothelial cells, increases IgG clearance, downregulates the activation and effector function of T and B cells, and inhibits complement activation and cytokine production. IVIG causes a rapid reduction in DSA, and has shown efficacy in clinical trials as part of desensitization strategies. The standard dose is 2 g/kg up to a maximum of 140 g in a single administration infused over 4 to 8 hours. Minor reactions, such as flushing, chills, headache, nausea, myalgia, and arthralgia, are common; these are reduced with premedication and by slowing the infusion rate. Hemolytic anemia, aseptic meningitis, and thrombotic complications are rare. Acute kidney injury, due to osmotic nephrosis from the sucrose or sorbitol vehicle, is usually self-limited.

Bortezomib (Velcade) is a 26S proteasome inhibitor that is approved for the treatment of multiple myeloma. Proteasomal inhibition results in the accumulation of misfolded IgG and causes apoptosis of plasma cells. Bortezomib also reduces NF-κB activity by inhibiting the degradation of IκB, which then leads to reduced transcription of IL-6, a potent plasma cell survival factor. Bortezomib has been used for desensitization, treatment of acute AMR, and in experimental protocols of transplant tolerance. It has been shown to significantly reduce anti-HLA antibody levels. The main toxicity of bortezomib is neurologic, with de novo or worsened peripheral neuropathy being common. Hematologic and GI toxicity can also occur.

Eculizumab (Soliris) is a monoclonal antibody to the complement protein C5, which blocks C5 cleavage and halts the formation of the membrane attack complex. It is approved for the treatment of paroxysmal nocturnal hemoglobinuria and is emerging as a novel therapy for the treatment of acute AMR due to its ability to arrest complement-mediated injury. This creates a window of opportunity for other therapies to clear DSA. Since eculizumab diminishes the defense against encapsulated bacteria, especially meningococci, patients should ideally undergo meningococcal vaccination before receiving the first eculizumab treatment.

BAFF (B cell–activating factor, also known as BLys, TALL-1, and THANK) belongs to the TNF family and is an important stimulator of B cell survival and expansion. Belimumab is a humanized monoclonal antibody that specifically inhibits BAFF, is approved for the treatment of systemic lupus, and may be useful for B cell depletion and to decrease antibody production. Ataticept is a fusion protein formed from TACI, the extracellular domain of one of the receptors for BAFF. It binds BAFF and APRIL (a proliferation inducing ligand), which also promotes B cell and plasma cell survival. Ataticept may be useful in sensitized patients with established plasma cells.

TREATMENT OF REJECTION

Maintenance immunosuppression is effective in preventing acute cellular rejection; however, it is less effective in blocking activated T cells and thus in treating established acute rejection or preventing chronic rejection. After the acute rejection episode has been treated, intensification of the maintenance regimen and closer monitoring are often indicated.

Treatment of acute cellular rejection requires the use of agents directed against activated T cells. These include glucocorticoids in high doses (pulse therapy), polyclonal antilymphocyte antibodies, or muromonab-CD3. Steroids reverse about 75% of first acute rejections, and are typically tapered down over a few weeks to maintenance doses of 5 to 10 mg/day. Thymoglobulin has largely replaced OKT3, and reverses about 90% of severe acute rejections. The treatment of acute AMR consists of strategies to remove DSA (plasmapheresis), decrease antibody production (IVIG, rituximab, and bortezomib), and inhibit complement activation (eculizumab).

The management of chronic allograft rejection is difficult because the histologic changes seen are often irreversible and lead to progression of kidney disease, regardless of the original injury. Intensification of calcineurin inhibition is generally not effective, and some studies have shown benefit with reduction/elimination of the CNI while maintaining or increasing adjunctive therapy. There is the most experience with MMF in these situations, although sirolimus may be an appropriate alternative in the absence of proteinuria. C4d positivity in patients with chronic rejection is a marker for ongoing humoral injury, and these patients may benefit from intensification of immunosuppression and IVIG. The risks and benefits of immunosuppression must be weighed carefully at every stage. If graft function continues to deteriorate, immunosuppression should be withdrawn in a stepwise fashion to avoid precipitating acute rejection, and the patient should be prepared for ESRD.

TOLERANCE

Operational transplant tolerance is defined as prolonged survival of a transplanted organ in the absence of immunosuppression, without evidence of a destructive response. In addition, the recipient should be able to respond normally to immune stimuli such as infection and tumors. Transplant tolerance is therefore an active state of antigen-specific nonresponsiveness, rather than a failure to respond to the allograft.

Chimerism (coexistence of cells from two genetic lineages in a single individual) can be induced by first dampening or eliminating immune function in the recipient and then providing a new source of immune function by adoptive transfer (transfusion) of bone marrow or hematopoietic stem cells. Upon reconstitution of immune function, the recipient no longer recognizes new antigens provided during a critical period as nonself. Early animal studies showed that fetal/neonatal exposure to donor blood cells led to hematopoietic chimerism and specific transplant tolerance. In the pre-cyclosporine era, improved kidney transplant outcomes were seen with donor-specific blood transfusions. These disappeared after the introduction of CsA, presumably due to the efficacy of this drug in blocking T cell activation. It is possible that the effect may have been from cell surface or soluble HLA molecules. Soluble HLA and peptides corresponding to linear sequences of HLA molecules have been shown to induce immunologic tolerance in animal models.

The creation of bone marrow chimeras as a tool for transplant tolerance was first demonstrated when patients who had undergone bone marrow transplantation (BMT) for treatment of hematologic malignancies subsequently underwent successful kidney transplantation for kidney failure from their original BMT donor, without the requirement for maintenance immunosuppression. However, the toxicity of the myeloablative therapy and the risk for lethal graft-versus-host disease (GVHD) precludes this protocol for routine transplantation. Two approaches to reduce toxicity involve the creation of a mixed allogeneic chimera using (a) cytotoxic drugs and thymic irradiation in combination with a limited course of immunosuppression or (b) total lymphoid irradiation (TLI), which targets the thymus, the spleen, and supradiaphragmatic lymph nodes. TLI, compared with total body irradiation, resulted in markedly reduced incidence of GVHD by sparing recipient NK cells, but neither approach has been reliable in achieving durable operational tolerance in HLA-mismatched patients.

One small study has used pretransplant, donor-specific blood transfusion to activate donor-reactive lymphocytes that were then selectively depleted by bortezomib. Initial results are encouraging, but further studies are needed to confirm the potential benefits of this approach. Several combinations of biologics can be envisioned as potentially inducing tolerance. Although preclinical trials of a monoclonal antibody to CD40 ligand (CD40L) with CTLA4Ig were promising, clinical trials were halted due to increased thromboembolic events. The combination of belatacept and anti-CD40 antibody may be useful.

Regulatory T cells (T_{regs}) were found to suppress the rejection response of naive T cells in adoptive transfer assays. T_{regs} express the transcription factor FOXP3 that is responsible for their suppressive functions, whereas activated effector T cells do not stably express FOXP3. Strategies to expand the population of natural and induced T_{regs} are currently being tested.

Operational tolerance in transplantation has not yet been routinely achieved. The development of new agents and improved understanding of transplant immunology are now allowing us to create simplified immunosuppressive regimens with low toxicities that have the potential to improve long-term patient and graft survival.

IMMUNE MONITORING

Current monitoring of kidney transplant recipients consists primarily of serial measurements of kidney function and of immunosuppressive drug levels. These tools have limited sensitivity and specificity for the diagnosis of rejection, which is usually made by kidney biopsy. However, a kidney biopsy is invasive, cannot be used for frequent monitoring, and only identifies an established rejection process.

Biomarkers may serve not only as diagnostic parameters but also as predictive tools that anticipate the subsequent development of subclinical and clinical acute rejection. The identification of biomarkers of immune alloreactivity in blood, urine, and tissue would allow early identification of patients at risk for rejection, optimization of drug regimens, monitoring responses to changes in therapy, and guiding the development of novel therapies. Studies in human kidney recipients suggest unique protein and genetic signatures that may identify biomarkers of injury, as well as potential targets of therapy.

Preformed and de novo anti-HLA antibodies are associated with both acute and chronic AMR and graft loss. Anti-HLA antibodies developed in a third of recipients at 5 years, and about 30% are donor-specific. Serial monitoring of DSA is used mostly in highly sensitized patients, and further studies are needed to identify their cost-effectiveness and clinical utility in broader populations, especially given the limited effect of current therapies on decreasing DSA.

Cell-based assays aim to measure recipient T cell reactivity. The cell-mediated lympholysis (CML) assay primarily measures class I alloreactivity through the direct pathway, whereas the mixed lymphocyte culture (MLC) test recognizes class II differences between the recipient and donor by both direct and indirect recognition pathways. Alloreactive T cells can be measured with flow cytometry-based assays, as well as by using HLA class I and class II tetramers. An enzyme-linked immunosorbent spot assay (ELISPOT) can measure the secretion of cytokines such as γ interferon from T cells after alloantigen stimulation and provides a useful means of assessing the indirect pathway. ELISPOT may identify recipients at risk for acute rejection posttransplant, and further testing is underway to establish its role. The ImmuKnow assay (Cylex) quantifies the amount of intracellular ATP that is released from CD4 T cells in response to a nonspecific mitogenic stimulus. It is less specific, and changes in test values may be more predictive than single time point assessments. Combining gene microarray with tandem mass spectroscopy of RNA and proteins extracted from peripheral blood mononuclear cells has also been reported to correlate with graft interstitial fibrosis and tubular atrophy (IF/TA). These transcripts and proteins are undergoing further validation in larger prospective clinical trials.

Urine proteomics, as well as mRNA isolation, have been proposed as another means of identifying acute rejection, graft IF/TA, and drug toxicity. Urinary mRNA levels of several cytolytic proteins such as granzyme B and perforin have been demonstrated to significantly discriminate acute rejection from stable allograft function or tubular necrosis, and are currently undergoing development in commercial assays.

Microarray analysis and real-time polymerase chain reaction (PCR) of candidate transcripts in allograft tissue obtained from kidney biopsy have demonstrated unique findings in clinical settings such as ischemia-reperfusion injury, stable graft function, acute rejection, subclinical rejection, and polyoma virus infection. Specific transcriptional patterns are currently being identified.

The development of reliable biomarkers is crucial for individualizing therapy aimed at extending allograft survival and improving patient health, particularly when incorporating novel immunosuppressive agents, implementing drug minimization protocols, and selecting patients for transplant tolerance trials.

KEY BIBLIOGRAPHY

Auphan N, DiDonato JA, Rosette C, et al: Immunosuppression by glucocorticoids: Inhibition of NF-κB activity through induction of IκB synthesis, *Science* 270:286-290, 1995.

Boffa DJ, Luan F, Thomas D, et al: Rapamycin inhibits the growth and metastatic progression of non-small cell lung cancer, *Clin Cancer Res* 10:293-300, 2004 Jan 1.

Brennan D, Daller J, Lake K, et al: Rabbit antithymocyte globulin versus basiliximab in renal transplantation, *N Engl J Med* 355:1967-1977, 2006.

Ekberg H, Grinyo J, Nashan B, et al: Cyclosporine sparing with mycophenolate mofetil, daclizumab and corticosteroids in renal allograft recipients: the CAESAR study, *Am J Transplant* 7:560-570, 2007.

Ekberg H, Tedesco-Silva H, Demirbas A, et al: for ELITE-Symphony Study. Reduced exposure to calcineurin inhibitors in renal transplantation, *N Engl J Med* 357:2562-2575, 2007 Dec 20.

Gloor JM, Sethi S, Stegall MD, et al: Transplant glomerulopathy: subclinical incidence and association with alloantibody, *Am J Transplant* 7:2124-2132, 2007.

Halloran PF: Immunosuppressive drugs for kidney transplantation, *N Engl J Med* 351:2715-2729, 2004.

Hanaway MJ, Woodle ES, Mulgaonkar S, et al: for INTAC Study Group-Alemtuzumab induction in renal transplantation, *N Engl J Med* 364:1909-1919, 2011 May 19.

Jordan SC, Vo AA, Peng A, et al: IVIG: a novel approach to improve transplant rates and outcomes in highly HLA-sensitized patients, *Am J Transplant* 6:459-466, 2006.

Knight S, Russell N, Barcena L, et al: Mycophenolate mofetil decreases acute rejection and may improve graft survival in renal transplant recipients when compared with azathioprine: a systematic review, *Transplantation* 87:785-794, 2009.

Li B, Hartono C, Ding R, et al: Noninvasive diagnosis of renal-allograft rejection by measurement of messenger RNA for perforin and granzyme B in urine, *N Engl J Med* 344:947-954, 2001.

Maluccio M, Sharma V, Lagman M, et al: Tacrolimus enhances transforming growth factor-beta1 expression and promotes tumor progression, *Transplantation* 76:597-602, 2003 Aug 15.

Patel R, Terasaki PI: Significance of the positive crossmatch test in kidney transplantation, *N Engl J Med* 280:735-739, 1969.

Scehna F, Pascoe M, Albaru J, et al: Conversion from calcineurin inhibitors to sirolimus maintenance therapy in renal allograft recipients: 24-month efficacy and safety results from the CONVERT trial, *Transplantation* 87:233-242, 2009.

Starzl TE: Immunosuppressive therapy and tolerance of organ allografts, *N Engl J Med* 358:407-411, 2008.

Vincenti F, Kirkman R, Light S, et al: Interleukin-2-receptor blockade with daclizumab to prevent acute rejection in renal transplantation. Daclizumab Triple Therapy Study Group, *N Engl J Med* 338:161-165, 1998.

Vincenti F, Larsen C, Durrbach A, et al: Costimulation blockade with belatacept in renal transplantation, *N Engl J Med* 353:770-781, 2005.

Vincenti F, Larsen CP, Alberu J, et al: Three-year outcomes from BENEFIT, a randomized, active-controlled, parallel-group study in adult kidney transplant recipients, *Am J Transplant* 12:210-217, 2012.

Vincenti F, Schena F, Paraskevas S, et al: for the FREEDOM Study Group. A randomized, multicenter study of steroid avoidance, early steroid withdrawal or standard steroid therapy in kidney transplant recipients, *Am J Transplant* 8:307-316, 2008.

Zachary AA, Montgomery RA, Ratner LE, et al: Specific and durable elimination of antibody to donor HLA antigens in renal transplant patients, *Transplantation* 76:1519-1525, 2003.

Full bibliography can be found on www.expertconsult.com

64

Infectious Complications of Kidney Transplantation

Robin K. Avery

Transplant infectious disease has increasingly evolved toward prevention and early detection of infections in order to prevent full-blown syndromes, which can entail multiorgan involvement and allograft dysfunction. Internationally accepted guidelines from transplant-related organizations now provide recommendations on prophylaxis and treatment for many pathogens, as well as donor and recipient screening, immunizations, and strategies for safer living (Box 64.1). Careful attention to detail can help preserve good health and allograft function for the long term.

IMMUNOSUPPRESSIVE AGENTS AND INFECTIOUS RISK

Although any immunosuppressive regimen carries risk for infection, there are specific risks conferred by particular agents. For example, antilymphocyte therapies such as thymoglobulin (particularly when administered for steroid-refractory rejection) deplete virus-specific cytotoxic T lymphocytes and increase the likelihood of reactivation of cytomegalovirus (CMV) and Epstein-Barr virus (EBV), among others. High doses of steroids affect a variety of aspects of immune function and predispose patients to bacterial, fungal, and viral infections. Sirolimus and everolimus are associated with relatively lower risk for viral infections, but increased risk for bacterial infections, including those associated with slower wound healing.

Rubin described the "net state of immunosuppression" decades ago; this is the concept that the immunosuppressed state of the patient derives from more than exogenously administered medications. The patient's age, underlying kidney disease, comorbidities, metabolic and nutritional factors, impairment of defenses such as skin and mucosal integrity, neutropenia, and other factors all may play a role. Methods of assessing this state of immunosuppression, either global or pathogen-specific, are an area of active research.

De novo posttransplant hypogammaglobulinemia is a recognized complication of immunosuppressive regimens and can increase risk for a variety of infections. Replacement with intravenous immune globulin (IVIG) for patients with extremely low IgG levels (e.g., <400 mg/dL) is a therapy that can aid in defense against infections without precipitating rejection.

TIMETABLE OF POSTTRANSPLANT INFECTIONS

The paradigm of three posttransplant periods of infection risk, articulated by Rubin and modified by Fishman, remains a useful construct. In this model, infections during the first posttransplant month are largely postsurgical, including surgical site infections, postoperative pneumonias, catheter-related infections, and urinary tract infections. Any technical or anatomic issues occurring during or after the transplant operation can predispose to infections (e.g., urinomas, hematomas, lymphoceles). Pretransplant colonization with multiresistant bacteria may lead to invasive infection in the setting of transplant immunosuppression. Also during the first month, reactivation of herpes simplex virus (HSV, usually oropharyngeal and sometimes anogenital) is very common if antiviral prophylaxis is not administered. Most patients who are not on CMV prophylaxis with valganciclovir will require acyclovir or valacyclovir during the first month for HSV prophylaxis. Oropharyngeal candidiasis (thrush) and urinary tract candidiasis are also common during the first month, and many centers administer prophylaxis with either topical or systemic antifungal medications. Finally, preexisting infections in the recipient or donor (unsuspected or partially treated) can appear in an active form in the recipient during this time frame, underscoring the need for a thorough screening of both donor and recipient before transplantation.

During the second time period, classically months 2 through 6 after transplant, the patient is at risk for a variety of opportunistic infections, particularly after intensified immunosuppression for rejection. These include all members of the herpesvirus family, as well as many other viruses, bacteria, fungi, and occasionally parasitic infections. This is the time period in which prophylaxis and monitoring are generally most extensive. In the era of antiviral prophylaxis, some of the infectious risk may be transferred to the time period of months 6 to 12.

In the third, or late, time period, recipients have varying risk depending on how successfully their immunosuppression has been tapered and how much rejection they have experienced. Those on lesser immunosuppressive regimens are less likely to experience opportunistic infections, but can still develop infection with community-acquired respiratory viruses, pneumococcal pneumonia, and urinary tract infections (including transplant pyelonephritis). Those requiring intensified immunosuppression remain at risk for all of the opportunistic pathogens seen during the second period. A third risk group reflects the effects of long-term viruses (hepatitis B or C, BK virus, human papillomavirus, and others). In kidney transplant recipients, BK virus has emerged as especially important because of its effects on long-term allograft function.

This model can help assess the risk for a transplant recipient who is seen in the office or hospital for fever and other symptoms of possible infection. Knowledge of the time posttransplant, prophylaxis, immunosuppression regimen,

575

Box 64.1   Guidelines and Resources in Transplant Infectious Disease

American Society of Transplantation (AST) Infectious Disease Guidelines, 2nd Edition. *American Journal of Transplantation,* Supplement 4, pages S1-S281, 2009. (http://onlinelibrary.wiley.com/doi/10.1111/ajt.2009.9.issue-s4/issuetoc)

Influenza Vaccination in the Organ Transplant Recipient: Review and Summary Recommendations. *American Journal of Transplantation,* October issue, pages 2020-2030, 2011

Kidney Disease in Global Outcomes (KDIGO) Guidelines. *American Journal of Transplantation,* Supplement 3, pages S1-S155, 2009 (http://www.kdigo.org/clinical_practice_guidelines/pdf/TxpGL_publVersion.pdf)

The Transplantation Society (TTS): International Consensus Guidelines on the Management of Cytomegalovirus in Solid Organ Transplantation. *Transplantation,* Volume 89, pages 779-795, 2010

Box 64.2   Donor Serologies and Cultures

For All Potential Deceased Donors

- FDA-licensed HIV-1 and HIV-2 (diagnostic testing not acceptable)
- HBsAg, HBcAb, and anti-HCV
- VDRL or RPR
- Anti-CMV
- EBV serologic testing
- Blood and urine cultures
- Urinalysis before cross clamp

Other Possible Testing for Deceased Donors

- Nucleic acid amplification testing (NAT) for HIV, HBV, HCV (recommendations under revision)
- HSV 1 and 2 IgG
- Toxoplasma IgG
- VZV IgG

Regionally Important Infections

- Chagas disease serology
- Coccidioidomycosis serology
- HTLV I, II serology

Additional Testing for Prospective Living Donors

- NAT testing for HIV, HBV, HCV (recommendations under revision)

From the Organ Procurement and Transplantation Network website Section 2.2.4.1. Available http://optn.transplant.hrsa.gov/Policiesand-Bylaws2/policies/pdfs/policy_2.pdf.

---

rejection history, and environmental exposures can help to limit the vast field of diagnostic possibilities and focus the evaluation.

DONOR-DERIVED INFECTIONS

Both deceased donors and living donors are assessed with a serologic panel, as well as a detailed medical and social history (Box 64.2). The serologic panel may be used in three ways. First, serology results may disqualify the donor, as in human immunodeficiency virus (HIV) seropositivity in the United States at this time. Second, the serology results may identify a subgroup of recipients to whom that donor might be restricted, such as hepatitis C–positive donors and recipients. Third, the serologic panel may influence posttransplant prophylaxis, as with CMV, EBV, and the hepatitis B virus (HBV) core–positive donor. For example, the HBV core-positive donor refers to one who is hepatitis B surface antigen (HBsAg)–negative but hepatitis B core antibody (HBcAb)–positive, usually reflecting past but not active HBV infection (although this can also occasionally reflect the "window period" of early HBV infection, or a false positive test). Whereas the risk for transmission of hepatitis C virus (HCV) from an HCV-seropositive donor to an HCV-seronegative recipient is high, the risk for transmission of HBV from a core-positive donor to an HBV-negative, nonliver recipient is far lower (about 1:30 to 1:60, and can be reduced by pretransplant HBV vaccination and by posttransplant prophylaxis with hepatitis B immune globulin and/or antiviral therapy). HBV core-positive donors are commonly used, with management according to current guidelines.

In addition to the serologic panel, the medical and social histories of the donor are important. High-risk behaviors including sexual promiscuity, injection drug use, and incarceration increase the likelihood that the donor may be harboring viruses such as HIV, HBV, or HCV and may be in the window period before antibody seroconversion. The availability of rapid molecular testing for viral loads of these three viruses (NAT testing) in the deceased donor time frame has changed the landscape, although a debate still exists over whether NAT testing should be confined to donors with high-risk behavior or extended to all donors.

In the United States, recently revised guidelines for living donors are based on a case in which HIV was transmitted from a previously seronegative donor. Since this case, repeat NAT testing within 1 week of anticipated donation is now recommended, along with education of prospective living donors on avoidance of risky behavior that could lead to acquisition of new infections in the period before donation.

Preexisting active infections may also be present in the donor; these may or may not be recognized at the time of organ harvest (e.g., bacteremias, pneumonias, viral encephalitis). For bacterial infections, many but not all these cases can be managed by pathogen-specific posttransplant antibacterial therapy. Blood cultures obtained from the donor that turn positive after transplantation should prompt consideration of prolonged antimicrobial therapy in the recipient, both to prevent sepsis and also mycotic aneurysms at vascular anastomotic sites. The presence of multidrug-resistant organisms in donor cultures should prompt extreme caution, since much of the literature validating the use of bacterially infected donors has involved community organisms such as *Pneumococcus* without multidrug resistance. Although donors with bacterial meningitis with community organisms are often acceptable, transplant clinicians should beware of possible viral infections of the central nervous system, which could include such untreatable infections as rabies, West Nile virus, and lymphocytic choriomeningitis virus. Encephalitis, meningitis, or other central nervous system infection without a definite positive bacterial culture should prompt rejection of the proposed donor. Finally, *Candida* species in the preservation fluid of the donor kidney can be associated with adverse outcomes such as fungal mycotic aneurysms at anastomotic sites and should thus be taken seriously and treated.

BACTERIAL INFECTIONS

As discussed previously, postsurgical infections with "conventional" bacteria are most common in the first month after transplantation (Box 64.3). Although bacteria such as *Staphylococcus aureus* or enteric gram-negative bacilli remain common pathogens in this setting, increasing numbers of multidrug-resistant bacterial isolates are being seen (e.g., vancomycin-resistant enterococci (VRE), ciprofloxacin-resistant *E. coli*, extended-spectrum beta-lactamase (ESBL) producing *E. coli* and *Klebsiella*, carbapenem-resistant *Klebsiella*, carbapenem-resistant *Acinetobacter*, multidrug-resistant *Pseudomonas*). Management of these infections is a challenge, reflecting both the tenacity of the pathogens and the nephrotoxicity of many of the agents used to treat them (e.g., amikacin and intravenous colistin). Risk factors for such infections include extended ICU and hospital stays, prolonged mechanical ventilation, postoperative bleeding and reoperations, extensive prior antibiotic use, and pretransplant colonization.

Transplant pyelonephritis is very common, especially in the first few months posttransplant. Enteric gram-negative bacilli and *Enterococcus* are frequently encountered. The hallmark of these infections is usually fever and chills; additionally, tenderness over the allograft and elevation of the serum creatinine (SCr) may be present, while voiding symptoms such as dysuria may be absent. At times, fever and chills may occur without any localizing signs. Protracted therapy (4 to 6 weeks of antibiotics) may be required to eradicate the kidney tissue focus. In this current era, gram-negative bacilli resistant to both sulfa and quinolones (e.g., ciprofloxacin) are common. Oral therapy with a quinolone can no longer be assumed to cover the organisms involved, and microbiologic identification with antimicrobial susceptibility testing is essential.

With so many reasons for administering antibiotics, it is not surprising that *Clostridium difficile* is common posttransplant, particularly since the introduction of the epidemic strain in 2005. *C. difficile*–associated diarrhea often manifests with severe frequent watery diarrhea and abdominal cramps. More ominous, however, is the presentation with abdominal distention and without diarrhea, since ileus and toxic megacolon can occur. Fever, elevated leukocyte count, abdominal distention, and ileus should prompt emergent evaluation and treatment for possible *C. difficile*.

Foodborne infections, such as salmonellosis, shigellosis, and listeriosis, may be more severe in transplant recipients than in others. In particular, *Listeria* can be transmitted by a wide variety of foods, including nonpasteurized dairy foods, soft cheese, deli meats, hot dogs, salmon, and many others. Meningitis, bacteremia, and rarely brainstem encephalitis can result.

Nocardia species can cause pulmonary nodular infiltrates and intracerebral abscesses, as well as localization in soft tissue and other organs. *Rhodococcus* can cause pulmonary nodules, especially in those exposed to farms and horses. Both of these bacterial organisms are more common, as in the case of fungal infections, in transplant recipients with extensive outdoor and environmental exposures such as gardening and farming.

Box 64.3 Bacterial Organisms Commonly Causing Infection in Transplant Recipients

Gram-Positive

- *Staphylococcus aureus,* including MRSA
- Coagulase-negative staphylococci
- *Enterococcus* spp (including VRE)
- *Streptococcus* spp
- *Nocardia* spp
- *Listeria monocytogenes*
- *Clostridium difficile*

Gram-Negative

Enteric gram-negative bacilli

- *E. coli* (including ESBL-producing isolates)
- *Klebsiella pneumoniae* and *K. oxytoca* (including ESBL-producing and carbapenemase-producing isolates)
- *Proteus, Providencia, Morganella* spp
- *Serratia marsescens*
- *Enterobacter* spp

Gastroenteritis pathogens

- *Salmonella, Shigella, Campylobacter, Vibrio* spp.

Nonenteric gram-negative bacilli

- *Pseudomonas aeruginosa*
- *Acinetobacter baumanii* (including carbapenemase-producing isolates)
- *Stenotrophomonas maltophilia*

Anaerobic gram-negative bacilli

- *Bacteroides* spp.

Mycobacteria

- *Mycobacterium tuberculosis*
- *M. avium* complex (MAC)
- *M. abscessus, M. chelonae, M. fortuitum* (rapid-growers)

Bacterial pneumonias may be community-acquired pneumonia (CAP), healthcare-associated pneumonia (HAP), and/or ventilator-associated pneumonia (VAP), with pathogens seen in other immunocompromised patients. Legionellosis deserves special mention because it may be severe, multilobar, and hard to diagnose (especially non–*Legionella pneumophila* species). The urine antigen test detects only *L. pneumophila* type 1, so *Legionella* pneumonia should be considered in any patient with unexplained pulmonary infiltrates, even despite negative initial cultures and *Legionella* urinary antigen testing. Hospital water systems, as well as domiciliary exposures, may lead to *Legionella* pneumonia.

Mycobacterial infections may occur after kidney transplantation in a localized (primarily pulmonary) or disseminated pattern. Tuberculosis (TB) is more likely to be military (disseminated) posttransplant, and it results most commonly from reactivation in the recipient. Donor-derived cases account for a small portion. Screening for latent TB infection (LTBI) in all transplant candidates is recommended, with consideration given to isoniazid prophylaxis for 9 months for those who screen positive but do not have evidence of active tuberculosis. Either the tuberculin skin test (TST) or the more recent interferon-gamma release assay (IGRA) may be used, although false negative results can occur in patients with impaired cellular immune function. LTBI prophylaxis may be completed before transplant, or may be commenced pretransplant and completed posttransplant. In some highly endemic areas, approaches may vary.

Nontuberculous mycobacterial infections (*Mycobacterium avium-intracellulare, M. fortuitum, M. chelonae, M. abscessus,* and others) may occur in patients with outdoor exposures, chronic lung disease, exposure to water sources such as hot tubs or jacuzzis, and/or intensive immunosuppression. Pulmonary nodular infiltrates with or without cavitation are the most common manifestation. Skin and soft tissue infections or occasionally surgical site infections may occur, particularly with rapid-grower mycobacterial species. Disseminated infection may present with fever, pancytopenia, elevated liver function tests, and/or pulmonary infiltrates. Diagnosis may be difficult because mycobacteria (except the rapid-growers) do not grow on routine bacterial culture media. Bronchoalveolar lavage, mycobacterial blood cultures, bone marrow biopsy, or liver biopsy may be necessary to make this diagnosis. If tissue is obtained, it should be sent for stains and cultures for mycobacteria, fungi, and other pathogens. Therapy is typically long (more than 6 months and often longer than 12 to 18 months) and involves combination therapy; toxicity of the agents may be an issue. Thus it is important to make a microbiologic diagnosis.

VIRAL INFECTIONS

CYTOMEGALOVIRUS

Cytomegalovirus remains one of the most important transplant-associated pathogens, although both prophylaxis and preemptive therapy have reduced its severity and incidence. Approximately two thirds to three fourths of the adult population is CMV seropositive, including most donors. CMV infection can occur through reactivation of CMV in the recipient, or by acquisition of the donor strain of CMV. Clinical manifestations include asymptomatic viremia, CMV syndrome (a flulike illness with fever, chills, myalgias, and often leukopenia, thrombocytopenia, and mild elevations of liver function tests), and tissue-invasive disease in which CMV can be found on histopathology or immunostaining of tissue (e.g., esophagitis, gastritis, colitis, pneumonitis, hepatitis). Occasionally, CMV meningoencephalitis or retinitis may also occur. The aforementioned categories of CMV infection, in order of increasing severity, roughly correspond with the blood viral load as detected by quantitative CMV polymerase chain reaction (PCR) or pp65 antigenemia. The highest viral loads are usually seen in patients with tissue-invasive CMV, although exceptions can occur, particularly in the gastrointestinal tract. In addition to these direct infectious consequences, CMV can also predispose to fungal and other opportunistic infections, as well as to allograft dysfunction. With any CMV prevention strategy, it is important to observe the direct and indirect consequences.

Major risk factors for CMV infection include the donor-seropositive (D+)/recipient-seronegative (R−) scenario in which the recipient has no preexisting anti-CMV immunity but acquires CMV from the donor. D+/R− patients often have the highest viral loads, risk for tissue-invasive disease, recurrences of CMV viremia, and ganciclovir resistance.

Table 64.1 CMV Prevention Recommendations*

Organ/Group	Recommendation/Options (see text for dose, evidence rating, and special pediatric issues)
Kidney, liver, pancreas, heart	• Prophylaxis: valganciclovir, oral ganciclovir, or intravenous ganciclovir (or valacyclovir in kidney) for 3 to 6 months. Some centers add CMV immune globulin for heart transplant.
D+/R−	• Preemptive therapy an option (see Figure 1). Many authorities prefer to use prophylaxis and reserve preemptive therapy for lower-risk populations (see text).
Kidney, liver, pancreas, heart	• Valganciclovir, oral ganciclovir, intravenous ganciclovir or valacyclovir (kidney) for 3 months. Some centers add CMV immune globulin for heart transplant *OR*
R+	• Pre-emptive therapy an option (see Figure 1).
Lung, heart-lung	• For D+/R− patients valganciclovir or intravenous ganciclovir for 6 months. Some centres will prolong prophylaxis beyond 6 months.
D+/R−, R+	• For R+ patients, valganciclovir, oral ganciclovir or intravenous ganciclovir for 3–6 months. • Some centers will add CMV immune globulin especially for D+/R−.

From Humar A, Snydman D: Cytomegalovirus in solid organ transplant recipients, Am J Transplant *Suppl 4:S81, 2009.*
*These guidelines do not represent an exclusive course of action. Several factors may influence the precise nature and duration of prophylaxis or preemptive therapy.

However, other patients (D+/R+, D−/R+) can also develop severe CMV infection, particularly after intensified immunosuppression. Treatment for rejection should prompt resumption of prophylaxis and/or viral load monitoring in order to treat CMV reactivation rapidly. Those who are both donor- and recipient-seronegative (D−/R−) are at low risk, but can acquire CMV through transfusions (which should be leukopore-filtered or CMV-screened), community exposures, or when the donor test is falsely negative.

Strategies for CMV prevention are divided into two main categories: prophylaxis and preemptive therapy. Prophylaxis refers to the administration of antiviral therapy to all patients at risk for CMV, whereas preemptive therapy refers to administration of antiviral therapy only to those who develop evidence of CMV infection on a sensitive early-detection test such as the CMV PCR or pp65 antigenemia assay (Table 64.1). Metaanalyses have demonstrated the efficacy of prophylaxis to prevent allograft dysfunction, as well as direct CMV effects and indirect effects, such as fungal and other opportunistic infections. Preemptive therapy can be logistically challenging and labor intensive for transplant coordinators, because all results must be received and acted on in a timely fashion. On the other hand, proponents of preemptive therapy cite advantages such as less cost, less toxicity, and possibly earlier reconstitution of CMV-specific immunity as reasons for choosing this strategy. Prophylaxis also carries the risk for "late CMV" occurring after discontinuation. Most centers use either prophylaxis, preemptive therapy, or a combination, but prophylaxis is often recommended for the high-risk D+/R− group. The IMPACT study has demonstrated benefits in CMV outcomes using a 6-month duration as compared with a 3-month duration of valganciclovir prophylaxis in D+/R− kidney transplant recipients.

EPSTEIN-BARR VIRUS AND POSTTRANSPLANT LYMPHOPROLIFERATIVE DISORDER

Epstein-Barr virus seropositivity is even more common in the adult population (>90%) than CMV. Reactivation of EBV can occur under the influence of immunosuppression, or it can be acquired from the donor in the case of an EBV D+/R− transplant. When the cellular immune system is unable to inhibit the proliferation of EBV-infected lymphocytes, a polyclonal lymphoproliferative process can occur that ultimately may progress to a monoclonal process, usually B cell lymphoma. This process has a histopathologic spectrum and is known as posttransplant lymphoproliferative disorder (PTLD). Risk factors for PTLD include EBV D+/R− status, intensified immunosuppression for rejection, younger age (children are more likely to be EBV-seronegative), and certain types of organ transplants such as intestinal and lung transplants (which involve transfer of lymphoid tissue).

The incidence of PTLD is biphasic, with one peak in the first 6 months posttransplant, often related to EBV, and a later peak some years posttransplant, occasionally unrelated to EBV. Clinical presentations of PTLD are varied and can involve the lungs, GI tract, liver, spleen, lymph nodes, bone marrow, central nervous system (CNS), and the allograft. Isolated presentation in the CNS can occur. For EBV-related PTLD, peripheral blood EBV DNA viral loads are often high. Tissue biopsy is important in the diagnosis of PTLD; in addition to characteristic histopathology, EBV in situ hybridization can help establish the diagnosis. Treatment of PTLD has been improved by the advent of rituximab (or rituximab plus combination chemotherapy). Reduction of immunosuppression is important and may result in regression of early PTLD without any other therapies. Surgery and radiation may be employed for certain cases of localized disease.

POLYOMAVIRUSES

Polyomaviruses (especially BK virus, or BKV) are particularly important in kidney and kidney-pancreas recipients because of implications for long-term kidney allograft dysfunction. JC virus, the agent of progressive multifocal encephalopathy, can also cause adverse effects, although less frequently than BKV. BKV causes an interstitial nephritis that is silent (generally no systemic symptoms) but gradually leads to replacement of kidney allograft tissue with fibrosis. In earlier years, BKV interstitial nephritis was sometimes confused with rejection and treated with enhanced immunosuppression, thus exacerbating BKV allograft nephropathy (BKVAN). If no preventive measures are taken, between 4% to 8% of all kidney allografts may be lost to BKV.

One of the most important advances in BKV control has been the introduction of routine screening of blood and urine, generally with quantitative molecular testing at intervals during the first year. When BKV levels are detected above a particular threshold, reduction of immunosuppression is employed with regression of BKV viremia in many cases, although it may take months to clear. In cases in which BKV viremia appears refractory to immunosuppression reduction, several therapies have been employed, including leflunomide, cidofovir, IVIG, and quinolones. The optimal therapy and timing of treatment have yet to be defined. However, in the screening era, BKV-associated graft loss has decreased up to eightfold. In the future, measurement of BKV-specific cellular immunity will likely be more widely available.

OTHER VIRUSES

Other viruses important in transplantation include other members of the herpesvirus family (herpes simplex virus, varicella-zoster virus, and human herpesvirus 6, 7, and 8), parvovirus, adenovirus, respiratory viruses, and gastrointestinal viruses such as Norwalk. Herpes simplex virus (HSV) reactivates most frequently during the first month posttransplant or at times of increased immunosuppression, and it can cause painful oroesophageal or anogenital ulcerations. Rarely, visceral disease such as HSV hepatitis or encephalitis can occur. Varicella-zoster virus (VZV) reactivation can cause either dermatomal or disseminated zoster, depending on the degree of immunosuppression. Primary varicella posttransplant is associated with significant morbidity and mortality. Human herpesvirus 6 and 7 may reactivate and cause pneumonitis, hepatitis, meningoencephalitis, and pancytopenia. Adults are commonly IgG seropositive, so a blood PCR is necessary for diagnosis. Finally, human herpesvirus 8 can occasionally reactivate in the form of Kaposi sarcoma.

Parvovirus is associated with severe anemia in the absence of bleeding, with bone marrow biopsy demonstrating an abnormal appearance of erythroid progenitor cells. Diagnosis is best made by blood PCR or bone marrow examination rather than serologic testing, and treatment is with intravenous immunoglobulin. Adenovirus can cause nephritis and fever, with hematuria and kidney dysfunction. Treatment with cidofovir has been used in some cases.

Respiratory viruses are a seasonal threat and may lead to diffuse pulmonary infiltrates and hypoxemia in highly immunosuppressed patients. Influenza, parainfluenza, respiratory syncytial virus (RSV), adenovirus, and metapneumovirus are among those that may have severe consequences. Avoidance of exposures is crucial, particularly during winter and early spring months. Yearly influenza vaccination is recommended for transplant candidates and recipients, as well as family members and health care providers, although immunization in the early posttransplant months may be less effective (see later).

Gastrointestinal viruses can cause chronic diarrhea in immunosuppressed populations. In particular, Norwalk virus (norovirus), which is well known for causing community outbreaks and mass diarrhea on cruise ships, may result in a long-lasting diarrheal syndrome in kidney transplant recipients rather than the short-lived illness usually seen in healthy individuals.

FUNGAL INFECTIONS

In addition to *Candida* species mentioned earlier, fungal infections posttransplant may include molds (e.g., aspergillosis, mucormycosis), cryptococcosis, endemic mycoses such as histoplasmosis and coccidioidomycosis, and *Pneumocystis jiroveci* pneumonia (PJP, formerly known as *P. carinii* pneumonia).

Regarding mold infections, kidney recipients are at a lower risk than lung recipients whose allograft is exposed to the external environment, but such infections may occur in the setting of enhanced immunosuppression or intense environmental exposures. Routine prophylaxis with mold-active antifungals is not generally employed in kidney transplant patients unless a special level of risk is identified. Patients who are gardeners, farmers, landscapers, marijuana smokers, or construction workers may have more extensive fungal spore exposure than others, and can be colonized before transplantation, placing them at risk for posttransplant reactivation. Mold infections most commonly present in the lungs or sinuses, reflecting areas of initial colonization, but may be widespread, including the CNS, skin, soft tissue, and other sites. The availability of newer azole antifungals such as voriconazole and posaconazole has improved the treatment of invasive mold infections, but these are still associated with high mortality. Immunosuppressant dose modification is necessary for patients receiving calcineurin inhibitors and requiring azole treatment due to inhibition of the cytochrome p450 system. Prevention through avoiding exposures is preferable by far.

Cryptococcus is a yeast associated with birds, bird droppings, and soil exposures. Cryptococcus most commonly causes meningitis, but can also be associated with pulmonary nodules, infection of abdominal ascites, cellulitis, undifferentiated fever, and many other presentations. Treatment of cryptococcosis may be associated with an immune reconstitution inflammatory syndrome (IRIS), in which manifestations of disease are transiently enhanced after cultures have turned negative.

Endemic mycoses, such as histoplasmosis in the American Midwest and coccidioidomycosis in the American Southwest, may reactivate after transplant. These endemic mycoses may also be donor-derived. Evidence of remote histoplasmosis in the form of calcified granulomata in the lungs and spleen is common in individuals residing in the Midwest, especially those with farming or other significant outdoor exposure. No specific prophylaxis is recommended, but individuals in endemic areas with serologic evidence or clinical history of coccidioidomycosis may require long-term prophylaxis with azole antifungals to avoid reactivation.

P. jiroveci pneumonia is now classified among fungal infections. Risk for PJP is highest during the first 6 to 12 months posttransplant and at times of enhanced immunosuppression. PJP can be a clinically devastating pneumonia, leading to pneumothoraces and long-term loss of lung function, with a protracted recovery period and debilitation. All individuals without allergies to sulfa should receive prophylaxis with trimethoprim-sulfamethoxazole for at least 6 months posttransplant, although some centers prefer 1 year or longer. Trimethoprim-sulfamethoxazole also provides some preventive activity against *Nocardia*, *Toxoplasma*, and *Listeria*. For sulfa-allergic patients, dapsone, aerosolized pentamidine, or atovaquone are alternatives. For patients taking dapsone, a G6PD screen must first be performed to avoid a hemolytic reaction.

PARASITIC INFECTIONS

Strongyloides is a parasite of worldwide distribution that can remain dormant for many years in the intestine, and then

Box 64.4   Summary of Immunizations Recommended for Adult Transplant Candidates and Recipients

Immunizations Recommended for Adult Pretransplant Candidates

- Yearly influenza vaccine (injected, nonlive)
- Pneumococcal polysaccharide vaccine (PSV-23), if not given within 5 years
- Tdap (tetanus-diphtheria-acellular pertussis), if not given within 10 years
- Hepatitis A vaccine series, if seronegative
- Hepatitis B vaccine series, if seronegative (consider enhanced-potency preparation)
- Varicella vaccine, if varicella-seronegative, not on immunosuppression, and more than 4 weeks from anticipated date of transplant
- Consider zoster vaccine according to current age eligibility guidelines, if not on immunosuppression, and more than 4 weeks from anticipated date of transplant
- Consider HPV vaccine according to current age eligibility guidelines

Immunizations Recommended for Adult Posttransplant Recipients

- Yearly influenza vaccine (injected, nonlive; more than 3 months posttransplant according to current guidelines, but this waiting period may be waived in an active influenza outbreak)
- Pneumococcal polysaccharide vaccine (PSV-23), if not given within 5 years
- Tdap (tetanus-diphtheria-acellular pertussis), if not given within 10 years
- Complete hepatitis A vaccine series and hepatitis B vaccine series, if not completed and if still seronegative
- No live vaccines
- For travel-specific vaccines and prophylaxis, visit a travel clinic at least 2 months in advance

*See guidelines listed in Box 64.1 for more details and pediatric recommendations.

cause a devastating syndrome of disseminated strongyloidiasis posttransplant. Individuals who have resided in tropical countries or the southeastern United States are frequently screened pretransplant with *Strongyloides* IgG serology, and treated with ivermectin preemptively if seropositive. Chagas disease (*Trypanosoma cruzi*) is a risk for both recipient reactivation and, occasionally, donor-derived infection in patients (or donors) from endemic areas of Central and South America. PCR monitoring can be helpful in long-term management of patients at risk.

IMMUNIZATIONS AND INFECTION PREVENTION

Recommended vaccinations are highlighted in Box 64.4. The reader is referred to the guidelines listed in Box 64.1 for full details (e.g., the AST Infectious Disease Guidelines contain sections on immunization and on strategies for safer living). The pretransplant evaluation is an important time to update immunizations in adults, including yearly influenza (injected form), pneumococcal, tetanus-diphtheria-acellular pertussis (Tdap), and hepatitis A and B vaccines. All of the aforementioned vaccines are nonlive and may be administered posttransplant, although their efficacy is likely greater in the pretransplant period. Yearly influenza vaccine (injected, nonlive) should be administered posttransplant to all recipients, with the exception of waiting until after 3 months posttransplant to maximize the likelihood of seroconversion. This requirement of waiting until 3 months posttransplant can be waived in the event of an active influenza outbreak.

Live vaccines are not currently recommended posttransplant, although a few pediatric studies have suggested safety in some patients. Varicella and zoster vaccines are live-attenuated vaccines. Varicella-seronegative transplant candidates should receive varicella vaccine if they are not on immunosuppression and not anticipated to receive a transplant within 4 weeks. Similarly, zoster vaccine can be given to patients who are 50 years or older if they are not on immunosuppression and not anticipated to receive a transplant within 4 weeks.

When the recipient has recovered enough to contemplate international travel, he or she should be referred to a specialized travel clinic for additional vaccines and/or malaria prophylaxis, destination-specific advice, and education regarding food and water precautions. Other advice regarding pets, community exposures, and outdoor exposures can be found in current guidelines, and this information should be shared with transplant candidates and recipients.

Although kidney and kidney-pancreas transplant recipients remain at risk for many infections, modern molecular diagnostic assays, along with highly developed strategies for prevention and monitoring, have improved the outlook from the infection perspective. Careful modulation of immunosuppression, timely immunizations, and avoidance of certain environmental exposures can be extremely helpful. In the future, more sophisticated understanding of risk factors, including polymorphisms of immune system function and testing for pathogen-specific immune responses, will help to guide individualized therapies.

BIBLIOGRAPHY

Asberg A, Humar A, Rollag H, et al: Oral valganciclovir is noninferior to intravenous ganciclovir for the treatment of cytomegalovirus disease in solid organ transplant recipients, *Am J Transplant* 7:2106-2113, 2007.

Braun WE, Avery R, Gifford RW Jr, et al: Life after 20 years with a kidney transplant: redefined disease profiles and an emerging nondiabetic vasculopathy, *Transplant Proc* 29:247-249, 1997.

Fishman JA, Rubin RH: Infection in organ-transplant recipients, *N Engl J Med* 338:1741-1751, 1998.

Hirsch HH, Brennan DC, Drachenberg CB, et al: Polyomavirus-associated nephropathy in renal transplantation: interdisciplinary analyses and recommendations, *Transplantation* 79:1277-1286, 2005.

Humar A, Lebranchu Y, Vincenti F, et al: The efficacy and safety of 200 days valganciclovir cytomegalovirus prophylaxis in high-risk kidney transplant recipients, *Am J Transplant* 10:1228-1237, 2010.

Humar A, Michaels M: American Society of Transplantation recommendations for screening, monitoring, and reporting of infectious complications in immunosuppression trials in recipients of organ transplantation, *Am J Transplant* 6:262-274, 2006.

Humar A, Snydman D: Cytomegalovirus in solid organ transplant recipients, *Am J Transplant* (Suppl 4):S78-S86, 2009.

Mawhorter S, Yamani MH: Hypogammaglobulinemia and infection risk in solid organ transplant recipients, *Curr Opin Organ Transplant* 13:581-585, 2008.

Singh N: Late-onset cytomegalovirus disease as a significant complication in solid organ transplant recipients receiving antiviral prophylaxis: a call to heed the mounting evidence, *Clin Infect Dis* 40:704-708, 2005.

HYPERTENSION

65 Pathogenesis of Hypertension

Christopher S. Wilcox

Hypertension implies an increase in either cardiac output or total peripheral resistance (TPR). Essential hypertension developing in young adults may be initiated by an increase in cardiac output, associated with signs of overactivity of the sympathetic nervous system; the blood pressure (BP) is labile, and the heart rate is increased. Later, the BP increases further because of a rise in TPR, with consequent return to a normal cardiac output. Most patients in clinical practice with sustained hypertension have an elevated TPR accompanied by constriction of resistance vessels. Through time, vascular remodeling contributes a structural component to vasoconstriction.

The abrupt left ventricular systole creates a shock wave that is reflected back from the peripheral resistance vessels and reaches the ascending aorta during early diastole. It is often visible in younger subjects as the dicrotic notch in tracings of aortic pressure. With aging, there is loss of elasticity and an increase in the tone of the resistance vessels. The pressure wave is transmitted more rapidly within the arterial tree. Eventually, this shock wave in the aorta coincides with the upstroke of the aortic systolic pressure wave, leading to an abrupt increase in the height of the systolic BP. This largely accounts for the frequent finding of isolated, or predominant, systolic hypertension in the elderly. In contrast, systolic hypertension in the young usually reflects an enhanced cardiac contractility and output.

PATHOPHYSIOLOGY OF HYPERTENSION

INTEGRATION OF CARDIORENAL FUNCTION

The integration of cardiorenal function is illustrated by the response of a normal person to standing. There is an abrupt fall in venous return and hence in cardiac output that elicits a baroreflex response, as resistance vessels contract to buffer the immediate fall in BP, and capacitance vessels contract to restore venous return. The outcome is only a small drop in the systolic BP, with a modest rise in diastolic BP and heart rate. During prolonged standing, increased renal sympathetic nerve activity enhances the reabsorption of sodium chloride (NaCl) and fluid by the renal tubules, as well as the release of renin from the juxtaglomerular apparatus. Renin release results in the subsequent generation of angiotensin II and aldosterone, which maintain the BP and the volume of the circulation. In contrast, the BP of patients with autonomic insufficiency declines progressively on standing, sometimes to the point of syncope. These patients with autonomic failure illustrate vividly the crucial importance of a stable BP for efficient function of the brain, heart, and kidneys. Therefore, it is no surprise that evolution has provided multiple, coordinated BP-regulatory processes. The understanding of the cause for a sustained change in BP, such as hypertension, requires knowledge of a number of interrelated pathophysiologic processes. The most important and best understood of these are discussed in this chapter.

RENAL MECHANISMS AND SALT BALANCE

The kidney has a unique role in BP regulation. Renal salt and water retention sufficient to increase the extracellular fluid (ECF) volume, blood volume, and mean circulatory filling pressure enhances venous return, cardiac output, and BP. The kidney is so effective in excreting excess NaCl and fluid during periods of surfeit, or retaining them during periods of deficit, that the ECF and blood volumes normally vary less than 10% with changes in salt intake. Consequently, the role of body fluids in hypertension is subtle. For example, a tenfold increase in daily NaCl intake in normal subjects increases ECF volume by only about 1 L (about 6%) and normally produces no change, or only a small increase, in BP. Conversely, a diet with no salt content leads to the loss of approximately 1 L of body fluid over 3 to 5 days and only a trivial fall in BP. Different effects can be seen in patients with chronic kidney disease (CKD) whose BP often increases with the level of salt intake. This "salt-sensitive" component to BP increases progressively with loss of kidney function in patients with vascular or glomerular kidney disease. Among normotensive subjects, a salt-sensitive component to BP is apparent in about 30% and appears to have a genetic component. Salt sensitivity is almost twice as frequent in patients with hypertension, and is particularly common among African Americans, the elderly, and those with CKD. It is generally associated with a lower level of plasma renin activity (PRA).

What underlies salt sensitivity? The normal kidneys are exquisitely sensitive to BP. A rise in mean arterial pressure (MAP) of as little as 1 to 3 mm Hg elicits a subtle increase in renal NaCl and fluid elimination. This "pressure natriuresis" also works in reverse and conserves NaCl and fluid during decreases in BP. It is rapid, quantitative, and fundamental for normal homeostasis. It is primarily a result of changes in tubular NaCl reabsorption rather than total renal blood flow (RBF) or glomerular filtration rate (GFR). Indeed, renal autoregulation maintains RBF and GFR remarkably constant during modest changes in BP. The pressure natriuresis mechanism accurately adjusts salt excretion and body fluids in persons with healthy kidneys across a range of BPs.

Two primary mechanisms of pressure natriuresis have been identified.

First, in some studies in rats, a rise in renal perfusion pressure increases blood flow selectively through the medulla, which is not as tightly autoregulated as cortical blood flow. This increase in pressure and flow enhances renal interstitial hydraulic pressure throughout the kidney, which reduces proximal tubule reabsorption and impairs fluid return to the bloodstream. Therefore, net NaCl and fluid reabsorption is diminished. Second, the degree of stretch of the afferent arteriole regulates the secretion of renin into the bloodstream and hence the generation of angiotensin II. Therefore, an increase in BP that is transmitted to this site reduces renin secretion. Angiotensin II coordinates the body's salt and fluid retention mechanisms by stimulating thirst and enhancing NaCl and fluid reabsorption in the proximal and distal nephron segments. By stimulating secretion of aldosterone and arginine vasopressin, and inhibiting atrial natriuretic peptide (ANP), angiotensin II further enhances reabsorption in the distal tubules and collecting ducts. Thus, during normal homeostasis, an increase in BP is matched by a decrease in PRA. It follows that a normal or elevated value for PRA in hypertension is effectively "inappropriate" for the level of BP, and is thereby contributing to the maintenance of hypertension.

The relationships between long-term changes in salt intake, the renin-angiotensin-aldosterone system (RAAS), and BP are shown in Figure 65.1. Normal human subjects regulate the RAAS closely with changes in salt intake. An increase in salt intake brings about only a modest and transient rise in MAP, because the RAAS is suppressed and the highly effective pressure natriuresis mechanism rapidly increases renal NaCl and fluid elimination sufficiently to restore a normal blood volume and BP. Expressed quantitatively in Figure 65.1, the slope of the long-term increase in NaCl excretion with BP is almost vertical. One factor contributing to the steepness of this slope, or the gain of the pressure natriuresis relationship, is the reciprocal changes in the RAAS with BP that dictate appropriate alterations in

salt handling by the kidney. Therefore, when the RAAS is artificially fixed, the slope of the pressure natriuresis relationship flattens resulting in salt sensitivity, displacement of the set point, and a change in ambient BP. For example, an infusion of angiotensin II into a normal subject raises the BP. Because angiotensin II is being infused, the kidney cannot suppress angiotensin II levels appropriately by reducing renin secretion. Therefore, the pressure natriuresis mechanism is prevented, and the BP elevation is sustained without an effective and complete renal compensation. In contrast, normal subjects treated with an angiotensin-converting enzyme (ACE) inhibitor to block angiotensin II generation or an angiotensin receptor blocker (ARB) to block AT_1 receptors have a fall in BP. Again, the kidney cannot stimulate an appropriate effect of angiotensin II and aldosterone that would be required to retain sufficient NaCl and fluid to buffer the fall in BP. Therefore, when the RAAS is fixed, the BP changes as a function of salt intake and becomes highly "salt sensitive" (see Fig. 65.1). These studies demonstrate the unique role of the RAAS in long-term BP regulation and its importance in isolating BP from NaCl intake.

Some recent findings add complexity to these simple relationships. Renin is also generated within the connecting tubule and collecting ducts. This renal renin may contribute to the very high level of angiotensin within the kidney that does not share the same relationship with dietary salt. Animal models of diabetes mellitus demonstrate an increase in local angiotensin generation and action in the kidneys that may contribute to the beneficial effects of ACE inhibitor and ARB therapy despite low circulating renin levels. Other studies have shown that prorenin, although not itself active, becomes activated after binding to a renin receptor in the tissues where novel signaling adds another component to the effects of the RAAS. This is important, because conventional RAAS antagonists may not block these actions. It is generally considered that the novel renin inhibitors do not block this renin receptor.

Four compelling lines of evidence implicate the kidney and RAAS in long-term BP regulation. First, kidney transplantation studies in rats showed that a normotensive animal

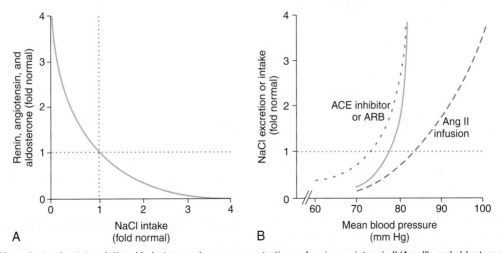

Figure 65.1 A, Normal, steady-state relationship between plasma concentrations of renin, angiotensin II (Ang II), and aldosterone and dietary salt intake. B, Relationships between sodium excretion relative to intake and mean arterial blood pressure in normal subjects (solid line), in subjects given an angiotensin-converting enzyme (ACE) inhibitor or angiotensin receptor blocker (ARB) (short dashes), and in subjects given an infusion of Ang II (long dashes) to prevent adaptive changes in Ang II levels. (Modified from Guyton AC, Hall JE, Coleman TG, et al: In Laragh JH, Brenner BM, editors: *Hypertension, pathophysiology, diagnosis and management,* New York, 1995, Raven, pp 1311–1326 with permission.)

that received a kidney from a hypertensive animal become hypertensive, and vice versa. Similarly, human kidney transplant recipients frequently become hypertensive if they receive a kidney from a hypertensive donor. Apparently, the kidney in hypertension is programmed to retain salt and water inappropriately for a normal level of BP, thereby resetting the pressure natriuresis to a higher level of BP and dictating the appearance of hypertension in the recipient even if the neurohumoral environment is that of normotension. Nevertheless, recent studies in gene-deleted or transgenic mice subjected to kidney transplantation concluded that the increase in BP during prolonged infusion of angiotensin II was mediated by the combined effects within the kidney and the systemic circulation, most likely involving the brain. A second observation was that the BP was normally reduced 5% to 20% by an ACE inhibitor, an ARB, an aldosterone receptor antagonist, or a renin inhibitor. The fall in BP was greatest in those with elevated PRA values, and it was enhanced by dietary salt restriction or concurrent use of diuretic drugs (see Fig. 65.1). Third, almost 90% of patients approaching end-stage renal disease (ESRD) have hypertension. Fourth, the major monogenetic causes of human hypertension involve genes that activate RAAS signaling (such as glucocorticoid remediable hypertension) or renal sodium transport (such as Liddle syndrome).

TOTAL-BODY AUTOREGULATION

An increase in cardiac output necessarily increases peripheral blood flow. However, each organ has intrinsic mechanisms that adapt its blood flow to its metabolic needs. Therefore, over time, an increase in cardiac output is translated into an increase in TPR. The outcome is that organ blood flow is maintained, but hypertension becomes sustained. This total-body autoregulation is demonstrated in human subjects who are given salt-retaining mineralocorticosteroid hormones. An initial rise in cardiac output is translated in most individuals into sustained hypertension and an elevated TPR over 5 to 15 days.

STRUCTURAL COMPONENTS TO HYPERTENSION

Hypertension causes not only hypertrophic or eutrophic remodeling in the distributing and resistance vessels and the heart, but also fibrotic and sclerotic changes in the glomeruli and interstitium of the kidney. Hypertrophy of resistance vessels limits the ratio of lumen to wall, and dictates a fixed component to TPR. This is evidenced by a higher TPR in hypertensive subjects during maximal vasodilatation. Moreover, thickened and hypertrophied resistance vessels have greater reductions in vessel diameter during vasoconstrictor stimulation. This is apparent as an increase in vascular reactivity to pressor agents. Remodeling of resistance arterioles diminishes their response to changes in perfusion pressure. This manifests as a blunted myogenic response contributing to incomplete autoregulation of RBF, thereby adding a component of barotrauma to hypertensive kidney damage. Sclerotic and fibrotic changes in the glomeruli and renal interstitium, combined with hypertrophy of the afferent arterioles, limit the sensing of BP in the juxtaglomerular apparatus and interstitium of the kidney. This blunts renin release and pressure natriuresis, thereby

contributing to salt sensitivity and sustained hypertension. Rats receiving intermittent weak electrical stimulation of the hypothalamus initially had an abrupt increase in BP followed by a sudden fall after the cessation of the stimulus. However, eventually the baseline BP increased in parallel with the appearance of hypertrophy of the resistance vessels. These structural components may explain why it often takes weeks or months to achieve maximal antihypertensive action from a drug, a reduction in salt intake, or correction of a renal artery stenosis or hyperaldosteronism. Vascular and left ventricular hypertrophy is largely, but usually not completely, reversible during treatment of hypertension, whereas fibrotic and sclerotic changes are not.

SYMPATHETIC NERVOUS SYSTEM, BRAIN, AND BAROREFLEXES

A rise in BP diminishes the baroreflex, reduces the tone of the sympathetic nervous system, and increases the tone of the parasympathetic nervous system. Paradoxically, human hypertension is often associated with an increase in heart rate, maintained or increased plasma catecholamine levels, and an increase in directly measured sympathetic nerve discharge despite the stimulus to the baroreceptors. What is the cause of this inappropriate activation of the sympathetic nervous system in hypertension? Studies in animals show that the baroreflex "resets" to the ambient level of BP after 2 to 5 days. Baroreflex no longer continues to "fight" the elevated BP, but defends it at the new higher level. Much of this adaptation occurs within the baroreceptors themselves. With aging and atherosclerosis, the walls of the carotid sinus and other baroreflex sensing sites become less distensible. Therefore, the BP is less effective in stretching the afferent nerve endings, and the sensitivity of the baroreflex is diminished. This may contribute to the enhanced sympathetic nerve activity and increased plasma catecholamines that are characteristic of elderly hypertensive subjects. Additionally, animal models have identified central mechanisms that alter the gain of the baroreflex process, and therefore the sympathetic tone, in hypertension. The importance of central mechanisms in human hypertension is apparent from the effectiveness of drugs, such as clonidine, that act within the brain to decrease the sympathetic tone. The kidneys themselves contain barosensitive and chemosensitive nerves that can regulate the sympathetic nervous system. Patients with ESRD on hemodialysis experienced an increased sympathetic nervous system discharge and increased BP that were not apparent after bilateral nephrectomy. This suggested that the renal nerves were maintaining enhanced sympathetic tone. Recently, the success of radiofrequency ablation of the renal nerves in improving BP control in patients with drug resistant hypertension further illustrates the importance of the renal nerves in setting the long-term level of BP in human subjects.

ENDOTHELIUM AND OXIDATIVE STRESS

Calcium-mobilizing agonists such as bradykinin or acetylcholine, as well as shear forces produced by the flow of blood, release endothelium-dependent relaxing factors, predominantly nitric oxide (NO). NO has a half-life of only a few seconds because of inactivation by oxyhemoglobin or reactive oxygen species (ROS) such as superoxide anion (O_2^-). Humans with essential hypertension have defects in endothelium-dependent relaxing factor responses of peripheral vessels and also diminished NO generation. One underlying mechanism is oxidative stress. Excessive O_2^- formation inactivates NO, leading to a functional NO deficiency. Another mechanism is the appearance of inhibitors of nitric oxide synthase (NOS), including asymmetric dimethyl arginine (ADMA). Finally, atherosclerosis, prolonged hypertension, or the development of malignant hypertension causes structural changes in the endothelium that limit NO generation further. In the kidney, NO inhibits renal NaCl reabsorption in the loop of Henle and collecting ducts. Therefore, NO deficiency not only induces vasoconstriction but also diminishes renal pressure natriuresis. Functional NO deficiency in large blood vessels contributes to vascular inflammation and atherosclerosis.

GENETIC CONTRIBUTIONS

The heritability of human hypertension can be assessed from differences in the concordance of hypertension between identical twins (who share all genes and a similar environment) versus nonidentical twins (who share only a similar environment). These studies suggested that genetic factors contributed less than half of the risk for developing hypertension in modern humans. Studies in mice with targeted disruption of individual genes or insertions of extra copies of genes provided direct evidence of the critical regulatory roles for certain gene products in hypertension. Deletions of the gene in mice for endothelial NOS leads to salt-dependent hypertension. The BP of mice decreases with the number of copies of the gene encoding ACE. These are compelling examples of circumstances in which a single gene can sustain hypertension. However, there is increasing recognition of the complexity and importance of gene–gene interactions and the crucial effects of the genetic background on the changes in BP that accompany insertion or deletion of a gene.

Currently, there is evidence that certain individual gene defects can contribute to human essential hypertension. However, the net effect on BP is small. Certain rare forms of hereditary hypertension are caused by single-gene defects. For example, dexamethasone-suppressible hyperaldosteronism is caused by a chimeric rearrangement of the gene encoding aldosterone synthase that renders the enzyme responsive to adrenocorticotropic hormone. Liddle syndrome is caused by a mutation in the gene encoding one component of the endothelial sodium channel that is expressed in the distal convoluted tubule. The mutated form has lost its normal regulation, leading to a permanent "open state" of the sodium channel that dictates inappropriate renal NaCl retention and salt-sensitive, low-renin hypertension (see Chapters 9, 39, and 67).

IMPLICATED MEDIATORS OF HYPERTENSION

Alterations in the synthesis, secretion, degradation, or action of numerous substances are implicated in certain categories of hypertension. The most important of these are described in the following paragraphs.

RENIN, ANGIOTENSIN II, AND ALDOSTERONE

The PRA is not appropriately suppressed in most patients with essential hypertension, and it is increased above normal values in approximately 15%. Subjects with normal or high PRA have a greater antihypertensive response to single-agent therapy with an ACE inhibitor, an ARB, or a β-blocker than patients with low-renin hypertension, who respond notably to salt restriction and diuretic therapy. The RAAS is particularly important in the maintenance of BP in patients with renovascular hypertension, although its importance wanes during the chronic phase when structural alterations in blood vessels or damage in the kidney dictate a RAAS-independent component to the hypertension.

SYMPATHETIC NERVOUS SYSTEM AND CATECHOLAMINES

Pheochromocytoma is a catecholamine-secreting tumor, often occurring in the adrenal medulla, that increases plasma catecholamines tenfold to 1000-fold. However, even such extraordinary increases in pressor amines are rarely fatal, because an intact renal pressure natriuresis mechanism reduces the blood volume, thereby limiting the rise in BP. Indeed, such patients can have orthostatic hypotension between episodes of catecholamine secretion (see Chapter 67).

An increased sympathetic nerve tone of resistance vessels in human essential hypertension causes α_1-receptor–mediated vasoconstriction of the blood vessels and β_1-receptor–mediated increases in contractility and output of the heart that are incompletely offset by β_2-receptor–mediated vasorelaxation of peripheral blood vessels. Increased sympathetic nerve discharge to the kidney leads to α_1-mediated enhancement of NaCl reabsorption and β_1-mediated renin release.

DOPAMINE

Dopamine is synthesized in the brain and renal tubular epithelial cells independent of sympathetic nerves. Dopamine synthesis in the kidney is enhanced during volume expansion and contributes to decreased reabsorption of NaCl in the proximal tubule. Defects in tubular dopamine responsiveness are apparent in genetic models of hypertension. Recent evidence relates single nucleotide polymorphisms of genes that regulate dopamine receptors to human salt-sensitive hypertension.

ARACHIDONATE METABOLITES

Arachidonate is esterified as a phospholipid in cell membranes. It is released by phospholipases that are activated by agents such as angiotensin II. Three enzymes principally metabolize arachidonate. Cyclooxygenase (COX) generates unstable intermediates whose subsequent metabolism by specific enzymes yields prostaglandins that are either generally vasodilative (e.g., prostaglandin I_2 [PGI_2]), vasoconstrictive (e.g., thromboxane), or of mixed effect (e.g., PGE_2). COX-1 is expressed in many tissues, including platelets, resistance vessels, glomeruli, and cortical collecting ducts. Inflammatory mediators induce COX-2. However, the normal kidney is unusual in expressing substantial COX-2, which is located in macula densa cells, tubules, renal medullary interstitial cells, and arterioles. The net effect of blocking COX-1 generally is to retain NaCl and fluid while raising BP and dropping PRA. Blockade of COX-2 has little effect on normal BP, but it can increase BP in those with essential hypertension. Nonsteroidal antiinflammatory agents exacerbate essential hypertension, blunt the antihypertensive actions of most commonly used agents, predispose to acute kidney injury during periods of volume depletion or hypotension, and blunt the natriuretic action of loop diuretics. In contrast, aspirin reduces BP in patients with renovascular hypertension, testifying to the prohypertensive actions of thromboxane and other prostanoids that activate the thromboxane-prostanoid receptor in this condition. Metabolism of arachidonate by cytochrome P-450 monooxygenase yields 19,20-hydroxyeicosatetraenoic acid (HETE), which is a vasoconstrictor of blood vessels but inhibits tubular NaCl reabsorption. Metabolism by epoxygenase leads to epoxyeicosatrienoic acids (EETs), which are powerful vasodilators and natriuretic agents. Arachidonate metabolites act primarily as modulating agents in normal physiology. Their role in human essential hypertension remains elusive.

L-ARGININE-NITRIC OXIDE PATHWAY

Nitric oxide is generated by three isoforms of NOS that are widely expressed in the body. NO interacts with many heme-centered enzymes. Activation of guanylyl cyclase generates cyclic guanosine monophosphate, which is a powerful vasorelaxant and inhibits NaCl reabsorption in the kidney. Defects in NO generation in the endothelium of blood vessels in human essential hypertension may contribute to increased peripheral resistance, vascular remodeling, and atherosclerosis, whereas defects in renal NO generation may contribute to inappropriate renal NaCl retention and salt sensitivity. NOS activity is reduced in hypertensive human subjects and in those with CKD.

REACTIVE OXYGEN SPECIES

The incomplete reduction of molecular oxygen, either by the respiratory chain during cellular respiration or by oxidases such as nicotinamide adenine dinucleotide phosphate (NADPH) oxidase, yields ROS including O_2^- and generates peroxynitrite ($ONOO^-$). $ONOO^-$ has long-lasting effects through oxidizing and nitrosylating reactions. Reaction of ROS with lipids yields oxidized low-density lipoprotein (LDL), which promotes atherosclerosis, and isoprostanes, which cause vasoconstriction, salt retention, and platelet aggregation. ROS are difficult to quantitate, but indirect evidence suggests that hypertension, especially in the setting of CKD, is a state of oxidative stress. Drugs that effectively reduce O_2^- reduce BP in animal models of hypertension, but they are largely unexamined in human hypertension.

ENDOTHELINS

Endothelins are produced primarily by cells of the vascular endothelium and collecting tubules. Discrete receptors mediate either increased vascular resistance (type A) or the release of NO and inhibition of NaCl reabsorption in the collecting ducts (type B). Endothelin type A receptors potentiate the vasoconstriction accompanying angiotensin II infusion or blockade of NOS. Endothelin is released by hypoxia, specific agonists such as angiotensin II, salt loading, and cytokines. Nonspecific blockade of endothelin receptors lowers BP in models of volume-expanded hypertension. The role of endothelin in human essential hypertension is unclear.

ATRIAL NATRIURETIC PEPTIDE

Atrial natriuretic peptide is released from the heart during atrial stretch. It acts on receptors that increase GFR, decrease NaCl reabsorption in the distal nephron, and inhibit renin secretion. ANP is released during volume expansion and contributes to the natriuretic response. Its role in essential hypertension is unclear. Endopeptidase inhibitors that block ANP degradation are natriuretic and antihypertensive, but also inhibit the metabolism of kinins. Although an increase in kinins may contribute to the fall in BP with endopeptidase or ACE inhibitors, kinins can cause an irritant cough or a more serious anaphylactoid reaction.

PATHOGENESIS OF HYPERTENSION IN CHRONIC KIDNEY DISEASE

With progression of CKD, the prevalence of salt-sensitive hypertension increases in proportion to the fall in GFR. Hypertension is almost universal in patients with CKD caused by primary glomerular or vascular disease, whereas those with primary tubulointerstitial disease may be normotensive or, occasionally, salt losing.

With declining nephron number, CKD limits the ability to adjust NaCl excretion rapidly and quantitatively during changes in intake. The role of ECF volume expansion is apparent from the ability of hemodialysis to lower BP in patients with ESRD.

Additional mechanisms besides primary renal fluid retention contribute to the increased TPR and hypertension in patients with CKD. The RAAS is often inappropriately stimulated. The ESRD kidney generates abnormal renal afferent nerve impulses, which entrain an increased sympathetic nerve discharge that is reversed by bilateral nephrectomy. Plasma levels of endothelin increase with kidney failure. CKD induces oxidative stress, which contributes to vascular disease and impaired endothelium-dependent relaxing factor responses. A decreased generation of NO from L-arginine follows the accumulation of ADMA, which inhibits NOS. The thromboxane-prostanoid receptor is activated and contributes to vasoconstriction and structural damage.

Clearly, hypertension in CKD is multifactorial, but volume expansion and salt sensitivity are predominant. Pressor mechanisms mediated by angiotensin II, catecholamines, endothelin, or thromboxane-prostanoid receptors become more potent during volume expansion. This fact may underlie the importance of these systems in the ESRD patients. Finally, many of the pathways that contribute to hypertension in ESRD (such as impaired NO generation and excessive production of endothelin, ROS, and ADMA) also contribute to atherosclerosis, cardiac hypertrophy, and progressive renal fibrosis and sclerosis. Indeed, in poorly treated hypertension, kidney damage leads to additional hypertension, which itself engenders further kidney damage, generating a vicious spiral culminating in accelerated hypertension, progressively diminishing kidney function, and the requirement for renal replacement therapy. Therefore, rational management of hypertension in CKD first entails salt-depleting therapy with a salt-restricted diet and diuretic therapy. Patients frequently require additional therapy to combat the enhanced vasoconstriction and to attempt to slow the rate of progression.

BIBLIOGRAPHY

DiBona GF: Sympathetic nervous system and the kidney in hypertension, *Curr Opin Nephrol Hypertens* 11:197-200, 2002.

Guyton AC, Hall JE, Coleman TG, et al: The dominant role of the kidneys in the long-term regulation of arterial pressure in normal and hypertensive states. In Laragh JH, Brenner BM, editors: *Hypertension: pathophysiology, diagnosis and management*, New York, 1990, Raven, pp 1029-1052.

Navar LG: The role of the kidneys in hypertension, *J Clin Hypertens* 7:542-549, 2005.

Wilcox CS: Oxidative stress and nitric oxide deficiency in the kidney: a critical link to hypertension? *Am J Physiol Regul Integr Comp Physiol* 289:R913-R935, 2005.

Wilcox CS: *Therapy in nephrology and hypertension*, 3rd ed, Philadelphia, 2008, WB Saunders.

66 Evaluation and Management of Hypertension

Yonghong Huan | Raymond R. Townsend

Hypertension remains the leading cause of cardiovascular morbidity and mortality, including stroke, heart disease, kidney disease, and other vascular disease. The relationship between blood pressure (BP) and cardiovascular risk is linear, continuous, and additive to other well-known risk factors such as diabetes, dyslipidemia, obesity, and cigarette smoking. For individuals aged 40 to 69 years, each increment of either 20 mm Hg in systolic BP or 10 mm Hg in diastolic BP doubles the mortality risk related to stroke, ischemic heart disease, and other vascular causes across the entire BP range from 115/75 to 185/115 mm Hg. The cardiovascular risk increases further in the presence of other risk factors.

The Joint National Committee (JNC 7) on Prevention, Detection, Evaluation, and Treatment of High Blood Pressure classified BP into four categories as listed in Table 66.1. Hypertension affects close to one third of the U.S. adult population, and the prevalence continues to increase steadily due to aging and increasing obesity. The lifetime risk for developing hypertension is about 90%. The category "prehypertension," which was created to reflect its association with higher cardiovascular risk compared with normal BP, affects on average about a quarter of the U.S. adult population.

Correctly assessing BP status and overall cardiovascular risk is the key to optimizing therapy to reduce cardiovascular morbidity and mortality. At first diagnosis, a comprehensive evaluation is usually undertaken in those with systolic BP higher than 140 mm Hg and/or diastolic BP higher than 90 mm Hg on repeat measurements.

EVALUATION OF HYPERTENSION

Three key questions must be addressed in assessing each hypertensive patient. The first question asks whether the elevated BP is essential (primary) or represents a secondary form of hypertension. Most hypertensive patients have primary, or essential, hypertension and are likely to remain hypertensive for life. However, some patients have identifiable, or secondary, causes for their elevated BP. This cause may warrant specific therapy in addition to antihypertensive medications to address the underlying specific or dominant pathology and offer possible cure. The common forms of secondary hypertension are listed by their involved organ systems in Table 66.2, and are discussed further in Chapter 67.

The second question assesses the presence of other cardiovascular risk factors, as summarized in Table 66.3. Defining overall cardiovascular risk is important in the choice of antihypertensive medications, BP target, and management of other treatable factors such as dyslipidemia.

The third question evaluates the presence of end-organ damage, defined as clinically evident cardiovascular diseases related to hypertension as summarized in Table 66.4. The presence of end-organ damage redirects the goal of BP treatment from primary prevention of target organ integrity to the more challenging realm of secondary prevention.

MEASURING BLOOD PRESSURE

Measuring BP correctly is the key to proper BP classification. Figure 66.1 lists steps recommended to obtain reliable BP readings, and Box 66.1 lists common mistakes leading to inaccurate BP measurements. During the initial visit, BP should be measured in both arms (and in the leg if aortic coarctation is suspected). For proper assessment, it is important to take the BP properly at least twice on any occasion and on at least two (preferably three) separate days for the initial diagnosis of hypertension.

Pseudohypertension is a problem occasionally encountered in examining patients with blood vessels that are difficult to compress as a result of arterial wall calcification. The pressure required to compress the stiff brachial artery and to stop the audible blood flow with a standard BP cuff can be much greater than the actual intraluminal pressure. Osler maneuver can be used to identify this condition by inflating the BP cuff at least 30 mm Hg above the palpable systolic pressure and then trying to "roll" the brachial or radial artery underneath the fingertips. Pseudohypertension may be present when something resembling a stiff tube is felt underneath the skin because a normal artery should not be palpable when empty. It is important to identify pseudohypertension because it tends to occur in the elderly and chronically ill. These patients are also more prone to orthostatic and postural hypotension, which can be aggravated by the unwarranted intensification of BP treatment.

Electronic devices are increasingly used to measure BP. Most of these devices work on oscillometric principles. The cuff is inflated until the disappearance of the brachial pulses is detected. Upon deflation, sensors detect the increasing amplitude in the brachial pulsation and measure the mean arterial pressure. The systolic and diastolic BP readings are then derived from the mean arterial BP. Typically, systolic BP is slightly lower and diastolic BP is slightly higher when measured by electronic devices compared to invasively measured arterial pressure.

Table 66.1   Classification of Blood Pressure Status

BP Classification	Systolic BP (mm Hg)		Diastolic BP (mm Hg)
Normal	<120	and	<80
Prehypertension	120-139	or	80-89
Stage 1 hypertension	140-159	or	90-99
Stage 2 hypertension	≥160	or	≥100

Table 66.2   Forms of Secondary Hypertension

Type	Examples
Endocrine disorders	Hyperaldosteronism (adrenal adenoma or hyperplasia), pheochromocytoma or paraganglioma, Cushing syndrome, hyperthyroidism, hypothyroidism, acromegaly, hyperparathyroidism, carcinoid syndrome
Renal	Chronic kidney disease, congenital or acquired salt-retention disorders
Vascular	Aortic coarctation, renal artery stenosis, fibromuscular dysplasia
Drug-induced	NSAIDs, oral contraceptives, sympathomimetic agents, illicit drugs, steroids, calcineurin inhibitors, erythropoietin, VEGF inhibitors, licorice, dietary supplements
Other comorbidities	Obstructive sleep apnea

NSAIDs, Nonsteroidal antiinflammatory drugs; *VEGF*, vascular endothelial growth factor.

Table 66.3   Other Cardiovascular Risk Factors in Hypertensive Patients

Risk Factors	Level Considered Abnormal	Approximate Frequency (%)
Obesity	BMI >30 kg/m^2	40
Increased total cholesterol	>240 mg/dL	40
Reduced HDL cholesterol	<35 mg/dL	25
Proteinuria*	Dipstick positive (≥1+)	
Diabetes	Type 1 and type 2 diabetes mellitus; fasting glucose >126 mg/dL	15
Insulin resistance	Elevated fasting insulin and/or impaired glucose tolerance	50
LVH*	Defined by various ECG or echocardiogram criteria	≈30†
Sedentary lifestyle	Arbitrary	≈30

BMI, Body mass index; *HDL*, high density lipoprotein; *LVH*, left ventricular hypertrophy.
*Proteinuria and LVH are risk factors as well as markers of target organ damage.
†Based on echocardiogram criteria.

ASSESSING OVERALL CARDIOVASCULAR RISK AND END-ORGAN DAMAGE

The evaluation of each hypertensive patient should include a detailed personal and family history, thorough physical examination, and selected tests focused on addressing the aforementioned three key questions. Key components of the history and physical examination are listed in Table 66.5.

A detailed personal history of hypertension includes its onset, duration, severity and related symptoms, cardiovascular risks, and complications. The presence of diabetes or cardiac, renal, or other vascular diseases suggests the need for more aggressive BP control. The medication history should include the prior and current use of any prescription and over-the-counter agents. Special attention should be paid to antihypertensive medications with their related clinical responses and adverse effects, as well as common offending agents as nonsteroidal antiinflammatory drugs (NSAIDs), oral contraceptive, and cold/cough remedies. For example, NSAIDs can increase BP on their own, but they also decrease the efficacy of antihypertensive medications by inhibiting vasodilatory and natriuretic effects of prostaglandins and potentiating vasoconstrictive effects of angiotensin II. Dietary salt intake, alcohol consumption, tobacco use, physical activity, and weight changes should be recorded. With the increasing prevalence of obesity, essential hypertension manifests at younger ages, often in the third decade. In addition, more older adult patients are expected to develop essential hypertension as systolic BP increases throughout life. Although essential hypertension is more common, the sudden onset of severe hypertension warrants consideration of secondary hypertension. Family history of hypertension, diabetes, and related cardiovascular complications should also be noted, because a positive family history further increases the individual's cardiovascular risk. Excluding monogenic causes of hypertension, available data suggest that the heritability of essential hypertension ranges from 20% to 40%.

Physical examination should start with measurement of height, weight, and waist circumference. BP is usually measured in supine, sitting, and standing positions on the initial evaluation, and at least once in both arms (and at least one leg if aortic coarctation is suspected). Subsequent BP measurements are obtained in the seated position from the arm with the higher initial BP reading.

The optic fundi are the only places where arterioles can be directly examined. The fundoscopic examination looks for arteriolar narrowing (grade 1), arteriovenous compression (grade 2), hemorrhages and/or exudates (grade 3), and papilledema (grade 4), which provides not only information on the degree of target organ damage but also important prognostic information on overall cardiovascular outcomes.

Bruits in the neck, abdomen, and groin should be noted. Bruits may simply result from vascular tortuosity, particularly with high flow. However, they may be a sign of vascular stenosis and irregularity, and a clue to vascular damage leading to future loss of target organ function. The radial artery is similarly distant from the heart as the femoral artery, and the pulse should arrive at approximately the same moment when palpating both sites simultaneously. In aortic coarctation, a palpable delay in the arrival of the femoral pulse compared with the radial pulse supports this diagnosis, as does an interscapular murmur heard during auscultation over the back of the patient. A systolic BP in the leg lower than the brachial value suggests the presence of aortic or iliac obstruction, but may also reflect more peripheral arterial disease in certain patients, such as smokers and those with target organ damage. Patients should be advised that measuring femoral BP may be uncomfortable, given the large cuff and the amount of pressure required to occlude the femoral artery.

Cardiac examination by palpation may reveal a displaced apical impulse, indicative of left ventricular enlargement. A sustained apical impulse may suggest left ventricular

Table 66.4   Target Organ Effects of Hypertension

Organ	History/Symptom(s)	Physical Examination	Laboratory
Retina	Blurry vision, headache, disorientation	Retinopathy	
Brain	Stroke, TIA, confusion/disorientation	Focal neurologic deficits, carotid bruits	MRI, CT, or ultrasound
Heart	Angina, MI, heart failure, cardiac arrest, atrial fibrillation	Cardiomegaly, S4, rales, irregular heart beats	ECG showing LVH and/or prior MI
Kidney	Chronic kidney disease, polyuria, nocturia, uremia, peripheral edema	Palpable kidneys, epigastric bruits	Elevated creatinine, proteinuria, hematuria, ultrasound showing small kidneys with increased echogenicity
Circulation	Peripheral arterial disease, claudication, ischemic digits	Femoral bruits, absent pedal pulses	Ankle-brachial index <0.9

CT, Computed tomography; *ECG,* electrocardiogram; *MI,* myocardial infarction; *MRI,* magnetic resonance imaging; *TIA,* transient ischemic attack.

1. Have patient relax for at least 5 minutes before taking blood pressure. Feet should be on the floor, with the back supported.

2. The patient's arm should be supported (i.e., resting on a desk) for the measurement.

3. The stethoscope bell, not the diaphragm, should be used for auscultation.

4. Blood pressure should first be checked in both arms with the patient sitting. Note which arm gives the higher reading. This arm (with the higher reading) should then be used for all other (standing, lying down) and future readings.

5. All measurements should be separately by 2 minutes.

6. Measure the blood pressure in the sitting, standing, and lying positions.

7. Use the correct cuff size and note if a larger or smaller than normal cuff size is used.

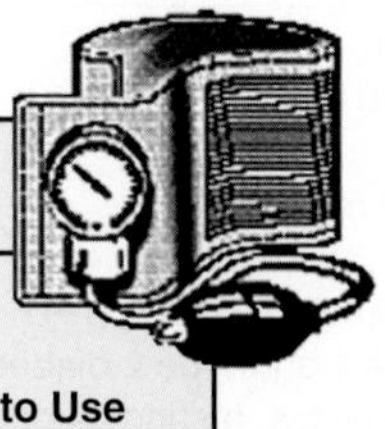

Blood Pressure Cuff Size Criteria			
Arm Circumference	Weight		Cuff Size to Use
	Female	Male	
24–32 cm	<150	<200	REGULAR
33–42 cm*	>150	>200	LARGE
38–50 cm*	–	–	THIGH
* Either cuff is acceptable in the overlap diameter zone			

8. Record systolic (onset of first sound) and diastolic (disappearance of sound) pressures.

9. Do not round off results to zeros or fives. Record exact results to nearest even number.

Figure 66.1   Instructions for taking blood pressure. Steps in obtaining accurate blood pressure measurements by aneroid sphygmomanometry

hypertrophy (LVH). Auscultation should focus on listening for an S4, indicating left ventricular stiffness. An S3 may indicate impairment in left ventricular function and underlying heart disease when rales are present on lung examination, though the presence of S3 and rales are uncommon on initial office evaluation of new hypertensive patients. The lower extremities should also be examined for peripheral arterial pulses and edema. The loss of pedal pulses is a sign of peripheral vascular disease, and is associated with higher cardiovascular risk.

Box 66.1   Common Causes Contributing to Inaccurate Blood Pressure Readings

Failure to sit quietly for 5 minutes before a reading is taken
Lack of arm and foot support
Too small a cuff size relative to the arm (cuff bladder should encircle ≥80% of upper arm circumference)
Overly rapid cuff deflation (i.e., more than 2 mm Hg/second)
Ongoing conversation
Recent caffeine intake or cigarette use

Finally, a brief neurologic examination for evidence of remote stroke should be documented, including gait, bilateral grip strength, speech, memory, and mental acuity. Given the link between hypertension and future loss of cognitive function, it is useful to establish the cognitive function status before starting antihypertensive medications because some patients may complain of memory loss after starting treatment.

Several laboratory studies are recommended in the routine evaluation of the hypertensive patient. Testing should include hemoglobin or hematocrit, urinalysis with microscopic examination, serum potassium, creatinine, glucose, fasting lipid profile, and 12-lead electrocardiogram (ECG). Assessing diabetes and albuminuria is important because both potentiate the cardiovascular risk associated with hypertension and call for tighter BP control. Assessing kidney function is also important because chronic kidney disease (CKD) is not only a sign of target organ damage but also a common cause of hypertension. Depending on the degree of glomerular filtration rate (GFR) loss, up to 90% of patients with advanced CKD or end-stage renal disease have hypertension. When CKD is present, a lower BP goal is currently recommended. Uric acid may be checked in those with a history of gout, as diuretics can increase uric acid level

---

Table 66.5   Key Elements of History and Physical Examination in Evaluating Hypertensive Patients

Key Elements	Evaluation
History	
Age of onset, duration, and severity	Onset at younger age (<25 years) or older age (>55 years) suggests secondary causes; new onset of severe hypertension also suggests a secondary cause
Contributing factors	Dietary salt intake, physical inactivity, psychosocial stress, symptoms of sleep apnea
Concomitant medications	Common offenders include NSAIDs, oral contraceptives, corticosteroids, licorice, cough/cold/weight-loss sympathomimetic agents (pseudoephedrine, Ma-Huang, ephedrine)
Risk factors for cardiovascular disease	Diabetes, smoking, family history of premature cardiovascular disease particularly in a first-degree relative (parent or sibling)
Symptoms suggestive of secondary causes	Palpitations or tachycardia, spontaneous sweating, paroxysmal migraine-like headaches (catecholamine excess); muscle weakness, polyuria (decreased potassium from aldosterone excess); personal or family history of kidney disease, proteinuria, hematuria, or ankle swelling (edema); thinning of skin and stigmata of corticosteroid excess; snoring and daytime somnolence (sleep apnea); heat intolerance and weight loss (hyperthyroidism)
Target organ damage	Chest pain or chest discomfort (possible coronary artery disease); neurologic symptoms consistent with stroke or transient ischemic attack; dyspnea and easy fatigue (possible heart failure); claudication (peripheral arterial disease)
Physical Examination	
General appearance, skin lesions, distribution of body fat	Patient may fit criteria for metabolic syndrome (increased cardiovascular risk); evidence of prior stroke from gait/station; rarely, striae (Cushing syndrome) or mucosal fibromas (MEN type II)
Funduscopy	See text for lesion grades; retinal changes reflect severity of hypertension (target organ damage to the eyes) as well as future cardiovascular risk
Neck	Diffuse multinodular goiter indicates Graves disease; presence of carotid bruits suggests potential stroke risk
Cardiopulmonary examination	Rales and cardiac gallops consistent with target organ damage (heart enlargement or heart failure), interscapular murmur for aortic coarctation
Abdominal examination	Palpable kidneys suggest polycystic kidney disease; midepigastric bruits indicate renal artery disease
Neurologic examination	Signs of previous stroke (reduced grip, hyperreflexia, spasticity, Babinski sign, muscle atrophy, and gait disturbances) reflect target organ damage
Pulse examination	Delayed or absent femoral pulses may reflect coarctation of the aorta or atherosclerosis

MEN, Multiple endocrine neoplasia; *NSAIDs*, nonsteroidal antiinflammatory drugs.

and lead to gouty flares. In some cases, checking calcium or thyroid-stimulating hormone (TSH) levels may be reasonable when clinically indicated.

Plasma renin activity and serum aldosterone levels are useful in screening for aldosterone excess and salt sensitivity. However, these measurements are usually reserved for patients with hypokalemia or those who fail to achieve blood pressure control on a three-drug regimen (which includes a diuretic). A suppressed renin activity level with an increased ratio of plasma aldosterone to renin supports a contribution of dietary sodium excess to hypertension, which should respond well to dietary salt restriction and diuretics. It is worth noting that primary hyperaldosteronism is much more common than previously thought. In patients who were referred to one hypertension center in Italy, 11% had primary hyperaldosteronism, with 5% having a potentially curable aldosterone-secreting adenoma and 6% having idiopathic hyperaldosteronism.

Additional testing may be indicated in some patients depending on the clinical situations. Limited echocardiography is more sensitive than an ECG for detection of LVH. The presence of LVH, a sign of target organ damage, can help establish the need for antihypertensive therapy, especially in those who have borderline BP and/or are reluctant to start antihypertensive medications.

AMBULATORY AND HOME BLOOD PRESSURE MONITORING

Since BP can be influenced by an environment such as an office or hospital, ambulatory BP monitoring (ABPM) or home BP monitoring (HBPM) is useful in establishing or excluding the diagnosis of hypertension from "white-coat hypertension" or masked hypertension (Fig. 66.2). ABPM and HBPM are also useful in assessing the adequacy of BP control in outpatients and in helping identify those with morning surges in BP (i.e., more than a 55 mm Hg increase in systolic BP during the early waking hours compared with sleeping). The morning surge has been associated with increased risk for cerebrovascular diseases such as white matter lesions and stroke. In addition, ABPM is helpful in screening for nocturnal hypertension, or nondipper status (i.e., less than a 10% reduction in nighttime BP compared with daytime). Data from large ABPM cohorts suggest that nighttime BP provides the greatest information regarding cardiovascular risk. Cardiovascular risks associated with elevated nighttime BP levels outweigh the risks associated with the elevated routine office BP measurements, as well as those of the cumulative daytime hours. In addition, data from ABPM suggest that the greater the degree of BP variability during the 24 hours of monitoring, the greater the risk for cardiovascular target organ damage. ABPM is typically programmed to take BP measurements every 15 to 20 minutes during daytime hours and every 30 to 60 minutes during the night. It is important for the patients to complete the diary correctly so that the hours of sleep (including naps) can be incorporated into the ABPM report.

Current estimates indicate that more than half of hypertensive patients measure their BP at home. Although not reimbursed by most insurers in the United States, home BP monitors are relatively inexpensive and reasonably accurate. Specific recommendations have been published on how to incorporate HBPM into overall BP assessment. For the diagnosis of hypertension, it is recommended to take two BP readings in the morning between 7 AM and 10 AM and two measurements in the evening between 7 PM and 10 PM for 7 consecutive days. Values from the first day are discarded, and the subsequent 6 days values are averaged. For the diagnosis of hypertension in untreated patients, hypertension is not present if the average is below 125/76 mm Hg, but hypertension is likely present if the value is above 135/85 mm Hg. For values in between, ABPM is recommended and hypertension is considered present when the ABPM 24-hour average is higher than 130/80 mm Hg.

The National Center for Health and Clinical Excellence (NICE) in the United Kingdom updated its hypertension guideline in the summer of 2011. NICE recommended using ABPM or HBPM to confirm all new diagnoses of hypertension. Since all the data for treating hypertension have been based on standard office BP measurement and ABPM is currently only reimbursed by Center for Medicare and Medicaid Services (CMS) for suspected untreated white-coat hypertension, it remains uncertain whether ABPM and HBPM will be used more widely to help diagnose and manage hypertension in the United States.

After the proper initial evaluation and correct staging of BP status, it is necessary to develop an appropriate follow-up plan guided by both BP readings (as shown in Table 66.6) and clinical judgment. If the systolic BP and diastolic BP fall into different categories, the follow-up plan should be based on the category requiring more frequent evaluations (i.e., shorter interval).

MANAGEMENT OF HYPERTENSION

TARGET BLOOD PRESSURE LEVELS

According to the JNC 7, in the absence of comorbidities or compelling indications, the BP goal is 140/90 mm Hg

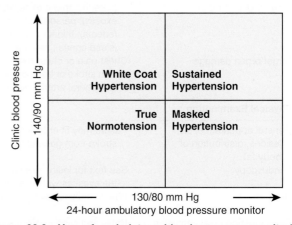

Figure 66.2 Use of ambulatory blood pressure monitoring in diagnosing hypertension. This grid helps to integrate ambulatory blood pressure (BP) monitor data with office BP results. Sustained hypertension is diagnosed if office BP is ≥140/90 mm Hg and 24-hour average of ambulatory BP is ≥130/80 mm Hg. White-coat hypertension is diagnosed when office BP is ≥140/90 mm Hg, but 24-hour average of ambulatory BP is <130/80 mm Hg. Masked hypertension is diagnosed when office BP is <140/90 mm Hg, but 24-hour average of ambulatory BP is ≥130/80 mm Hg.

for patients under 80 years of age. In 2011, the American College of Cardiology in collaboration with the American Heart Association and other major societies with an interest in hypertension released a comprehensive review of hypertension management in older adults, defined as older than 64 years of age. It recommended measuring standing BP in older adults to assess orthostasis, with a BP goal of lower than 140/90 mm Hg.

In patients with diabetes and chronic kidney disease, a BP goal below 130/80 mm Hg is currently recommended by the American Diabetic Association (ADA) and the National Kidney Foundation (NKF). Existing evidence strongly supports the benefits of treating systolic BP ≥160 mm Hg in people age 60 years or above and diastolic BP ≥90 mm Hg in people age 30 years or above in reducing cardiovascular risk, including heart attack, heart failure, stroke, and cardiovascular death. In patients with isolated systolic BP between 140 to 159 mm Hg or patients under 30 years of age, the benefit of treating BP is less clear, although most guidelines recommend lifestyle modification and initiation of drug therapy if systolic BP is persistently higher than 140 mm Hg.

For the very elderly (age 80 years or older), a reasonable systolic BP goal is less than 150 mm Hg based on the

Hypertension in the Very Elderly Trial (HYVET). Regarding the BP goal in the very elderly group, a metaanalysis in 2010 summarized the data from the HYVET feasibility trial, the HYVET main trial, and the subgroups of six trials in the United States and Europe. The pooled analyses demonstrated the benefits of treating hypertension in lowering risk for heart failure, cardiovascular events, and stroke, but failed to show the benefits in reducing coronary events and overall mortality. HYVET and the Swedish Trial in Old Patients with Hypertension (STOP-hypertension) are the only two trials that have shown a mortality benefit of treating hypertension in the very elderly group, but both trials were stopped prematurely due to perceived benefits at the early phase of the trials.

LIFESTYLE MODIFICATIONS

Several nonpharmacologic approaches are used in lowering BP. The most effective method to reduce BP is weight loss in obese patients. The second most effective measure is reducing dietary sodium intake to less than 100 mmol/day (2300 mg of sodium), followed by an increase in physical activity to at least 30 minutes daily on most days of the week. Finally, limiting alcohol intake to two drinks a day for men (one drink a day for women) helps to control BP. Other approaches, including supplementation of potassium, magnesium, and calcium, fish oil, garlic, and green tea, have had variable success in managing BP. Although they do not appear harmful, these approaches do not have robust data to support their widespread use in the management of prehypertension and hypertension. Table 66.7 summarizes the effects of various lifestyle modifications on BP.

PHARMACOLOGIC AGENTS

Many patients with hypertension find it difficult to lose weight or adjust their dietary intake and physical activity to effectively lower their BP. Treatment with antihypertensive medications is recommended when BP remains higher than 140/90 mm Hg in patients younger than 80 years of age. In patients aged 80 years or older, a systolic BP of 150 mm Hg

Table 66.6 Recommended Follow-Up Based on Initial Blood Pressure

Initial BP (mm Hg)		
Systolic	Diastolic	Follow-Up Recommended
<130	<85	Recheck in 2 years
130-139	85-89	Recheck in 1 year (provide lifestyle modification advice)
140-159	90-99	Confirm within 2 months (provide lifestyle modification advice)
160-179	100-109	Evaluate or refer to appropriate provider within 1 month
≥180	≥110	Evaluate or refer to appropriate provider immediately or within 1 week, depending on clinical situation

Table 66.7 Lifestyle Modification to Manage Hypertension*

Modification	Recommendation	Approximate SBP Reduction
Weight reduction	Maintain normal body weight (BMI 18.5-24.9)	5-20 mm Hg/10 kg weight loss
DASH eating plan	Consume a diet rich in fruits, vegetable, and low-fat dairy products with a reduced content of saturated and total fat	8-14 mm Hg
Dietary sodium reduction	Reduce dietary sodium intake to no more than 100 mmol/L (2.3 g sodium or 6 g sodium chloride)	2-8 mm Hg
Physical activity	Engage in regular aerobic physical activity, such as brisk walking (at least 30 min per day, most days of the week)	4-9 mm Hg
Moderation of alcohol consumption	Limited consumption to no more than two drinks per day (1.2 oz or 28 g alcohol—e.g., 24 oz beer, 10 oz wine, or 3 oz 80-proof whiskey) for most men and no more than one drink per day for most women and lighter-weight persons	2-4 mm Hg

BMI, Body mass index; DASH, dietary approaches to stop hypertension.
*For overall cardiovascular risk reduction, stop smoking. The effects of implementing these modifications are dose- and time-dependent, and could be higher for some individuals.

is recommended as the threshold for initiating antihypertensive medications.

Major classes of antihypertensive medications with their mechanism of actions, common side effects, and compelling indications are listed in Table 66.8. Heart failure and stroke are the target organs protected to the greatest extent by long-term antihypertensive therapy. A recent metaanalysis suggests that all five classes of antihypertensive agents (angiotensin converting enzyme [ACE] inhibitors, angiotensin II receptor blockers [ARB], beta blockers, calcium channel blockers [CCB], and diuretics) can reduce target organ damage when used to control BP effectively. Choosing an agent should take into account the patient's demographics (age and ethnicity), the cost of the drug, and the

---

Table 66.8   Major Classes of Available Antihypertensive Medications With Their Mechanisms and Side Effects

Class	Mechanisms	Side Effects	Compelling Indications for Comorbidities
Diuretics	Reducing renal sodium absorption		Heart failure, high CAD risk, diabetes, stroke
Thiazide diuretics	Inhibiting sodium and chloride cotransporter in the renal distal convoluted tubule; more effective in BP control than loop diuretics	Hypokalemia, hyponatremia, hypomagnesemia, hyperuricemia, photosensitivity, and metabolic effects including dyslipidemia and impaired glucose tolerance	
Loop diuretics	Inhibiting sodium, potassium, and chloride cotransporter in the thick ascending limb of the loop of Henle	Hypokalemia, but fewer other metabolic side effects	
Potassium-sparing diuretics	Inhibiting the epithelial sodium channel in the renal distal tubule	Hyperkalemia	
Renin-Angiotensin System Blockers	Dampening arterial wave reflections, increasing aortic distensibility, and venodilation		Heart failure, post-MI, high CAD risk, diabetes, CKD, stroke
Angiotensin converting enzyme (ACE) inhibitors	Blocking the conversion of angiotensin I to angiotensin II	Cough, hyperkalemia, elevated creatinine, angioedema, and fetal toxicity	
Angiotensin II receptor type I blockers (ARB)	Blocking binding of angiotensin II to the type 1 angiotensin receptor	Similar to ACE inhibitors, except no cough	
Direct renin inhibitors	Blocking the conversion of angiotensinogen to angiotensin I	Similar to ARB; diarrhea at high doses	
Calcium Channel Blockers	Inhibiting the L-type voltage-gated plasma membrane channel		High CAD risk, diabetes
Dihydropyridine	Vasodilation	Dependent edema, gingival hyperplasia	
Diltiazem	Vasodilation and AV nodal blockade	Bradycardia	
Verapamil	Vasodilation and AV nodal blockade	Bradycardia, constipation	
Beta Blockers	Inhibiting adrenergic receptors	Reduced exercise tolerance, depression, and bronchospasm	Heart failure, post-MI, high CAD risk, diabetes, stroke
Nonselective beta blockers	Inhibiting both beta 1 and 2 receptors	More bronchospasm	
Selective beta blockers	Blocking beta 1 receptors	Less bronchospasm	
Combined alpha and beta blockers	Blocking both beta and alpha receptors		
Aldosterone Blocker	Blocking aldosterone receptor		Heart failure, post-MI
Spironolactone		Androgen blocking effect, including irregular menses, gynecomastia, and impotence	
Eplerenone		Less potent, but fewer side effects related to androgen blocking	
Direct Vasodilators	Smooth muscle relaxant	Peripheral edema	
Alpha-1 Blockers	Vasodilatation	Postural hypotension	
Central Adrenergic Agonists	Inhibiting central adrenergic tone	Drowsiness, fatigue, and dry mouth	

CAD, Coronary artery disease; *CKD*, chronic kidney disease; *MI*, myocardial infarction.

anticipated side effect profile. The usual response to a single antihypertensive agent is a reduction in systolic BP of 12 to 15 mm Hg and diastolic BP of 8 to 10 mm Hg. Follow-up visits for BP assessment and dose titration are often scheduled in 2 to 4 weeks for single agent therapy because most agents will exert their antihypertensive effects by then.

In patients with systolic BP more than 20 mm Hg and/or diastolic BP more than 10 mm Hg above the goal, beginning treatment with combination drug therapy can shorten the time to achieve BP goal, require less dose titration of antihypertensive agent, and increase the likelihood of achieving BP goal. Combination therapy is often more desirable than a stepwise approach of maximizing one agent before adding another agent because of the better efficacy in BP control and reduced side effect profile.

A useful approach in building an effective combination therapy is based on a convenient model shown in Fig. 66.3. This approach is similar to the popular "Birmingham Square" used in the United Kingdom to develop combination regimens. The art in building or adjusting a combination antihypertensive regimen is to use medications with complementary and not overlapping mechanisms of action, and to try to minimize side effects by leveraging known pharmacology. Examples include adding an ACE inhibitor to a diuretic to reduce occurrence of hypokalemia, or adding an ACE inhibitor (or an ARB) to a CCB to reduce CCB-dependent edema.

MAJOR CLASSES OF ANTIHYPERTENSIVE AGENTS AND ASSOCIATED CARDIOVASCULAR BENEFITS

DIURETICS

Diuretics are proven antihypertensive agents and play a key role in building a successful combination regimen. They work mostly by inhibiting renal sodium absorption. Abundant evidence supports the benefit of diuretics compared with placebo in reducing cardiovascular morbidity and mortality, including ischemic heart disease, heart failure, stroke, other vascular disease, and death. Data from the Antihypertensive and Lipid Lowering Treatment to Prevent Heart Attack Trial (ALLHAT) suggest that thiazide diuretics are as effective as CCBs and ACE inhibitors in lowering BP and reducing coronary events. Despite the concern of higher incidence of new-onset of diabetes with diuretics, secondary analyses from ALLHAT found diuretics to be equally effective as ACE inhibitors and CCBs in reducing cardiovascular risk, including ischemic heart disease, heart failure, stroke, kidney disease, and death in both diabetic and nondiabetic patients. The recently published data on long-term outcomes in the Systolic Hypertension in the Elderly Program (SHEP) affirm the benefits of diuretic therapy in reducing cardiovascular endpoints.

RENIN-ANGIOTENSIN-ALDOSTERONE SYSTEM BLOCKADE

ACE inhibitors, ARBs, direct renin inhibitors, and spironolactone/eplerenone block the conversion of angiotensin I to II (ACE inhibitors), the binding of angiotensin II to its receptor (ARBs), the conversion of angiotensinogen to angiotensin I (direct renin inhibitors), and the binding of aldosterone to the mineralocorticoid receptor (spironolactone/eplerenone). ACE inhibitors and ARBs have been shown in many studies to reduce cardiovascular events, prevent stroke, improve kidney outcomes, and lower the incidence of new onset diabetes.

Aliskiren, a direct renin inhibitor, is an effective antihypertensive agent with a side effect profile that appears similar to ARBs, but lacks evidence of benefit in hard endpoint outcome trials. Aliskiren should not be used in patients with diabetes or CKD also treated with ACE inhibitors or ARB due to concern for worsening kidney function, hypotension, and hyperkalemia. Although spironolactone and eplerenone both have potential benefits in congestive heart failure, they are currently used as third- or fourth-line antihypertensive agents.

CALCIUM CHANNEL BLOCKERS

Calcium channel blockers inhibit the L-type voltage gated channels resulting in vasodilation. Nondihydropyridine CCBs are also associated with decreased cardiac output. Data from ALLHAT suggest that dihydropyridine CCBs are as effective as thiazide diuretics and ACE inhibitors in lowering BP and reducing cardiovascular events including MI, stroke, and overall mortality. In addition, data from Anglo-Scandinavian Cardiac Outcomes Trial (ASCOT) showed that a combination of CCB with ACE inhibitor was more effective in reducing stroke than a combination of beta blocker with ACE inhibitor. Data from the Avoiding Cardiovascular Events through Combination Therapy in Patients Living with Systolic Hypertension (ACCOMPLISH) trial demonstrated that despite identical BP control, combination therapy with ACE inhibitor and CCB seemed superior to the combination of ACE inhibitor and diuretic in hypertensive patients with high cardiovascular risk.

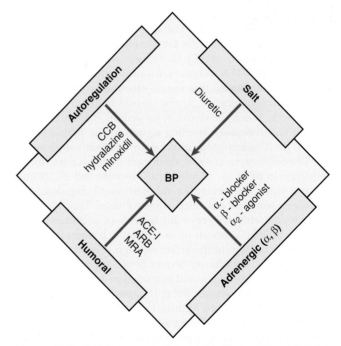

Figure 66.3 Building successful combination antihypertensive therapy. The diagram emphasizes four basic physiologic processes that regulate blood pressure and places the major classes of antihypertensive medications along the side, corresponding to the process responsible for the primary antihypertensive effect of the class. Combining agents to control hypertension is usually more effective when drugs are chosen from different sides (e.g., diuretic plus ARB) as opposed to the same side (e.g., β-blocker plus α₂-agonist) of the diagram. *ACE-I,* Angiotensin converting enzyme inhibitor; *ARB,* angiotensin receptor blocker; *CCB,* calcium channel blocker; *MRA,* mineralocorticoid antagonist.

BETA BLOCKERS

Beta blockers generally decrease cardiac output, but many show vasodilatory effects either from a combined alpha blockade (labetalol and carvedilol) or through nitric oxide potentiation (nebivolol). Beta blockade is useful in treating ischemic heart disease and congestive heart failure. However, beta blockers in older patients have been increasingly replaced by other classes of agents, including diuretics, ACE inhibitors, ARBs, and CCBs, because of concerns that beta blockade does not prevent stroke as effectively as other agents. Although the ASCOT trial suggests the combination of dihydropyridine CCB plus ACE inhibitor is better than the selective beta blocker atenolol plus diuretic, the newer generation of beta blockers with combined alpha and beta blocking activities or nitric oxide potentiating effect may provide more benefit in lowering cardiovascular events, although this remains speculative at present.

OTHER AGENTS

Alpha-1 blockers and other direct vasodilators are still used as add-on therapy in resistant hypertension. The alpha-1 blocker arm using doxazosin in ALLHAT was terminated early because of its inferior cardiovascular outcomes, particularly for new heart failure, compared with the diuretic, ACE inhibitor, and CCB arms.

NOVEL ANTIHYPERTENSIVE THERAPIES

Two device-based interventions are under investigation to treat hypertension refractory to therapy with standard antihypertensive medications. The first approach, the Rheos® System (CVRx), utilizes the known effects of carotid baroreceptor activation (BAT) to reduce sympathetic output and lower BP. This requires surgical implantation of a pacemaker-like device that has an electrode tunneled from its subclavicular location to the carotid body on each side of the neck. When the device is turned on, it stimulates the carotid baroreceptors, sending signals to the brainstem to reduce BP. The European multicenter feasibility study using the Rheos® System showed significant and sustained mean reduction in BP of 21/12 mm Hg at 3 months and 33/22 mm Hg at 2 years. The recently published double-blinded, randomized, placebo-controlled Rheos Pivotal Trial enrolled 265 patients with drug-resistant hypertension and assigned them to BAT at 1 month or at 6 months postimplantation of the device. Despite the relatively high procedure-related adverse events, the Rheos® System device appears to be safe, and provided significant and sustained reductions of more than 30 mm Hg in systolic BP at 12 months.

Another device-based approach, the Symplicity® System (Medtronic), directly ablates renal nerves using radiofrequency energy directly applied through the lumen of both renal arteries using a femoral catheter. The procedure usually takes less than an hour to complete and reduces sympathetic flow into (efferent) and out of (afferent) the kidneys. The Symplicity HTN-1 trial, a proof-of-concept study without a control arm, demonstrated a significant reduction in both systolic and diastolic BP in patients with drug-resistant hypertension following renal denervation. The Symplicity HTN-2 trial was a randomized controlled trial enrolling 106 patients with drug-resistant hypertension (systolic BP >160 mm Hg or >150 mm Hg with diabetes). It confirmed the

progressive BP reduction in the 6 months following renal denervation with a mean reduction of 32/12 mm Hg in systolic and diastolic BP at 6 months, and showed no significant procedure or device-related adverse events. The Simplicity HTN-3 trial, a multicenter, randomized, controlled trial currently ongoing in the United States, will likely provide more information on the role of renal denervation in the treatment of drug-resistant hypertension.

SPECIAL POPULATIONS

WOMEN

When compared with men, women show similar BP response to antihypertensive agents in randomized clinical trials. Before menopause, women have lower BP than men of a similar age. This tends to reverse after menopause, with black women tending to have the highest BP. In women of childbearing age, ACE inhibitors and ARBs are avoided because of the risk for fetal malformations. Women tend to have a higher risk for hypokalemia when treated with diuretics and greater risk for hyponatremia when treated with thiazide diuretics, but in general show similar benefits from antihypertensive agents as men.

BLACKS

Hypertension is more prevalent in blacks and tends to be more closely connected to salt intake, thus responding better to diuretics and CCBs than to ACE inhibitors, ARBs, and beta blockers. In addition, blacks tend to experience higher rates of target organ damage than do whites at any level of BP. The reason is not entirely clear, but the intense search for genetic predisposition continues to attract much attention. Compared with whites, blacks have more frequent cardiovascular complications such as heart failure, and about a fourfold higher risk for end-stage kidney disease. The International Society of Hypertension in Blacks (ISHIB) recently released a consensus statement on the recommendations for managing hypertension in black patients. It recommends a goal BP below 135/85 mm Hg in patients without target organ damage and a goal BP lower than 130/80 mm Hg in patients with evidence of target organ damage, although robust evidence is lacking for this recommendation.

OLDER ADULTS

The pattern of BP elevation in older patients is characterized predominantly by systolic BP. This relates in large part to the significant role of vascular stiffness in the elevated BP of older patients, which in addition to raising systolic BP also contributes to a decline in the diastolic BP and an increase in the pulse pressure. Clinical trials have documented the value of reducing systolic BP when it exceeds 160 mm Hg. Although the target BP of 140/90 mm Hg is generally accepted for most patients, fewer data are available on patients over the age of 80 years to guide therapy. The HYVET enrolled patients of at least 80 years of age and used a target systolic BP of 150 mm Hg. The HYVET trial was stopped early by its safety monitoring board because of excessive deaths in the control arm compared with the ACE inhibitor with diuretic arm. Although the trial failed to show a significant benefit for the primary endpoint of reducing stroke, it demonstrated benefits in reducing mortality and heart failure. For patients between 60 and 79 years of age, a target BP of 140/90 remains a reasonable goal in the absence of other comorbidities (diabetes, coronary artery disease, CKD) and significant side effects, particularly orthostatic hypotension. Treating systolic BP above 160 mm Hg can result in less stroke and cardiovascular disease. However, further lowering of diastolic BP in patients with existing coronary artery disease is not recommended because of increasing cardiovascular events below a certain threshold of BP. Current recommendations are to avoid lowering diastolic BP below 70 mm Hg in those with active coronary artery disease at any age.

PATIENTS WITH DIABETES MELLITUS

The presence of both diabetes and hypertension represents a substantial cardiovascular risk. Treating hypertension is an effective way of reducing this risk, although the goal BP in diabetic patients remains debatable. Based largely on the Hypertension Optimal Treatment (HOT) trial, which showed that the subgroup of diabetics assigned to the lowest diastolic goal (<80 mm Hg) had about half the cardiovascular events as those assigned to a standard goal of 90 mm Hg, the ADA and the NKF recommend a target BP below 130/80 mm Hg, irrespective of age. In the recently completed Action to Control Cardiovascular Risk in Diabetes (ACCORD) trial, the intensive group with an SBP goal below 120 mm Hg did not experience an improvement in the primary composite outcome of fatal and nonfatal cardiovascular events, despite an SBP that was 14 mm Hg lower than the standard group. However, stroke (a prespecified secondary outcome) was significantly reduced in the group with the lower BP goal. It is important to note that the increased medication requirement in the lower BP group resulted in more side effects, including reduced kidney function.

PATIENTS WITH CHRONIC KIDNEY DISEASE

The goal BP for patients with CKD has progressively decreased from 140/90 mm Hg to the current 130/80 mm Hg in the past decade by recommendations of several major societies, including JNC, ADA, and NKF. However, the recent systematic review by Upadhyay and colleagues suggests that the evidence to support the current goal BP of 130/80 in CKD is lacking.

Abundant evidence supports the current recommendation of using ACE inhibitors and ARBs in patients with CKD, especially with proteinuria. The ACCOMPLISH trial compared the cardiovascular outcomes of combination therapy with ACE inhibitor plus CCB to ACE inhibitor plus thiazide diuretic. ACCOMPLISH was terminated early because of the significantly lower risk for cardiovascular endpoints in the ACE inhibitor plus CCB group compared with the ACE inhibitor plus thiazide diuretic group. A prespecified subgroup analysis of the ACCOMPLISH trial compared kidney outcomes, including doubling of serum creatinine, reaching an estimated GFR less than 15 mL/min, or initiating dialysis, with results showing that the combination therapy of ACE inhibitor plus CCB had a 48% reduction in renal endpoints (mostly related to reduced kidney function, not initiation of dialysis) when compared with the combination of ACE inhibitor plus thiazide diuretic.

PATIENTS WITH HEART DISEASE

Beta blockers and renin-angiotensin system blockers have been shown to reduce morbidity and mortality associated with acute MI and high-risk ischemic heart disease. Although beta blockers may worsen acute congestive heart failure, beta blockade remains a key agent in managing chronic congestive heart failure. Diuretics also play an essential role in managing patients with congestive heart failure.

PATIENTS WITH STROKE

Treatments of hypertension with diuretics, renin-angiotensin blockers, calcium channel blockers, and beta blockers are all beneficial for reducing the risk for recurrent stroke. As mentioned before, beta blockade may not provide *as much* benefit in stroke reduction as other forms of antihypertensive drug therapy. However, BP targets in the acute phase of stroke remain less clear. The recent Scandinavian Candesartan Acute Stroke Trial (SCAST) showed that treatment with candesartan to a target SBP below 120 mm Hg after acute stroke did not improve the primary outcome, including a composite cardiovascular death, MI, stroke, and functional status. The American Stroke Association recommendations suggest reducing blood pressure to <185/110 mm Hg in acute stroke patients, and maintaining such reduction when thrombolysis is indicated. With completed stroke, the PROGRESS trial showed that a combination of indapamide (diuretic) and perindopril (ACE inhibitor) substantially reduced risk for recurrent stroke compared with placebo in both hypertensive and nonhypertensive subjects.

CONCLUSION

Hypertension is common, and the prevalence continues to rise with an increasingly older and obese population. Adequate treatment of hypertension remains the key in lowering cardiovascular morbidity and mortality. Although many effective therapies are available, control of BP remains suboptimal, in part related to noncompliance and provider inertia, along with the growth of comorbidities complicating treatment, such as obesity, sleep apnea, and diabetes. New developments in BP lowering devices may provide additional options in managing the truly resistant hypertension.

BIBLIOGRAPHY

ALLHAT Officers and Coordinators for the ALLHAT Collaborative Research Group: Major outcomes in high-risk hypertensive patients randomized to angiotensin-converting enzyme inhibitor or calcium channel blocker versus diuretic: the Antihypertensive and Lipid-Lowering Treatment to Prevent Heart Attack Trial (ALLHAT), *JAMA* 288:2981-2997, 2002.

Appel LJ, Wright JT Jr, Greene T, et al: Intensive blood-pressure control in hypertensive chronic kidney disease, *N Engl J Med* 363:918-929, 2010.

Aronow WS, Fleg JL, Pepine CJ, et al: ACCF/AHA 2011 expert consensus document on hypertension in the elderly: a report of the American College of Cardiology Foundation Task Force on Clinical Expert Consensus documents developed in collaboration with the American Academy of Neurology, American Geriatrics Society, American Society for Preventive Cardiology, American Society of Hypertension, American Society of Nephrology, Association of Black Cardiologists, and European Society of Hypertension, *J Am Coll Cardiol* 57:2037-2114, 2011.

Bakris GL, Sarafidis PA, Weir MR, et al: Renal outcomes with different fixed-dose combination therapies in patients with hypertension at high risk for cardiovascular events (ACCOMPLISH): a prespecified secondary analysis of a randomised controlled trial, *Lancet* 375:1173-1181, 2010.

Beckett NS, Peters R, Fletcher AE, et al: Treatment of hypertension in patients 80 years of age or older, *N Engl J Med* 358:1887-1898, 2008.

Bisognano JD, Bakris G, Nadim MK, et al: Baroreflex activation therapy lowers blood pressure in patients with resistant hypertension: results from the double-blind, randomized, placebo-controlled rheos pivotal trial, *J Am Coll Cardiol* 58:765-773, 2011.

Cushman WC, Evans GW, Byington RP, et al: Effects of intensive blood-pressure control in type 2 diabetes mellitus, *N Engl J Med* 362:1575-1585, 2010.

Dahlöf B, Sever PS, Poulter NR, et al: Prevention of cardiovascular events with an antihypertensive regimen of amlodipine adding perindopril as required versus atenolol adding bendroflumethiazide as required, in the Anglo-Scandinavian Cardiac Outcomes Trial-Blood Pressure Lowering Arm (ASCOT-BPLA): a multicentre randomised controlled trial, *Lancet* 366:895-906, 2005.

Esler MD, Krum H, Sobotka PA, et al: Renal sympathetic denervation in patients with treatment-resistant hypertension (The Symplicity HTN-2 Trial): a randomised controlled trial, *Lancet* 376:1903-1909, 2010.

Flack JM, Sica DA, Bakris G, et al: Management of high blood pressure in Blacks: an update of the International Society on Hypertension in Blacks consensus statement, *Hypertension* 56:780-800, 2010.

Jamerson K, Weber MA, Bakris GL, et al: Benazepril plus amlodipine or hydrochlorothiazide for hypertension in high-risk patients, *N Engl J Med* 359:2417-2428, 2008.

Krause T, Lovibond K, Caulfield M, et-al. Management of hypertension: summary of NICE guidance, *BMJ* 343: d4891.

Lenfant C, Chobanian AV, Jones DW, et al: Seventh report of the Joint National Committee on the Prevention, Detection, Evaluation, and Treatment of High Blood Pressure (JNC 7): resetting the hypertension sails, *Hypertension* 41:1178-1179, 2003.

Ogihara T, Saruta T, Rakugi H, et al: Target blood pressure for treatment of isolated systolic hypertension in the elderly: valsartan in elderly isolated systolic hypertension study, *Hypertension* 56:196-202, 2010.

Sandset EC, Bath PM, Boysen G, et al: The angiotensin-receptor blocker candesartan for treatment of acute stroke (SCAST): a randomised, placebo-controlled, double-blind trial, *Lancet* 377:741-750, 2011.

Upadhyay A, Earley A, Haynes SM, et al: Systematic review: blood pressure target in chronic kidney disease and proteinuria as an effect modifier, *Ann Intern Med* 154:541-548, 2011.

Yusuf S, Teo KK, Pogue J, et al: Telmisartan, ramipril, or both in patients at high risk for vascular events, *N Engl J Med* 358:1547-1559, 2008.

Secondary Hypertension

67

Rory F. McQuillan | Peter J. Conlon

Hypertension is a risk factor for cardiovascular disease including myocardial infarction and stroke, and it is a worldwide public health concern. In 2000, one quarter of the world's population was estimated to have hypertension. In the United States, one in three adults is hypertensive. The majority of cases are the result of a complex interaction of genetic traits with lifestyle factors such as weight, sodium intake, and stress, and are termed essential or idiopathic hypertension. Ten to fifteen percent of cases reflect a specific underlying pathophysiology and are considered secondary hypertension. It is important that physicians identify patients for whom screening for secondary hypertension is appropriate so as to minimize overinvestigation of essential hypertension while not failing to diagnose a readily treatable underlying condition. Many causes of secondary hypertension are reversible, and specific treatment may allow significant improvement or normalization of the blood pressure.

Box 67.1 lists some clinical clues that may suggest the presence of secondary hypertension. Box 67.2 summarizes the many causes of secondary hypertension. This chapter provides a concise overview of these conditions, and suggests a practical clinical approach to the diagnosis and treatment of the patient with suspected secondary hypertension.

KIDNEY CAUSES OF SECONDARY HYPERTENSION

RENOVASCULAR HYPERTENSION

Renovascular disease is the most common correctable cause of secondary hypertension. Its prevalence varies according to the clinical circumstances; it is relatively rare in patients with mild hypertension, but accounts for 10% to 45% of severe or refractory hypertension.

Renovascular hypertension is mediated by activation of the renin-angiotensin-aldosterone system (RAAS) resulting from unilateral or bilateral renal artery stenosis (RAS). To trigger renin release, the stenosis must cause a translesional peak systolic gradient of 15 to 25 mm Hg. This generally only occurs with lesions that result in greater than 70% occlusion of the artery. Because of RAAS activation and sympathetic overactivity, patients with renovascular hypertension have a high incidence of end-organ damage compared to those with essential hypertension. In addition to renovascular hypertension, RAS may cause kidney function impairment and otherwise unexplained episodes of acute pulmonary edema.

The majority of cases of RAS are caused either by atherosclerotic renal artery stenosis (ARAS) or fibromuscular dysplasia (FMD). Rarely, RAS may be caused by extrinsic renal artery compression, neurofibromatosis type 1, or Williams syndrome.

ARAS is usually found in patients older than 50 years with other cardiovascular risk factors or known cardiovascular disease. It constitutes more than 85% of all renovascular disease. Lesions tend to progress, and there is often a coexistent reduction in kidney function. The optimal treatment of ARAS remains controversial. FMD is a nonatherosclerotic, noninflammatory vascular disease that causes stenosis in medium-sized and small arteries, most commonly in the renal and carotid arteries. Renovascular hypertension is the most common clinical manifestation, usually occurring in 30- to 50-year-old women. The progression of stenosis is slow, and renal kidney function is usually well preserved. The most common subtype of the disease causes medial dysplasia of the affected artery, with multiple contiguous stenoses creating the appearance on imaging of a string of beads. FMD has an estimated prevalence among hypertensive patients of less than 1%, but this may be an underestimate because many cases likely go undetected. FMD can be a familial disease. Diagnosis of renal artery FMD should prompt screening of the carotid arteries for associated lesions. Revascularization with percutaneous angioplasty generally improves the associated hypertension.

DIAGNOSIS

Several well-recognized clinical situations that suggest the presence of renovascular disease are summarized in Box 67.3. Clinical examination may show evidence of systemic atherosclerotic disease, such as carotid or femoral bruits or absent pedal pulses. The presence or absence of abdominal bruits is not particularly useful. The urine sediment is usually bland, with mild to moderate proteinuria. A kidney ultrasound may show a discrepancy in size between the two kidneys. Renal artery narrowing is often an incidental finding, particularly in elderly patients, and may coexist with essential hypertension. It is important therefore that investigation only be pursued in patients who are potential candidates for revascularization of the renal arteries.

The imaging modalities available for evaluating renovascular disease are summarized in Table 67.1. Most centers do not proceed directly to intraarterial angiography (Fig. 67.1) because of the risk of contrast nephrotoxicity, cholesterol embolization, and damage to the renal or femoral arteries, but first perform one of several available screening tests.

Box 67.1   Clues to the Presence of Secondary Hypertension

Young age at onset (less than 30 yr)
Sudden onset of hypertension
Uncontrolled or refractory hypertension
Malignant hypertension
Features of a recognized underlying cause

Box 67.2   Causes of Secondary Hypertension

Kidney Causes

Renovascular hypertension
Renal parenchymal hypertension

Endocrine Causes

Primary hyperaldosteronism
Cushing syndrome
Pheochromocytoma
Renin secreting tumor
Hypothyroidism or hyperthyroidism
Acromegaly
Hyperparathyroidism

Cardiovascular or Cardiopulmonary Causes

Coarctation of the aorta
Obstructive sleep apnea

Drugs

Glucocorticoids
Nonsteroidal antiinflammatory drugs
HAART
Combined oral contraceptive pills
VEGF inhibitors, e.g., Bevacizumab, Sunitinib
Venlafaxine
Calcineurin inhibitors
Phenylephrine
Caffeine
Excess alcohol
Erythrocyte stimulating agents
Licorice

Inherited Causes

Glucocorticoid-remediable aldosteronism
SAME
Gordon syndrome (i.e., type 2 pseudohypoaldosteronism)
Liddle syndrome

HAART, Highly active antiretroviral therapy; *SAME,* syndrome of apparent mineralocorticoid excess; *VEGF,* vascular endothelial growth factor.

Box 67.3   Clinical Clues to the Presence of Renovascular Disease

Abrupt onset of or accelerated hypertension at any age
Episodes of flash pulmonary edema with normal ventricular function
Acute, unexplained rise in the serum creatinine level after use of an angiotensin-converting enzyme inhibitor or ARB
Elevated serum creatinine level in patients with severe or refractory hypertension
Asymmetric kidney size

ARB, Angiotensin receptor blocker.

SCREENING TESTS

The most commonly used screening tests are duplex ultrasonography, magnetic resonance angiography (MRA), and computed tomography angiography (CTA). Duplex ultrasonography of the renal arteries reliably detects RAS when performed by an experienced ultrasonographer. However, its accuracy is operator dependent; the sensitivity and specificity of Doppler ultrasonography are estimated at about 80% to 85% in most published trials, but they have been as high as 97% to 99% in a trial enrolling patients who later underwent conventional angiography. Duplex ultrasound allows the operator to predict the severity of stenosis based on the peak systolic velocity (PSV) in the renal artery, which may then be expressed in relation to the PSV in the aorta, termed the *renal-aortic ratio* (RAR). Renal PSV greater than 200 cm/s, RAR greater than 3.5, and the presence of post-stenotic turbulence in the renal artery are highly suggestive of significant RAS. A related measurement is the resistive index, which is calculated by subtracting the peak diastolic velocity (PDV) in the renal artery from the PSV, and dividing by the PSV. As the PDV falls, the resistive index increases. A low resistive index has been suggested as a predictor of response to revascularization, with a resistive index greater than 0.8 predictive of a poor response.

MRA has been the screening investigation of choice for RAS in most centers (Fig. 67.2). It is noninvasive, avoids ionizing radiation, and uses a nonnephrotoxic contrast agent (gadolinium). Recently, nephrogenic systemic fibrosis (NSF) has been linked to gadolinium exposure in patients with GFR less than 30 mL/min. The causal link is based on research showing gadolinium in skin biopsies of patients with NSF. NSF is a rapidly progressive, debilitating condition that causes cutaneous and visceral fibrosis for which there is no well-defined treatment. Gadolinium should therefore be avoided in patients with GFR less than 30 mL/min (see Chapter 6). Improvements in MR technology may allow for vascular imaging without gadolinium.

The accuracy of CTA is reduced in patients with serum creatinine levels greater than 2 mg/dl, probably because of reduced renal blood flow. The need for a significant contrast load in patients with coexistent reduced kidney function is also a limitation. The accuracy of CTA and MRA for detecting RAS is debatable. Metaanalyses have estimated sensitivity and specificity at 97% and 93% for MRA, and 96% and 99% for CTA. This is contradicted, however, by a large, well-designed, prospective study showing that, although both tests had reasonable specificity (88% for MRA and 94% for CTA), sensitivity was relatively poor at 78% and 77%, respectively. We therefore recommend catheter angiography in the setting of high clinical suspicion despite inconclusive noninvasive imaging.

Captopril renography was formerly used extensively. However, it is cumbersome, does not provide images of the renal artery, and has poor predictive value in identifying significant RAS. It is no longer commonly used.

Table 67.1 Investigations to Evaluate Renal Artery Stenosis

	Advantages	Disadvantages
Duplex Ultrasound	Noninvasive No radiation Highly sensitive/specific if operator has appropriate expertise Resistive index may predict response to revascularization	Highly operator dependent Utility of resistive index not universally accepted
MRA	Noninvasive Not nephrotoxic	Gadolinium a risk for NSF in patients with GFR < 30 mL/min Questionable accuracy
CTA	Noninvasive	Nephrotoxicity Sensitivity reduced in advanced CKD
Captopril Renography	Noninvasive Theoretically provides information about functional effect of stenosis	Poor predictive value for degree of stenosis
Intraarterial Angiography	Most accurate determination of stenosis Allows for measurement of transstenotic gradient	Invasive Nephrotoxicity Damage to femoral and renal arteries and other mechanical complications Cholesterol emboli
Renal Vein Renin Sampling	Lateralization in bilateral disease	Inaccurate unless complete occlusion

CKD, Chronic kidney disease; *CTA,* computed tomography angiography; *MRA,* magnetic resonance angiography; *NSF,* nephrogenic systemic fibrosis.

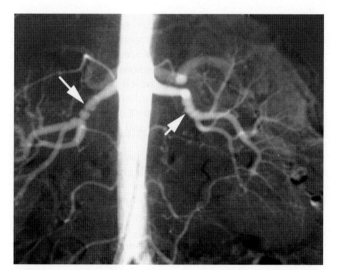

Figure 67.1 Conventional renal angiography demonstrates the classic beadlike appearance of fibromuscular dysplasia in both renal arteries *(arrows).* (Courtesy Professor Mick Lee, Beaumont Hospital, Dublin, Ireland.)

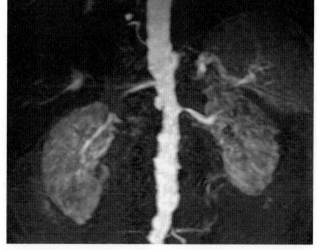

Figure 67.2 Magnetic resonance angiography shows diffuse atherosclerotic disease of the aorta and right renal artery, and a tight ostial stenosis of the left renal artery. (Courtesy Professor Mick Lee, Beaumont Hospital, Dublin, Ireland.)

CONFIRMATORY TESTS

Conventional intraarterial angiography is considered the gold standard for detecting and quantifying the degree of RAS. Newer techniques allow for the measurement of transstenotic pressure gradients. One study that measured the transstenotic gradient after intraarterial infusion of papaverine showed a gradient of at least 21 mm Hg to be highly predictive of an improvement in hypertension at 1 year following revascularization, having a predictive value of 84% compared to only 69% for visual estimation of stenosis as greater than 60%.

Renal vein renin sampling is no longer commonly used in the evaluation of RAS, as it performs poorly at lateralizing lesions unless the renal artery is completely occluded.

TREATMENT

All patients with RAS should receive appropriate antihypertensive therapy. Given the role of the RAAS in mediating hypertension, an angiotensin converting enzyme (ACE) inhibitor or angiotensin receptor blocker (ARB) should be the first-line choice of therapy. Treatment with lipid-lowering drugs and antiplatelet agents is advised in the setting of ARAS

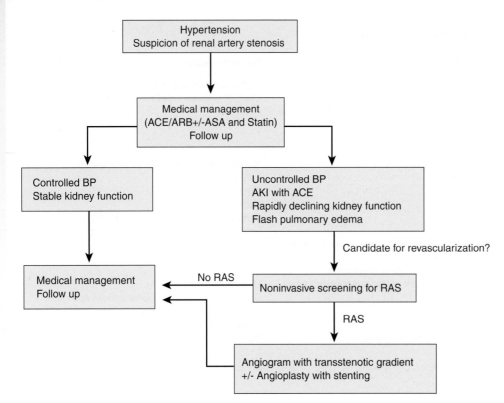

Figure 67.3 Algorithm for investigation and management of renal artery stenosis. *ACE,* Angiotensin converting enzyme; *AKI,* acute kidney injury; *ARB,* angiotensin receptor blockers; *ASA,* aspirin; *BP,* blood pressure; *RAS,* renal artery stenosis.

given the high burden of cardiovascular disease. Figure 67.3 presents a management algorithm for renovascular disease.

Hypertensive patients with FMD should initially be treated with an ACE inhibitor or ARB. If they remain hypertensive, the treatment of choice is revascularization with percutaneous transluminal renal angioplasty (PTRA). PTRA in patients with FMD is almost always technically successful with a low restenosis rate, minimal risk, and usually an improvement, though not complete "cure," of the associated hypertension. There is sparse literature addressing the use of stenting in this disease, presumably because of the high rate of prolonged success with angioplasty alone. Stenting is an option in cases of restenosis, although in view of the young age of many of these patients, surgical revascularization should also be considered.

Revascularization for ARAS is not as straightforward. Although intuitively attractive, restoration of blood flow to the kidneys in unselected patients has had disappointing results. Several randomized controlled trials (Table 67.2) have compared angioplasty with and without stenting to medical management alone. None have demonstrated any benefit in terms of blood pressure control, kidney function, or cardiovascular events with intervention compared to medical management. Revascularization may cause serious adverse events. There are several important limitations to these trials. First, patients included were, by and large, clinically stable: The Angioplasty and Stent Therapy for Renal Artery Lesion (ASTRAL) trial, the largest to date, used physician uncertainty as its key inclusion criterion leading to the recruitment and randomization to intervention of patients with nonsignificant degrees of stenosis that might be less likely to benefit from revascularization. The STent placement for Atherosclerotic Renal-artery stenosis (STAR) trial was similarly compromised. These results must therefore not be extrapolated to patients with ARAS and malignant range hypertension, rapidly advancing

kidney failure, or flash pulmonary edema. The ASTRAL, Dutch Renal Artery STenosis Intervention Cooperative study group (DRASTIC), and Essai Multicentrique Medicaments vs. Angioplastie (EMMA) trials all allowed crossover from the medical to interventional arms, which reduced their ability to detect a difference between treatments. The medical management of hypertension was not well defined in these trials, RAAS blockade was not universal, and the control of BP was often inadequate in both groups.

The DRASTIC and EMMA trials used angioplasty without stenting, which is associated with higher rates of restenosis and is not recommended. Figure 67.4 shows a stent in the left renal artery after percutaneous intervention.

For patients with significant disease in whom there is clinical uncertainty regarding treatment, the ongoing Cardiovascular Outcomes in Renal Artery Lesions (CORAL) trial may provide some guidance. CORAL is a randomized trial that seeks to recruit 1080 patients to determine whether stenting is superior to medical management in terms of controlling hypertension, arresting the decline in kidney function, and preventing cardiovascular events. Its inclusion criteria, which either include more than 80% stenosis on catheter angiography or more than 60% with a demonstrable transstenotic pressure gradient of greater than 20 mm Hg, should ensure that only patients with hemodynamically significant RAS are included. All patients will be treated with RAAS blockade.

Pending results from CORAL, management of patients with ARAS must be evaluated on a case-by-case basis with careful consideration given to the clinical situation and correlation with investigations. It is helpful to decide before recommending revascularization procedures whether the indication for intervention is treatment of renovascular hypertension, preservation of kidney function, or both. Renovascular hypertension typically manifests as an abrupt onset of severe hypertension or a marked deterioration from

Table 67.2 Prospective Randomized Control Trials Comparing Percutaneous Transluminal Angioplasty to Medical Management in Renal Artery Stenosis

Trial	Number of Patients	Year of Publication	Inclusion Criteria	Primary Outcome	Treatment in Revascularization Group	Treatment in Comparison Group	Outcome	Limitations
ASTRAL	806	2009	Significant RAS and physician uncertainty regarding benefit of revascularization	Reciprocal creatinine concentration over time	Medication plus PTA with or without stent	Antihypertensive medication	No difference in primary outcome, BP, or cardiovascular events	Enrollment bias Not standardized imaging (42% of patients less than 70% stenosis) 6% crossover
STAR	140	2009	RAS greater than 50% GFR 15 to 80 mL/min Stable BP	Decrease in GFR ≥20%	Medication plus PTA with stent	Antihypertensive medication	No significant difference in primary outcome or BP	Included patients with minor disease 28% of treatment group did not receive stent due to trivial nature of stenosis
DRASTIC	106	2000	Unilateral or bilateral RAS ≥50% Diastolic BP ≥95 mm Hg on 2 drugs or an increase in creatinine ≥20 μmol/L on ACE inhibitors	Office BP	PTA	Antihypertensive medication	No difference in BP or creatinine Reduction in defined daily doses of antihypertensive drugs	44% crossover No stents Short follow-up Inadequate BP control in both groups
EMMA	49	1998	Unilateral RAS ≥75% or ≥60% plus a positive renography	24 hr ambulatory BP	PTA (2 patients received a stent)	Antihypertensive medication	No difference in BP or creatinine clearance reduction in defined daily doses of antihypertensive drugs	27% crossover Few stents Short follow-up RAAS blockade avoided
Webster et al.	55	1998	Unilateral or bilateral RAS Diastolic BP greater than 95 mm Hg on 2 drugs	Office BP	PTA	Antihypertensive medication	No significant difference in cardiovascular events, BP, or GFR	No stents Short follow-up Inadequate BP control in both groups Excluded patients on ACE inhibitors

ACE, Angiotensin converting enzyme; *ASTRAL,* the Angioplasty and Stent Therapy for Renal Artery Lesion; *BP,* blood pressure; *DRASTIC,* Dutch Renal Artery Stenosis Intervention Cooperative study group; *EMMA,* Essai Multicentrique Medicaments vs. Angioplastie; *GFR,* glomerular filtration rate; *PTA,* percutaneous transluminal angioplasty; *RAAS,* renin-angiotensin aldosterone system; *RAS,* renal artery stenosis; *STAR,* Stent placement for Atherosclerotic Renal-artery stenosis.

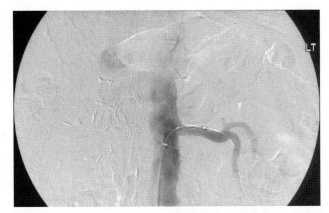

Figure 67.4   A stent can be seen in the ostium of the left renal artery. (Courtesy Professor Mick Lee, Beaumont Hospital, Dublin, Ireland.)

a previously stable baseline. Chronic stable hypertension present for many years is unlikely to be caused by progressive RAS, and is therefore unlikely to respond to intervention. Data suggest that revascularization cannot improve blood pressure in patients who have already lost more than 60% of kidney function.

Although ischemic nephropathy is a significant cause of end-stage renal disease, the issue of revascularization for preservation of kidney function is controversial. Patients (especially those with serum creatinine levels of ≥2.5 mg/dl) often already have significant, irreversible renal parenchymal disease, and kidney function is unlikely to be improved by revascularization. Other signs of poor response to intervention include kidney size less than 9 cm, a renal resistive index greater than 80 on Doppler ultrasonography, significant proteinuria, evidence of another kidney disease, or findings of marked chronicity on kidney biopsy. In patients with known RAS greater than 60%, following serial serum creatinine measurements can identify those who are progressively losing kidney function that may still be salvaged. There is some evidence that this group responds better to intervention than those with chronic, stable kidney function impairment.

ARAS may also manifest as recurrent episodes of flash pulmonary edema. There is evidence from small, nonrandomized trials that this subgroup of patients benefit from renal artery stenting, and treatment is strongly recommended by the American College of Cardiology.

RENAL PARENCHYMAL HYPERTENSION

Hypertension is a common feature of acute and chronic kidney disease (CKD), particularly in glomerular and vascular disorders. Hypertension results from a combination of a positive salt balance, increased activity of the RAAS, and overactivity of the sympathetic nervous system. Treatment of hypertension in CKD consists of dietary salt restriction and promotion of salt excretion with diuretics, blockade of the RAAS system with ACE inhibitors and ARBs, and inhibition of the sympathetic nervous system. The recent Simplicity HTN-2 Trial demonstrated that catheter-based renal sympathetic denervation can be used to reduce blood pressure substantially in treatment-resistant hypertensive patients. Clues to the presence of renal parenchymal disease in

hypertensive patients are elevated serum creatinine levels and abnormal urinalyses. A kidney ultrasound is a useful noninvasive screening test to assess kidney size and asymmetry, and to rule out major kidney structural abnormalities or obstructive lesions. The varied disorders have many treatments available, and a discussion of each is beyond the scope of this chapter.

ENDOCRINE CAUSES OF SECONDARY HYPERTENSION

Hypertension is a feature of several endocrine conditions (see Box 67.2) with the best-characterized associations being primary hyperaldosteronism, Cushing syndrome, and pheochromocytoma.

PRIMARY HYPERALDOSTERONISM

Primary hyperaldosteronism is the most common endocrine cause of hypertension, and its incidence increases with the severity of hypertension. Among patients with resistant hypertension, the prevalence of primary hyperaldosteronism is estimated to be 17% to 20%.

As a group, African-American patients tend to have lower renin levels, but no ethnic differences in the prevalence of primary hyperaldosteronism have been described. No difference between the sexes has been reported.

Primary hyperaldosteronism may be caused by bilateral adrenal hyperplasia (65% of cases), aldosterone producing adenoma (30% of cases), or, rarely, a secretory adrenal carcinoma or inherited endocrinopathy (discussed later). Patients with adrenal adenomas tend to be younger and have a more severe clinical picture than those with adrenal hyperplasia.

CLINICAL SYNDROME

Conn first described the clinical syndrome of primary hyperaldosteronism in 1955 in a 34-year-old woman with hypertension, episodic paralysis, hypokalemia, and metabolic alkalosis. She was subsequently cured by the removal of an adrenal adenoma.

DIAGNOSIS

Although hypokalemia may arouse suspicions of hyperaldosteronism, the latter is not present in most cases. Testing for hyperaldosteronism should be considered in any of the following circumstances: hypertension and spontaneous hypokalemia (or hypokalemia induced by low-dose diuretic), severe hypertension (i.e., systolic pressure greater than 160 mm Hg, diastolic pressure greater than 100 mm Hg, or both); a patient requiring three or more antihypertensive drugs; hypertension manifesting at a young age (less than 40 years); hypertensive patients with an incidental adrenal mass; and hypertensive relatives of a patient with primary hyperaldosteronism. Figure 67.5 is an algorithm to evaluate suspected primary hyperaldosteronism.

SCREENING TESTS

Measurement of the ratio of plasma aldosterone concentration (PAC) to plasma renin activity (PRA) is the screening test of choice for patients with suspected primary

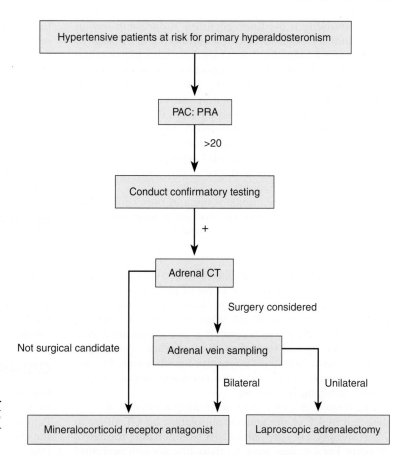

Figure 67.5 Algorithm for the evaluation and management of suspected primary hyperaldosteronism. *CT,* Computed tomography; *PAC,* plasma aldosterone concentration; *PRA,* plasma renin activity.

hyperaldosteronism. A PAC/PRA ratio greater than 20 in combination with a PAC greater than 15 ng/dl (416 pmol/L) is considered a positive screening test result. The test is performed in the morning on an ambulatory patient. Hypokalemia, if present, should be first corrected, as it may suppress aldosterone secretion. Aldosterone antagonists and amiloride should be stopped 6 weeks before testing. As ACE inhibitors, ARBs, and diuretics can falsely elevate the PRA value, the presence of a detectable PRA or a low PAC/PRA ratio in patients taking these agents does not exclude a diagnosis of primary hyperaldosteronism. However, if the PRA is undetectable in a patient taking an ACE inhibitor or ARB, then a diagnosis of primary hyperaldosteronism should be considered, and the ACE inhibitors or ARB need not be stopped. Adrenergic inhibitors (i.e., β-blockers and, to a lesser extent, α_2-agonists) suppress renin and reduce aldosterone levels, although to a lesser degree, in normal individuals. The PAC/PRA ratio may be increased in hypertensive patients without hyperaldosteronism who are taking adrenergic antagonists, but the PAC will not be greater than 15 ng/dl, and the diagnostic power of the test is therefore unaffected. Table 67.3 summarizes how some commonly used antihypertensive medications may affect the interpretation of the PRA/PAC. Verapamil (a nondihydropyridine calcium channel blocker), hydralazine, and α-adrenergic agents such as prazosin, doxazosin, and terazosin have little or no effect on PRA/PAC, and may be used to control hypertension during testing.

CONFIRMATORY TESTS

The PAC/PRA ratio is a screening tool, and confirmatory tests are necessary to confirm autonomous adrenal

Table 67.3 Commonly Used Antihypertensive Agents Affecting the Plasma Aldosterone Concentration to Plasma Renin Activity Ratio

	PAC	PRA	PAC:PRA	Clinical Consequence
ACE inhibitor	↓	↑	↓	False negative
ARB	↓	↑	↓	False negative
β Blockers	↓	↓↓	↑	False positive
Central α-blockers	↓	↓↓	↑	False positive
Diuretics	↑	↑↑	↓	False negative
Dihydropyridine Ca Channel Blockers	↓	↑	↓	False negative

ACE, Angiotensin converting enzyme; *ARB,* angiotensin receptor blocker; *Ca,* calcium; *PAC,* plasma aldosterone concentration; *PRA,* plasma renin activity.

production of aldosterone. The hallmark of primary hyperaldosteronism is nonsuppressible aldosterone secretion with nonstimulable renin secretion. In principle, administration of a sodium load should result in suppression of aldosterone in normal individuals, whereas in patients with hyperaldosteronism, suppression will not occur. This may be achieved by means of oral sodium chloride load over several days, or by administration of intravenous saline over several hours.

An alternative is the fludrocortisone suppression test, in which fludrocortisone acetate is administered at a dosage of 0.1 mg every 6 hours for 4 days together with a high-sodium diet. In the normal individual, aldosterone is suppressed.

These tests have potential risks, particularly for patients with poor left ventricular function. An alternative is the captopril suppression test, in which oral administration of captopril does not suppress aldosterone levels below 15 ng/dl in patients with primary hyperaldosteronism. This test has the advantage of avoiding salt loading in individuals in whom this is contraindicated, but it may cause profound hypotension in some patients.

All of these tests are cumbersome and time consuming, and many centers now directly proceed to imaging after a positive biochemical screening test result.

IMAGING

The adrenal glands are best imaged with computed tomography (CT) to determine the cause of primary hyperaldosteronism. Adenomas 10 mm in diameter and sometimes even smaller can be detected. Magnetic resonance imaging (MRI) is less attractive, because it is more expensive than CT with less spatial resolution. Radionuclide scintigraphy with [^{131}I]iodocholesterol is sensitive for adenomas, but not widely available. There have also been several case reports documenting missed lesions.

Incidentally detected nonfunctioning adenomas may be detected in 4% of the general population on CT, rising to 7% at autopsy. They are particularly common after the age of 40 years. For a patient younger than 40 years with profound hyperaldosteronism (e.g., PAC greater than 30 ng/dl or 832 pmol/L), an adenoma found on CT that is larger than 1 cm, of uniform diameter, and hypodense (less than 10 Hounsfield units), and a contralateral adrenal gland that appears normal on imaging, it is reasonable to proceed to adrenalectomy, because the chance of an aldosterone-producing adenoma is high. In older individuals, adrenal vein sampling should be performed if an adenoma is detected, because aldosterone-producing adenomas become increasingly rare with advancing age. If the adrenal glands appear normal on imaging, patients should proceed directly to adrenal vein sampling. This technique can strongly predict a therapeutic response to unilateral adrenalectomy. An experienced radiologist must perform adrenal vein sampling, and it is more accurate when performed after adrenocorticotropic hormone (ACTH) stimulation. The position in the adrenal vein is confirmed by simultaneously measuring adrenal vein and peripheral vein cortisol levels. A greater than five-fold increase in PAC compared with the contralateral side is expected on the side of an active adenoma. In adrenal hyperplasia, there should be little difference between the two adrenal vein levels. Occasionally, the adenoma may be extraadrenal, and the result of adrenal vein sampling is normal. If imaging and adrenal vein sampling are negative, the rare diagnosis of glucocorticoid-remediable aldosteronism (discussed later) should be considered.

TREATMENT

Patients with adenomas should be referred for unilateral laparoscopic adrenalectomy as removal of well-localized unilateral lesions is very successful. Embolization of adenomas with ethanol may be an option in patients medically unfit for surgery. Selective hypoaldosteronism may occur for some months after surgery, and potassium should be supplemented cautiously during this period. The drugs of choice for medical management of adrenal hyperplasia and preoperative management of adenomas in the past have been spironolactone, amiloride, and ACE inhibitors. Eplerenone, a newer selective aldosterone receptor antagonist, is popular because it causes much less gynecomastia than spironolactone. However, a recent well-powered double-blinded randomized controlled trial demonstrated that eplerenone is less effective than spironolactone for controlling blood pressure.

HYPERRENINISM

Renin-secreting tumors are rare. Affected patients are typically hypertensive and hypokalemic, with high PRA along with elevated aldosterone levels and urinary potassium excretion. These tumors usually originate from the juxtaglomerular apparatus in the kidney, but renin production has been reported with other malignancies, including teratomas and ovarian tumors.

CUSHING SYNDROME

Cushing syndrome is a clinical condition resulting from excess effects of exogenous or endogenous glucocorticoids. Patients develop a characteristic clinical appearance, with the classic cushingoid *moon facies* related to facial fat deposition, along with truncal obesity, abdominal striae, hirsutism, and kyphoscoliosis. Patients have varying degrees of multiorgan involvement, with diabetes mellitus, cataracts, neuropsychiatric disorders, proximal myopathy, avascular necrosis of humeral and femoral heads, osteoporosis, and secondary hypertension among the more prominent. The original syndrome described by Cushing related to a patient with pituitary ACTH excess driving excess cortisol production. As a consequence, pituitary-dependent disease is known as Cushing disease. Hypertension resulting from the mineralocorticoid effect of the glucocorticoids is a common feature. Causes of Cushing syndrome are listed in Box 67.4. The most common cause of endogenous glucocorticoid excess is a pituitary adenoma.

DIAGNOSIS

The presence of cortisol excess must be confirmed biochemically. This can be achieved with the low-dose dexamethasone suppression test, measurement of 24-hour urinary free-cortisol levels, or assessment of the circadian pattern

---

Box 67.4   Causes of Cushing Syndrome

Exogenous glucocorticoid administration
Endogenous glucocorticoid excess
ACTH excess
    Ectopic production
    Pituitary secretory adenoma (Cushing disease)
Cortisol excess

ACTH, Adrenocorticotropic hormone.

of cortisol secretion. In the overnight, low-dose dexamethasone suppression test, a 2-mg dose of dexamethasone is taken at 11 PM, and a plasma cortisol sample is drawn at 9 AM the next morning. Suppression is defined as a cortisol level of less than 5 mg/dl. To assess circadian cortisol secretion, cortisol levels are measured at 9 AM and 11 PM. They are usually highest in the morning and lowest at night.

Other causes of abnormally high cortisol secretion include stress, major depression, and chronic excess alcohol consumption. A normal response to an insulin suppression test suggests major depression.

When cortisol excess is confirmed, further testing to elucidate a pituitary, adrenal, or ectopic source should follow. Extremely high plasma or urinary cortisol levels suggest adrenal carcinoma or ectopic ACTH secretion. An adrenal carcinoma often causes marked virilization and severe hypokalemic metabolic alkalosis.

If there is an adrenal source of glucocorticoids, plasma ACTH levels should be suppressed below the normal range. A normal or moderately raised level suggests pituitary disease. High levels suggest ectopic disease.

The high-dose dexamethasone suppression test is performed by administering dexamethasone 2 mg every 6 hours for 2 days. Cortisol levels are measured at 9 AM on day 1 and day 3. Reduction of cortisol to less than 50% of the day 1 level is defined as suppression. Pituitary-dependent Cushing disease should respond in this way, whereas ectopic ACTH production should not.

IMAGING

CT or MRI of the adrenals or the pituitary, depending on the clinical suspicion, should be performed. If ectopic ACTH is diagnosed, a bronchial neoplasm should be aggressively ruled out.

TREATMENT

If the cause is exogenous steroid use, efforts should be made to withdraw the medication dose carefully and slowly if the patient is able and the clinical condition being treated allows. Steroid-sparing agents may help.

Endogenous Cushing syndrome is best treated by surgical excision. In patients who are not deemed surgical candidates, or in those with recurrent disease after resection, radiation is an alternative therapy. If there is adrenal overactivity without tumor localization or ectopic ACTH activity, symptoms may be relieved by suppressing the adrenal gland with medications such as metyrapone, aminoglutethimide, or mitotane.

PHEOCHROMOCYTOMA

Pheochromocytoma is a secretory tumor of neurochromaffin cells in the adrenal medulla. It is a rare condition responsible for less than 0.2% of all hypertensive cases. Symptoms result from catecholamine hypersecretion.

Patients classically present with the triad of episodic headache, sweating, and tachycardia; most have at least two of these symptoms. Pallor, paroxysmal hypotension, orthostatic hypotension, visual blurring, papilledema, high erythrocyte sedimentation rate, weight loss, polyuria, polydipsia, psychiatric disorders, hyperglycemia, dilated cardiomyopathy, and, rarely, secondary erythrocytosis are less common clinical features. About one half of patients have paroxysms of hypertension, whereas most of the remainder have apparent essential hypertension. Many have no symptoms and are detected serendipitously with abdominal radiology, at surgery, or at postmortem examination.

When referring to these tumors, the "10% rule" is often cited, and is still clinically useful: approximately 10% of cases are extraadrenal, 10% are malignant, 10% are bilateral, and 10% are associated with familial syndromes. There are two main familial syndromes associated with pheochromocytoma:

1. In patients with von Hippel-Lindau syndrome, pheochromocytoma occurs in 10% to 20% of cases.
2. Multiple endocrine neoplasia syndrome type 2 is associated with medullary thyroid carcinoma and hyperparathyroidism. Pheochromocytoma occurs in 20% to 50% of affected individuals.

Pheochromocytoma is found in less than 5% of patients with neurofibromatosis type 1. Genetic screening is recommended in patients younger than 21 years of age, with extraadrenal or bilateral disease, or multiple paragangliomas.

DIAGNOSIS

A classic history of the typical triad of symptoms or a family history may suggest the diagnosis. The screening tests used are measurements of urinary and plasma catecholamines or their metabolites.

Urinary, Plasma, and Platelet Catecholamine Levels

A study based on prospective data from 152 consecutive patients with pheochromocytoma compared the relative diagnostic sensitivities of the various catecholamine and catecholamine metabolite levels. It showed that the most sensitive tests were urinary normetanephrine and platelet norepinephrine levels, with sensitivities of 96.9% and 93.8%, respectively. For patients in whom a pheochromocytoma is clinically suspected but cannot be confirmed by urinary, plasma, or platelet catecholamine levels, a ^{131}I-labeled metaiodobenzylguanidine (MIBG) radioisotope scan may be performed. MIBG is an analogue of epinephrine. It improves the sensitivity of platelet epinephrine to 100%. When combined with an MIBG plasma norepinephrine assay, it has a sensitivity of 97.1% in predicting the presence of pheochromocytoma. The likely reason for the increased sensitivity of platelet epinephrine is that the neurosecretory granules in the platelets concentrate the catecholamines that are intermittently secreted by the pheochromocytoma. Measurement of platelet epinephrine should be part of the standard screening for pheochromocytoma.

Clonidine Suppression Test

The clonidine suppression test is an alternative method for confirming a diagnosis when catecholamine levels are suggestive but not diagnostic of pheochromocytoma. Clonidine is administered after all antihypertensives have been withheld for at least 12 hours; plasma catecholamines are measured 3 hours later and should fall to less than 500 pg/mL in normal individuals. This test is 90% sensitive for pheochromocytoma.

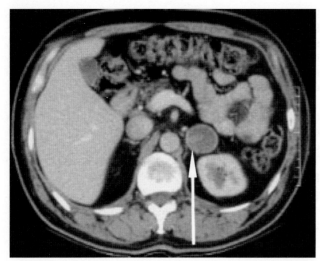

Figure 67.6   Computed tomography shows a pheochromocytoma arising from the left adrenal gland (arrow). (Courtesy Professor Mick Lee, Beaumont Hospital, Dublin, Ireland.)

Imaging

Imaging should be performed after biochemical confirmation of the diagnosis using the assays already described. Ninety-five percent of pheochromocytomas are intraabdominal, with 90% located in the adrenal glands. CT or MRI is the initial modality of choice (Fig. 67.6); both are up to 98% sensitive but only about 70% specific because of the high prevalence of nonfunctional adrenal adenomas, particularly with increasing age.

If CT or MRI imaging is negative despite positive screening assays, the diagnosis should be reconsidered. If pheochromocytoma is still strongly suspected, an MIBG or total-body MRI should be performed. In addition to the role previously described, MIBG scans can be used to detect pheochromocytomas when the result of CT or MRI is negative or extraadrenal or metastatic disease is suspected. Positron emission tomographic (PET) scanning may have a future role in detecting metastatic disease.

TREATMENT

The definitive treatment for a pheochromocytoma is surgical excision, but medical treatment to control the effects of catecholamine excess is crucial preoperatively. There are several accepted approaches. The most widely used is administration of the α-blocker phenoxybenzamine, starting at a dose of 10 mg once daily and increasing the dose every few days until blood pressure and symptoms are controlled. A β-blocker may then be added to control tachycardia. Using this approach, a patient should be ready for surgery in 10 to 14 days.

A β-blocker should never be administered first, as the subsequent unopposed α-agonist vasoconstrictive action can markedly worsen hypertension. A hypertensive crisis precipitated by β-blockade may be a clue to the presence of a pheochromocytoma in a patient with hypertension.

Surgery for pheochromocytoma has a perioperative mortality rate of 2.4% and a morbidity rate of 24%. Associated metastases should be resected if possible, and skeletal lesions irradiated. Chemotherapy may be used in selected patients.

PROGNOSIS

Long-term follow-up is indicated in all patients because of the high incidence of recurrent hypertension, even with complete tumor removal. The tumor recurs in about 10% of patients. Recurrences are more common in familial cases, and a significant proportion of recurrences are malignant.

CARDIOVASCULAR AND CARDIOPULMONARY CAUSES OF SECONDARY HYPERTENSION

COARCTATION OF THE AORTA

Coarctation is a congenital narrowing of the aortic lumen occurring most commonly just distal to the origin of the left subclavian artery. Clinically, patients have hypertension when blood pressure is measured in the upper limbs, with reduced or unmeasurable blood pressure in the legs. If the coarctation is proximal to the origin of the left subclavian artery, the blood pressure and brachial pulsation in the left upper limb may be reduced. The femoral pulses may be delayed or diminished compared with the radial or brachial pulses, and there may be an audible bruit over the patient's back. Diagnosis is confirmed with aortic imaging, and treatment is surgical.

SLEEP APNEA SYNDROME

The association of obesity, obstructive sleep apnea, and hypertension has long been recognized. Owing to a combination of factors inherent to sleep apnea, including apnea, hypoxia, hypercapnia, and arousal from sleep, activation of the sympathetic nervous system leads to hypertension. Many cases of obstructive sleep apnea go undiagnosed unless the physician is alert to the possibility. In most studies of patients with sleep apnea and hypertension, daytime and nighttime levels of blood pressure improved significantly after treatment with continuous positive airway pressure (CPAP) or related modalities.

INHERITED CAUSES OF SECONDARY HYPERTENSION

Several monogenetic disorders are associated with hypertension. Although all are probably significantly underdiagnosed, each is rare. They are all associated with upregulation of sodium reabsorption in the distal nephron with accompanying expansion of extracellular volume. The PRA is uniformly suppressed. These conditions may be divided into primary disorders of the distal nephron and primary adrenal disorders. They are summarized in Table 67.4.

DISTAL NEPHRON DISORDERS

LIDDLE SYNDROME

In 1963, Liddle and colleagues described a familial syndrome of severe hypertension, hypokalemia, and metabolic alkalosis mimicking hyperaldosteronism. This disorder affects the handling of sodium in the distal nephron. Reabsorption of sodium in the collecting duct depends on the

Table 67.4   Inherited Causes of Hypertension

Inherited Disorder	Mode of Transmission	Chromosome	Defective Protein	OMIM Number
Liddle Syndrome	Autosomal dominant	16p12.2	β and γ subunits of ENaC	177200
Gordon Syndrome	Autosomal dominant	17q21.31	WNK 4	601844
	Autosomal dominant	12p13.33	WNK 1	605232
Syndrome of AME	Autosomal recessive	16q22.1	11β-hydroxysteroid dehydrogenase type II	614232
Autosomal Dominant Early Onset Hypertension Exacerbated by Pregnancy	Autosomal dominant	4q31.23	Mineralocorticoid receptor S810L	605115
Glucocorticoid Remediable Hyperaldosteronism	Autosomal dominant	8q24.3	11β-hydroxylase:fusion of CYP11B2 CYP11B1	103900
Familial Hyperaldosteronism Type 2	Autosomal dominant	17p22	Unknown	605635
Congenital Adrenal Hyperplasia	Autosomal recessive	8q24.3	11β-hydroxylase	610613
	Autosomal recessive	10q24.32	17α-hydroxylase	202110

AME, Apparent mineralocorticoid excess; *ENaC,* epithelial sodium channel; *OMIM;* Online Mendelian Inheritance in Man. www.ncbi.nlm.nih.gov/omim.

activity of the amiloride-sensitive epithelial sodium channel (ENaC). The activity of ENaC is based on recycling of the channel between the apical membrane and subapical vesicles. Mutations in the genes coding for either the beta or gamma subunits of ENaC result in deletion of the binding site necessary for degradation or recycling, leading to an increased number of functional sodium transport channels.

Hypertension usually begins in childhood but may not be diagnosed until early adulthood. Hypokalemia and alkalosis occur as the electronegativity of the collecting duct lumen is increased by excess sodium reabsorption. This favors potassium and hydrogen ion excretion, although the actual presence of metabolic alkalosis and hypokalemia is variable. PRA and PAC are suppressed. Treatment involves a low-salt diet and an agent that directly inhibits ENaC, such as amiloride or triamterene. Mineralocorticoid receptor antagonists do not have an effect since the defective sodium transport is independent of aldosterone.

GORDON SYNDROME: TYPE 2 PSEUDOHYPOALDOSTERONISM

Gordon and colleagues first described this syndrome of hypertension and hyperkalemia in 1970. It has since been characterized as an autosomal dominant disorder caused by mutations in two members of the WNK family of serine-threonine kinases, a group of enzymes involved in regulating the activity of the thiazide-sensitive NaCl cotransporter (NCCT) in the distal convoluted tubule. WNK4 phosphorylates NCCT, preventing incorporation of the transporter into the apical membrane. Missense mutations in the WNK4 gene (chromosome 17) produce mutant proteins that allow increased NCCT expression, a lesion complementary to the deficiency of NCCT expression in Gitelman syndrome. WNK1 is predominantly a cytoplasmic protein that inhibits WNK4 function. Mutations in the WNK1 gene (chromosome 12) that increase WNK1 production lead to excess WNK4 inhibition and to increased NCCT expression. Both WNK kinase mutations cause overactivity of the NCCT, with resultant excess salt reabsorption. This causes volume-dependent hypertension and suppression of the RAAS.

Augmented absorption at this site reduces collecting duct sodium delivery to the ENaC channel, leading to a reduction in lumen electronegativity with consequent potassium and acid retention, and thus development of a hyperkalemic metabolic acidosis. The hyperkalemia may be exacerbated by the fact that the same mutation in WNK4 that releases NCCT from suppression has an inhibitory effect on the secretory renal outer medullary potassium channels (ROMK). The PRA value is low. Aldosterone levels vary, and may be increased by hyperkalemia, although not enough to correct it. The metabolic abnormalities tend to precede the onset of hypertension, which often does not manifest until adult life. Spitzer-Weinstein syndrome, which consists of hyperkalemia, metabolic acidosis, and growth failure but not hypertension, is thought to be an early manifestation of Gordon syndrome. Treatment typically involves a combination of dietary salt restriction with a low-dose thiazide or loop diuretics, and is usually very effective. WNK kinases and their targets may offer novel targets for future antihypertensive agents.

SYNDROME OF APPARENT MINERALOCORTICOID EXCESS

Apparent mineralocorticoid excess (AME) is a rare autosomal recessive disorder in which the enzyme 11β-hyroxysteroid dehydrogenase type 2 (11HD2) is inactive. In aldosterone-sensitive tissues, this enzyme usually converts cortisol to inactive cortisone and prevents its mineralocorticoid effect. In AME, cortisol acts on the mineralocorticoid receptor, causing apparent hyperaldosteronism despite suppressed aldosterone levels. Because of the lack of 11HD2, the conversion of cortisol to cortisone is impaired, resulting in an abnormal ratio of cortisol metabolites (i.e., tetrahydrocortisol and allotetrahydrocortisol) to cortisone metabolites (e.g., tetrahydrocortisone) in the urine. The disease was thought to be invariably present from childhood, with patients presenting with low birth weight, failure to thrive, hypokalemia, and metabolic alkalosis. It has been associated with end-organ damage and a high mortality rate if untreated. However, milder phenotypes with only partial inactivation of 11HD2 have been described. Mineralocorticoid receptor blockers, potassium supplementation, and dietary sodium restriction are the mainstays of treatment. A mild acquired variant may be encountered in patients with excessive licorice intake. The principal metabolite of licorice, glycyrrhizic acid, inhibits 11HD2 causing a weak mineralocorticoid effect. Carbenoxolone, a licorice derivative previously used for treatment of peptic ulcers was also associated with hypertension.

AUTOSOMAL DOMINANT EARLY ONSET HYPERTENSION EXACERBATED BY PREGNANCY

Autosomal Dominant Early Onset Hypertension Exacerbated by Pregnancy is a recently described rare genetic condition in which an activating mutation of the mineralocorticoid receptor renders it especially sensitive to non-mineralocorticoid steroids such as progesterone. Since progesterone levels increase 100-fold during pregnancy, this condition typically is detected in pregnant women, although affected individuals are often hypertensive before conception and males can also be affected. The mineralocorticoid receptor in these patients can also be activated by spironolactone, and this agent is contraindicated in this condition.

ADRENAL DISORDERS

GLUCOCORTICOID-REMEDIABLE ALDOSTERONISM: FAMILIAL HYPERALDOSTERONISM TYPE 1

Glucocorticoid-remediable aldosteronism is a rare subtype of primary hyperaldosteronism in which the hyperaldosteronism can be reversed with steroid administration. Glucocorticoid-remediable aldosteronism is inherited as an autosomal dominant trait and should be suspected in patients with onset of hypertension before the age of 21 years along with a family history of early hypertension or intracerebral hemorrhage. Individuals are otherwise phenotypically normal. The plasma potassium concentration may be low, but is often normal. One clue indicating this condition is severe hypokalemia after administration of a thiazide diuretic, which is due to increased sodium delivery to the aldosterone-sensitive potassium-secretory site in the cortical collecting tubule. As many as 18% of patients suffer a cerebrovascular complication, mainly hemorrhage from ruptured berry aneurysms. The incidence of aneurysm is similar to that among patients with autosomal dominant polycystic kidney disease. Surveillance MRA has been recommended, but the benefit of this approach has not been proved. Mean age of onset of cerebral hemorrhage if an aneurysm is present is 32 years.

In the adrenal cortex, aldosterone is normally synthesized in the zona glomerulosa, whereas glucocorticoids are predominantly synthesized in the adjacent zona fasciculata. Two isozymes of 11β-hydroxylase, encoded by chromosome 8, are responsible for the synthesis of aldosterone and cortisol. The isozyme in the zona glomerulosa (aldosterone synthase or CYP11B2) mediates aldosterone production under the influence of potassium and angiotensin II, whereas the isozyme in the zona fasciculata (CYP11B1) induces cortisol production under the influence of ACTH. In glucocorticoid-remediable aldosteronism, the promoter region for CYP11B1 fuses with the coding sequences of the aldosterone synthase enzyme, CYP11B2, resulting in ACTH-dependent aldosterone synthesis in the zona fasciculata.

The diagnosis is made by dexamethasone suppression testing demonstrating the production of 18-carbon oxidation products of cortisol. However, a genetic test demonstrating the pathologic chimeric gene is recommended since there is a significant false-positive rate for patients with primary hyperaldosteronism when tested with dexamethasone.

Corticosteroids suppress ACTH and lower the blood pressure to normal. The target dose should be enough to suppress aldosterone levels sufficiently without causing debilitating side effects.

FAMILIAL HYPERALDOSTERONISM TYPE II

In familial hyperaldosteronism type II, excess mineralocorticoid production is responsible for hypertension, but it is not suppressible by dexamethasone. Autosomal dominance suggests a single gene mutation, and the locus has been narrowed to a band on chromosome 7. Familial hyperaldosteronism type II is clinically and biochemically indistinguishable from sporadic primary hyperaldosteronism, and can be detected only by a positive family history.

CONGENITAL ADRENAL HYPERPLASIA

Congenital adrenal hyperplasia is an autosomal recessive disorder that results in an inability to synthesize cortisol. In this condition, defects in the final steps of steroid biosynthesis cause excess mineralocorticoid and androgen effects, with coincident signs of glucocorticoid deficiency. The most common forms, 17α-hydroxylase deficiency and 11β-hydroxylase deficiency, may induce hypertension through overproduction of cortisol precursors that are metabolized to mineralocorticoid agonists.

BIBLIOGRAPHY

Bax L, Woittiez AJ, Kouwenberg HJ, et al: Stent placement in patients with atherosclerotic renal artery stenosis and impaired renal function: a randomized trial, *Ann Intern Med* 150:840-848, 2009. W150-1.

Conlon PJ, O'Riordan E, Kalra PA: New insights into the epidemiologic and clinical manifestations of atherosclerotic renovascular disease, *Am J Kidney Dis* 35:573-587, 2000.

Funder JW, Carey RM, Fardella C, et al: Case detection, diagnosis, and treatment of patients with primary aldosteronism: an endocrine society clinical practice guideline, *J Clin Endocrinol Metab* 93:3266-3281, 2008.

Guller U, Turek J, Eubanks S, et al: Detecting pheochromocytoma: defining the most sensitive test, *Ann Surg* 243:102-107, 2006.

Mattsson C, Young WF Jr: Primary aldosteronism: diagnostic and treatment strategies, *Nat Clin Pract Nephrol* 2:198-208, 2006. quiz, 1 p following 30.

Parthasarathy HK, Menard J, White WB, et al: A double-blind, randomized study comparing the antihypertensive effect of eplerenone and spironolactone in patients with hypertension and evidence of primary aldosteronism. *J Hypertens;* 29:980–990.

Plouin PF, Chatellier G, Darne B, et al: Blood pressure outcome of angioplasty in atherosclerotic renal artery stenosis: a randomized trial. Essai Multicentrique Medicaments vs Angioplastie (EMMA) Study Group, *Hypertension* 31:823-829, 1998.

Radermacher J, Chavan A, Bleck J, et al: Use of Doppler ultrasonography to predict the outcome of therapy for renal-artery stenosis, *N Engl J Med* 344:410-417, 2001.

Radermacher J, Weinkove R, Haller H: Techniques for predicting a favourable response to renal angioplasty in patients with renovascular disease, *Curr Opin Nephrol Hypertens* 10:799-805, 2001.

Slovut DP, Olin JW: Fibromuscular dysplasia, *N Engl J Med* 350:1862-1871, 2004.

Tan KT, van Beek EJ, Brown PW, et al: Magnetic resonance angiography for the diagnosis of renal artery stenosis: a meta-analysis, *Clin Radiol* 57:617-624, 2002.

van Jaarsveld BC, Krijnen P, Pieterman H, et al: The effect of balloon angioplasty on hypertension in atherosclerotic renal-artery stenosis. Dutch Renal Artery Stenosis Intervention Cooperative Study Group, *N Engl J Med* 342:1007-1014, 2000.

Vasbinder GB, Nelemans PJ, Kessels AG, et al: Accuracy of computed tomographic angiography and magnetic resonance angiography for diagnosing renal artery stenosis, *Ann Intern Med* 141:674-682, 2004. discussion 682.

Vehaskari VM: Heritable forms of hypertension, *Pediatr Nephrol* 24:1929-1937, 2009.

Webster J, Marshall F, Abdalla M, et al: Randomised comparison of percutaneous angioplasty vs continued medical therapy for hypertensive patients with atheromatous renal artery stenosis. Scottish and Newcastle Renal Artery Stenosis Collaborative Group, *J Hum Hypertens* 12:329-335, 1998.

Wheatley K, Ives N, Gray R, et al: Revascularization versus medical therapy for renal-artery stenosis, *N Engl J Med* 361:1953-1962, 2009.

Wilson FH, Disse-Nicodeme S, Choate KA, et al: Human hypertension caused by mutations in WNK kinases, *Science* 293:1107-1112, 2001.

Wittenberg G, Kenn W, Tschammler A, et al: Spiral CT angiography of renal arteries: comparison with angiography, *Eur Radiol* 9:546-551, 1999.

Index

Page numbers followed by *f* indicate figures; *t*, tables; *b*, boxes.